The Thalassaemia Syndromes

The Thalassaemia Syndromes

Fourth edition

D.J. Weatherall and J.B. Clegg

With contributions by:
R. Gibbons
D.R. Higgs
J.M. Old
Nancy F. Olivieri
Swee Lay Thein
W.G. Wood

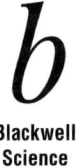

Blackwell
Science

© 2001
Blackwell Science Ltd
Editorial Offices:
Osney Mead, Oxford OX2 0EL
25 John Street, London WC1N 2BS
23 Ainslie Place, Edinburgh EH3 6AJ
350 Main Street, Malden
  MA 02148 5018, USA
54 University Street, Carlton
  Victoria 3053, Australia
10, rue Casimir Delavigne
  75006 Paris, France

Other Editorial Offices:
Blackwell Wissenschafts-Verlag GmbH
Kurfürstendamm 57
10707 Berlin, Germany

Blackwell Science KK
MG Kodenmacho Building
7–10 Kodenmacho Nihombashi
Chuo-ku, Tokyo 104, Japan

Iowa State University Press
A Blackwell Science Company
2121 S. State Avenue
Ames, Iowa 50014-8300, USA

First published 1965
Second edition 1972
Third edition 1981
Fourth edition 2001

Set by Best-set Typesetter Ltd., Hong Kong
Printed and bound in Italy
by Rotolito Lombarda SpA, Milan

The Blackwell Science logo is a
trade mark of Blackwell Science Ltd,
registered at the United Kingdom
Trade Marks Registry

A catalogue record for this title
is available from the British Library

ISBN 0-86542-664-3

Library of Congress
Cataloging-in-publication Data
Weatherall, D.J.
    The thalassaemia syndromes /
D.J. Weatherall and J.B. Clegg, with
contributions by
    R. Gibbons . . . [et al.]. – 4th ed.
      p.; cm.
    Includes bibliographical references
and index.
    ISBN 0-86542-664-3
    1. Thalassemia. I. Clegg, J. B. II.
Title.
    [DNLM: 1. Thalassemia. WH 170
W362t 2001]
RC641.7.T5 W4 2001
616.1'52–dc21   00-056465

DISTRIBUTORS
Marston Book Services Ltd
PO Box 269
Abingdon, Oxon OX14 4YN
(*Orders*: Tel: 01235 465500
            Fax: 01235 465555)

USA
Blackwell Science, Inc.
Commerce Place
350 Main Street
Malden, MA 02148-5018
(*Orders*: Tel: 800 759 6102
                781 388 8250
            Fax: 781 388 8255)

Canada
Login Brothers Book Company
324 Saulteaux Crescent
Winnipeg, Manitoba R3J 3T2
(*Orders*: Tel: 204 837 2987)

Australia
Blackwell Science Pty Ltd
54 University Street
Carlton, Victoria 3053
(*Orders*: Tel: 3 9347 0300
            Fax: 3 9347 5001)

For further information on
Blackwell Science, visit our website:
www.blackwell-science.com

Contents

Authors and contributors, vi

Preface to the fourth edition, vii

Preface to the first edition, ix

Acknowledgements, x

Part 1
Historical background

1 Historical perspectives: the many and diverse routes to our current understanding of the thalassaemias, 3

Part 2
The biology of the thalassaemias
Contributors: D.R. Higgs,
Swee Lay Thein, W.G. Wood

2 Human haemoglobin, 65

3 Thalassaemia: classification, genetics and relationship to other inherited disorders of haemoglobin, 121

4 The molecular pathology of the thalassaemias, 133

5 The pathophysiology of the thalassaemias, 192

6 Distribution and population genetics of the thalassaemias, 237

Part 3
Clinical features of the thalassaemias
Contributors: R. Gibbons, D.R. Higgs,
Nancy F. Olivieri, W.G. Wood

7 The β thalassaemias, 287

8 The δβ and related thalassaemias, 357

9 The β and δβ thalassaemias in association with structural haemoglobin variants, 393

10 Hereditary persistence of fetal haemoglobin, 450

11 The α thalassaemias and their interaction with structural haemoglobin variants, 484

12 α Thalassaemia with mental retardation or myelodysplasia, 526

13 Thalassaemia intermedia, 550

Part 4
Diagnosis and management of thalassaemia
Contributors: J.M. Old, Nancy F. Olivieri,
Swee Lay Thein

14 Avoidance and population control, 597

15 Management and prognosis, 630

16 The laboratory diagnosis of the thalassaemias, 686

Part 5

The future, 727

References, 733

Appendix: Addresses of patient support organizations, 823

Index, 827

Authors and contributors

J.B. Clegg, *MRC Molecular Haematology Unit, Institute of Molecular Medicine, University of Oxford*

D.R. Higgs, *MRC Molecular Haematology Unit, Institute of Molecular Medicine, University of Oxford*

R. Gibbons, *Institute of Molecular Medicine, University of Oxford*

J.M. Old, *National Haemoglobin Reference Laboratory, Institute of Molecular Medicine, University of Oxford*

Nancy F. Oliveri, *Hospital for Sick Children and the Toronto General Hospital, Toronto, Ontario*

Swee Lay Thein, *MRC Molecular Haematology Unit, Institute of Molecular Medicine, University of Oxford*

D.J. Weatherall, *MRC Molecular Haematology Unit, Institute of Molecular Medicine, University of Oxford*

W.G. Wood, *MRC Molecular Haematology Unit, Institute of Molecular Medicine, University of Oxford*

Preface to the fourth edition

Why has there been a gap of 20 years between the third and fourth editions of this book? Although this is in part a reflection of our indolence, together with pressures from other scientific, literary and administrative activities, this is not the whole story. The first three editions covered the period between 1965 and 1981, a time of rapid evolution of research into human genetic disease. Indeed, work in the globin field over that period led the way towards the development of molecular medicine. The haemoglobin disorders had been well defined at the clinical and genetic levels and were custom-made for the new tools of molecular biology, as they became available in the late 1970s. In addition to haematologists, scientists from many different disciplines descended on the field, offering as it did the first opportunity to analyse disease at the DNA level. Hence there was a need for an extensive review of the genetics and phenotypic variability of the thalassaemias and related disorders, to direct these workers through this complicated maze. This is almost certainly why, much to our surprise, the third edition became a Citation Classic in *Current Contents* in August 1987. During this period the rate of discovery was so great that there never seemed to be a time when it was possible to write any review of the field which was not out of date before it was published! More recently the speed of development in the thalassaemia field has slowed down and we thought that it was now appropriate to take stock again, and to try to see what has been achieved and where the future lies.

It is now apparent that the thalassaemias are not only the commonest monogenic diseases in humans, but that, because of major demographic changes in the pattern of disease in many of the developing countries, they will pose an increasingly serious health problem in the new millennium. Hence, the great challenge for the future, and one that extends right across the uncertain field of molecular medicine, is how to translate our remarkable knowledge of the molecular pathology of these diseases into better ways for their control and treatment. For, as well as

clarifying the many different mutations that underlie the thalassaemias, work over the last 15 years has underlined the complexity of the many genetic and acquired factors which may modify the phenotype of these disorders. In this new edition we have tried to guide clinicians who are responsible for the care of patients and their families through this maze, highlight our continuing areas of ignorance and define priorities for developing programmes for the control and treatment of thalassaemia in the future.

Because of the vast amount of information which has been obtained about the genetic control of haemoglobin in general, and the thalassaemias in particular, and also because of our increasing senility, we have invited some younger colleagues with whom we have worked for many years to help us with this new edition. We must make it absolutely clear, however, that any deficiencies of this book are due entirely to our idiosyncrasies and prejudices as editors, reflecting as they do the tolerance rather than lack of competence of our colleagues.

As this book goes to press the whole future of clinical research is being subjected to debate on both sides of the Atlantic. It is felt by many that the complexities of the biomedical sciences in the post-genome period will be such that it will not be possible for clinicians to make major contributions which require the increasingly complex tools of molecular and cell biology. The development of the thalassaemia field, which has probably told us more about the relationship between molecular pathology and what we see in our patients than any other family of diseases, has, apart from some of its early foundations based on the structure and genetic control of haemoglobin, depended on the work of clinical scientists who are able to apply the tools of molecular biology, or teams of clinicians and basic scientists who could communicate with each other. This is the only way in which translational research of this type can be pursued; the critical evaluation of clinical phenotypes and their subtleties is, in its own way, no less demanding than their analysis at the molecular level.

If the thalassaemia field has taught us anything, it is of the importance of scientists, be they clinical or basic, who can sit astride the field, linking the findings in patients to those in the laboratory. Indeed, one of the disappointments of our review of the current state of this field is the frequency with which detailed molecular studies are accompanied by limited clinical data. Hence although we now know more about phenotype/genotype relationships for the thalassaemias than for any other genetic diseases, there is still a long way to go. This information will become of increasing importance as we move to more experimental and invasive forms of therapy in the future; it will be vital to offer parents an accurate account of the likely course of their child's illness before embarking on these journeys into the unknown.

D.J. Weatherall
J.B. Clegg
Oxford, February 2001

Preface to the first edition

During the last few years there has been a rapid increase of knowledge about the genetic control of haemoglobin synthesis in health and disease. This has resulted in a marked revival of interest in thalassaemia and associated disorders of haemoglobin production. It is now clear that these conditions occur much more frequently, and in many more racial groups, than was previously realized. Furthermore the study of these disorders promises to answer some fundamental questions about the genetic mechanisms involved in defective protein synthesis. For these reasons thalassaemia has become the field of interest for workers of many different disciplines and there is a widening gap in communication between the clinical responsible for recognizing and treating these disorders and the basic scientist, whose studies of the molecular control of protein synthesis have so many applications to these clinical problems. In this book, by presenting evidence from several of these disciplines, an attempt has been made to summarize present knowledge about this important group in inherited disorders of haemoglobin synthesis.

In a work of this size it has not been possible to cover the vast literature of the thalassaemia field. The subject has been covered in several excellent reviews, both in English and Italian, and the present work has been designed to summarize the evidence which suggests that the clinical picture of thalassaemia may result from several different inherited defects of globin synthesis, very similar in type to the other inherited haemoglobinopathies.

Acknowledgements

As in the case of previous editions, this book could not have been written without the help of our friends and colleagues in the thalassaemia field, both in this country and overseas. Lack of space prevents us from mentioning all of them by name; they encompass the entire subject and, indeed, the whole field of human genetics. We are also extremely grateful for the forbearance of our many patients who have allowed us to study them and their families. Because of the critical importance of the facial appearances in thalassaemia we have not followed the common custom of covering part of the face in our clinical figures. We have made every possible effort to obtain permission to reproduce these figures, and are particularly grateful to these patients for helping other sufferers from thalassaemia in this way.

We are also very grateful to the colleagues who have joined us in writing parts of this new edition, particularly for their forbearance with our editorial quirks and constant pressure.

It is also a pleasure to acknowledge the help of many colleagues, editors and publishers who have allowed us to reproduce material for this edition. As far as possible we have cited these sources under individual captions. We are particularly grateful to Dhira Sonakul for sending us copies of her beautiful atlas on the pathology of thalassaemia and for allowing us to borrow freely from it to illustrate parts of this book. Similarly, we thank Professors Caterina Borgna-Pignatti and Guido Lucarelli for preparing and allowing us to reproduce graphs of survival data in their patient populations, and Professor Ida Bianco for providing us with some information about early Italian publications which may have preceded the formal descriptions of thalassaemia in the early part of the twentieth century. We also acknowledge valuable discussions on the population control of thalassaemia over the years with Professor Bernadette Modell, and on population screening with Dr Elizabeth Letsky.

We are indebted to our many overseas colleagues who have enabled us to work in their countries and helped us to understand the particular problems of thalassaemia in different populations: Professor Graham Serjeant (Jamaica); Drs Shanthimali de Silva, Windsor Perera, Anuja Premawardhena and Mr Adrian Basnayake (Sri Lanka); Dr Michael Alpers (Papua New Guinea); Dr Donald Bowden (Vanuatu); Dr Abdul Salam Sofro (Indonesia); Professors Prawase Wasi, Suthat Fucharoen and Sornchai Looareesuwan (Thailand); Professor Georgi Efremov (Macedonia); Professor Antonio Cao (Sardinia); Dr Richard Perrine (Saudi Arabia); Professors Eliezer Rachmilewitz and Chaim Hershko (Israel); Professors Phaedon Fessas and Christos Kattamis (Greece); and Drs David Nathan, Elliot Vichinsky and Gary Brittenham (USA).

We also acknowledge with gratitude the continued support from the Medical Research Council, Wellcome Trust and Department of Health without whose financial support none of this work would have been carried out.

Finally, we are grateful to Blackwell Science for their encouragement and forbearance with the slow gestation of this edition. It would never have seen the light of day without the enormous efforts and patience of our secretaries Janet Watt, Liz Rose and Milly Graver, and David Lockett for his computing skills. The fact that they are still with us after this edition is a miracle.

Notice to all readers

The authors have made every effort to ensure that the drug dosages in this book are accurate. They are, however, subject to change and may have been revised so we urge you, as a matter of routine and safe-practice, to check the recommended dosages before administering any drug. You should consult:
- your local hospital formulary;
- your national formulary; or
- the pharmaceutical company's literature.

Part 1
Historical background

Chapter 1
Historical perspectives: the many and diverse routes to our current understanding of the thalassaemias

It is indeed so. Nature is nowhere wont to reveal her innermost secrets more openly than where she shows faint traces of herself away from the beaten track. Nor is there any surer route to the proper practice of medicine than if someone gives his mind over to discerning the customary law of Nature through the careful investigation of diseases that are of rare occurrence.

WILLIAM HARVEY (1578–1657)

Introduction

The story of the accumulation of knowledge about the thalassaemias and other inherited diseases of haemoglobin poses some intriguing questions for historians of science and medicine in the twentieth century. In particular, they will ask how it was that the study of what, at least at first, appeared to be a group of rare genetic anaemias turned out to be the forerunner of a completely new era of medical science and practice. For, in effect, it was the elucidation of their molecular basis that was to lead to the notion of 'molecular disease', and, later, molecular medicine; that is, a change of emphasis from the study of illness in patients or their organs to a description of its pathology at the level of cells and molecules.

It is beyond the scope of this book to provide a comprehensive account of the history of haemoglobin and its disorders. However, because of the central importance of thalassaemia in paving the way to unravelling the molecular basis of human single-gene disorders, and, in particular, explaining the reasons for their remarkable phenotypic diversity, we thought it worthwhile to begin with a brief account of some of the events that led up to, and formed the foundation for, our present understanding of the field. Various aspects of the history of thalassaemia and sketches of the lives of some of the physicians who played a prominent part in its investigation are given by Bannerman (1961), Weatherall (1980) and Wintrobe (1985).

Any account of how we arrived at our present state of knowledge about thalassaemia is, of necessity, rather involved, based as it is on such an extensive literature from Europe, North America and elsewhere. Because of difficulties of language, and lack of scientific communication during the Second World War, it has often proved difficult to give correct priorities for key discoveries and to develop an accurate historical picture of the precise order in which events occurred. Overall, however, the development of the field seems to fall into several distinct phases.

The period between 1925 and 1940 saw the first descriptions of the clinical features of several different types of thalassaemia. From 1940 to 1960 there was an amalgamation of information from Europe and the United States that gave a clearer picture of their inheritance. By 1960 it was apparent that 'thalassaemia' is not one disease, but a very diverse group of genetic disorders, all of which result from abnormalities of haemoglobin synthesis. Furthermore, they were found to have a widespread distribution and not to be localized to the Mediterranean region, from where the name 'thalassaemia' is derived.

Over the next 20 years there was steady progress on several fronts. Careful studies of families with different haemoglobin disorders led to an understanding of the genetic control of haemoglobin and, remarkably, to an almost complete description of the clusters of genes on different chromosomes that are involved. Much was learnt about the synthesis of haemoglobin and its abnormalities in the different forms of thalassaemia, information which led to a better appreciation of the pathophysiology of the disease and, incidentally, to improvements in its symptomatic treatment. It also became possible to make some educated guesses about its molecular pathology, so that by the late 1970s the thalassaemia field was, in effect, custom-built for the new tools of recombinant DNA technology.

Not surprisingly, therefore, thalassaemia became the subject of intense interest to molecular biologists in the 1980s. Because the genetics of haemoglobin was already so well understood, the globin genes were an obvious target for some of the first attempts at isolating human genes; it soon became apparent that the picture of the arrangement of the globin genes that had evolved from earlier family studies was correct in almost every detail. Against this background, and because of the many different well-characterized disorders of haemoglobin synthesis that had been found in particular types of thalassaemia, several groups of research workers began a systematic analysis of the molecular basis for the disease. Over the next 10 years this work was to yield a remarkable picture of the diversity of human molecular pathology, and, as a bonus, provided some extremely valuable insights into how human genes are regulated and how these functions may break down in different inherited diseases. Happily, much of this information also had valuable practical applications for the population control, diagnosis and, at least to some extent, the management of many forms of thalassaemia.

In the following sections we shall examine briefly these different threads in the development of knowledge about thalassaemia that came together at about the time the last edition of this book was written, and that underpinned the remarkable successes of the last decade.

The early history of thalassaemia

Introduction

Thalassaemia is such a common condition, particularly in the Mediterranean region and south-east Asia, that it must have been frequently seen by physicians before the first clinical descriptions in 1925. However, there is very little evidence that it was recognized as a specific entity before that time.

Some suggested early descriptions

The Greek physician Caminopetros noted one possible reference to thalassaemia in Hippocrates' Coan Prognosis. Bannerman (1961) quotes an English translation as follows: 'When children of seven years of age show weakness, a bad colour, and rapid respiration on walking, together with a desire to eat earth, it denotes destruction of the blood and asthenia.' However, it is more likely that this was a description of iron-deficiency anaemia in early childhood; a desire to eat dirt, a condition known as pica, occurs in iron-deficiency anaemia and is not characteristic of children with thalassaemia.

Menke (1973) has made the more plausible suggestion that there is a description of sickle-cell thalassaemia in a volume of the Hippocratic Collections: Concerning Internal Diseases, entry 32. He quotes a Latin version given by Ermerins as follows:

> Another disease of the spleen. It begins indeed in the time of Spring but more especially from the blood. For when the spleen is filled with blood it bursts out into the abdomen, and sharp pains (then) attack the spleen, the breast, the shoulder, and under the shoulder blades. The entire body is of a leaden colour and over the shins are minor scratches from which originate large ulcers . . .

Although this interesting clinical description might do almost equally well for other haemolytic anaemias such as favism (which Pythagoras recognized as resulting from the ill effects of the broad bean, and which is seasonal), generalized pains and leg ulcers are particularly characteristic of the sickle-cell disorders; enlargement of the spleen in older patients is more in keeping with sickle-cell thalassaemia than sickle-cell anaemia.

Porotic hyperostosis

Another approach to the question of whether thalassaemia occurred in historic or prehistoric times is the study of peculiar thalassaemia-like bone changes in skulls found in ancient burial places, or mummies in a good state of preservation (Hart 1980). There is a condition well known to anthropologists called 'porotic hyperostosis' in which the structural and radiological changes in the skull are very similar to those of severe thalassaemia. Bone changes of this type have been found in skulls excavated in Sicily and Sardinia as well as in those of the ancient native populations of America, the Incas of Peru, Indians from Colombia, Aztecs from Mexico, Mayan Indians from the Yucatan, and from many other sites (Chini & Valeri 1949). Indeed, several students of palaeontology believe that one contribution to the extinction of some of these ancient populations might have been a high incidence of a blood disease, possibly a genetic anaemia like thalassaemia. It should be remembered, however, that many of these skulls are from adults and that there are probably other genetic haemolytic anaemias, or even nutritional anaemias, that might produce bone changes consistent with porotic hyperostosis.

In a recent analysis of a sample of skeletons from the 4000-year-old site of Khok Phanom Di on the coast of central Thailand, Tayles (1996) identified several with bone changes suggestive of severe anaemia. In a detailed and scholarly review of the differential diagnosis of the possible causes of these changes, she makes a very strong case for a form of thalassaemia, probably one of intermediate severity, which might have allowed survival into late childhood or early adult life. Convincing though these arguments are, the case for skeletal changes of thalassaemia in these ancient burial grounds will only be proven when it is possible to isolate DNA from the bones and identify thalassaemia mutations directly.

Splenic anaemia

By the beginning of this century, clinicians were becoming aware of the syndrome of splenic anaemia of infancy. One such clinical disorder became known as 'anaemia infantum pseudoleucaemica'. It was first described by Rudolf von Jaksch-Wartenhorst (1855–1947), who spent most of his professional life in Prague and was one of the first clinicians to appreciate the importance of chemical and radiological investigations. His original paper (von Jaksch 1889) concerns a young boy with anaemia, leucocytosis, splenomegaly and fever in whom a subsequent autopsy did not show changes of leukaemia. He observed further cases later (von Jaksch 1890). It seems unlikely, however, that he was seeing thalassaemia in Prague at that time. Many other accounts of 'von Jaksch's anaemia' appeared over the next 25 years (see, for example, those of Whitcher (1930) and Capper (1931)), but on reviewing these clinical descriptions the reader is struck by their extraordinary heterogeneity. There is little doubt that some of them deal with different varieties of leukaemia, while others may have been forms of nutritional deficiency, tuberculosis, congenital syphilis, or other infections. However, for 30 years or more after the turn of the century it was common practice to describe any unusual anaemia in infancy as 'von Jaksch's anaemia', particularly if the spleen was enlarged.

Early Italian writings on familial splenic anaemia of children may have included cases of thalas-

saemia. Bannerman (1961) has investigated some of the reports in the literature that the Italian workers (Silvestroni & Bianco 1959) thought might be descriptions of thalassaemia which predated that of Thomas Cooley in 1925. He concludes that most of them dealt with conditions such as leishmaniasis, tuberculosis or congenital syphilis, and in no case was there clear evidence that the authors had identified a disease that would be accepted today as a form of thalassaemia. While this is true, Dr Ida Bianco has recently analysed some further published material from the period coming up to the turn of the century (Dr Ida Bianco, personal communication), particularly that of Cardarelli (1880, 1890) and Somma (1884). In these and similar reports of children with splenic anaemia written at about this time, in some cases there is more than one affected family member, bone changes similar to thalassaemia, and generalized osteoporosis; the latter finding is particularly difficult to reconcile with an infective origin. These authors were clearly puzzled by this disease and, although they included malaria, tuberculosis and other infections in their differential diagnosis, they recognized that there might be constitutional factors involved.

However, it was not until 1925 that the condition which later became known as thalassaemia was clearly separated from this heterogeneous collection of anaemias of infancy.

The first clinical descriptions of severe thalassaemia

Although the credit for the first clinical description of thalassaemia is given to the American paediatrician Thomas B. Cooley (Fig. 1.1) it is quite clear that the disease was identified as a distinct entity at about the same time by several Italian clinicians. Undoubtedly, Cooley was responsible for the first description of the severe, life-threatening form of thalassaemia, while the Italian workers described a milder variety of the condition. This raises another particularly interesting set of questions for students of the history of the disease. Why was the first clinical description of the severe form of thalassaemia made in the United States, where the disease is rare, instead of the Mediterranean, where it is extremely common? And why did the Italian clinicians identify the milder varieties of thalassaemia yet fail to recognize the severe forms, which must have been much more common in their population?

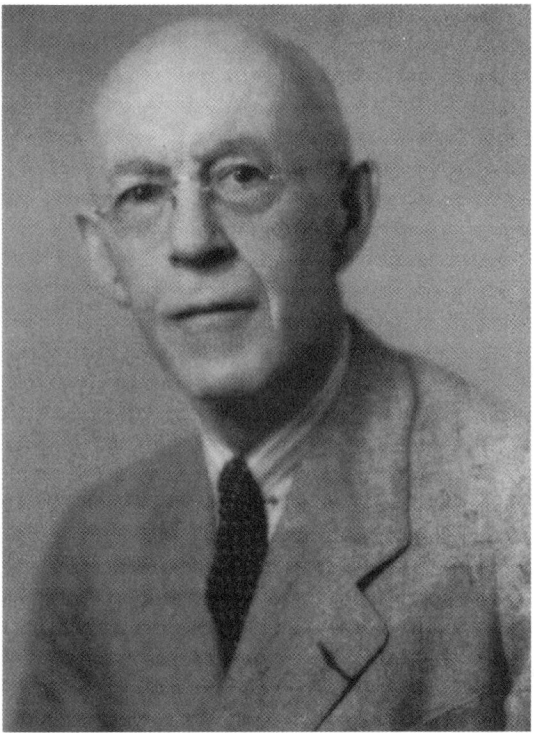

Fig. 1.1 Thomas B. Cooley (1871–1945). Cooley was born at Ann Arbor, Michigan, graduated MD in 1895 and interned at the Boston City Hospital. After studying in Germany he returned to Boston to work in contagious disease. After further appointments in Ann Arbor and Detroit, and a period of service in France during the First World War, he settled in Detroit, where he spent the rest of his life in paediatric practice.

Childhood illness in the Mediterranean region in the late nineteenth century

A possible explanation for this interesting conundrum is to be found in the pattern of illness in infancy and childhood in Italy and other Mediterranean countries in the latter half of the nineteenth and early twentieth centuries. In the present context malaria is of particular importance. An excellent account of the problem posed by malaria during this period is given by Bruce-Chwatt and de Zulueta (1980) (Figs 1.2 and 1.3). Reasonable frequency and mortality data for malaria in Italy are available from 1887 onwards. At the turn of the century and up to the mid-1930s there were over 200 000 cases notified each year, and

between 2000 and 10 000 deaths. The disease was originally present in 2600, or one-third, of the municipalities in Italy. About 4–5 million hectares of land remained uncultivated because of the ravages of the disease, which was particularly severe in the south of the country, in the Latium and in Sardinia (Fig. 1.4). It seems likely that these figures are a minimal estimate; it has been suggested that at the turn of the century malaria may have been affecting as many as two million out of a population of approximately 30 million (Pampana 1944). In Greece, during the period 1921–32, the number of deaths attributed to malaria varied between 3000 and 8000 per annum, and constituted, on average, 5.6% of total mortality in the population.

Since malaria causes anaemia and splenomegaly in early life, it is not surprising that severe thalassaemia was not recognized as a distinct entity in Mediterranean countries during the early part of this century. Furthermore, there were other common infections which would have produced a similar clinical picture. Leishmaniasis was widespread in the Mediterranean populations; this disease is also characterized by severe anaemia and splenomegaly. There was also a high infant mortality due to other infectious diseases, particularly tuberculosis, and malnutrition and nutritional iron deficiency were widespread. A genetic anaemia, even though it might be affecting close to one per cent of the population in parts of Italy and some of the islands of the Mediterranean, would easily have been overlooked against this background of childhood illness.

Thalassaemia in Cyprus

The history of thalassaemia in Cyprus provides a particularly telling example of why this condition was not recognized in the Mediterranean region until malaria control programmes and other public health improvements had decreased the rate of infant and childhood mortality from infectious disease. Thalassaemia was not known to occur on the island until 1944, when Alan Fawdry, a District Medical Officer of the Colonial Service, reported the clinical findings in 20 patients. This paper, remarkable for its scholarly discussion of the differential diagnosis of 'splenic anaemia', highlights the difficulty in identifying this disease in the island population against the background of chronic malaria. It was published at the end of an extremely successful three-year programme to

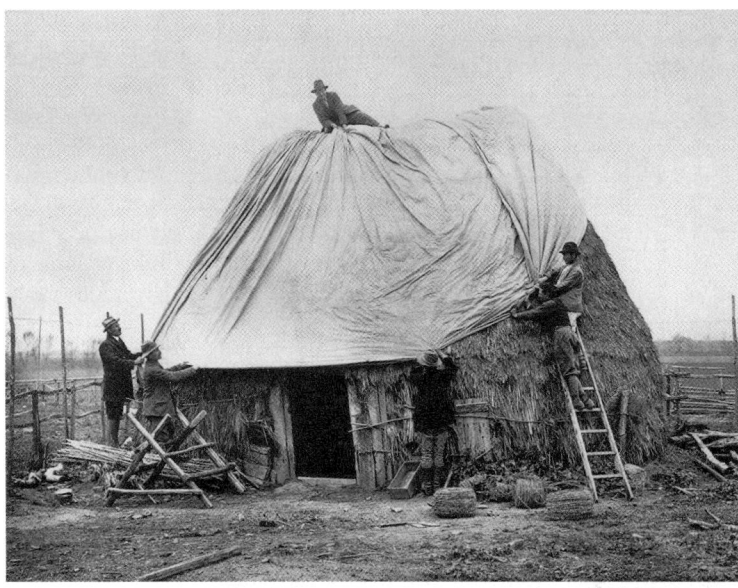

Fig. 1.2 Malaria control in Italy by fumigation of houses. One of the earliest attempts by Missiroli (1883–1951) to control adult anopheles by fumigation of houses after covering the roof with tarpaulin. This photograph appears in *The Rise and Fall of Malaria in Europe* by Bruce-Chwatt and de Zulueta (Oxford University Press, 1980) and is reproduced by permission of the publishers and the Wellcome Institute Library, London.

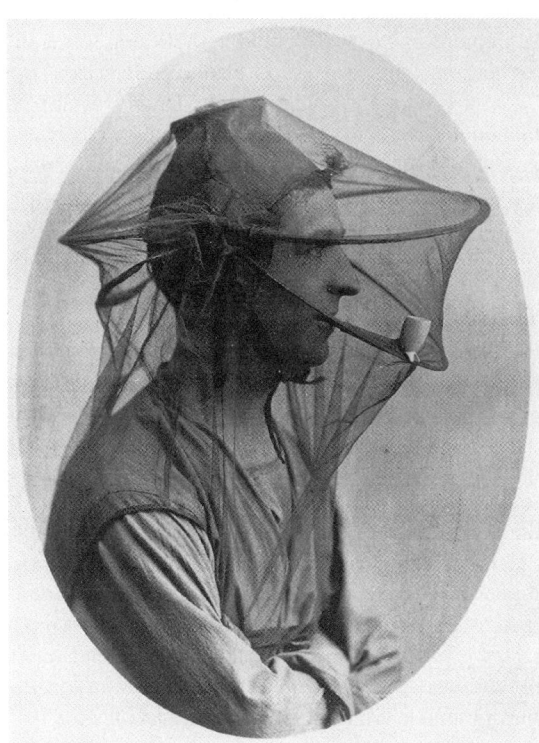

Fig. 1.3 Malaria control in Europe in the 1920s. A postcard showing mosquito nets worn as veils. Reproduced from *The Rise and Fall of Malaria in Europe* by Bruce-Chwatt and de Zulueta (Oxford University Press, 1980) with permission of the publishers and the Wellcome Institute Library, London.

control anopheline breeding, during which time Fawdry found that anaemia secondary to malaria had almost disappeared; within this remarkably short period it became clear that there was a high frequency of a genetic anaemia with features of thalassaemia in the island population.

It is not surprising therefore that the severe form of thalassaemia which kills children during the first years of life was first recognized in Mediterranean immigrants in the United States, where, in the 1920s, anaemia and splenomegaly due to infection would have been quite unusual. On the other hand, the milder form that was described independently in Italy at the same time is compatible with survival into late childhood and even into adult life. Hence it would have been identifiable, even in a population with a high frequency of death or morbidity resulting from infection in infancy.

Haematology in Italy

There may be other reasons why thalassaemia was not identified as a separate entity in Italy at the beginning of this century. Although haematology was a rapidly developing field, most of the Italian haematologists who were concerned with the study of the morphology of the blood cells were most active in Pavia and Siena, where there is little thalassaemia (Baserga 1958). And, although it is clear from many

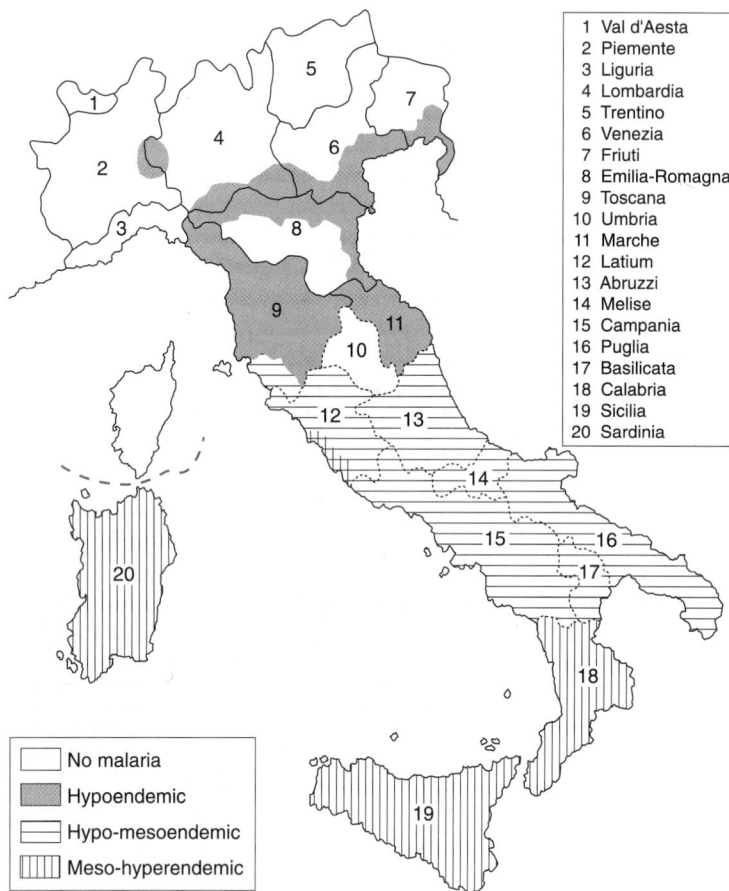

1 Val d'Aesta
2 Piemente
3 Liguria
4 Lombardia
5 Trentino
6 Venezia
7 Friuti
8 Emilia-Romagna
9 Toscana
10 Umbria
11 Marche
12 Latium
13 Abruzzi
14 Melise
15 Campania
16 Puglia
17 Basilicata
18 Calabria
19 Sicilia
20 Sardinia

☐ No malaria
■ Hypoendemic
≡ Hypo-mesoendemic
▥ Meso-hyperendemic

Fig. 1.4 Epidemiological stratification of the levels of endemic malaria in Italy based on pre-operational malarial control data of 1946. Reproduced from *The Rise and Fall of Malaria in Europe* by Bruce-Chwatt and de Zulueta (Oxford University Press, 1980), with permission.

of the early reports of splenic anaemia in the Italian population that there was a familial aggregation of cases, this would not in itself have aroused the suspicions of the clinicians of the time; it was only many years later that the importance of inheritance in the causation of disease came to be appreciated.

The first description of severe thalassaemia

Cooley's first account of what became known as thalassaemia appears in a single-page abstract in the *Transactions of the American Pediatric Society* in 1925 (Fig. 1.5), entitled 'A Series of Cases of Splenomegaly in Children, with Anemia and Peculiar Bone Changes'. Co-authored by Dr Pearl Lee, it describes four young children with anaemia and splenomegaly, enlargement of the liver, discoloration of the skin and of the sclerae, and no bile in the urine. Their red cells showed increased resistance to hypo-

tonic solutions and there was a moderate leucocytosis with nucleated red cells in the peripheral blood. In addition there was a peculiar mongoloid appearance caused by enlargement of the cranial and facial bones. In one case a splenectomy had been performed, without improvement. In this report, and in a more detailed version in a later paper, Cooley gave a complete description of what was almost certainly severe β thalassaemia (Cooley & Lee 1925; Cooley *et al.* 1927). He thought that the disease was congenital but probably not hereditary. Cooley's great contribution was to describe a series of children with a specific clinical syndrome and to separate clearly this disorder from the heterogeneous groups of childhood anaemias which hitherto had gone under the general name of 'von Jaksch's anaemia'. Readers interested in learning more about the life and work of this austere and enigmatic character should read a delightful essay written by Zuelzer (1956).

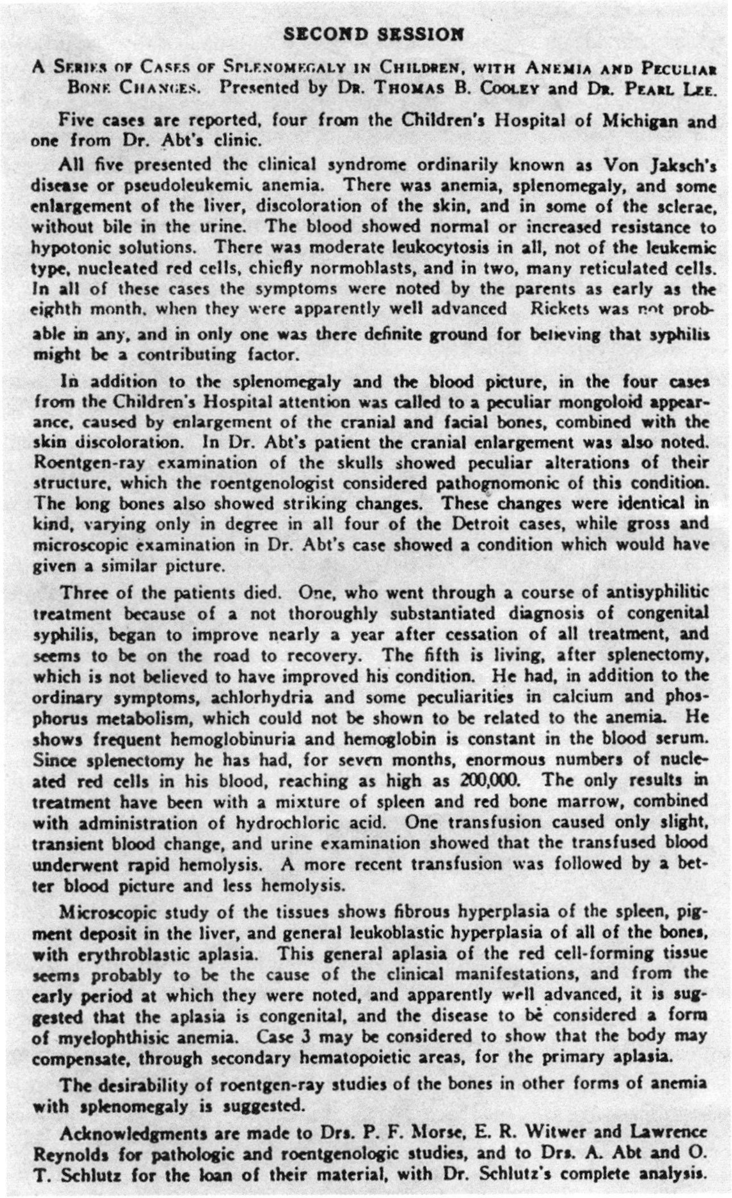

SECOND SESSION

A Series of Cases of Splenomegaly in Children, with Anemia and Peculiar Bone Changes. Presented by Dr. Thomas B. Cooley and Dr. Pearl Lee.

Five cases are reported, four from the Children's Hospital of Michigan and one from Dr. Abt's clinic.

All five presented the clinical syndrome ordinarily known as Von Jaksch's disease or pseudoleukemic anemia. There was anemia, splenomegaly, and some enlargement of the liver, discoloration of the skin, and in some of the sclerae, without bile in the urine. The blood showed normal or increased resistance to hypotonic solutions. There was moderate leukocytosis in all, not of the leukemic type, nucleated red cells, chiefly normoblasts, and in two, many reticulated cells. In all of these cases the symptoms were noted by the parents as early as the eighth month, when they were apparently well advanced Rickets was not probable in any, and in only one was there definite ground for believing that syphilis might be a contributing factor.

In addition to the splenomegaly and the blood picture, in the four cases from the Children's Hospital attention was called to a peculiar mongoloid appearance, caused by enlargement of the cranial and facial bones, combined with the skin discoloration. In Dr. Abt's patient the cranial enlargement was also noted. Roentgen-ray examination of the skulls showed peculiar alterations of their structure, which the roentgenologist considered pathognomonic of this condition. The long bones also showed striking changes. These changes were identical in kind, varying only in degree in all four of the Detroit cases, while gross and microscopic examination in Dr. Abt's case showed a condition which would have given a similar picture.

Three of the patients died. One, who went through a course of antisyphilitic treatment because of a not thoroughly substantiated diagnosis of congenital syphilis, began to improve nearly a year after cessation of all treatment, and seems to be on the road to recovery. The fifth is living, after splenectomy, which is not believed to have improved his condition. He had, in addition to the ordinary symptoms, achlorhydria and some peculiarities in calcium and phosphorus metabolism, which could not be shown to be related to the anemia. He shows frequent hemoglobinuria and hemoglobin is constant in the blood serum. Since splenectomy he has had, for seven months, enormous numbers of nucleated red cells in his blood, reaching as high as 200,000. The only results in treatment have been with a mixture of spleen and red bone marrow, combined with administration of hydrochloric acid. One transfusion caused only slight, transient blood change, and urine examination showed that the transfused blood underwent rapid hemolysis. A more recent transfusion was followed by a better blood picture and less hemolysis.

Microscopic study of the tissues shows fibrous hyperplasia of the spleen, pigment deposit in the liver, and general leukoblastic hyperplasia of all of the bones, with erythroblastic aplasia. This general aplasia of the red cell-forming tissue seems probably to be the cause of the clinical manifestations, and from the early period at which they were noted, and apparently well advanced, it is suggested that the aplasia is congenital, and the disease to be considered a form of myelophthisic anemia. Case 3 may be considered to show that the body may compensate, through secondary hematopoietic areas, for the primary aplasia.

The desirability of roentgen-ray studies of the bones in other forms of anemia with splenomegaly is suggested.

Acknowledgments are made to Drs. P. F. Morse, E. R. Witwer and Lawrence Reynolds for pathologic and roentgenologic studies, and to Drs. A. Abt and O. T. Schlutz for the loan of their material, with Dr. Schlutz's complete analysis.

Fig. 1.5 The first description of Cooley's anaemia. From the *Transactions of the American Pediatric Society*, **37**, 29–30, 1925.

Why 'thalassaemia'?

The term 'thalassaemia' was first used by Whipple and Bradford in 1932 in their classical paper on the pathology of the condition. The word is taken from the Greek 'θαλασσα', meaning 'the sea'. The purist might have preferred 'thalassanaemia', but thalassaemia has stuck. Indeed, Whipple and Bradford were not too happy with their invention, preferring the term 'Mediterranean disease'. In an account of the work of George Whipple, Diggs (1976) leaves the reader in no doubt that it was Whipple who invented the word. He writes:

I have always blamed Bradford rather than Whipple for suggesting a seemingly erudite but less meaningful and less understood word. Bradford was from a small town in Missouri. He knew the batting averages of the St. Louis

Cardinals, was quite familiar with the north end of southbound mules and the ways of quail and pheasant. He was a sluggish left-handed first base in the Strong Memorial baseball team in Rochester while I covered the left field. In addition I knew that he did not know a word of Greek. When I wrote recently to ask him why in the name of heaven he changed the name of the disease to 'thalassaemia', a term which did not identify the sea involved, he replied that a good baseball player does not argue with the umpire.

The story of how thalassaemia received its name was related to Maxwell Wintrobe and the authors by George W. Corner, who was at Rochester at the time when Whipple and Bradford were doing their early pathological work on Cooley's anaemia (Weatherall 1980). He wrote:

> Because I was perhaps the most bookish of the young Rochester faculty, Dean Whipple made me his informal consultant on literary matters, several times asking my opinion on questions of nomenclature and etymology. Wishing to avoid the eponymic title 'Cooley's anaemia', he sought a name that would associate the disease with the Mediterranean area, all the cases known at that time having occurred in families originating there. He had studied Greek at Phillips-Andover Academy, and he recalled the great story in the Anabasis of Xenophon's army coming over the mountain and gazing at last upon the sea, the Ten Thousand shouting as one man, 'thalassa, thalassa!'. Whipple sent for me and asked whether I thought the name 'thalassic anaemia' correct and appropriate. I had in fact never studied Greek, but of course I knew about the retreat of the Greek army from Persia and could at least tell the Dean that both words of his proposed name were from Greek roots and therefore properly associated. I gave no thought to the geographical aspects of the problem. Not until long afterward did I learn that the view hailed so joyfully by the homeward-bound Greeks was actually the Black Sea. The weary men still had a voyage before them, and the Bosphorus to pass before reaching the Mediterranean Sea.

As it turned out, however, the minor classical deficiencies of the Rochester School were not to matter. Later work was to show that the Black Sea is a very suitable location to give its name to thalassaemia;

it is (unlike the Mediterranean) surrounded by the disease on all sides!

Further description

During the decade following the original report by Cooley many cases of severe thalassaemia were described in the literature, in both North America and Europe. Although some of them continued to use the term 'von Jaksch's anaemia', it is clear that many of them were describing Cooley's anaemia. Interestingly, in the second edition of Janet Vaughan's *The Anaemias*, published in 1936, there is a very comprehensive section entitled 'Erythroblastic Anaemia of Cooley', which, incidentally, contains a description of the bone and marrow pathology which has never been bettered, and an account of the disease in an English girl (Vaughan 1936). During this time it became widely accepted that the condition is found predominantly in Mediterranean peoples; where such ancestry could not be proved it was usually assumed! An extensive bibliography of the literature of this period is given in the review of Chini and Valeri (1949).

Early descriptions of milder forms of thalassaemia

In 1925, Fernando Rietti of Ferrara (Fig. 1.6) (Rietti 1925) described a mild form of haemolytic jaundice in which the red cells showed increased osmotic resistance. This was a very important observation because it clearly distinguished the disorder from hereditary spherocytosis. Indeed, the increased osmotic resistance of thalassaemic red cells has been an important diagnostic tool ever since Cooley's and Rietti's first observations. Similar descriptions were published shortly afterwards by other Italian workers, including Greppi (1928) and Micheli et al. (1935). Interestingly, Micheli mentions that he had noted abnormalities of the red cells of this type in the parents of a child with Cooley's anaemia. But, although the latter was recognized for the first time in Italy one year previously, as Bannerman (1961) points out, it is very unlikely that these early Italian authors understood the true relationship of what became known as La Malattia di Rietti–Greppi–Micheli, or 'haemolytic jaundice with decreased red-cell fragility', to Cooley's anaemia. The large body of Italian literature on the form of anaemia described by Rietti, Greppi and Micheli is reviewed by Chini and Valeri (1949). A condition

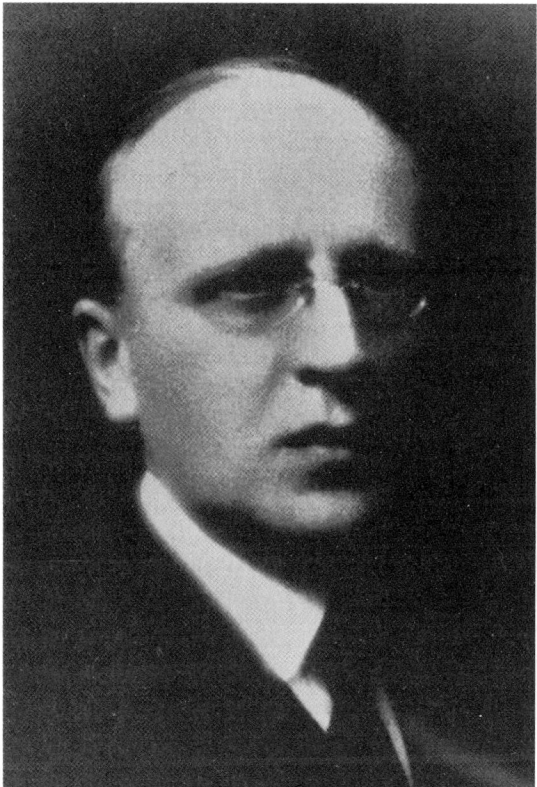

Fig. 1.6 Fernando Rietti (1890–1954). Rietti was born in Ferrara and studied in Florence, where he obtained his doctorate in 1914. He spent the rest of his life at Ferrara, working at the Arcispedale Di Sant' Anna. He published widely in the field of neurology and haematology. Reproduced from *Thalassemia. A Survey of Some Aspects* by Robin Bannerman (Grune and Stratton, New York, 1961), with permission.

which seems to have had many of the features of this disorder was also described by Silvestroni and Bianco (1945). They called it 'anaemia microcitica constituzionale', or constitutional microcytic anaemia, and subsequently wrote extensively on its clinical and genetic aspects (see Silvestroni & Bianco 1948, 1951; Silvestroni *et al.* 1957).

In reviewing the literature on these milder forms of thalassaemia it is clear that they show considerable clinical and genetic heterogeneity. The degree of anaemia is variable, but in most cases splenomegaly is reported. Unlike those with Cooley's anaemia many of these patients survived into adult life. The genetics was equally varied; in some cases both parents showed evidence of mild thalassaemia while in other families the condition appeared to be inherited as a single gene. However, it should be remembered that the diagnostic criteria for thalassaemia at the time were entirely dependent on red-cell morphology and osmotic-fragility testing.

There seems little doubt therefore that most of these early reports of milder forms of thalassaemia dealt with what today would be called 'thalassaemia intermedia', a term that only started to appear in the literature in the 1950s (Sturgeon *et al.* 1955).

1940–1950: first descriptions of the pattern of genetic transmission of thalassaemia

Early observations in Greece and Italy

The first definite evidence that Cooley's anaemia is genetically determined was reported by Caminopetros in Greece in his important papers in 1938 (Caminopetros 1938a,b) (Fig. 1.7), and by Angelini in Italy at about the same time (Angelini 1937). Both these workers noticed that relatives of patients with Cooley's anaemia, though not anaemic, have red cells with increased osmotic resistance. The work of Caminopetros was particularly important although, as pointed out by Fessas (1992), the results of his family studies were strange, because he usually found increased osmotic resistance in only one parent of children with thalassaemia major. On the other hand, he was certainly very explicit in his conclusions:

> The increased osmotic resistance is found constantly among seemingly healthy parents and siblings of the deceased . . . These findings speak for accepting the hereditary transmission of the pathologic element. The only possible explanation is a lesion of haemopoiesis, which is hereditary and idiopathic. Therefore, the disease must be considered as being transmitted by heredity, in fact as a recessive carrier, according to the laws of Mendel, as can be concluded by the transmission through seemingly healthy individuals (Caminopetros 1938a).

Consolidation of genetic data from the USA and Europe

In the early 1940s steady progress was made in establishing the genetic basis for thalassaemia. This impor-

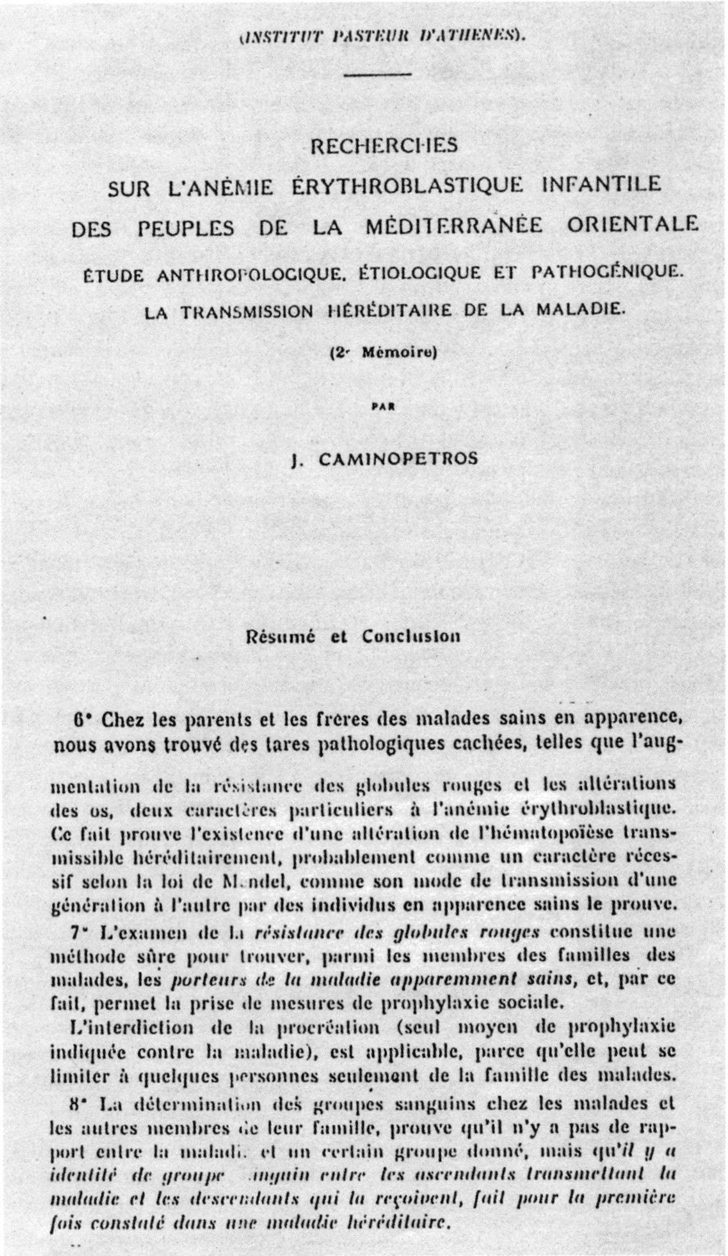

(INSTITUT PASTEUR D'ATHENES).

RECHERCHES

SUR L'ANÉMIE ÉRYTHROBLASTIQUE INFANTILE

DES PEUPLES DE LA MÉDITERRANÉE ORIENTALE

ÉTUDE ANTHROPOLOGIQUE, ÉTIOLOGIQUE ET PATHOGÉNIQUE.

LA TRANSMISSION HÉRÉDITAIRE DE LA MALADIE.

(2ᵉ Mémoire)

PAR

J. CAMINOPETROS

Résumé et Conclusion

6° Chez les parents et les frères des malades sains en apparence, nous avons trouvé des tares pathologiques cachées, telles que l'aug-

mentation de la résistance des globules rouges et les altérations des os, deux caractères particuliers à l'anémie érythroblastique. Ce fait prouve l'existence d'une altération de l'hématopoïèse transmissible héréditairement, probablement comme un caractère récessif selon la loi de Mendel, comme son mode de transmission d'une génération à l'autre par des individus en apparence sains le prouve.

7° L'examen de la *résistance des globules rouges* constitue une méthode sûre pour trouver, parmi les membres des familles des malades, les *porteurs de la maladie apparemment sains*, et, par ce fait, permet la prise de mesures de prophylaxie sociale.

L'interdiction de la procréation (seul moyen de prophylaxie indiquée contre la maladie), est applicable, parce qu'elle peut se limiter à quelques personnes seulement de la famille des malades.

8° La détermination des groupes sanguins chez les malades et les autres membres de leur famille, prouve qu'il n'y a pas de rapport entre la maladie et un certain groupe donné, mais qu'il y a *identité de groupe sanguin entre les ascendants transmettant la maladie et les descendants qui la reçoivent, fait pour la première fois constaté dans une maladie héréditaire.*

Fig. 1.7 The paper by Caminopetros (1938b) in which he describes the Mendelian transmission of thalassaemia.

tant work was carried out quite independently in the USA and in Italy. It was only after the end of the War, when scientific communication became possible and several new haematology journals with a truly international flavour were established, that it was possible to amalgamate information from Europe and the USA.

In 1940 Wintrobe and colleagues described typical thalassaemic blood changes in some of the relatives of Italian patients with moderately severe thalassaemia attending the Johns Hopkins Hospital, Baltimore. They realized that this was a mild form of thalassaemia, and in a footnote pointed out that they had seen this haematological picture in both parents of a child with Cooley's anaemia. The story of this important observation is reviewed by Conley and

Wintrobe (1976) and by Wintrobe (1985). Similar findings were published independently at about the same time in the USA by Dameshek (1940) and by Strauss *et al.* (1941). A series of more extensive genetic studies followed, notably by Smith (1948) and Valentine and Neel (1944, 1948). Valentine and Neel, whose work on the genetic transmission of thalassaemia was seminal, named the mild form of Cooley's anaemia 'thalassaemia minor', and the severe type described by Cooley 'thalassaemia major'. Dameshek pointed out that the microcytic anaemia in these cases is often accompanied by the presence of large, pale macrocytes and target cells and called the condition 'leptocytosis', or 'target-cell anaemia'. James Neel has written an interesting account of how he was stimulated to carry out his important studies on the genetics of thalassaemia by reading Wintrobe's account of the Baltimore family (Neel 1994).

At about the same time, and without any knowledge of the activities of the American workers, important studies on the genetic transmission of thalassaemia were carried out in Italy (Gatto 1942; Silvestroni & Bianco 1944, 1946a,b). An extensive bibliography of this work was published by Silvestroni (1949). At first it appeared as if one parent might be affected, particularly in families of patients with 'anaemia microcitica constituzionale'. In retrospect this is not surprising; these intermediate forms of thalassaemia are now known to result from interactions with 'silent' forms of β thalassaemia (see Chapter 13). But, when large numbers of patients with typical Cooley's anaemia were studied in Ferarra, both parents were found to have mild red-cell abnormalities and decreased red-cell osmotic fragility. Silvestroni and Bianco named this condition microcytaemia. By the end of the 1940s scientific communication had been freely established between Europe and the USA and it was possible for the results of these different studies to be more fully assessed and reviewed (Neel 1950; Bianco *et al.* 1952). By then it was clear that Cooley's anaemia is the homozygous state for a recessive or partially dominant Mendelian gene and that the heterozygous state is characterized by extremely mild anaemia with osmotically resistant red cells. Different nomenclature for the carrier state was used in Italy and the United States. Gatto called it 'thalassaemia minima', while Silvestroni and Bianco used the term 'microcytemia'. In English-speaking countries Valentine and Neel's 'thalassaemia minor' was favoured.

Thus by the early 1950s there was a genuine understanding of the genetic transmission of Cooley's anaemia. It was also clear that the milder, or intermediate, forms of thalassaemia are inherited, but their genetic relationship to thalassaemia major and minor remained unclear.

Thalassaemia is a heterogeneous disorder

Reviews of the work of this period, those of Marmont and Bianchi (1948) and Chini and Valeri (1949) for example, leave no doubt that the Italian workers of the time were extremely puzzled by the clinical variability of thalassaemia. They invoked 'modifying factors' and other mechanisms which might somehow lead to variation in the thalassaemic phenotype. Hence, by 1949 it was already apparent that thalassaemia is not a single disorder but a complex syndrome characterized by wide phenotypic diversity, ranging from profound anaemia in early infancy, through milder anaemia with splenomegaly, to symptomless conditions identified only by morphological or osmotic abnormalities of the red cells. This complexity is mirrored in Chini and Valeri's use of the term 'Mediterranean haemopathic syndromes' to describe these diverse disorders.

The stage was now set for the further analysis of thalassaemia by studies of the haemoglobin of patients with different forms of the condition.

1949–1960: thalassaemia as a genetic disorder of haemoglobin

The period after the late 1940s was a time of rapid progress in all aspects of the human haemoglobin field. By 1959 it was possible for Ingram and Stretton to set out their important theoretical model for the genetic basis of thalassaemia. The background information which allowed them to develop this hypothesis was derived from many different sources. There was already a large body of knowledge about the structure and genetic control of human haemoglobin, and studies of the haemoglobins of patients with different types of thalassaemia had been reported from many parts of the world. The field developed so quickly during the 1950s, and on so many different fronts, that in some cases it is difficult to give priorities for major discoveries.

The genetic control of human haemoglobin

It is beyond the scope of this book to recount the

early history of haemoglobin. This fascinating story, which starts with the observation by Michael Servetus in 1533 of how blood changes colour when it passes through the lungs, is recounted in several extensive reviews (Cournand 1964; Edsall 1972, 1980) and is summarized by Bunn and Forget (1986) and Weatherall and Clegg (1999).

Heterogeneity of human haemoglobin

It had been known since 1866, when Korber showed that human placental blood is more resistant to alkali denaturation than that of adults, that normal human haemoglobin is heterogeneous (Korber 1886). In 1949 Pauling and his associates, following a suggestion by William Castle of Boston, studied the haemoglobin of patients with sickle-cell disease, a condition that had been recognized by Herrick as far back as 1910, and showed that it had different electrophoretic properties from that of normal adult human haemoglobin. Moreover, all the haemoglobin of individuals with sickle-cell disease was abnormal, whereas that of symptomless carriers was a mixture of both normal and abnormal types; these were called 'haemoglobin (Hb) A' and 'HbS', respectively. Pauling and colleagues recognized that their findings must mean that the structures of Hbs A and S are different, and hence used the term 'molecular disease' to describe sickle-cell anaemia. An excellent account of this seminal discovery is given by Conley (1980).

Early genetic studies

The elegant genetic studies of Neel (1949), Beet (1949) and the Lambotte-Legrands (1951), taken together with the findings of Pauling and colleagues, suggested that the structure of human haemoglobin is controlled by a pair of genes, and that the sickle-cell gene is a mutant allele of the HbA gene. Soon afterwards HbC was described by Itano and Neel (1950) and later shown by Ranney (1954) to be an allele of HbS. There followed a spate of new electrophoretic haemoglobin variants whose inheritance appeared to follow a simple Mendelian pattern (Fig. 1.8). Several of them were also shown to be allelic with haemoglobin S. At first each new variant was named by a letter of the alphabet; when there were none left place names of the origins of the persons in whom the variant was first found were used.

In 1958 Smith and Torbert described a large Balti-

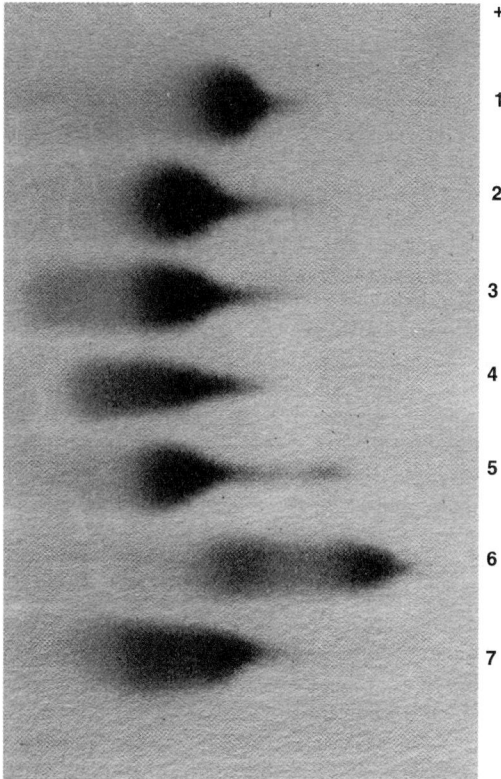

Fig. 1.8 Filter-paper electrophoresis of haemoglobin. This technique, used in the 1950s, was the main approach to identification of abnormal haemoglobins before methods were developed which gave better resolution. The anode is on the right and the following samples are analysed (top to bottom): 1, normal adult; 2, normal cord blood with Hbs F and A; 3, cord blood with HbC trait; 4, cord blood with HbS; 5, cord blood with Hb Bart's; 6, an adult with HbI and HbA (HbI α thalassaemia); 7, sickle-cell trait.

more family in which several members carried two abnormal haemoglobins, S and Hopkins 2, in addition to HbA. This important pedigree (Fig. 1.9) suggested that the genes for HbS and Hb Hopkins 2 were non-allelic, and hence that there must be two genetic loci involved in the control of adult haemoglobin synthesis. Furthermore, the patterns of segregation of these variants suggested that these two loci are not linked and, in fact, might be on separate chromosomes.

Further heterogeneity

In 1955, Kunkel and Wallenius described a minor

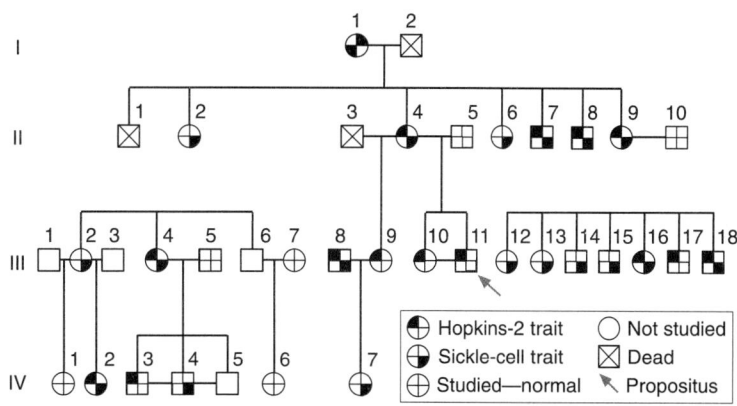

Fig. 1.9 The family pedigree published by Smith and Torbert (1958) which showed the independent segregation of two haemoglobin variants, Hopkins-2 and S. This was the first indication that there were at least two separate loci for the regulation of haemoglobin production. Later it was shown that Hb Hopkins-2 is an α-chain variant and hence this family demonstrated that the α- and β-globin genes are unlinked and probably on different chromosomes.

haemoglobin fraction in adult red cells which they called HbA$_2$. Later, a variant of this haemoglobin was described by Ceppellini (1959a,b), suggesting the existence of a third locus involved in the genetic control of adult haemoglobin.

Structural studies

While these genetic studies were being carried out, rapid progress was being made towards the elucidation of the chemical structure of haemoglobin. In 1956 Ingram showed that globin consists of two identical half-molecules. These findings agreed beautifully with X-ray crystallographic evidence (Perutz *et al.* 1960); in short, both approaches suggested that each half-molecule is made up of two different peptide chains. Further structural work confirmed that human adult haemoglobin consists of two pairs of identical peptide chains, which were called α and β (Rhinesmith *et al.* 1957; Braunitzer 1958; Braunitzer *et al.* 1961). Schroeder and Matsuda (1958) established that human fetal haemoglobin, although having a grossly similar structure to adult haemoglobin, has a different subunit composition. One pair of peptide chains is identical to the α chains of HbA; the others, which are quite unlike the β chains, were called γ chains. By the early 1960s technical advances in protein sequencing had enabled the complete amino-acid sequences of the α, β and γ chains to be determined. Furthermore, it was found that HbA$_2$ contained a fourth type of globin chain, δ, similar in structure to β, again combined with α chains (Ingram & Stretton 1961).

Ingram's demonstration that sickle-cell haemoglobin differs from normal by a single amino-acid substitution in the β chain, reviewed by Ingram (1989), together with increased knowledge of the inheritance of the sickle-cell gene, was an elegant demonstration of the extension of Beedle and Tatum's 'one-gene–one-enzyme' hypothesis to the concept of 'one-gene–one-peptide-chain'. In the context of haemoglobin this meant that the primary products of the globin genes would be single peptide chains and hence, since haemoglobin is composed of different subunits, it must be regulated by more than one pair of genes.

In 1960 Itano and Robinson re-examined the Baltimore family with Hbs S and Hopkins 2, and, using an ingenious method for dissociating and re-associating haemoglobin subunits in buffers of different pH, were able to show that Hb Hopkins 2 is an α-chain variant. Thus it appeared that the α and β chains of human haemoglobin are determined by distinct gene loci which are some distance apart on the same chromosome, or on different chromosomes.

An early synthesis

A picture of the genetic control of human haemoglobin was beginning to emerge. Four different loci, controlling the structures of the α, β, γ and δ chains, are involved. In fetal life the α-chain and γ-chain loci are active and produce HbF. Later, γ chains are replaced by β and δ chains, which, on combination with α chains, form Hbs A and A$_2$.

Haemoglobin patterns in patients with thalassaemia

The first observation that the haemoglobin constitution of thalassaemic patients might be abnormal predated Pauling's discovery of sickle-cell haemoglobin by several years. In 1946 Vecchio noted that the haemoglobin of patients with Cooley's anaemia was more alkali-resistant than normal adult haemoglobin. This suggested that these patients have more fetal haemoglobin than is usually found after the first year of life. Vecchio and colleagues extended and confirmed these findings, and Rich (1952) suggested that thalassaemia might result from a defect in HbA synthesis with persistent production of HbF. The fact that patients with thalassaemia major usually have elevated levels of fetal haemoglobin was confirmed by many workers over the next few years, and the chemical identity of the alkali-resistant haemoglobin of thalassaemia with that of genuine fetal haemoglobin was established.

Sickle-cell thalassaemia

The next clue to the general nature of thalassaemia came from the study of the haemoglobin patterns of patients with sickle-cell thalassaemia. This condition was first described by Silvestroni and Bianco in Italy (Silvestroni & Bianco 1944–45, 1946b) and called 'microdrepanocytic disease', and later recognized in the United States (Powell *et al.* 1950). The haemoglobin pattern of patients with this condition was first analysed by Sturgeon *et al.* (1952) and by Singer *et al.* (1955). They found that the red cells of patients who received the thalassaemia gene from one parent and the sickle-cell gene from the other have more HbS than HbA; that is, the *reverse* of what is found in the sickle-cell trait. This critically important observation suggested that the action of the thalassaemia gene was to *reduce* the amount of HbA relative to HbS, i.e. there was 'interaction' between the two genes.

However, it soon became evident that interaction of this kind between haemoglobin variants and thalassaemia did not always occur, an observation which gave an important insight into the genetic heterogeneity of thalassaemia. In 1954 Zuelzer and Kaplan described a patient with HbC thalassaemia, in whom the relative amounts of Hbs A and C were similar to those found in the heterozygous state for HbC alone. Cohen *et al.* (1959) later reported a family in which there was a form of sickle-cell thalassaemia which did

not result in reversal of the haemoglobin A/S ratio. Furthermore, whereas in most families with sickle-cell thalassaemia the thalassaemia gene appeared to behave as an allele of the sickle-cell gene, this was not the case in this family, in which the two genes segregated independently. The recognition of this 'non-interacting form' of thalassaemia, and its possible non-allelism with the sickle-cell gene, indicated that there must be at least two genetic loci involved in the generation of thalassaemia.

Another key observation on the alteration of the haemoglobin patterns in patients with thalassaemia was made in 1955, when Kunkel and Wallenius reported that levels of HbA_2 were raised in thalassaemia heterozygotes. This was confirmed by Gerald *et al.* (1961) and by many other workers subsequently. However, in a later paper, Kunkel and colleagues noted that in two out of 34 parents of children with thalassaemia major there were normal levels of HbA_2 (Kunkel *et al.* 1957), again pointing to the heterogeneity of thalassaemia.

Haemoglobins composed of homotetramers

Further evidence that thalassaemia is not a single genetic entity was gathered during the mid-1950s. In 1955, Rigas and colleagues observed an electrophoretically 'fast' haemoglobin variant in the blood of two members of a Chinese family, both of whom had the clinical picture of thalassaemia. At that time new haemoglobins were still being assigned letters of the alphabet and so the variant was called HbH. A similar haemoglobin was noted independently in a Greek patient with thalassaemia by Gouttas and colleagues in Athens in the same year (Gouttas *et al.* 1955). Further reports of the association of HbH with thalassaemia came from south-east Asia in 1958 and it was noted that the form of thalassaemia in these families was not usually associated with elevated HbA_2 levels (Minnich *et al.* 1958).

Chemical analysis of HbH showed that it consists of a tetramer of four apparently normal β chains (Jones & Schroeder 1963); that is, it has the molecular formula β_4. Hence HbH was, up to that time, a unique variant in that it had no α chains. However, in 1957 Fessas and Papaspyrou described an abnormal haemoglobin in the umbilical cord blood of an infant whose parents showed evidence of thalassaemia. Pending further identification it was called 'F and P'. A similar variant was reported in 1958 by Ager and

Lehmann in a nine-month-old infant with the blood picture of thalassaemia who was a patient in St Bartholomew's Hospital, London. Because by now there were no letters of the alphabet left for new haemoglobins this was called Hb Bart's. It was realized subsequently that this and the variant described by Fessas and Papaspyrou, 'HbF and P', are identical. Chemical studies showed that Hb Bart's is a γ-chain tetramer (γ_4) (Hunt & Lehmann 1959; Kekwick & Lehmann 1960). Haemoglobin Bart's thus appeared to be the fetal counterpart of HbH, i.e. a fetal haemoglobin variant without α chains.

The heterogeneity of thalassaemia

Hence several apparently unrelated observations about the haemoglobin of patients with thalassaemia were made between 1950 and 1960. First, it was established that many thalassaemia carriers, but not all, have raised HbA_2 levels. The thalassaemia gene associated with an increased level of HbA_2 'interacts' with the sickle-cell gene. However, there are forms of thalassaemia with normal levels of HbA_2 which do not interact with the sickle-cell gene, nor, or so it appeared, do their genetic determinants behave as though they are alleles of the sickle-cell gene. Finally, Hbs H and Bart's seemed to be associated with a form of thalassaemia with low levels of HbA_2, and both these variants were unusual in that they have no α chains and consist of tetramers of normal β or γ chains.

What was needed was a working hypothesis to explain these observations and hence to describe the general nature of the defect in thalassaemia and to account for its genetic heterogeneity.

The concept of α and β thalassaemia

Itano (1953) was the first to discuss the significance of the finding that the level of HbS in the sickle-cell trait is less than that of HbA. He had observed that the level of HbS in carriers falls into several modes which appear to be genetically determined, a finding that led him to propose his 'structure/rate' hypothesis. In short, he suggested that the rate of synthesis of a particular haemoglobin is in some way related to its primary structure. Pauling (1954) developed the idea that thalassaemia might result from the production of an abnormal haemoglobin with properties so closely similar to those of normal adult haemoglobin that the

differences might have escaped detection. He suggested that because the thalassaemia allele interferes with the manufacture of normal haemoglobin, but does not seriously affect the manufacture of abnormal haemoglobins, as observed in patients with sickle-cell thalassaemia, it must occupy the same locus on the chromosome as the alleles for other abnormal haemoglobins. He went on to suggest that the 'thalassaemia gene' might be responsible for the production of an abnormal haemoglobin of such a nature as to interfere with the inclusion of haem into the molecule. He further postulated that it should be possible to show a chemical difference between 'thalassaemia haemoglobin' and normal adult haemoglobin. Itano extended and refined the 'structure/rate' hypothesis and its relationship to thalassaemia and, in 1957, wrote 'thalassaemia mutants at the haemoglobin locus are analogous to the mutants for abnormal haemoglobins, differing in their failure to alter the net charge of adult haemoglobin and in the greater inhibition they exert on the net rate of synthesis' (Itano 1957).

In 1959 Ingram and Stretton extended these ideas in an important paper which proposed a model for the genetic basis of thalassaemia. They suggested that there are two major classes, α and β, in the same way as there are two major types of structural haemoglobin variants; that is, with abnormal α or β chains. They examined published pedigrees and explained quite elegantly the interaction between β thalassaemia and β-chain haemoglobin variants and α thalassaemia and α-chain variants. Furthermore, they went on to interpret the synthesis of HbH as resulting from an inherited defect in α-chain synthesis, resulting in excess β-chain production. While, like Pauling and Itano, they believed that the reduced rate of α- or β-chain synthesis might be due to a 'silent' (i.e. undetectable) mutation of the haemoglobin genes, they also proposed an alternative explanation, the 'tap hypothesis'. In essence, this suggested that the defect might not lie in the structural gene, but in the area of DNA in the connecting unit preceding it. They concluded that the genetic data available at that time were compatible with either hypothesis.

It is difficult to give clear-cut priorities for the elegant concepts and experimental work carried out in the late 1950s which culminated in the theoretical paper of Ingram and Stretton. In 1961, Itano and Pauling wrote a letter to *Nature* in which they claimed that the genetic and chemical studies on haemoglobin reported since 1957 had not substantially altered their inferences regarding the general nature of thalassaemia. This, they argued, was evidenced from the conclusions expressed by Ingram and his associates in their papers in the late 1950s. Incidentally, their paper had a sting in its tail; they added that Ingram's papers were remarkable for the extent to which the custom of giving pertinent references to the ideas and findings of previous workers had been ignored!

The ideas set out by Ingram and Stretton were undoubtedly influenced by other workers in the field at the time. Their paper was published in *Nature* on 19 December 1959. In May of the same year the Ciba Foundation had organized a symposium on 'Human Biochemical Genetics in Relationship to the Problem of Gene Action', in Naples, attended by many of the key workers in the haemoglobin field (Wolstenholme & O'Connor 1959). The structure/rate hypothesis and the likely genetic heterogeneity of thalassaemia were aired in great detail. From the lengthy published discussion after a paper by Hunt and Ingram on abnormal haemoglobins (which, incidentally, did not mention the notion of α and β thalassaemia) it is clear that many workers were thinking about the disease in this way. Indeed, Ceppellini, discussing the genetics of thalassaemia, said 'thus two genetically independent varieties of thalassaemia, α type and β type, could be visualized'. During the same discussion Neel summarized such limited evidence as existed at the time for allelism between β thalassaemia and the β-globin genes. And later in the same year Lehmann's group in London described α-chain deficiency in two generations of a family from Israel (Ramot *et al.* 1959).

In short, the seminal ideas about the nature of thalassaemia that evolved during the late 1950s were the product of many talented scientists. Undoubtedly, Itano and Pauling were responsible for the concept, first hinted at by Rich (1952), that thalassaemia results from a defect in the production of adult haemoglobin. But it was the extension of this idea, particularly in the framework of what was being learnt about the genetic control of haemoglobin, to trying to interpret the changes in the haemoglobin pattern in patients with thalassaemia, by workers such as Lehmann, Gerald, Neel, Ceppellini and colleagues, that culminated in the theoretical summary published at the end of 1959 by Ingram and Stretton.

This interpretation of events is supported by the generous acknowledgement made to the ideas of others at the end of their paper.

Thalassaemia is not confined to the Mediterranean region

Even as early as the 1930s sporadic case reports had started to appear that suggested that thalassaemia-like disorders are not confined to patients of Mediterranean background. Chernoff, in an extensive review in 1959, gave a very complete historical picture of the distribution of thalassaemia up to that time. By then it was quite clear that it occurs at a high frequency in south-east Asia, the Indian subcontinent and in parts of the Middle East.

Mediterranean anaemia in Asia

Some of the early studies in south-east Asia were the forerunners of a further level of complexity in the thalassaemia field that was to have important implications as attempts were made to relate genotype to phenotype. In 1954 Chernoff and colleagues described a new haemoglobin variant which was called 'HbE'. As more was learnt about this abnormal haemoglobin, it became apparent that, in homozygotes, it is associated with the phenotype of a very mild form of β thalassaemia, similar to the trait. Furthermore, it can interact with β thalassaemia to produce a severe form of thalassaemia, haemoglobin-E thalassaemia (Chernoff *et al.* 1956) (Fig. 1.10). Later work was to show that it is extremely common in parts of India, Burma and south-east Asia. In this sense HbE is a 'thalassaemic haemoglobin', that is, a structural variant that is associated with a thalassaemic phenotype. Over the next decade several more examples of haemoglobin variants with these properties were discovered. It is curious that Itano and Pauling, in their discussions of thalassaemia as a special form of haemoglobinopathy, never mentioned this work. Perhaps it was published just too late to add substance to their hypothesis.

Many workers throughout the world began to attempt to estimate thalassaemia gene frequencies in their populations. An early start was made in Thailand by Chernoff, Minnich, Wasi and Na-Nakorn and their colleagues. They carried out extensive population surveys in the 1950s, and by the end of the decade

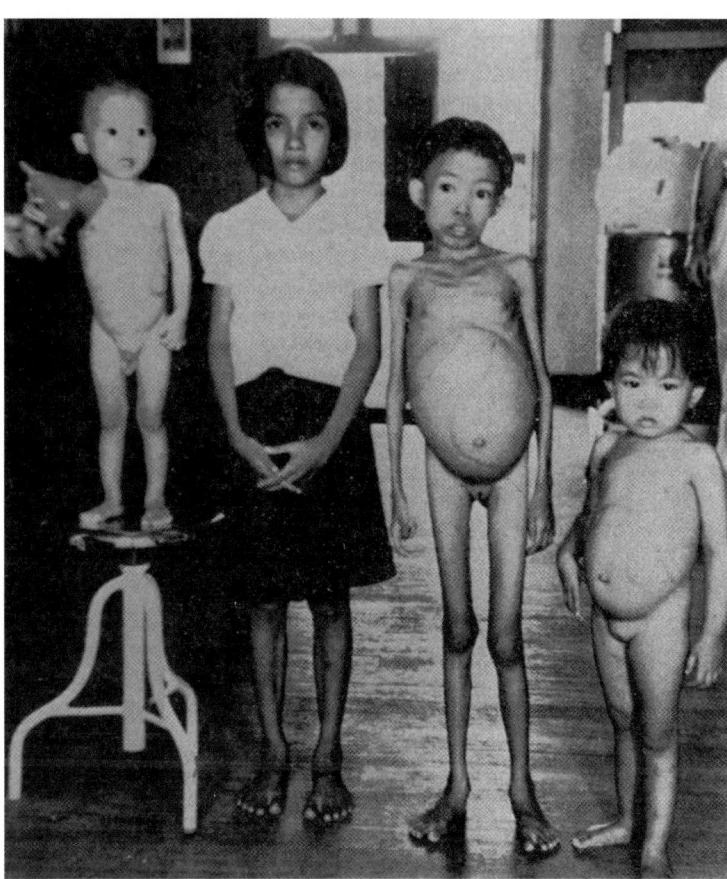

Fig. 1.10 The first children to be described as having haemoglobin E β thalassaemia. From Chernoff *et al.* (1956) with permission.

an extraordinary picture had emerged, both of the frequency and heterogeneity of thalassaemia in Thailand; indeed the Thais were later able to describe over 50 different genotypes of interactions of various α- and β-thalassaemia genes and HbE (Wasi *et al.* 1969). Other workers in south-east Asia, notably Vella and Wong in Singapore and Lie-Injo in Indonesia, obtained further evidence that both α and β thalassaemia are relatively common disorders in the populations of the Malay peninsula and Indonesia. Chatterjee and colleagues in Calcutta showed that the β-thalassaemia genes occur frequently in various Indian populations and Aksoy characterized the disease in Turkey. Details of some of these early population studies are given by Chernoff *et al.* (1956), Minnich *et al.* (1954, 1958), Vella (1958b), Weatherall and Vella (1960), Chernoff (1959), Lie-Injo (1959b), Aksoy (1959), Chatterjea (1959) and Wong (1966).

The frequency of the thalassaemias

Meanwhile, work continued on the analysis of the frequency and heterogeneity of thalassaemia in the Mediterranean region. Over many years Silvestroni and Bianco carried out extensive population surveys in various parts of Italy (Fig. 1.11), and Fessas and colleagues in Greece both estimated the gene frequencies and characterized the different forms of thalassaemia in several Greek populations (see Fessas 1959; Silvestroni & Bianco 1959). Beta thalassaemia had been recognized in the American black population in the mid-1950s (Schwartz & Hartz 1955) and it became evident that both α and β thalassaemia occurs in individuals of African origin (Weatherall 1964a,b).

During the late 1950s and early 1960s information about the occurrence of thalassaemia in the different

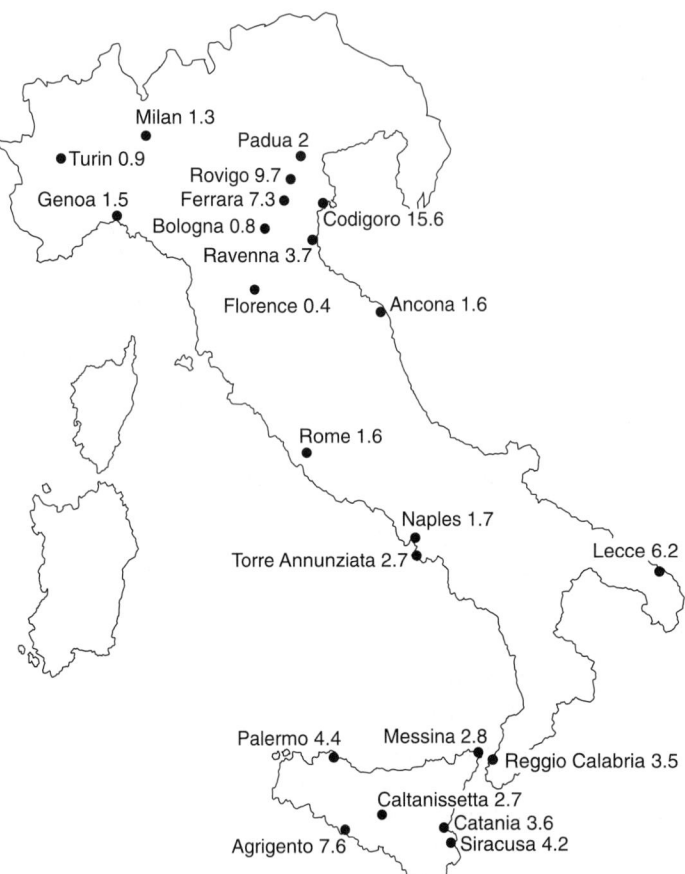

Fig. 1.11 The distribution of thalassaemia in Italy (percentage of population). Results of surveys using osmotic fragility screening. From Silvestroni and Bianco (1959).

populations of the world started to become widely disseminated. There are several reasons why this happened. Between 1958 and 1964 there were at least three major international meetings on the abnormal haemoglobins and thalassaemia, and several new journals were founded, the contents of which were restricted to diseases of the blood. It is not surprising therefore that the next 20 years were to see a dramatic increase in the thalassaemia literature and, in particular, the publication of surveys which attempted to establish the gene frequency of thalassaemia in different populations.

It should be remembered, however, that it was not easy to carry out large-scale, accurate population surveys during the 1960s and early 1970s. Although an elevated level of HbA$_2$ had been established as the diagnostic yardstick for the carrier state for β thalassaemia, the methods that were available for its estimation during this time were both tedious and difficult to apply to large population studies. Starch-block electrophoresis, described by Kunkel and Wallenius (1955), remained the only reliable method for many years, until it was superseded by more rapid chromatographic and electrophoretic approaches. Since electronic red-cell counters were not widely available until the 1970s, and morphological changes of the red blood cells in thalassaemia could be easily confused with those of iron-deficiency anaemia, screening using haematological criteria was impractical. These problems were not new, however. As early as 1943, Silvestroni and Bianco had developed a one-tube osmotic-fragility test to enable them to identify the increased osmotic resistance of thalassaemic cells. The story of this rapid screening method, and its application to large populations in different parts of Italy (Fig. 1.11), is recounted by Silvestroni and Bianco (1959).

The osmotic-fragility screening test was used

widely in the 1950s and 1960s and undoubtedly gave some indication of the frequency of thalassaemia in many different populations (Fig. 1.11). However, this technique was quite difficult to standardize and, at least in some studies, gave erroneously high figures for the frequency of thalassaemia. For example, Vella (1962b) estimated that about 25% of the population in Malta are thalassaemia carriers. But when the same population was studied using HbA_2 levels estimated by starch-block electrophoresis an incidence of only 3.5% was obtained (Cauchi 1970). And even those who attempted to study large populations by measuring HbA_2 levels ran into some difficulties. Although there was a reasonable separation of thalassaemic from normal values, every population that was analysed in this way showed some overlap, with varying numbers of individuals with HbA_2 values in the region of 3.5%, which were difficult to categorize (Weatherall 1964b; Weatherall *et al.* 1971).

By the early 1960s therefore it was clear that different forms of thalassaemia are distributed throughout the Mediterranean region, the Middle East, parts of Asia, India and Burma, and in south-east Asia. Because of the difficulties of accurate diagnosis many of the published figures for the frequency of thalassaemia may not have been entirely accurate, but there was now no doubt about the common occurrence of the disorder and the public health problem that it was likely to pose, particularly once the high infant and early-childhood mortality caused by malaria, malnutrition and other infections came under control in the developing world.

1960–1980

The stage was now set for rapid progress on many different fronts. A good working model of the genetics of the disease had been established and relatively simple analytical techniques had been developed for analysing the levels of Hbs A_2 and F and for detecting Hbs H and Bart's. Hence, haematologists in hospital laboratories throughout the world could study the haemoglobin of thalassaemic patients. It soon became apparent that not only are the thalassaemias extremely common, but both in their clinical manifestations and patterns of inheritance they are remarkably heterogeneous. During the early 1960s considerable progress was made towards a better understanding of their pathophysiology and a start was made in attempting to understand their underlying molecular pathology, work that was to culminate in a relatively complete understanding of their molecular basis during the 1980s.

The evolution of knowledge about the genetic control of the human haemoglobins

Work directed towards a better understanding of the genetic control of the different human haemoglobins progressed side by side with thalassaemia research throughout the 1960s and 1970s; the two fields of study were very closely related and fed off each other on more than one occasion. There were several long periods of uncertainty about the genetics of the thalassaemias which reflected gaps in an understanding of the numbers and arrangement of the globin genes. In the event it took nearly 15 years from the first description of the structures of the different human haemoglobins before a reasonably clear picture of their genetic control was obtained.

The association and assembly of the globin gene products

By 1960 it was clear was that there must be separate genes for the α, β, γ and δ chains and that the loci controlling the α and β chains are almost certainly on different chromosomes. During the early 1960s, studies of families with different haemoglobin variants clarified how the products of these genes interact to produce different fetal and adult haemoglobins. Several individuals were encountered who were doubly heterozygous for HbG, an α-chain variant, and the β-chain variant HbC (Atwater *et al.* 1960; Raper *et al.* 1960; Baglioni & Ingram 1961; McCurdy & Pearson 1961; Weatherall *et al.* 1962). In each case four major haemoglobin components were found. Since the genotype of such persons is α^A, α^G, β^A, β^C, and four types of dimer subunits are produced, α_2^A, α_2^G, β_2^A and β_2^C, their random combination should produce four molecular species: $\alpha_2^A\beta_2^A$; $\alpha_2^G\beta_2^A$; $\alpha_2^A\beta_2^C$; and $\alpha_2^G\beta_2^C$. This is precisely what was found in the red cells of these individuals. These observations provided clear evidence that, after synthesis of the globins, there is random combination of haemoglobin subunits.

Further information about the control of the assembly of the peptide chains of haemoglobin was obtained from studies of the HbA_2 and F of individuals who had inherited α-chain variants. Shooter *et al.*

(1960) and Weatherall & Boyer (1961) found that adult heterozygotes of this kind had two minor haemoglobin components, with the molecular formulae $\alpha_2\delta_2$ and $\alpha_2{}^X\delta_2$. Similarly, Minnich *et al.* (1962), Weatherall and Boyer (1962) and Weatherall and Baglioni (1962) found that in newborn infants who were heterozygous for the α-chain variant, HbG, there were four distinct haemoglobins, $\alpha_2\gamma_2$, $\alpha_2{}^G\gamma_2$, $\alpha_2\beta_2$ and $\alpha_2{}^G\beta_2$. These observations suggested that α-chain synthesis in fetal and adult life is controlled by the same genetic locus, α chains combining *in utero* with γ chains to produce HbF and in adult life with β chains to produce HbA; the switch from fetal to adult haemoglobin therefore involves a change from γ- to β-chain synthesis; α-chain production continues under the control of the same locus during intrauterine and adult life.

The embryonic haemoglobins

For a while, and largely because of the difficulty in obtaining blood samples from small fetuses, there was some doubt about the existence of a haemoglobin which precedes HbF in young embryos. However, in 1961 Huehns and his associates at University College Hospital in London described two embryonic haemoglobins which they called Hbs Gower 1 and Gower 2 (University College Hospital is in Gower Street). It turned out that Hb Gower 2 has normal α chains, the non-α chains, later called ε chains, differing in several places from the γ chains of HbF (Huehns *et al.* 1964b). Haemoglobin Gower 1, at first thought to be a homotetramer consisting of one type of globin chain, was later shown to consist of ζ chains (see below) and ε chains.

Some years later it was found that embryonic red cells and even cord-blood cells contain traces of a haemoglobin component with the formula $x_2\gamma_2$, which was named Hb Portland (Hecht *et al.* 1967). When it became clear that babies with certain forms of α thalassaemia have relatively large amounts of Hb Portland the characterization of this variant became possible. It was found that the 'x' chains differ from all the other normal globin chains (Capp *et al.* 1970; Todd *et al.* 1970; Weatherall *et al.* 1970). This work suggested that the 'x' chains of Hb Portland are the products of another normal haemoglobin locus that is only expressed early in fetal life. Hence the 'x' chains were designated ζ chains (Capp *et al.* 1970).

The numbers and order of the globin genes

During the 15 years or so that were required to define all the normal human globin chains there was slow but steady progress towards placing them in order on their respective chromosomes. As we shall see when we consider the genetic heterogeneity of thalassaemia, one of the most useful approaches to test for allelism or linkage is to examine children born of matings between a normal parent and one heterozygous for two variants at the globin-gene loci, different abnormal haemoglobins or one type of haemoglobin and a thalassaemia allele, for example. If the mutations of the two genes that we wish to investigate in this way are on the same chromosome, that is in *cis*, then, if the genes are linked, children born of a mating between a doubly affected person and a normal person should show either both variants or neither. On the other hand, if the two mutations of the linked genes are on opposite chromosomes, that is the linkage is in *trans*, the children will show one or other of the mutations, but never both or neither. Early studies of children born of matings between persons heterozygous for both β- and δ-chain haemoglobin variants provided unequivocal evidence that the β- and δ-globin-chain loci are linked (Ceppellini 1959a; Horton *et al.* 1961; Boyer *et al.* 1963b; Horton & Huisman 1963; Ranney *et al.* 1963). At about the same time Baglioni (1962) showed that the Hb Lepore variant, which we shall describe later, has non-α chains which consist of part δ and part β chains, that is they are the product of a $\delta\beta$-fusion gene. These observations, taken together, indicated that the δ- and β-globin genes are closely linked, in the order $\delta\beta$.

Throughout the early 1960s it was assumed that each of the human globin chains is under the control of a single gene. However, careful chemical studies of γ chains prepared from the blood of infants showed that position 136 is occupied not only by glycine, as had been reported in earlier structural studies, but also by alanine (Schroeder *et al.* 1968). Schroeder and colleagues also observed that, in infants heterozygous for an abnormal fetal haemoglobin, the abnormal fraction contained only glycine or alanine at position 136 in the γ-chain variant, a finding that was soon confirmed for other fetal haemoglobin variants (Cauchi *et al.* 1969). These results suggested that there are at least two γ-chain loci on each chromosome; one directs the production of $^G\gamma$ chains, that is, γ

chains containing glycine at position 136, the other the production of $^A\gamma$ chains, chains containing alanine at position 136.

Up until the early 1970s it was not clear whether the γ-chain genes were close to the β- and δ-chain genes, although the close linkage of the β-chain locus to the genetic determinant for hereditary persistence of fetal haemoglobin, a condition that we shall consider later, suggested that they might be. This problem was resolved in 1972 when Huisman and colleagues described Hb Kenya, a γβ fusion variant associated with the production of HbF containing only $^G\gamma$ chains (Huisman *et al.* 1972). By analogy with the haemoglobin Lepores it was suggested that the γβ chain had arisen by unequal crossing over between misaligned chromosomes, such that the DNA coding for the N-terminal part of the $^A\gamma$ gene had become fused to that coding for the C-terminal end of the β gene. In the process the DNA coding for the other ends of the $^A\gamma$ and β genes and the entire δ gene had been deleted. This interpretation suggested that the most likely order for the non-α-globin genes is $^G\gamma$–$^A\gamma$–δ–β.

When it was discovered that the human γ-gene loci are duplicated, thoughts turned to whether any of the other human gene loci might have undergone the same process. Hints that this might be the case first came from the study of other species. Kilmartin and Clegg (1967) found that in the horse there are four different α chains which seemed to be the product of allelic genes and which were later shown to direct the synthesis of different quantities of gene products (Clegg 1970). At about the same time Huisman *et al.* (1967) found that the α-chain locus is duplicated in the goat. Based on these observations, and the curious finding that, overall, α-globin-chain variants tend to occur at lower levels than β-chain variants in humans, Lehmann and Carrell (1969) suggested that the human α-chain loci might be duplicated. In 1970 there were reports of families which, initially, provided evidence both for and against this suggestion. Two individuals of Hungarian origin were found to be heterozygous for two α-chain variants. In addition to the two variants, they were both found to have considerable quantities of HbA (Brimhall *et al.* 1970). This could only occur if there are two α-chain loci (or more) on each chromosome. Since one of these individuals had a child with neither α-chain variant, the possibility was raised that the loci are not closely linked. On the other hand, in the same year an

individual homozygous for the α-chain variant HbJ Tongariki was described. In this case no HbA was found (Abramson *et al.* 1970).

During the 1970s a number of other individuals homozygous for α-chain variants, or compound heterozygous for two α-chain variants, were encountered, all of whom also had HbA in their red cells. The variants included Hb Constant Spring (Lie-Injo *et al.* 1974), Hbs Koya Dora and Rampa (de Jong *et al.* 1975) and HbJ Mexico (Trabuchet *et al.* 1976–77). The puzzle of HbJ Tongariki was not solved until some years later when it was found that this variant occurs at an α-chain locus on a chromosome on which its partner α-globin gene has been lost by one of the deletions that gives rise to α thalassaemia. These findings, taken together with the slow accumulation of information about the genetics of α thalassaemia that we shall describe later, left little doubt that in humans there are two α-globin genes per haploid genome and, furthermore, it seemed highly probable that they are closely linked.

The chromosomal location of the globin-gene clusters

In the late 1970s it was finally possible to determine the chromosomal location of the human globin-gene clusters. This work depended on the application of methods of somatic cell genetics. Fused human and mouse fibroblasts were used to obtain hybrid cell lines devoid of various human chromosomes. Correlation of the chromosome content with the presence or absence of human globin genes detected by nucleic-acid hybridization led to the assignment of the α gene to chromosome 16 and the γδβ-gene cluster to chromosome 11 (Deisseroth *et al.* 1977, 1978).

Thus by the late 1970s the order of the human haemoglobin genes in the α- and non-α-gene clusters was known, together with an approximate chromosomal location of the clusters. There was still no information about the relationship of the embryonic ζ and ε genes to these clusters, although, based on no better evidence than that the other genes were in the order in which they were expressed during development, it was guessed that they would lie upstream, that is, to the left of the clusters. When direct gene mapping was used to analyse these clusters in the early 1980s, these predictions were found to be correct.

The genetic heterogeneity of the β thalassaemias

Characterization of β thalassaemia

By the early 1960s sufficient numbers of homozygous and heterozygous β thalassaemics had been studied to establish a reasonably clear picture of the haemoglobin findings in this disorder. Those in homozygotes were not easy to interpret because their transfusional status was not always clear. However, it appeared that the fetal haemoglobin level could range widely, between 10 and over 90% of the total haemoglobin. Furthermore, although HbA$_2$ values ranged from low normal to those found in heterozygotes, the mean level in most series was within the normal range (Carcassi *et al.* 1957a; Kunkel *et al.* 1957; Marinone & Bernasconi 1957; Silvestroni *et al.* 1957; Josephson *et al.* 1958; Fessas 1959; Went & MacIver 1961; Sitarz *et al.* 1963).

The findings in β-thalassaemia heterozygotes were much more consistent. The mean HbA$_2$ level in several large series ranged from about 3.5 to 6.5%, though in many of the early series there appeared to be a few patients with values in the normal range (Carcassi *et al.* 1957b; Kunkel *et al.* 1957; Silvestroni *et al.* 1957; Josephson *et al.* 1958; Fessas 1959; Vella 1959; Gerald *et al.* 1961; Weatherall 1964a). There were several extensive studies of fetal haemoglobin levels in heterozygotes published at about this time. In 130 cases of mixed ethnic background reported by Beaven *et al.* (1961) about half had no demonstrable increase in HbF, while the remainder fell into the 1–5% range, with a mean level of 2.1%; only seven cases had levels of 5% or over. Similar results were obtained in 50 Greek patients studied by Fessas (1959) and in 90 black patients reported by Weatherall (1964a).

It appeared therefore that homozygous β thalassaemia is usually a transfusion-dependent disorder characterized by the production of very high levels of fetal haemoglobin and a variable amount of HbA$_2$; the HbA$_2$ level appeared to be of little diagnostic help. On the other hand, the level of HbA$_2$ is almost invariably elevated to about twice normal in heterozygotes, while the fetal haemoglobin levels may be raised, but rarely to more than 5% of the total haemoglobin. And there were increasing hints that there might be forms of β thalassaemia with normal levels of HbA$_2$.

The β-thalassaemia determinant is an allele of the β-globin gene

One of the key issues at about this time was whether the genetic determinant for β thalassaemia is an allele of the structural locus for the β-globin chains. Evidence that this might be the case depended on studies of the children of matings between compound heterozygotes for β thalassaemia and β-globin structural variants, sickle-cell thalassaemia or HbC thalassaemia for example, and normal persons. If the β-thalassaemia and structural loci are alleles the offspring of such matings should either have β-thalassaemia trait or carry the β-haemoglobin variant; there should be no normal or compound heterozygous children. In 1959, at the time of Ingram and Stretton's paper on α and β thalassaemia, there were very few data of this type available. This important problem was addressed by both Ceppellini and Neel in the discussion session at a Ciba Foundation Symposium on the Biochemistry of Human Genetics in Naples (Wolstenholme & O'Connor 1959). Ceppellini presented several families which showed evidence of allelism, while Neel described one family with apparent non-allelism, which was published later that year (Cohen *et al.* 1959). Interestingly, the form of thalassaemia which segregated independently from the β-globin locus in this family was one which was not associated with an elevated level of HbA$_2$. Weatherall (1964a) provided strong evidence for allelism for β thalassaemia and the β-globin locus in an extensive study of black families, and in the first edition of this book, published in 1965 (Weatherall 1965), it was possible to collate observations on 62 offspring of matings between sickle-cell thalassaemics and normals. Of the five offspring who were reported as normal, three came from the family of Cohen *et al.* (1959) and in two cases there were insufficient data to be certain about the type of thalassaemia involved. These findings, together with essentially similar data from studies of children born of patients with HbC thalassaemia (McCurdy & Pearson 1961; Weatherall 1964a), seemed to leave little doubt that the β-thalassaemia and β-structural genes are alleles.

β thalassaemia is heterogeneous with respect to the level of β-chain production

In the thalassaemia field, as in many branches of

science, important advances have followed the development of new techniques at least as commonly as new ideas. In the early 1960s improved methods for separating and analysing haemoglobin variants became available. Fessas and Karaklis (1962), using a two-dimensional paper–agar electrophoretic system demonstrated the absence of HbA in cases of homozygous β thalassaemia. Starch gel electrophoresis, developed by Oliver Smithies for the separation of serum proteins (Smithies 1959), was first adapted for haemoglobin analysis by Shooter *et al.* (1960) and Weatherall and Boyer (1961). Although these workers used slightly different modifications it was clear that this technique offered major advantages over filter-paper electrophoresis, particularly for detecting minor haemoglobin variants. Applying this approach to the study of patients with sickle-cell and HbC thalassaemia, Weatherall (1964b) found that they fell into two clear-cut groups: those who produce HbA, usually in the 20 to 30% range, and those in whom no HbA can be detected. It appeared that the former group might be heterogeneous; in a few cases much lower levels of HbA were found. Furthermore, the ability to produce HbA always ran true within families.

It appeared therefore that there must be two main forms of β thalassaemia, HbA- and non-HbA-producing. These observations were presented in 1963 at the first Cooley's Anaemia Conference in New York. During the discussion that followed, Fessas mentioned that he had made similar observations in Greek patients with sickle-cell thalassaemia, data which were presented at the Ibadan symposium in 1963 (Fessas 1965). It seemed therefore that there are two distinct forms of β thalassaemia in different populations, in which there is either a reduced level of β-chain production or no β-chain production at all. During the late 1960s these were given the names β^0 and β^+ thalassaemia, respectively; the term β^{++} thalassaemia also came into limited use to describe β thalassaemia with relatively high levels of HbA (Fessas 1968).

The discovery of δβ thalassaemia

Further evidence for the heterogeneity of β thalassaemia stemmed from studies of the haemoglobin patterns of heterozygotes. During the early 1960s several workers observed thalassaemia carriers who had normal levels of HbA_2 and levels of F in the 5 to 15% range; that is, much higher than usually observed in β-thalassaemia heterozygotes (Zuelzer *et al.* 1961; Fessas & Stamatoyannopoulos 1962; Weatherall 1964a). Because this condition 'interacted' with high HbA_2 β thalassaemia to produce a more serious clinical disorder in compound heterozygotes, it appeared to be a form of β thalassaemia. Initially it was called the 'high fetal haemoglobin variety of β thalassaemia', or 'F thalassaemia'. While these early descriptions were mainly in Mediterraneans and Africans it soon became apparent that it also occurs in Orientals (Flatz *et al.* 1965b; Wasi *et al.* 1969; Mann *et al.* 1972). By the mid-1960s this disorder had collected further synonyms, including normal HbA_2 β thalassaemia and β thalassaemia type 2.

Later, the homozygous state for F thalassaemia was observed (Brancati & Baglioni 1966; Fessas 1968; Silvestroni *et al.* 1968b; Ramot *et al.* 1970). All these patients, who had the clinical picture of a mild form of Cooley's anaemia, had 100% fetal haemoglobin, and no Hbs A or A_2. Thus this condition could now be defined as a variant of β thalassaemia in which there is complete absence of β- and δ-chain production; therefore it was called δβ thalassaemia.

The first description of hereditary persistence of fetal haemoglobin

Evidence that there is another condition resembling thalassaemia, with similarities to δβ thalassaemia, came from a completely different source. In 1955 Edington and Lehmann described a Nigerian patient with a mild form of sickle-cell anaemia characterized by unusually high levels of fetal haemoglobin. This appeared to be the result of the inheritance of the sickle-cell gene from one parent and a gene associated with the production of approximately 25% fetal haemoglobin from the other. Surprisingly however, the heterozygous parent with the high level of fetal haemoglobin seemed otherwise haematologically normal. Similar families were reported from Uganda by Jacob and Raper (1958), who, emphasizing the absence of thalassaemic red-cell changes in the individuals with high levels of HbF, suggested the name 'hereditary persistence of fetal haemoglobin (HPFH)' for this condition.

Similar forms of HPFH were subsequently observed in Ghana (Thompson & Lehmann 1962), Nigeria (Watson-Williams 1965), Jamaica (Went & MacIver 1958a; MacIver *et al.* 1961) and in Afro-

Americans (Herman & Conley 1960; Bradley *et al.* 1961; Kraus *et al.* 1961; Oliva & Myerson 1961). The most complete description of HPFH in Blacks was reported by Conley *et al.* (1963), who summarized the findings in 19 Baltimore families. It was now clear that the heterozygous state for HPFH is characterized by fetal haemoglobin levels in the 15 to 25% range and slightly reduced levels of HbA$_2$. There are no haematological abnormalities. In compound heterozygotes for HPFH and Hbs S or C there is no HbA, but again, the levels of HbF are unusually high—in the 20 to 30% range. The offspring of matings between such persons and normals are heterozygous for either HPFH or the β-globin variant, suggesting allelism or close linkage between the β structural gene and that for HPFH.

Further information about the nature of HPFH came from the study of three Black homozygotes (Wheeler & Krevans 1961; Ringelhann *et al.* 1970; Siegel *et al.* 1970). These people all had 100% fetal haemoglobin with no Hbs A or A$_2$. Although they appeared to be clinically and haematologically normal, their red cells were both small and poorly haemoglobinized. Thus it appeared that HPFH is an extremely mild form of δβ thalassaemia in which defective β-chain production is almost, but not entirely, compensated by increased HbF synthesis.

Further heterogeneity of δβ thalassaemia: the identification of haemoglobin Lepore

There were further twists to the story of defective δ- and β-chain synthesis. In 1961 Gerald *et al.* had discovered a haemoglobin variant associated with a thalassaemia-like disorder. One parent and four relatives of a child with the clinical picture of thalassaemia major carried about 10% of an abnormal haemoglobin which migrated in a similar position to HbS. This variant was named Hb Lepore, after the family in which it was first found. The first definitive chemical studies of Hb Lepore were reported by Baglioni (1962). He showed that it has normal α chains combined with non-α chains which consist of portions of both δ and β chains. He suggested that the non-α chain of Hb Lepore has arisen by unequal crossing over at the closely linked δ and β loci, with the production of a δ–β fusion gene. It was assumed that it was a property of the δ gene sequences that caused the product of the fusion gene to be produced

at a reduced rate, thus leading to the phenotype of β thalassaemia.

There followed descriptions of Hb Lepore in other Italians (Pearson *et al.* 1959; Silvestroni & Bianco 1963; Wolff & Ignatov 1963; Barkham *et al.* 1964; Labie *et al.* 1966), Greeks (Fessas *et al.* 1962), Papuans (Neeb *et al.* 1961), Turkish Cypriots (Beaven *et al.* 1964), American blacks (Ranney & Jacobs 1964; Ostertag & Smith 1969), Yugoslavs (Duma *et al.* 1968), Romanians (Rowley *et al.* 1969), Indians (Chouhan *et al.* 1971), and others. Further chemical studies of Hb Lepore from these different population groups showed that there were at least three distinct varieties, Hb Lepore Washington Boston, the first variant to be studied chemically, Hb Lepore Hollandia (Barnabus & Muller 1962) and Hb Lepore Baltimore (Ostertag & Smith 1969). These variants differed from Hb Lepore Washington Boston in the position of the crossover event which generates the δβ fusion gene.

Patients homozygous for Hb Lepore were discovered in Greece (Fessas & Stamatoyannopoulos 1964), New Guinea (Neeb *et al.* 1961), Yugoslavia (Duma *et al.* 1968), and Italy (Quattrin *et al.* 1967). As might be expected they produced only Hbs Lepore and F, with no Hbs A or A$_2$.

Although, with the possible exception of Yugoslavia, the forms of thalassaemia associated with Hb Lepore are uncommon, this chapter of the thalassaemia story is of considerable importance. First, it confirmed genetic studies that were carried out in the early 1960s which suggested that the δ- and β-globin genes are closely linked, and it established the order of these genes along the chromosome. And, of course, the Hb Lepore disorders were the first forms of thalassaemia in which the molecular basis was understood, at least in outline.

β Thalassaemia shows even greater heterogeneity

As well as these well defined variants of β and δβ thalassaemia, during the 1960s and early 1970s there was growing evidence for even further heterogeneity. Much of this information came from unexpected findings in the parents or relatives of children with different clinical forms of β thalassaemia. As mentioned earlier, it had long been suspected that there must be at least some forms of β thalassaemia in which the HbA$_2$ level is not elevated. Since in some cases there were no associated haematological changes the only evidence for the existence of a β-thalassaemia gene lay in the consequences of its interaction with typical forms of thalassaemia associated with a raised HbA$_2$ level. In other words, a family study of a patient with β thalassaemia intermedia would reveal that one parent had typical β-thalassaemia trait, while the other was 'normal'. It was from studies of families of this kind that the concept of a 'silent' β-thalassaemia gene arose (Silvestroni & Bianco 1951; Silvestroni *et al.* 1957; Aksoy 1959; Aksoy *et al.* 1961; Bernini *et al.* 1962; Schwartz 1969). However, as time went on it became apparent that there were other forms of 'normal HbA$_2$ β thalassaemia', in which the red-cell findings in heterozygotes were indistinguishable from those with a raised HbA$_2$ (Aksoy *et al.* 1975; Silvestroni *et al.* 1978; Kattamis *et al.* 1979). In order to describe these different types of β thalassaemia they were designated 'normal HbA$_2$' β thalassaemia, types 1 and 2. Later genetic studies hinted that the more severe form, type 2, might often result from the inheritance of both β and δ thalassaemia (Silvestroni *et al.* 1978).

But this was not the end of the heterogeneity of the β thalassaemias. Rare reports had appeared over this period which suggested that there is yet another form of high HbA$_2$ β thalassaemia with unusually high HbF levels in heterozygotes (Weatherall 1964a; Schokker *et al.* 1966), or unusually high levels of HbA$_2$ (Braverman *et al.* 1973; Schroeder *et al.* 1973b, 1974). The situation was complicated further by observations that in a few European families there was a thalassaemia-like disorder with many of the features of β thalassaemia intermedia which was inherited in a dominant fashion, that is, the result of a single mutant gene (Weatherall *et al.* 1973; Stamatoyannopoulos *et al.* 1974; Friedman *et al.* 1976a).

Thus in the 20 years that followed the classification of the thalassaemias into α and β forms, substantial evidence for the heterogeneity of the β thalassaemias was obtained. It became apparent that there must be many different types of mutation that can affect the β-globin genes themselves, and another and equally diverse set of lesions that can underlie defective synthesis of both δ and β chains. There was also some progress towards an understanding of how these different disorders can lead to such diverse clinical phenotypes. However, to understand how this came about we need to leave β thalassaemia for the moment and discuss the development of knowledge about α thalassaemia and how the thalassaemias mediate their effects at the level of the red-cell precursors. Because, in the event, it turned out that all these pieces of the jigsaw had to be in place before it was possible to appreciate the many factors that can modify the action of mutations at the β- or β- and δ-globin-gene loci.

The accumulation of knowledge about α thalassaemia

The exploration of the α thalassaemias between 1960 and their first analyses by the tools of molecular biology in the late 1970s is a good example of the confusion that can arise in a research field if some of the critical premises on which it is based are uncertain (or wrong). Had the family that provided the first real evidence that humans have two α-globin genes per haploid genome, and not one, been discovered 10 years earlier, a great deal of hard work, not to mention many hours of speculation and review writing, would not have been necessary. But this was not to be; those who worked on α thalassaemia had to do the best that they could with the incomplete information that was available about the genetic control of human α globin.

We shall not subject our readers to a blow-by-blow recapitulation of the tortuous discussions about the genetics of α thalassaemia of previous editions of this book, but simply outline the main steps that led to its clarification in the late 1970s and early 1980s.

Haemoglobin Bart's as a 'marker' of α thalassaemia

There are several threads to the early part of this story. We have already recounted the first, that is, the discovery of Hbs H and Bart's and the suggestion that they reflect accumulation of excess γ and β chains due to defective α-chain synthesis. After its discovery, Hb Bart's was found subsequently in newborn infants from many population groups (Vella 1958b; Tuchinda *et al.* 1959; Hendrickse *et al.* 1960; Minnich *et al.* 1962; Weatherall & Boyer 1962). Based on its structure it was reasonable to assume that it is the fetal counterpart of HbH and that, like the latter, it occurs when there is a deficiency of α chains, in this case in intrauterine life. Further evidence in favour of this notion came from the finding that the red cells of some adults with HbH disease also have traces of Hb Bart's (Fessas 1960; Huehns *et al.* 1960; Sturgeon *et al.* 1961).

A curious feature that puzzled many workers who found increased levels of Hb Bart's in cord blood was the observation that the variant usually disappeared over the first six months of life and was not replaced by HbH (Minnich *et al.* 1962; Weatherall & Boyer 1962; Weatherall 1963, 1964b; Pootrakul *et al.* 1967b, 1970). This unexpected finding suggested that babies with a moderate increase in Hb Bart's at birth might have milder forms of α thalassaemia. An argument was developed along the following lines. During the neonatal period, at the time of the switch from fetal to adult haemoglobin production, both γ and β chains are competing for available α chains. Hence a mild deficiency of α chains will become evident during this time and will be reflected by a small excess of γ chains, particularly if α chains bind β chains in preference to γ chains. Once the switch from γ- to β-chain production is complete, the deficiency of α chains might be too small to lead to the production of detectable amounts of HbH (Weatherall 1963). It was reasoning along these lines that led to the notion that the neonatal period might be the most useful time to demonstrate the milder forms of α thalassaemia. This concept led to many surveys of newborn infants for increased Hb Bart's levels and hence to a crude assessment of α-thalassaemia gene frequencies.

The haemoglobin Bart's hydrops syndrome

The third strand in the α-thalassaemia story also dates from 1960, when Lie-Injo and Jo (1960a,b) described a stillborn Indonesian infant whose haemoglobin consisted largely of haemoglobin Bart's. Further cases were reported from Malaya by Lie-Injo *et al.* (1962), and this condition, which became known as the Hb Bart's hydrops fetalis syndrome, subsequently became widely recognized in south-east Asia (Wong 1965; Pootrakul *et al.* 1967a; Todd *et al.* 1967). It appeared that these babies had inherited an extremely severe form of α thalassaemia which caused them to produce very high levels of Hb Bart's and led to stillbirth with the clinical picture of intrauterine hypoxia and hydrops fetalis.

α Thalassaemia inherited together with haemoglobin variants

The final thread that was to complete the background to the later and more successful studies of α thalassaemia came from the gradual accumulation of information about the haemoglobin patterns of individuals who had inherited α thalassaemia together with α- or β-haemoglobin variants. Although this approach had been seminal in the first studies of the genetics of β thalassaemia, it proved to be much more complicated in the case of α thalassaemia. During the early 1960s several patients were reported who had inherited the α-chain variant HbQ together with α thalassaemia (Vella *et al.* 1958; Dormandy *et al.* 1961; Lie-Injo & de V. Hart 1963). These individuals had the clinical picture of HbH disease; their haemoglobin consisted of Hbs Q and H and there was no HbA. This was important information, because, taken together with the findings in babies with the Hb Bart's hydrops syndrome, it suggested that a severe form of α thalassaemia exists that is associated with no α-chain production. However the picture was soon complicated by the findings in a Black patient with HbI thalassaemia, described by Atwater *et al.* (1960). This patient was healthy, but had mild thalassaemic blood changes associated with a haemoglobin pattern consisting of about 70% HbI, the rest being HbA with a low level of HbA_2. Clearly, if this patient had inherited an α-thalassaemia gene, and the finding of Hb Bart's in several of their children suggested that she had (Baglioni & Ingram 1961), it must be milder and not characterized by a complete absence of α-chain production. This suggested that there might be a less severe form of α thalassaemia, at least in African populations.

As mentioned earlier, Cohen and colleagues had reported a Black family with sickle-cell thalassaemia in 1959 in which the thalassaemia determinant segregated independently from the sickle-cell gene and did not interact with it, that is, the level of HbS in the doubly affected patient was similar to or even lower than that in the sickle-cell trait. The first evidence that this might be a form of α thalassaemia was obtained by Weatherall (1963, 1964b), who followed up a group of infants who had had increased levels of Bart's in infancy and who had also inherited either the sickle-cell or HbC traits. As they grew older and the Hb Bart's disappeared these infants developed the picture of non-interacting sickle-cell or HbC thalassaemia, very similar to that described earlier by Cohen and colleagues. It appeared therefore that the 'non-interacting' form of thalassaemia which occurs in Black populations is a mild type of α thalassaemia.

Hypotheses on the genetics of α thalassaemia based on observations up to 1965

By the late 1960s, certain facts about α thalassaemia had been established. It was known that the Hb Bart's hydrops fetalis syndrome results from the inheritance of two severe α-thalassaemia genes. Although the genetics of HbH disease was confusing there was enough evidence to conclude, in the first edition of this book, that 'HbH disease appears to result from the interaction of one α-thalassaemia gene with a second gene which is not detectable by present techniques in the absence of the α-thalassaemia gene. It may well be that this 'silent' gene itself is an α-thalassaemia gene, another factor suggesting heterogeneity of the α thalassaemias' (Weatherall 1965). It was also clear that α thalassaemia is widespread in Black populations, but the absence of HbH disease or the Hb Bart's hydrops fetalis syndrome suggested that it must be a mild form. Hence the scene was set for workers in a population with a high incidence of the different clinical types of α thalassaemia to put all these apparently disconnected facts together.

Further clarification of the genetics of α thalassaemia

The critical studies came from the group in Bangkok (Wasi *et al.* 1964; Pootrakul *et al.* 1967a,b; Na-Nakorn *et al.* 1969; Pornpatkul *et al.* 1969; Na-Nakorn & Wasi 1970). These workers took two different though related approaches to the problem. First, they made extensive studies of the level of haemoglobin Bart's in Thai newborns to see if, with large numbers of cases, they could demonstrate any segregation of values of levels of the variant at birth. In their earlier papers they had found increased haemoglobin Bart's levels in 6.2% of newborns in Thailand, but later, using a more sensitive technique, found the figure was 20% (Pootrakul *et al.* 1967b, 1970). In the latter study they suggested that the relative amount of Hb Bart's could be 'graded' into: traces, small amounts and moderate amounts, corresponding to 1 to 2, 5 to 6 and 25% of Hb Bart's, respectively. Using the term 'α

thalassaemia 1' for the more severe α-thalassaemia allele, and 'α thalassaemia 2' for the milder one, they suggested that concentrations of Hb Bart's in cord blood of 100, 25, 5 and 1 to 2% represent α-thalassaemia-1 homozygosity, α thalassaemia 1/α thalassaemia 2 (HbH disease), α-thalassaemia-1 trait and α-thalassaemia-2 trait, respectively.

With this working hypothesis the Thai group went on to investigate the frequencies of different α-thalassaemia genes in northern Thailand. Using the Hardy–Weinberg distribution the frequencies that they obtained were compatible with α-thalassaemia-1 and α-thalassaemia-2 loci being alleles, or closely linked. Furthermore, their findings provided strong evidence that HbH disease follows the interaction of these genes. Further evidence that this is the case was obtained by Na-Nakorn *et al.* (1969) who examined 31 offspring of HbH disease patients and found that all of them had Hb Bart's; there was a tendency for the levels of Hb Bart's to fall into two groups, with vales of 1 to 2 and 5 to 6%, respectively.

One of the difficulties in understanding the genetics of HbH disease had been the many well-documented examples of parent-to-child transmission of this disorder. If the two α-thalassaemia genes are alleles this must result from a mating between a patient with HbH disease and a carrier of either α thalassaemia 1 or 2. Wasi and colleagues estimated that, in order to account for the observed incidence of parent-to-child transmission in Thailand, the overall incidence of the two α-thalassaemia genes must be about 21%; in the cord-blood surveys cited above, there is an overall incidence for α thalassaemia 1 and 2 of 20.4%, a remarkably close agreement to the predicted figure.

α Thalassaemia associated with an α-chain termination mutation

A further twist to the α-thalassaemia story occurred in 1970 with the discovery of the elongated α-chain variant, Hb Constant Spring (Clegg *et al.* 1971b; Milner *et al.* 1971). This novel haemoglobin was first identified in a Chinese family in Jamaica (Constant Spring is a district of Kingston) and genetic analysis suggested that it was associated with the clinical phenotype of α thalassaemia 2; that is, when it is inherited together with α thalassaemia 1 it produced HbH disease (Fig. 1.12). Later studies in Thailand suggested that at least 1 to 2% of the population carry a haemoglobin variant similar to Constant Spring and there-

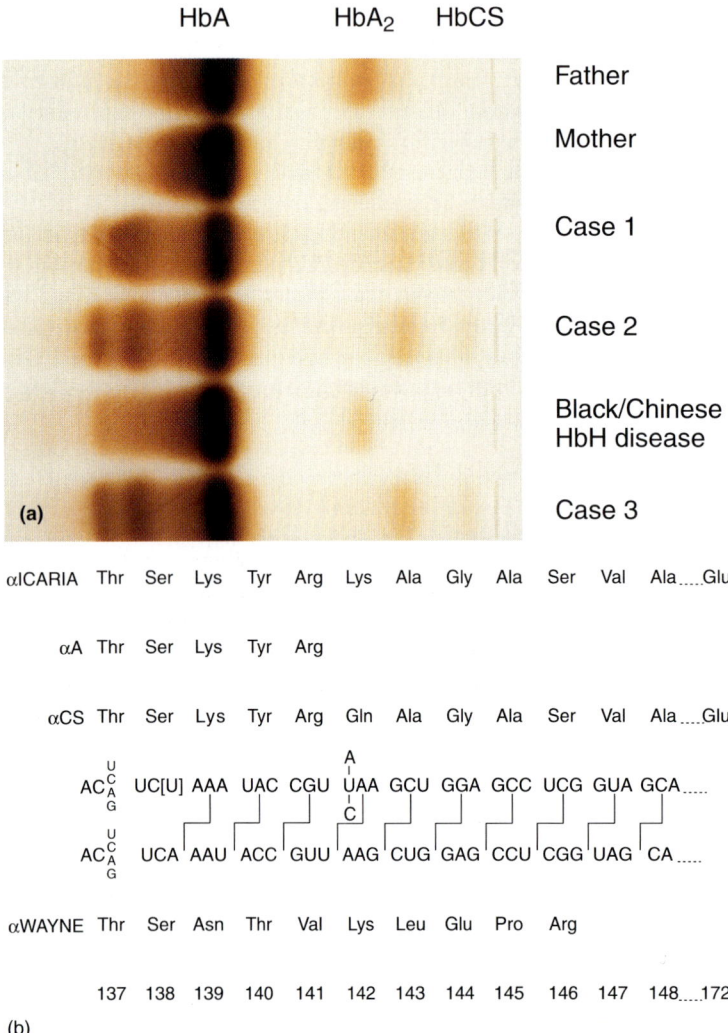

(a)

αICARIA   Thr Ser Lys Tyr Arg Lys Ala Gly Ala Ser Val Ala ....Glu

αA   Thr Ser Lys Tyr Arg

αCS   Thr Ser Lys Tyr Arg Gln Ala Gly Ala Ser Val Ala ....Glu

AC$^{U}_{A}$$^{C}_{G}$ UC[U] AAA UAC CGU UAA GCU GGA GCC UCG GUA GCA.....

                                   A
                                   |
                                   C

AC$^{U}_{A}$$^{C}_{G}$ UCA AAU ACC GUU AAG CUG GAG CCU CGG UAG CA ....

αWAYNE Thr Ser Asn Thr Val Lys Leu Glu Pro Arg

         137 138 139 140 141 142 143 144 145 146 147 148....172

(b)

Fig. 1.12 Haemoglobin Constant Spring (HbCS). (a) Starch gel electrophoresis of the first family with this disorder to be identified, sent to the authors by Dr Paul Milner. The two HbCS components can be seen in the three cases of HbH disease, migrating between HbA$_2$ and the origin. (b) When it was found that the α chain of Hbs Constant Spring and Icaria has an elongated C-terminal end it was apparent that it might result from a point mutation in the α-globin gene termination codon. With the amino acid sequence of the extended α chain, together with information derived from an elongated α-chain variant due to a frameshift mutation, Hb Wayne, it was possible to deduce the structure of the region of α-globin mRNA after the chain termination codon, which is not normally translated. This structure was later shown to be correct by nucleotide sequencing. From Clegg *et al.* (1974).

fore, in Thailand at least, there must be two genetic forms of HbH disease, α thalassaemia 1/α thalassaemia 2, and α thalassaemia 1/Hb Constant Spring. A similar variant was found in Greece at about this time and, when samples from Greece, Thailand and Jamaica were compared in the authors' laboratory, they were found to be identical (Fessas *et al.* 1972).

Studies of the structure of Hb Constant Spring suggested that it results from a mutation of the α-globin-gene chain termination codon, UAA→CAA, which leads to the insertion of an amino acid (glutamine) instead of the termination of chain synthesis (Fig. 1.12). The elongated α chain was thought to result from the translation of mRNA beyond the termination codon, which is not normally utilized, thus destabilizing the α-globin mRNA and leading to defective α-chain synthesis (Clegg *et al.* 1971b). It was anticipated that a family of such variants might exist, due to different substitutions in the α-chain termination codon. This was subsequently found to be the case (Weatherall & Clegg 1975). Thus the α-chain termination mutations joined the Hb Lepores as forms of thalassaemia in which the molecular pathology was anticipated, at least in outline, well before the molecular era.

Models of α thalassaemia based on lesions of one or other of a pair of linked α-globin genes

As mentioned earlier, much of the work of the late

1960s was put on a more solid basis by the discovery of the family in which the presence of two structural α-globin variants showed that, beyond any reasonable doubt, there must be two α-globin loci per haploid genome. During the late 1960s and early 1970s several workers produced models for the genesis of the different forms of α thalassaemia based on the deletion or inactivation by other mechanisms of one or both of the putative linked α-globin genes as the basis for α thalassaemias 1 and 2, respectively. Although other models had to be considered, particularly if the two α-globin genes were not linked, the data that were available at the time were more compatible with the two α genes being closely linked (Lehmann & Carrell 1968; Lehmann 1970; Wasi 1970; Weatherall & Clegg 1972).

Thus by the early 1970s there was a reasonable understanding of the genetics of α thalassaemia, at least in Oriental populations. But many questions remained. For example, there was genetic evidence that forms of HbH disease might occur in other parts of the world that were due to homozygosity rather than compound heterozygosity for α thalassaemia (McNiel 1967, 1971). Furthermore, it was still not clear how the milder forms of α thalassaemia in Black populations were related to the different forms in Orientals. And there remained some equally perplexing problems about the haemoglobin constitution of patients who had inherited both α thalassaemia and α-globin structural variants.

However, many of the fundamental genetic problems had been solved. The field was ready for these models and hypotheses to be verified by the methods of molecular biology, which were to become available in the mid-1970s; gratifyingly to those who had struggled through the morass of uncertainties of the preceding years, most of them were!

The classification of α thalassaemia

The nomenclature of α thalassaemia also changed in the late 1960s; at the 12th Congress of the International Society of Haematology in 1968 Fessas suggested that, to keep in line with the descriptive β^0- and β^+-thalassaemia classification, it would be sensible to change the term 'α thalassaemia 1', which was now thought to result from the loss of both linked α-globin genes, to α^0 thalassaemia. Similarly, α thalassaemia 2 should be called 'α^+ thalassaemia', since it was assumed that one of the two α genes had been lost or inactivated, and hence there is still α-chain

synthesis directed by the affected chromosome. Although subsequent molecular studies were to show that these predictions about the molecular pathology of α thalassaemia were correct, it took a long while for the α^0/α^+-thalassaemia notation to come into wide usage. We made a strong plea for this in the last edition of this book, but α thalassaemia 1 and 2 still keep turning up in the literature. Indeed the α^0/α^+-thalassaemia nomenclature has been heavily criticized recently (Huisman *et al.* 1997), though we find the arguments unconvincing.

Why is thalassaemia so common? Early progress in population genetics

Earlier, we discussed the remarkable explosion of information in the 1940s and 1950s that enabled Chernoff to write an extensive review in 1959, describing the world distribution of the thalassaemias. As the heterogeneity and genetics of thalassaemia was worked out in the 1960s and early 1970s, and with gradual improvement in techniques for population screening, these early impressions about the high frequency of the thalassaemias in many parts of the world were confirmed and extended. It gradually became apparent that these disorders must represent the commonest single-gene diseases in humans, and that they have a particularly high frequency in the Mediterranean region, the Middle East, the Indian subcontinent and Burma, and in south-east Asia in a line starting in southern China, passing down the Malay peninsula, and ending in the island populations of Melanesia. Although they were also found sporadically in every population group, it was soon apparent that there are no particularly high-frequency populations outside this tropical belt. And, surprisingly, this disease did not seem to be common in the indigenous populations of the New World.

The extraordinarily high gene frequencies for the sickle-cell and β-thalassaemia traits puzzled population geneticists, particularly those who had become interested in mutation rates as a result of their investigations of the survivors of the atomic bombs which had been dropped on Hiroshima and Nagasaki. From their first population studies in the USA, and assuming that the fitness of a thalassaemia homozygote is zero and that the heterozygote is selectively neutral, Neel and Valentine (1947) calculated a mutation rate for thalassaemia of 1 in 2500. An even higher rate was proposed by Silvestroni (1949), who also suggested that some form of positive selection must have operated to maintain the frequency of thalassaemia heterozygotes.

The malaria hypothesis

In 1948, J.B.S. Haldane, addressing the Eighth International Congress of Genetics in Stockholm, proposed that the selective agent for maintaining the high frequency of thalassaemia might be malaria. He spoke as follows:

> Neel and Valentine believe that the thalassaemia heterozygote is less fit than normal, and think that the mutation rate is above 4×10^{-4} rather than below it. I believe that the possibility that the heterozygote is fitter than normal must be seriously considered. Such increased fitness is found in the case of several lethal and sublethal genes in *Drosophila* and *Zea*. A possible mechanism is as follows. The corpuscles of the anaemic heterozygotes are smaller than normal, and more resistant to hypotonic solutions. It is at least conceivable that they are also more resistant to attacks by the sporozoa which cause malaria, a disease prevalent in Italy, Sicily and Greece, where the gene is frequent . . . Until more is known about the physiology of this gene in various environments I doubt if we can accept the hypothesis that it arises very frequently by mutation in a small section of the human species. (Haldane 1949b)

In a recent and not over-generous review of Haldane's contribution, Lederberg (1999) suggests that the concept of genetic resistance to infection was already well known by this time. He does not reference the paper that we have just quoted, but discusses a paper published in the same year based on a lecture given by Haldane at the Symposium on Ecological and Genetic Factors in Speciation among Animals, held in Milan (Haldane 1949a). Haldane does not mention thalassaemia or malaria in this paper. It is possible that Montalenti may have brought his attention to the work of Silvestroni and colleagues in Italy at this meeting. However, in a footnote recording the discussion, Montalenti acknowledges a verbal communication from Haldane to the effect that carriers of thalassaemia may be more resistant to malaria. Haldane is recorded as suggesting that they may also be advantaged in an environment in which iron defi-

ciency is common. Since the Milan meeting followed the one in Stockholm, it is clear that Haldane had already formulated his ideas on heterozygote advantage before these discussions. Certainly his account of what became known as the 'malaria hypothesis' in his paper that followed the meeting in Stockholm was the first clear exposition of this concept—one that was to become central to our later understanding of the population genetics of thalassaemia.

According to Haldane's hypothesis the high frequency of thalassaemia might therefore reflect an example of balanced polymorphism. P.M. Sheppard, in his excellent book *Natural Selection and Heredity*, describes, in simple language, the work of quantitative geneticists like R.A. Fisher and E.B. Ford, whose ideas formed the basis for our understanding of how genes achieve their frequencies in different populations. Ford defined polymorphism as 'the occurrence together in the same habitat at the same time of two or more distinct forms of the species in such proportions that the rarest of them cannot be maintained merely by recurrent mutation'. Sheppard points out that this type of phenomenon usually reflects a situation of particular genetic and evolutionary interest, because the presence of two or more distinct forms means that there is a balance of selective forces maintaining each of them in the population. R.A. Fisher showed that, if this were not the case, one of the forms would increase in frequency to the exclusion of the other, because it is very unlikely that two variants that are morphologically or physiologically different would be equally well fitted to the environment in which they exist. The term 'balanced polymorphism' intimates that the gene frequency for the advantageous heterozygous state for a condition like thalassaemia will increase until its incidence is balanced by the loss of homozygotes from the population. For no better reason than that nobody has ever come up with a better idea, Haldane's hypothesis has stood the test of time, though until the molecular era it was extremely difficult to obtain solid evidence to either confirm or refute it.

Early attempts to test the malaria hypothesis

As early as 1946 Vezzoso suggested that the distribution of thalassaemia in Italy is correlated with that of malaria. Certainly, this tended to hold true in the extensive population surveys for the distribution of the gene in Italy which were cited earlier in this chapter (see also Bannerman & Renwick 1962). But perhaps the most impressive evidence for the association between β thalassaemia and endemic malaria was obtained by Carcassi *et al.* (1957b) and Siniscalco *et al.* (1966) from population studies in Sardinia. In some ways Sardinia provides an ideal population for this type of study, since it has many villages which are of great antiquity and which have remained isolated for long periods. Furthermore, because of the high altitude of some of these villages, there are malaria-free populations of similar ethnic background to the lower-lying high malaria populations. Carcassi and Siniscalco and their colleagues showed a reasonably clear correlation between the frequency of malaria and β thalassaemia in the Sardinian population. Subsequently this work was subjected to heavy criticism, mainly based on uncertainties about the origins of the populations in the mountains and villages, although it is still far from clear whether all these concerns were justified.

Unfortunately, however, when such correlations were sought in other parts of the world they were not found. There seemed to be little relationship between the distribution of thalassaemia and present or past malaria in Greece (Fraser *et al.* 1964; Stamatoyannopoulos & Fessas 1964), Cyprus (Plato *et al.* 1964), Malta, Sudan and New Guinea (Gilles *et al.* 1967; Livingstone 1967). Similar negative or equivocal results were obtained in Thailand (Kruatrachue *et al.* 1969, 1970). At the same time as these studies were being carried out, a body of evidence regarding the putative protection of sickle-cell heterozygotes against *P. falciparum* malaria was growing. This has been reviewed extensively at different stages of its evolution and we shall not discuss it further here (Allison 1954; Rucknagel & Neel 1961; Allison 1964; Motulsky *et al.* 1964; Allison 1965; Livingstone 1967, 1971). In short, extensive population studies provided suggestive though not unequivocal evidence that the sickle-cell trait might protect against severe malarial infection. Later on, a number of *in vitro* studies of this protective effect were reported, though again many uncertainties remained about the precise mechanism involved (Luzzatto *et al.* 1970; Friedman 1978; Pasvol *et al.* 1978; Friedman *et al.* 1979).

The origins of thalassaemia

As well as trying to understand the mechanisms for the high frequency of the thalassaemias many workers began to wonder why the disease is so widespread among so many different populations. Not surprisingly perhaps, it was many years before the idea that it might have arisen independently in many parts of the world was considered. Thus there was much speculation about where thalassaemia might have first arisen. Some of the early ideas of this once hotly debated topic are summarized by Bannerman (1961). One of the first, and one that gained particular popularity, was the idea that the disease originated in an ancient race, 'Palaeoinsulara Mediterranea', which inhabited Sicily, Greece and parts of Italy, and from whence it spread by migration to other parts of the world. A number of variations on this theme were proposed. For example, it was suggested that thalassaemia was distributed by the Greeks of the 6th and 7th centuries BC who colonized Magna Grecia, including Sicily and southern Italy, and perhaps later spread eastwards within the empire of Alexander the Great. On the other hand, several writers who had observed thalassaemia in Persians proposed that the gene had arisen in the Orient and spread to the Mediterranean from the east; others, sitting firmly on the fence, suggested an Armenian origin with spread in both directions!

Speculations along these lines continued for many years. In 1978, Todd, in his inaugural lecture to the University of Hong Kong, entitled 'Genes, Beans and Marco Polo' (Todd 1978), gave an absorbing, and often lurid, account of the movements of the Mongoloid peoples and concluded that it is likely that the thalassaemia genes had followed these populations.

Until the new technology of the molecular era made it possible to re-examine the whole question of the world distribution and population genetics of the thalassaemias, little further progress was made. The story of the notions about the origins and distribution of the thalassaemias is, like Galen's interpretation of cardiovascular physiology, an interesting example of how, when incorrect ideas become widespread, they are extremely difficult to eradicate. As we shall see in Chapter 6, for the last 15 years it has been abundantly clear that the many different forms of thalassaemia are widespread in their distribution and have arisen independently in different populations throughout the world. Yet the *Cambridge World History of Human Disease*, published as recently as 1993, in its short insert on thalassaemia, states 'It has been suggested that thalassaemia originated in Greece and spread to Italy when it was colonized by Greeks between the 8th and 6th century BC. At present, it is most frequent in areas where ancient Greek immigration was most intense.'

Haemoglobin synthesis in thalassaemia

Although the analysis of the haemoglobin patterns of patients with different forms of thalassaemia was of enormous value in defining the thalassaemias as inherited disorders of globin production, it had its limitations. In the early 1960s it was realized that to understand the pathophysiology of the disease, that is, how abnormal gene action at the globin loci could result in the protean clinical manifestations of the thalassaemias, and to try to make some progress in understanding the types of mutations that might underlie the disease, a more dynamic approach was needed. Hence thoughts turned to the possibility of trying to study haemoglobin synthesis in the red-cell precursors of thalassaemic patients using some of the *in vitro* experimental systems that were being developed at the time to study normal haemoglobin synthesis.

It had been known for many years, since the pioneering experiments of London, Shemin, Borsook and colleagues, that it is possible to incorporate radioactive amino acids into haemoglobin in red cells incubated *in vitro,* provided there are sufficient numbers of reticulocytes present in the blood sample. Several groups of workers in the late 1950s and early 1960s made use of these techniques to try to pinpoint the defect in haemoglobin synthesis in thalassaemia. The earliest studies were carried out by Bannerman and Grinstein, working with Carl Moore in St Louis (Bannerman *et al.* 1959; Grinstein *et al.* 1960). These workers showed that there was a defect in haem synthesis in thalassaemic red cells, but it was difficult to equate this finding with the observed interaction between the thalassaemia and sickle-cell genes, which was much more in keeping with the idea that thalassaemia results from a primary defect in globin synthesis. For this reason it seemed likely that the defect in haem production was secondary to defective globin production.

Globin synthesis in thalassaemia

The earliest attempts to study the mechanism of defective globin synthesis in thalassaemic red-cell precursors were made by Marks and colleagues at Columbia University. Although they were able to study some aspects of *in vitro* haemoglobin synthesis,

and to rule out abnormal ribosomal function as the basis for thalassaemia (Marks & Burka 1964a,b; Marks *et al.* 1964), a story that we shall continue later, further progress was held up by the lack of a method for quantifying the relative rates of α- and β-chain production in thalassaemic red-cell precursors.

It was quite clear by the early 1960s that, because globin could be labelled with radioactive amino acids in an *in vitro* reticulocyte system, it should be possible to measure the relative rates of α- and β-chain synthesis, provided that a reliable method for separating these globins could be found which would give a quantitative recovery and which required relatively small quantities of starting material. At that time methods for separating the different globins were tedious, required large amounts of globin, often resulted in poor yields of either the α or β chains, and were quite unsuitable for analysis of the relatively small blood samples which were available from thalassaemic patients. In the early 1960s attempts were made by one of us to measure globin synthesis in thalassaemic reticulocytes by separating the chains by countercurrent distribution or by symmetrical recombination of the human α and β chains with canine globin chains. While equal labelling of α and β chains was obtained in experiments with normal reticulocytes, and there was clear evidence of unequal labelling of thalassaemic α and β chains, the results were not quantitative. In 1964 Heywood and colleagues also demonstrated unequal labelling of the α and β chains of haemoglobin after incubation of thalassaemic reticulocytes with radioactive amino acids. These workers separated the globin chains chromatographically, but the method they employed also made it impossible to quantify the relative rates of production of the α and β chains.

The technique which enabled further progress to be made was developed by Clegg *et al.* (1965, 1966), who showed that the peptide chains of globin could be quantitatively fractionated by chromatography on carboscymethyl (CM) cellulose in 8 M urea. At the same time these workers found that if human reticulocytes were labelled *in vitro* and then lysed and the whole lysate converted to 'globin' it was possible to measure the total amounts of α and non-α chains synthesized, with a recovery of radioactivity and protein in excess of 95% (Weatherall *et al.* 1965) (Fig. 1.13). As this technique was further refined it became possible to separate the γ and β chains and hence to provide an accurate assessment of the relative rates

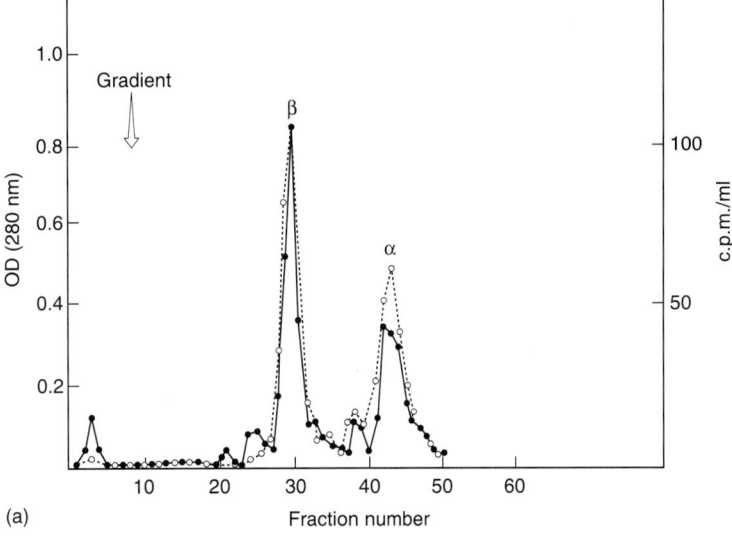

(a)

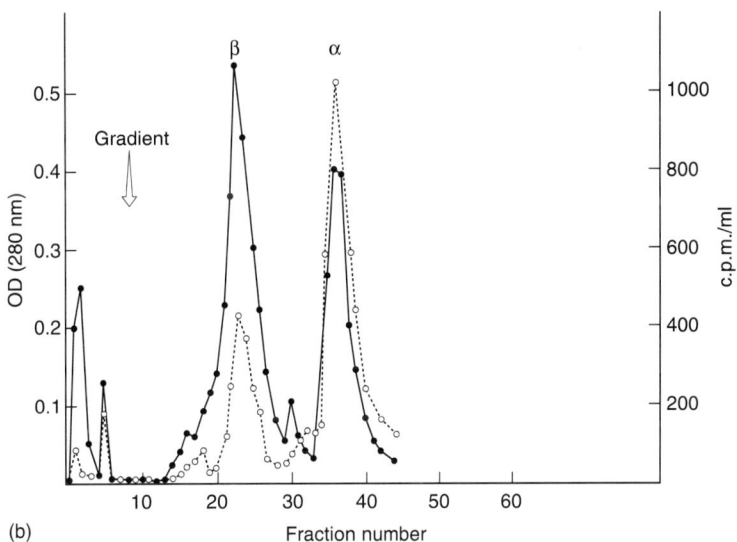

Fig. 1.13 Globin synthesis in β thalassaemia. These were the first experiments to demonstrate imbalanced globin production in β thalassaemia by *in vitro* labelling and separation by carboxymethyl cellulose chromatography. (a) Incorporation of radioactivity (open circles) into the α and β chains from a patient with hereditary spherocytosis. (b) The same experiment carried out on the red cells of a patient with β thalassaemia major, showing excess α-chain production. In these early experiments the conditions had not yet been developed in which the γ and β chains could be separated. Weatherall *et al.* (1965).

(b)

of globin synthesis, first in reticulocytes and, later, in bone-marrow red-cell precursors.

In the first description of the application of this technique to the study of thalassaemia it was possible to provide a fairly complete picture of the pattern of normal globin synthesis and of abnormal globin production in α and β thalassaemia. It was found that in normal reticulocytes α- and β-chain production is almost synchronous, although there is a very slight excess of α-globin production. In HbH disease a marked defect in α-chain synthesis was demonstrated. Furthermore, it appeared that as well as $β_4$ molecules the red-cell precursors of patients with this condition contain a relatively large pool of free β chains which are available to combine with newly synthesized α chains to produce HbA. In β thalassaemia there is also marked globin imbalance and, overall, a large excess of α chains are produced. It was also found that there is defective δ-chain compared with β-chain production in normal red cells (Weatherall *et al.* 1965).

In these early experiments it was often observed that, after incubation of reticulocytes from normal or β-thalassaemia patients, the δ or β globins had a lower specific activity than the α chains. At first we wondered if this reflected a 'block' of δ- or β-globin synthesis at the ribosomal level, with an accumulation of finished globin. However, this idea had to be revised when it was demonstrated that there is rapid exchange of newly made α chains with Hbs A or A_2. Hence it was difficult to learn much about the assembly of globin polypeptide chains by examining the patterns of radioactivity in completed haemoglobin molecules.

Over the next few years this type of approach was used by several workers and these results were confirmed and extended. By using a combination of gel filtration and chromatographic techniques it was possible to demonstrate a pool of free α chains in the cells of β thalassaemics that exchange freely with unlabelled α chains in HbA. It was also found that excess α chains undergo two fates; some are rapidly degraded by proteolysis, while others become associated with the red-cell membrane. It was confirmed that in some forms of β thalassaemia there is a complete suppression of β-chain synthesis, while in others there is only a partial defect (Bank & Marks 1966; Bank & O'Donnell 1969; Modell *et al.* 1969; Pontremoli *et al.* 1969; Weatherall & Clegg 1969; Weatherall *et al.* 1969b). It was also found that there is marked globin imbalance in other common forms of thalassaemia such as sickle-cell and HbE thalassaemia (Weatherall *et al.* 1969b).

Subsequently, *in vitro* globin synthesis was applied to study heterozygous forms of thalassaemia, particularly β thalassaemia. Several groups found that there is imbalanced globin synthesis in the reticulocytes, with α/β-chain production ratios ranging from 1.5 to 2.5 (Vigi *et al.* 1969; Schwartz 1970; Clegg & Weatherall 1972; Kan *et al.* 1972c; Shchory & Ramot 1972; Knox-Macaulay *et al.* 1973; Chalevelakis *et al.* 1975, 1976). About this time some puzzling observations were reported which suggested that globin synthesis might be more or less balanced in the bone marrow (Schwartz 1970; Kan *et al.* 1972c; Shchory & Ramot 1972; Gallo *et al.* 1975). However, Clegg and Weatherall (1972) found that there was some degree of globin imbalance in the bone-marrow precursors, together with a larger pool of free α chains than in normal bone marrow. When this problem was re-examined in detail by Chalevelakis *et al.* (1975, 1976) it became clear that there is imbalanced globin synthesis in bone marrow in heterozygous β thalassaemia and that previous reports of more balanced synthesis

probably resulted from the authors not taking into account the very rapid proteolysis of excess α chains in the marrow during the time in which the rates of globin synthesis were being measured.

In 1970 Weatherall *et al.* were able to study the pattern of haemoglobin synthesis in an infant with the Hb Bart's hydrops fetalis syndrome and could detect no α-globin synthesis or fragments of α-globin chains. Thus it appeared that the homozygous state for the severe form of α thalassaemia is characterized by a complete absence of α-chain production. At about this time several workers attempted to measure the relative rates of α- and β-chain production in heterozygotes for different forms of α thalassaemia (Kan *et al.* 1968; Schwartz *et al.* 1969). It was found that there is a significant reduction in α-chain synthesis in both 'silent' carriers and individuals with the α-thalassaemia trait, but that there is considerable overlap between the two groups. In a later study by workers in Thailand it was possible to obtain a reasonable separation between the α/β-chain synthesis ratios of heterozygotes for $α^0$ or $α^+$ thalassaemia, although the numbers reported were small (Pootrakul *et al.* 1975a). In the last edition of this book we concluded that, though many heterozygous α thalassaemics have significantly reduced α/β-globin synthesis ratios, because of the marked overlap between $α^0$ and $α^+$ thalassaemia, and between $α^+$ thalassaemia and normal, it is unlikely that this technique is precise enough to determine accurately which type of α-thalassaemia gene is present in any individual case; unfortunately, time has proved us right. However, until the advent of DNA technology this remained the only approach for attempting to define the α-thalassaemia carrier states.

Globin synthesis in fetal blood

Another application of the analysis of globin synthesis, and one which was to have important practical implications for the control of thalassaemia, followed in the early 1970s. From earlier studies of the electrophoretic patterns of fetal blood it appeared that small quantities of HbA might be present very early in fetal life (Walker & Turnbull 1955; Huehns *et al.* 1964b). As methods for analysing globin synthesis were improved in the early 1970s it became clear that β-chain synthesis is activated by the 8th week or even earlier, and reaches a steady level of about 10% of total non-α globin up to 30 to 34 weeks

(Hollenberg *et al.* 1971; Kan *et al.* 1972a; Pataryas & Stamatoyannopoulos 1972; Kazazian & Woodhead 1973; Wood & Weatherall 1973). In the study of Wood and Weatherall (1973) it was found that the relative rates of β- and γ-chain synthesis are synchronized throughout the different haemopoietic organs in the fetus; that is, the amounts of γ- and β-chain production do not differ between red cells produced in the fetal liver, spleen or bone marrow. Further work, by Kazazian and Woodhead (1974), Cividalli *et al.* (1974a) and Alter *et al.* (1976a,b), suggested that β-chain synthesis makes up about 7% of total globin synthesis at five weeks, and increases to approximately 11% at 20 weeks.

Prenatal diagnosis

These observations led to the important notion that if small blood samples could be obtained from fetuses between 10 and 20 weeks' gestation, and subjected to globin synthesis analysis, it might be possible to diagnose homozygous β thalassaemia *in utero*, assuming of course that the β-thalassaemia mutation is expressed early in fetal life. Reasoning along these lines led Chang *et al.* (1975) to examine globin synthesis in small blood samples obtained from aborted fetuses who were at risk of being homozygous for β thalassaemia. They found two cases in which the β/γ-chain synthesis ratios were approximately half of the value expected for the gestational ages, and one fetus in which there was no β-chain production. This study suggested that it might be possible to use this approach for prenatal diagnosis of β thalassaemia. Interestingly, the same method was used for the prenatal diagnosis of sickle-cell anaemia a year or two earlier (Kan *et al.* 1972a).

Of course a major difficulty remained; how to obtain fetal blood samples. Two ways were explored—placental aspiration and direct aspiration of samples from the chorionic plate by fetoscopy. Unfortunately, many of the blood samples obtained by these methods contained mixtures of fetal and maternal red cells. Not daunted, several workers explored a number of ingenious ways to separate them, or at least to try to calculate the degree of contamination of one by the other. They included suppression of maternal reticulocyte production by transfusion (Alter *et al.* 1976b), a variety of mathematical corrections to allow for maternal–fetal admixture of red cells (Cividalli *et al.* 1974a; Chang *et*

al. 1975), and the application of physical or chemical methods for separation of fetal and adult cells (Kan *et al.* 1974b; Furbetta *et al.* 1978; Alter *et al.* 1979a). Although all these methods were used in some of the early attempts at prenatal diagnosis, they proved difficult, and hence thoughts turned to direct fetal blood sampling. As the technique of fetoscopy improved it became possible to obtain fetal blood directly, an advance which greatly facilitated the prenatal diagnosis of thalassaemia (Valenti 1973; Hobbins *et al.* 1974; Hobbins & Mahoney 1975; Benzie & Pirani 1977). The problem of contamination of fetal blood samples with small amounts of maternal blood remained, however. In the end it was solved by using methods based on the difference in size between fetal and adult red cells (Kan *et al.* 1974b), together with the acid-elution technique of Kleihauer *et al.* (1957) for identifying the relative numbers of maternal cells in fetal blood samples.

By the end of 1978 groups of workers in the USA, England, Sardinia and Italy were able to publish the results of these early attempts at the prenatal diagnosis of β thalassaemia (Kan *et al.* 1975b,c; Alter *et al.* 1976a,b; Cividalli *et al.* 1976; Kan *et al.* 1976, 1977b; Alter & Nathan 1978; Fairweather *et al.* 1978; Furbetta *et al.* 1978). It appeared that, based on experience of well over 100 attempts, the technique seemed to be feasible for identifying homozygous β thalassaemia and sickle-cell anaemia; there had been remarkably few errors in diagnosis, and the only worrying feature was the relatively high fetal loss attributable to the procedure.

This was a particularly pleasing chapter in the story of the exploration of the thalassaemias. For, in little over 10 years, an experimental technique that had been developed to explore the rates of globin synthesis, and hence the pathogenesis of the disease, had been applied in several countries for its effective prenatal diagnosis. It was to be another 10 years before this approach was largely superseded by fetal DNA analysis, a time during which *in vitro* globin biosynthesis was applied widely in many populations and led to a major decline in the number of births of infants with severe forms of thalassaemia.

The pathophysiology of thalassaemia

The early literature on thalassaemia stressed the haemolytic basis for the anaemia. Indeed Cooley first described the condition as a haemolytic anaemia.

However, as pointed out by Bannerman (1961), Cooley and Lee soon felt that this was not a sufficient explanation and elaborated it a few years later, adding that some of the other features involving the bone marrow 'may be the result of some metabolic disturbance which compels the tissues to make bricks without straw' (Cooley & Lee 1932). In their early papers on the pathology of thalassaemia, Whipple and Bradford (1932, 1936) suggested that the disorder might result from a defect in the metabolism of pigment, similar to haemochromatosis, although they did not expand on this idea. Dameshek (1943) wrote: 'the fundamental inherited abnormality appears to lie in a disturbance of the haemoglobin metabolism', while a few years later Perosa (1949) listed the possible causes as either an impaired union of iron with porphyrin, defective porphyrin synthesis, or a lack, or abnormal synthesis, of globin. Indeed, Perosa, in a very detailed analysis of the evidence that was available at the time, came to the conclusion that an abnormality of globin synthesis was the most likely possibility.

In their extensive review of the clinical and haematological findings and aetiology of Mediterranean anaemia, written in 1948, Marmont and Bianchi stressed the diverse manifestations of the disease, including iron loading of the tissues, faulty red-cell production in the bone marrow, high iron levels in the blood associated with hypochromic red blood cells, excess ferritin in the tissues, and a shortened red-cell survival. They also stressed the increased rate of fragmentation of the red blood cells. Though they tried, they found it impossible to ascribe these diverse findings to a single mechanism. In the end the best they could do was to describe the disorder as a form of 'metabolic dyserythropoiesis', a term first used by the British haematologist Janet Vaughan (1948).

Once it was realized that the thalassaemias result from defective α- or β-chain production, thinking about their pathophysiology moved in two different though often overlapping directions. On the one hand workers in the field wanted to understand how mutations at the α- or β-globin gene loci could result in the widespread clinical manifestations, which seemed to affect nearly every system of the body and which were not confined to the red cells in which the globin genes are expressed. On the other, it seemed equally important to try to determine the different kinds of mutations that might underlie the defective production of α and β chains. Although both aspects of thalassaemia research moved along together after

the early 1960s, it turned out to be easier to answer the first set of questions; a definitive answer to the second had to await the molecular era in the late 1970s and early 1980s.

Ineffective erythropoiesis

Little progress towards a genuine understanding of the pathophysiology of thalassaemia was made until techniques became available for the study of red-cell survival and turnover with radioactive isotopes. Sturgeon and Finch in Seattle were the first workers to carry out careful iron and erythrokinetic studies on patients with thalassaemia major. Their work showed that there was a marked degree of ineffective erythropoiesis of a very similar pattern to that found in pernicious anaemia (Sturgeon & Finch 1957). This was confirmed by *in vivo* studies of haemoglobin turnover by Grinstein, Bannerman and colleagues (Bannerman *et al.* 1959). Later, Finch *et al.* (1970) found that the degree of ineffective erythropoiesis in thalassaemia is probably greater than in any other disorder. These findings implied that there is extensive destruction of red-cell precursors in the bone marrow as well as a shortened survival of red cells in the peripheral blood. Taken together with the massive expansion of the bone marrow, this work suggested that there is a major drive to erythropoiesis, but that the expanded bone marrow is incapable of effective red-cell maturation and production.

Globin precipitation and inclusions in red-cell precursors

A clue to the basis for the destruction of the red cells and their precursors came in 1963 from the elegant studies of Fessas in Athens. He showed that there are large, ragged inclusion bodies in the red-cell precursors of patients with β thalassaemia (Fig. 1.14). They were also found in the peripheral blood, but only after splenectomy, and their staining properties suggested that they contained haemoglobin. Fessas suggested that these inclusions might be precipitated α chains; in β thalassaemia, he reasoned, there could be an excessive production of α chains which might precipitate and produce intracellular inclusions. Because it was not yet known whether there was imbalanced globin production, he also suggested that they might be aggregates of abnormal β chains or complete haemoglobin molecules (Fessas 1963).

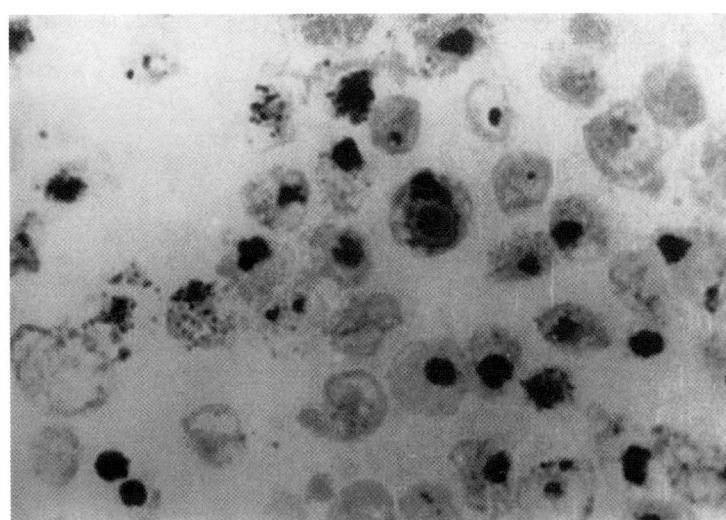

Fig. 1.14 The demonstration of red-cell inclusions in β thalassaemia. Kindly supplied by Professor Phaedon Fessas.

The work of Fessas, which shows how much can be achieved by an astute observer with a microscope and a few simple stains, was absolutely seminal in our understanding of the pathogenesis of β thalassaemia, particularly since imbalanced globin production was demonstrated shortly after he had made these observations. The inclusion bodies in the bone marrow, and in the peripheral blood after splenectomy, are so large and well defined that it is difficult to understand why it took nearly 40 years from the first description of the disease for them to be recognized. A careful reading of earlier papers that deal with the morphology of the marrow and blood shows very little evidence that they were observed before 1963, however. It is possible that the unusual structures described in earlier electron-microscopic studies (Hoffman *et al.* 1956; Bessis *et al.* 1958) may have been inclusions of this kind. In reviewing their Italian patients, Silvestroni and Bianco touched on the phenomenon of erythrocytic inclusions and pointed out that they are not restricted to HbH disease and are seen in other forms of thalassaemia (see Fig. 7 of Silvestroni & Bianco 1959). However, these are brilliant cresyl blue preparations of peripheral blood cells from patients with both thalassaemia major and intermedia. The preformed inclusions described by Fessas are best demonstrated with methyl violet, and, although they can sometimes be seen on brilliant cresyl blue preparations, those shown in Silvestroni and Bianco's paper do not resemble α-chain inclusions. In fact, they mentioned that they had published descriptions

of 'intracorpuscular crystallization' of haemoglobin as early as 1956. They concluded their discussion by saying 'it is evidently a non-specific phenomenon of microcythaemic syndromes. Its appearance in severe microcythaemic syndromes indicates, as in other haemoglobinopathies, only a generic instability of many abnormal haemoglobins.'

Large, single inclusion bodies had also been observed in the red cells of patients with HbH disease after splenectomy (Rigas *et al.* 1955). They were first described in Thai patients by Minnich *et al.* (1954) although, because HbH disease had not been diagnosed at that time, they were not recognized as such. It was suggested that HbH precipitates in older red cells and that the haemolysis of this disorder is due to the trapping of cells containing large inclusion bodies in the spleen (Rigas & Koler 1961). A similar mechanism presumably occurs in β thalassaemia and hence this is why inclusion bodies are only seen in the blood after splenectomy.

The notion that the major mechanism for damage to the red-cell precursors in the thalassaemias is globin precipitation was, of course, strongly supported by the finding of imbalanced globin synthesis, in both α and β thalassaemia (Weatherall *et al.* 1965). Furthermore, experiments of this kind showed that the free α chains which are produced in β thalassaemia are unstable and rapidly precipitate to become associated with the red-cell membrane (Bargellesi *et al.* 1968; Weatherall *et al.* 1969b). Subsequently it was found that some free α chains are destroyed by proteolysis. Thus it appeared that inclusion-body formation must reflect a balance between the magnitude of the excess of α chains and the red-cell precursors' capacity to cope with them by proteolysis (Bank & O'Donnell 1969; Clegg & Weatherall 1972).

The further consequences of unbalanced globin synthesis

During the early 1960s there was a gradual accumulation of evidence that there is remarkable heterogeneity in the amount and constitution of haemoglobin in the red cells of β thalassaemics. Using the acid-elution technique of Kleihauer *et al.* (1957) to stain red cells for fetal haemoglobin, several groups showed that the distribution of fetal haemoglobin is extremely heterogeneous (Frazer & Raper 1961; Mitchiner *et al.* 1961; Shepherd *et al.* 1962; Silvestroni *et al.* 1968a). The uneven distribution of HbF in sickle-cell anaemia and thalassaemia, compared with its more homogeneous distribution in hereditary persistence of fetal haemoglobin, was stressed by Shepherd *et al.* (1962) and Conley *et al.* (1963). Elegant *in vivo* labelling studies by Gabuzda *et al.* (1963) suggested that the relative turnover rates of HbA and F are different in β thalassaemia, and that HbF-containing cells survive relatively longer than those that contain predominantly HbA. These findings were confirmed by differential centrifugation studies which showed a greater proportion of HbF in the older, more dense red-cell populations (Loukopoulos & Fessas 1965).

By now it was clear therefore that all the thalassaemias are associated with imbalanced globin production, that both excess α and β chains precipitate to form red-cell inclusions, and that there is marked heterogeneity of haemoglobinization of the red blood cells in β thalassaemia, with the more rapid destruction of those that contain relatively less HbF.

The idea that the clinical haematological manifestations of thalassaemia are primarily a reflection of imbalanced globin production was refined and extended in l966 by Nathan and Gunn, who suggested that the abnormalities of red-cell maturation and survival could all be ascribed to the effects of unbalanced globin production, with precipitation of the particular globin subunits which are produced in excess. They argued that in β thalassaemia those cells which continue to produce γ chains will be relatively

protected from the deleterious effects of α-chain precipitation because some of the excess α chains combine with γ chains to make HbF ($\alpha_2\gamma_2$). This would account for the observation that HbF-containing cells survive relatively longer than HbA-containing cells in the blood. Nathan and Gunn also suggested that, in addition to causing abnormalities of cellular maturation, precipitating globin might interfere with membrane function and cause 'leakiness' of the red cells. This, together with the mechanical effects of inclusions on red cells in the microcirculation and spleen, might explain the haemolysis observed in all the thalassaemia syndromes. Although these concepts had to be refined and extended as more was learnt about the mechanisms of haemoglobin precipitation, work carried out over subsequent years confirmed that this general concept of the basis for the anaemia of thalassaemia is correct. In effect, all the important manifestations of thalassaemia are the result of globin imbalance and a complex combination of ineffective erythropoiesis and haemolysis.

'Experiments of nature' confirm importance of unbalanced globin production

As we have seen, it has been a recurring theme throughout the thalassaemia story that careful study of the unusual experiment of nature is likely to yield results which may have much wider implications. There is no better example than the discoveries that provided incontrovertible evidence that the thalassaemias are primarily disorders of imbalanced globin synthesis. If globin imbalance is the major cause of the anaemia in severe β thalassaemia, individuals with this condition who had also been fortunate enough to inherit α thalassaemia might have less severe anaemia. In effect, the two conditions should cancel each other out; the red cells would be hypochromic, but because there would be less α-chain excess there would be less globin precipitation, and hence more effective erythropoiesis.

In 1970 Kan and Nathan described a patient with a mild form of β thalassaemia intermedia whose parents both had raised levels of HbA_2. However, globin synthesis studies showed that one of them had the expected imbalance associated with β thalassaemia, while the other had balanced synthesis. The authors suggested that the latter person might be carrying an α-thalassaemia determinant and that the patient's mild course might result from the reduced amount of excess α-chain production consequent on the action of this α-thalassaemia gene. Interestingly, later analysis of this patient's α-globin genes failed to demonstrate any evidence of α thalassaemia (Dr David Nathan, personal communication)! Similar individuals were reported later by Musumeci *et al.* (1979a) and Weatherall *et al.* (1980). Of course these observations depended on the interpretation of balanced globin synthesis ratios as indicating the presence of α thalassaemia in β-thalassaemia heterozygotes, but as soon as it was possible to analyse the DNA of families of this type it became clear that α thalassaemia can undoubtedly modify the clinical course of homozygous β thalassaemia (Weatherall *et al.* 1981b).

A working model for the pathophysiology of thalassaemia

By the end of the 1970s, therefore, a reasonable working model of how mutations at the α- or β-gene loci can produce the remarkably diverse phenotypic effects of the thalassaemias had been developed. The severe globin imbalance of β thalassaemia leads to α-chain precipitation, intramedullary destruction of red-cell precursors, and haemolysis. The latter is associated with progressive splenomegaly and its consequences, including trapping of red cells and haemodilution. The selective survival of red-cell precursors that synthesize relatively more γ chains results in relatively large amounts of HbF in the blood of β-thalassaemic patients. The profound anaemia stimulates increased erythropoietin production, leading to expansion of the bone marrow and subsequent skeletal deformities. The widespread iron deposition in the organs is the result of increased iron absorption in the face of the marked dyserythropoietic anaemia, together with the effects of blood transfusion. Thus it became unnecessary to ascribe mysterious 'pleotrophic effects' to the action of the thalassaemia genes; a primary defect in globin production could explain most of the widespread clinical manifestations, and, incidentally, at least some of the phenotypic heterogeneity.

Greater knowledge of the pathophysiology of thalassaemia leads to improved treatment

The early textbook pictures of severe thalassaemia, showing children with gross skeletal deformities, growth retardation and massive enlargement of the spleen and liver, are a sad reflection on how little could be done for this disease up until the early 1960s. In countries in which blood transfusion services were available, transfusions were given, usually when the patient's haemoglobin level had fallen to an extremely low value. Otherwise children with severe thalassaemia died early in life. And even those who were transfused, usually when they were symptomatic, tended to succumb early to infections or other complications (see Bannerman 1961).

This chaotic and completely unsatisfactory state of the management of thalassaemia is well exemplified in a series of papers presented at a meeting in New York in 1963 organized by the Medical Advisory Board of the Cooley's Anemia Blood and Research Foundation for Children, Inc., and the New York Academy of Sciences. The current practices for transfusion of thalassaemic children were assessed from an enquiry sent to more than a dozen centres, caring in all for more than 150 patients with Cooley's anaemia. The results showed that there were no consistent criteria for determining when a child with thalassaemia should be transfused. Overall, transfusions appeared to be administered either when a particular haemoglobin level was reached, or when patients became symptomatic. In centres at which blood was administered for symptomatic treatment, the pre-transfusion haemoglobin level was often as low as 3.0 g/dl. And even if a particular haemoglobin level was chosen, it tended to be somewhere between 5 and 7 g/dl (Schorr & Radel 1964). It seems likely that these practices would have reflected those at almost any centre that was treating thalassaemic children up to the early 1960s.

High-level transfusion regimens

At the same meeting, Irving Wolman, of the Children's Hospital of Philadelphia, presented findings from a preliminary study that set out to determine whether thalassaemic children who had been maintained at a near-normal haemoglobin level were better off than those who had been transfused only when symptomatic. Wolman suggested, albeit tentatively, that children in the highest haemoglobin group were taller, had smaller livers and spleens, showed less skeletal deformities and fewer fractures, had better dental development, and appeared to have smaller hearts. It appeared therefore that a high transfusion regimen might be capable of reversing many of the more distressing features of severe thalassaemia (Wolman 1964). Though these observations were encouraging, Wolman was quick to point out that the children who had received more transfusions, though they were more healthy, would have received considerably more iron than those maintained at a lower haemoglobin level. On the other hand, he speculated that, by maintaining a high haemoglobin level, there might be less stimulus to increased iron absorption from the intestine so that, in the long term, they might accumulate less iron than those who grow up with consistently low haemoglobin levels.

At a similar meeting in New York 5 years later Wolman was able to present a further follow-up of this group of patients (Wolman & Ortolani 1969). By now it was clear that the children maintained on a high transfusion rate had grown well during their early years, although it appeared that they did not exhibit the normal adolescent growth spurt. On the other hand they continued to have less skeletal deformity and bone disease, and their spleens and livers were smaller. Worryingly, however, of a total 17 children who had been on the high-transfusion regimen for a sufficient number of years to warrant adequate evaluation, 6 had died, all from disorders which appeared to be related to the effects of iron loading. At the same meeting, Wolman's results were confirmed by similar studies on other groups of children with β thalassaemia (Beard *et al.* 1969; Piomelli *et al.* 1969). Further follow-up studies, both in the United States (Necheles *et al.* 1974; Piomelli *et al.* 1974) and in Europe (Kattamis *et al.* 1970; Loukopoulos 1976; Rotoli 1976; Modell 1977; Esposito *et al.* 1978), left little doubt that children maintained on a high-transfusion regimen fared much better than those who are transfused on demand. In short, maintaining a high haemoglobin level depressed ineffective erythropoiesis and thereby appeared to retard the development of hepatosplenomegaly and skeletal deformity.

However, while the high transfusion regimen was a major advance in the management of thalassaemia in childhood, it soon became apparent that Wolman's early hopes that reducing intestinal iron absorption might result in less iron accumulation were not to be fulfilled. By the early 1960s there was growing literature on transfusion haemochromatosis in thalassaemia (see Fink 1964), and all the centres that used the high transfusion programme during the late 1960s and early 1970s were observing deaths due to iron loading, particularly of the myocardium, once their patients reached their late teens or early 20s.

Iron chelation

Clearly, if further progress was to be made, a way of removing excess iron which accumulated as the result of blood transfusion had to be developed. In the early 1960s scientists working for the drug company Ciba Ltd. (later Novartis) introduced a potent iron-chelating agent desferrioxamine, a sideramine obtained from *Streptomyces pilosus*. Desferrioxamine was introduced for the treatment of transfusion-dependent thalassaemia by Sephton-Smith (1962, 1964). Early experiences with this drug (reviewed by Waxman & Brown 1969) were disappointing. It appeared to be incapable of achieving a negative iron balance, and because it had to be given by intramuscular injection it was poorly tolerated by thalassaemic children. Indeed, Waxman and Brown questioned the validity of its use as a chelating agent in iron-loading anaemias.

However, an important study by Barry *et al.* (1974) at Great Ormond Street Hospital for Children, London, revived interest in the use of desferrioxamine. Barry and colleagues described the results of a 7-year trial in which a group of patients were treated with regular intramuscular desferrioxamine together with an intravenous injection at the time of transfusion. A control group was maintained simply on blood transfusion at a similar level to those that were receiving the drug. When the two groups were analysed after 7 years the serum ferritin level — a reasonable if imprecise indicator of the body-iron load — was significantly lower in the treated group, and, even more importantly, the liver iron concentration in the treated group was lower than in the controls (Letsky *et al.* 1973; Barry *et al.* 1974; Letsky 1976). Later analysis of the two groups approximately 10 years after the initiation of the trial suggested that there might be a significant decrease in the number of deaths in the treated group, although the numbers were too small to draw any dogmatic conclusions (Modell & Berdoukas 1984). However, it was undoubtedly this study, and the encouraging results obtained by high-transfusion regimens, which, in the mid-1970s, led several groups to review the whole question of the best way to administer desferrioxamine.

In his pioneering study on the use of desferrioxamine for the removal of iron in thalassaemic children, Sephton-Smith (1962) had found that much more iron can be removed by continuous intravenous infusion of the drug, an observation that was later confirmed by Modell and Beck (1974). In 1976 Propper and colleagues in Boston found that if they gave an intramuscular dose of desferrioxamine they removed only 15–26 mg of iron; after continuous intravenous administration of the same dose over 24 h they were able to remove 74 mg of iron, almost the theoretical maximum that the drug can chelate.

Because of the impracticability of using intravenous desferrioxamine, several groups of workers, stimulated by Propper and colleagues, examined the patterns of iron excretion after continuous infusions of the drug given subcutaneously (Hussain *et al.* 1976, 1977; Propper *et al.* 1977; Pippard *et al.* 1978a,b). In these studies it was found that there is marked variability in individual dose–response curves to desferrioxamine given subcutaneously. However, it was clear that, whether given by the subcutaneous or intravenous routes, a plateau of iron excretion is achieved during the period of the infusion and is maintained until the infusion is stopped. Based on these observations Pippard *et al.* (1978b) suggested that the drug could be given as a 12-hour subcutaneous infusion during sleep. It appeared that for many patients there was no real advantage in using a longer continuous infusion because the same amount of iron could be removed by doubling the dose of desferrioxamine, up to a dose of 4 g over 12 h, as by doubling the infusion time. Furthermore, administering the drug overnight was much more convenient and acceptable to young patients. During some of these studies it was also found that the administration of ascorbic acid significantly increased the urinary iron excretion in response to desferrioxamine (Modell & Beck 1974; O'Brien 1974; Nienhuis *et al.* 1976; Propper *et al.* 1977; Pippard *et al.* 1978b).

Using these improved regimens, together with a variety of different pumps for the slow infusion of desferrioxamine, genuine progress was made towards controlling the iron loading of transfusion-dependent thalassaemics, at least in those countries that could afford this expensive form of treatment. But problems remained, notably difficulties of compliance for a regimen that meant a nightly infusion of a drug via a clockwork pump. Although, as we shall see in later chapters, this type of regimen undoubtedly was capable of prolonging the lives of transfusion-dependent thalassaemics indefinitely, the relatively low compliance rate meant that many patients still died in their late teens or early 20s. Hence a search for an effective and safe oral chelating agent was started, a problem which, as we shall see, has still not been solved satisfactorily.

Splenectomy

The other major form of treatment for thalassaemia, splenectomy, has an even longer and more chequered history. This operation has been performed on patients with thalassaemia major for almost as long as the disease has been recognized (see Penberthy and Cooley (1935) and early reviews of the effects of splenectomy by Bouroncle and Doan (1964)). Over the years a rather confusing literature amassed round this subject, but, by and large, most studies seemed to demonstrate that a proportion of children with severe β thalassaemia have a reduction in transfusion requirements after the operation (Lichtman *et al.* 1953; Smith *et al.* 1955; Reemsta & Elliot 1956; Smith *et al.* 1960; Bouroncle & Doan 1964; Engelhard *et al.* 1975; Montouri *et al.* 1975; Modell 1977). Modell attempted to anticipate the development of hypersplenism by drawing a series of 'standard curves' for blood transfusions (Modell 1976, 1977). From these studies it appeared that the rate of fall of haemoglobin levels might be a useful guide to whether a splenectomy would be helpful; of 58 splenectomized patients analysed in this way, all but three had a permanent reduction in blood requirement.

It had been known for many years that splenectomy, particularly if carried out early in life, made children more prone to serious infection (see Perla & Marmorston 1941). In a series of careful observations Carl Smith and colleagues in New York collected extensive evidence during the early 1960s that post-splenectomy infection was a frequent and serious complication in thalassaemic children (Smith *et al.* 1964). Since it was particularly common if the splenectomy had been carried out in early childhood, it became common practice to withhold the operation until children had reached at least the age of 5 years. Later, prophylactic penicillin and vaccination programmes were introduced to try to reduce the frequency of overwhelming infections in these children.

As high-transfusion regimens were established, it soon became clear that splenomegaly was being seen less frequently (Smith *et al.* 1964; O'Brien *et al.* 1972; Necheles *et al.* 1974; Piomelli *et al.* 1974; Modell 1977). Indeed, it appeared that the presence of a large spleen in a transfusion-dependent thalassaemic child might well indicate that the transfusion regimen was inadequate.

Improved management but problems remain

These forms of symptomatic treatment undoubtedly transformed the lives of many thalassaemic children after the mid-1960s. But they did not completely overcome the problem of iron-loading and many young people with the disease continued to die. And for many countries in the developing world, where blood transfusion was difficult to organize and the prohibitive costs of desferrioxamine meant that it was not available for most of their patients, there was little genuine improvement in the outlook for thalassaemic children. The first report of a genuine 'cure' for thalassaemia came in 1982 when Thomas and colleagues from Seattle reported a successful bone-marrow transplant. Thus began a new era in the management of thalassaemia, a story which is still not complete.

1980 and after: the final unravelling of the molecular pathology of thalassaemia

Background

The story of the unravelling of the complex molecular pathology of the thalassaemias falls naturally into two periods. Up until the second half of the 1970s the cell nucleus remained an impenetrable black box, and it was only possible to try to make educated guesses about what might be going on at the level of the genes by studying protein synthesis, or, in the present context, haemoglobin synthesis, in the cytoplasm. In a few cases it was possible to deduce the molecular pathology from structural changes in haemoglobin associated with thalassaemia, the Lepore haemoglobins and the α-globin-chain termination mutations, for example. But for the most part all that could be done was to analyse the patterns of protein synthesis in thalassaemic cells, and, from what was found, speculate what might be happening at the DNA level. This all changed in the late 1970s when it became possible to isolate human messenger RNA and, later, the globin genes themselves.

Model building and globin synthesis

Although, in retrospect, it might be said that we learnt relatively little about the molecular pathology of thalassaemia in the protein synthesis era, at least some clues emerged about its general nature. We shall not attempt to give a detailed account of the work of this period, but rather highlight just a few of the major findings (and blind alleys) which set the scene for the RNA and DNA work of the late 1970s. Much of it was directed at trying to explore a number of models of the molecular basis for thalassaemia which had been proposed in the early 1960s.

The previous decade was a time of enormous excitement and productivity in the fields of molecular genetics and protein synthesis. By the early 1960s the general steps in protein synthesis had been worked out, and a great deal of research was directed at trying to understand the mechanisms of initiation, elongation and termination of peptide-chain synthesis. A variety of new techniques for studying *in vitro* protein synthesis were developed and the availability of relatively efficient cell-free protein synthesis systems enabled a start to be made at investigating the properties of globin messenger RNA.

Structure/rate hypothesis

It is not surprising therefore that thoughts about the molecular basis of the thalassaemias during this period tended to reflect current progress in the analysis of the complexities of protein synthesis. As mentioned earlier in this chapter, the first hypothesis that attempted to account for defective globin production in thalassaemia revolved round the notion that this disorder might be very similar to sickle-cell disease or the other haemoglobinopathies resulting from structural haemoglobin variants—the only difference being that the amino acid substitution in thalassaemia would not alter the charge of the haemoglobin molecule and therefore might make it difficult to identify. Since some structural haemoglobin variants seemed to be synthesized relatively ineffectively compared with normal haemoglobin, it seemed reasonable to suppose that a structural change of this type might be responsible for thalassaemia. The main references to these ideas and to the work of their protagonists, Harvey Itano and Linus Pauling, were cited earlier.

Perhaps the most complete statement of what

became known as the structure–rate hypothesis was presented at a symposium on abnormal haemoglobins held in Ibadan in 1963 (*Abnormal Haemoglobins in Africa*, CIOMS 1965). There, Itano recapitulated the original hypothesis, and, based on work on the properties of the genetic code that had been published a year or two earlier, set out a number of possible mechanisms for how a structural change in a globin subunit might alter its rate of synthesis. One idea that he explored in considerable detail was the possibility of varying affinity of putative, abnormal thalassaemic β chains for α chains. After posing several alternatives, including rate-limiting steps in variant globin polypeptide chain assembly, Itano finished by suggesting that, because of the degeneracy of the genetic code, it is possible that a base substitution could generate a messenger-RNA codon that is identified by a transfer RNA that is in relatively low abundance. This, he argued, might lead to a reduced rate of globin production.

In summarizing this important 'state of the art' lecture, Itano concluded that a mechanism involving degeneracy of the genetic code is the most likely explanation for defective globin synthesis in thalassaemia. This was a novel and interesting approach to the problem. Not only did it offer a possible explanation for the apparent inefficiency of synthesis of some structural haemoglobin variants, but it went further. In effect it left open the possibility that, even in the absence of an amino-acid substitution in a globin chain, there might still be a base change which altered a codon such that, although the normal amino acid is inserted in the right position, this process might be rate-limiting in globin synthesis because the altered codon now had to be recognized by a transfer RNA that is in short supply. At least it was an idea that could be tested, always provided that ways could be found to study the rates of assembly of globin polypeptide chains.

There was no mention at the Ibadan symposium in 1963 that, at another haemoglobin meeting at Arden House in 1962, Guidotti had announced that he had sequenced a considerable number of the tryptic peptides of the β globin of a patient with β thalassaemia and found no abnormality in the amino-acid composition or sequence (Guidotti 1962). As far as we know this work was never formally published, although it was widely quoted in the years that followed as sounding the death knell of the structure–rate hypothesis.

Other models

In October 1963 a meeting on thalassaemia was held in New York under the auspices of the New York Academy of Sciences. In one of the main presentations Vernon Ingram reviewed all the previously proposed molecular models for thalassaemia, and added a few new ones for good measure (Ingram 1964). Quoting Guidotti's work as effectively seeing off the structure–rate hypothesis, and finding his own earlier (tap) hypothesis less appealing, Ingram went on to present a new model that attempted to explain both the diminished production of adult haemoglobin in thalassaemia and the persistence of fetal haemoglobin in hereditary persistence of fetal haemoglobin (HPFH). In a rather complex series of speculations Ingram borrowed freely from the elegant operon model for the regulation of enzyme production which had been worked out so beautifully in microbial systems by Jacob and Monod (1961). Noting that at least two authors had already speculated that HPFH might be due to an operator gene mutation (Neel *et al.* 1961; Motulsky 1962), he suggested that, normally, the β, δ and γ genes might be under the regulation of an operator gene which is also involved in the regulation of the switch from γ- to β-chain production. He postulated that β thalassaemia might result from a mutation at the β-globin locus such that abnormal messenger RNA is produced, which, in turn, results in a blockage of the ribosomes and defective globin synthesis. Except for restating Itano's suggestions about degeneracy of the code he did not speculate further on what the abnormality of β-globin messenger RNA might be. But, using the operon model, he suggested that HPFH could be pictured as a mutation of a repressor molecule, such that it is incapable of combining with an environmental modifier of globin-gene switching.

It is not surprising that the operon was freely adapted by many other workers in the early 1960s as a possible model for the regulation of globin-gene expression (Neel *et al.* 1961; Guidotti 1962; Motulsky 1962; Sturgeon *et al.* 1963; Zuckerkandl 1964). The sheer elegance of the work of Jacob and Monod suggested that, though *E. coli* is a long evolutionary step from human beings, it is possible that similar mechanisms might be responsible for the regulation of protein synthesis in higher organisms. In essence, an operon consists of a group of linked genes of similar metabolic function, the activity of which is controlled by a closely linked operator gene. The action of the operator is always in *cis*, that is, on the same chromosome. The operator itself is under the control of what was originally called a regulator gene, the product of which is a specific repressor that acts in both *cis* and *trans*, and when bound to the operator inhibits the expression of all the genes in the operon. Because of its steric properties the repressor can exist in several different states, depending on its interaction with various metabolites, thus allowing induction or repression of sets of genes of related function. The only thing that the globin-gene cluster had in common with an operon was that it consisted of a group of linked genes of related function! But, given the wonderful versatility of the operon it was possible, of course, to ascribe almost any observation in the haemoglobin field to a putative mutation involving either the operator itself, the regulator or its repressor product. The major problem was, of course, that none of these ideas were open to any form of experimental verification!

In 1963 Nance proposed quite a different mechanism for the cause of thalassaemia, based largely on Smithies' work on haptoglobin genetics (Smithies 1964) and Baglioni's interpretation of how Hb Lepore had arisen (Baglioni 1962). In short, Nance suggested that there might have been a series of unequal but homologous crossovers at the γδβ-gene complex. From this model he was able to derive many of the thalassaemia genotypes and phenotypes.

Thus by the mid-1960s, although there was no shortage of models and hypotheses for the molecular basis of the thalassaemias, it was not obvious where to go next. The only hope for further progress seemed to rest on studies of haemoglobin synthesis.

Globin synthesis in thalassaemia

In the early 1960s several groups made a start at attempting to dissect some of the steps in haemoglobin synthesis in the thalassaemias, in either intact cells or cell-free systems. Some of the most important initial studies were made by Paul Marks and colleagues in New York (Burka & Marks 1963; Marks & Burka 1964a,b; Marks *et al.* 1964). They found that the distribution of radioactivity among polysomes isolated from labelled reticulocytes of normals and β-thalassaemics was essentially the same, indicating that, in general, similar-sized polysomes were active in protein synthesis in both cases. Later, Bank and

Marks (1966) found that β-thalassaemia polysomes in a cell-free system respond to the addition of poly(U) by directing polyphenylalanine synthesis in the same way as normal polysomes. Furthermore, a cell-free system containing β-thalassaemia polysomes was not significantly stimulated by supernate fractions from either normal or rabbit reticulocytes. It was concluded that the defect in $β^+$ thalassaemia was probably in the mRNA/ribosome complex, either a qualitative reduction in β-globin mRNA, or a reduced rate of initiation or translation. Further confirmation that $β^+$-thalassaemia ribosomes are normal came several years later from the work of Gilbert *et al.* (1970) and Nienhuis *et al.* (1971), who showed that messenger RNA prepared from rabbit reticulocytes directs the synthesis of rabbit α and β chains in a cell-free system, using either normal or β-thalassaemia ribosomes.

Globin assembly in thalassaemia

When methods for measuring the relative rates of α- and β-globin-chain synthesis were developed in the mid-1960s (Weatherall *et al.* 1965) it was hoped that it might be possible to learn something about the assembly of the globin polypeptide chains by studies of their relative specific activities after incubation of reticulocytes for short periods with radioactive amino acids. However, because of rapid exchange of globin subunits in experiments of this type it soon became clear that a more direct approach was required. In the early 1960s one of us had been fortunate enough to hear a seminar by Howard Dintzis describing his elegant experiments in rabbit reticulocytes, in which he proved unequivocally that globin polypeptide chain synthesis begins at the amino-terminal end and extends sequentially to the C terminus. By labelling reticulocytes, Dintzis was able to plot the growth of a globin chain, both in the soluble cell fraction and on the ribosomes (Dintzis 1961). Not only was it possible to determine, albeit approximately, the time it takes to synthesize a peptide chain but it was also feasible to describe the pattern of addition of amino acids to a growing globin polypeptide chain (Fig. 1.15).

It occurred to us that these methods could be applied to human reticulocytes, and, in particular, to the reticulocytes of thalassaemic patients. In this way, we reasoned, it might be feasible at least to exclude some of the models that were currently being aired

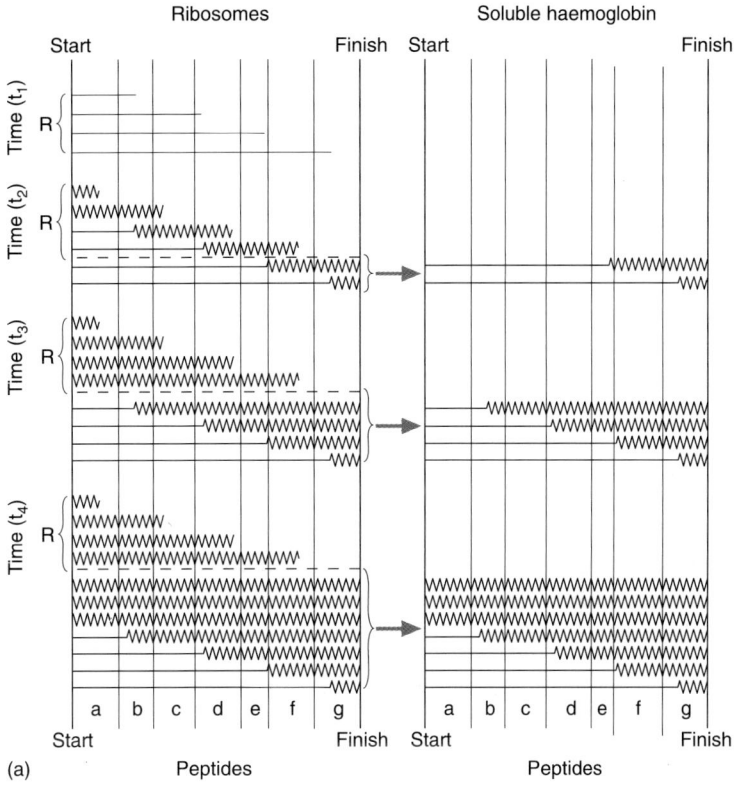

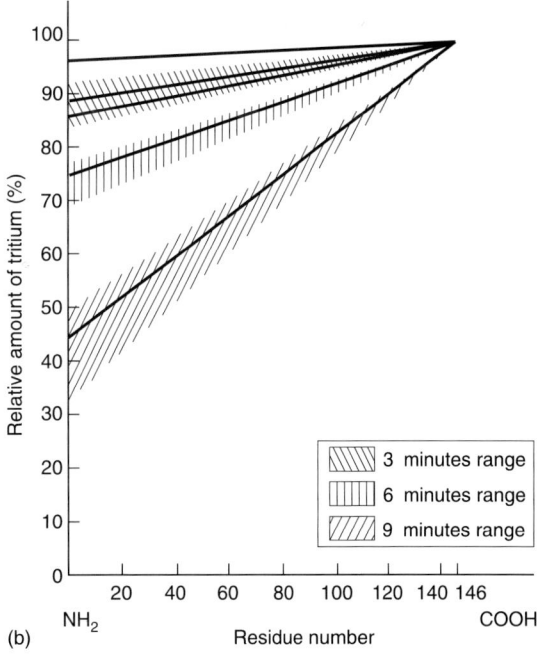

Fig. 1.15 Assembly of the α- and β-globin chains in normal and β-thalassaemic red cells. (a) The classical experiment of Dintzis (1961) to demonstrate that peptide chains are synthesized sequentially from the N terminus. The wavy lines represent the addition of radioactivity to growing peptide chains at different times of incubation of reticulocytes with radioactive amino acids. If peptide chains are synthesized sequentially from the N terminus, in the soluble haemoglobin the C-terminal ends will be labelled first, and vice versa on the ribosomes. (b) Normal globin-chain initiation and assembly in β thalassaemia. The hatched regions show the normal range of assembly and the dark line shows the results obtained from the red cells of patients with β thalassaemia. From Clegg *et al.* (1968b).

about the molecular pathology of thalassaemia—rate-limiting steps in mRNA translation or termination, for example. In the event it took almost 5 years to adapt experiments designed to study globin synthesis in the numerous reticulocytes of phenylhydrazine-treated rabbits to the relatively small numbers available from normal humans and thalassaemics.

The results of these difficult experiments, which used reticulocytes from patients with β thalassaemia, showed that the patterns and times of assembly of the β-globin polypeptide chains did not differ from normal. Since in this experimental system the pattern of globin labelling depends on the translation times for the α- or β-globin mRNAs and the release of finished peptide chains from the ribosomes, it appeared that the mechanisms of translation and chain termination were not affected by β+-thalassaemia mutations, at least those that were analysed in this way (Clegg & Weatherall 1967; Clegg et al. 1968b; Weatherall & Clegg 1969) (Fig. 1.15). These findings essentially ruled out many of the previously suggested models for the pathogenesis of the thalassaemias and suggested that the primary defect was most likely to be a reduced amount of messenger RNA for the affected globin. (In retrospect it is interesting to reflect that from what is known now about the molecular pathology of the β+ thalassaemias in Thailand, from where the reticulocytes for these experiments were obtained, this conclusion was correct.) But it still remained possible that some forms of β thalassaemia result from defective initiation of globin polypeptide-chain synthesis.

The measurement of peptide-chain initiation rates presented even greater problems, but evidence was obtained that this phase of protein synthesis, too, is normal in β+ thalassaemia. Careful studies of normal human reticulocytes suggested that β chains are made on larger polysomes than α chains (Hunt et al. 1968; Clegg et al. 1971a), a curious fact that was later explained when it was found that the rate of initiation on β-globin messenger RNA is faster than that on α (Lodish 1974). It was found that in β+ thalassaemia the distribution of nascent globin polypeptide chains on polysomes is identical to normal (Cividalli et al. 1974b; Lodish 1974). These findings, and further studies of globin-chain initiation in the β thalassaemias, suggested that this process is normal (Crystal et al. 1973).

All these experiments had attempted to determine the level of the defect in protein synthesis in forms of β thalassaemia in which some β globin was synthesized. In 1969 Baglioni and colleagues pursued the idea that β thalassaemias in which there was no β-chain production might be caused by mutations that generate premature chain termination codons. If this were the case, it was reasoned, it might be possible to demonstrate short peptide fragments which would have resulted from the premature termination of peptide-chain synthesis. Several investigators followed this lead but no such fragments were identified (Baglioni et al. 1969; Dreyfus et al. 1972).

A frustrating interlude: Ferrara β⁰ thalassaemia

To this extent the results of these difficult studies were undoubtedly correct and were borne out by later molecular work. The only exception was the extraordinary saga of what became known as 'Ferrara β⁰ thalassaemia'. In a series of biosynthetic and *in vivo* studies workers from Ferrara showed that the local form of β⁰ thalassaemia seemed to be unique in that the underlying defect could, at least in part, be corrected by a soluble factor from normal reticulocytes. And, even more remarkably, it appeared that patients with this disorder started to synthesize small amounts of normal β globin after blood transfusion (Conconi et al. 1972; Conconi & del Senno 1974). Intrigued by these findings many workers attempted to reproduce at least the *in vitro* results but this never proved possible (Pritchard et al. 1976; Ramirez et al. 1976; Ottolenghi et al. 1977). Many years later the form of β⁰ thalassaemia which is common in Ferrara was found to be the result of a simple premature chain-termination mutation. It is very difficult, even in retrospect, to understand how these findings arose; this brief and frustrating diversion constitutes one of the few still unexplained mysteries of the thalassaemia story.

The end of the protein-synthesis era

The end of the 1960s saw, to all intents and purposes, the last attempts to identify the molecular defects in the thalassaemias by means of studies of protein synthesis. It had been a period of difficult and frustrating experimentation, and most of those who were left in the field were by now fairly confident that the defect lay in globin messenger RNA, either that it is quantitatively deficient or that it is rendered sufficiently abnormal to be unable to participate in protein synthesis.

Messenger RNA analysis in β thalassaemia

Defective messenger RNA function

In the early 1970s several groups attempted to measure the role of messenger RNA (mRNA) in β thalassaemia by isolating mRNA from thalassaemic reticulocytes and assaying it for β-globin-synthesizing activity in heterologous cell-free systems. The first experiments of this type were carried out by Nienhuis and Anderson (1971) using a rabbit reticulocyte lysate system, and by Benz and Forget (1971) using a mouse ascites tumour system. Both these groups showed that, whereas mRNA isolated from normal reticulocytes directed the synthesis of equal amounts of α and β chains, mRNA from reticulocytes of patients with β thalassaemia made fewer β chains than α chains. These observations were confirmed and extended by many other workers using similar or other cell-free systems (Dow *et al.* 1973; Kan *et al.* 1973; Natta *et al.* 1973; Nienhuis *et al.* 1973; Benz *et al.* 1974; Forget *et al.* 1974a; Gambino *et al.* 1974; Benz *et al.* 1975; Pritchard *et al.* 1976).

While these studies clearly demonstrated that there is a deficiency of functional β messenger RNA in β-thalassaemic cells, because the cell-free systems used measured activity and not quantity, they were unable to clarify whether the observed reduction in biological activity of the mRNA was due to its being present in decreased amounts. The possibility still remained that β-thalassaemic cells contained normal amounts of β mRNA with a greatly impaired or non-existent capacity to function normally in protein synthesis. The methods which allowed these questions to be finally resolved, and, incidentally, to move the thalassaemia field into the molecular era, came from a completely different direction.

Quantification of messenger RNA

In the early 1970s the discovery of an enzyme called reverse transcriptase in certain tumour viruses made it possible to synthesize complementary DNA (cDNA) from mRNA templates (Baltimore 1970; Temin & Mizutani 1970). By obtaining DNA from reticulocytes, it was possible to synthesize radioactively labelled α- and β-globin cDNAs which could

then be used to analyse the levels of mRNA in the reticulocytes of patients with thalassaemia by molecular hybridization. In the early experiments cDNAs were made from rabbit mRNA templates, and relied on cross-hybridization between rabbit and human nucleic acid sequences for their success. Later, highly purified cDNAs specific for individual α-, β- and γ-globin mRNA sequences were made.

The first workers to use these new methods successfully were Kacian *et al.* (1973) and Housman *et al.* (1973). Using reasonably pure cDNA hybridization probes Kacian examined five β⁺- and two β⁰-thalassaemic patients. In five cases, considerably reduced levels of β-globin mRNA were observed, although in two the reduction was less than expected on the basis of cell-free experiments, raising the possibility that substantial levels of inactive β-globin mRNA might be present. Housman *et al.* (1974) and Forget *et al.* (1975), using purer cDNA probes, obtained similar results. These early hybridization experiments were thus in broad agreement that β mRNA levels are reduced in β⁺ thalassaemia and the results were more or less in line with the amount of globin imbalance seen in cell-free and whole-cell protein synthesis experiments.

Encouraged by these findings, many workers attempted to analyse the reticulocytes of patients with β⁰ thalassaemia for β-globin mRNA. Although it was assumed that very little would be found, these studies turned out to be much more complicated, and, incidentally, gave the first real indication of the remarkable diversity of the molecular defects which were likely to underlie the β thalassaemias.

Initial findings suggested that very little or no β-globin mRNA is present in β⁰ thalassaemias (Forget *et al.* 1974b; Housman *et al.* 1974; Ottolenghi *et al.* 1975; Forget *et al.* 1976; Ramirez *et al.* 1976; Tolstoshev *et al.* 1976; Comi *et al.* 1977; Godet *et al.* 1977; Benz *et al.* 1978; Old *et al.* 1978b; Ramirez *et al.* 1978). In some cases, however, low levels of hybridization to β cDNA probes were observed which could not always with certainty be ascribed to contaminating δ mRNA sequences (Forget & Hillman 1977). On the other hand, Old *et al.* (1978b) and Benz *et al.* (1978) showed clearly that, given the availability of highly purified cDNA probes and the use of stringent hybridization conditions, β-globin mRNA levels were less than one per cent in some β⁰ thalassaemias.

In 1975 Kan *et al.* (1975e) reported that substantial amounts of β-globin mRNA were present in reticulocytes and bone marrow of two Chinese patients with β^0 thalassaemia, a finding that had been presaged in a paper by Kacian *et al.* (1973), in which a much less sophisticated hybridization analysis had been used. In the same paper, Kan *et al.* also described an Italian patient with β^0 thalassaemia in whose red-cell precursors there appeared to be considerable amounts of β-globin mRNA. Further evidence that this was genuine β-globin mRNA came from work of Temple *et al.* (1977). Other workers also observed that some cases of β^0 thalassaemia might have variable levels of non-functional β-globin mRNA. Old *et al.* (1978b) and Benz *et al.* (1978) analysed mRNA isolated from a number of patients from a wide variety of ethnic groups and found considerable heterogeneity at the molecular level. The overall results fell into three main categories: (1) no β-globin mRNA detectable; (2) significant amounts of (apparently) full-length but non-functional β-globin mRNA; and (3) structurally abnormal β-globin mRNA.

Messenger RNA structure

Attempts were now made to try to characterize the defective β-globin mRNAs found in some of these patients with β^0 thalassaemia. Using cDNA probes specific for RNA sequences in the 5' and 3' non-coding regions of β-globin mRNA, Old *et al.* (1978b) were able to demonstrate that, in the case of a British homozygote with full-length β mRNA, the 3' and 5' non-coding sequences were intact, but that a hexa-nucleotide primer specific for the Met Val His coding sequence at the 5' (N-terminal) end of the β-chain mRNA bound very inefficiently to the β-thalassaemia RNA. This suggested a defect in or near the chain initiation site. In contrast, a Saudi Arab and an Indian β^0-thalassaemic had β-globin mRNAs which hybridized incompletely to the β-globin cDNA at the 3' non-coding sequences, suggesting a deletion or insertion of approximately 150 bases in the extreme 3' coding and non-coding sequences.

These extremely encouraging findings were extended by Chang and Kan (1979), who determined the nucleotide sequence of non-functional β mRNA from a Chinese patient with β^0 thalassaemia. They found that the AAG codon for lysine at position $\beta 17$ had mutated to the chain termination codon UAG, thus leading to premature chain termination with the production of short, 16-residue N-terminal fragments

of the β chain. These findings were elegantly confirmed by translating the defective β-globin mRNA in a cell-free system in the presence of a UAG tyrosine suppressor tRNA; under these conditions full length β-globin polypeptide chains were synthesized (Chang *et al.* 1979).

The final twist to this important period of exploration of the β thalassaemias came in the late 1970s when two groups of workers found substantial amounts of β-globin-like RNA sequences in the nucleus but not in the cytoplasm of red-cell precursors (Comi *et al.* 1977; Benz *et al.* 1978). These findings suggested that in these cases of β^0 thalassaemia there might be a defect in processing, or, alternatively, extreme instability of β-globin mRNA.

Messenger RNA in α thalassaemia

Globin synthesis studies carried out in the mid-1960s and early 1970s established conclusively that α-chain synthesis is reduced in α^+ thalassaemia and totally abolished in α^0 thalassaemia. In the α^0-thalassaemia homozygote studied by Weatherall *et al.* (1970), an exhaustive search for α-chain fragments also failed to provide any evidence for a nonsense mutation leading to premature chain termination. In α^+ thalassaemia (studied in the form of HbH disease) the reduced rate of α-chain synthesis did not appear to be due to any defects at the translational level, since translation times measured by pulse labelling experiments were in the normal range (Weatherall & Clegg 1974). Later work showed that α-chain polysomes in α thalassaemia were the normal size, indicating normal rates of chain initiation (Cividalli *et al.* 1974b).

These early studies thus provided indirect evidence that a deficiency or absence of functional α-globin mRNA is the cause of the reduced synthesis of α chains. Direct evidence that this is the case was obtained when it became possible to isolate globin mRNA and assay it in a variety of different heterologous cell-free systems (Benz *et al.* 1973; Grossbard *et al.* 1973; Pritchard *et al.* 1974; Natta *et al.* 1976; Pritchard *et al.* 1976).

Although these experiments with cell-free systems showed that there is deficiency of functional α-globin mRNA in HbH disease, the possibility remained that substantial amounts of non-translatable α-globin mRNA might be present. However, with the development of quantitative assays for globin mRNAs it was shown conclusively by DNA hybridization that there is no α-globin mRNA in α⁰-thalassaemia homozygotes (Kan *et al.* 1974d; Ramirez *et al.* 1975). Similarly, a reduced amount of α-globin mRNA was found consistently in reticulocytes from patients with HbH disease (Housman *et al.* 1973; Kacian *et al.* 1973; Natta *et al.* 1976; Hunt *et al.* 1980). Further corroboration of these findings came from experiments in which α and β mRNAs in HbH disease were fractionated by gel electrophoresis in 99% formamide, characterized by nucleotide sequencing and quantified (Forget *et al.* 1975; Kazazian *et al.* 1975).

Many of these experiments also showed that α-globin mRNA is present in excess in globin mRNA obtained from normal reticulocytes (Old *et al.* 1978a; Hunt *et al.* 1980). These findings were, of course, consistent with the studies mentioned earlier which indicated that β-globin mRNA is initiated at a faster rate than α-globin mRNA, necessitating an excess of α-globin mRNA to achieve balanced globin synthesis (Hunt *et al.* 1968; Clegg *et al.* 1971a; Lodish 1971; Lodish & Jacobsen 1972; Lodish 1974)—if, as seemed likely, translation rates for α- and β-globin mRNAs are similar. This observation was of particular importance when attempts were made to determine the magnitude of the deficiency of α-globin mRNA in different forms of thalassaemia.

The purity of the probes and sensitivity of these techniques were developed to such a degree that, by 1980, Hunt and colleagues were able to show a clear separation of levels of α-globin mRNA between normals, α⁺-thalassaemia or α⁰-thalassaemia carriers, and patients with HbH disease.

Probing the globin genes in thalassaemia

Gene deletions in α thalassaemia

In the early 1970s thoughts were already turning to the possibility of exploring the notion that some forms of thalassaemia could be caused by gene deletions by using cDNA/DNA hybridization to probe for the presence or absence of globin genes. After demonstrating the complete absence of α-globin synthesis or α-globin fragments in a baby with the Hb Bart's hydrops syndrome (Weatherall *et al.* 1970), we approached Dr John Paul's group in Glasgow, who had had some experience of this type of molecular

hybridization, to discuss whether such an experiment might be feasible using blood and tissues from an infant with the same syndrome. A sample of fetal liver was obtained from an affected infant from Bangkok in whom we had been able to confirm that there was a complete absence of α-chain synthesis. DNA was isolated from the liver and hybridized with specific α- and β-cDNA probes complementary to human α- and β-globin mRNA (DNA) sequences. It was found that the hydropic fetal liver cells contained normal amounts of β-globin DNA, but a more or less complete absence of α-chain DNA. In DNA prepared from the tissues of normal infants, the expected amounts of α- and β-DNA sequences were present (Fig. 1.16). It turned out that Y.W. Kan had set up a similar collaboration with Harold Varmus in San Francisco at about the same time and had obtained an identical result using the tissues of a Chinese baby with the Hb Bart's hydrops fetalis syndrome. The results of these experiments were published side by side in 1974 (Ottolenghi *et al.* 1974; Taylor *et al.* 1974). These studies were the first direct demonstration of a gene deletion as the cause of human disease and were subsequently confirmed (Ramirez *et al.* 1975) and extended using more stringent techniques; Old *et al.* (1977) showed that there are less than 0.2 α genes/diploid genome in homozygous α⁰-thalassaemia DNA. As there were known to be structural similarities between the α and ζ chains, it was suggested that this residual binding represented cross hybridization of the α-cDNA probe to ζ-chain genes.

These encouraging results were soon augmented by some elegant experiments by Kan *et al.* (1975a), who found that the hybridization pattern of HbH disease DNA to specific α-cDNA probes was indistinguishable from that of an artificial 1/3 mixture of normal and Hb Bart's hydrops DNA, indicating that HbH disease DNA has only one-quarter of the normal complement of α genes. Since there are no α genes on the chromosome derived from the α⁰-thalassaemia parent, these results suggested that the chromosome derived from the α⁺-thalassaemia parent must only have one α gene, instead of the normal two. This experiment established conclusively that two of the common forms of α thalassaemia, α⁰ thalassaemia and α⁺ thalassaemia, seen in Oriental populations are the result of deletions of one or both α-chain genes from the haploid genome, respectively.

Normal   Bart's hydrops

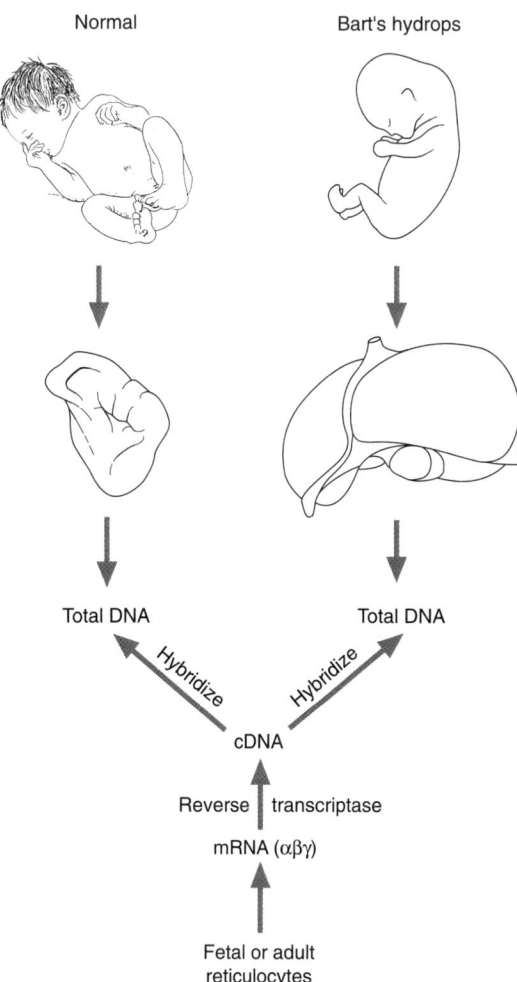

Total DNA   Total DNA

Hybridize   Hybridize

cDNA

Reverse | transcriptase

mRNA (αβγ)

Fetal or adult
reticulocytes

Fig. 1.16 The experimental design to probe the α-globin genes by cDNA/DNA hybridization. This experiment by Ottolenghi *et al.* (1974) and a similar experiment by Taylor *et al.* (1974), which showed a major deletion of the α-globin genes in babies with the Hb Bart's hydrops fetalis syndrome, were the first to demonstrate directly a deletion as the basis for a human genetic disease. The details of the experiment are described in the text.

While these seminal results from the application of cDNA/DNA hybridization to the study of α thalassaemia were being obtained, similar approaches were being applied to β thalassaemia. Although the findings were less spectacular they provided some valuable information in the period just before globin genes could be examined directly by mapping and sequencing.

Globin genes in β thalassaemia

As mentioned earlier, β-globin mRNA studies had already pointed to considerable molecular heterogeneity of the β thalassaemics. Using β-globin cDNA probes it was soon possible to verify that in the Chinese cases described by Kan *et al.* (1975e) and Temple *et al.* (1977), in which there were considerable levels of non-functional β-globin mRNA, the β-globin genes were intact. Subsequently a number of cases of homozygous β^0 thalassaemia which were completely lacking in β-globin mRNA were analysed by solution hybridization. In each case the globin genes were found to be largely intact (Ramirez *et al.* 1976; Tolstoshev *et al.* 1976; Godet *et al.* 1977).

Gene deletions in δβ thalassaemia and related disorders

During this period molecular hybridization was also applied to some of the variants of β thalassaemia, notably δβ thalassaemia and hereditary persistence of fetal haemoglobin (HPFH). Globin synthesis studies in the homozygous state for δβ thalassaemia showed that there was a complete absence of δ- and β-globin production (Russo *et al.* 1973a) and it was subsequently found that there is no δ- or β-globin mRNA in reticulocytes from these patients (Forget *et al.* 1974b). Globin gene analysis was carried out on three Sicilian δβ-thalassaemia homozygotes by Ottolenghi *et al.* (1976) and repeated on one of them by Ramirez *et al.* (1976). The results of these experiments suggested that at least 75% of the normal β- and δ-gene complement is deleted from the diploid genome.

Similar studies were applied to some forms of HPFH at about the same time. Before describing them we must remind ourselves about what was known about this condition by the mid-1970s. In 1976 globin synthesis studies carried out by the authors in collaboration with Samuel Charache showed that HPFH homozygotes have imbalanced α- and β-globin synthesis and a complete absence of δ- and β-chain production (Charache *et al.* 1976). This observation suggested that this form of HPFH is an extremely mild form of δβ thalassaemia in which the absence of δ- and β-chain production is almost but not entirely compensated for by the production of γ chains. Further clues to the likely molecular mechanisms involved in HPFH were obtained by studies of the structure of the associated HbF. In the type found in black populations, both $^G\gamma$ and $^A\gamma$ chains were present (Huisman *et al.* 1969; Ringelhann *et al.* 1970; Huisman *et al.* 1971; Ringelhann *et al.* 1977). However, a less common form of HPFH was identified in black populations a little later in which only $^G\gamma$ chains were present in the HbF and, in addition, there appeared to be some β-globin synthesis directed by the same chromosome as the HPFH determinant (Huisman *et al.* 1975b; Friedman & Schwartz 1976; Tatsis 1978; Higgs *et al.* 1979a). And, to complicate the situation even further, Huisman *et al.* (1970b) found that the HbF in a form of HPFH that had been first described in Greece by Fessas and Stamatoyannopoulos (1964) has non-α chains that consisted entirely of $^A\gamma$ chains.

As mentioned earlier, another form of HPFH had been reported by Huisman *et al.* (1972) which was associated with the presence of Hb Kenya, a variant that turned out to have normal α chains combined with non-α chains that are γβ-fusion chains. When the non-α globin of fetal haemoglobin was analysed it turned out to consist only of $^G\gamma$ chains. Thus it appeared that this variant had resulted from an abnormal crossover between the $^A\gamma$- and β-globin genes, which had deleted the 3′ end of the $^A\gamma$ gene, the entire δ-chain gene and the 5′ end of the β gene. Taken together, all these observations suggested that many forms of HPFH might result from different-sized gene deletions.

By applying the cDNA/mRNA and cDNA/DNA hybridization techniques outlined earlier, several groups found there was a complete absence of β-globin mRNA in HPFH homozygotes and that at least two-thirds of the δ- and β-globin gene sequences had been deleted (Kan *et al.* 1975d; Forget *et al.* 1976; Ramirez *et al.* 1976). In attempting to further extend these findings Ramirez *et al.* (1976) showed that DNA from a Sicilian δβ-thalassaemia homozygote hybridized to β cDNA to a slightly higher extent than the black HPFH DNA, suggesting that the latter has a bigger deletion. However, further refinement of these studies, achieved by using cDNA probes specific for the 5′ and 3′ ends of the β(δβ)-globin genes, showed that there was no hybridization with either probe in the homozygous HPFH DNA, suggesting a complete deletion of the β- and δ-chain genes.

The end of the analysis of globin genes by indirect approaches

Towards the end of the 1970s, techniques for direct analysis of the globin genes were becoming available. In effect this brought to an end a period of over 20 years in which the molecular pathology of the thalassaemias was studied by the indirect phenotypic approaches of globin synthesis and mRNA analysis. Considering the difficulties involved it had been a remarkably successful phase in the exploration of these diseases. By now it was known that the common Oriental α thalassaemias result from the deletion of either one or both of the linked α-globin genes. The other common form of α thalassaemia in Orientals had been identified as a mutation in the α-globin-chain termination codon. It was known that the β thalassaemias are highly heterogeneous at the molecular level, that very few of them result from gene deletions, and that, at least in one case, the disease is caused by a mutation which produces a premature chain termination codon. And it had also been established that the δβ thalassaemias and some forms of HPFH are due to deletions of different sizes that involve the β- and δ-globin genes and, in some cases, the $^A\gamma$ genes.

The scene was set therefore for the direct exploration of the globin genes and for the final elucidation of the molecular pathology of the many different forms of thalassaemia.

New technology: the structure and diversity of the human globin genes

During the late 1970s and early 1980s several new analytical techniques were developed that were to revolutionize the study of the globin disorders and, later, the whole of human genetics.

Southern blotting

The discovery of restriction enzymes, that is, enzymes that cut DNA at specific base sequences, allowed DNA to be fractionated precisely and reproducibly. In 1975 Southern introduced a form of hybridization in which one of the components in the reaction, the DNA under study, is immobilized on a cellulose nitrate filter. The beauty of this method was that it made it possible to transfer DNA from gel electrophoresis to these filters by blotting (Southern

1975). Hence fragments of DNA separated on the basis of their size by electrophoresis could be assayed for the presence or absence of specific genes. In this way it became feasible to produce maps of genes and their surrounding regions of DNA (Fig. 1.17). And the advent of recombinant DNA technology made it possible to clone, that is, selective purify and amplify, a chosen DNA sequence. These methods soon became extremely sophisticated, to the point that whole 'libraries' of cloned DNA fragments representing the entire human genome were available for study.

By gene mapping it was possible to build up a picture of the physical organization and linkage of genes on chromosomes. Using this general approach a detailed map of the order and linkage of the globin genes was constructed in the late 1970s. This work provided direct physical evidence that, gratifyingly, confirmed all the gene arrangements which had been tentatively surmised from earlier genetic studies. What could not have been deduced from these studies, however, was that all the globin genes, and most mammalian genes for that matter, turned out to contain one or more non-coding inserts, or intervening sequences (Flavell *et al.* 1978; Lawn *et al.* 1978;

Mears *et al.* 1978b; Smithies *et al.* 1978; Bernards *et al.* 1979b; Little *et al.* 1979; Proudfoot & Baralle 1979). Since the intervening sequences were not found in mature messenger RNA it followed that they would have to be removed from the primary transcript during the maturation of mRNA in the cell nucleus.

The structure of the globin genes

Following the advent of gene cloning and sequences, by the beginning of the 1980s the complete nucleotide sequence of the five human non-α-globin genes and parts of their flanking regions had been determined (Baralle *et al.* 1980; Lawn *et al.* 1980; Slightom *et al.* 1980; Spritz *et al.* 1980). These studies showed that the 5′ non-coding regions of these genes contain a number of regulatory regions that are homologous with those found in genes of other species. They also demonstrated that within the non-α-globin gene cluster there are at least two genes with significant sequence homology to functional β genes but which have mutations that prevent their expression. Such pseudogenes, as they were called, were also found in corresponding places in the β-globin gene clusters of other species. At the same time equally

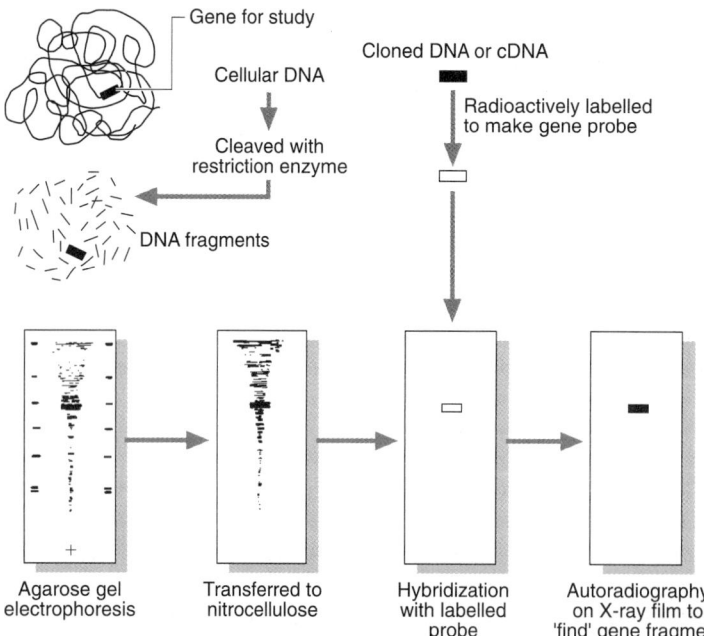

Fig. 1.17 Southern blotting. The principle behind the technique which made it possible to analyse the structure of the globin genes for the first time.

rapid progress was made in analysing the arrangements of genes in the ζ/α-globin-gene cluster and in determining the sequence of the linked α-globin genes and of the DNA which surrounds them (Lauer *et al.* 1980; Liebhaber *et al.* 1980; Michelson & Orkin 1980; Proudfoot & Maniatis 1980). It is beyond the scope of this book to give detailed reference for the extraordinary amount of work that went into defining the fine structure of the globin genes during this extremely productive period. Excellent reviews of progress over this time are given by Proudfoot *et al.* (1980), Maniatis *et al.* (1980, 1981) and Bunn and Forget (1986).

Restriction-fragment-length polymorphisms

Another important discovery that was made at about this time was that sequence variations might be relatively common among the globin gene clusters (Jeffreys 1979). Jeffreys found two polymorphisms for the enzyme *Hind* III in the γ genes of a number of individuals and estimated that perhaps one percent of nucleotide sites might be polymorphic. Subsequent work showed that although such restriction-fragment-length polymorphisms (RFLPs) are spread throughout the globin-gene clusters, they do not occur in a random fashion. Rather, it was established that they are present in linked groups called haplotypes (Antonarakis *et al.* 1982; Higgs *et al.* 1986). Within any particular population there are usually a small number of haplotypes that are common and a much larger number that are rare. As well as providing a valuable approach to studying population affinities and evolution, it turned out that linkage of particular haplotypes to different forms of thalassaemia offered a valuable approach to the study of thalassaemia mutations, both within individual families and in populations.

In the event, as several research groups started to explore the globin genes by gene mapping in the late 1970s, one of the first observations that was to be of considerable clinical importance related to RFLPs. Kan and Dozy (1978b), using the restriction enzyme *Hpa* I, found that the β-globin gene of normal individuals is located on a fragment of DNA approximately 7.6 kb (kilobase or 1000 nucleotide bases). However, using the same enzyme for cutting the DNA of patients with sickle-cell disease, they found that the β globin was on a larger piece of DNA, approximately 13 kb. It appeared therefore that the sickle-cell mutation was on a chromosome which also carried a polymorphism of the DNA outside the coding area for the β chain, and further studies showed that this was a very strong association. The same workers proceeded to study the DNA from amniotic-fluid fibroblasts of a fetus at risk for sickle-cell disease. The DNA had both 7.6- and 13-kb β-globin gene-containing fragments, indicating that the fetus had sickle-cell trait (Kan & Dozy 1978a). It was clear that, if other polymorphisms of DNA could be found which are associated with particular mutations of the β-globin genes, the β thalassaemias for example, this approach might have more general application for the early prenatal diagnosis of these conditions. These predictions were found to be correct by Little *et al.* (1980), and over subsequent years this approach was used widely for the prenatal detection of at least some forms of β thalassaemia.

Mapping the globin genes in thalassaemia

α *Thalassaemia*

The scene was now set for the direct identification of some of the mutations that underlie different forms of thalassaemia. Since it was already known that at least some common forms of α thalassaemia are due to gene deletions it is not surprising that, during the first year or two that gene mapping was applied to the study of thalassaemia, progress in sorting out the molecular pathology of α thalassaemia was more rapid than for β thalassaemia.

In 1978 Orkin *et al.* found that the α-gene-containing fragments generated by *Eco*R1 or *Hind* III digestion of normal DNA are missing in Hb Bart's hydrops DNA. In fact, no fragments of any size in digests of restriction endonuclease-treated hydrops DNA hybridized to α-specific probes, confirming the earlier soluble hybridization studies that indicated that the α-gene sequences are completely deleted in homozygous α^0 thalassaemia. It was subsequently found, using DNA from south-east Asian patients with HbH disease, that one of the pair of α genes in the haploid genome is deleted in α^+ thalassaemia (Embury *et al.* 1979; Orkin *et al.* 1979b). Some discrepancies between the mapping data in these two studies suggested that there might be heterogeneity of the deletions which cause α^+ thalassaemia. These predictions were confirmed when it was demonstrated that α^+ thalassaemia can arise by at least two different mechanisms, both similar to that which generates the Lepore haemoglobins; these different variants appeared to have resulted from unequal crossing over between the two linked α-globin genes, resulting in two different-sized deletions, 3.7 and 4.2 kb, respectively (Embury *et al*. 1980). A consequence of unequal crossing over between mispaired α genes is that one of the chromosomes produced should contain three α genes, while the other would have a single α gene. Examples of haplotypes containing three α genes were discovered in the same year (Goossens *et al*. 1980; Higgs *et al*. 1980a).

As soon as gene mapping became available it was used to investigate some of the long-standing puzzles about the nature of α thalassaemia in other populations, notably Africans. It was found that individuals of this ethnic background who have the clinical phenotype of heterozygous α^0 thalassaemia are, in fact, homozygotes for deletional forms of α^+ thalassaemia (Dozy *et al*. 1979b; Higgs *et al*. 1980a,b). It turned out that the prevalence of α^+ thalassaemia in some African populations is about 25%, and that the homozygous state for α^+ thalassaemia is responsible for the presence of approximately 5–10% of Hb Bart's in cord blood (Higgs *et al*. 1980b). These observations explained the results of earlier studies that had demonstrated a clearly definable α-thalassaemia-like disorder in association with the presence of Hb Bart's in blacks. The reason for the lack of HbH disease in this population was also now clear; α^0 thalassaemia is extremely rare.

During this extremely productive period in α-thalassaemia research it also became apparent that α^0 thalassaemia is very heterogeneous. By 1980 Lauer *et al*. had determined the overall structure of the ζ/α-globin gene cluster and had found that the ζ genes, like the α genes, are duplicated. At the time, the order of genes appeared to be $\zeta2$–$\zeta1$–$\psi\alpha$–$\alpha2$–$\alpha1$. When ζ-gene probes became available it was possible to study the extent of the long deletions that give rise to α^0 thalassaemia. Pressley *et al*. (1980c) found that the two common α^0 determinants seen in south-east Asia and the Mediterranean are due to different-sized deletions; while the former removes both α genes and the $\psi\alpha$ gene, but spares the two ζ genes, the latter, in addition, involves the $\zeta1$ gene. This was a particularly interesting observation since, in the Greek hydropic infants studied by Pressley *et al*. (1980a), there was a significant amount of Hb Port-

land ($\zeta_2\gamma_2$) present in the peripheral blood. Thus the ζ chains could only have been derived from the expression of the $\zeta2$ gene. It was suspected at the time, and later confirmed, that the $\zeta1$ gene is, in fact, a pseudogene.

Two other α^0-thalassaemia determinants were characterized at about the same time and these appeared to be different from the common southeast Asian and Mediterranean varieties. Orkin *et al*. (1979b) and later Orkin and Michelson (1980) described a long deletion, extending for at least 25 kb, which started at codon 57 of the $\alpha1$ gene and removed all the other genes in the α-globin-gene cluster. Another example of a chromosome containing a dysfunctional α gene was reported by Pressley *et al*. (1980a); in this case a deletion of 5.2 kb removed the $\alpha2$ gene and 5' end of the $\alpha1$ gene, leaving the 3' end of the latter intact.

These seminal gene-mapping studies also demonstrated that there were at least some heterozygous α-thalassaemics in different populations in whom both α-globin genes are intact (Orkin *et al*. 1979b; Pressley *et al*. 1980b). It was assumed that these 'non-deletion' forms of α thalassaemia might result from point mutations or other changes that could not be detected by restriction-enzyme mapping. A year or two later, when cloning and sequencing technology was adapted to the study of the haemoglobin genes, these predictions turned out to be correct. As we shall see in later chapters there are many different non-deletional forms of α thalassaemia, as there are many different deletional forms of α^0 and α^+ thalassaemia.

It is remarkable to reflect that in less than 3 years a relatively complete picture of the molecular pathology of the α thalassaemias was obtained by Southern blotting technology. Although many details remained to be worked out, and there were still some surprises to come, the basis for a genuine understanding of the reasons for the remarkable diversity of α thalassaemia had been laid. Interestingly, as these experiments were being carried out, a new and completely unexpected twist to the α-thalassaemia story emerged. In 1981 Weatherall *et al*. (1981a) described three children of North European extraction with moderate-to-severe mental retardation and dysmorphic features who also had a mild form of HbH disease. The family findings were quite unlike those observed in any other form of HbH disease. The authors suggested that the underlying molecular pathology which led to defective α-chain synthesis might also be involved in causing mental retardation. Although it was to be another 10 years before the heterogeneity and molecular basis of these conditions was clarified, the original predictions turned out to be correct, and opened up an interesting new chapter in the exploration of the genetic basis of mental retardation.

β Thalassaemia

Analysis of the β thalassaemias by gene mapping was not to be so productive, largely because very few of them turned out to be due to gene deletions. As mentioned earlier, work in the authors' laboratory had suggested that in the case of a patient of North Indian origin there might be a defect at the 3′ end of the β-globin gene. We reasoned therefore that this might be a good candidate for a partial deletion of the β-globin gene and subsequent restriction-enzyme mapping showed that this was the case; Orkin et al. (1979c) found that approximately 600 nucleotide bases had been lost from this region. Similar results were also obtained by Flavell et al. (1979), working on DNA from the same patient. Although subsequent work suggested that this particular mutation is common in individuals from North India, extensive mapping studies of other DNA samples obtained from patients with β thalassaemia showed no other cases that were due to deletions of the size which could be identified by this approach.

δβ Thalassaemia and hereditary persistence of fetal haemoglobin

Unlike the β thalassaemias, mapping of the δβ thalassaemias and different forms of hereditary persistence of fetal haemoglobin (HPFH) turned out to be more productive. By now, from studies of the fetal haemoglobin found in these conditions, together with solution hybridization analyses, it was already clear that many of them must result from deletions of the γδβ-globin-gene cluster that either leave both the $^G\gamma$ and $^A\gamma$ genes intact, or remove the $^A\gamma$ genes as well as the δ and β genes. Studies of DNA from $^G\gamma^A\gamma\delta\beta$-thalassaemia homozygotes showed that part of the δ- and the whole of the β-globin genes had been deleted (Mears et al. 1978a,b; Bernards et al. 1979a; Fritsch et al. 1979; Ottolenghi et al. 1979). On the other hand, the DNA of a $^G\gamma\delta\beta$-thalassaemia homozygote showed a much more extensive deletion involving

the $^A\gamma$-, δ- and β-globin genes (Orkin et al. 1978; Fritsch et al. 1979; Orkin et al. 1979a). After some early uncertainties it was also found that the form of $^G\gamma^A\gamma$ HPFH that is found in Afro-American populations also results from a long deletion which removes the δ- and β-globin genes, and that the condition is heterogeneous in that at least two different-sized deletions are responsible for a similar clinical phenotype (Mears et al. 1978b; Fritsch et al. 1979; Ottolenghi et al. 1979; Bernards & Flavell 1980; Tuan et al. 1980). In 1981 Jones et al. described the molecular basis for a form of $^G\gamma\delta\beta$ thalassaemia found in an Indian patient. In this case a novel lesion was found, consisting of two short deletions and a complete inversion of sequences between the γ- and β-globin genes. This was the first example of an inversion to be described in humans.

The elucidation of the molecular basis for non-deletional forms of HPFH, that is, conditions in which there were no major deletions of the γδβ-globin gene cluster, took longer and required cloning and sequencing the particular γ genes involved. In 1984 Collins et al. found that the Greek form, in which there is persistent $^A\gamma$-chain synthesis, almost certainly results from a point mutation in the 5′ non-coding region of the $^A\gamma$-globin gene. Many other mutations of this type involving these regions of the $^G\gamma$- or $^A\gamma$-globin genes were found later.

Cloning and sequencing thalassaemia globin genes

Once it was established that restriction-enzyme maps of the β-globin genes of the majority of β-thalassaemics were normal it was clear that it would be necessary to clone and sequence the β-globin genes in order to identify the molecular pathology of β thalassaemia. The first successful identification of a mutation causing β^+ thalassaemia by gene sequencing was reported by Spritz et al. (1981) and by Westaway and Williamson (1981). Both these groups, working on samples from Cypriot patients, identified a single nucleotide base substitution, G→A, at nucleotide 110 of the first intervening sequence (IVS1) of the β-globin gene. At first this was a surprising result because it was not clear how a mutation in an intron could result in defective globin-gene function. It seemed possible, however, that it might lead to abnormal processing of precursor globin mRNA; that is, the new intron sequence might lead to abnormal splicing of mRNA during the process in which introns are removed and exons joined together to form the definitive mRNA template. This hypothesis was soon proved to be correct (Busslinger *et al.* 1981; Fukumaki *et al.* 1982).

Despite this encouraging start, a major problem remained for workers who wished to define particular forms of β-thalassaemia mutations. Cloning and sequencing of thalassaemic globin genes from different, random individuals would be likely to lead to the repeated identification of genes with the same mutation, particularly if certain forms of thalassaemia are prevalent in the same population. This concern was soon found to be justified; within a period of only one year, six different groups found the same nonsense mutation at position 39 in the β-globin gene from unrelated individuals of Mediterranean background! Clearly it was important to try to avoid such a fruitless duplication of effort. This problem was soon solved by Orkin and colleagues. As mentioned earlier, Antonarakis *et al.* (1982) observed that the polymorphic restriction-enzyme sites in the β-globin cluster are not arranged in a random fashion but in a series of patterns, or haplotypes, that vary in frequency between different populations. Orkin and his coworkers reasoned that the different types of β-thalassaemia mutations were likely to be found in association with particular haplotypes. Furthermore, these haplotypes could be used within families to 'mark' particular β-globin genes, and hence provide a way of sequencing the appropriate gene. These predictions turned out to be correct. For example, it was found that, in Mediterranean populations, different β-thalassaemic mutations are associated with particular haplotypes. Using this approach the definition of β-thalassaemia mutations moved extremely quickly, and, by the end of the 1980s, almost 100 different mutations had been determined. It became clear that in any population in which there was a high frequency of β thalassaemia, one or two mutations predominate. And, even more importantly, the pattern of mutations is quite different in different parts of the world.

The definition of the different β-thalassaemia mutations, and those responsible for the non-deletional forms of α thalassaemia, has provided a wealth of information about abnormal gene action. As well as those that cause premature chain termination or scrambling of the genetic code as a result of the generation of shifts in the reading frame, many different mechanisms for abnormal RNA processing

were established and a variety of different mutations in the promoter or chain termination regions were found. Thus in a relatively short period work in the thalassaemia field had provided a remarkable picture of the repertoire of mutations that can underlie abnormal gene action in humans. Furthermore, a start could be made in trying to unravel the complex interactions of the β-thalassaemia mutations, and those of the α-globin genes, which form the basis for some of the remarkable clinical diversity of the thalassaemias (Weatherall *et al.* 1981b).

Further technical advances

There was another extremely encouraging development in the thalassaemia field during the 1980s which followed rapid improvements in the technology for analysing mutant globin genes. As we have seen, this started with Southern blotting and evolved to gene cloning and sequencing, methods that at first were quite time-consuming and cumbersome. Once mutations had been identified, a variety of methods were developed for their rapid detection. In some cases the base change itself might produce a new restriction-enzyme site and hence it could be identified directly by Southern blotting (Phillips *et al.* 1979; Little *et al.* 1980; Chang & Kan 1981; Geever *et al.* 1981). This was not always the case, however, and another approach to the rapid identification of single-base mutations was required. This problem was solved by synthesizing short oligonucleotide probes which, if labelled, could be used to identify point mutations directly (Wallace *et al.* 1981; Conner *et al.* 1983; Orkin *et al.* 1983a).

These methods for mutation analysis were still quite time-consuming, however. But in the mid-1980s the field was revolutionized by the development of the polymerase chain reaction (PCR), which made it possible rapidly to amplify any DNA sequence that needed to be studied (Saiki *et al.* 1985). The application of this approach to the analysis of the haemoglobin genes soon allowed specific mutations to be identified within a few hours. And further modification of PCR for the development of rapid methods of DNA sequencing made it feasible to sequence individual genes for diagnostic purposes.

Clinical applications

As methods for the diagnosis of different forms of

thalassaemia evolved, they were soon used in day-to-day practice for carrier detection or prenatal diagnosis. Initially, fetal DNA was obtained from amniotic fluid cells, but the development of chorion villus sampling made it possible to obtain DNA much earlier in pregnancy. The methods used for prenatal diagnosis changed every few years from the late 1970s, reflecting the rapid improvement in the techniques of gene analysis over this period. The first diagnoses of sickle-cell anaemia or β thalassaemia used restriction-fragment-length polymorphism linkage analysis to 'track' the thalassaemia genes from both sides of the family (Kan & Dozy 1978a; Kan *et al.* 1980; Little *et al.* 1980). This was followed by the direct identification of mutations by Southern blotting, an approach which was feasible in cases in which there was a gene deletion, or the mutation produced a new restriction-enzyme cutting site, or removed a previously existing one (Orkin *et al.* 1978; Dozy *et al.* 1979a). Later, specific oligonucleotide probes were used to identify particular mutations in fetal DNA (Orkin *et al.* 1983a; Pirastu *et al.* 1983a; Old *et al.* 1989). Finally, a variety of methods for prenatal diagnosis were developed, based on the use of the polymerase chain reaction or a variant of this technique (Saiki *et al.* 1985; Old *et al.* 1990).

Centres that had established prenatal diagnosis programmes using globin synthesis switched to fetal DNA analysis, and in several countries, notably Sardinia, Cyprus, Greece, Italy and Great Britain, there was a major decline in the numbers of babies born with severe forms of thalassaemia.

Not surprisingly, the molecular era of investigation of thalassaemia also raised the expectation that the disease might be amenable to gene therapy; that is, the definitive correction of the molecular defect of the globin genes (Cline *et al.* 1980; Mercola *et al.* 1980; Mulligan & Berg 1980). In 1979 Martin Cline, unable to obtain permission from an ethics committee in the USA to perform an experiment of this kind, attempted to transfer normal β-globin genes into the marrow cells of two patients, one in Israel, the other in Italy. Since at that time very little was known about the regulation of the globin genes, there were no efficient methods for gene transfer, and there were considerable doubts about the safety of the procedure, this story was viewed with deep concern by the scientific community (Anderson & Fletcher 1980). However, no harm was done, and at least this premature experiment had the effect of jolting scientists on both sides of the Atlantic into the realization that, in the future, any form of gene therapy would have to come under close scrutiny by properly constituted control bodies.

Nobody has attempted gene therapy for thalassaemia since this episode. The fact that this disease can be cured by marrow transplantation suggests that sooner or later this will be achieved. Much has been learnt about the regulation of globin genes, and about the properties of the haemopoietic stem cells which must be the target for successful gene transfer. But many problems remain, and early attempts at gene therapy have been restricted to diseases in which tighter regulation of the inserted genes is not so important as it is in the haemoglobin disorders.

Postscript

This account of some of the major advances in the thalassaemia field over the last 70 years has taken us from the first descriptions of the disease to the beginnings of its exploration at the molecular level (Table 1.1); the complete story of what has followed will be told in subsequent chapters. The speedy progress in thalassaemia research is a remarkable reflection of the way in which the medical sciences have progressed over this period. Medical research has, in essence, moved from the study of patients and their diseased organs to the definition of disease at the molecular and cellular level. The molecular analysis of the haemoglobin disorders undoubtedly opened up the field of human molecular genetics, and studies of the molecular pathology of thalassaemia have yielded some remarkable insights into the repertoire of mutations that underlie human monogenic disease. As other single-gene disorders have been dissected in the same way, very similar patterns of mutations have turned up. But, perhaps most importantly, a careful analysis of the relationships between the genotype and phenotype in thalassaemic patients has yielded some valuable insights into the molecular mechanisms for the phenotypic diversity of monogenic disease.

Future historians of twentieth-century medicine will undoubtedly ask why the haemoglobin disorders, which are not common in the more advanced countries in which research in molecular biology was established, were among the first to be defined at the molecular level—work that, in effect, opened up the era of molecular medicine. Although this is a difficult

Table 1.1 Chronology of some landmarks in the haemoglobin field up to 1981. Adapted from Weatherall and Clegg (1999).

Year	Discovery	Authors
1628	Circulation of the blood	Harvey
1664	The '*vital quintessence*' of air	Boyle, Hooke
1669	Function of the pulmonary circulation	Lower
1772	Dephlogisticated air	Priestley
1775	Oxygen	Lavoisier
1862	Oxygen-binding pigment is named 'haemoglobin'	Hoppe-Seyler
1866	Spectral change on deoxygenation of blood	Stokes
1866	Fetal blood is alkali-resistant	Körber
1884	Stoichiometry of oxygen binding	Von Hufner
1904	Sigmoid oxygen dissociation curve Curve modified by carbon dioxide	Bohr
1910	Equation for oxygen binding	Hill
1910	Sickle-cell anaemia	Herrick
1913	Structure of haem	Kuster
1925–27	Molecular weight of haemoglobin	Adair, Svedberg
1925	Kinetics of oxygen binding	Roughton, Hartridge
1925	Description of 'thalassaemia'	Cooley, Rietti
1932	Term 'thalassaemia' first used	Whipple & Bradford
1936	Cooperative behaviour of haemoglobin	Pauling
1937–44	Inheritance of thalassaemia	Caminopetros, Neel, Valentine, Silvestroni, Bianco, Gatto, Smith
1944–46	Sickle-cell thalassaemia	Silvestroni, Bianco
1948	Alkali-resistant haemoglobin in thalassaemia	Vecchio
1949	Sickle-cell haemoglobin	Pauling *et al.*, Castle
1949	Malaria hypothesis	Haldane
1949–50	Genetics of sickle-cell anaemia	Neel, Beet, Lambotte-Legrand
1950	Tactoid formation in sickle-cell disease	Harris
1954	Sickle-cell trait protects against malaria	Allison
1955	HbA_2 is raised in some thalassaemias	Kunkel & Wallenuis
1955	Haemoglobin-H disease	Rigas *et al.*
1955	Hereditary persistence of fetal haemoglobin	Eddington & Lehmann
1956	Haemoglobin consists of subunits	Ingram
1956	Structure of haemoglobin S	Ingram
1957	Ineffective erythropoiesis in thalassaemia	Sturgeon & Finch
1958	Adult haemoglobin controlled by two gene loci	Smith & Torbert
1958	Hb Bart's	Ager & Lehmann
1959	Three-dimensional structure of haemoglobin	Perutz
1959	α- and β-thalassaemia hypothesis	Ingram & Stretton
1960	Hb Bart's hydrops	Lie-Injo & Jo
1960–63	Structure of α, β, γ and δ chains	Konigsberg *et al.*, Schroeder *et al.*, Jones *et al.*, Braunitzer *et al.*, Hill *et al.*
1962	Hb Lepore; a δβ-fusion variant	Baglioni
1962	Chelation therapy. Desferrioxamine	Sephton-Smith
1963	Inclusion bodies in thalassaemia	Fessas
1964	High-level transfusion for thalassaemia	Waldman
1965	Imbalanced globin synthesis in α and β thalassaemia	Weatherall, Clegg, Naughton
1966	Fibre formation in sickle cells	Stetson, Murayama
1966	Consequences of globin imbalance	Nathan, Gunn
1967–69	Assembly of globin peptide chains in thalassaemia	Clegg, Weatherall *et al.*
1968	Multiple γ-globin genes	Schroeder *et al.*
1970	Genetics of α thalassaemia	Na-Nakorn & Wasi
1971	Globin mRNA function in thalassaemia	Nienhuis & Anderson, Benz & Forget
1971	Chain-termination mutations in α thalassaemia	Milner, Clegg, Weatherall

Continued

Table 1.1 *Continued.*

Year	Discovery	Authors
1972	Prenatal diagnosis of sickle-cell anaemia by globin synthesis	Kan *et al.*
1972	Hb Kenya; a βγ-fusion variant	Huisman *et al.*
1973	Globin mRNA quantification	Kacian *et al.*, Housman *et al.*
1973	Dominantly inherited β thalassaemia	Weatherall *et al.*
1974	Liver iron level controlled by desferrioxamine	Barry *et al.*
1974	Deletion of α-globin genes in thalassaemia	Ottolenghi *et al.*, Taylor *et al.*
1976–78	Desferrioxamine infusions; iron balance in transfused patients	Propper *et al.*, Hussain *et al.*, Pippard *et al.*
1976–77	Structure of globin mRNA	Baralle, Forget *et al.*, Proudfoot and Longley, Chang *et al.*, Wilson *et al.*, Marotta *et al.*
1979	Restriction-fragment-length polymorphism for prenatal diagnosis	Kan & Dozy
1979	Stop-codon mutation in β-globin mRNA	Chang & Kan
1979	β thalassaemia due to gene deletion	Orkin *et al.*
1979–81	Heterogeneity of α-gene deletions	Embury *et al.*, Orkin *et al.*, Pressley *et al.*, Higgs *et al.*, Kan *et al.*
1980–81	Globin genes sequenced	Lawn *et al.*, Spritz *et al.*, Barralle *et al.*, Slightom *et al.*, Lauer *et al.*, Maniatis *et al.*
1981	α thalassaemia/mental retardation	Weatherall *et al.*
1981	Mutations in β thalassaemia in cloned DNA	Spritz *et al.*, Westaway & Williamson

question, the answer must, at least in part, reflect the chance coming together of several disciplines at the right time. Haemoglobin, because its function is so important and because it is easy to obtain relatively pure from red cells, was of particular interest to protein chemists and those who wanted to study protein synthesis and structure–function relationships. The seminal work of Pauling and the equally important studies on the genetics of sickle-cell anaemia came at a time when haematology and human genetics were just emerging as potentially exciting branches of medical research. It is not surprising therefore that the haemoglobin diseases attracted some of the most able workers in many parts of the world. Thus throughout the period after the early 1960s a handful of young clinical scientists in the USA, Europe and south-east Asia developed a dialogue with the relevant basic sciences, and were able themselves to apply each new technical advance as it was developed. This close relationship survived into the molecular era and was, in effect, the main reason why a number of talented molecular biologists were briefly attracted to the haemoglobin field in the 1980s.

Against this background it is not surprising that the haemoglobin field led the way in the evolution of molecular medicine. For the thalassaemias were already so well characterized by the mid-1970s that, once methods for isolating and sequencing human genes became available, it was already clear which genes should be looked at and, in some cases, what was likely to be found.

Another important feature of the thalassaemia story is how quickly advances in the research laboratory have been applied in the clinic, both for the diagnosis of different forms of thalassaemia and for their prenatal detection. Unfortunately, the story is not complete. Early hopes that the thalassaemias might be among the first disorders that would be amenable to correction at the molecular level by gene therapy have not been fulfilled. The globin genes require particularly tight regulation; more research towards a better understanding of these complex processes is required before this will be achieved.

Thalassaemia provides yet another interesting lesson for biomedical research. By studying the abnormal it is often possible to clarify normal biological functions. A great deal has been learnt from work on the abnormal haemoglobins about how haemoglobin functions as an oxygen carrier. Similarly, by recognizing that several different types of thalassaemia are the result of mutations of key regulatory sequences, it has been possible to identify regions of DNA at considerable distances from the globin genes that are involved in their normal activation and control.

The thalassaemia story is therefore a fine example of what can be achieved when the basic biological and clinical sciences freely interact. In the chapters that follow we shall try to provide our readers with a summary of our current state of knowledge of this complex syndrome. No doubt there are still new forms of thalassaemia to be discovered.

Haematologists and colleagues who care for patients with these diseases should be on a constant lookout for the unusual. For, if this brief survey of the story of thalassaemia has told us anything, it is that it is the unexpected finding in a patient with this kind of disorder which, if investigated in depth, is likely to lead to a genuine advance in our understanding of the complex mechanisms that underlie the clinical diversity of inherited disease, and which, as a bonus, may tell us a great deal about normal function.

Part 2
The biology of the thalassaemias

Contributors:
D.R. Higgs
Swee Lay Thein
W.G. Wood

Chapter 2
Human haemoglobin

Introduction

Since the thalassaemias are genetic disorders of haemoglobin synthesis, and because they are often co-inherited with different abnormal haemoglobins, this chapter introduces the principles of the structure, function, synthesis and genetic control of haemoglobin and discusses some of its more important structural variants. It is beyond our scope to deal with this subject in detail. Various aspects are covered more extensively in several recent reviews and monographs (Steinberg *et al.* 2001; Stamatoyannopoulos *et al.* 2001; Weatherall *et al.* 2001) and further references to the literature on some of the important structural haemoglobin variants are given in Chapters 9 and 11. In addition to the account in Chapter 1, those who wish to learn more about how the human haemoglobin field developed should consult the essays of Perutz (1998) and the reviews of Weatherall *et al.* (2000) and Weatherall and Clegg (1999).

We are aware that some of our readers may not be familiar with the principles of protein structure and the genetic control of protein synthesis. For this reason we are prefacing this chapter with a brief introduction to this topic. Others may wish to bypass this section and move on to the description of the structure and function of haemoglobin, on p. 72.

An introduction to the structure and synthesis of proteins

This short account is directed to those who are coming to this field for the first time. There are several excellent monographs and reviews which deal with protein structure and the genetic control of protein synthesis in greater detail (Perutz 1991; Alberts *et al.* 1994; Kyte 1995; Creighton 1997; Lewin 1997).

Protein structure

Proteins are the basic building blocks of all living organisms. In humans, it has been estimated that there are about 10^5 different proteins, which perform functions ranging from maintaining the architecture of tissues, through ion membrane transport and defence against infection, to mediating the myriad of complex chemical reactions that drive our metabolism. Proteins can perform this diverse set of functions because they have widely differing structures. Remarkably, they are made up of the same backbone and the same 20 amino acids. It is the sequence in which the amino acids are linked together that distinguishes one protein from another and which determines their structure.

The structure of proteins can be viewed at various levels of complexity, from primary, to tertiary or quaternary.

Primary structure

The basic structure of all proteins is a string of between 50 and as many as 5000 amino acids, linked together to form a polypeptide chain. As shown in Fig. 2.1, the links in the chain result from the formation of peptide bonds between each amino acid, with the loss of one water molecule per bond. These polypeptide chains are, in effect, simply repetitions of the basic amino acid unit, and hence they have a free amino group at one end, the N-terminus, and a free carboxyl group at the other, the C-terminus (Fig. 2.1). Each amino acid along the chain is called a 'residue', and individual residues are numbered sequentially, starting at the N-terminus.

When the sequence of amino acids is written to describe the structure of a polypeptide chain, they appear either in an abbreviated form, 'Ala' for alanine for example, or in a one-letter code in which each amino acid is represented by a different letter; in this form alanine would be written 'A'. The one-letter codes for amino acids are shown in Table 2.1.

The reason that polypeptide chains do not exist as linear structures is that the side-chains of the individual amino acids all have different properties and tend to interact with one another to produce complex

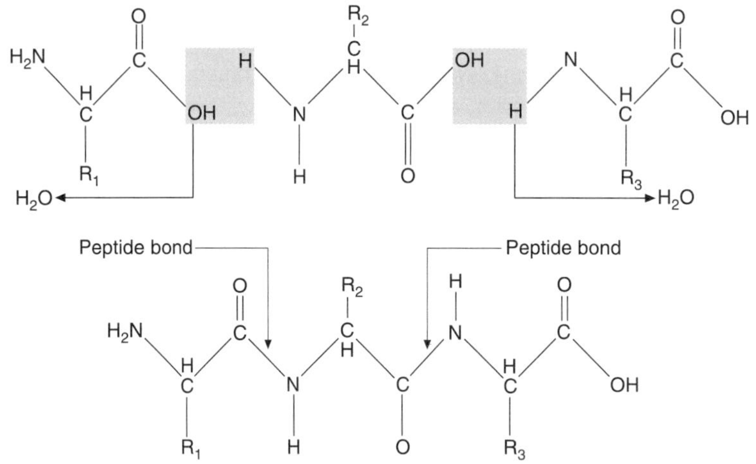

Fig. 2.1 Peptide-bond formation. This is a covalent amide linkage between amino-acid residues in a polypeptide chain which is formed by linking the α-carboxyl carbon of one residue with the α-amino nitrogen of another.

Table 2.1 One-letter code and abbreviated forms for amino acids.

A	Alanine (Ala)	M	Methionine (Met)
C	Cysteine (Cys)	N	Asparagine (Asn)
D	Aspartic acid (Asp)	P	Proline (Pro)
E	Glutamic acid (Glu)	Q	Glutamine (Gln)
F	Phenylalanine (Phe)	R	Arginine (Arg)
G	Glycine (Gly)	S	Serine (Ser)
H	Histidine (His)	T	Threonine (Thr)
I	Isoleucine (Ile)	V	Valine (Val)
K	Lysine (Lys)	W	Tryptophan (Trp)
L	Leucine (Leu)	Y	Tyrosine (Tyr)

three-dimensional configurations. Amino acids are classified into different groups, depending on a variety of properties of their side-chains, in particular whether they are charged (acidic or basic) or whether they are uncharged (polar or non-polar). Amino acids with uncharged polar groups tend to be relatively hydrophilic (interact with water) and are usually found on the outside of proteins, while the side-chains on non-polar amino acids tend to be hydrophobic (repel water) and to cluster together on the inside. Amino acids with basic or acidic side-chains are especially polar, and hence they are nearly always found on the outside of protein molecules.

Secondary and tertiary structure

As the result of complex interactions between the side-chains of their constituent amino acids, polypeptide chains tend to fold into a complex tertiary configuration, with straight regions interspersed with numerous bends. The straight segments in proteins that fold often develop some secondary structures, the commonest of which are the α helix and β strand. The α helix is a right-handed helix with about 3.6 amino-acid residues per turn. In β strands, the polypeptide chain is almost fully extended, with the CO and NH groups of each residue pointing to one side. Multiple β strands aggregate side by side, forming bonds between the CO of one strand and the NH of another, to form what are called 'β sheets'. Some proteins, such as haemoglobin, are composed only of α helices and turns, others consist entirely of β sheets and turns, and yet others contain both conformations. In helical proteins, the helices are often designated by letters of the alphabet.

The shapes of the complex tertiary structures, which are most easily characterized by X-ray crystallography or nuclear magnetic resonance analysis, are absolutely critical for the stability and function of proteins. Their interiors are compact, with few cavities. The surfaces and interiors vary in their structure, depending on whether they exist in aqueous solutions or are embedded in membranes. As we discussed earlier, for water-soluble proteins like haemoglobin, amino acids with side-chains that are normally ionized occur only on the surface, where they interact with water, and not in the interior, which is occupied almost entirely by amino acids with non-polar side-chains.

Quaternary structure

Many proteins consist of multiple copies of the same or different polypeptide chains. In these structures individual peptide chains are referred to as 'subunits', and designated by Greek letters. Human adult haemoglobin, for example, has two different pairs of subunits, called α and β; it is written $\alpha_2\beta_2$.

The stability of the folded states of individual subunits and their interactions with others depend on the action of many different forces. Among the most important are hydrogen bonds between polar groups, and van der Waals interactions between non-polar atoms. Hydrogen bonds are weak, non-covalent, bonds in which a hydrogen atom covalently bonded to a very electronegative atom interacts with another atom. On the other hand, van der Waals forces are non-specific attractive forces which occur between two atoms, strongest when the atoms are 3–4 Å apart.

Protein function

Many proteins, particularly those which subserve different types of transport, contain binding sites for other molecules, or ligands, with which they interact. In some cases these simply consist of small regions on the surface of the protein that are complementary, both sterically (in shape) and physically, to the ligand. For binding very small ligands, oxygen for example, which could not be recognized in this way, proteins carry additional, or prosthetic, groups which are incorporated into their structure for this purpose. For example, in the case of haemoglobin, each polypeptide chain carries one haem, a ring of carbon, nitrogen and hydrogen atoms called porphyrin, with an iron atom at its centre.

The binding of ligands to proteins is often expressed as a dissociation constant; that is, the concentration of free ligand at which the protein binding site is occupied half the time at equilibrium. Some proteins bind multiple ligands. In many cases the binding of one ligand changes the binding affinity of another at a different site, a phenomenon called 'allostery'. As we shall see later in this chapter, haemoglobin is a prime example of an allosteric protein, in that the binding of oxygen to one of its four subunits increases the affinity of each of the others.

From these simple considerations it is clear that the structure and function of proteins is entirely dependent on having the appropriate order of amino acids in its constituent polypeptide chains, and, of course, on their being synthesized at the appropriate level in the right place at the right time. These critical factors depend on the genes that are involved in determining their structure and synthesis.

Gene action and protein synthesis

Essentially, genes are lengths of DNA which contain the information required to make their protein product. Although there are more complicated situations, the primary product of most genes is a single polypeptide chain. This means that, for proteins such as haemoglobin, in which there are different subunits, more than one gene must be involved in determining their structure. The information that genes carry includes not only the appropriate order of amino acids in a particular polypeptide chain, but also the directions required to ensure that it is synthesized in the appropriate cells at the correct time of development and in the right amount. The instructions required to synthesize a polypeptide chain are transported from the nuclei of cells to the cytoplasm by means of a type of ribonucleic acid (RNA) called 'messenger RNA' (mRNA) which has a structure exactly complementary to that of the DNA from which it is copied, or transcribed. The process whereby a protein chain is synthesized on an mRNA template is called translation. Thus, the flow of genetic information in cells can be written

$$\text{DNA} \xrightarrow{\text{transcription}} \text{RNA} \xrightarrow{\text{translation}} \text{protein}$$

Gene structure

DNA consists of two chains of nucleotide bases wrapped around each other in the form of a double helix (Fig. 2.2). There are four bases, adenine (A), guanine (G), cytosine (C) and thymine (T). The building-blocks of each chain are deoxyribonucleotides, which consist of a base, deoxyribose and phosphate, covalently joined. The backbone of DNA, which is constant throughout the molecule, consists

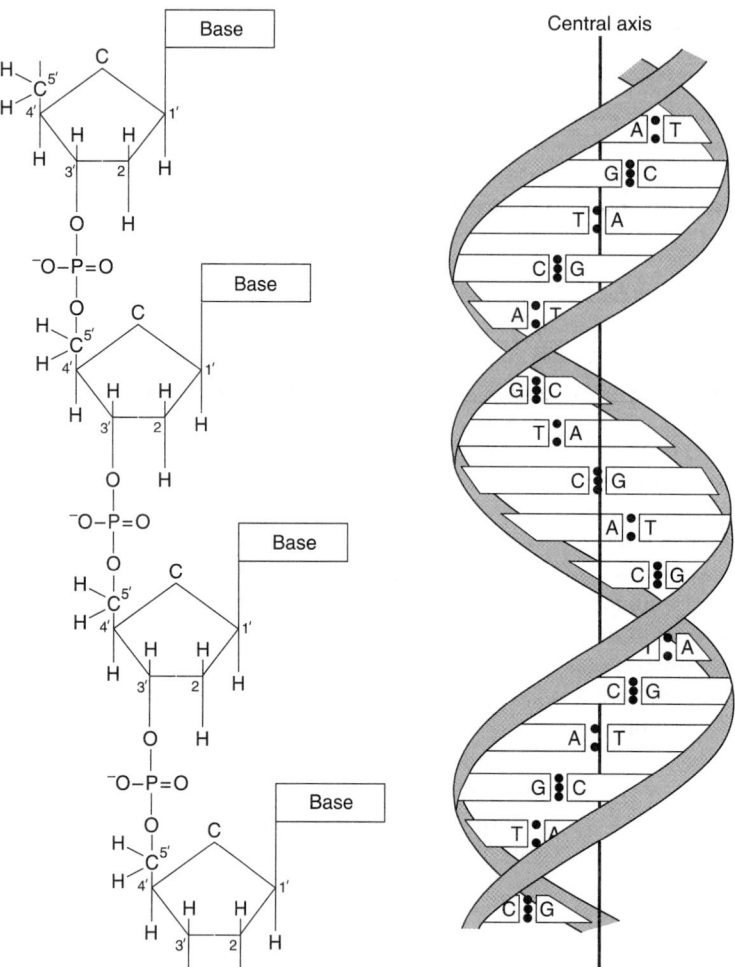

Fig. 2.2 The structure of DNA. From Weatherall, D.J. *The New Genetics and Clinical Practice*, 3rd edn, Oxford University Press (1991).

of deoxyribose sugars linked by phosphates. The variable part of a DNA chain is the sequence of bases, which can be in any order along a sugar–phosphate backbone. Because of their particular shapes, A always pairs with T, and C with G in the double helix; the bases, and hence the two chains, or strands, are linked by hydrogen bonds.

When DNA replicates, the strands separate and each acts as a template to produce two new, double-stranded identical copies. Genetic information is encoded by the order of the bases as a triplet, non-overlapping code in which three bases determine a particular amino acid. It follows therefore that a gene must contain three times the number of nucleotide bases as the number of amino acids in its polypep-

tide-chain product. However, things are more complicated than this. The coding sequences, called exons, are interrupted by sequences of various lengths which do not have any coding function, called 'intervening sequences' (IVS), or introns. Furthermore, the genes contain other sequences at their 5′ (left-hand, as conventionally written in single-strand form) and 3′ (right-hand) ends which subserve important regulatory functions.

Transcription and processing of messenger RNA

When a gene is transcribed, mRNA is synthesized on one strand of its DNA template in a 5′ → 3′ fashion by the action of an enzyme called RNA polymerase. This process is initiated by formation of a complex containing the enzyme and a large number of regulatory proteins, or transcription factors, at a region at the 5′ end of the gene called the promoter (see below). Chemically, RNA is similar to DNA with two exceptions; the sugar of DNA is deoxyribose while in RNA it is ribose, and instead of thymine RNA contains the closely related pyrimidine, uracil (U). The synthesis of RNA on DNA templates involves the formation of complementary base pairs so that, as in the case of DNA replication, G pairs with C, though when mRNA is being made on a DNA template, A pairs with U instead of T. The primary transcript is a large mRNA precursor which contains a copy of the entire gene complex, both exons and introns. This molecule undergoes a series of processing steps before it is ready for delivery to the cell cytoplasm. The introns are excised, the exons joined together and a number of structural modifications are made at both ends.

The processes of excision and splicing are complex and multistep, and involve highly conserved donor and acceptor sequences at the 5′ and 3′ exon/intron junctions. The initial step is cleavage of the 5′ splice site to produce a lariat structure which contains the intron and the 3′ exon. This is followed by the joining together of the two exons and release of the now free intron. Although this seems simple enough, it requires the formation of a complex called a spliceosome, which consists of five small ribonuclear particles (snRNPs) and a large number of protein-splicing factors; its assembly is achieved through a series of intermediate complexes called E, A, B and C.

Immediately after initiation of transcription, the 5′ end of the newly synthesized mRNA molecule is modified by the addition of a 7-methylguanosine residue linked to the terminal nucleotide by a 5′–5′ triphosphate bond. This process and the associated methylation of nearby bases and ribose residues are referred to as 'capping'; thus the start site for RNA transcription on the gene is referred to as the 'CAP'. The mRNAs are also modified at the 3′ end by the addition of a string of adenylic acid residues (poly(A)).

Protein synthesis

Once mRNA has been processed, it moves into the cell cytoplasm to act as a template for protein synthesis. Because amino acids cannot interact directly with nucleic acids they are brought to the RNA template on carrier molecules called transfer RNAs (tRNAs) (Fig. 2.3). There is a family of different tRNAs, each specific for a different amino acid by virtue of the three bases (anticodons) that they carry, which are complementary to the appropriate mRNA codons for their particular amino acids. There is a specific mRNA codon (AUG) for initiation of protein synthesis. This involves the formation of a complex consisting of several initiation factors, two ribosomal subunits and an initiator tRNA. Once this is in place, a second tRNA binds to the next codon along and a peptide bond is formed between the two amino acids carried by these tRNAs. The first tRNA is then released. This cyclical process, which involves the shifting of the growing chains of amino acids between specific donor and acceptor sites on the ribosomes, is then repeated in a 5′ → 3′ direction from codon to codon, until the termination codon is reached. The completed chain is then released from the last tRNA molecule and the ribosome units fall off the mRNA. Most mRNAs carry several ribosomes at any one time; the mRNAs with ribosomes attached along their length (polysomes) resemble a string of beads (Fig. 2.3).

The term 'genetic code' is used to describe the relationship between the sequence of the bases in DNA or its RNA transcript and that of the amino acids in polypeptide chains. As mentioned earlier, amino acids are encoded by groups of three bases called codons. Of the 64 possible coding triplets, 61 identify particular amino acids, whereas the three others, UAA, UAG and UGA are signals for chain termination (Table 2.2). Thus, since only 20 different amino acids occur naturally in proteins, most of them must have one or more code words; in other words, the genetic code is degenerate.

Regulation

One of the most important questions that we shall be addressing in subsequent sections of this chapter, and indeed throughout this book, is how genes are regulated. For, as we shall see, many forms of thalassaemia reflect a breakdown of this function. Some genes are expressed at very low levels in almost every tissue. However, unlike these so-called 'housekeeping genes', globin genes are much more specialized and are only expressed in the red-cell precursors of the bone marrow. Indeed, many genes are only active in specific tissues and at particular times during development. How this is brought about, and the way in

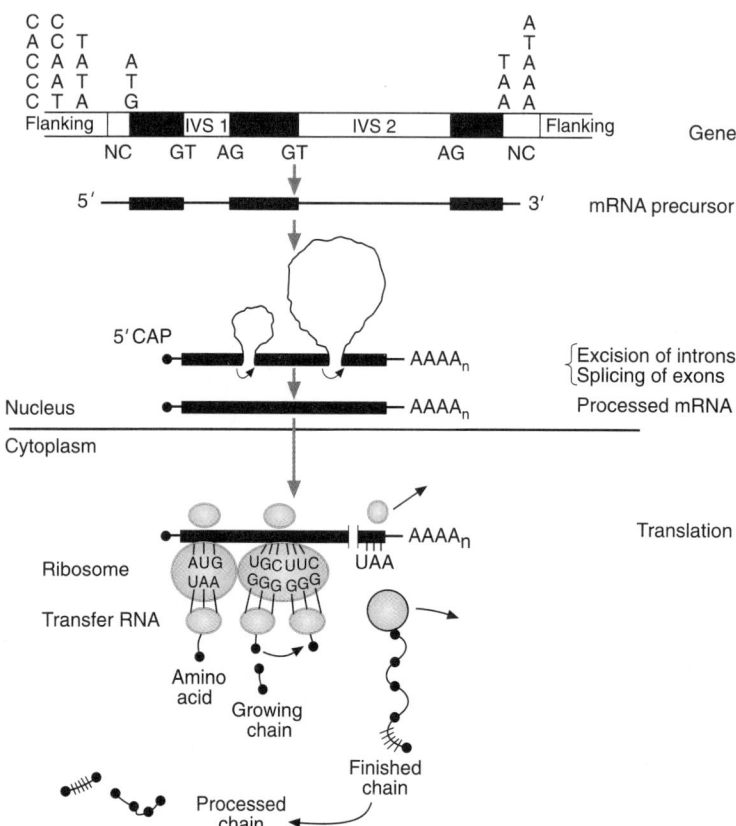

Fig. 2.3 A schematic representation of gene action and protein synthesis.

Table 2.2 The genetic code. The codons are given as they appear in mRNA. The abbreviations for the different amino acids are shown in Table 2.1.

First position (5′ end)	Second position				Third position (3′ end)
	U	C	A	G	
U	Phe	Ser	Tyr	Cys	U
	Phe	Ser	Tyr	Cys	C
	Leu	Ser	Stop	Stop	A
	Leu	Ser	Stop	Trp	G
C	Leu	Pro	His	Arg	U
	Leu	Pro	His	Arg	C
	Leu	Pro	Gln	Arg	A
	Leu	Pro	Gln	Arg	G
A	Ile	Thr	Asn	Ser	U
	Ile	Thr	Asn	Ser	C
	Ile	Thr	Lys	Arg	A
	Met	Thr	Lys	Arg	G
G	Val	Ala	Asp	Gly	U
	Val	Ala	Asp	Gly	C
	Val	Ala	Glu	Gly	A
	Val	Ala	Glu	Gly	G

which our hundred thousand or so genes are orchestrated, will be one of the major questions for biology in the next millennium. But a little is known already, and this information has major relevance to an understanding of the rapid progress which has been made in the thalassaemia field.

Although the standard pictures of DNA (Fig. 2.2) give the impression of long, linear strings of bases, in fact, as it exists in living organisms, it is in a highly compact state; every cell in the body contains approximately 2 m! Each DNA molecule is packaged to form a chromosome. The structure of chromosomes, and the nomenclature used to describe them, is summarized in Fig. 2.4. Chromosomes are composed of chromatin. In this form, DNA is complexed with a family of positively charged proteins called histones, together with smaller amounts of other DNA binding proteins, called, collectively, nonhistone proteins. The histones organize DNA into a regular, repeating structure, the basic unit of which is the nucleosome.

Each nucleosome contains a characteristic length

has been determined to a resolution of 1.7 Å by X-ray crystallography by Perutz and colleagues in Cambridge (Muirhead & Perutz 1963; Perutz 1963, 1965; Perutz *et al.* 1965, 1968a,b; Baldwin 1980a,b; Fermi *et al.* 1984) (Figs 2.6 and 2.7). The subunits in the molecule (an ellipse measuring approximately 64 × 55 × 50 Å) are orientated in a unit with a twofold symmetry axis which runs down a water-filled cavity in the centre of the molecule.

Three-quarters of the polypeptide chains of the haemoglobin molecule are in the form of an α helix. At places where the helical structure is interrupted — by proline residues for example — the chains can turn corners, enabling them to fold and form the compact fit characteristic of the tetrameric molecule. In this, the individual polypeptide chains have relatively few contact sites; consequently, there is relatively little interaction between them compared with the forces that are responsible for maintaining their individual secondary and tertiary structures.

The individual subunit chains of haemoglobin have quite similar three-dimensional structures.

Eight helical regions (lettered A–H) are present in the β chain, and the α chain has analogous regions except that it lacks the residues of the D helix. Amino acid residues can thus be identified by their helical positions (Fig. 2.8).

The interiors of the subunits are made up almost entirely of non-polar (hydrophobic) residues, which are in contact nearly everywhere with neighbouring residues by van der Waals forces. As described earlier, these are weak attractive forces arising from the induced fluctuating charges caused by the close proximity of atoms. They operate over only relatively short distances and have low energies. Hence they are only an effective force under physiological conditions when several atoms in a molecule interact. All the side-chains that are ionizable under physiological conditions are on the surface of the subunits. This is true also of most of the polar (hydrophilic) side-groups. The surface of the molecule is thus covered with polar groups, and in general these make contact with water rather than other charged side-chains.

The prosthetic group of haemoglobin, haem, is fer-

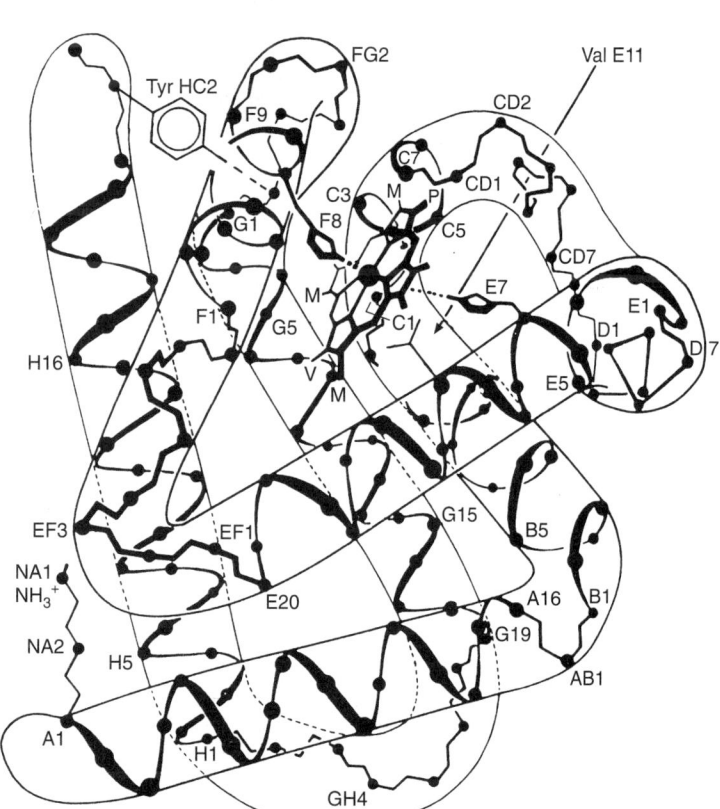

Fig. 2.7 The α subunit of human haemoglobin showing the haem pocket and the position of the haem molecule. By permission of Dr M.F. Perutz and editors of the Cold Spring Harbor Symposium on Quantitative Biology.

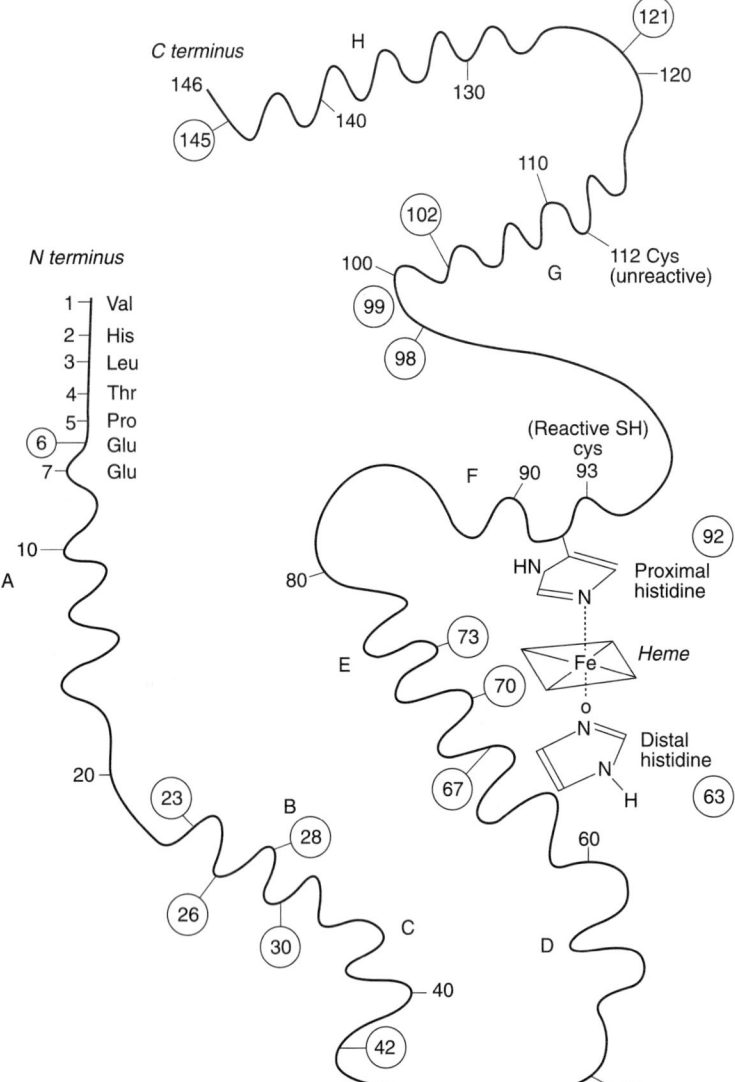

Fig. 2.8 The human β chain. The relationship of the haem molecules to the proximal and distal histidines are shown together with the helical and non-helical segments. In addition, the position of the reactive (β93) and unreactive (β112) cysteines is shown. By permission of Dr E.S. Giblett and Blackwell Science.

roprotoporphyrin IX in which the iron atom is located at the centre of the porphyrin ring (Fig. 2.9). The haem residues lie in clefts in the surface of the globin subunits (Fig. 2.8). These pockets are lined with non-polar residues, and the haem is located between two histidines, one of which (the proximal histidine) is bonded directly through the imidazole nitrogen to the haem iron atom, while the other (the distal histidine) lies opposite to the site of combination with oxygen, but is not directly attached to the haem. The orientation of the haem in the cleft is such

that its non-polar vinyl groups are deeply buried in the hydrophobic interior, while the polar propionic acid groups are presented to the hydrophilic surface of the globin subunit. A large number of inter-atomic contacts (within 4 Å) between the haem and amino-acid side-chains of the E and F helices act to stabilize this structure. The residues surrounding haem are invariant throughout the animal kingdom, suggesting that this particular structure is essential for the normal functioning of haemoglobin as an oxygen carrier.

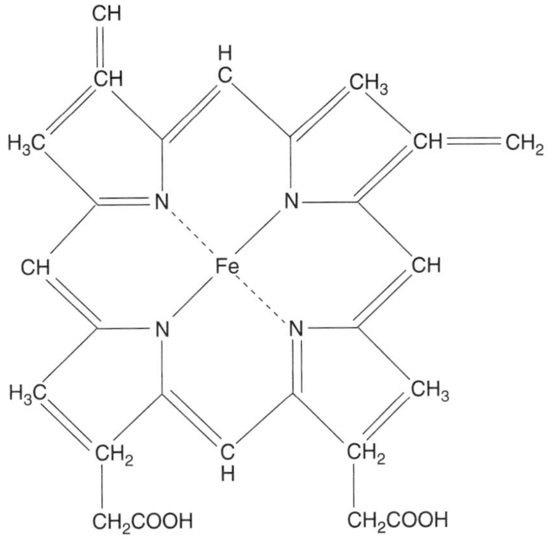

Fig. 2.9 The haem molecule.

As will become apparent in a later section, mutations in the haem pocket can lead to profound alterations in oxygen-binding properties, and, indeed, in the stability of the entire haemoglobin molecule.

The oxygenated and deoxygenated forms of haemoglobin have markedly different three-dimensional structures, a consequence of the changes in relative orientation of the subunits during binding and release of oxygen. In the HbA tetramer each α chain is in contact with two β chains, contacts that are defined as $\alpha_1\beta_1$ and $\alpha_1\beta_2$. Because of the twofold symmetry, there are also the structurally identical $\alpha_2\beta_1$ and $\alpha_2\beta_2$ contacts. During oxygenation/deoxygenation most of the subunit movement takes place at the weaker $\alpha_1\beta_2$ ($\alpha_2\beta_1$) interfaces, while the stronger (40 contacts vs. 17) $\alpha_1\beta_1$ ($\alpha_2\beta_2$) interfaces remain relatively static (Perutz 1970a).

Haemoglobin can exist in two quaternary states

Effective contacts between subunits depend upon key regions of the two αβ dimers being in the same relative orientation. This favours the formation of two specific quaternary states: oxy or 'relaxed' (R), and deoxy or 'tense' (T), without any stable intermediates (Baldwin 1980a,b; Perutz 1980). The nature and number of contacts change during oxygenation/deoxygenation because of movement that

occurs at the $\alpha_1\beta_2$ and $\alpha_2\beta_1$ interfaces. In the deoxy (T) state there are about 40 contacts overall, of which 19 are hydrogen bonds: this drops to 22 and 12, respectively, in the oxy (R) state. The structure of the $\alpha_1\beta_2$ contact, like the haem pocket, has been highly conserved throughout evolution, and mutations in this region can have serious functional consequences.

The more stable quaternary structure of the deoxy-haemoglobin that follows from the larger number of $\alpha_1\beta_2$ and $\alpha_2\beta_1$ contacts is augmented by other inter- and intra-subunit salt linkages that are not present in oxyhaemoglobin. The most prominent are between the COO⁻ group of the C-terminal arginine of one α chain to the ε-amino side-chain of lysine 132 (H10) in the other α chain, and an α–α link between the C-terminal arginine–guanidinium group and the COO⁻ of aspartate 131 (H9). There is also a chloride ion-mediated link between the C-terminal guanidinium and the opposing α-N-terminal amino group. In oxyhaemoglobin, steric hindrance prevents any of these links from forming (Baldwin 1980a,b). The β chains form similar deoxy-specific links. Two involve the C-terminal histidine: one with the imidazole group and aspartate 94 (FG1) of the same β chain, the second with the carboxyl group and the ε-amino group of lysine α40 (C5), which forms a salt bridge across the $\alpha_1\beta_2$ ($\alpha_2\beta_1$) interface. In oxyhaemoglobin the distances between the residues are too great to allow salt bridges to form.

Function and structure–function relationships

It has been known for many years that haemoglobin has a sigmoid-shaped oxygen dissociation curve (Fig. 2.10). In practical terms this means that it can absorb and release large quantities of oxygen in response to relatively small changes in partial pressure in the physiological range. This property is dependent upon interaction, or cooperation, between the haem groups; the oxygenation of one haem enhances the reactivity of the remainder, a phenomenon known as haem–haem interaction. Haemoglobin is thus an allosteric protein; combination of oxygen at one site facilitates combination at others. Furthermore, the oxygen affinity of haemoglobin is affected by the binding of small molecules such as 2,3-diphosphoglycerate (2,3-DPG); it is also sensitive to small changes in pH, a phenomenon known as the Bohr effect, and to the intracellular Cl⁻-ion concentration. The molecular bases for these effects have become

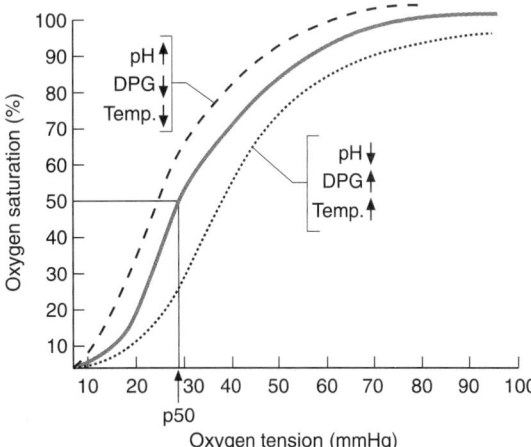

Fig. 2.10 The oxygen dissociation curve of human adult haemoglobin. The left and right shifts in relationship to changes in pH, 2,3-DPG concentration and temperature are shown.

clear from the structural studies of Perutz and colleagues (Perutz 1970a,b, 1972; Perutz *et al.* 1994).

Changes in conformation with oxygenation of haemoglobin

It seems likely that the haem–haem interaction is dependent on small rearrangements which occur between subunits when oxygen is taken up or released. The iron atoms of the β-chain haems move apart about 7 Å during oxygenation, reorientations which depend on interactions between the α and β chains, since they do not occur in the abnormal haemoglobin, HbH, a tetramer of β chains which exhibits no haem–haem interaction or Bohr effect (see Chapter 5), and which consequently cannot act as an oxygen carrier under normal physiological oxygen tensions (Benesch *et al.* 1961).

There are several reasons for believing that the $\alpha_1\beta_2$ (and $\alpha_2\beta_1$) contacts are particularly important in these cooperative interactions. First, the three-dimensional structure shows that interaction between the α_1 and β_2 (or α_2 and β_1) subunits can be more direct than between the α_1 and β_1 or α_2 and β_2 subunits. Furthermore, oxygenation of the β_2 subunit causes it to rotate further with respect to the α subunit than does oxygenation of the β_1 subunit. The amino acid residues in the $\alpha_1\beta_2$ ($\alpha_2\beta_1$) contact have

remained invariant throughout mammalian evolution, whereas more than a third of those in the $\alpha_1\beta_1$ ($\alpha_2\beta_2$) contact have changed. Indeed, in most cases of an abnormal haemoglobin with impaired haem–haem interaction the mutation is usually found in, or near, the $\alpha_1\beta_2$ ($\alpha_2\beta_1$) contact.

The molecular basis for these conformational changes in the subunits during oxygenation has been proposed by Perutz (1970a,b, 1972). When there is no oxygen bound to haem the atomic diameter of the iron atom is too great to allow it to align with the plane of the porphyrin ring; it sits 0.6 Å displaced towards the proximal F8 histidine residue. When an oxygen molecule is bound to the haem iron, the resulting changes in distribution of electrons orbiting the iron atom nucleus lead to an effective reduction in its atomic diameter, and hence it can move flush into the plane of the porphyrin ring. This movement results in a tilt of the haem in its pocket and this is amplified as a change in the tertiary structure of the subunit.

Deoxyhaemoglobin has a more stable quaternary structure than oxyhaemoglobin, probably because of the presence of additional inter- and intra-subunit salt linkages (strong ionic bonds between charged residues, such as $NH_3^+ \ldots COO^-$). Thus the C-terminal β-chain carboxyl groups are linked to the ε-amino groups of the lysine residues at α40. Similarly the imidazoles of the C-terminal β-chain histidines are salt-bridged to the carboxyl residues of aspartic acid at position 94 of the same β chain.

Physiological measurements indicate that the free-energy change in going from the deoxy to the oxy conformation is about 10 to 12 cal/mol/tetramer, and this accords well with the total amount of energy locked up in the salt bonds (assuming 1 to 2 cal/bond) stabilizing the deoxyhaemoglobin molecule. The salt bonds thus represent a considerable amount of energy holding the deoxyhaemoglobin molecule in a high-energy or 'tense' (T) conformation (which has, in a graphic analogy, been likened to a set trap (Bunn *et al.* 1977)).

The 0.6 Å movement of the iron atom into the plane of the haem upon oxygenation is the trigger which releases this energy. The movement of the iron is associated with the movement of the attached histidine. This in turn squeezes the haem pocket, which pushes out the penultimate tyrosine from its pocket between the F and H helices and rupture of the C-terminal salt bridges results. The transition of the quaternary structure from the tense (T) to the relaxed (R) oxy conformation occurs abruptly as these salt bridges successively rupture, and constraints at the $\alpha_1\beta_2$ ($\alpha_2\beta_1$) contact area are relaxed. Since the α-chain haems are relatively more accessible to oxygen they are probably oxygenated first. The shift from the T to R structure then opens up the pockets of the unliganded β-chain haems, greatly increasing their affinity for oxygen.

Modification of haemoglobin function by 2,3-diphosphoglycerate

Organic phosphates also enhance the stability of deoxyhaemoglobin. In human red cells the major cofactor of this type is 2,3-diphosphoglycerate (2,3-DPG) (Benesch & Benesch 1967; Chanutin & Curnish 1967; Benesch & Benesch 1968, 1969). This binds specifically to the β chains of deoxyhaemoglobin (Benesch *et al.* 1968a) (more strictly to haemoglobin in the T state) through electrostatic bonds between the phosphates of the 2,3-DPG and the N-terminal amino groups and imidazole groups of the β143 histidines, and between the 2,3-DPG carboxyl group and the ϵ-amino group of β86 lysine (Arnone 1972). When the quaternary state of haemoglobin changes from the T to the R state, bound 2,3-DPG molecules are ejected. Thus the binding of oxygen and 2,3-DPG are mutually exclusive, and the effect of this is that 2,3-DPG lowers the affinity of haemoglobin for oxygen (Fig. 2.10) as it acts to maintain or stabilize the deoxy configuration of the molecule.

It is clear therefore that the level of 2,3-DPG is critical in determining the oxygen affinity of haemoglobin. Differences in oxygen affinity between fetal and adult blood are largely dependent on the fact that 2,3-DPG has only a weak affinity for fetal deoxyhaemoglobin (Bauer *et al.* 1968; Tyuma & Shimizu 1969). Other situations where the interaction between haemoglobin and 2,3-DPG is important include the change in oxygen affinity which follows prolonged storage of blood, the adaptive changes which occur with increasing altitude or in response to anaemia and the relationship of sodium transport across the red-cell membrane to the oxygenation of haemoglobin (Benesch & Benesch 1969). In Chapter 5 we shall see how the relative lack of interaction of 2,3-DPG with fetal haemoglobin may have important implications for oxygen transport in the blood of patients

Table 2.4 Some conditions that modify 2,3-disphosphoglycerate (2,3-DPG) levels and the oxygen dissociation curve of haemoglobin.

Increased 2,3-DPG; increased p50, reduced oxygen affinity
Anaemia
Alkalosis
Hyperphosphataemia
Renal failure
Hypoxia
Pregnancy
Congenital heart disease
Thyrotoxicosis
Some red-cell enzyme deficiencies
Decreased 2,3-DPG; decreased p50, increased oxygen affinity
Acidosis
Cardiogenic or septicaemic shock
Hypophosphataemia
Hypothyroidism
Hypopituitarism
Replacement with stored blood

with severe forms of β thalassaemia. Some other clinical situations in which 2,3-DPG plays an important role are summarized in Table 2.4.

The Bohr effect

We have already mentioned that the binding of O_2 to haemoglobin is sensitive to changes in pH, an effect that was first observed many years ago by Bohr (1904). Its physiological importance lies in its effect on the transportation of CO_2 in the blood. Carbon dioxide released on respiration is too insoluble to be transported in any quantity except in the form of bicarbonate, by reaction with water:

$$CO_2 + H_2O \rightleftharpoons HCO_3^- + H^+$$

The protons released can combine with deoxyhaemoglobin, thus forcing the reaction in the direction of bicarbonate formation. The released protons lower the O_2 affinity of the haemoglobin by stabilizing the deoxyhaemoglobin configuration and thus facilitate O_2 unloading in the tissues (Perutz 1978). Conversely, in the lungs the opposite occurs. Oxygen binds to haemoglobin and displaces protons which drive the CO_2–HCO_3^- reaction to the left, thereby facilitating the unloading of CO_2 from the plasma.

Hence, because of the Bohr effect, CO_2 promotes O_2 exchange, and vice versa.

In addition to its role as O_2 carrier, haemoglobin is also responsible for the direct transport of some (approximately 10%) of the CO_2 in the blood. It has been shown by Kilmartin and Rossi-Bernardi (1969, 1971) that CO_2 combines reversibly at physiological pH and temperature with the N-terminal amino groups of haemoglobin to form a carbamate ion:

$$RNH_2 + CO_2 \rightleftharpoons RNH\ COO^- + H^+$$

Carbon dioxide binds more readily to deoxy- than to oxyhaemoglobin, and thus facilitates the reciprocal transport of O_2 and CO_2 through the circulation. The combination of CO_2 with haemoglobin is, like the binding of 2,3-DPG and the Bohr effect, another example of an oxygen-linked reaction. These mutual interactions are all examples of allosteric effects. Indeed, haemoglobin can be considered as the model allosteric protein *par excellence*.

The chloride effect

Chloride also behaves as an allosteric effector, reducing the oxygen affinity of haemoglobin by stabilizing the deoxy (T) structure. It thus behaves in a similar fashion to 2,3-DPG. Unlike 2,3-DPG, however, chloride does not have specific binding sites within the haemoglobin molecule. Rather it appears to function by neutralizing electrostatic repulsion by excess positive charges in the central cavity of the tetramer (Perutz *et al.* 1994).

Globin-gene organization

How did our present-day globin genes evolve?

Globin genes arose early in evolution and are found in some fungi, plants and invertebrates as well as in all vertebrate species. Gene duplication, followed by selection of adaptive sequence changes, resulted in the production of diverse globins with specialized functions, allowing the original monomeric forms of haemoglobin to evolve into the tetrameric proteins that are now found in all higher animals. Structurally distinct α and β globins are found in all vertebrates, suggesting that they originated before ~450 million years ago (MYA). In fish and amphibians that have been examined, the genes for these two types of globin are linked together in a single cluster. Chromosomal rearrangements resulted in separation of the α- and β-gene clusters by the time that birds evolved.

Gene duplication and subsequent regulatory changes also allowed developmental-stage-specific expression of the globin genes. In the α-globin gene cluster, duplication, leading to a specialized embryonic (ζ)-globin chain, occurred around 400 MYA, while the α gene underwent at least three separate duplications, first in birds about 400 MYA, subsequently in early eutherian mammalian evolution, and lastly in the higher primates after their divergence from prosimians. In many species, repeated gene-conversion events, that is, non-reciprocal genetic exchange, have maintained homology between the duplicated adult α genes. Duplication of the primitive β-globin gene occurred independently in birds and mammals (~180–200 MYA) to give rise to the embryonic ε gene. Prior to the divergence of the mammals (~85 MYA) further duplication events of both genes gave rise to ε and γ protogenes in one case and the adult proto-δ and -β genes in the other. A further duplication of the ε gene at around this time gave rise to a pseudogene which is present in most mammalian species examined and which is known as ψβ in humans. In most mammals the proto-γ gene has remained as an embryonically expressed gene and was only recruited to the fetal stage of development after the emergence of the primates (55–60 MYA). Duplication of this gene occurred 35–55 MYA and has been maintained in the lineages leading to the apes — gene conversions again maintaining the sequence identity of the two copies.

The human haemoglobin genes are organized into clusters

The genes that regulate the synthesis and structures of the different globins are organized in two separate clusters (Fig. 2.11). The α-like globin genes, which are encoded on chromosome 16, are found in the order $5'–ζ–ψζ–ψα2–ψα1–α2–α1–θ–3'$. The β-like globin genes, on chromosome 11, occur in the order $5'–ε–^Gγ–^Aγ–ψβ–δ–β–3'$.

In understanding the genetic control of haemoglobin we have to try to account for how the expression of these genes is regulated in a tissue- and developmental-stage-specific fashion, and how the production of the different gene products determined on two different chromosomes is synchronized in such a way that there is no major excess of one or other pair of globin subunits at any stage during human

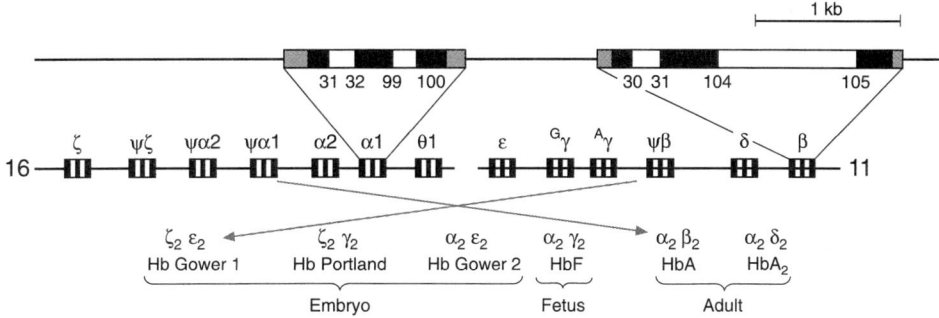

Fig. 2.11 The α- and β-globin gene clusters on chromosomes 16 and 11, respectively. In the extended α- and β-globin genes the introns are shaded dark, the 5′ and 3′ non-coding regions are hatched, and the exons are unshaded.

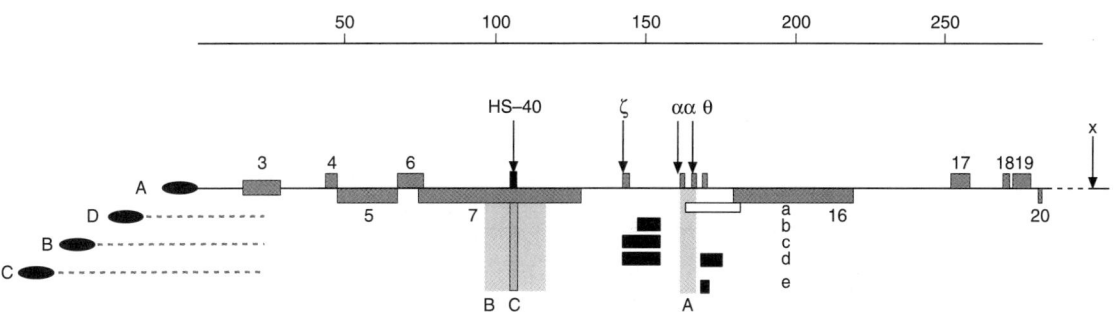

Fig. 2.12 The telomeric and subtelomeric region of chromosome 16p including the α-globin-gene cluster. The major polymorphic, telomeric variants (A–D) of 16p, as described in the text, are indicated with dotted lines (not to scale). Beyond the subtelomeric region the diagram shows the α-globin-gene cluster located at the tip of 16p, surrounded by non-globin genes including: the IL9 receptor pseudogene (3); genes of unknown function (4, 5, 16, 17); a DNA repair enzyme MPG (6); Rho-GDl-R (18), an inhibitor of the dissociation of GDP from Rho; and PDl (19), a protein disulphide isomerase. Further details given in Flint *et al.* (1997).

    Genes illustrated above the line are transcribed towards the centromere and those below towards the telomere. The ψζ1, ψα2 and ψα1 pseudogenes within the α cluster are not shown. Erythroid-specific DNase-l-hypersensitive sites are shown as arrows above the line. X denotes the position of chromosomal translocation (Higgs *et al.* 1990). The shortest region of overlap for α-globin deletions (A) and natural deletions of the regulatory element (HS-40) are shown as shaded boxes. The area removed in the knockout experiment described in the text is indicated (C). The α-ZF deletion is marked as (a) and four rearrangements that do not perturb α-globin expression are indicated. Sources: b–e; summarized in Higgs *et al.* (1989); b is also described in Fei *et al.* (1989). The scale is in kilobase pairs and coordinate 1 is the first nucleotide in the sequence described by Flint *et al.* (1997).

development. Since an understanding of these issues is so central to an appreciation of the molecular basis for the different forms of thalassaemia, we shall describe the structure and functions of each of these clusters of globin genes in the sections that follow. It should be emphasized, particularly for newcomers to the field, that there is considerable normal variation within both globin-gene clusters. The extent of this structural heterogeneity must be appreciated by those who wish to explore the structure of the globin genes and their flanking regions to search for abnormalities in patients with different forms of thalassaemia.

The α-globin gene cluster

General structure

In humans, the α-globin gene cluster (Fig. 2.12) occupies a region of about 70 kilobases (kb: 1000 nucleotide bases) close to the tip of the short arm of chromosome 16, band 16p13.3. For convenience in describing the positions of the genes, the CAP site of the ζ gene is designated 0, distances towards the telomere are given minus prefixes, and distances towards the centromere are denoted with plus prefixes. Thus the α2 gene, at +20 kb, lies 20 kb away from the ζ gene on the centromeric side, and the α1 gene lies a further 3.7 kb away, at +24 kb (Fig. 2.12). Sequences which are essential for α-globin expression, notably the major α-globin-gene regulatory element, HS –40, are centred on a region 40 kb upstream of the ζ-globin gene. In addition to the three functional α-like genes, the cluster contains three pseudogenes (ψζ, ψα2, ψα1) and another gene, θ. The latter is transcribed at a low level in erythroid cells, but so far no protein product has been identified; the protein predicted from its sequence is unlikely to be a functional globin (Clegg 1987).

The complete DNA sequence of the terminal 300-kb region of chromosome 16p has been determined (Flint *et al.* 1997). It shows that the α-globin gene cluster lies between 170 and 430 kb from the telomere, the variability depending on the length of the subtelomeric repetitive sequences (see below). The sequence is unusually GC-rich and also has a high density of genes. On the telomeric side of the cluster lies an interleukin-9 pseudogene (~125 kb away), a gene involved in DNA repair, 3-methyl-adenine DNA glycosylase (~74 kb), and three genes of unknown function (at –14, –70, –89 kb). Four further genes have been located on the centromeric side. Most of these genes are expressed in a wide variety of tissues and must therefore be regulated independently of the erythroid-cell-specific α-globin genes.

The region around the α-globin cluster is rich in Alu repetitive sequences. Large numbers of these repeats flank the cluster and several copies are interspersed within it. Other families of repetitive sequences are less represented, although several partial L1 repeats are found within the cluster.

Normal structural variation

Variation at the 16p telomere

The α-globin locus lies very close to the telomere of the short arm of chromosome 16 (Fig. 2.12). There are four polymorphic, subtelomeric alleles in which the α-globin genes lie 170 kb (A), 245 kb (D), 350 kb (B) or 430 kb (C) from the 16p telomeric repeats (Wilkie *et al.* 1991a; Higgs *et al.* 1993). Their structures are quite different. For example, beyond the region of divergence the A and B alleles are more closely related to non-homologous chromosomes than to each other. The A allele is related to the subtelomeric regions of Xqter and Yqter whereas the B allele is more like 9qter, 10pter and 18pter. Despite these major structural differences at the 16p telomere, the haematological findings in individuals with A and B alleles are indistinguishable.

Rarely, chromosomal translocations involving 16p13.3 place the α-globin locus at the tip of another chromosome, as seen, for example, in some parents of patients with the ATR-16 syndrome (see Chapter 12). To date we know of 15 individuals with such balanced translocations, none of whom has α thalassaemia. Hence, since the centromeric breakpoints of these translocations lie 102 Mb from the α-globin genes, it follows that the *cis*-acting sequences required for full α-globin regulation are not perturbed by rearrangements on this scale. Similarly, in two individuals with unbalanced translocations, and three copies of 16p13.3, the α/β-globin synthesis ratios were 1.5 and 1.6 (Wainscoat *et al.* 1981; Buckle *et al.* 1988; unpublished data), indicating that the additional, misplaced copy of the α-gene complex is expressed even though its genomic position has been altered. Ultimately, it will be of great interest to know exactly where these breakpoints lie with respect to the α-globin genes and how close other breakpoints would have to be to affect their expression.

Variation in the number of globin genes

As a result of unequal genetic exchange, otherwise normal persons may have 4, 5 or 6 α-globin genes (Goossens *et al.* 1980; Higgs *et al.* 1980a; Galanello *et al.* 1983c; Gu *et al.* 1987) and 3, 4, 5 or 6 ζ-like genes (Winichagoon *et al.* 1982; Felice *et al.* 1986; Trent *et al.* 1986a; Titus *et al.* 1988) (see Chapter 4). A surprisingly high frequency of the ααα chromosome (gene frequency ~0.01 to 0.08) is found in most populations that have been studied; the reason is not yet clear, although it is possible that an ααα chromosome offers a selective advantage. Although there appears to be an excess of α mRNA produced from the ααα arrangement (Higgs *et al.* 1980a; Liebhaber & Kan 1981) and excess α globin (Higgs *et al.* 1980a; Sampietro *et al.* 1983; Higgs *et al.* 1984a; Henni *et al.* 1985; Camaschella *et al.* 1987a; Kulozik *et al.* 1987b), homozygotes ($\alpha\alpha\alpha/\alpha\alpha\alpha$) seem to be haematologically normal (Galanello *et al.* 1983c; Trent *et al.* 1985). As we shall see in Chapter 13, however, additional α-globin genes may have important phenotypic effects in those with β thalassaemia.

Several members of a single reported family have a complex rearrangement in which three α-gene clusters are on one copy of chromosome 16 (Fichera *et al.* 1994); provisional data suggest that at least two and possibly all three are fully active. A carrier for this abnormal chromosome ($\alpha\alpha$: $\alpha\alpha$: $\alpha\alpha/\alpha\alpha$) has an α/β-globin synthesis ratio of 2.7. Patients who co-inherit this type of chromosome ($\alpha\alpha$: $\alpha\alpha$: $\alpha\alpha$) with a mild form of β thalassaemia produce sufficient excess α chains to have β thalassaemia intermedia (Fichera *et al.* 1994) (see Chapter 13).

Chromosomes bearing a single ζ gene, $\zeta 2$ rather than the normal $\zeta 2$–$\psi\zeta 1$ arrangement, are relatively common, with a gene frequency of ~0.05 in West Africans (Winichagoon *et al.* 1982; Rappaport *et al.* 1984; Felice *et al.* 1986; Higgs *et al.* 1986; our unpublished data), and occur sporadically in other populations. There is no discernible phenotype associated with the $-\zeta/\zeta\zeta$ genotype (Winichagoon *et al.* 1982; Felice *et al.* 1986; Trent *et al.* 1986a) and, to date, only one homozygote ($-\zeta/-\zeta$) has been identified; there was no haematological abnormality.

The triplicated ζ gene arrangement ($\zeta\zeta\zeta$) has the structure $\zeta 2$–$\psi\zeta 1$–$\psi\zeta 1$ (Hill *et al.* 1985) and was originally identified in south-east Asia, where its frequency is 0.09 to 0.20 (Winichagoon *et al.* 1982; Chan *et al.* 1986a; Higgs *et al.* 1986). It is also particularly common throughout Melanesia, Micronesia and Polynesia, where phenotypically normal homozygotes ($\zeta\zeta\zeta$–$\zeta\zeta\zeta$) have been described (Higgs *et al.* 1986; Trent *et al.* 1986a; Hill *et al.* 1987a). Elsewhere $\zeta\zeta\zeta$ is uncommon. Structural analysis of the $\zeta\zeta\zeta$ arrangement shows that it has arisen by an unusual interchromosomal recombination event (Hill *et al.* 1985, 1987a) between Ia and IId haplotypes (see later section). All of the $\zeta\zeta\zeta$ chromosomes studied from south-east Asia and the Pacific have this unusual structure (Hill *et al.* 1987a), suggesting that they have a common, single origin. Some of these chromosomes appear to have been subsequently modified, as indicated by the presence of a *Bgl* II polymorphism in 8–15% of cases (Hill *et al.* 1987a) and the occasional presence of the Hb Constant Spring mutation on the linked $\alpha 2$ gene (Winichagoon *et al.* 1982) (see Chapters 4 and 11). A very rare example of a chromosome with four ζ genes ($\zeta\zeta\zeta\zeta$) was described by Titus *et al.* (1988).

VNTRs and CA repeats

The different classes of repeat sequences are described in Chapter 4. At least 10 variable-number tandem repeats (VNTRs, also known as hypervariable regions, HVRs) have been identified in and around the α-globin locus (Flint *et al.* 1997). These include the 5' HVR at ~–70kb (Jarman & Higgs 1988), HVRs within the ζ genes (Proudfoot *et al.* 1982), an interzeta HVR (Goodbourn *et al.* 1983) and one at the 3' end of the cluster (Jarman *et al.* 1986). In addition there are a number of dinucleotide CpA repeats around the cluster, including one within the $\psi\alpha 1$ gene (Fougerousse *et al.* 1992). The number of repeats in these arrays may be altered at mitosis or meiosis, producing highly polymorphic segments of the cluster. In the α-gene complex there appears to be no relationship between the structure of such regions and the associated phenotype. Whatever their function, if any, they are of great value as genetic markers throughout the genome and have been used to produce individual-specific genetic fingerprints (Jeffreys 1987; Fowler *et al.* 1988).

Polymorphic base substitutions

A large number of single-base polymorphic sites have been described in the α-globin-gene cluster, often affecting restriction-enzyme sites and hence producing restriction-fragment-length polymorphisms (RFLPs) (Higgs *et al.* 1986). Rather than being associated with each other in a random fashion, groups of polymorphisms are linked together in particular patterns, referred to as 'RFLP haplotypes'. Haplotypes exist because their constituent polymorphic sites are in very strong linkage disequilibrium; in other words, they are so close together that they are rarely disrupted by recombination. For practical purposes, only the most common variants are currently incorporated into haplotypes. In the α complex, for example, 9 sites are used, 7 single-site restriction enzyme polymorphisms and two length variants (Fig. 2.13). Of the possible 768 combinations, only about 70 have been observed in world-wide surveys (reviewed by Flint *et al.* 1998). The practical value of these hap-

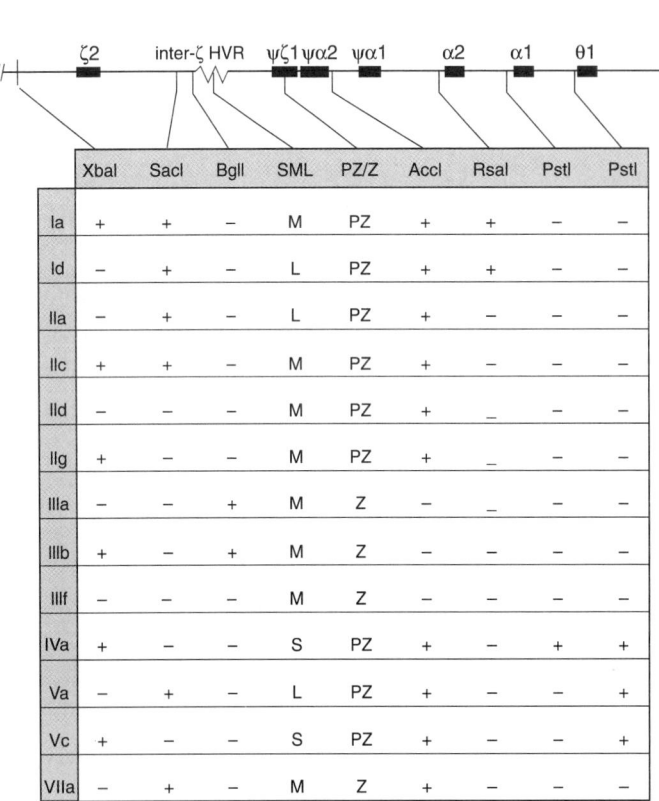

	XbaI	SacI	BglI	SML	PZ/Z	AccI	RsaI	PstI	PstI
Ia	+	+	–	M	PZ	+	+	–	–
Id	–	+	–	L	PZ	+	+	–	–
IIa	–	+	–	L	PZ	+	–	–	–
IIc	+	+	–	M	PZ	+	–	–	–
IId	–	–	–	M	PZ	+	_	–	–
IIg	+	–	–	M	PZ	+	_	–	–
IIIa	–	–	+	M	Z	–	_	–	–
IIIb	+	–	+	M	Z	–	–	–	–
IIIf	–	–	–	M	Z	–	–	–	–
IVa	+	–	–	S	PZ	+	–	+	+
Va	–	+	–	L	PZ	+	–	–	+
Vc	+	–	–	S	PZ	+	–	–	+
VIIa	–	+	–	M	Z	+	–	–	–

Fig. 2.13 The positions of polymorphic restriction-enzyme sites (RFLPs) and hypervariable regions (HVRs) used in the construction of different α-globin haplotypes. Some individuals carry a variant of the ψζ1 gene; the sequence has been corrected by gene conversion and it is designated ζ1. PZ/Z refers to the presence of either the ψζ1 (PZ) or the ζ1 (Z) variants. Three allele sizes of the inter-ζ HVR are included in the haplotype: small (S), medium (M) or large (L). From Higgs *et al.* (1986).

lotypes in population genetics and prenatal diagnosis is described in Chapters 6 and 14.

DNA sequence analysis has also revealed six minor variants of the HS –40 regulatory element (Harteveld 1998). Again, these polymorphic variants are found in normal people and provide informative examples of *in vivo* mutagenesis, which makes it possible to relate the structure of this important regulatory region to its function.

Gene conversions

The DNA strand exchanges involved in misaligned but reciprocal recombination mentioned earlier may also resolve with non-reciprocal genetic exchange, a mechanism which is known as gene conversion (Strachan & Read 1996). During this process genetic information may be exchanged between allelic or non-allelic homologous sequences without any crossovers or chromosomal rearrangements. Gene conversion between both the α1/α2 pair and the ζ2/ψζ1 pair may occur quite frequently. Sequence analysis suggests that it has occurred between the α1 and α2 (Michelson & Orkin 1983) and ζ2 and ψζ1 genes (Proudfoot *et al.* 1982; Hill *et al.* 1985) throughout evolution. A probable example of a conversion between the α2 and α1 genes has been documented in persons expressing an unexpectedly high level of HbI, an α-chain variant ($\alpha^{16Lys \rightarrow Glu}$), in whom the same mutation is present on both α2 and α1 genes in *cis* (Liebhaber *et al.* 1984). Other possible examples of non-reciprocal exchange were described by Molchanova *et al.* (1994a), who observed identical sequence mutations affecting the α1 and α2 genes on independent chromosomes; one possibility is that they arose by conversion from one gene to another.

Analysis of the downstream ζ-like gene in several populations has shown that its exists in two distinct forms (Hill *et al.* 1985). In one, its structure is clearly that of a pseudogene (ψζ1), and in the other (ζ1) the ψζ1 gene has undergone a gene conversion by the ζ2 gene such that it becomes more similar to the functional ζ gene, although it still appears not to be expressed *in vivo*. The frequency of the ζ2–ζ1 chromosome varies from one population to another (0.14 to 0.57), and phenotypically normal persons homozygous for either ζ2–ψζ1 or ζ2–ζ1 chromosomes have been observed (Hill *et al.* 1985). Conversions of the ζ2 gene by ψζ1 have not yet been described, although several candidate chromosomes have been identified.

In addition to these examples of gene conversion, it seems likely that, as occurs in other mammalian multigene families (Collier *et al.* 1993; Flint *et al.* 1998), short segmental conversions may also be responsible for transferring thalassaemic and non-thalassaemic variants within and between different chromosomal backgrounds.

Deletions and insertions

Two uncommon deletions involving the θ1 gene remove either 1.8 kb or 6.0 kb from between the intact α1 gene and the α-globin 3′ HVR (Fei *et al.* 1988a) (Fig. 2.12). Neither variant is associated with any phenotypic abnormalities in the neonatal period, and an adult heterozygous for the 1.8-kb deletion also appears to be normal. The individual with the 6.0 kb deletion also had a –ζ chromosome (Fei *et al.* 1988a). We have also studied a person who apparently has the same 6.0-kb deletion and in this case the –ζ arrangement is present in *cis* to the θ1 gene deletion (Higgs *et al.* 1989). Similarly, Ballas *et al.* (1989a) found that both of these rearrangements may exist on the same chromosome. Thus these individuals have

deletions at both the 5′ (10 kb) and 3′ (6 kb) ends of the cluster, with no discernible effect on α-gene expression. Finally, in a large survey of newborn babies (Fei *et al.* 1989a), a small (2.5 kb) deletion between the ζ and ψζ genes was observed in two haematologically normal babies from Sardinia (see Fig. 2.12).

Phenotypically 'silent' insertions also occur in the α-gene complex. An insertion of 0.5 to 0.7 kb between the α2 and α1 genes was identified in the non-thalassaemic chromosome of a Chinese individual (Nakatsuji *et al.* 1986). Most probably this arose from a reciprocal crossover between a normal chromosome (αα) and the common α-thalassaemia determinant (–α³·⁷, see below). In addition we have observed an insertion/deletion polymorphism in the 5′-flanking region of the α complex that appears to involve members of the *Alu* family of repeats (Higgs *et al.* 1989).

The β-globin gene cluster

The β-globin gene cluster (Fig. 2.14) is on the short arm of chromosome 11, band 11p15.4. The two fetal γ genes lie 15 and 20 kb downstream from the embryonic ε gene, while the δ and β genes are 35 and 43 kb further downstream. Upstream of the ε gene, lies the locus-control region (LCR), the regulatory region that is essential for expression of all the genes in the complex. It spans ~15 kb and contains four elements (HS1 to HS4) which are marked by erythroid-cell-specific DNase1-hypersensitive sites. There are two other hypersensitive sites, one 5′ to the LCR and one ~20 kb 3′ to the β-globin gene. It has been suggested that they mark the boundaries of a β-globin gene domain. The β-gene clusters of man and mouse (and possibly chicken) are embedded in an array of olfac-

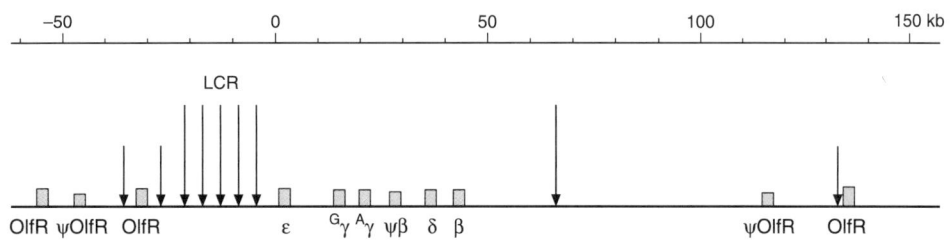

Fig. 2.14 The β-globin gene cluster. The cluster is set among several genes for olfactory receptors (OlfR). The arrows indicate DNase-sensitive sites. LCR = locus-control region.

tory receptor genes (Bulger *et al.* 1999). This is a large family of ~1000 genes, widely distributed throughout the genome and expressed in the olfactory epithelium. Two olfactory receptor genes and a pseudogene lie 10–35 kb upstream of the human β LCR, while 3' of the cluster there are at least another two genes found close to breakpoints of HPFH 1 and HPFH 6 (see Chapter 4).

General structure

The entire β-globin complex has been sequenced. Microsatellite repeats of $(CA)_n$, where n is usually 17 dinucleotides, are found within the cluster, while there is an $(ATTTT)_n$ repeat between the δ and β genes. Both *Alu* and L1 families of repeat DNA sequences (see Chapter 4) are found within and around the cluster. Inverted pairs of *Alu* repeats occur 5' to the ε gene and on either side of the γ-gene pair; similar pairs also occur upstream of the δ gene and downstream from the β-globin gene. There are two long stretches, each 6 kb, of L1 repeat sequences, one between the ε and the $^{G}\gamma$ gene and the other downstream from the β gene. Their role is not known.

Structural variation

Chromosomal translocations

Translocations involving the short arm of chromosome 11 are relatively common, but there have been few reports of any effect on β-globin production. A complex balanced translocation involving a breakpoint on chromosome 11 close to the β locus was observed in a mother and daughter with increased HbF levels of 5 and 8% (Jensen *et al.* 1984). As the mother's parents were karyotypically and haematologically normal, it is possible that the altered chromosomal structure may have resulted in abnormal regulation of the cluster. A second example, in which the end of the short arm of chromosome 11, including the β-gene locus, was translocated close to the centromere of chromosome 22, was also associated with a stable red-cell dimorphism in which a small proportion of the cells were hypochromic and microcytic (Rees *et al.* 1994). It was suggested that the centromeric sequences may have caused position-effect variegation on the expression of the β cluster, resulting in its suppression in a small number of cells.

Variation in the number of globin genes

As within the α-gene cluster, variations are frequently observed in the structure of the β-gene complex, most often involving the γ genes. Unequal crossing over has resulted in chromosomes with one, three, four or five γ genes rather than the normal $^{G}\gamma^{A}\gamma$ arrangement. Loss of one gene ($-^{A}\gamma$) occurs with a low incidence world-wide and has little effect other than lowering the $^{G}\gamma^{A}\gamma$ ratio of HbF in newborn infants (Trent *et al.* 1981; Huisman *et al.* 1991). Lower haemoglobin levels and a reduced proportion of HbF are found at birth in homozygotes for a γ-gene deletion (Huisman *et al.* 1983).

Triplicated γ genes are widespread, and four different types have been identified, all of the general structure $^{G}\gamma^{G}\gamma^{A}\gamma$. They differ depending on the position of the crossover point and on the presence or absence of an *Xmn* I site –158 to the $^{G}\gamma$ gene (Liu *et al.* 1988). Adults who are *Xmn* I positive on both chromosomes have slightly raised levels of HbF and a very high proportion of $^{G}\gamma$ chains. Quadruplicated γ genes have been reported in Japanese, Turkish and Sri Lankan populations, and one individual with five γ genes on a chromosome was described in an Afro-American (Fei *et al.* 1989a). Adults with additional γ genes are haematologically normal, demonstrating that the insertion of up to an extra 15 kb of DNA between the LCR and the β-globin gene does not appreciably alter the regulation of the cluster. The genes are arranged $^{G}\gamma^{G}\gamma^{G}\gamma^{A}\gamma$ and $^{G}\gamma^{G}\gamma^{G}\gamma^{G}\gamma^{A}\gamma$ and, depending on where the crossover occurred, the inner genes are different $^{A}\gamma^{G}\gamma$ hybrids. Just as in the normal $^{G}\gamma^{A}\gamma$ arrangement, the 5' gene is preferentially transcribed, so in chromosomes with additional γ genes there is polarity of expression, production decreasing from the 5' to the 3' gene.

The quadruplicated γ-gene arrangement has also been found in *cis* to a β^{0}-thalassaemia allele. Interestingly, a homozygote for this condition, i.e. homozygous β thalassaemia with eight γ-globin genes, was only mildly affected and maintained a haemoglobin level of over 10 g/dl after splenectomy (Yang *et al.* 1986). This suggests that the additional γ genes can result in a higher production of γ chains in adults than the normal two-gene arrangement, even in the presence of a normal promoter on the β gene.

Unequal crossing over can also occur between the γ and β genes and the δ and β genes. This leads to the production of the fusion variants Hb Kenya and anti-

Kenya and Hb Lepore and anti-Lepore, respectively. These haemoglobins are described, together with their clinical and haematological associations, in Chapters 9–10.

Gene conversions

Gene conversions between the two γ genes occur quite frequently, and are probably responsible for the overall similarity in their structure (Slightom *et al.* 1980; Shen *et al.* 1981; Metzenberg *et al.* 1991). Analyses of cord-blood samples from many populations have identified a small proportion of babies with unusually low (0.4–0.5) or unusually high (>0.8) ${}^{G}\gamma^{A}\gamma$ ratios, which reflect gene conversions that have generated ${}^{A}\gamma^{A}\gamma$ or ${}^{G}\gamma^{G}\gamma$ gene arrangements (Powers *et al.* 1984).

Polymorphic base substitutions

There are numerous polymorphic base substitutions within the β-globin-gene cluster. As with the α-gene cluster, many of them produce RFLPs which are combined in a limited number of haplotypes (Fig. 2.15) that are in linkage disequilibrium with β-globin-gene mutations (Antonarakis *et al.* 1982).

Haplotype analysis provides information on the chromosomal background on which the β-thalassaemia mutations have occurred (Orkin *et al.* 1982a) and was of considerable value for their identification and prenatal diagnosis before it became possible to identify them directly. In addition, identical thalassaemic mutations on different haplotypes may be associated with small differences in clinical phenotype, indicating that modifying sequence elements, probably factors that affect HbF production, may also be in linkage disequilibrium with the β-globin gene (see later section and Chapter 10).

Based on haplotype analysis, it became apparent that non-random association of polymorphic restriction sites in the β-gene cluster occurs within two regions, a 5′ segment from the ε gene to the 5′ end of the δ gene, and a 3′ segment extending 19 kb in a 3′ direction from the 5′ end of the β gene. Between the 5′ and 3′ clusters there is a 9-kb region that displays random association with either segment and is therefore thought to be a recombination 'hot spot' (Chakravarti *et al.* 1984; Flint *et al.* 1998) (Fig. 2.15b). To date, five families showing recombination within this region have been observed (Gerhard *et al.* 1984; Old *et al.* 1986b; Camaschella *et al.* 1988; Hall *et al.* 1993a; Smith *et al.* 1998).

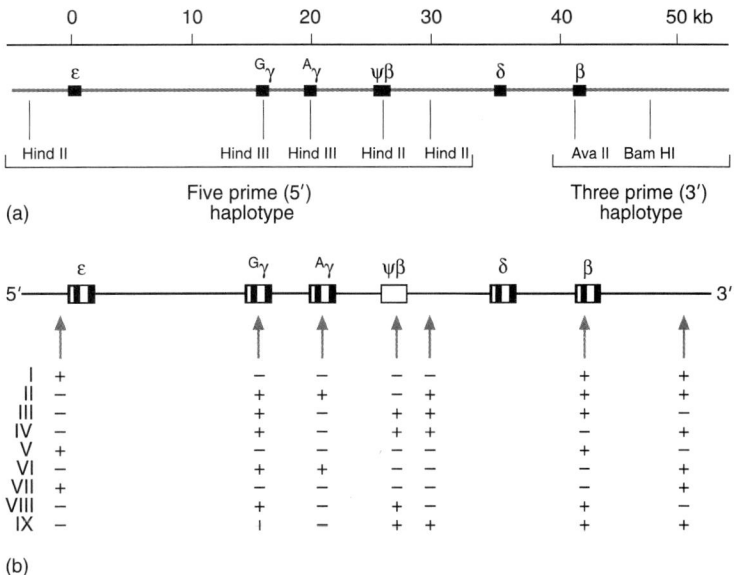

Fig. 2.15 The restriction-fragment-length polymorphisms and haplotypes of the β-globin gene cluster. (a) The organization of the common haplotypes. An increased rate of recombination in the region between the δ- and β-globin genes has led to the subdivision of the full haplotype into 5′ and 3′ subhaplotypes. (b) Some of the common haplotypes of the β-globin gene cluster.

Globin-gene structure, function and regulation

General structure

The structure of globin genes has been highly conserved throughout evolution. Their transcribed regions are contained in three exons, separated by two introns, or intervening sequences (IVS), of variable length (Fig. 2.16). From the CAP site, the start of transcription, the first exon encompasses ~50 bp of 5′ untranslated sequence (UTR) and the codons for amino acids 1–31 in the α- and 1–29 together with the first two bases of codon 30 in the β-globin genes. Exon 2 encodes amino acids 32–99 and 31–104, respectively, the portion of the globin polypeptide that is involved in haem binding and the $\alpha_1\beta_2$ ($\alpha_2\beta_1$) contacts. The third exon encodes the remaining amino acids, 100–141 for α, 105–146 for β, together with a 3′ untranslated region of ~100 bp (Fig. 2.16). In the α-globin genes both introns are small, 117–149 bp, while in the ζ gene IVS1 is ~886 and IVS2 is ~239 bp. The IVS1 intron varies in length from one allele to another, as a result of differences in the number of copies of a 14-bp tandem-repeat sequence. The first intervening sequence in the β-like genes is also small, 122–130 bp, while IVS2 is much larger, 850–904 bp.

The removal of the intervening sequences from the initial transcript and joining the exon sequence to form mRNA is dependent on sequences at the border between the exons and introns. A survey of a large number of eukaryotic genes has demonstrated consensus sequences in these regions. At the 5′ end of each intron the consensus is ^C_AAG/**GT**^A_GAGT, where the oblique line denotes the excision site immediately preceding the invariant GT residues, shown in bold. At the 3′ end, there is a rather looser consensus (^C_T)N ^C_T**AG**/G, in which an invariant AG dinucleotide precedes the excision site. Among the globin genes, there is strong adherence to these consensus sequences (Table 2.5) and in all cases GT and AG dinucleotides are maintained. As mutations in these sequences frequently lead to thalassaemia (see Chapter 4), the globin genes provide excellent examples of their functional importance.

The processing of globin mRNA involves the addition of a poly(A) tract of 75 to a few hundred residues at the 3′ end of the mRNA. This poly(A) tail is involved in stability of the mRNA. A poly(A) additional signal, AAUAAA, is conserved in the 3′ untranslated region of the RNA, approximately 10-30 nucleotides upstream of where the initial transcript is cut and the poly(A) tract is added. This signal sequence is found in all of the transcribed human

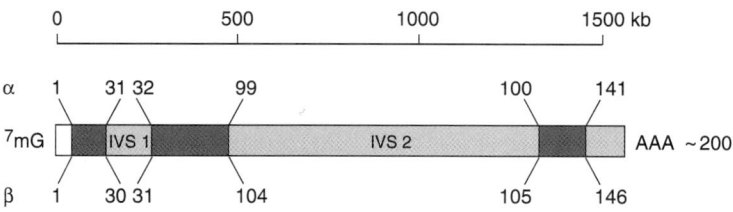

Fig. 2.16 A schematic representation of the α- and β-globin genes showing the position and size of the introns (IVS1 and IVS2). ^{7}mG represents the site of modification by the CAP structure, and AAA indicates the poly(A) addition site.

Table 2.5 Consensus sequences at the donor and acceptor splice sites in the human globin genes.

Gene	5′ UTR region (nts)	Donor splice site	IVS1 (nts)	Acceptor splice site	Donor splice site	IVS2 (nts)	Acceptor splice site	3′ UTR region (nts)	Poly(A) signal
ζ	58	GAG'**GT**GAGT	866–	CCAG'G	AAG'**GT**GCGC	239–	CCA**G**'C	108	AATAAA
α2	40	GAG'**GT**GAGG	117	GCAG'G	AAG'**GT**GAGC	142	ACA**G**'C	113	AATAAA
α1	40	GAG'**GT**GAGG	117	GCAG'G	AAG'**GT**GAGC	149	ACA**G**'C	113	AATAAA
ε	53	CAG'**GT**AAGC	122	TTTCAT**AG**'ACT	AAG'**GT**GAGT	855	CCTAACA**G**'CTC	99	AATAAA
$^G\gamma$	53	AAG'**GT**AGGC	121	TCTCAC**AG**'ACT	AAG'**GT**GAGT	886–904	CTCAACA**G**'CTC	66	AATAAA
$^A\gamma$	53	AAG'**GT**AGGC	121	TCTCAC**AG**'ACT	AAG'**GT**GAGT	866–876	CTCAACA**G**'CTC	66	AATAA
δ	48	CAG'**GT**TGGT	138	ACCCTCA**G**'ATT	AGG'**GT**GAGT	898	CTCCGCA**G**'CTC	111	AATAAA
β	50	CAG'**GT**TGGT	130	ACCCTT**AG**'GCT	ACG'**GT**GAGT	850	TCCCACA**G**'CTC	113	AATAAA

globin genes except θ, where the sequence is AGUAAA.

These general features of the α- and β-globin genes are shared by the other genes of the α- and β-globin-gene clusters. Such differences as there are are summarized in Table 2.5. Both sequence analysis and hybridization studies have shown that, despite the homology of their coding sequences, the sequences of the different introns have diverged considerably and share very little homology except for the duplicated $^G\gamma$- and $^A\gamma$-globin genes. There has been considerably more conservation of a sequence of IVS1 between some though not all of the non-α-globin genes; there is undoubted homology between IVS1 sequences for the β and δ, γ and ε, and β and ε gene-pair comparisons, but not in the case of the β/γ genes. In the α-globin genes there has been considerable conservation of the sequences of IVS1 and IVS2 between α2 and α1 and the ψα genes, but there is little homology between the intron sequences of these genes and those of the ζ and ψζ genes.

The regulation of globin-gene function

The expression of globin genes and their regulation seem to depend on the interactions of a variety of different *trans*-acting regulatory proteins with specific sequences both adjacent to and at a distance from particular genes. The critical regulatory sequences for the globin genes include their promoters, a series of enhancer elements and a 'master' regulatory region which is involved in regulating the entire α- or β-globin gene complex. Although we have learnt a great deal about the different interactions of these sequences with both erythroid-specific and more generally active regulatory proteins, many of the details of how these complex interactions underlie the control of the globin-gene clusters remain to be worked out.

Promoters

Transcription of genes is dependent on the attachment of a transcription complex, including RNA polymerase, at their 5' ends. Correct positioning of the transcription machinery is brought about by recognition of specific DNA sequences in the region upstream of the transcriptional start site known as the promoter. In many tissue-specific genes, including all the globin genes, TATA and CCAAT homology boxes are found 30 and 70 bp upstream of the mRNA CAP site (Fig. 2.17) and are critical for the correct siting of initiation and a high level of transcription (Anagnou *et al.* 1985; Myers *et al.* 1986; de Boer *et al.* 1988; Antoniou & Grosveld 1990). The CCAAT site is duplicated in the two γ-globin genes and both sites are necessary for maximum rates of initiation. The modification of the CCAAT sequence to CCAAC may be partially responsible for the low level of transcription of the δ-globin gene (see Chapter 8).

In addition to these two homology boxes, many erythroid-specific genes have a CACCC box in the

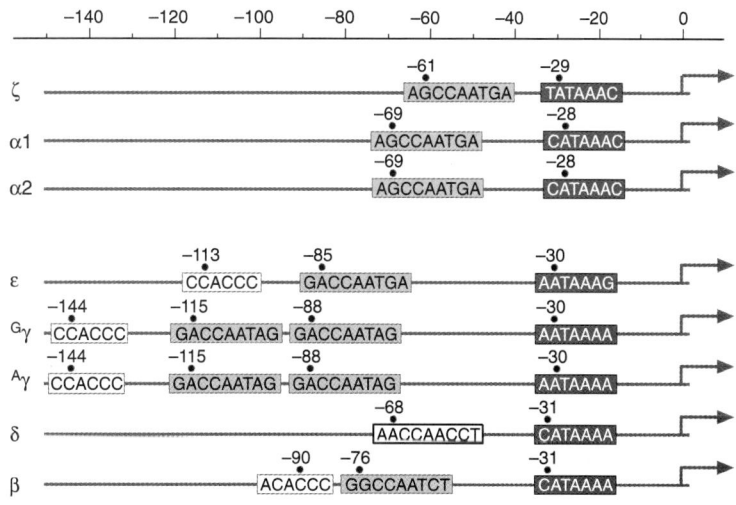

Fig. 2.17 The human globin-gene promoters.

promoter, upstream of the CCAAT box. CACCC-box homologies are found in most of the β-globin promoters and are duplicated in the β gene itself but are not found in the α-globin promoters. The sequence is also missing from the promoter of the δ gene; insertion of the β-gene CACCC box considerably upregulates its expression (Donze *et al.* 1996). Some naturally occurring mutations in the human β-gene promoter have confirmed the importance of the TATA and CACCC sequences for globin-gene expression (see Chapter 4).

Additional sequence motifs are commonly found in the more distal regions of the promoters of these genes, including binding sites for the erythroid transcription factors GATA-1 and NF-E2 and sites for the ubiquitous factors YY1, Sp1 and Oct-1 (see later section). Their precise role is not fully understood but it is believed that the combination of multiple factors is necessary for maximum rates of transcription.

Enhancers

In addition to the promoter sequences at the 5′ end of genes, more distal sequences are frequently found to increase the levels of gene transcription in experimental expression systems. These 'enhancers' may lie 5′ or 3′ to the gene or within the gene itself. They are detected by transient transfection studies in which DNA constructs are transferred into appropriate cell types by electroporation, calcium phosphate precipitation or lipofection, that is, packaged in fatty envelopes. The DNA fragments remain as episomal structures in the nucleus and the rate of transcription can be monitored. Analyses of the α- and β-globin complexes have revealed regions with typical enhancer activity, as defined in this way. These include the regulatory region of the α cluster (HS −40) and one of the elements of the β LCR (HS2) but not the other elements.

A small region (800 bp) lying 3′ of the $^A\gamma$ gene (Bodine & Ley 1987; Purucker *et al.* 1990; Balta *et al.* 1994) and two segments around the β-globin gene, one in the large intervening sequence and one 3′ to the gene (Behringer *et al.* 1987; Kollias *et al.* 1987; Trudel & Costantini 1987; Antoniou *et al.* 1988; Wall *et al.* 1988), have enhancer properties. Loss of the $^A\gamma$ enhancer from the human cluster has no effect on the level or developmental regulation of the genes in transgenic mice (Liu *et al.* 1998) while deletion of the

enhancer 3′ to β significantly reduces expression of the β gene in this system (Liu *et al.* 1997). Additional enhancer sequences have been identified 30 and 100 kb 3′ to the β cluster, immediately beyond the 3′ breakpoints of deletions which cause hereditary persistence of fetal haemoglobin (Feingold & Forget 1989; Anagnou *et al.* 1995) (see Chapters 4 and 10). It has been suggested that these sequences may play a role in the increased γ-gene expression in this condition.

Major regulatory elements

After cloning the human globin genes, experimental systems were developed to study the control of gene expression, including both transient and stable transfection of erythroid cell lines and transgenic mice. When individual human globin genes were stably transfected into cell lines, mouse erythroleukaemia (MEL) lines for example, expression was detectable but the levels were low and variable from clone to clone. Similarly, in transgenic mice the expression of the human β gene was only detectable in some lines, was not always erythroid-specific and, even in the highest expressing lines, did not approach the levels of the endogenous globin genes. No α-globin gene expression could be detected in any of the transgenic lines generated.

It is now clear that the reason for this low and inconsistent expression was the lack of major regulatory elements in the DNA that was transferred in these experiments. The identification of a series of erythroid-specific DNase1-hypersensitive sites in the region upstream of the β-globin genes (Tuan *et al.* 1985; Forrester *et al.* 1987) suggested that this area might be of regulatory importance, a notion that was given further weight by the identification of forms of thalassaemia in which this region was deleted (Orkin *et al.* 1981b; Taramelli *et al.* 1986; Driscoll *et al.* 1989). Its importance was demonstrated conclusively when Grosveld *et al.* (1987) produced transgenic mice which contained this region attached to a β-globin gene. The mice not only exhibited erythroid-specific, copy-number-dependent β-globin gene expression in lines containing the transgene but the levels of expression were very high, more or less equivalent to the endogenous levels of RNA. These results were rapidly confirmed by others (Enver *et al.* 1989; Forrester *et al.* 1989; Ryan *et al.* 1989) and the upstream sequences, originally termed the dominant control region or locus-activating region, were renamed the β-globin locus control region, or β LCR.

Within the α-globin cluster, a major regulatory element, termed HS –40, has also been identified, 40 kb upstream of the ζ-globin gene (Higgs *et al.* 1990). Several deletions of this region, which spare the α-globin genes, all result in α thalassaemia with minimal output of α globin from the affected chromosome (Hatton *et al.* 1990; Liebhaber *et al.* 1990; Wilkie *et al.* 1990b) (see Chapter 4). Attachment of the HS –40 element to an α-globin gene results in high-level expression of the gene in transgenic mice, although copy-number dependence is not observed and expression frequently declines during development (Sharpe *et al.* 1992, 1993; Gourdon *et al.* 1994).

The β-globin locus control region

Five DNase-hypersensitive sites have been identified upstream of the β-globin genes (Fig. 2.14). The most 5′ site (HS5) does not show tissue specificity, while HSs1–4, which together form the LCR, are largely erythroid-specific, although HS2 has been observed in several non-erythroid cell lines and HS4 has been found in an embryonic carcinoma cell line (Dhar *et al.* 1990). Maximum expression of a linked β-globin gene is obtained when the whole LCR is present intact, but if each site is excised as a 1–3-kb fragment and joined together as a mini- or micro-LCR, high levels of expression are still obtained (Forrester *et al.* 1989; Talbot *et al.* 1989; Collis *et al.* 1990). When each of the four HSs is assayed individually for their ability to direct β-globin gene expression, the major activity is found in sites 2 (Curtin *et al.* 1989; Ryan *et al.* 1989; Fraser *et al.* 1990; Talbot *et al.* 1990; Caterina *et al.* 1991), 3 (Fraser *et al.* 1990; Philipsen *et al.* 1990, 1993) and 4 (Fraser *et al.* 1990; Pruzina *et al.* 1991), each of

which expressed at 15–40% of the activity of the whole LCR; levels of expression directed by HS1 are less than 5% (Forrester *et al.* 1989; Collis *et al.* 1990; Fraser *et al.* 1990). Similar results are obtained when individual sites are deleted from the mouse LCR in its normal chromosomal environment, with reductions in globin-gene expression of 10–30% (Fiering *et al.* 1995; Hug *et al.* 1996).

Structure. The major activity of each of the HS elements lies in a core region of 200–400 bp. Sequence analysis shows multiple binding sites for erythroid or ubiquitous transcription factors in each of the cores (Fig. 2.18). The HS2 element contains duplicated sites for the erythroid transcription factors NF-E2 and GATA-1 as well as sites for the ubiquitous factors USF and YY1, together with a G-rich site, which may bind Sp1 or a related factor. Deletion of each of these sites individually does not prevent position-independent expression but reduces the level of expression, particularly when the NF-E2 sites are affected (Ney *et al.* 1990a,b; Talbot *et al.* 1990; Caterina *et al.* 1991; Talbot & Grosveld 1991; Liu *et al.* 1992; Caterina *et al.* 1994). It appears therefore that multiple combinations of binding sites can confer position-independent expression and that a combination of sites is necessary for maximum expression.

HS3 consists of duplicated units of GATA-1 sites flanking G-rich sites (Philipsen *et al.* 1990, 1993) (Fig. 2.18); EKLF appears to be the important factor that binds to the G-rich region (Gillemans *et al.* 1998). Unlike HS2, a single copy of HS3 can activate a linked globin gene, suggesting that this element contains a dominant chromatin-opening function (Ellis *et al.* 1996).

HS4 contains binding sites for the erythroid factors GATA-1 and NF-E2 and, in addition, binds a number

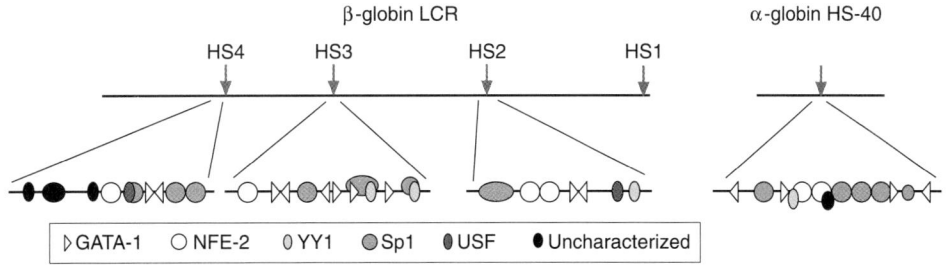

Fig. 2.18 The structures of the β-globin gene cluster locus control region (LCR) and the α-globin gene cluster HS-40.

of ubiquitous proteins, Sp1, J-BP and the CACC box binding protein TEF-2 (Pruzina *et al.* 1991; Lowrey *et al.* 1992). Again, it appears that the GATA-1 and NF-E2 sites are essential for the functioning of this element (Stamatoyannopoulos *et al.* 1995).

Function. The LCR could function by providing an entry site for RNA polymerase, which would then track along the cluster until the appropriate gene promoter was reached, when transcription would begin (Tuan *et al.* 1992). Alternatively, it might simply keep the genes in an open chromatin conformation (Forrester *et al.* 1990), transcription being determined by localized factors at the relevant promoters (Martin *et al.* 1996). In contrast to these indirect mechanisms, a more widely favoured model suggests that the LCR loops round and physically interacts with the promoter through DNA binding proteins at each site or bridging proteins (Choi & Engel 1988; Dillon & Grosveld 1993; Engel 1993). These interactions could occur between the promoter and individual LCR elements or, alternatively, the four HS elements might combine into a single holocomplex which contacts the promoter (Fraser *et al.* 1993; Wijgerde *et al.* 1995). As yet there is no direct evidence to support direct interaction between the LCR and the promoter.

Analysis of globin-gene transcription in transgenic mouse erythroid cells at the time of switching from γ- to β-gene transcription using labelled oligonucleotides to the primary transcripts has suggested that, on each chromosome, only one gene is transcribed at a time (Wijgerde *et al.* 1995; Milot *et al.* 1996; Gribnau *et al.* 1998; Trimborn *et al.* 1999). This appears to preclude the possibility that different HS elements can interact with separate promoters in synchrony and is more compatible with the notion that the elements combine to form a holocomplex.

Clearly, the precise mechanism of action of the LCR remains to be determined. A critical review of the possibilities, based on the results of studies which suggest that it might not be required for the activation of the murine β-globin locus (Epner *et al.* 1998; Reik *et al.* 1998), raises the question as to whether it may have different functions in mouse and man (Bulger & Groudine 1999; Grosveld 1999).

The α-globin major regulatory element, HS –40

Mapping of DNase1-hypersensitive sites around the α-globin genes identified erythroid-specific sites at the globin-gene promoters, as well as five sites in the upstream region at –4, –8, –10, –33 and –40 kb relative to the ζ-globin gene. Testing of each of these sites for their ability to enhance α-globin gene transcription in MEL cells or transgenic mice showed that only the element at HS –40 is active (Higgs *et al.* 1990). This site coincides with the region of overlap of several naturally occurring deletions which remove parts of the upstream region and inactivate the remaining globin genes (see Chapter 4). These observations suggest that the major regulatory element of the α-globin cluster is HS –40. However, whether this is the only regulatory element is as yet unclear. In transgenic mice bearing DNA fragments containing the human HS –40 element together with an α-globin gene, levels of expression are not copy-number dependent, do not reach the levels of the endogenous α-globin genes and do not remain developmentally stable (Sharpe *et al.* 1992, 1993; Gourdon *et al.* 1994). By these criteria therefore HS –40 is not equivalent to the β LCR, suggesting that additional α-globin regulatory elements may still remain to be found; since fragments containing 150 kb of the α-globin cluster do not show complete regulation, they must be a considerable distance from the gene themselves.

Structure and function. The structure of HS–40 closely resembles HS2 of the β LCR (Jarman et al. 1991). A 350-bp core fragment retains most of the activity and contains a duplicated NF-E2 binding site flanked by GATA-1 sites, as well as several CACCC motifs and a YY1 binding site (Fig. 2.18). This structure is largely conserved in the mouse (Gourdon et al. 1995).

The mechanism by which HS –40 activates the α-globin gene is not known. The chromatin structure of the whole region from the telomere to downstream of the α-globin cluster is in an open conformation in all tissues. The genes in the upstream region are widely transcribed, including a gene which contains HS –40 within one of its introns (Vyas *et al.* 1995). It is unnecessary therefore for there to be a major change in chromatin structure, as must occur with the β-globin cluster, in order to activate the α-globin genes in their normal chromosomal environment. Indeed, no differences have been observed in chromatin structure in the α-globin region between a normal chromosome 16 and one lacking HS –40 in an erythroid cell (Craddock *et al.* 1995). Nevertheless, HS –40 must contain some chromatin-opening function since all transfected MEL cells and transgenic mice express the α-globin gene when, and only when, HS −40 is present. There is no evidence as to whether HS −40 interacts with the globin-gene promoters.

Transcription

Transcription of the globin genes requires the formation of a transcription complex on the promoter region of the gene. This is a multiprotein complex which includes the enzyme RNA polymerase II (pol II), which transcribes DNA into an mRNA copy. Details of how this is brought about are rather sketchy at present and the early events may well differ between the α- and β-globin gene complexes. The α-globin genes lie in a region of open chromatin, surrounded by housekeeping genes that are transcribed in all tissues. The chromatin structure of this whole region is in an open conformation in all tissues and thus does not require any prior unpacking from the type of highly condensed structure that the β cluster adopts in non-erythroid cells. The stage in haemopoietic/erythroid cell differentiation at which the β-globin gene cluster becomes decondensed is not known for certain but is likely to be early, possibly before erythroid commitment (Jimenez *et al.* 1992). It is clear that the LCR is involved in this process since, when it is deleted, the whole cluster remains tightly repressed in erythroid cells over a distance of more than 150 kb (Forrester *et al.* 1990). Decondensation is associated with the appearance of DNase1-hypersensitive sites in the β LCR, which are believed to involve the displacement of one or more nucleosomes and the attachment of various *trans*-acting factors. Hypersensitive sites at the promoter may not be present at this initial stage but they appear at the time the gene is actually transcribed.

The complex interplay between networks of transcription factors and the mechanisms of chromatin modification that underlie eukaryotic transcription is reviewed in detail by Kadonaga (1998).

Basal transcription machinery

Once an open chromatin structure is produced, and in the presence of the appropriate erythroid transcription factors, transcription can proceed. The mechanism of transcription is under investigation by both biochemical and genetic approaches using a variety of organisms, particularly yeast. As this process is well conserved in eukaryotes, many of the findings are likely to apply to higher organisms although the precise details may differ. The basal transcription apparatus (see Buratowski 1994) recognizes the core promoter and consists of RNA polymerase II, TATA binding protein (TBP) and the general transcription factors TFIIB, TFIIE, TFIIF and TFIIH. TBP binds the TATA box, TFIIH contains a helicase for separation of the DNA strands and a kinase to phosphorylate the C-terminal tail of pol II, while TFIIB forms a bridge between TBP and pol II to correctly position the start site of transcription. RNA pol II itself consists of 12 well conserved subunits. TBP is also multipart, consisting of TFIID and eight or more TBP-associated factors (TAFs), many of which have been characterized.

It is not yet clear whether these complexes are put together in a stepwise fashion, as originally suggested by biochemical assays of *in vitro* transcription, or whether within the cells there is a relatively stable holocomplex in which many of these factors remain bound. There is also uncertainty about whether such a complex is bound to the nuclear matrix or whether it is free to diffuse within the nucleus.

In addition to this preinitiation complex, tissue-specific and gene-specific activator proteins bind to upstream promoter elements and flanking enhancer sequences, and interface with the transcription complex. This interaction appears to be via the TAFs during transcription in *Drosophila*, while in yeast it occurs through a 'mediator' complex consisting of an alternative set of proteins known as SRB (or SSNs). The precise details remain to be determined and as yet little or nothing is known about the interactions responsible for globin-gene transcription.

Once transcription is initiated, the preinitiation complex is dissociated. TBP and, possibly, associated TAFs remain associated with the promoter and may provide the basis for the next round of initiation, while the other factors may be released individually or as a subcomplex. It is likely that additional factors may be required for elongation as the polymerase transcribes the DNA at a rate of ~2 kb per minute (Bentley 1995). Transcripts terminate downstream of the gene, not at a defined point but in a heterogeneous array, possibly as a concomitant of processing of the 3′ end of the nascent transcript.

Erythroid-specific transcription factors

Current knowledge about the transcription factors that are involved in erythropoiesis and the regulation

Table 2.6 Some transcription factors involved in the regulation of erythropoiesis and globin synthesis.

GATA-1	Binds to (A/T)GATA(A/G) sequence elements Contains two zinc fingers (N and C)
FOG	'Friend of GATA–1' Multi-zinc-finger protein Interacts with GATA-1 to enhance transcription
NF-E2	Nuclear factor erythroid 2 B ZIP transcription factor Heterodimer: subunits p45 and p18 Binds to (T/C)TGCTGA(C/G)TCA(T/C)
EKLF	Erythroid Krüppel-like factor Zinc-finger transcription factor Binds to CCACACC element
SSP	Stage-selector protein A protein complex that binds to γ-gene promoter

of haemoglobin synthesis has been reviewed extensively (Orkin 1996; Orkin & Zon 1997; Orkin 1998).

In addition to the basic transcription machinery both the major regulatory regions, β LCR and α HS −40, and the globin-gene promoters contain sequence motifs for various ubiquitous and erythroid-restricted transcription factors (Table 2.6). Binding of the various factors to these sequences has mainly been demonstrated by *in vitro* 'footprinting' and electrophoretic mobility-shift assays. In these studies, nuclear proteins are extracted from erythroid or non-erythroid cells and allowed to interact with oligonucleotide fragments containing the sites of interest. The interactions are monitored by the ability of the bound proteins to protect the sites from digestion by DNase1 or by the altered mobility of the bound fragment after polyacrylamide gel electrophoresis. Many of these *in vitro* observations have been confirmed by '*in vivo* footprinting' in which the protection of sequences in the region of interest against DNase1 or restriction-enzyme cleavage is assayed in intact nuclei.

Binding sites for transcription factors have been identified in each of the globin-gene promoters and at the hypersensitive-site regions of the various regulatory elements. A number of the factors which bind in these areas are found in all cell types. They include Sp1, YY1 and USF. In contrast, transcription factors such as GATA-1, EKLF and NF-E2 are restricted in

their distribution, which may, in addition to erythroid cells, include megakaryocytes and mast cells. The overlapping of erythroid-specific and ubiquitous-factor binding sites in several cases suggests that competitive binding may play an important part in the regulation of erythroid-specific genes. The balance of competition could be affected by either quantitative changes in the various factors or post-translational modifications.

GATA-1

GATA-1 is an X-linked member of the GATA family of zinc-finger proteins, of which there are at least six members. GATA-2 and GATA-3 are also found in erythroid cells but at a lower concentration and, like other GATA factors, have a wider tissue distribution. GATA-1 sites are found in the promoters of all of the globin genes except α, and in the regulatory elements as well as in the promoters of all other erythroid-specific genes that have been studied. The importance of this factor for erythropoiesis was demonstrated by 'knocking out' its gene in embryonic stem cells and creating chimeric embryos containing cells that are either GATA-positive or negative (Pevny *et al.* 1991). The negative cells could contribute to most of the tissues of the developing embryo but were not present among the definitive erythroid cells. When lines of mice were developed in which the GATA-1 gene has been 'knocked out' it was shown that GATA-1-negative males died *in utero* at about 10.5–11.5 days of gestation (Fujiwara *et al.* 1996). The function of this gene in erythropoiesis therefore cannot be compensated by any other member of this family. Over-expression of GATA-1 in mice transgenic for the human β-globin gene cluster resulted in marked reduction of ε-globin gene expression but no change in the γ-to-β-gene switch (Li *et al.* 1997).

NF-E2

NF-E2 is a heterodimer of two basic leucine zipper subunits, p45 and p18 (Andrews *et al.* 1993a; Ney *et al.* 1993). Binding sites for this factor are common in erythroid genes and their regulators. The p18 protein has a ubiquitous distribution and is a member of the *maf* family of transcription factors (Andrews *et al.* 1993b), while p45 is restricted to erythroid, megakaryocytic and mast cells. The genes for both of these subunits have been 'knocked out' in embryonic stem cells, and lines of mice lacking each factor have been produced. The loss of p18 has no phenotypic effect and presumably can be substituted by another family member (Kotkow & Orkin 1996). 'Knockout' of p45 has a profound downregulatory effect on globin-gene transcription in MEL cells (Kotkow & Orkin 1995). Surprisingly, it has little effect on erythropoiesis *in vivo*; mice that lack NF-E2 have only slightly reduced haemoglobin levels but are severely thrombocytopenic (Shivdasani *et al.* 1995).

EKLF

EKLF is an erythroid-specific zinc-finger protein which binds to the CACCC box of β-globin genes and may interact with GATA-1 to permit transcriptional activation (Gregory *et al.* 1996). Mice in which EKLF has been 'knocked out' have a characteristic β-thalassaemic blood picture, and β-gene transcription, but not α, is reduced to about 10% of normal (Nuez *et al.* 1995; Perkins *et al.* 1995). Other CACCC-box-containing, erythroid-specific genes, including carbonic anhydrase 1, porphobilinogen deaminase, pyruvate kinase, GATA-1 and mouse βh1 globin are unaffected in these mice. This suggests that EKLF is specific for the β-globin gene. However, it is expressed throughout development, including yolk-sac erythroid cells in which the β gene is inactive, indicating that either the β gene is inaccessible to the factor at this stage or that its structure has to be modified, by phosphorylation or the binding of another protein for example, before it becomes fully functional (Donze *et al.* 1995). Its presence in yolk-sac cells may be related to the requirement of LCR HS3 for EKLF for its function (Tewari *et al.* 1998). Over-expression of EKLF in mice transgenic for the β-globin cluster results in an earlier switch from γ- to β-gene expression (Tewari *et al.* 1998).

FKLF

Screening of a fetal liver cDNA library for EKLF-related proteins produced a transcription factor, FKLF, that preferentially activated ε- and γ-gene promoters. Higher levels of the factor were found in fetal liver than in adult marrow and it appeared to be predominantly expressed in erythroid cells (Asano *et al.* 1999). As this protein appears to be identical to TIEG2, which was reported to be widely expressed (Cook *et al.* 1998), functional *in vivo* assays will be required to determine its importance in differential globin-gene expression.

SSP

SSP, the stage selector protein, which may play a part in globin-gene switching, was originally identified by competition between γ- and β-gene expression in transiently transfected K562 cells (Jane *et al.* 1992, 1993). Constructs containing an intact γ-gene promoter suppressed the activity of a linked β gene. Deletion of −53 to −35 bp relative to the CAP site derepressed the β gene, suggesting that this sequence is important in mediating the preferential interaction of the γ promoter with the LCR element, HS2. Purification of a nuclear protein that binds to this sequence demonstrated that it is a heterodimer consisting of the ubiquitous factor CP2, first identified from its binding to the murine α-globin CCAAT box, and two molecules of an erythroid-specific 22 kDa protein called NF-E4 (Jane *et al.* 1995; Zhou *et al.* 2000). NF-E4, like EKLF, is not developmental stage specific, but appears to specifically activate ε and γ genes.

RNA processing

The primary RNA transcript of a gene is short lived; for globin genes it has been estimated to have a half-life of about 5 min. Its further processing involves modifications at both its 5′ and 3′ ends together with removal of the intervening sequences and uniting the exons to form a definitive template for protein synthesis. All these events take place in the nucleus.

Capping

At the 5′ end of the mRNA, a 7-methylguanosine residue is added in a 5′–5′ linkage to the first base, a process known as capping (see pp. 69, 97). This may play a role in its stability and in ribosomal binding to the mRNA during translation.

Poly(A) addition

The 3′ end of the primary transcript is cleaved at a specific point that is usually 10–25 nucleotides downstream of a highly conserved AAUAAA motif, after which a 200–300-bp tract of poly(A) residues is added to the end. The importance of the AAUAA/poly(A) addition signal to this process is illustrated by α- or β-globin genes in which mutations in this sequence lead to thalassaemia (see Chapter 4). This process is carried out by another protein complex consisting of a cleavage and polyadenylation specificity factor (CPSF), a cleavage stimulation factor (CstF), poly(A) polymerase (PAP) and poly(A) binding protein (PABII) (Keller 1995). CPSF, which consists of at least three polypeptides, binds to the AAUAAA sequence and links up with CstF, which also contains three polypeptides, which binds to U or G+U-rich sequences downstream of the cleavage site. The bound RNA is cleaved by an unidentified ribonuclease, after which a short tract of poly(A) is added by PAP, followed by a rapid burst of poly(A) addition until the poly(A) tail is ~250 bp long.

Although poly(A) addition may play a role in transcription termination and transport of the RNA from the nucleus to the cytoplasm, its major importance appears to lie in determining the stability of mRNA. Loss of the poly(A) tail is associated with rapid destruction of the mRNA, both *in vitro* and *in vivo* (Ross 1995).

Splicing

The other major goal of mRNA processing is the removal of the intervening sequences. This process is understood in greater detail than many other intranuclear events (Newman 1998; Misteli 1999). The initial step is cleavage of the 5′ splice site after a nucleophilic attack by the 2′ OH group on an A residue 10–60 nucleotides upstream of the 3′ acceptor site. This forms a 2′–5′ phosphodiester bond to produce a 'lariat' structure containing the intron and the 3′ exon. The 3′ OH group on the 5′ exon is now free to attack the 3′ splice site, resulting in the joining of the two exons and release of the free lariat intron.

Splicing is carried out by a large, multisubunit complex, the spliceosome, consisting of several proteins, some of which have been purified to homogeneity, and a number of small nuclear ribonucleoprotein particles (snRNPs). The snRNPs contain a small RNA (snRNA) of 56–217 nucleotides which is rich in uracil, together with a common set of proteins as well as those unique to each complex. The initial step in splicing is the binding of the UI snRNP to the 5′ end of the splice site, brought about by the complementarity of the 5′ end of the UI RNA to the splice con-

sensus sequence. In the second step, U2 snRNP binds to the sequence around the branch site of the lariat. Finally, U4/U6 and U5 snRNPs are added together with additional proteins to form the spliceosome, after which splicing can take place.

Many β-thalassaemia mutations involve the splicing mechanism. Indeed, they provide excellent natural models for the consequences of incorrect mRNA processing. Their effects are considered in detail in Chapter 4.

Transportation of mRNA to the cytoplasm

Once the primary transcript has been processed to mRNA, it is exported from the nucleus to the cytoplasm. Little is known about how this occurs, although, by analogy with other systems, it seems likely to be an active process, possibly involving carrier proteins as well as the protein complexes of the nuclear pore. There are hints that it may be linked to translation. The level of β-globin mRNA containing a premature stop-codon mutation (nonsense mutation) in exon 1 or 2 in the cytoplasm is reduced to less than 10% of normal. Such mRNA as survives appears to have normal stability (Humphries *et al.* 1984; Takeshita *et al.* 1984). It is not clear whether destruction takes place in the cytoplasm, in the nucleus or during transit between the two. Normal levels of primary transcript are found in the nucleus, but the levels of processed nuclear mRNA are reduced (Takeshita *et al.* 1984; Kugler *et al.* 1995), a situation that has also been reported for triosephosphate isomerase genes containing nonsense codons in the first few exons (Belgrader *et al.* 1994). Others, however, have reported that, when human β-globin genes containing nonsense codons are expressed in mice, the mRNAs appear to be degraded in the cytoplasm rather than the nucleus (Lim *et al.* 1992; Lim & Maquat 1992). As these experiments have involved different genes, species and tissues, it is not yet possible to reconcile these results. However, the suggestion that translation-linked transport from the nucleus to the cytoplasm is involved in producing the low levels of mRNA containing nonsense codons warrants further investigation. We shall return to this question in Chapters 4 and 13, when we discuss its relevance to the molecular basis of dominant β thalassaemia.

Globin mRNAs

The general structure of globin mRNA is shown in Fig. 2.19, illustrating the features of human β-globin mRNA elucidated by Forget, Proudfoot, Kan and coworkers (Proudfoot & Longley 1976; Chang *et al.* 1977; Forget 1977; Marotta *et al.* 1977; Proudfoot 1977). All globin mRNAs contain the modified 5′ end CAP structure and the 3′ poly(A) tail. In addition there are non-coding sequences at the 5′ and 3′ ends. For example, β globin has 53 nucleotides before the AUG initiation codon, and a further 132 nucleotides between the termination codon and the poly(A). Thus, although the β chain has 146 amino acids (which require $3 \times 146 = 438$ nucleotides to code for them, in addition to the AUG initiator and UAA terminator, a total of 444 nucleotides in all), the β-globin mRNA is approximately 650–750 nucleotides long, depending on the exact size of the poly(A) tail.

Many animal and viral mRNAs have a 5′ structure containing methylated nucleotides (Shatkin 1976). Several versions, CAP-0, CAP-1 and CAP-2, have been found. CAP-2 is present in all globin mRNAs and, in general, appears to be present only in cytoplasmic mRNAs. CAP-1 is found in both nuclear and cytoplasmic mRNA, and it is probable that CAP-2 is derived from CAP-1. Enzymic removal of the CAP reduces the translational efficiency of globin mRNA in cell-free systems (Lodish 1976; Revel & Groner 1978), and CAP analogues inhibit its translation. Thus, it is likely that CAP is necessary for the maximum translational efficiency of globin mRNA. There is some evidence for a direct interaction between the CAP and a reticulocyte initiation factor (Shafritz *et al.* 1976), although whether it is truly involved in the regulation of chain initiation is not yet known. We shall discuss the effects of mutations of the CAP site in Chapter 4.

A string of adenylic acid residues at the 3′ end of mRNA is found in all globin mRNAs (Lim & Canel-lakis 1970; Burr & Lingrel 1971). The exact length seems to vary with the age of the mRNA, being longest in newly synthesized RNA and shortest in mRNA isolated from 'old' reticulocytes. Its functions were discussed earlier. Although deadenylated mRNA will function in a cell-free system (Sippel *et al.* 1974), its lifetime is much shorter than poly(A)-containing mRNA when it is incubated in *Xenopus* oocytes over a period of several days (Marbaix *et al.* 1975; Maniatis *et al.* 1976).

The nucleotide sequences of the human α, β and γ messenger RNAs (and, by extrapolation from the DNA sequences of the cloned genes, those δ and ε mRNAs) are now known in considerable detail (Proudfoot & Longley 1976; Baralle 1977; Chang *et al.* 1977; Forget 1977; Marotta *et al.* 1977; Wilson *et al.* 1977; Chang *et al.* 1978; Forget *et al.* 1979; Proudfoot & Baralle 1979). There is little overall homology in the non-coding sequences, although certain features, such as the CUUPyUG sequence found near to the 5′ CAP, which may be involved in ribosome recognition, and the AAUAAA sequence found in all eukaryotic messengers about 20 bases from the poly(A) addition site, recur. The function of these non-coding regions is not clear. Obviously those at the 5′ end include the ribosome binding site, and the differences between α and β mRNA 5′ non-coding sequences presumably account, at least in part, for the fact that α chains are initiated more slowly than β chains on these messengers. It may also be relevant that the potential exists for forming hairpin loop structures in parts of these non-coding regions, which may help to stabilize the molecules by preventing degradation by exonucleases.

Globin synthesis

Globin chains are synthesized in the cytoplasm by the interaction of mRNA, ribosomes, transfer RNAs and various cofactors in a series of reactions proceeding

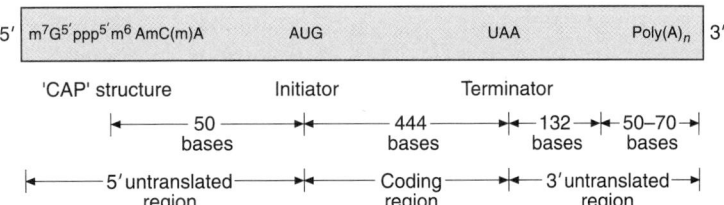

Fig. 2.19 The structure of a typical globin messenger RNA.

through three separate phases: initiation; elongation; and termination (Fig. 2.3). A detailed description of the mechanisms of protein synthesis is given by Lewin (1997). Here, we outline the major steps in globin synthesis.

Initiation

The initial step involves the formation of a tertiary complex between the initiation factor eIF-2, GTP and the initiation transfer RNA, tRNAmet, which subsequently binds to the small 40S ribosomal subunit. With the help of other initiation factors, globin mRNA and the large ribosomal subunit are added to this complex so that, in its final configuration, the mRNA is aligned with the ribosome with the AUG initiation codon opposite the UAC anticodon of the tRNAmet. AUG is the only codon for the amino acid methionine. Thus in all mammalian systems, just as in bacteria, the first amino acid incorporated into a protein chain is methionine; in bacterial systems the methionine has a blocked, formylated amino group but this is not found in mammalian cells. Once translation starts the initiation factors dissociate to participate in another initiation cycle.

Elongation

Protein synthesis now proceeds by stepwise addition of amino acids from the N-terminal end to form the growing peptide chain. This cycle involves at least three distinct stages. The first is a codon-directed binding of an aminoacyl-tRNA to a ribosome site next to that occupied by the initiator tRNAmet. Peptide transfer then takes place between the newly bound aminoacyl-tRNA and the tRNAmet. Lastly, the newly made peptidyl-tRNA and the mRNA are both shifted from the acceptor to the donor site on the ribosome. In this way the acceptor site is freed and the process can be repeated. At the same time the tRNA that donated the growing peptide chain is released. Two protein factors, EF-1 and EF-2, are involved in the elongation process. EF-1 participates in a GTP-dependent reaction by which aminoacyl-tRNAs bind to ribosomes, while EF-2, or translocase, catalyses the translocation step in another GTP-dependent reaction. The N-terminal methionine incorporated during initiation is removed enzymatically from the globin chain after the addition of about 20 amino acids.

Most mRNAs are long enough to support a number of ribosomes active in synthesis along their length. Once a ribosome has moved away from the initiation site, another can bind and start synthesis, so forming polyribosome complexes.

Termination

Globin synthesis stops when the ribosome reaches a chain termination codon (UAA, UAG, UGA) in the message. At this point the polypeptide chain is split from the tRNA in another GTP-dependent hydrolytic reaction, which involves at least one protein cofactor. The ribosome is released from the mRNA and dissociates into subunits, which are then free to participate in another round of synthesis.

Regulation

Although, as mentioned earlier, it is now apparent that globin synthesis is regulated mainly at the level of transcription, there appears to be some fine-tuning at the level of translation; β mRNA is a much more efficient initiator than α by a factor of about 1.5 (Lodish 1976). However, this imbalance is compensated by there being more α-globin mRNA than β in red-cell precursors. The net effect is that the number of α and β chains synthesized are almost equal but not quite; there is usually a slight over-production of α chains in normal precursors (Weatherall *et al.* 1965), which, presumably, are disposed of proteolytically to achieve a final balance.

As mentioned earlier, the output of the α2-globin gene exceeds that of the α1 gene, probably reflecting the different levels of mRNA production at these two loci. Assessment of the ribosome loading of α2- and α1-globin mRNA has shown that they have identical translational profiles and therefore should be translated with equal efficiencies, predicting a dominant role for the α2-globin locus (Shakin & Liebhaber 1986). It follows that, in heterozygotes, naturally occurring structural mutations of the α2 gene should represent ~37% of the peripheral blood haemoglobin, and α1-gene mutants ~13%. However, two studies addressing this point came to different conclusions. In the first, it was found that α2-gene variants represented 24–40%, whereas α1-gene variants represented 11–23%, suggesting a predominant role for the α2 gene at both mRNA and protein levels (Liebhaber *et al.* 1986). In contrast, a more extensive survey of α-globin variants by Molchanova *et al.* (1994a) found that in heterozygotes the average proportion of stable variants resulting from α2-gene mutants (23.5%) was only slightly higher than from α1-gene mutations (19.7%), suggesting a less efficient translation of the α2-globin mRNA and a more equal contribution from the two genes at the protein level. Further work will be needed to resolve this issue since this is clearly of importance in understanding the pathophysiology of the non-deletional forms of α thalassaemia (see Chapter 4).

Haem synthesis

The biosynthesis of haem in red-cell precursors (reviewed by Sassa 1995) takes place in a series of enzymatically controlled steps, beginning with the condensation of glycine and succinyl-CoA to form α-amino β-keto adipic acid, which is then rapidly decarboxylated to form δ-aminolaevulinic acid (ALA) (Fig. 2.20). This reaction, which is catalysed by the enzyme ALA synthase and requires pyridoxal phosphate and ferrous ion as cofactors, is the only step in the whole chain which requires energy (to convert succinate to succinyl-CoA), all the rest being essentially irreversible (with the possible exception of the formation of uroporphyrinogen III). Next, two molecules of ALA combine to form the monopyrrole porphobilinogen by the action of the enzyme ALA dehydratase, and then four of these porphobilinogen molecules are condensed to form the basic tetrapyrrole ring, uroporphyrinogen. After side-chain modifi-

cations this is converted to protoporphyrinogen, which, on oxidation by oxygen in the presence of coproporphyrinogen oxidase, is finally converted to the red protoporphyrinogen molecule. Iron is then inserted by the enzyme ferrochelatase to form haem.

The first and last two enzymes of this pathway are present in the mitochondria while the rest are found in the cell cytoplasm, and it is interesting to note that both oxidation steps take place in the mitochondria. Regulation is mediated mainly by the level of haem; increasing levels result in feedback inhibition of ALA synthase.

Haem–globin interactions and the assembly of haemoglobin

Although the differential regulation of globin synthesis is achieved against a background of predetermined cytoplasmic mRNA levels, the overall level of protein synthesis in red-cell precursors may be modified to a considerable extent by haem, which is a powerful stimulator of globin synthesis (Lodish 1976). In conditions of haem deficiency a protein kinase specifically phosphorylates, and thereby inactivates, the initiation factor eIF-2 (Farrell *et al.* 1977; Revel & Groner 1978). Although haem deficiency is not relevant to the thalassaemias, it is worth noting that the excess haem which is liberated in thalassaemic red cells from the dissociation of globin subunits plays an important role in generating pathological changes in their membranes (see Chapter 5).

As mentioned earlier, there is usually a small pool

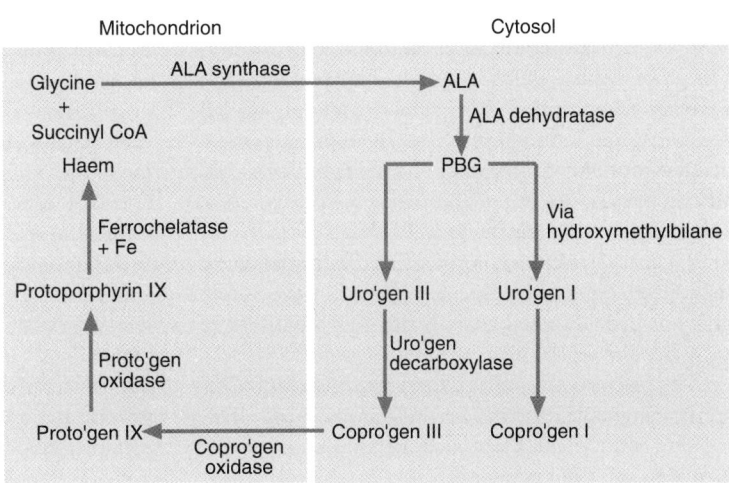

Fig. 2.20 The pathway of haem synthesis. The abbreviations uro'gen and copro'gen represent uroporphyrinogen and coproporphyrinogen, respectively. ALA, δ aminolaevulinic acid; PBG, porphobilinogen.

of excess α chains in red-cell precursors. It was suggested that α chains from this pool associate with β chains on ribosomes to await their release as αβ dimers (Baglioni & Campana 1967). While these may be true intermediates in haemoglobin assembly (Winterhalter *et al.* 1969), and kinetic studies indicate this is probably the case, it seems unlikely that their formation on ribosomes is obligatory, because in certain conditions, such as HbH disease (see Chapters 5 and 11), β chains can be freely released from ribosomes into the cell cytoplasm.

Haem is probably incorporated into the α and β chains after their release into the cytoplasm (Felicetti *et al.* 1966), and tetramer formation follows immediately after their association into dimers (Winterhalter & Huehns 1964).

It is often the case that the levels of β-chain haemoglobin variants in heterozygotes depart considerably from the expected 50%. At least some of these discrepancies undoubtedly reflect differential affinity of α chains for β chains of different structure. Indeed, there is clear evidence that α chains bind γ chains less effectively than β chains. Throughout this book we shall see how the differential affinity of globin subunits one for another may have a profound effect on the relative levels of particular haemoglobin variants in individuals with different forms of thalassaemia in which one or other globin subunit is found in reduced amounts. We shall take up this story again in Chapter 3 and in greater detail in Chapters 9 and 11.

Developmental regulation of the globin genes

The developmental changes in haemoglobin production are brought about by differential activation of the globin genes, which is largely determined at the level of transcription. This series of events, called 'haemoglobin switching', has been extensively studied, not only for its innate biological interest but also because a better understanding of its regulation might lead to its manipulation, which could be of therapeutic benefit to those with β thalassaemia or sickle-cell disease. However, despite all the effort that has been directed towards this end, we still have only the flimsiest of ideas about how switching is regulated. Because this information is so central to our better understanding of the thalassaemias, we shall outline some of the approaches that are being followed to solve this problem.

Haemoglobin production during development

Human haemoglobin is heterogeneous at all stages of development, beginning with the youngest embryos that have been studied and continuing throughout adult life (Fig. 2.21). In embryos, haemoglobin synthesis is confined to the yolk sac, where Hbs Gower 1 ($\zeta_2\varepsilon_2$), Gower 2 ($\alpha_2\varepsilon_2$) and Portland ($\zeta_2\gamma_2$) are produced. At 5 weeks' gestation, the $\zeta/\zeta +\alpha$-chain synthesis ratio is 0.82 ± 0.04; by 6 weeks it has declined to 0.03 ± 0.02 (Peschle *et al.* 1985). The $\varepsilon/\varepsilon +\gamma$ ratio is 0.83 ±0.05 at 5 weeks and declines more slowly to 0.31 ± 0.10 at 6 weeks, and 0.03 ± 0.02 at 7 weeks. Synthesis of β chain becomes detectable at about 6 weeks, when it comprises ~1.5% of the non-α chains, increasing to 5% at 7 weeks and ~10% by 10 weeks. At around 7–8 weeks' gestation the liver becomes the major site of erythropoiesis, producing large enucleated red cells. Using more sensitive mRNA assays, θ-gene transcripts are detected in yolk sac, fetal liver (Leung *et al.* 1987), adult blood (Albitar *et al.* 1989) and bone marrow (Ley *et al.* 1989). Very small amounts of ζ mRNA are also present throughout fetal life (for example, see Hill *et al.* 1985) and ζ globin (as Hb Portland) is present in the cord bloods of non-thalassaemic newborns (for example, see Chui *et al.* 1989).

Throughout most of fetal life HbF production predominates, with a small amount (<10%) of HbA. The different γ chains are produced in a ratio of $^G\gamma$ to $^A\gamma$ of 3:1, which remains constant until late in gestation (Nute *et al.* 1973). At mid-term the bone marrow begins to take over as the major site of red-cell production, though erythropoiesis is also found in the spleen, as well as in other tissues (Kelemen *et al.* 1981). There are no differences in the relative proportions of fetal and adult haemoglobins produced in these sites (Wood & Weatherall 1973).

Towards the end of gestation there is a gradual and reciprocal switch from HbF to A production. At birth, the cord blood normally contains ~70% HbF and this declines to ~20% by 3 months, 7.5% at 6 months, and less than 2% by the age of 1 year. At the same time there is a differential decline in $^G\gamma$- and $^A\gamma$- chain production, so that their relative proportions become closer to equal. Both fetal and adult haemoglobins are produced in the same cell during the switching period, with a gradual increase in the proportion of cells containing predominantly HbA. The proportion of HbF continues to decline throughout childhood and probably throughout adult life

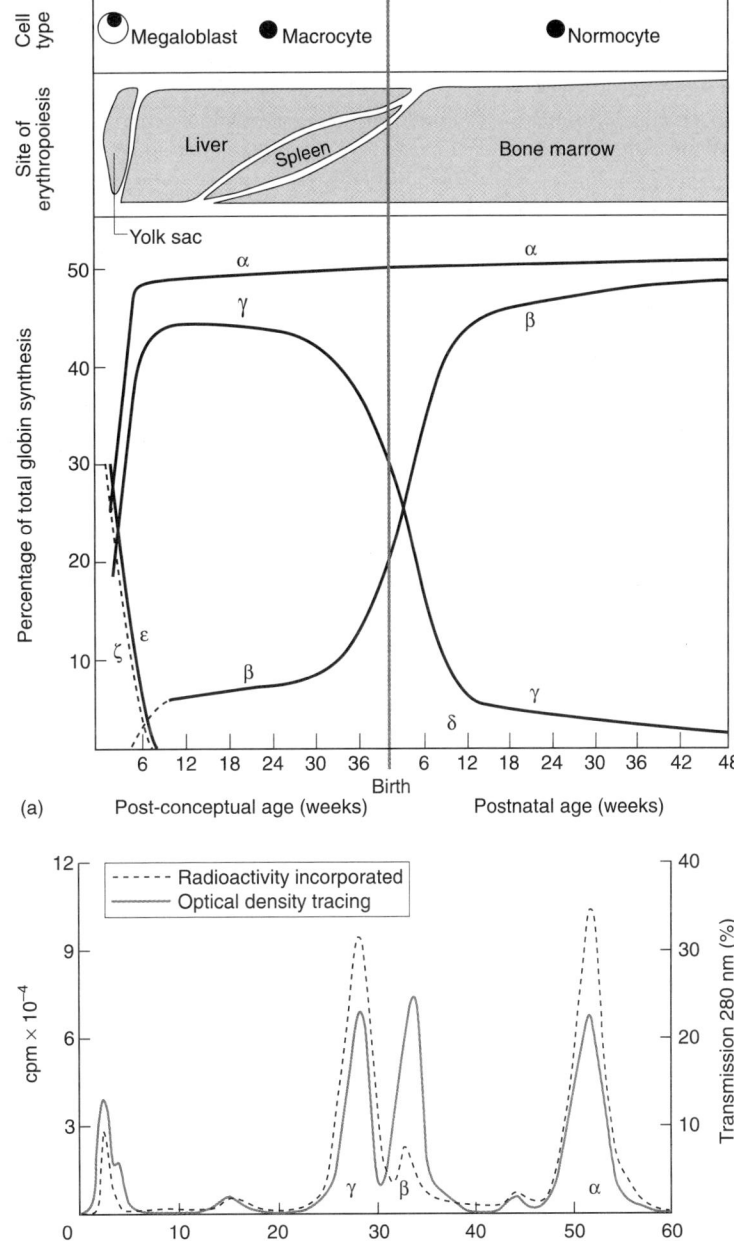

Fig. 2.21 Developmental changes in haemoglobin production. (a) The sites of erythropoiesis during development and the different globins produced at each stage. (b) Globin synthesis in blood obtained from a 20-week-old fetus. The cells were incubated with radioactive amino acids and the globins separated. Adult haemoglobin was added as 'carrier'. There is approximately 10% β-chain synthesis at this gestational age.

(Rutland *et al.* 1983), at which time the small amount of HbF is only detectable in 3–5% of red cells, known as F cells (Fig. 2.22). The latter do not have any other features of fetal erythroid cells and the HbF constitutes no more than 20% of the haemoglobin content.

Although the products of the α2 and α1 genes are identical, two methods exploiting the sequence divergence in their 3′ non-coding regions have enabled the relative amounts of their mRNAs to be determined in reticulocytes (Liebhaber & Kan 1981; Orkin & Goff 1981a). In both fetal and adult life the steady-state level of α2-globin mRNA predominates over

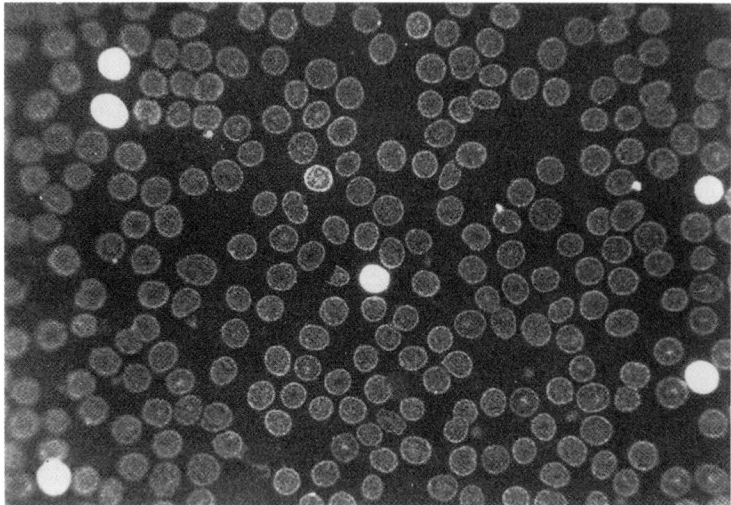

Fig. 2.22 F cells in normal adult blood. Normal adult blood treated with a fluorescently labelled anti-HbF antibody.

α1-globin mRNA by approximately 3:1, probably as a result of differences at the level of transcription of the two genes. More recently, these findings have also been confirmed using quantitative RT-PCR analyses (Molchanova *et al.* 1994a).

Cellular aspects of haemoglobin switching

Timing

Theoretically, haemoglobin switching could reflect the replacement of one haemopoietic cell population by another, or, alternatively, changes in gene expression within the same cell lineage (Wood 1984). In the latter case, switching could result from an autonomous cellular programme or a response to an external signal supplied by other cells or by a circulating regulator, a hormone for instance.

Haematopoiesis begins in the embryo in a region known as the 'para-aortic splanchnopleura' or the 'aorta-gonad-mesonephros' (Dzierzak *et al.* 1998). During early development, there are two waves of red-cell production, one in the yolk-sac cells, the other in the fetal liver and bone marrow (Cumano *et al.* 1996; Medvinsky & Dzierzak 1996). The lineage relationships between these populations have not yet been established. The switch from embryonic to fetal haemoglobin production may be principally the result of the replacement of one cell lineage programmed for embryonic haemoglobins by another

which is independently programmed for fetal and adult haemoglobins. Unlike fetal-to-adult haemoglobin switching, which only occurs in ruminants and primates, the embryonic switch occurs in all vertebrates. It is possible therefore that the regulatory mechanism involved in embryonic-to-postembryonic switching may be fundamentally different from the relatively recently evolved fetal-to-adult haemoglobin switch.

The fetal-to-adult haemoglobin switch reflects a change from γ- to β-gene expression within the same haemopoietic lineage, both genes being expressed in the same cell at the time of switching (Wood 1984). The process is protracted, beginning several weeks before birth and largely completed three to six months later. The timing is unaffected by birth, and although tens of thousands of blood samples from newborn infants have been examined world-wide, very few examples of premature or delayed switching have been reported. Infants of diabetic mothers show a delay, probably as a result of high fetal butyrate levels (Perrine *et al.* 1985, 1988). Whether this is due to a change in the time of onset of switching or a secondary chemical effect on γ-gene expression has yet to be determined.

Experimental approaches to modifying the time of switching have shown that, in sheep, fetal thyroidectomy or nephrectomy have little or no effect, while hypophysectomy, which results in a generalized developmental delay, retards switching although the time of onset appears to be unaffected (Wood *et al.* 1976a). Similar delays are observed in adrenalec-tomized fetuses and can be reversed by injections of cortisol (Wintour *et al.* 1985). Thus the rate, if not the time of onset, of switching can be modified by hor-monal factors.

When adult marrow is injected into fetal sheep there is no reversion to fetal haemoglobin production (Zanjani *et al.* 1982). The converse experiment, trans-plantation of fetal liver haemopoietic cells to adult sheep, results in the production of fetal, and later adult, haemoglobin (Zanjani *et al.* 1979; Bunch *et al.* 1981; Wood *et al.* 1985). Similar results are obtained when human fetal liver is transplanted to adults (Delfini *et al.* 1983; Papayannopoulou *et al.* 1986). The time of switching is not related to the time after trans-plantation, but rather to the age of the fetal cells (Wood *et al.* 1985). These results suggest that the fetal and adult 'environments' do not play a major role in determining the type of haemoglobin that is made. Rather, they imply that the time of switching is an inbuilt property of haemopoietic cells, as if they have their own 'developmental clock'.

However, the time taken for switching to occur in these transplantation experiments is sufficiently short for the results to reflect the activities of long-lived, committed progenitor cells. Therefore, further work is required before the timing of switching can be ascribed unequivocally to an inherent pro-gramme within haemopoietic cells. Indeed, it has been shown recently that, when such cells obtained from adult bone marrow are injected into mouse blastocysts, they can give rise to red cells later in development that contain embryonic rather than adult globins (Geiger *et al.* 1998). This observation suggests that the developmental potential of the adult stem cell may be more plastic than previously thought.

At which stage in haemopoietic-cell development is switching determined?

It appears likely that the decision about whether a cell produces fetal or adult haemoglobin is taken early in erythropoiesis. The most primitive progenitor cell that is committed to the erythroid lineage is the early burst-forming-unit erythroid (BFU-E), a cell with a large proliferative capacity which can give rise to several thousand mature red blood cells in *in vitro* colonies (Fig. 2.23). When these cells are isolated from fetal tissues and cultured in serum-free medium in the absence of accessory cells, but with growth factors that allow their proliferation and maturation, they give rise to large, haemoglobinized colonies that contain fetal haemoglobin (Stamatoyannopoulos & Papayannopoulou 1981; Peschle *et al.* 1984). Similar colonies from adult bone marrow grown under the same conditions contain adult haemoglobin. It appears therefore that information about the haemo-globin type of red cells is already programmed into a cell that is 10 or more divisions away from activating its globin genes. It follows that the critical events which mediate differential globin-gene expression need not necessarily occur when genes are tran-scribed in early erythroblasts, but may happen much earlier in erythroid differentiation and in cells which are rare and difficult to isolate.

The molecular basis for gene switching

The role of cis-active sequences

An analysis of the sequences that might be involved in haemoglobin switching requires either a series of naturally occurring mutations or an experimental model in which manipulations can be made. Initially, the mutations associated with persistent HbF pro-

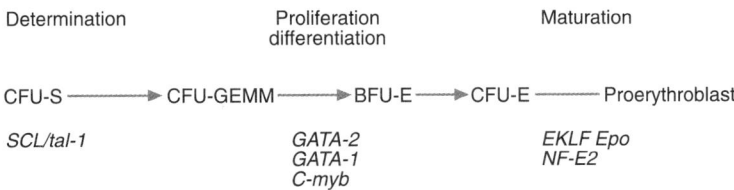

Fig. 2.23 The different classes of progenitors during red-cell maturation. Below, some of the regulatory proteins are also shown. CFU = Colony-forming unit. BFU = burst-forming unit. E = erythroid. The action of the different regulators is described in the text (see pp. 93–5).

duction appeared to offer valuable models, but, in the event, they have been surprisingly uninformative (see Chapters 4 and 10). Therefore it has been necessary to develop other systems to attack this problem.

Early studies of globin-gene expression were limited to transfection of human DNA into cell lines. While this was useful for identifying essential regulatory elements such as promoters and enhancers, developmental regulation could not be achieved, appropriate cell lines were not always available, and there were concerns that results obtained from cells in culture might stem from artefacts and not reflect events in normal cells.

Among the many technical advances of modern biology, the ability to incorporate human genes into mice has been among the most important, particularly for examining gene expression. Injection of cloned human DNA into the pronuclei of fertilized mouse eggs, at a time before the gametic nuclei fuse, results in its integration into the mouse genome in a random fashion. After transfer of the injected eggs to pseudopregnant females, up to 30% of the fetuses or newborn animals contain the injected DNA. In most cases, the human DNA fragment is incorporated as multiple copies in a tandem 5′ to 3′ or 'head to tail' array, although occasionally single copies are found. In some cases, integration takes place after the first cell division, resulting in mosaicism in which the human DNA is present in some but not all cells; the proportion may vary from tissue to tissue. However, breeding from these 'founder' mice usually generates transgenic lines in which inheritance of the transgene is Mendelian.

The first globin-gene fragments used to generate transgenic mice consisted of the γ- and β-globin genes, together with a small amount of flanking sequence. When their tissues were examined for human gene expression by RNA analysis, the levels were usually low, only a few per cent of the endogenous mouse mRNA, or there was none at all (Magram *et al.* 1985; Townes *et al.* 1985; Chada *et al.* 1986; Kollias *et al.* 1986). However, when a gene was expressed, it was usually in the appropriate tissue and both γ and β genes were developmentally regulated. These experiments, while giving disappointing levels of expression, nevertheless led to the important conclusion that sequences involved in globin-gene expression at different developmental stages must lie in and around the genes themselves.

The variably low or absent expression of the human genes in these cell lines is now believed to reflect the site of integration; in an open region of chromatin, expression is possible, whereas, if the region is inactive in erythroid cells, so is the transgene. With the discovery of the LCR (see earlier), this problem was overcome. Constructs containing the LCR are highly expressed, the level being proportional to the copy number of the transgenes and equivalent per copy to that of the endogenous mouse genes (Grosveld *et al.* 1987; Ryan *et al.* 1989). This advance paved the way for detailed dissection of the *cis* regulation of the β-globin gene cluster.

Expression of the entire human β-globin-gene cluster in mice

In transgenic mice containing the whole β-globin gene complex, either as a 70-kb DNA fragment (Strouboulis *et al.* 1992) or in a yeast artificial chromosome (Gaensler *et al.* 1993; Peterson *et al.* 1993), a tightly regulated pattern of developmental regulation is observed. The ε-globin gene is expressed largely in yolk-sac cells and is switched off by about day 12.5. The γ genes are highly expressed in yolk-sac cells and their expression persists in the fetal liver until about day 16.5. They also show a switch from $^G\gamma$ to $^A\gamma$ expression during this period, as occurs during human development. The β-globin gene is virtually inactive in yolk-sac cells and is expressed in parallel with the mouse β genes. It appears therefore that many aspects of developmental regulation of human genes are reproduced in these mice; the major difference lies in the embryonic expression of the γ genes and the fact that they are transcribed at a level five- to 10-fold greater than the ε transgene. This probably reflects the fact that the mouse has no γ genes of its own, making it a less than perfect model.

ε-Gene expression

Studies of human ε-gene expression in transgenic mice have shown a similar pattern when it is attached to LCR elements, on its own or together with the rest of the complex. In other words, the presence of other genes does not affect its transcription, indicating that it is autonomously regulated. The particular sequences responsible appear to lie within the 5′ end of the gene (Shih *et al.* 1993), a region containing a number of positive and negative regulatory sequences (Cao *et al.* 1989; Trepicchio *et al.* 1993, 1994; Dyer *et al.* 1996).

Deletion of the region from −392 to −177 relative to the CAP site, a region that contains a negative regulator that may possibly overlap a positive element, prevents complete downregulation of the gene, resulting in continued low-level ε-gene activity in adult life. Thus, one of the regulatory sites involved in its post-embryonic suppression has been identified (Raich *et al.* 1990, 1992, 1995). Surprisingly, deletion of the part of this sequence believed to contain the element responsible for silencing the gene in adult cells (−304 to −179) from a yeast artificial chromosome (YAC) containing the whole β-globin cluster results in marked suppression of ε-gene transcription in embryonic yolk-sac cells. Furthermore, the loss of this sequence also downregulates expression of the γ genes (Liu *et al.* 1997). Clearly, both expression and repression of the ε gene is subject to several *cis* regulatory elements.

γ-Gene expression

While the γ genes are highly expressed in embryos and almost entirely repressed in adult mice containing the whole human globin-gene complex, with smaller constructs, γ-gene repression in adults is more variable. When the LCR or micro LCR is attached to a 3.3-kb fragment containing the ^{A}γ gene (extending to +1951 bp from the CAP site, but lacking the downstream enhancer element), γ mRNA levels decline between fetal liver and adult blood stages but continue to be expressed at relatively high levels. With micro LCR ^{A}γδβ or ^{G}γ^{A}γδβ constructs, a further reduction in adult levels of γ-gene expression is observed, suggesting that the presence of a β gene downstream may be important in suppressing γ-gene expression (Behringer *et al.* 1990; Enver *et al.* 1990). On the other hand, complete repression of γ-gene expression in adults is observed when the LCR is attached to an ^{A}γ gene extended to +4308, as long as only low-copy-number mice are utilized (Dillon & Grosveld 1991). This fragment includes the ^{A}γ 'enhancer', and hence a role for this element in γ-gene silencing was implicated. However, when other γ-gene fragments that include this element are analysed, they are incompletely switched off in adults (Lloyd *et al.* 1992; Roberts *et al.* 1997b; Stamatoyannopoulos *et al.* 1997). An element lying between 3342 and 4308 has been reported to act as a silencer in

transient assays (Kosteas *et al.* 1996) and could also be involved in suppressing γ genes in adults.

What are these complex and apparently contradictory findings telling us about γ-gene regulation? As some constructs containing the γ gene alone show complete repression in adults, the γ genes, like the ε gene, appear to be largely autonomously regulated, a conclusion which is supported by evidence from transgenic mice containing rearranged β-globin loci from YAC inserts (Peterson *et al.* 1995). It also appears, however, that the presence of the β-globin genes must play at least some role in their developmental expression.

β-Gene expression

The main regulatory regions that have been defined within or adjacent to the β-globin genes were described earlier. They show appropriate developmental regulation in the absence of the LCR (Magram *et al.* 1985; Kollias *et al.* 1986) but, in an LCR-β gene construct, the β gene is also expressed in yolk-sac cells and stays on at a similar level throughout development (Behringer *et al.* 1990; Enver *et al.* 1990). As we have already seen, correct developmental regulation of the β gene is reacquired when a γ-globin gene is placed between it and the LCR or one of its elements (Behringer *et al.* 1990; Enver *et al.* 1990). These findings suggest that upstream γ-globin genes are necessary to keep the β gene silenced in embryonic cells, and indicate that there may be competition between the two genes, presumably for activation by the LCR. In fact, any gene in this position can fulfil this function; an α-globin gene (Hanscombe *et al.* 1991; Peterson & Stamatoyannopoulos 1993) or a non-globin gene (Anderson *et al.* 1993) can prevent the embryonic expression of the β gene. In the embryonic environment, the γ genes are favoured in this competition, silencing the β gene, but if the γ genes are absent the LCR is free to activate the β gene.

The role of the different LCR elements

The major functions of the LCR, together with the effects of deletion of its different components, were outlined earlier in this chapter. When HS2, 3 or 4 was individually linked to a 35-kb ^{G}γ^{A}γδβ fragment in transgenic mice, some differences were observed in the relative levels of γ- and β-gene expression at different stages of development, HS3 appearing to favour β, and HS4 γ, levels (Fraser *et al.* 1993). However, the lack of major developmental differences in mouse or human globin-gene expression when different sites are 'knocked out' of the complex suggests that individual HSs do not play a major selective role in activating individual genes (Fiering *et al.* 1995; Hug *et al.* 1996).

The role of gene order

As we have seen, it appears that the ε and γ genes are autonomously regulated, while β-gene expression requires competition from the γ genes for its silencing in embryonic erythropoiesis. This might imply that gene-specific transcription factors mediate the expression of these genes by facilitating their activation by the LCR. However, there is compelling evidence that expression from within the β-globin gene is dependent on the order of genes and their proximity to the LCR. The closer the gene is to the LCR, the more likely it is to be expressed, even to the degree of overcoming normal developmental regulation (Hanscombe *et al.* 1991; Peterson & Stamatoyannopoulos 1993; Dillon *et al.* 1997).

The role of trans-acting factors

It has long been believed that the differential gene expression that underlies haemoglobin switching must reflect difference in protein transcription factors between embryonic, fetal and adult cells. Thus in fetal erythroblasts there may be a set of factors which bind to the γ-gene promoters and facilitate transcription via an interaction with the LCR. In adult erythroblasts, an alternative set of factors might stabilize the interaction of the β-gene promoter with the LCR and hence result in expression of the β rather than γ genes. Furthermore, some of these factors, when bound to DNA, might prevent or repress expression; fetal cells would contain β-gene repressors and adult cells γ-gene repressors, for example.

Stage-specific globin-gene regulatory proteins with these properties have proved to be extremely elusive, however. Candidates such as the stage-selector protein have been identified in chick and human cells (see earlier section), but even the erythroid-specific component of this complex is not developmental stage specific and hence its role in selective gene

expression remains to be ascertained. EKLF, which has been shown specifically to activate the β-globin gene (see p. 95), is clearly necessary for β-globin-gene-expression but it does not appear to be sufficient on its own. For example, it is present in embryonic cells, yet the β gene is inactive. This observation suggests that searching for novel nuclear protein factors between embryonic, fetal and adult cells may not necessarily identify stage-specific factors. Post-translational modification may be needed to activate a factor for binding to a specific sequence. Alternatively, it may be that relatively small quantitative differences in several factors, rather than the appearance of new factors, may effect differential gene expression. As some transcription factors can act as either activators or repressors, dependent on their concentration and the presence of other factors, the differences between cells from various developmental stages could be quite subtle. Furthermore, critical regulatory events may occur at a much earlier stage in erythroid differentiation than the time at which transcription of the genes actually begins.

It is important to emphasize that stage-specific factors are not essential for the expression of a gene at the appropriate time. High levels of γ-gene expression can occur in adult cells in conditions such as hereditary persistence of fetal haemoglobin (HPFH) (see Chapter 10). Many HPFH mutations are due to deletions of the δ and β genes and therefore do not involve a change in the *trans*-acting factors. Nevertheless, levels of γ globin in adult cells in these conditions are not much less than those of β chains in normal cells. Furthermore, when a chromosome from a fetal cell expressing its γ but not its β genes is transferred to an 'adult' mouse erythroleukaemia cell line, it continues to express the γ genes and does not switch on the β gene (Papayannopoulou *et al.* 1986; Stanworth *et al.* 1995). This suggests that in these circumstances, the chromatin conformation of the genes may be more important than the *trans*-acting environment in determining stage-specific expression. When these observations are taken together with the results from transgenic mice that demonstrate that switching is dependent on the structure of the globin-gene construct (Roberts *et al.* 1997b), it is clear that *trans*-acting factors cannot be solely responsible for switching, although they may be important to maximize expression of the appropriate gene.

Developmental regulation of the α-globin gene cluster

In the α-globin cluster, both the embryonic ζ gene and the adult α genes are expressed together in the earliest embryonic cells, at least in mice (Leder *et al.* 1992) and probably in humans (Peschle *et al.* 1985). Regulation of the ζ-globin gene, like the ε gene, is autonomous in that it is unaffected by the presence or absence of α genes (Spangler *et al.* 1990; Albitar *et al.* 1991). As this applies when the gene is controlled by HS–40, the β LCR or HS2, it appears that the critical regulatory sequences must lie in or around the ζ-globin gene itself. Sequences within the ζ-gene promoter, the transcribed sequence and the 3′-flanking sequences may be necessary for complete silencing of the gene (Sabath *et al.* 1993; Liebhaber *et al.* 1996; Pondel *et al.* 1996; Russell *et al.* 1998; Wang & Liebhaber 1999), but the individual elements involved have yet to be identified. Small amounts of ζ mRNA can be found in fetal life and in cord blood (Hill *et al.* 1985; Chui *et al.* 1989).

Although the α-globin genes are expressed at all stages of development, their level of transcription may be upregulated when the ζ gene is silenced. There is no change in α2:α1-globin mRNA ratio between fetal and adult life and the steady-state level of α2-globin mRNA predominates over α1-globin mRNA by approximately 3:1, probably as a result of differences at the level of transcription of the two genes. These findings have been confirmed using quantitative RT-PCR analyses (Molchanova *et al.* 1994a).

Postscript

We have considered some of the experimental systems that have been utilized to attempt to help us to understand how the human globin genes are regulated at different stages of development. After struggling through this account readers will be left in no doubt about the complexity of these issues. But this should not come as a surprise. The changes in the globin genes are but one of a series of alterations in the pattern of protein production during the different developmental stages of erythropoiesis. Furthermore, they are occurring at a time when an extraordinarily wide range of similar changes are taking place through every organ system. Thus, while the reductionist approach that has been used to study

this problem has told us something of the cellular and molecular mechanisms involved, it seems likely that they are but the tip of the iceberg of a series of complex interactions which are orchestrated throughout the developing organism. Defining all the genes involved, and their interplay during development, will undoubtedly be a long haul, and require new technologies and mathematical modelling of cellular circuitry of a kind that has yet to be developed.

The inherited disorders of haemoglobin

The genetic disorders of haemoglobin can be broadly classified into three groups (Table 2.7): (1) haemoglobin variants, in which there is a structural alteration in one of the globin chains; (2) the thalassaemias, in which there is impaired synthesis of normal globins; and (3) a diverse group of conditions, which have the general title 'hereditary persistence of fetal haemoglobin' (HPFH), in which there is a defect in the developmental progression from fetal to adult haemoglobin production. As might be expected however, any simple classification is likely to have exceptions: in particular, some forms of thalassaemia are due to structural haemoglobin variants. And even the most uncomplicated forms of thalassaemia, in which normal α- or β-chain synthesis is affected, are

Table 2.7 General classification of genetic disorders of haemoglobin.*

Structural variants

Common variants associated with disease
  Hbs S, C and E

Rare variants
  Associated with disease
  'Silent'

Thalassaemias
  α thalassaemia
  β thalassaemia
  δβ thalassaemia
  εγδβ thalassaemia

Structural variants that result in a thalassaemic phenotype

Hereditary persistence of fetal haemoglobin (HPFH)

---

*More detailed classifications of the thalassaemias are given in Chapter 3 and in subsequent chapters which deal with individual varieties.

ultimately the result of abnormal globin structure. Whereas normal tetrameric haemoglobin is a highly stable, very soluble protein, the individual α or β chains, which accumulate in excess in β or α thalassaemia, respectively, are not. They precipitate in developing red-cell precursors and their progeny, leading to their premature destruction, and it is this, rather than the reduced amount of haemoglobin made, that is responsible for the ineffective erythropoiesis and haemolysis characteristic of all the thalassaemias.

Although this book deals primarily with the thalassaemias and HPFH we thought it important to include a short outline of the main properties and clinical associations of the structural haemoglobin variants. Their pathophysiology has much in common with the thalassaemias and because some of them are so common they are frequently inherited together with different forms of thalassaemia; in these compound heterozygous conditions, which are described in detail in Chapters 9 and 11, it is often the properties of the haemoglobin variant that determine the nature of the clinical manifestations.

Structural haemoglobin variants

As of early 1998, 750 haemoglobin variants had been described (Huisman *et al.* 1998), 90% of which are single amino-acid substitutions in the α, β, γ or δ chains; no embryonic variants are known. The remaining 10% are abnormal haemoglobins with two substitutions in the same globin chain, deletions or insertions, N-terminal or C-terminal elongations, or hybrid globins. Not surprisingly, the majority (~75%) of structural variants described are due to mutations in the α or β chains of the major adult component, HbA. Even so, it has been calculated that only about 20% of all possible HbA variants have been discovered. The use of increasingly sophisticated electrophoretic methods for mass screening has resulted in the detection of large numbers of these variants, most of which have normal, or near-normal, functional properties. The ones that concern us here have, for the most part, come to light because of the clinical disorders that they cause.

The structural haemoglobin variants have evolved a complex and at times exotic terminology. At first they were named by letters of the alphabet, and when these were all used up they were usually called by the

place names in which they were first discovered. Occasionally, it has not been possible to reach a compromise in cases in which there was uncertainty about the origin of the first patient. Similarly, it was at one time thought that it might be better to use the family names of the person from whom the variant was first isolated; fortunately this notion was soon dropped. This rather chequered history of the nomenclature of haemoglobin has left some interesting, if not confusing, names behind it. For example Hb Lepore Washington/Boston reflects the fact that Lepore was the family name of the patient in whom this variant was first isolated, while the two American cities are glorified because of uncertainties about the origins of the material on which the first structural studies were carried out.

As for the haemoglobinopathies in general, structural variants can be classified into three overlapping groups (Table 2.8). By far the most important are Hbs S, C and E. These three variants are all thought to provide protection against *P. falciparum* malaria in the carrier state and so have reached very high frequencies in regions where malaria is, or was, endemic (Flint *et al.* 1993b, 1998). The carrier (heterozygous) states for all three are, for the most part, symptomless. But, because of their high frequency in many populations, homozygotes are common and, in the case of HbS especially, may suffer serious clinical symptoms. The other clinically important variants are much rarer, and fall into two major groups: those that alter oxygen affinity with resulting polycythaemia or methaemoglobinaemia, and unstable haemoglobins that cause haemolytic anaemia. In addition, there are

Table 2.8 Diseases resulting from structural haemoglobin variants.

Haemolytic anaemia
HbS, HbC
Unstable haemoglobins
Hereditary polycythaemia
High-oxygen-affinity haemoglobins
Hereditary cyanosis
M haemoglobins
Low-oxygen-affinity variants
Thalassaemia phenotype
Highly unstable haemoglobins
Chain-termination haemoglobin variants
Fusion-chain haemoglobin variants

a few structural variants that, for one reason or another, are synthesized ineffectively and so have a thalassaemic phenotype.

Sickle-cell disorders

Haemoglobin S is found commonly in either the homozygous state or in the compound heterozygous state together with other structural haemoglobin variants or β thalassaemia.

This, the first variant to be characterized at the amino-acid-sequence level (Ingram 1956), is found throughout sub-Saharan Africa, parts of the Mediterranean, Middle East and India, and in populations derived therefrom (Flint *et al.* 1993b, 1998). In the homozygous state it causes considerable morbidity and mortality in these populations (Serjeant 1992), yet despite over 40 years' research the links between the β6 glutamic acid-to-valine substitution and the pathophysiological sequelae are still not fully understood.

Pathophysiology

It is beyond the scope of this chapter to deal in detail with the molecular pathogenesis of sickling and the properties of sickle-cell haemoglobin, a topic which has been reviewed extensively in recent years (Noguchi *et al.* 1993; Bunn 1997; Hebbel 1997; Hebbel & Vercellotti 1997; Dover & Platt 1998; Steinberg 1998).

Concentrated solutions of HbS form birefringent gels containing fibres of HbS molecules when deoxygenated (Edelstein *et al.* 1973; Finch *et al.* 1973). They result in reduced deformability of the red cell, and seriously affect its passage through the microcirculation (Fig. 2.24). This is the basis for the vaso-occlusion that characterizes sickle-cell disease. In addition, the altered structural properties of sickle red cells lead to a chronic haemolytic anaemia due to a shortened red-cell lifespan.

Considerable effort has been made to characterize the fibre bundles seen in deoxy HbS solutions. X-ray diffraction techniques reveal that crystals of deoxy HbS have a double-stranded structure with haemoglobin tetramers arranged in staggered pairs (Wishner *et al.* 1975). Their three-dimensional structure is constituted by a rope-like polymer composed of 14 strands. The different conformations of sickle cells, banana-shaped or resembling a holly leaf, for

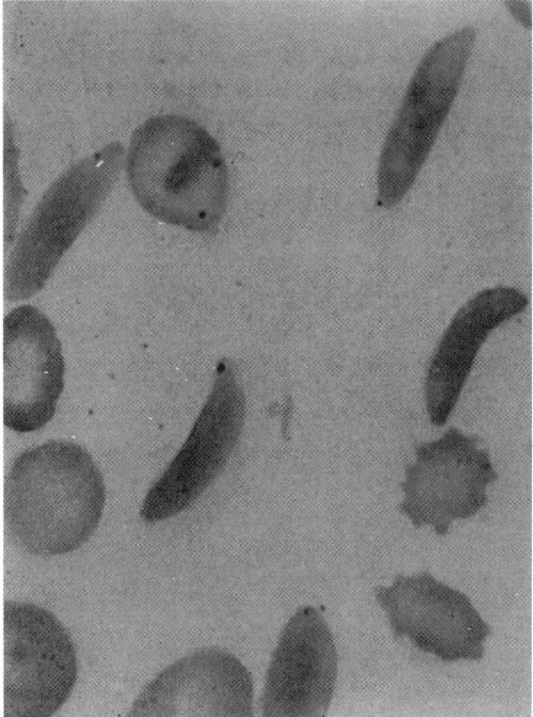

Fig. 2.24 A peripheral blood film from a patient with sickle-cell anaemia showing sickled erythrocytes (Wright's stain ×340).

example, reflect different orientations of bundles of fibres along the long axis of the red cell. Of the many intertetramer contacts in these strands, one, between the β6 valine side-chain of one β^S subunit and a hydrophobic pocket constituted by β85 phenylalanine and β88 leucine of a β^S subunit of an adjacent HbS molecule (Fig. 2.25), is sufficiently strong to stabilize the unique HbS double-stranded structure (Mirchev & Ferrone 1997). In HbA the glutamate in the β6 position is too large and strongly charged to enable it to fit into the hydrophobic β85/88 pocket. The likely relationship of the double-stranded structures seen in deoxy HbS crystals and the fibre bundles seen in solution is still unclear, although evidence drawn from physicochemical studies on the particular residues affecting HbS solubility are consistent with the unique contacts seen in the crystal structure.

HbS monomers are stable in solution under certain specific conditions of HbS concentration, pH, ionic strength and temperature. Nevertheless, quite small

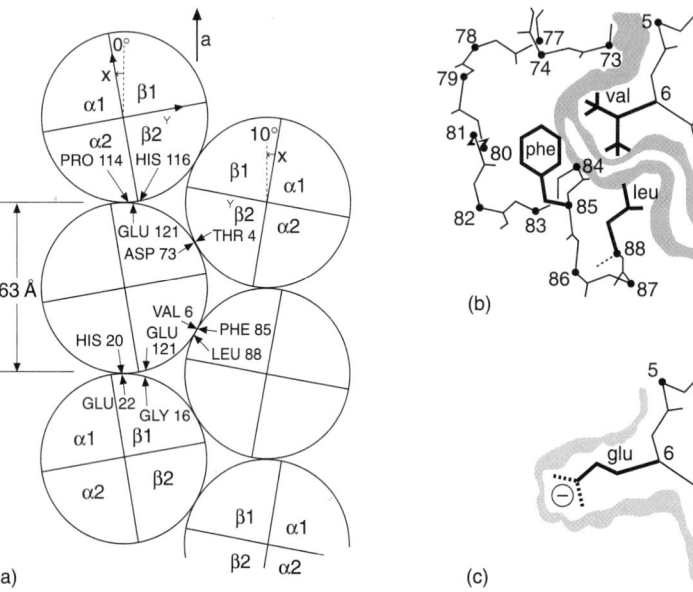

Fig. 2.25 A representation of the deoxy haemoglobin S polymer. (a,b) A single β-chain $β^6$ valine residue interacting with the $β^{85}$ phenylalanine and the $β^{88}$ leucine residue of an adjoining tetramer. (c) The normal $β^6$ glutamic acid residue, because of its charge and size, cannot make the same contact as the valine residue of HbS. From Schechter and Noguchi, *Sickle Cell Disease: Basic Principles and Clinical Practice*, New York, Raven (1999), with permission.

changes in conditions away from the ideal can lead to rapid gel formation in a manner which is not fully understood. When a solution of HbS is deoxygenated, there is a delay before polymer formation occurs; the time is inversely dependent on HbS concentration to the 30–50th power. The transition therefore appears to occur in two stages which have been related to a double nucleation mechanism (Eaton & Hofrichter 1990). Gelation is initiated by a process called homogenous nucleation, during which single deoxy-HbS molecules aggregate. Aggregation of a few molecules is thermodynamically unstable, but once a certain number of molecules aggregate, called the critical nucleus, addition of further molecules produces a more stable aggregate, or polymer. The second nucleation phase, called heterogeneous nucleation, appears to take place on the surface of pre-existing polymer. As polymerization progresses, more surface area becomes available and therefore the reaction becomes autocatalytic. Oxygenation and deoxygenation of a red cell take about the same time as the sol-to-gel transition for HbS in solution (Eaton *et al.* 1976). Thus in the high-oxygen partial pressures of the arterial circulation deoxy HbS will quickly dissolve and remain in solution until it reaches the microcirculation, where O_2 tension falls rapidly and deoxy HbS forms, haemoglobin solubility diminishes and sickle fibres form.

Polymerization of sickle haemoglobin produces damage to the red-cell membrane, the end result of which is an irreversibly sickled cell. The most important mechanism is cellular dehydration consequent on abnormalities of potassium/chloride cotransport and Ca^{++}-activated potassium efflux. Sickled cells contain increased amounts of calcium and when the cell membrane is distorted there is a transient increase in its cytosolic concentration. This is sufficient to trigger the calcium-dependent (Gardos) potassium channel, providing a mechanism for the loss of potassium and water and leading to cellular dehydration. The latter is also enhanced by increased activity of the potassium/chloride cotransport system. These complex interactions combine to produce dehydrated, rigid red cells.

The haemolytic component, which is mainly extravascular, has a complex pathophysiology. There is increasing evidence that the red-cell membrane undergoes damage by haemoglobin polymerization and by oxidation by the same mechanisms that occur in thalassaemia (see Chapter 5). This results in clustering of band 3, the anion transporter. This, in turn, results in IgG binding to membrane and the removal of red cells by macrophages with receptors for the Fc fragment of immunoglobulins.

The vascular pathology of sickling is not entirely related to the rigidity of sickled erythrocytes however; abnormal interactions between these cells and the vascular endothelium play a major role (Bunn 1997; Hebbel 1997). A variety of measurements have shown that sickle cells have sticky surfaces and that they attach themselves more readily than normal cells to cultured endothelial cells. Reticulocytes from patients with sickling disorders have, on their surface, the integrin complex α4β1, which binds to both fibronectin and a vascular-cell adhesion molecule which is expressed on the surface of endothelial cells, particularly after activation by inflammatory cytokines. Thrombospondin also binds to particular glycans on sickle cells. Other molecules, including von Willebrand factor, may also play an important role in the increased adhesion of sickled cells to the vascular endothelium.

The rate and extent of polymer formation, and hence the rate of sickling, depend on many factors including the degree of oxygenation, the cellular haemoglobin concentration and the presence or absence of HbF. The latter inhibits polymerization primarily because of a particular glutamine residue, γ87, which in some way prevents a critical natural contact in the double strand of the sickle fibre. We shall return to this question when we consider the interactions of the sickle-cell gene with β thalassaemia, in Chapter 9.

This outline summary of the pathophysiology of sickling has only touched on the tip of the iceberg of the complexity of this dynamic process. There is remarkable cellular heterogeneity with respect to polymer content, delay time and membrane damage, set in an equally variable and changing environment, in which the vascular endothelium, white cells, platelets, coagulation pathways and balance of local vasodilators and vasoconstrictors may all play a role in the sickling processes (Fig. 2.26).

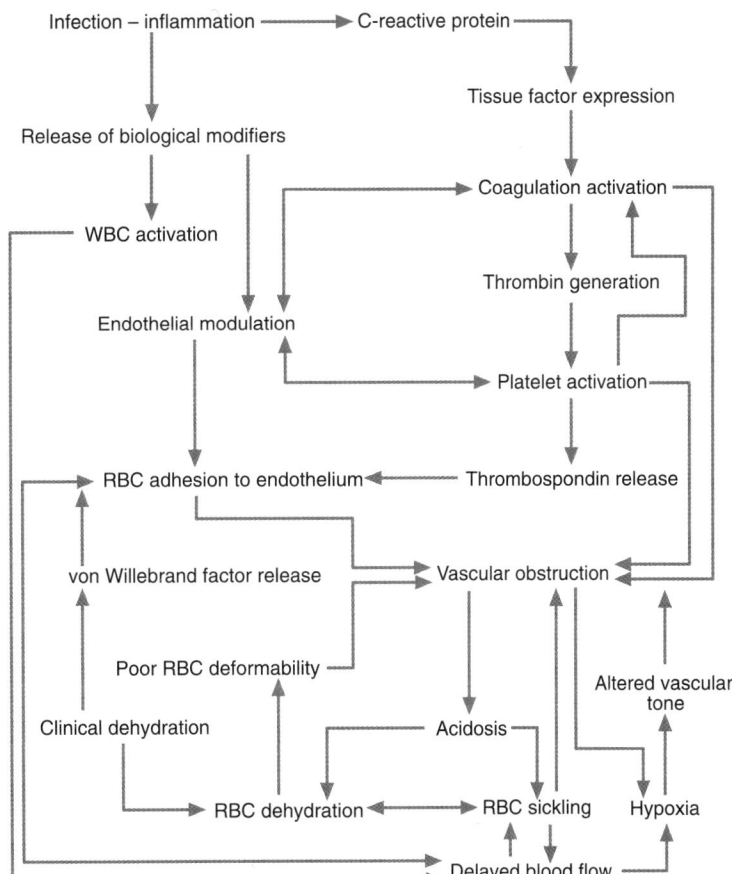

Fig. 2.26 The complexity of the numerous factors which interact to generate vaso-occlusion in sickle-cell anaemia. RBC = red blood cells; WBC = white blood cells. Reproduced from Embury *et al. Sickle Cell Disease; Basic Principles and Clinical Practice*, New York, Raven (1999), with permission.

Clinical features

It is beyond the scope of this chapter to deal in detail with the protean clinical manifestations of the sickling disorders. Some of them are described in detail in Chapter 9, as they relate to sickle-cell β thalassaemia, and readers who wish to learn more about this complex disease are referred to the monographs of Serjeant (1992) and Embury *et al.* (1996) and to the extensive review of Dover and Platt (1998). Here we simply outline the main features of the disease to form a basis for the descriptions of the interaction of the sickle-cell gene with the different forms of thalassaemia that are described in later chapters.

In describing the clinical features of the sickling disorders it is necessary to consider the sickle-cell trait, sickle-cell anaemia, and the interactions of the sickle-cell gene with other structural haemoglobin variants, particularly HbC.

Sickle-cell trait

Except in conditions of extreme oxygen deprivation, there are no clinical abnormalities which can be ascribed with certainty to the sickle-cell trait. Manifestations of intravascular sickling have been reported in persons exposed to low oxygen tensions in unpressurized aircraft or in other extreme conditions, but, otherwise, there are no clinical associations.

Sickle-cell anaemia

The homozygous state for the sickle-cell gene is characterized by chronic haemolytic anaemia, an increased propensity to infection, a number of complications due to chronic vascular occlusion, and acute exacerbations, or crises, which may take several different forms.

Patients with sickle-cell anaemia are anaemic from the first few months of life. Pallor and mild icterus may be the presenting symptom, or the disease may be heralded by one or other form of vaso-occlusive crisis. One of the commonest in early life is the so-called 'hand-and-foot' syndrome, in which there is painful swelling of the phalanges as a result of an underlying dactylitis involving the growing ends of the small bones of the hands and feet. While there are often no sequelae, occasionally these episodes may lead to lifelong shortening of one of the digits. Some-

times, the presenting symptom may be an overwhelming infection, which is a major cause of morbidity and mortality at all ages.

Remarkably, patients with sickle-cell anaemia seem to function extremely well at haemoglobin values of 6–9 g/dl, and although there may be some abnormalities of growth and development, overall, they go through a normal puberty and do not develop the skeletal deformities of under-treated patients with thalassaemia. This effective adaptation to their anaemia is due, at least in part, to the fact that HbS has a relatively low oxygen affinity with a right-shifted oxygen dissociation curve.

There are relatively few physical signs in patients with uncomplicated sickle-cell anaemia. There are pallor and mild icterus and, in early life, splenomegaly. However, probably due to repeated bouts of infarction, the spleen regresses and is rarely palpable after childhood. Apart from some non-specific cardiac signs associated with a hyperdynamic circulation resulting from the anaemia, there are no other characteristic findings.

Acute and life-threatening complications occur during the course of the illness. As already mentioned, serious infections, possibly related to hyposplenism, may occur at any time; these patients are prone to infection by a variety of organisms, particularly *Salmonella, Klebsiella, H. influenzae* and *M. pneumoniae*. Crises take several forms (Table 2.9). In *vaso-occlusive crisis* there is widespread bone pain, which probably results from marrow infarction with an overlying inflammatory reaction. Precipitating factors include cold, dehydration and infection. These episodes, which usually last for several days, are self-limiting. *Lung crises* are a common cause of mortality and are characterized by dyspnoea, hypoxaemia, pulmonary infiltrates on the chest X-ray and a falling haemoglobin and platelet count. They are thought to

Table 2.9 Sickle-cell crises.

Hand-and-foot syndrome
Painful
Lung
Brain
Sequestration
Spleen
Liver
Aplastic

reflect sequestration of sickled erythrocytes in the pulmonary circulation. The *brain syndrome*, which reflects strokes related to hypertrophic changes in the carotid circulation or cerebral haemorrhages, may present with almost any variety of acute neurological defect. In young children especially, acute sequestration of sickled erythrocytes in the spleen may cause the rapid splenic enlargement and anaemia characteristic of the *splenic sequestration syndrome*. A similar condition occurs in adults, in whom the red cells are sequestered into the liver, leading to its rapid enlargement and severe anaemia. Finally, patients may become rapidly anaemic as part of an *aplastic crisis*, a temporary period of red-cell aplasia often associated with parvovirus infection. Another distressing acute complication, though not usually classified as a 'crisis', is recurrent priapism, which may, if not adequately treated, lead to permanent deformity of the penis.

As well as these acute complications, there are a number of serious long-term disabilities associated with chronic vascular occlusion. These include aseptic necrosis of the femoral or humeral heads, progressive renal failure, intractable leg ulcers and a characteristic proliferative retinopathy. Chronic osteomyelitis due to infection with *S. typhi* also occurs in some populations.

The haematological findings are characterized by moderate to severe anaemia, with haemoglobin levels in the 6–10 g/dl range, reticulocytosis in the 10–20% range, and the presence of variable numbers of sickled cells on the blood film. The haemoglobin consists of Hbs S and A_2, with variable levels of HbF, ranging from a few per cent to over 25% of the total haemoglobin (Fig. 2.27). The laboratory findings are considered further in Chapter 9. The reasons for the variable levels of HbF are similar to those for β thalassaemia, and are discussed in Chapters 5, 10 and 13.

The clinical course of this disease varies widely and there is very limited information about the reasons for this remarkable heterogeneity. Factors which seem to ameliorate the disease, at least to some degree, include unusually high levels of HbF, the coexistence of α thalassaemia, and, perhaps most importantly, the environment, climate and availability of adequate health care. These issues are reflected in the prognosis of the disease. While little is known about the mortality in the developing countries, it is

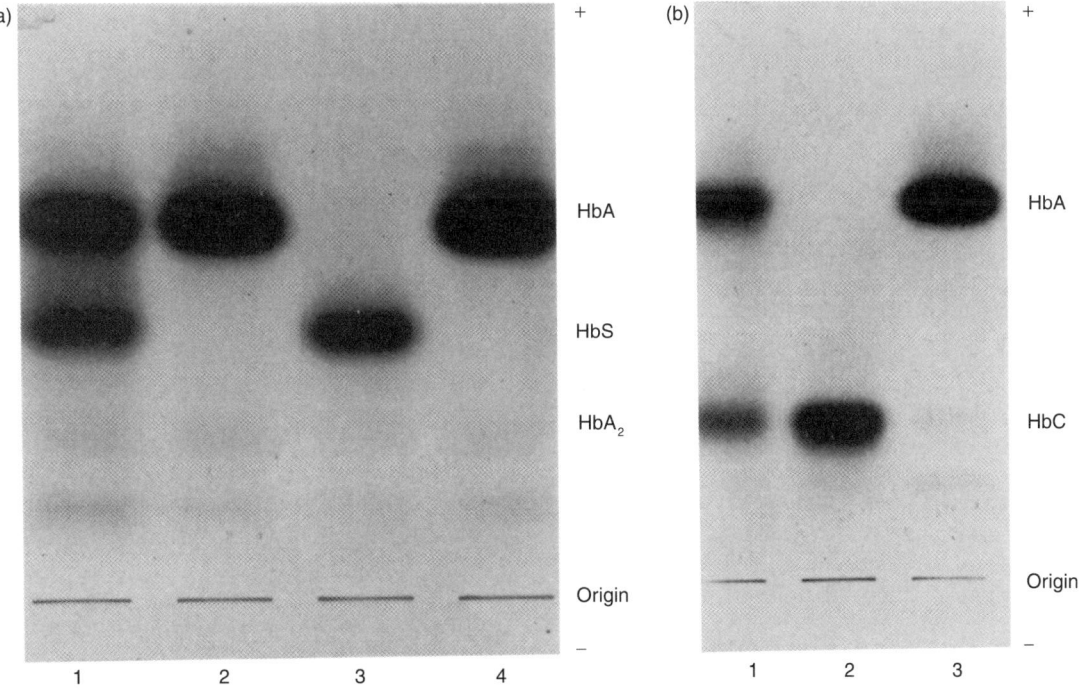

Fig. 2.27 Starch gel electrophoresis of haemoglobin variants. (a) (Left to right) 1. Sickle-cell trait; 2. normal; 3. sickle-cell disease; 4. normal. (b) (Left to right) 1. HbC trait; 2. HbC disease; 3. normal.

clear that in sub-Saharan Africa many children die early in life. Both in the USA and in Jamaica there appears to be a peak incidence of death between 1 and 3 years, usually as a result of infection. Recent data from the United States suggest that, in adults, the median age of death is 42 years for males, and 48 years for females. Among adults, those with the lowest levels of fetal haemoglobin and highest rates of painful crises and chest syndrome appear to have the greatest risk of dying at an early age. There is increased morbidity during pregnancy and a higher than normal rate of fetal loss.

Haemoglobin SC disease

After sickle-cell anaemia, this is the most important of the sickling disorders (Serjeant 1992). It is characterized by a much milder anaemia and fewer crises than sickle-cell anaemia. Indeed, many patients with this disorder pass through childhood and early adult life undetected. However, there are some important complications, including a high frequency of aseptic necrosis of the femoral and humoral heads, haematuria, proliferative retinopathy leading to diminution of vision or blindness, and a thrombotic tendency which, particularly in pregnancy and the puerperium, may lead to massive pulmonary thromboembolic disease and death.

There are no major clinical findings except for splenomegaly. The blood picture shows a mild degree of anaemia with striking morphological abnormalities of the red cells characterized by many target forms and intracellular crystals, sickled forms, and a modest reticulocytosis, much lower than that which occurs in sickle-cell anaemia.

Other interactions of the sickle-cell gene

The sickle-cell gene has been found in association with many other β-globin variants. The clinical features are reviewed by Serjeant (1992) and Dover and Platt (1998). The interactions of the sickle-cell gene with β thalassaemia are described in detail in Chapter 9 and with α thalassaemia in Chapter 11.

Haemoglobins C and E

Haemoglobin C

This variant (β6 glu→lys) occurs mainly in West Africa (Itano 1951; Ranney 1954). *In vitro* studies show that haemoglobin C is less soluble, with a tendency to crystal formation, than HbA (Diggs *et al.* 1954; Hirsch *et al.* 1985). It also has a lower oxygen affinity than HbA. In HbC homozygotes the red cells contain less water and export higher levels of K^+ ions than normal red cells. Possibly these changes result from the interaction of HbC crystals with the inner membrane surface, with consequential reduced deformability of the cell (Reiss *et al.* 1982). This in turn probably causes the associated haemolysis and increased red-cell turnover. Heterozygotes in which the proportion of HbC is about 30% are symptomatic.

The homozygous state for HbC, HbC disease, is characterized by a mild haemolytic anaemia associated with moderate splenomegaly. It is rarely symptomatic, except during periods of stress, such as pregnancy. The haematological changes are characterized by a moderate reduction in the haemoglobin level, a reticulocytosis and a characteristic appearance of the peripheral blood film, which shows large numbers of target cells and intracellular crystals.

This variant migrates in the same position as HbA_2 on most of the commonly used electrophoretic media (Fig. 2.27), though the two can be separated by isoelectric focusing or HPLC.

Haemoglobin E

This is probably the most common haemoglobin variant in the world population, notwithstanding its confinement to parts of the Indian subcontinent and south-east Asia (Chernoff *et al.* 1954; Sturgeon *et al.* 1955). Its pathophysiology is not fully understood, partly because the phenotype results from a combination of mild thalassaemia (Traeger *et al.* 1980) and abnormal haemoglobin. The β-chain codon 26 Glu→Lys mutation (GAG→AAG) partially activates a cryptic splice site towards the 3′ end of exon 1, resulting in a proportion of abnormally spliced mRNA (Orkin *et al.* 1982b). Thus, less β^E globin is synthesized and a mild thalassaemia phenotype results. In addition, *in vitro* experiments have shown that HbE is mildly unstable and may be susceptible to oxidant damage.

Haemoglobin-E heterozygotes, with about 30% HbE, are clinically normal and have only minor haematological changes. Homozygotes have a very mild anaemia, but are otherwise well; their haematological changes are similar to those of heterozygous β thalassaemia (see Chapter 7). It is the compound heterozygous state between HbE and β thalassaemia that gives rise to really serious clinical disease (Weatherall & Clegg 1981), with a phenotype ranging from mild anaemia to the most severe form of β thalassaemia major. This important and neglected condition is discussed in detail, together with a more extensive account of the properties of HbE, in Chapter 9.

Unstable haemoglobin variants

The story of the discovery and first characterization of these variants is outlined in the reviews of White & Dacie (1971) and White (1976). These disorders have usually only been described in the heterozygous (carrier) state. At a gross level, then, they have a dominant phenotype. It seems likely that some of the most severely abnormal variants of this kind would be incompatible with survival in the homozygous state.

Many haemoglobin variants show some features of instability, but a clear definition is not straightforward. From a clinical point of view the term 'unstable haemoglobin disorder' is reserved for those variants that cause clinically recognizable haemolysis. In the laboratory, they can be identified by a number of methods, such as the presence of Heinz bodies in red cells after splenectomy, heat instability of the variant in red-cell lysates, or instability in the presence of organic compounds such as isopropanol. Not all these methods detect all variants, so that qualifications such as 'mild' or 'severe' often accompany their description.

Pathophysiology

A number of different mechanisms result in instability (Carrell & Lehmann 1969; White 1976; Bunn & Forget 1986; Winterbourn 1990), but the majority of variants fall broadly into four categories: (1) substitutions that result in the replacement of an interior hydrophobic residue by a hydrophilic one; (2) disruption of secondary structure of one of the subunit chains; (3) replacement of residues in and around the haem pocket; and (4) gross alterations to subunit structure as, for example, occurs with some large deletions or C-terminal elongations of globins (Fig. 2.28).

As noted earlier, the interior of a globin subunit is largely a non-polar environment, with inter-residue contacts made via van der Waals forces. The consequence of introducing a polar residue into this hydrophobic milieu can, and often does, have drastic consequences for the tertiary structure of the haemoglobin molecule, especially if it allows water to enter the interior of the subunit. More subtle changes, even involving neutral-for-neutral changes, may cause instability if the stereochemical relationships between residues are substantially altered. Some of the most severe changes in subunit structure involve proline substitutions. About 75% of the globin subunits are α helix, and proline cannot form part of an α helix except in the first three residues. Almost 40 variants have been reported involving substitutions to proline and almost all are severely unstable. In contrast, substitution of a proline often does not result in instability, although there may be associated functional changes.

The haem–globin association involves very specific interactions with non-polar residues in the pocket formed by parts of the CD, E, F and FG helical regions. Most of the residues are invariant; substitutions at them almost inevitably result in changes in the orientation of the haem relative to the globin subunit. In the worst cases (the majority) these changes are sufficiently pronounced to alter haem binding and affect the stability of the entire subunit.

Unstable haemoglobins precipitate in red cells with the formation of rigid Heinz bodies, which affects cell deformability and ultimately leads to their premature destruction (Miller *et al.* 1971; Rachmilewitz 1974; Winterbourn & Carrell 1974; Milner & Wrightstone 1981; Flynn *et al.* 1983; Winterbourn 1990). Although the precise mechanism is unclear, it appears that an increased tendency to auto-oxidation to methaemoglobin may be the initial change that leads to haemoglobin precipitation. The formation of methaemoglobin (when the normal Fe^{++} iron of the haem is converted to Fe^{+++}) is associated with the production of a superoxide ion. This, and the superoxide reduction product, H_2O_2, can then generate more methaemoglobin. Unstable haemoglobins show a greater inherent tendency to oxidize. Moreover, the methaemoglobin so formed can be converted into insoluble haemichromes by a two-stage process that ultimately forms irreversible bonding of amino side-chains to the normally unbonded (distal) side of the haem moiety. These properties, and the effects of these changes on red-cell membrane function, have

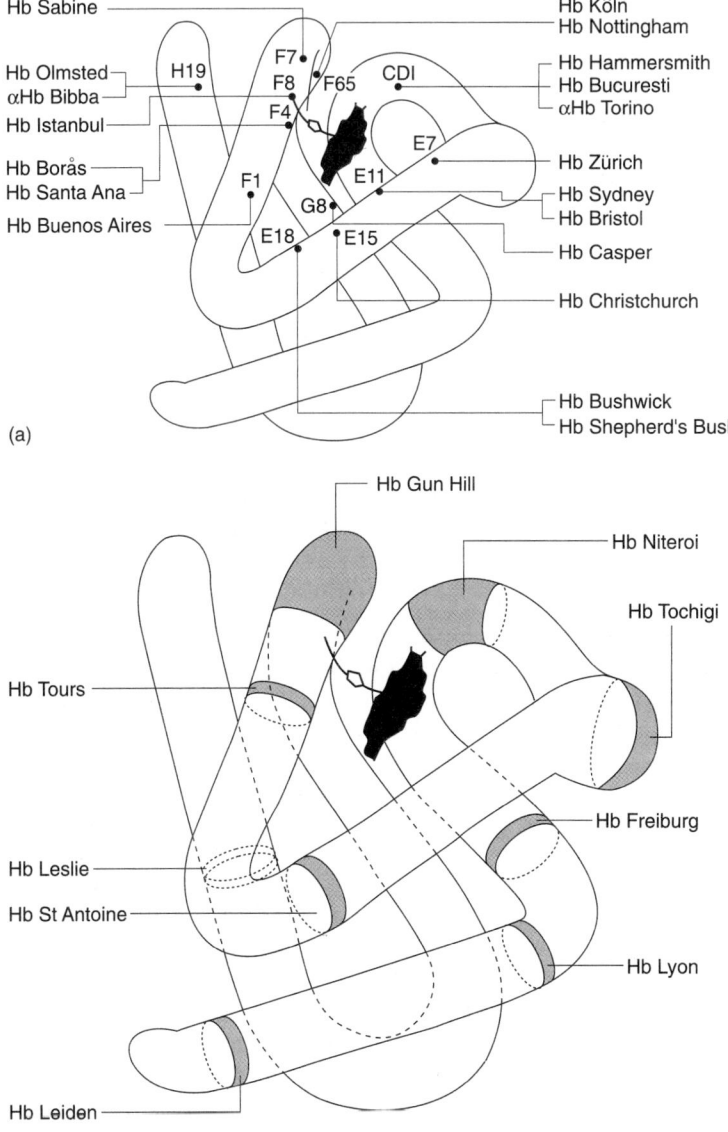

Hb Sabine

Hb Köln
Hb Nottingham

F7
Hb Olmsted
αHb Bibba
H19
F8   F65   CDI
F4
Hb Istanbul

Hb Hammersmith
Hb Bucuresti
αHb Torino

E7

Hb Borås
Hb Santa Ana
F1
G8
E11

Hb Zürich

Hb Sydney
Hb Bristol

Hb Buenos Aires

E18   E15

Hb Casper

Hb Christchurch

Hb Bushwick
Hb Shepherd's Bush

(a)

Hb Gun Hill

Hb Niteroi

Hb Tochigi

Hb Tours

Hb Freiburg

Hb Leslie

Hb St Antoine

Hb Lyon

Hb Leiden

(b)

Fig. 2.28 Unstable haemoglobin variants. (a) A three-dimensional representation of the β chain showing sites of amino-acid substitutions and the haem pocket. (b) A three-dimensional representation of the β chain, showing sites of amino-acid deletions that cause unstable haemoglobins. From Milner and Wrightstone, *The Function of the Red Blood Cells*; *Erythrocyte Pathobiology*, p. 197, Alan R. Liss, New York (1981), with permission.

much in common with those of excess α or β chains that are produced in different forms of thalassaemia and hence they are discussed in more detail in Chapter 5.

Clinical features

Patients with unstable haemoglobin variants have a mild to moderately severe haemolytic anaemia asso-

ciated with splenomegaly. Although this is usually compatible with a normal life, a few are so severely affected as to necessitate regular blood transfusion. The anaemia is exacerbated by intercurrent infection, the administration of oxidant drugs or, in some cases, by an elevated body temperature. Although there have been a few reports of splenectomy in this condition the numbers are too small to provide clear guidance as to its effectiveness. The blood picture shows a variable reduction in the haemoglobin level, a reticulocytosis and non-specific morphological abnormalities of the red cells. Preformed Heinz bodies are only seen after splenectomy. Many unstable haemoglobin variants cannot be identified by conventional haemoglobin electrophoresis, but they can be demonstrated by their heat instability or the other tests mentioned earlier.

Highly unstable globins

As we shall see in later chapters, the clinical results of the synthesis of highly unstable globins, or truncated or elongated globin chains, vary considerably (Adams & Coleman 1990; Weatherall *et al.* 2000). Because of their extreme instability, the existence of the 'variants' has had to be inferred from radio-labelling studies or, in extreme cases, from DNA analysis. Whether these highly unstable globins cause the phenotype of haemolytic anaemia or the hypochromic red-cell characteristics of thalassaemia seems to depend on their degree of instability.

As we shall see in Chapter 4, many forms of thalassaemia are due to mutations which cause premature termination of β-chain production. It turns out that those which would produce truncated β chains of up to about 72 amino acids long have the relatively mild phenotype of β-thalassaemia trait. Although originally this was thought to be because intracellular proteolytic mechanisms would be effective in degrading these truncated proteins and the resulting excess of α chains, it now appears that mutations of this type may actually interfere with the movement of messenger RNA into the cell cytoplasm and hence there may be no gene product synthesized. This is not the case for mutations which cause chain termination in exon 3 or are associated with the synthesis of some elongated globin chains. In this case, relatively long and highly unstable globin-gene products may be produced which are capable of binding haem, but not of combining with α chains to produce any kind of stable haemoglobin tetramer. Hence these large truncation products tend to precipitate in the red-cell precursors, together with excess α chains, to produce large inclusion bodies. This is the basis for the dominant forms of β thalassaemia that we shall describe in more detail in later chapters.

If the unstable globin products are able to combine with normal α- or β-globin subunits to produce a tetramer that is sufficiently stable to survive through the different stages of erythropoiesis and to appear in mature red cells, then its instability is reflected in a shortened red-cell survival and a haemolytic anaemia, rather than the ineffective erythropoiesis characteristic of the dominant forms of β thalassaemia. There may well be conditions with phenotypes which show a mixture of both characteristics.

In short, highly unstable haemoglobin disorders show a wide spectrum of phenotypes ranging from severe dyserythropoiesis characteristic of thalassaemia, through intermediate disorders with mixed dyserythropoiesis and haemolysis, to haemolytic anaemias of varying severity (Thein 1999). We shall discuss these heterogeneous conditions again in Chapters 4, 7, 11 and 13.

Haemoglobin variants with altered oxygen affinity

High-oxygen-affinity variants

The first evidence that some forms of hereditary polycythaemia might result from haemoglobin variants was reported by Charache *et al.* (1966). Some of the unstable variants described in the previous section have an increased oxygen affinity; nevertheless, the accompanying clinical manifestations result from haemolysis and not from the functional alterations. A much larger group of variants are now known, however, in which increased oxygen affinity is not associated with instability. Many of them result in polycythaemia (Charache *et al.* 1966; Adamson 1975; Bunn & Forget 1986; Huisman *et al.* 1998), a condition characterized by erythrocytosis and an elevated haemoglobin level. Under normal physiological conditions of pH and temperature, normal red cells *in vivo* have a p50 (the partial O_2 pressure at which haemoglobin is half-saturated with oxygen) of 26 mmHg. In individuals with polycythaemia due to an abnormal variant p50s may be as low as 10 mm. If, as is usually the case, the red-cell 2,3-DPG levels are normal, there is thus a substantial left shift to the oxygen-dissociation curve (Fig. 2.29).

Pathophysiology

As we have seen, haemoglobin can exist in two quaternary states, R and T, characteristic of the oxy and deoxy forms, respectively. When fully deoxygenated, haemoglobin assumes the T (tense) configuration,

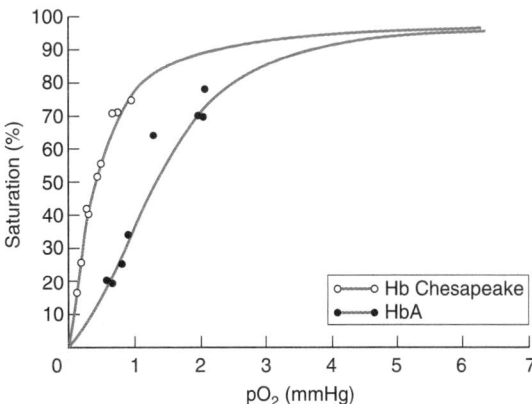

Saturation (%) — pO$_2$ (mmHg)

○——○ Hb Chesapeake
●——● HbA

Fig. 2.29 The oxygen dissociation curve of the high-affinity variant, haemoglobin Chesapeake, compared with that of haemoglobin A.

which has a relatively low oxygen affinity and a high affinity for allosteric effectors such as 2,3-DPG and Bohr protons. In oxyhaemoglobin, the converse applies; high oxygen affinity and low affinity for protons and 2,3-DPG. The transition between the two involves the intersubunit cooperation that is the basis of the haem–haem interaction (see p. 78). Most high-affinity variants thus involve substitutions that affect the R–T equilibrium. The majority of them occur at the $\alpha_1\beta_2$ ($\alpha_2\beta_1$) interface, 2,3-DPG binding sites or at the C-terminal end of the β chain.

If an amino acid substitution in haemoglobin decreases the stability of the deoxy (T) structure, the transition to the R state will occur earlier during oxygenation and the tetramer will have a higher oxygen affinity. An example that has been well studied is Hb Kempsey (Bunn *et al.* 1974), a β-chain variant with an Asp→Asn substitution at the $\alpha_1\beta_2$ contact residue β99 (G1). In HbA this residue is hydrogen-bonded to α42 (C7) tyrosine in the deoxy (T) state. During oxygenation, the α and β subunits in this region shift relative to one another so that the β99–α42 bond is broken and replaced by a link between β102(G4)Asn and α94(G1)Asp. In Hb Kempsey, the β99–α42 bond cannot form, resulting in a reduced stability of the T structure, so that even when fully deoxygenated the tetramer is still partly in the R state.

Many high-oxygen-affinity variants have a decreased Bohr effect. For example, substitutions at the C-terminal end of the β chain may affect the formation of the important salt bridge between the β146

(HC3) histidine and the COO⁻ group of β94(FG1) aspartate in deoxyhaemoglobin, a link that is responsible for 50% of the alkaline Bohr effect. Hb Hiroshima, β146 (HC3) His→Asp, is one such example (Imai *et al.* 1972). Also, variants that cannot fully assume the T structure upon deoxygenation, Hb Kempsey for example, fail to liberate all Bohr protons on deoxygenation.

Several variants with increased oxygen affinity have substitutions that interfere with 2,3-DPG binding. 2,3-DPG stabilizes the deoxy (T) structure. In Hb Rahere β82 (EF6) Lys→Thr, one of the crucial 2,3-DPG binding sites is lost, and the deoxyhaemoglobin has little affinity for the ligand (Lorkin *et al.* 1975). Thus, in contrast to normal haemoglobin, 2,3-DPG cannot reduce (right shift) the oxygen affinity of Hb Rahere. Consequently, the whole blood oxygen affinity curve is shifted to the left.

Clinical features

All these variants are associated with a moderate degree of polycythaemia. This can be easily distinguished from the myeloproliferative forms of polycythaemia by the lack of changes in the white cells and platelets and absence of splenomegaly. It may occasionally be confused with secondary polycythaemias due to cardiac or pulmonary disease or erythropoietin-producing neoplasms. There is also another rare group of hereditary polycythaemias caused by various abnormalities of erythropoietin regulation. None of these other forms of polycythaemia are associated with an increased oxygen affinity of haemoglobin.

The polycythaemia associated with haemoglobin variants of this type very rarely requires treatment. There is no evidence that these patients develop vascular occlusive disease. Although it might be expected that these variants might be associated with fetal hypoxia, there does not seem to be an increased frequency of stillbirth in affected families.

Low-affinity variants

There are far fewer variants with reduced oxygen affinity. Many of the unstable variants fall into this group (but, as above, their primary clinical disorder results from haemolysis) and some of the Hbs M (see below) also have low affinities. Hb Kansas β102(G4)Asn→Thr is one of the best studied (Reismann *et al.* 1961; Bonaventura & Riggs 1968). Interestingly, this substitution is in the $\alpha_1\beta_2$ ($\alpha_2\beta_1$) interface, as are many of the substitutions in high-affinity variants. Although the mechanism is not clear, it appears that the Hb Kansas mutation destabilizes the R structure. Two other variants at this position, Hbs Beth Israel and St Mandé, have similar clinical phenotypes. Low-affinity variants have a right-shifted O_2-dissociation curve and in the worst cases carriers are cyanosed from birth. These patients are not usually symptomatic, but the cause of their cyanosis has to be distinguished from that due to haemoglobin M or the family of red-cell enzyme defects that may cause this symptom; the latter can be excluded by a simple family history since they are inherited in a recessive fashion.

Haemoglobins M

This group of variants, 22 of which have been identified (Huisman *et al.* 1998), result in congenital cyanosis associated with methaemoglobinaemia (Nagel & Bookchin 1974; Bunn & Forget 1986). As shown in Figs 2.6 and 2.7, the haem moiety sits in a pocket between the E and F helices, with the iron atom of the haem linked to a histidine residue (the 'proximal histidine') of the α- and β-chain F helixes. On the opposite side of the haem, near the 6th coordination position of the iron atom where oxygen binds, lies another histidine (the distal histidine). This residue is not bonded to the iron, except in those conditions where irreversible haemichromes are formed.

Pathophysiology

Many of the M haemoglobins result from mutations at the proximal or distal histidines, to tyrosine residues. These and related substitutions stabilize the haem iron in the Fe^{+++} form, and it is then resistant to reduction. Perhaps surprisingly, in view of the homology between the structures of the α- and β-globin subunits, the His→Tyr substitutions at the proximal (F8) haem binding sites do not have similar functional consequences; likewise, mutations at the E7 distal binding site. The major factor is which type of globin subunit is affected. The α-chain variants (M Boston: 58(E7)His→Tyr and M Iwate 87(F8)His→Tyr) in which only the β chains can bind oxygen have a reduced oxygen affinity, whereas the β-chain variants (M Saskatoon 63(E7) and M Hyde

Park 92(F8)), in which only α globin binds O_2, have a near-normal oxygen-dissociation curve.

X-ray crystallographic analyses go some way to explain these paradoxical findings. In the deoxy state, both variants with the proximal (F8)His→Tyr mutation are structurally isomorphous with deoxy HbA. Thus, even though the haems of the affected subunits are oxidized, they must be in the 'T' state. In the β-chain variant M Iwate, the molecule retains the T state even when fully oxidized, and it is likely that this is the case when it is fully oxygenated. This explains why it has a low O_2 affinity and reduced Bohr effect (both characteristic of the T state in normal HbA). The α-chain variant M Hyde Park differs in that it can switch to the R state when fully oxidized. Since it displays a substantial Bohr effect it also seems likely that HbM Hyde Park can switch from the T to R state upon full oxygenation.

In HbM Boston, which has a tyrosine substitution in the α-globin *distal* histidine, the deoxyhaemoglobin molecule is again isomorphous with deoxy HbA. Remarkably, X-ray data show that the α haem Fe^{+++} has bonded to the E7 tyrosine phenolate group (i.e. the substituent side-chain); that is, it is no longer bonded to the F8 proximal histidine, having shifted its position toward the distal side of the porphyrin ring. In the oxy form, HbM Boston is probably fully in the T state; consequently its oxygen affinity is low and the Bohr effect diminished.

Clinical features

Individuals heterozygous for the M haemoglobins are cyanosed from early in life; if the mutation involves the α-globin genes, cyanosis is present at birth, whereas in the β-chain variants it only becomes manifest after the second or third month of life. These conditions can often be distinguished from congenital methaemoglobinaemia resulting from an enzyme defect, simply from the family history; the pattern of inheritance for HbM is typically dominant, whereas methaemoglobinaemia due to enzyme deficiency is always recessive. Overall, individuals with one or other of the M haemoglobins are not symptomatic although they may be embarrassed by the persistent cyanosis.

The M haemoglobins give a characteristic spectral abnormality provided that the haemoglobin is completely oxidized to the Fe^{+++} state. They cannot be demonstrated by haemoglobin electrophoresis under routine conditions, but they do separate if the red-cell lysate is first oxidized with ferricyanide.

Haemoglobin variants with elongated or shortened globin chains

Although most haemoglobin variants are the result of single amino-acid substitutions (and thus single base changes), a few have arisen by more complex mutation processes such as unequal crossing over producing insertions or deletions. In addition, there is a small group of variants which, although due to single base changes, have extensions at the N-terminal or C-terminal ends (Table 2.10).

For the most part, variants with internal deletions in a globin chain have impaired function or stability, some severely so, usually because of alterations in the helical (secondary) structure of the subunit.

Table 2.10 Examples of shortened and elongated globin variants. From Huisman *et al.* (1998).

Elongated chains

Single base-pair mutations or frameshifts at the 3′ end of exon 3

Hb Wayne	Codon 139 (−A) α1 or α2
Hb Constant Spring	Codon 142 T→A α2
Hb Cranston	Codons 144–145 (+CT) β
Hb Tak	Codon 147 (+AC) β

Single base-pair mutations or frameshifts at the 5′ end of exon 1

Hb Thionville	+1 (GTG→GAG) α2 or α1
Hb Doha	+1 (GTG→GAG) β
Hb S. Florida	+1 (GTG→ATG) β
Hb Marseille	+2 (CAC→CCC) β

Insertions

Hb Catonsville	α37–α38 +˙Glu
Hb Zaïre	α116–α117 +˙His-Leu-Pro-Ala-Glu
Hb Grady	α118–α119 +˙Glu-Phe-Thr

Shortened chains

Deletions of one or more amino-acid residues

Hb Taybe	α38 or 39 Thr→O
Hb Leiden	β6 or β7 Glu→O
Hb Freiburg	β23 Val→O
Hb Vicksburg	β75 Leu→O
Hb Gun Hill	β91–95 Leu-His-Cys-Asp-Lys→O

Longer or shorter chains due to deletions and insertions
Hb Montreal˙–˙Asp-Gly-Leu at β73–75˙+˙Ala-Arg-Cys-Gln
Hb Galicia˙–˙His-Val at β97–98˙+˙Leu

Mutations in the first or second codons of the α or β chains sometimes result in an N-terminal extension of methionine, in addition to the altered N-terminal or second residue, because the new N-terminal sequence prevents removal of the initiator methionine. None of these variants has had functional studies reported. Of more interest are those variants with C-terminal extensions (Huisman *et al.* 1998). One or two, such as Hbs Wayne and Saverne result from single base deletions close to the end of the last exon; the resulting frame-shifted mRNA is then read until the first in-phase termination codon is reached, resulting in α and β globins with altered C-terminal sequences beyond residues 139 and 142, respectively. In Hb Wayne the α chain is extended to 146 residues, while in Saverne the β chain has an added 11 amino acids. Both these variants have increased oxygen affinities, and Hb Saverne is also unstable. Similar functional changes accompany two β-chain variants, Hbs Cranston and Tak, with 2-base insertions close to the end of the third exon. Both have 11-residue C-terminal extensions, and are characterized by increased oxygen affinity and slight instability.

Finally, there is a group of variants that have 31 amino acid extensions to the normal α-globin sequence. These all result from mutations in the normal termination codon, leading to readthrough of α mRNA until the next in-phase termination codon is reached. Although stable, these variants are synthesized at very low levels, with a resulting thalassaemic phenotype (Weatherall & Clegg 1975). The most common of these chain-termination variants, Hb Constant Spring, is found throughout South-East Asia and, when it interacts with an α⁰-thalassaemia determinant, leads to a particularly severe form of HbH disease, a topic we shall consider further in Chapters 4 and 11.

The structural haemoglobin variants and thalassaemias form a phenotypic continuum

Clearly, the structural haemoglobin variants and different forms of thalassaemia form a continuum of complex phenotypes. In the next chapter we shall outline how thalassaemia is classified, and how this is based on the interactions of the different varieties of the disease with the structural haemoglobin variants.

Chapter 3
Thalassaemia: classification, genetics and relationship to other inherited disorders of haemoglobin

A useful working definition of the thalassaemias is that they are a family of genetic disorders, all characterized by a reduced rate of production on one or more of the globin subunits of haemoglobin. Like the other major class of inherited disorders of haemoglobin, the structural variants, nearly all the thalassaemias result from mutations at or close to the genes that encode for the different globins. Taken together, these two groups constitute the haemoglobinopathies (see Table 2.7, p. 107). Like most biological classifications, the division of these diseases into two watertight compartments is not entirely satisfactory. In reality, they form a continuum; at least a few common forms of thalassaemia result from structural haemoglobin variants that are either synthesized ineffectively or are so unstable that they cause a severe deficiency of one or other globin subunit, and hence a thalassaemic phenotype.

This chapter outlines how the thalassaemias are classified and the principles of their genetic transmission, and therefore serves as an introduction to later sections which describe each of the different types in detail and provide references to the original work on which these concepts are based, in addition to those found in Chapter 1. Because structural haemoglobin variants often occur commonly in the same populations as the thalassaemias, and a wide spectrum of disorders result from their co-inheritance, we shall also introduce the principles of the genetic basis for these important interactions. As well as their clinical importance, because of their central role in clarifying the genetics of the thalassaemias, and hence in setting the scene for their subsequent investigation at the clinical and molecular level, they must be thoroughly understood by anyone who is approaching this increasingly complex field for the first time.

The structural haemoglobin variants were discussed in the previous chapter. The information about their pathophysiology and clinical manifestations that is required to understand the consequences of their interactions with the thalassaemias will be found in later chapters. Readers who wish to learn more about them are referred to recent monographs and reviews which cover the abnormal haemoglobin field in more detail (Higgs & Weatherall 1993; Huisman et al. 1997; Steinberg et al. 2001; Weatherall et al. 2001).

General characteristics of the thalassaemias

As we saw in Chapter 1, studies of the interactions between different thalassaemia alleles and structural haemoglobin variants, later combined with in vitro analysis of the relative rates of synthesis of the different globins, allowed the thalassaemias to be subdivided into two broad groups, α and β thalassaemia. Although each can be further classified into different subgroups, all these disorders have one thing in common; there is always imbalanced globin synthesis. This is the hallmark of thalassaemia, and it is the deleterious consequences of the globin that is produced in excess that are responsible for the ineffective erythropoiesis and shortened red-cell survival that characterizes all the severe forms of the disease.

These principles are summarized in Fig. 3.1. Since β-chain synthesis is only fully activated after birth, it follows that β thalassaemia is not expressed as a disease in intrauterine life, but only becomes manifest as γ-chain synthesis declines during the first year after birth. It is characterized by persistent γ-chain, that is HbF, production and an elevated level of HbA_2 in heterozygotes. Since there is defective β-chain synthesis, it might be expected that there would be a relative increase in δ-chain production and therefore the increased level of HbA_2 would be expected. However, the reasons for persistent γ-chain production in β thalassaemia, and its marked variability from case to case, are much more difficult to explain, reflecting as it does both selective survival of cells with HbF and increased HbF production. It clearly distinguishes β thalassaemia from almost every other genetic or acquired haematological dis-

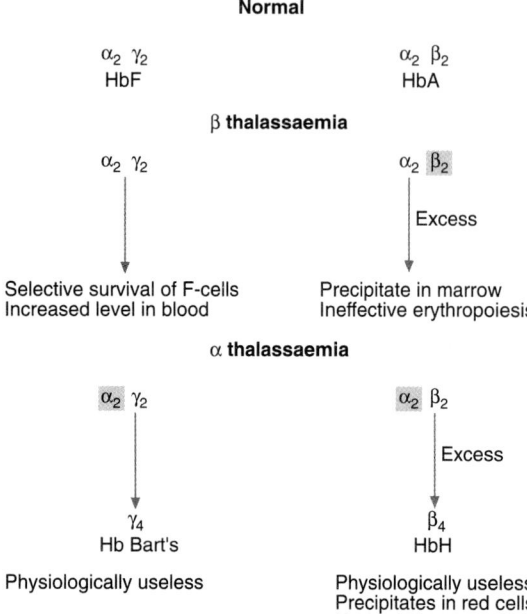

Normal

$\alpha_2\ \gamma_2$
HbF

$\alpha_2\ \beta_2$
HbA

β thalassaemia

$\alpha_2\ \gamma_2$

$\alpha_2\ \beta_2$

Excess

Selective survival of F-cells
Increased level in blood

Precipitate in marrow
Ineffective erythropoiesis

α thalassaemia

$\alpha_2\ \gamma_2$

$\alpha_2\ \beta_2$

Excess

γ_4
Hb Bart's

β_4
HbH

Physiologically useless

Physiologically useless
Precipitates in red cells
Haemolytic anaemia

Fig. 3.1 The α and β thalassaemias. A simplified representation of the differences in the haemoglobin patterns between the two main forms of thalassaemia. Shaded boxes indicate defective globin synthesis.

order and is of prime importance in determining the severity of its phenotype. We shall discuss in detail what little is understood about this tantalizing problem in Chapters 5 and 10.

Unfortunately, however, persistent γ-chain production is insufficient to compensate for the deficit of β chains in the more severe forms of β thalassaemia. Hence there is always an excess of α chains, aggregates of which cause damage both to developing red-cell precursors and to mature red cells. Thus the central pathophysiological mechanism of β thalassaemia is α-chain excess and the damage that it causes at every stage of erythropoiesis (Fig. 3.1).

Since α chains are shared by both fetal and adult haemoglobin, it is not surprising that the α thalassaemias are manifest in both fetal and adult life. However, unlike the surfeit of α chains that is produced in β thalassaemia, excess γ and β chains that result from defective α-chain production (Fig. 3.1) are able to form soluble homotetramers, γ_4 (or Hb Bart's) and β_4 (or HbH). These molecules are

physiologically useless because of their very high oxygen affinity and, at least in the case of HbH, instability. Thus the clinical features of the more severe forms of α thalassaemia are a reflection of the properties of haemoglobins Bart's and H and their effects on erythropoiesis, and in particular on red-cell survival. Although we shall consider the properties of these haemoglobins in detail in Chapters 5 and 11, it is worth pointing out here that their generation does not seem to be related directly to the deficit of α-chain production. In milder forms of α thalassaemia it may be difficult to demonstrate HbH, for example. It appears that a critical level of β-chain excess is needed before viable β_4 molecules are formed.

These general principles of the pathophysiology of the thalassaemias apply to all the different types of the disease that we shall encounter later in this book.

Classification

As knowledge about the thalassaemias has grown, different approaches to their classification have evolved and gradually become more sophisticated. The disease can now be described at several levels. First, there is a phenotypic classification based on its severity: this classification says nothing about the genetic constitution of a particular patient, but simply describes, in very general terms, a constellation of clinical features. Second, the thalassaemias can be defined by the particular globin(s) that is (are) synthesized at a reduced rate. In effect, this constitutes a genetic classification in that, in most cases, it describes the gene (or genes) that must be affected by the thalassaemia mutation. Finally, it is now often possible to subclassify many thalassaemias according to the particular mutation that is responsible for defective globin synthesis.

In clinical practice it is very useful to retain each of these classifications. Much of our approach to treatment is still determined by characterization of the disease at a clinical level. However, for an accurate assessment of the likely outcome it is becoming increasingly important to go to at least the next step, that is, a genetic classification by the particular globins involved. Indeed, in current day-to-day management of thalassaemia it is often extremely helpful to be able to analyse the disorder at the molecular level, particularly if its prenatal detection is contemplated.

Clinical classification

Based on clinical assessment, the thalassaemias can be divided into the *major* forms of the illness, which are severe and transfusion dependent, and the symptomless *minor* forms, which can only be identified haematologically and usually represent the carrier states, or traits. Although β thalassaemia major usually results either from the homozygous inheritance of a particular mutation or from the compound heterozygous state for two different mutations, it has become apparent that there are rare forms of moderately severe β thalassaemia that result from the action of a single mutant gene; that is, they are dominantly inherited.

Another term, 'thalassaemia intermedia', though it has an old-fashioned ring about it, is still retained and is extremely useful in clinical practice. It describes conditions which, though not as severe as the major forms, are associated with a more severe degree of anaemia than is found in the trait. In practice, this term encompasses a wide spectrum, ranging from disorders which are almost as serious as major forms to asymptomatic conditions which are only slightly more severe than the trait.

Finally, some heterozygotes for thalassaemia mutations are clinically and haematologically normal; they are sometimes designated 'silent' carriers.

Genetic classification

The thalassaemias are classified according to their genetic basis by describing the globin subunit which is synthesized at a reduced rate. A classification of the syndromes at this level is shown in Table 3.1.

The genetic classification of the thalassaemias divides them broadly into α, β, γ, δβ, δ and εγδβ varieties, depending on which globin or globins are underproduced. Newcomers to the field may be confused when they see that, as well as the thalassaemias, Table 3.1 includes 'hereditary persistence of fetal haemoglobin'. As we shall see in Chapter 10, it seems reasonable to include this heterogeneous collection of conditions with the thalassaemias since many of them are, in effect, forms of β or δβ thalassaemia in which globin imbalance is almost entirely compen-

Table 3.1 Genetic classification of the thalassaemias and related disorders.

α Thalassaemia
  α^0
  α^+
    Deletion $(-\alpha)$
    Non-deletion (α^T)

β Thalassaemia
  β^0
  β^+
    Variants with unusually high level of HbF or A_2
    Normal HbA_2
    'Silent'
    Dominant
    Unlinked to β-gene cluster

δβ Thalassaemia
  $(\delta\beta)^+$
  $(\delta\beta)^0$
  $(^A\gamma\delta\beta)^0$

γ Thalassaemia

δ Thalassaemia
  δ^0
  δ^+

εγδβ Thalassaemia

Hereditary persistence of fetal haemoglobin
  Deletion
    $(\delta\beta)^0$
  Non-deletion
    Linked to β-globin-gene cluster
      $^G\gamma\beta^+$
      $^A\gamma\beta^+$
    Unlinked to β-globin-gene cluster

sated by a genetically determined persistence of relatively high levels of fetal haemoglobin production.

In each of the later chapters that deal with particular forms of thalassaemia in detail, their classification is considered at greater length. But as a general introduction it may be helpful to outline the main features of the different genetic forms here.

α Thalassaemia

As we saw in Chapter 2, there are two α-globin genes per haploid genome, four in all. For this reason the α thalassaemias are classified according to the *total* output of each of the α-chain genes that constitute the haploid pairs. A normal α-globin genotype can be represented as $\alpha\alpha/\alpha\alpha$. When both α-globin genes on a chromosome are deleted or otherwise inactivated, the condition is called α^0 thalassaemia; the heterozygous genotype can be written $--/\alpha\alpha$. This is called α^0 thalassaemia because there is no output of α globin from the affected chromosome. When one of the linked α genes is inactivated, the condition is called α^+ thalassaemia, and the genotype is written $-\alpha/\alpha\alpha$ in cases in which one of the α-globin genes is deleted, or $\alpha^T\alpha/\alpha\alpha$ if one of them is inactivated by a mutation. In other words, the terms α^0 and α^+ thalassaemia describe an α-globin *haplotype*; that is, the state of the two linked α-globin genes on a particular chromosome; in α^0 thalassaemia there is no output of α globin, and in α^+ thalassaemia there is some output but usually only the product of a single α-globin locus. Previously, α^0 and α^+ were called α thalassaemia 1 and 2. However, as discussed in Chapter 1, we believe that classifying α thalassaemia into α^0 and α^+ varieties is simpler, more informative, and, as we shall see later, has the further advantage of being consistent with the way in which other forms of thalassaemia are treated.

β Thalassaemia

There are two main varieties of β thalassaemia, β^0 thalassaemia, in which no β globin is produced, and β^+ thalassaemia, in which some β globin is produced, but less than normal. Less severe forms of β thalassaemia are sometimes designated β^{++} to indicate that the defect in β-chain production is particularly mild.

The diagnostic feature of β thalassaemia is an elevated level of HbA_2 in heterozygotes, which is found in most forms of β^0 and β^+ thalassaemia. There are, however, less common forms of β thalassaemia in which the HbA_2 level is normal in heterozygotes. These so-called 'normal HbA_2 β thalassaemias' are themselves heterogeneous. Broadly, they are classified into two varieties: type 1, in which there are no associated haematological changes, and type 2, in which the haematological findings are typical of β-thalassaemia trait with a raised HbA_2. Type 1 is also called 'silent β thalassaemia'. As we shall see in Chapters 4 and 7, both varieties are heterogeneous at the molecular level.

$\delta\beta$ Thalassaemia

The $\delta\beta$ thalassaemias, which differ fundamentally from the β thalassaemias by virtue of the greater propensity for HbF production, are also heterogeneous. They are described in detail in Chapter 8. In some cases, no δ or β chains are synthesized (($\delta\beta$)^0 thalassaemia). At one time it was customary to further classify these conditions according to the structure of the γ chains of the HbF that is produced. Using this approach the two main forms were described, $^G\gamma^A\gamma$ and $^G\gamma$ ($\delta\beta$)^0 thalassaemia. To keep in line with other varieties of thalassaemia they are best described by the globin subunits which are defectively synthesized, that is, ($\delta\beta$)^0 and ($^A\gamma\delta\beta$)^0 thalassaemia.

There are also ($\delta\beta$)$^+$ varieties of $\delta\beta$ thalassaemia. In most of these conditions an abnormal haemoglobin is produced that has normal α chains combined with non-α chains that are constituted by the N-terminal residues of the δ chains fused with the C-terminal residues of the β chain. These $\delta\beta$-fusion variants, called collectively the 'Lepore haemoglobins', are synthesized inefficiently to produce the clinical phenotype of severe $\delta\beta$ thalassaemia.

δ Thalassaemia

Many different mutations cause a reduced output of δ chains and hence a low level of HbA_2. Like the other thalassaemias, these can be divided into δ^0 and δ^+ thalassaemias. All the δ thalassaemias are clinically silent and are of importance only in so far as when they are inherited together with β thalassaemia they may prevent an elevation of the level of HbA_2.

$\varepsilon\gamma\delta\beta$ Thalassaemia

This is a rare disease that results from loss of either the whole or a major part of the β-like globin-gene cluster and its regulatory regions. Strictly speaking, therefore, it should be described as ($\varepsilon^G\gamma^A\gamma\delta\beta$)^0 thalassaemia. Homozygotes have not been encountered, presumably because the condition would not be compatible with life; heterozygotes have the clinical phenotype of β thalassaemia with a normal HbA_2 level.

γ Thalassaemia

There have been several reports of deletions involving one or more of the γ-globin genes. They have only been identified during surveys of the relative levels of $^G\gamma$ and $^A\gamma$ chains in HbF and do not appear to be of clinical significance. As far as we know they are not associated with imbalanced globin production.

Hereditary persistence of fetal haemoglobin (HPFH) as a form of β or δβ thalassaemia

These diverse conditions, described in Chapter 10, are all characterized by persistent fetal haemoglobin synthesis in adult life in the absence of major haematological abnormalities. As we shall see later, by virtue of their interactions with the β thalassaemias and from other evidence, it is apparent that many of them are extremely well compensated forms of β or δβ thalassaemia. They are important in the thalassaemia field because they can modify the clinical phenotype of the β thalassaemias and reduce their severity.

As shown in Table 3.1, HPFH is best classified along similar lines to the thalassaemias. First, there are forms in which no δ or β chains are produced, but in which there is almost complete compensation by a high output of γ chains; these conditions are therefore designated $(\delta\beta)^0$ HPFH. Second, there is a family of HPFH variants in which there is β- and probably δ-chain synthesis *cis*, i.e. directed by genes on the same chromosome, to the HPFH determinant. Hence these conditions are designated $^G\gamma\beta^+$ or $^A\gamma\beta^+$ HPFH, depending on the structure of the HbF. Finally, there is a group, undoubtedly heterogeneous, in which much lower levels of HbF are found in otherwise normal individuals. Evidence is mounting that the genetic determinants for at least some types of this form of HPFH are not linked to the β-globin gene cluster.

In the first two groups of HPFH, relatively high levels of HbF are produced in heterozygotes, usually 5–25% of the total haemoglobin; HbF in these conditions is relatively homogeneously distributed among the red cells. In the third group, levels of persistent HbF production are much lower, in the 2–5% range, and the HbF is usually heterogeneously distributed among the red cells. Thus, HPFH is also classified as either pancellular or heterocellular, although, as knowledge of its molecular pathology increases, this subdivision is becoming less useful.

Molecular classification

As their molecular pathology has been elucidated, as described in Chapter 4, a more accurate approach to the description of the different types of α and β thalassaemia has been possible. For example, in many cases the genotype of a patient with a clinical picture of β thalassaemia major can be described according to the particular mutation at the homologous pair of β-globin loci. Homozygotes for a common Mediterranean nonsense mutation would have the following genotype: $\alpha\alpha/\beta^{39C\rightarrow T}\beta^{39C\rightarrow T}$. This tells us that, in this particular mutation, thymine has replaced cytidine in the 39th codon in the β-globin gene. Alternatively, compound heterozygotes for this mutation and an RNA-processing mutation that is found in the same population would have the genotype $\alpha\alpha/\beta^{39C\rightarrow T}\beta^{IVS1-1(G\rightarrow A)}$. The latter mutation is a replacement of guanine by adenine at the first position in the first intervening sequence (intron) in the β-globin gene.

The α thalassaemias can also be described at the molecular level. The α^0 thalassaemias are often designated by the particular length of the deletion that removes both α-globin genes. For example, the deletion that is common in Mediterranean populations (MED) is different from that which is common throughout south-east Asia (SEA); these different α^0 thalassaemias can therefore be described as $--^{MED}$ and $--^{SEA}$. Similarly, there are two common forms of α^+ thalassaemia, in which single α-gene deletions are due to loss of 3.7 or 4.2 kb of DNA from within the linked pair of α genes; they are written $-\alpha^{3.7}$ or $-\alpha^{4.2}$. Finally, if α^+ thalassaemia results from the inactivation of one α-globin gene by a mutation, $\alpha^T\alpha$, when the nature of the mutation is known, the T can be replaced by the precise molecular abnormality, in the same way as β thalassaemia.

These molecular classifications are considered in more detail in the next chapter and in subsequent chapters which deal with particular varieties of thalassaemia.

Inheritance

All the thalassaemias have a similar pattern of inheritance. The severe, symptomatic varieties usually result from the interaction of more than one genetic determinant. In most cases they are transmitted in a Mendelian autosomal fashion. In its simplest form the inheritance of thalassaemia is similar to that of sickle-cell anaemia and related disorders. Children with β thalassaemia major are homozygotes or compound heterozygotes for β-globin-gene mutations that cause only mild haematological abnormalities in their heterozygous parents. The offspring of matings between thalassaemia heterozygotes may be normal, thalassaemia carriers or homozygotes, in ratios expected of a Mendelian pattern of inheritance.

The inheritance of α thalassaemia is more complicated because it involves the products of a linked pairs of α genes (αα). Both the important clinical forms of α thalassaemia, the Hb Bart's hydrops syndrome and HbH disease, can be ascribed to the interactions of the different forms of α^0 and α^+ thalassaemia; the former results from the homozygous inheritance of α^0 thalassaemia, $--/--$, while the latter often, though not always, is due to the compound heterozygous inheritance of α^+ and α^0 thalassaemia, $--/-\alpha$ or $--/\alpha^T\alpha$ (Fig. 3.2). Less commonly, HbH disease results from the homozygous inheritance of a non-deletional form of α^+ thalassaemia, $\alpha^T\alpha/\alpha^T\alpha$. Overall, the output of α chains from an $\alpha^T\alpha$ pair is less than from $-\alpha$; the homozygous state for the latter, $-\alpha/-\alpha$, results, like the heterozygous state for α^0 thalassaemia, $--/\alpha\alpha$, in α-thalassaemia trait, a symptomless mild anaemia. The carrier states for the α^+ thalassaemias, $-\alpha/\alpha\alpha$ or $\alpha^T\alpha/\alpha\alpha$, are usually clinically and haematologically 'silent', or almost so. These conditions are described in detail in Chapter 11.

The statement that the heterozygous states for α^+ thalassaemia are haematologically 'silent' is true only after the first 6 months of life. This raises another important principle in the thalassaemia field. Just as there are important changes in haemopoiesis during normal development, so the haematological picture of thalassaemia may vary at different stages. We have already seen how β thalassaemia may be 'masked' by γ-chain synthesis during the first months of life. The opposite situation exists in the case of the carrier states for α thalassaemia. In newborns, probably because there is normally a mild overall deficit of α chains during the period of the switch from γ- to β-chain production, some babies heterozygous for α^+ thalassaemia, and all α^0-thalassaemia carriers, have elevated levels of Hb Bart's, which, as they grow older, is not replaced by an equivalent amount of HbH. In short, thalassaemia phenotypes are not 'fixed', but have to be described and interpreted in the context of the age of the affected individual.

A semantic question which is often raised about the genetic disorders of haemoglobin production is whether they should be referred to as 'dominant' or

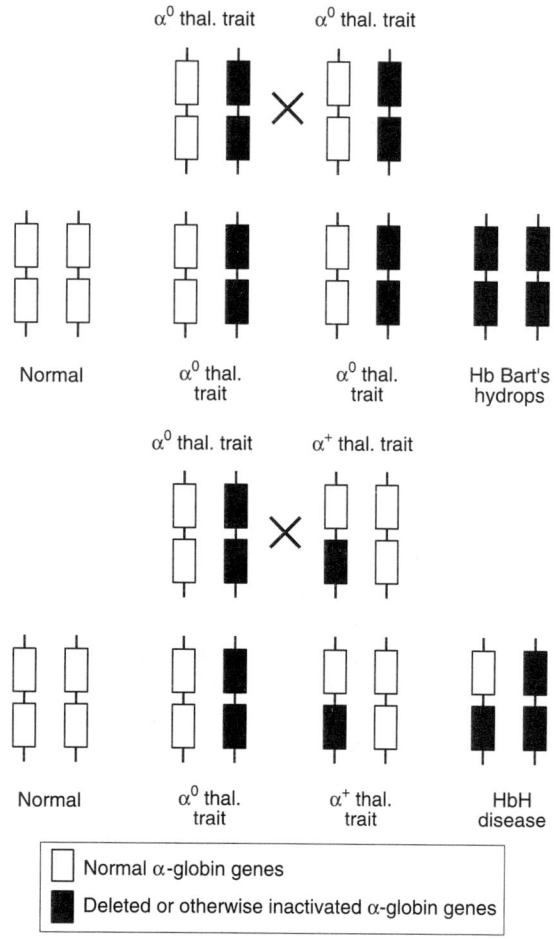

Fig. 3.2 A representation of the interactions of α^0 and α^+ thalassaemia. The unshaded boxes represent normal α-globin genes; the dark-shaded boxes represent deleted or otherwise inactivated α-globin genes.

'recessive'. A dominantly inherited disorder is one which is expressed in heterozygotes, whereas a recessive condition is completely silent. In fact, the sickling diseases and thalassaemias could be defined as 'dominant' or 'co-dominant', or 'recessive', depending on the particular techniques employed for pedigree analysis! If the latter relied on clinical manifestations then clearly these disorders would be classified as recessive, whereas if haematological criteria or haemoglobin analyses are applied they could be called co-dominant. However, since there are excellent methods for identifying carrier states for most of the haemoglobin disorders and thalassaemias, this question becomes relatively unimportant.

Another genetic concept which is often raised in discussions about thalassaemia revolves round expressivity or penetrance of genes, terms that are often confused and used rather loosely. When geneticists talk of 'penetrance' they usually refer to a percentage that expresses the probability that an abnormal gene will exert at least one of its phenotypic effects in the person who inherits it. If penetrance is less than 100% it is said to be incomplete; this may result from variation between unrelated affected persons with respect to the precise genetic defect, or it may reflect the interaction of other genetic and environmental modifiers. On the other hand, expressivity describes variability in the severity and other phenotypic manifestations between those carrying the same genetic defect.

As we shall see in later chapters, in thalassaemia pedigrees it is not unusual to encounter variable expressivity or penetrance. However, one of the great success stories of research in thalassaemia of recent years is how it has been possible to dissect the reasons for phenotypic variability, at both the clinical and molecular levels. We shall see that many of the apparent differences in expression can be explained by the interaction of other variant genes or acquired mechanisms which may modify the primary action of thalassaemia genes. While we are not always able to explain why there is variability of expression of a thalassaemia gene in a particular family, overall we probably know more about the mechanisms involved in such phenotypic diversity than for any other human single-gene disorder.

The inheritance of thalassaemia together with structural haemoglobin variants

As we saw in Chapter 1, studies of the haemoglobin patterns of patients who have inherited both thalassaemia and structural haemoglobin variants have been of seminal importance in the development of the concept of thalassaemia as a disorder of globin synthesis encoded at the globin-gene loci. And because in many populations there is a high frequency of the genes for different forms of thalassaemia and those for structural haemoglobin variants, and the two may interact to cause a variety of disorders of different degrees of severity, these complex conditions are of considerable clinical importance. They are described in detail in Chapters 9 and 11. Here we shall briefly consider the genetic principles involved in their interactions.

Interactions of α or β thalassaemia with β- or δ-chain haemoglobin variants

Although many different structural haemoglobin variants have been found together with the β thalassaemias only three β-chain variants, Hbs S, C and E, occur at a sufficiently high frequency to make their interactions of particular clinical importance.

In heterozygotes for β-chain haemoglobin variants it is usual to find that the level of HbA exceeds that of the abnormal haemoglobin. For example, in the sickle-cell trait ($\beta^A \beta^S$) HbS usually makes up about 35% of the total haemoglobin. In an individual who has inherited the sickle-cell gene from one parent and a β-thalassaemia gene (β^T) from the other (β^T/β^S) this pattern changes; the level of HbS is now considerably *greater* than that seen in the sickle-cell trait; this tells us that the β-thalassaemia mutation has reduced the output of β^A chains compared with β^S chains. In the case of β^+ thalassaemia this reversal may result in a level of HbA of 5–30%, depending on the severity of the β-thalassaemia allele. If, on the other hand, a β^0-thalassaemia allele is inherited together with the sickle-cell gene, no HbA is produced in the compound heterozygote and the haemoglobin pattern resembles that of sickle-cell anaemia. In all these cases there is said to be 'interaction' between the genes for the structural haemoglobin variant and thalassaemia (Fig. 3.3).

Thus compound heterozygotes inherit β thalassaemia from one parent and HbS from the other. Since the mutant genes are alleles, it follows that the offspring of a mating between a patient with sickle-cell β thalassaemia and a normal partner will either show the sickle-cell trait or the β-thalassaemia trait; there can be no normal or doubly affected children (Fig. 3.4) because the genes for β^S and β thalassaemia are on opposite homologous chromosomes. The reader might be curious to know, as we were for many years, what might happen if a sickle-cell gene and a β-thalassaemia gene were found together on the *same* chromosome, i.e. the β-chain locus carried *both* mutations. In fact this unusual gene has now been encountered (see Chapter 9), and, as might have been guessed, the haemoglobin pattern is quite different from that usually seen in sickle-cell β thalassaemia. In

Normal

Genotype	αα/αα		γγ/γγ	δ/δ	β/β
Haemoglobins		$\alpha_2\beta_2$		$\alpha_2\delta_2$	
(%)		97.0		3.0	

Sickle-cell trait

Genotype	αα/αα		γγ/γγ	δ/δ	β/β^S
Haemoglobins		$\alpha_2\beta_2$	$\alpha_2\beta_2^S$	$\alpha_2\delta_2$	
(%)		67	30	3	

Sickle-cell β thalassaemia

Genotype	αα/αα		γγ/γγ	δ/δ	β^T/β^S
Haemoglobins	$\alpha_2\gamma_2$	$\alpha_2\beta_2$	$\alpha_2\beta_2^S$	$\alpha_2\delta_2$	
(%)	Variable	0–25	70–95	5	

(a)

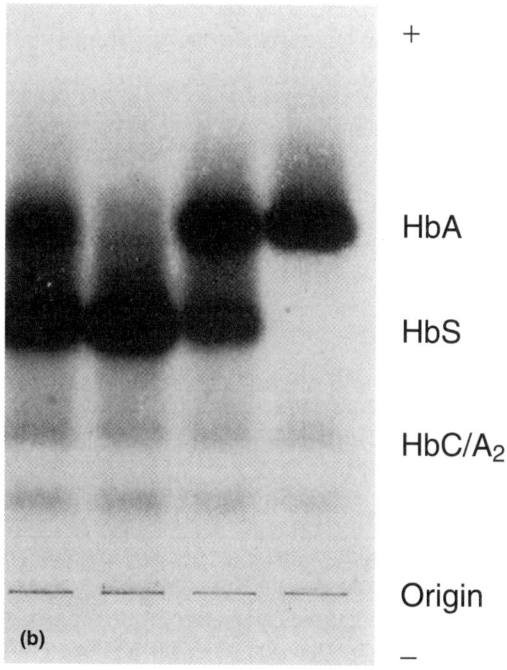

(b)

+

HbA

HbS

HbC/A₂

Origin

−

Fig. 3.3 The interaction of the sickle-cell and β-thalassaemia genes. (a) The genotypes of normal individuals, those with the sickle-cell trait and those with sickle-cell β thalassaemia. The action of the β-thalassaemia gene is to reduce the output of HbA compared with HbS in those with sickle-cell β thalassaemia. (b) A starch-gel electrophoretic pattern (Tris-EDTA-borate system, pH 8.5) of red-cell lysates prepared from persons with the following: 1, sickle-cell thalassaemia; 2, sickle-cell anaemia; 3, sickle-cell trait; 4, normal adult. The relatively low amount of HbA in sickle-cell β⁺ thalassaemia compared with the sickle-cell trait is shown.

β-globin genotypes	β/β × β^T/β^S
Offspring	β^T/β or β^S/β

Fig. 3.4 The genetics of sickle-cell β thalassaemia. A mating between a patient with sickle-cell β thalassaemia and a normal person results in offspring who have either β-thalassaemia trait or sickle-cell trait; no normal or doubly affected individuals are observed.

this case it is more like that of the sickle-cell trait except that there is an extremely low level of β^S because the action of the β^+-thalassaemia gene is to reduce the output of β^S chains (Fig. 3.5).

The situation is quite different if a person inherits the sickle-cell trait together with various forms of α thalassaemia. Here there is no interaction, in that, because defective α-chain synthesis is shared equally between haemoglobins A and S, the level of HbA exceeds that of HbS at approximately the ratio seen in the sickle-cell trait alone (Fig. 3.6). We use the word 'approximately' for a good reason. Curiously, what happens is that in those with the sickle-cell trait and α thalassaemia the level of HbS is *lower* than that usually found in the sickle-cell trait alone. Although it is not absolutely certain why, it seems likely that it reflects the differential affinity of β^A and β^S chains for α chains; when the latter are in limited supply they bind preferentially to β^A rather than β^S chains, and hence the relative level of HbA is increased over that of HbS. Because in some populations there are many different forms of α thalassaemia, this results in a variety of different abnormal haemoglobin levels in patients with the trait for a β-chain haemoglobin variant and α thalassaemia; this is well exemplified by the interactions of HbE with α thalassaemia that are described in Chapter 11.

It follows that the genetic consequences for children of persons who have both a β-haemoglobin variant, such as HbS, and α thalassaemia are quite dif-

Trans				
Genotype	$\alpha\alpha/\alpha\alpha$	$\gamma\gamma/\gamma\gamma$	β^T/β^S	δ/δ
Haemoglobins		$\alpha_2\beta_2$	$\alpha_2\beta_2^S$	$\alpha_2\delta_2$
(%)		25	70	5
Cis				
Genotype	$\alpha\alpha/\alpha\alpha$	$\gamma\gamma/\gamma\gamma$	β/β_S^T	δ/δ
Haemoglobins		$\alpha_2\beta_2$	$\alpha_2\beta_2^S$	$\alpha_2\delta_2$
(%)		85	10	5

Fig. 3.5 The different haemoglobin patterns in individuals with sickle-cell β thalassaemia depending on whether the two genes are in *trans* or *cis*. The β thalassaemia is the β^+ variety.

Genotype	$-\alpha/-\alpha$	$\gamma\gamma/\gamma\gamma$	β/β^S	δ/δ
Haemoglobins	$\alpha_2\gamma_2$	$\alpha_2\beta_2$	$\alpha_2\beta_2^S$	$\alpha_2\delta_2$
(%)	γ_4	78	20	2
	Newborn			

Fig. 3.6 The haemoglobin pattern in individuals with the sickle-cell trait who are also homozygous for α^+ thalassaemia. Unlike sickle-cell β thalassaemia there is no interaction and the pattern is of the sickle-cell trait with a slightly lower level of HbS than normal and hypochromic microcytic red cells. Haemoglobin Bart's is present at birth, but not during later development (shaded).

Genotypes	$\alpha\alpha/-\alpha \; \beta/\beta^S$		×		$\alpha\alpha/\alpha\alpha \; \beta/\beta$	
Offspring	$\alpha\alpha/\alpha\alpha \; \beta/\beta$	$\alpha\alpha/\alpha\alpha \; \beta/\beta^S$		$\alpha\alpha/-\alpha \; \beta/\beta$		$\alpha\alpha/-\alpha \; \beta/\beta^S$

Fig. 3.7 The genotypes in children born of a mating between a normal individual and one with the sickle-cell trait and the α^+-thalassaemia trait. Unlike the same kind of mating between a person with sickle-cell β thalassaemia and a normal person (Fig. 3.4) the two traits segregate independently in the offspring.

Trans			
Genotype	$\beta^T\delta/\beta\delta^X$	×	$\beta\delta/\beta\delta$
Offspring	$\beta^T\delta/\beta\delta$	or	$\beta\delta/\beta\delta^X$
	(β thal. trait)		(Hb δ^X trait)
Cis			
Genotype	$\beta^T\delta^X/\beta\delta$	×	$\beta\delta/\beta\delta$
Offspring	$\beta^T\delta^X/\beta\delta$	or	$\beta\delta/\beta\delta$
	(β thal. trait Hb δ^X trait)		(Normal)

Fig. 3.8 Findings in the children of individuals heterozygous for both β thalassaemia and a δ-chain structural variant (haemoglobin X, $\alpha_2\delta_2^X$). The findings in the children depend on whether the variants are in *cis* or *trans*.

ferent from those with sickle-cell β thalassaemia. Since the α- and β-globin genes are on different chromosomes the children of individuals with sickle-cell α thalassaemia born of normal partners may have any combination of the traits that are present in their affected parent, or they may be normal (Fig. 3.7).

Just as there are β-chain variants so there is a family of structurally abnormal δ-chain haemoglobin variants. In persons who are heterozygous for both β thalassaemia and a δ-chain variant, the levels of both HbA_2 *and* the abnormal form of HbA_2 ($\alpha_2\delta_2^x$) are elevated. This tells us that the output of the δ-chain genes on *both* pairs of homologous chromosomes, i.e. *cis* and *trans* to the β-thalassaemia determinant, is increased. It follows therefore that the augmented output of δ chains in β thalassaemia is not a direct result of the gene carrying the thalassaemia mutation being next to the δ-chain locus on the same chromosome, but is part of a more general 'compensatory' mechanism involving both homologous chromosomes. In short, a simple genetic observation has been of great value in clarifying the cellular consequences of the thalassaemia mutations; although their primary action is to reduce the output of α or β chains in *cis* they may have effects on other haemoglobin gene loci in both *cis* and *trans*.

The δ-chain mutation may be on the same chromosome as the β-thalassaemia mutation (*cis*) or on the opposite pair of homologous chromosome (*trans*). Because the δ- and β-globin genes are closely linked, the findings in the children of such doubly affected persons will vary depending on the site of the two mutations. If they are in *cis* the children will either all be normal or doubly affected, while if in *trans* they will either have the δ-chain mutation or β thalassaemia; there will be no normal and no doubly affected children (Fig. 3.8).

Interactions of α or β thalassaemia with α-chain haemoglobin variants

Before considering these complex phenotypes we should remind ourselves about the differences in the haemoglobin constitution of carriers for α- or β-chain haemoglobin variants. Unlike the β-globin genes, for which there is only one per haploid genome, there are two linked α-globin genes on each chromosome 16. If one of the α genes in the diploid pair of chromosomes carries a mutation for a structural variant, HbG Philadelphia for example, the genotype is written $\alpha^G\alpha/\alpha\alpha$. It follows that the abnormal haemoglobin will constitute approximately 25% of the total haemoglobin; that is, significantly lower than that usually found in persons heterozygous for a β-chain variant. The level of the α-chain variant is not always exactly 25% of the total haemoglobin; the two α-globin genes have different outputs and some haemoglobin variants are synthesized less effectively than normal haemoglobin. But, *on average,* carriers for β-haemoglobin variants have higher levels of abnormal haemoglobin than those for α-chain variants, an observation that provided the first clue to the possibility that the α-globin genes are duplicated. It follows, of course, that homozygotes for α-chain variants, in the example we have used with the genotype $\alpha^G\alpha/\alpha^G\alpha$, the haemoglobin consists of both Hbs A ($\alpha_2\beta_2$) and G ($\alpha^G_2\beta_2$), in roughly the same amounts.

There is a further twist to the genetics of α-globin variants. Although some are found on a chromosome with a normal α-globin gene partner, others may involve the only α-globin gene on the chromosome, the partner having been deleted as part of the mechanism for producing α^+ thalassaemia. In the case of HbG Philadelphia, it turns out that the mutation may be found on a chromosome with two intact α genes or with only a single α gene. Heterozygotes for the latter type of chromosome ($\alpha^G-/\alpha\alpha$) have higher levels of the abnormal α-chain variant than those in which the mutation occurs on a chromosome with two intact α-globin genes ($\alpha^G\alpha/\alpha\alpha$). Homozygotes for mutations on chromosomes of this kind (α^G-/α^G-) produce no HbA or A_2, but only Hbs G ($\alpha^G_2\beta_2$) and G_2 ($\alpha^G_2\beta_2$). Indeed, some α-globin chain variants, Hbs Q, Hasharon and J Tongariki for example, are always found on chromosomes with one α gene. These different α-globin genotypes are illustrated in Fig. 3.9.

It also follows, of course, that if an α-chain variant is encoded on a chromosome that also carries an α^+-thalassaemia deletion, α^G- for example, the co-inheritance of α-thalassaemia alleles on the partner chromosome will lead to an even greater deficit of normal α globin and hence an even higher relative level of the α-chain variant. For example, the inheritance of HbG on chromosomes in which the linked $\alpha-$ gene is deleted, together with α^0 thalassaemia, leads to the genotypes $\alpha^G-/--$. In these cases there is a moderately severe form of thalassaemia characterized by the presence of only HbG and G_2, together with HbH (β_4) resulting from the relatively large excess of β chains; this disorder is therefore called 'HbGH disease' (Fig. 3.9).

It is clear therefore that because of the duplication of the α-globin genes, and the fact that α-globin gene mutations can exist on chromosomes with or without a partner α-globin gene, a broad spectrum of phenotypes exist, characterized by increasing amounts of a particular α-chain variant associated with more marked thalassaemic phenotypes, at the most severe end of which is the characteristic phenotype of HbH disease associated with no HbA production. These conditions, which are described in Chapter 11, provide an excellent example of gene dosage effects, evidenced by a wide spectrum of different ratios of normal to abnormal haemoglobin. Indeed, before it was possible to explore the α-globin genes directly, analyses of the levels of mutant α-chain haemoglobin variants were the only way that it was possible to try to guess at what was happening at the molecular level.

Occasionally, persons with β thalassaemia are found who have also inherited α-chain structural haemoglobin variants. As might be expected, there is no interaction in this case, and the level of α-chain variants in heterozygotes remains much the same as it is in those without β thalassaemia. There are slight differences in the relative amounts of the normal and variant haemoglobin consequent on the presence of the β-thalassaemia gene, probably reflecting varying affinities of different α-globin subunits when there is a paucity of β chains (see Chapter 9).

Variation in the numbers of globin genes as a modifier of the thalassaemia phenotype

Variation in the numbers of α-globin genes, while it may have no effect in normal persons, may have important phenotypic consequences for those with different forms of thalassaemia (see Chapter 13). For example, it is not uncommon to find that the α-globin genes are triplicated, and hence the genotypes $\alpha\alpha\alpha/\alpha\alpha$ or $\alpha\alpha\alpha/\alpha\alpha\alpha$ are generated. Rarely, individu-

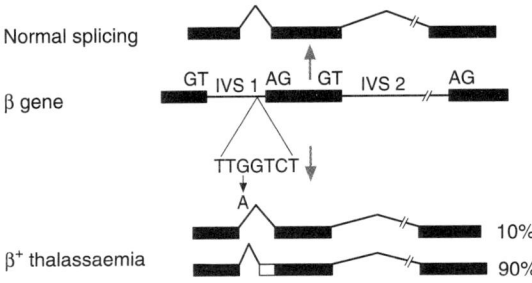

Fig. 4.2 A mutation resulting in both normal and abnormal messenger RNA due to the generation of a new splice site in an intron. The new splice site is used in preference to the normal site, resulting in only 10% of normal messenger RNA and gene product.

messenger RNA. As outlined above, nonsense or frameshift mutations result in translation of an abnormal protein; the process of translation may also be affected by point mutations that involve the initiation or termination codons.

Most mutations which involve transcription, processing or translation of messenger RNA cause a reduction or absence of the protein product of a particular gene. In the case of mis-sense mutations the product is usually synthesized normally but has an abnormal structure. While this may be harmless, in some cases the change in protein structure results in its instability or abnormal function and hence in a disease phenotype.

Larger gene rearrangements

Although point mutations are by far the commonest cause of molecular pathology, there are a number of larger disruptions which, as we shall see later in this chapter, underlie inherited diseases. They include deletions (that is, partial or complete loss of genes, gene fusions, insertions of new genetic material) and inversions (that is, lengths of DNA which are in the opposite orientation to normal). Clearly, lesions of this size will have a major effect on gene function and, indeed, in many cases they completely inactivate genes or even entire gene clusters.

Many of these larger genetic lesions result from inappropriate recombinational events. Genetic recombination (the formation of new combinations of linked genes by crossing over following breakage and rejoining between their loci) is, of course,

nature's way of redistributing genes during meiosis. Despite the fundamental importance of this process its precise mechanisms are still not fully understood.

Homologous unequal recombination

As we saw in Chapter 2, the linked α-globin genes, α1 and α2, have evolved by gene duplication and they also have flanking regions of homology, the sequences of which may have been maintained during evolution by the process of gene conversion and unequal crossing over. Such regions tend to potentiate homologous unequal recombination by chromosomal slippage at meiosis. As described in further detail later in this chapter, unequal crossing over following chromosomal misalignment can give rise to a single α gene on one chromosome and three on the homologous partner. There are other examples of this type of mechanism in regions of the genome which contain closely linked homologous loci. There are also examples of unequal recombination of this type between repetitive-sequence elements (see below).

Gene fusion products resulting from homologous unequal recombination

As discussed later in this chapter, chromosomal slippage and homologous unequal recombination can give rise to a fusion gene on one chromosome and a mirror image on the opposite pair. This is the basis for the Lepore haemoglobin variants and for different types of colour-blindness.

Non-homologous recombination

Major DNA rearrangements occurring in regions of minimum sequence homology also occur. Several types of junction have been observed: 'flush junctions', in which there is simple breakage and rejoining; insertional junctions, which contain novel nucleotides; and junctions with limited homology (see Cooper and Krawczak (1993) for a more detailed discussion).

Repetitive sequences

Later in this chapter we shall see that some of the abnormal recombinational events that have given rise to large deletions of the globin genes have been related to repetitive DNA sequences. There are many types of repetitive DNA in the human genome. For example, there are frequent stretches of simple dinucleotide repeats $(CA)_n$. In addition, there are long stretches of tandemly repeated DNA segments containing many copies of oligonucleotide (10–30 bp) repeats. These form useful genetic markers known as variable-number tandem repeats (VNTRs). Some stretches of repetitive DNA consist of much longer repeats, spanning many hundreds of kilobases. In addition to these tandemly repeated sequences, there are two major types of interspersed repeats in humans. These are called SINES (short interspersed elements) and LINES (long interspersed elements). The most abundant family of SINES are *Alu* elements, which make up 3–6% of the entire genome. The characteristic LINE family is *Kpn* I, or L1, repeats. The designation *Alu* or *Kpn* I refers to the restriction enzymes that were originally used to identify these repeats, while L1 is a characteristic transposable element, as described below.

Repetitive sequences tend to encourage recombinational instability. There are now many examples of deletions which involve *Alu* repeats.

Transposable elements

Although some gene insertions are the result of simple reduplication of sequences within particular genes, there is another family that results from the insertion of transposable, or mobile, genetic elements. Although at first these were thought to be restricted to maize they have now been found in a wide range of organisms, including humans. Both LINES and SINES are examples of transposable elements. Some of them act through an RNA intermediate, others directly from DNA to DNA. The former, sometimes called retrotransposons, encode polypeptides that have reverse transcriptase activity, that is, the potential to synthesize DNA on an RNA template. In other words they have the properties of retroviruses, which are able to insert their genetic material into the genomes of their hosts. While in lower organisms these elements have been viewed as a vehicle for the rapid generation of adaptive change, it is not clear what their function is, if any, in higher organisms. But there are several examples of the insertion of genetic material, apparently by mechanisms similar to these, as the basis for human molecular pathology (reviewed by Kazazian 1998).

Regulatory mutations

Most of the mutations that have been described so far, though they may be expressed at different levels of gene function, involve the gene itself or its immediate flanking regions. There are, however, mutations that involve important regulatory elements, which may have profound effects on the function of genes at some distance away on the same chromosome or on another chromosome. For example, we saw in Chapter 2 how the globin-gene clusters are regulated by elements that lie some distance upstream, the LCR in the case of the β-globin gene cluster and HS −40 for the α-globin genes. As we shall see later, deletions of these regions severely downregulate (<1%) their associated gene clusters. We also saw how there are families of regulatory DNA binding proteins, which are often encoded on other chromosomes and which may be either tissue-specific or ubiquitous in action. There are a number of examples of diseases that result from mutations of regulatory proteins of this type. As would be expected, since they may be involved in the regulation of many different genes, they may have widespread effects and cause extremely complex phenotypes. We shall encounter an excellent example of a family of mutations of this type when we discuss the syndrome of α thalassaemia and mental retardation in Chapter 12.

The α thalassaemias

In Chapter 3 we saw how the α thalassaemias are currently classified according to the output of α chains from the linked pair of α-globin genes on chromosome 16. In the α^0 thalassaemias there is no output of α globin from the linked pair, while in α^+ thalassaemia there is a reduced output. Here we shall describe the molecular lesions which give rise to these different forms of α thalassaemia. The clinical disorders that result from their interactions are described in Chapter 11.

As we saw in Chapter 2, analysis of the human α-globin cluster has revealed a remarkable degree of structural variability due to point mutations, deletions and insertions of DNA. These polymorphisms, which do not seem to interfere with α-globin production, are found in all populations. Variants that cause α thalassaemia are largely limited to tropical and subtropical countries in which malaria is, or has been, endemic (see Chapter 6). However, some rare and very informative mutations have been found outside these regions. In contrast to the β thalassaemias, which, as we shall see later, usually result from point mutations in the β-globin genes, the α thalassaemias are most often due to deletions involving one or both of the α-globin genes. Rarely, deletions that remove the α-globin gene regulatory element (HS –40) are responsible. This contrast in molecular pathology represents another difference between the properties of the α and β clusters, which may reflect their different chromosomal environments (see Chapter 2).

α+ *Thalassaemia resulting from deletions*

Heterogeneity

The α-globin genes are embedded within two highly homologous 4 kb duplication units, the sequence identity of which has been maintained throughout evolution by gene conversion and unequal crossover events (Lauer *et al.* 1980; Zimmer *et al.* 1980; Michelson & Orkin 1983; Hess *et al.* 1984). These regions are divided into homologous subsegments (X, Y and Z) by non-homologous elements (I, II and III, Figs 4.3 and 4.4). Unequal crossing over between Z segments (Fig. 4.3), which are 3.7 kb apart, produces a chromosome with only one α-globin gene ($-\alpha^{3.7}$, rightward

deletion) (Embury *et al.* 1980), that is, a deletional form of α+ thalassaemia, and one with three α-globin genes ($\alpha\alpha\alpha^{anti3.7}$) (Goossens *et al.* 1980; Higgs *et al.* 1980a). There are three varieties of this type of α+ thalassaemia, depending on exactly where within the Z box the crossover took place, that is $-\alpha^{3.7I}$, $-\alpha^{3.7II}$ and $-\alpha^{3.7III}$ (Higgs *et al.* 1984b) (Fig. 4.4). These subregions are defined by sequence differences in the Zα2 and Zα1 boxes that can be detected by Southern blot hybridization.

Non-reciprocal crossovers between homologous X boxes, which are 4.2 kb apart, also gives rise to an α-thalassaemia determinant ($-\alpha^{4.2}$) (Embury *et al.* 1980) and an $\alpha\alpha\alpha^{anti4.2}$ chromosome (Trent *et al.* 1981). Further recombination events between the resulting chromosomes (α, αα, ααα) give rise to quadruplicated α genes ($\alpha\alpha\alpha\alpha^{anti3.7}$, $\alpha\alpha\alpha\alpha^{anti4.2}$) (Trent *et al.* 1981; De Angioletti *et al.* 1992) or to other unusual rearrangements.

Three additional rare deletions that produce α+ thalassaemia have also been described (Fig. 4.4). One that removes the entire α1 gene and its flanking DNA ($-\alpha^{3.5}$) has been observed in two Asian Indians (Kulozik *et al.* 1988a); the breakpoints have not yet been reported in detail and thus it is not clear whether this represents a non-homologous recombination event (see later) or whether further sequences homologous to the Z box lie downstream of the α1 gene. Another deletion, referred to as $(\alpha)\alpha^{5.3}$, was

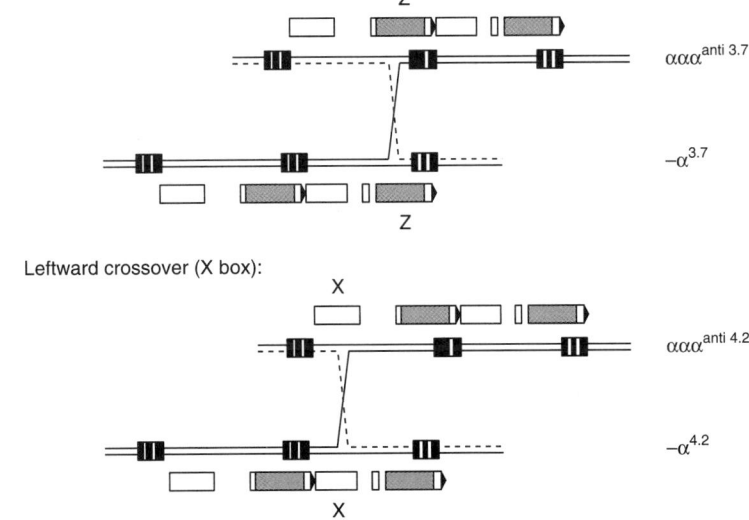

Fig. 4.3 The mechanism by which the common deletions underlying α+ thalassaemia occur. Crossovers between misaligned Z boxes give rise to the $-\alpha^{3.7}$ and $\alpha\alpha\alpha^{anti3.7}$ chromosomes. Crossovers between misaligned X boxes give rise to $-\alpha^{4.2}$ and $\alpha\alpha\alpha^{4.2}$ chromosomes.

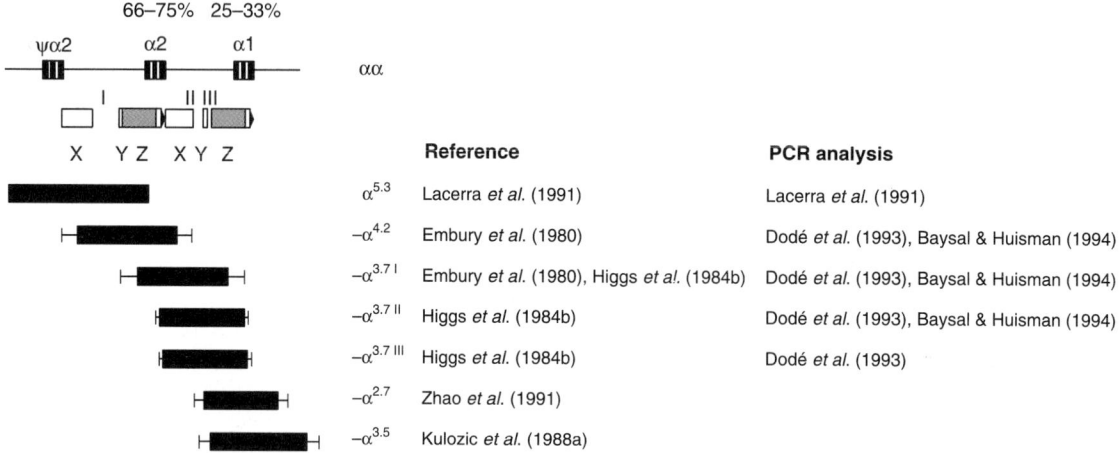

Fig. 4.4 Deletions that cause α⁺ thalassaemia. Above: the α-globin genes are shown with the duplication units divided into X, Y and Z boxes with regions of non-homology (I, II, III). Below: the extent of each deletion, represented by a black bar. The thin bar at the end of each thick bar denote the regions of uncertainty for the deletion breakpoints. Primary references for the characterization and examples of PCR analysis of these deletions are shown on the right-hand side of the diagram.

observed in a family from Italy (Lacerra *et al.* 1991). It removes the 5′ end of the α2 gene; the 5′ breakpoint lies 822 bp upstream of the mRNA CAP site of the ψα1 gene, while the 3′ breakpoint is located in IVS1 of the α2 gene. Sequence analysis indicates that this deletion has arisen by illegitimate recombination. A third rare allele was described in a Chinese patient with HbH disease (Zhao *et al.* 1991). This 2.7-kb deletion removes the α1 gene, but, since the breakpoints have not been sequenced, the mechanism by which it occurred is unknown.

How often have the deletional forms of α⁺ thalassaemia arisen?

The variety of independent recombination events giving rise to −α and ααα chromosomes identified in extant human populations suggest that recombination between the homologous X boxes and homologous Z boxes is relatively frequent. Several indirect observations support this notion. Both −α and ααα chromosomes are present in most populations. Moreover, the −α determinant is associated with many different α-globin variants in *cis* (Higgs *et al.* 1989), as well as different HVR alleles and α-globin restriction-fragment length-polymorphism (RFLP) haplotypes (Goodbourn *et al.* 1983; Winichagoon

et al. 1984; Flint *et al.* 1986) (the RFLPs and haplotypes of the α-globin genes are described in Chapter 2). In population isolates such as Papua New Guinea and Vanuatu the −α determinants are only found on the common α-globin haplotypes for that population, suggesting that they have arisen *de novo* (Flint *et al.* 1986). Some α-globin variants (e.g. HbG Philadelphia, $α^{68 \ \text{Asn}→\text{Lys}}$) are found on both normal (αα) chromosomes and those bearing an α-thalassaemia determinant (−α), suggesting a connection between the two through recombination or gene conversion (Strachan & Read 1996). Similar observations have been made for the poly(A) signal mutation found in Saudi Arabia (see later section), which is present on both αα and ααα chromosomes (Thein *et al.* 1988b).

It is interesting that the relative frequencies of the various types of α⁺ thalassaemia observed throughout the world correlate with the length of the homologous segments that serve as target areas for the crossovers involved ($-α^{3.7I}$ {1436 bp} > $-α^{4.2}$ {1339 bp} > $-α^{3.7II}$ {171 bp} > $-α^{3.7III}$ {46 bp}). Correlations between frequency of recombination and target size have been noted in other systems (Jinks-Robertson *et al.* 1993). However, since the α⁺-thalassaemia determinants have come under intense selection in many areas (Flint *et al.* 1986), these observations may not truly reflect recombination rates.

Direct evidence for a high rate of recombination between the duplicated α genes has recently been obtained using sperm typing by PCR (Lamb & Clegg 1996). Analysis of DNA extracted from the spermatozoa of a Caucasian donor indicated a frequency of $\sim 1.7 \times 10^4$.

Expression from the deletion α⁺-thalassaemia chromosomes

Although the relative expression of mRNA from the α2- and α1-globin genes on a normal chromosome is approximately 3:1, there are several lines of evidence that the α gene in the various −α chromosomes behaves like neither α1 nor α2. For example, homozygotes for the $-\alpha^{4.2}$ determinant, who essentially have two α1 genes ($-\alpha^{4.2}/-\alpha^{4.2}$), appear to express more α globin than the predicted 25% of normal (Bowden *et al.* 1987a), and homozygotes for $-\alpha^{3.7III}$, with the equivalent of two α2 genes ($-\alpha^{3.7}/-\alpha^{3.7}$), express less than the predicted 75% of normal (Bowden *et al.* 1987a). Direct measurements of α mRNA levels in patients with the $-\alpha^{3.7}$ determinant also suggest that the remaining α gene is expressed at a level roughly halfway between a normal α2 and α1 gene (Liebhaber *et al.* 1985). Since the transcriptional units of all the recombined genes ($-\alpha^{3.7I}$, $-\alpha^{3.7II}$, $-\alpha^{3.7III}$, $-\alpha^{4.2}$) are virtually identical to either the native α1 or α2 genes, the alteration in expression probably results from a change in the rate of transcription. Assuming that this is a *cis* effect, it could be brought about by the new combinations of flanking sequences, a release of transcriptional interference from the upstream gene (Proudfoot 1986), or by a change in chromosome conformation as a result of the deletions.

Another possibility is that the promoters of the α2 and α1 genes compete for interaction with the regulatory α-globin element (HS −40), similar to the way in which the γ and β genes are thought to compete for the β-globin gene LCR (see Chapter 2 and later in this chapter). In this case a single promoter in the −α chromosome would have continuous access to HS −40 and might, consequently, be expressed more efficiently.

Although there is no a priori reason to anticipate changes in ζ-globin expression in patients with the −α haplotype, it is useful to know that none of the −α mutations is associated with any significant change in ζ-globin expression (Chui *et al.* 1986).

α⁰ Thalassaemia due to deletions of the α-globin genes

Heterogeneity

As shown in Figs 4.5 and 4.6 many different length deletions have been found in patients with α⁰ thalassaemia. Unfortunately, these different mutations have attracted a rather complex and inconsistent nomenclature. Some of them are characterized by the name of the individual in whom they were first discovered, some by population origin and yet others by the particular size of the deletion. Though many of them are extremely rare or have only been observed on one occasion, two, those found in the Mediterranean region (MED) and in south-east Asia (SEA), reach high frequencies. This probably reflects both the time at which the lesions first occurred and intense heterozygote selection, presumably by *P. falciparum* malaria (see Chapter 6).

Extent of deletions

Recently, all of the DNA stretching for 300 kb from the 16p telomere was cloned, characterized and sequenced (Flint *et al.* 1997). This enabled us to define the full extent of several deletions that include the ζ, α and θ genes. They extend from 100 kb to over 250 kb (Fig. 4.6) and remove other genes that flank the α cluster, including a DNA repair enzyme (methyl adenine DNA glycosylase), an inhibitor of GDP dissociation from Rho (RhoGDIγ), a protein disulphide isomerase (PDI-R), and several anonymous housekeeping genes. Despite this, patients with these deletions appear phenotypically normal, apart from having α thalassaemia. In patients with more extensive deletions of 16p13.3, α thalassaemia is associated with developmental abnormalities and mental retardation (see Chapter 12).

Functional consequences

All of the deletions described in this section either completely or partially ($-(\alpha)^{5.2}$ and $-(\alpha)^{20.5}$) delete both α-globin genes (Figs 4.5 and 4.6), and therefore no α-chain synthesis is directed by these chromosomes *in vivo*. Homozygotes have the Hb Bart's hydrops fetalis syndrome (see Chapter 11). Several deletions remove both α-globin genes and the ζ gene

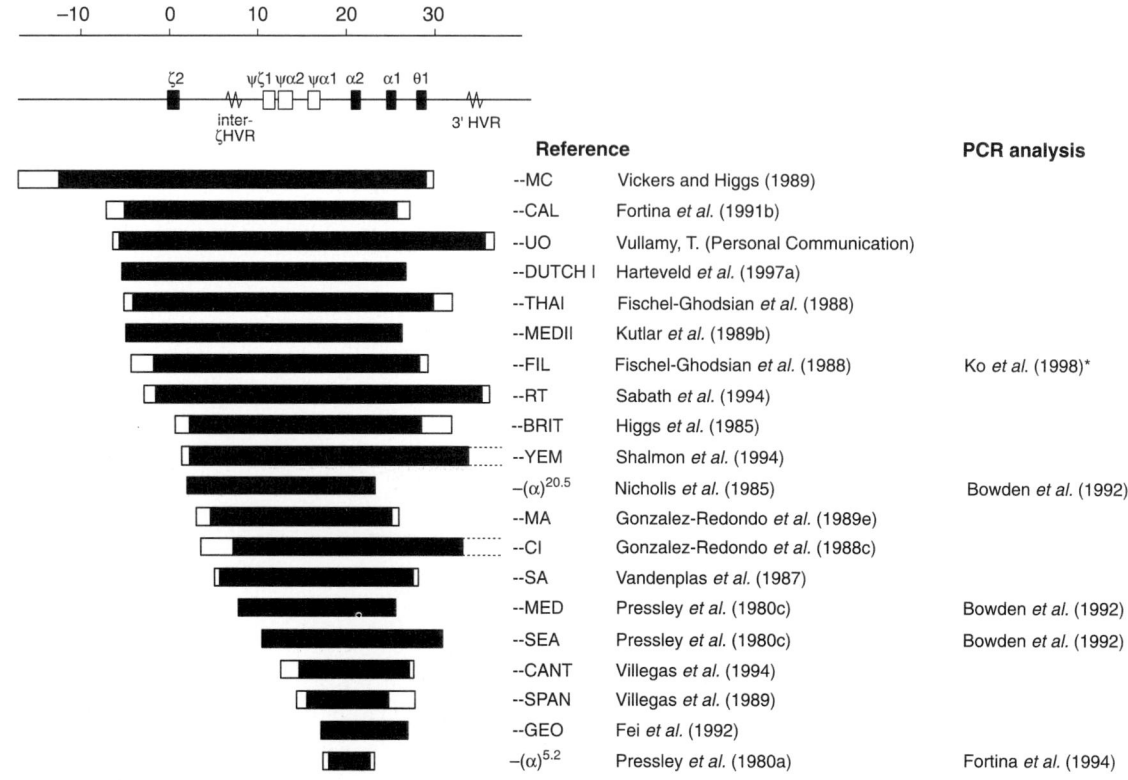

Fig. 4.5 Deletions that cause α° thalassaemia. Above: the α-gene complex is shown (scale in kilobases, 0 indicates the ζ2-globin mRNA CAP site). Below: the extent of each deletion is shown by a black bar. Regions of uncertainty for each breakpoint are shown by white boxes. To the right are the shorthand notations, primary references for the characterization and examples of PCR analysis for each deletion. *Although Ko *et al.* (1998) originally reported that their primers amplified the --THAI deletion it has subsequently been shown that, in fact, these deletions inadvertently characterized the --FIL mutation (Higgs *et al.* 1999). The --BRIT deletion may be the same as a rare α⁰-thalassaemia defect described in an Afro-American patient by Steinberg *et al.* (1986).

(Felice *et al.* 1984; Chan *et al.* 1985; Di Rienzo *et al.* 1986; Fischel-Ghodsian *et al.* 1988; Fortina *et al.* 1988; Vickers & Higgs 1989; Fortina *et al.* 1991b; Fei *et al.* 1992; Waye *et al.* 1992); although heterozygotes survive and appear to develop normally, homozygotes could not survive even the early stages of gestation, since neither embryonic ($\zeta_2\gamma_2$, $\zeta_2\varepsilon_2$, $\alpha_2\varepsilon_2$) nor fetal ($\alpha_2\gamma_2$) haemoglobin can be made (see Chapter 11).

Some, but not all, heterozygotes for deletions in which the embryonic gene remains intact continue to produce very small amounts of ζ globin in both fetal (Chui *et al.* 1989) and adult life (Kutlar *et al.* 1989b; Tang *et al.* 1992). This may be analogous to the persistent γ-globin production documented in

patients with downstream deletions of the β complex (see later in this chapter and Chapter 10). However, the amount of ζ globin in adults with these types of α thalassaemia is considerably less than that of γ globin in patients with comparable deletions of the β-gene complex. It seems that this increase of embryonic globin expression is not simply due to an increased rate of erythropoiesis since, in one study, no ε- or ζ-globin transcripts were detected in several patients with erythroid hyperplasia (Ley *et al.* 1989).

At the 3′ end of the complex most of these deletions include the θ1 gene, the function of which is not yet known. In one child homozygous for --SEA, who has been treated with blood transfusion, both θ1

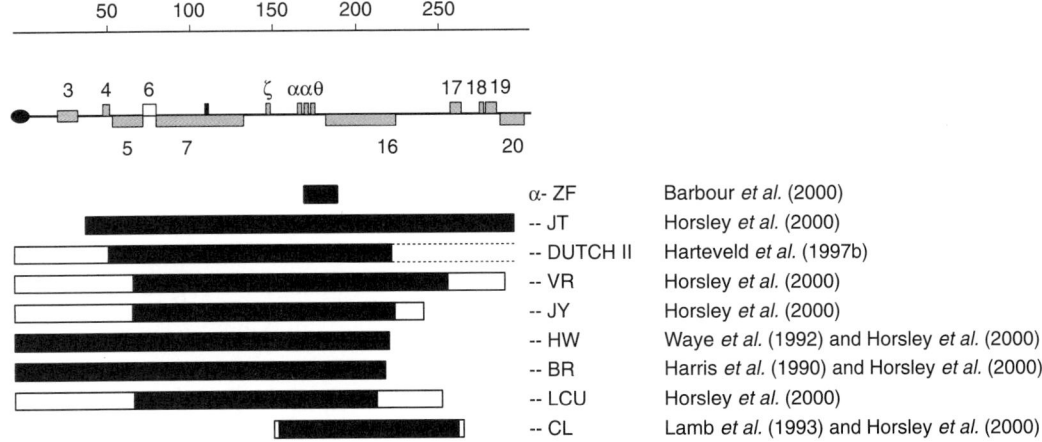

Fig. 4.6 Rare, large deletions that cause α thalassaemia but no associated abnormalities. Above the terminal 300 kb of chromosome 16p, as described in the legend to Fig. 2.12 (Chapter 2) (scale in kilobases). Below, black bars indicate the extent of each deletion. Regions of uncertainty for the breakpoints are shown by white boxes. To the right are the shorthand notations and primary references for each deletion.

genes are deleted, yet development appears to be normal (Fischel-Ghodsian *et al.* 1987).

How did the α⁰-thalassaemia deletions arise?

Detailed analyses of several determinants of α^0 thalassaemia have shown that they often result from illegitimate or non-homologous recombination (Nicholls *et al.* 1987). Such events may involve short regions of partial sequence homology where the breakpoints are rejoined, but they do not involve the extensive sequence matching required for the kind of homologous recombination that underlies the α^+ thalassaemias.

Sequence analysis has shown that members of the dispersed family of *Alu* repeats are frequently found at or near the breakpoints of these deletions. *Alu*-family repeats occur frequently in the genome (3×10^5 copies) and are particularly common in and around the α-globin gene cluster, where they make up ~25% of the entire sequence (Flint *et al.* 1997) (see earlier section). They may simply provide partially homologous sequences that facilitate DNA strand exchanges during replication, or possibly a subset may be more actively involved in the process. To date at least eight deletions causing α thalassaemia have been found to have one or both breakpoints lying in *Alu* sequences. Similar illegitimate recombination

events in the β locus less frequently involve *Alu* sequences, suggesting that this type of recombination may be, to at least some extent, locus specific (Henthorn *et al.* 1990).

Sequence analysis of the junctions of the α-globin deletions has revealed a number of interesting features, including palindromes, direct repeats, regions of weak homology and the frequent occurrence of the motif GAGG. One of the deletions ($--^{MED}$) also involves a more complex rearrangement that introduces a new piece of DNA bridging the two breakpoints. The inserted DNA originates from upstream of the α cluster and appears to have been incorporated into the junction in a manner which suggests that the upstream segment lies close to the breakpoint regions during replication (Fig. 4.7) (Nicholls *et al.* 1987).

At least two of the largest deletions ($--^{HW}$ and $--^{BR}$, Fig. 4.6) result from chromosomal breaks in the 16p telomeric region that have been 'healed' by the direct addition of telomeric repeats $(TTAGGG)_n$. This mechanism is described in further detail below.

Deletions of the α-globin-gene regulatory element

It has been shown that expression of the α-globin genes is critically dependent on a segment of DNA that lies 40 kb upstream of the ζ2-globin gene (Higgs

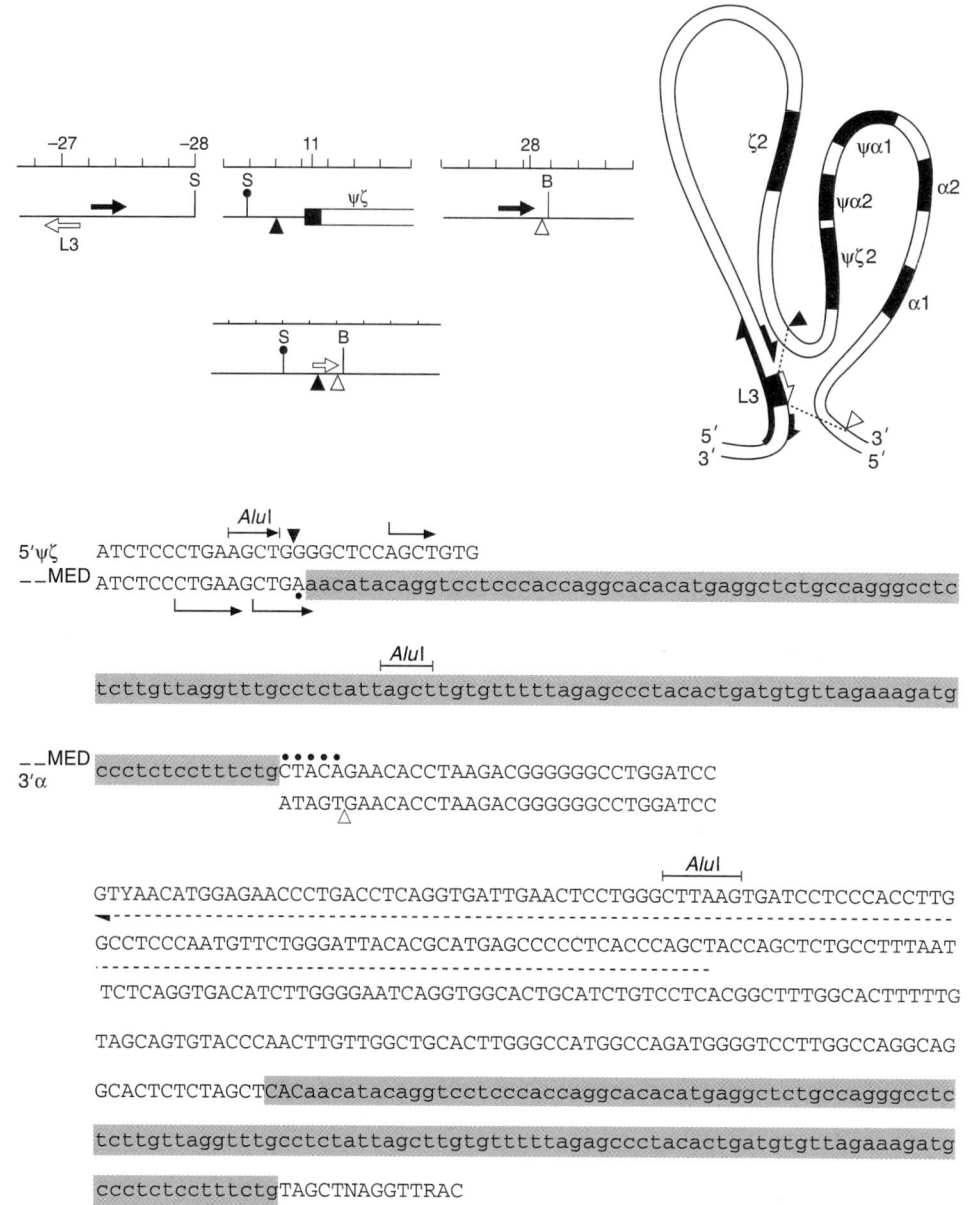

Fig. 4.7 A mechanism for the generation of the deletion which underlies a form of α⁰ thalassaemia. This deletion, −−^{MED} shown in Fig. 4.5, involves a complex rearrangement and introduces a new piece of DNA bridging the two breakpoints. As shown, the inserted DNA originates from upstream of the α cluster and appears to have been incorporated into the junction in a manner that suggests that the upstream segment lies close to the breakpoint regions during replication. From Nicholls *et al.* (1987).

et al. 1990). This region is associated with an erythroid-specific DNase1-hypersensitive site and is referred to as HS −40. It is described in detail in Chapter 2.

The first hint that such a remote regulatory sequence might exist came from studies of a patient with α thalassaemia (Hatton *et al.* 1990). Analysis of the abnormal chromosome (αα)^{RA} from this patient

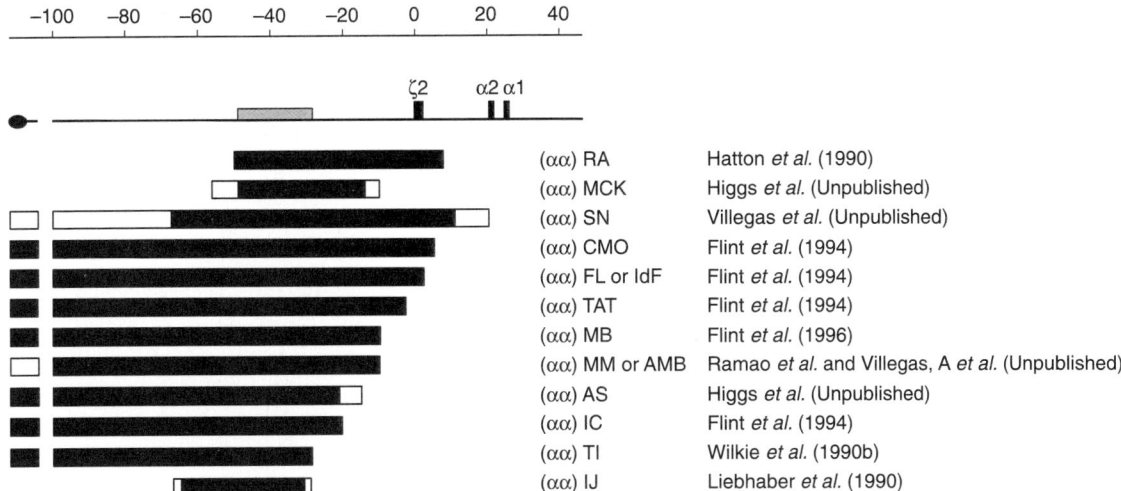

Fig. 4.8 Deletions extending upstream of the α cluster that cause α thalassaemia by removing the α-globin regulatory element (HS –40). Above: the α-gene cluster is shown (scale in kilobases; 0 indicates the ζ2 globin mRNA CAP site). The stippled box represents the shortest region of overlap between all deletions, including HS –40. The oval represents the 16p telomere. The extent of each deletion is indicated by black bars and the uncertainty of breakpoints is shown by white boxes. Primary references and shorthand notations are shown on the right.

demonstrated a 62-kb deletion from upstream of the α complex, which includes HS –40 (Fig. 4.8). Although both α genes on this chromosome are intact and entirely normal they appear to be non-functional. Since this observation, 10 more patients with α thalassaemia due to a deletion of HS –40 and a variable amount of the flanking DNA have been described (see Fig. 4.8 for references). A 20–24 kb segment of DNA containing HS –40 is deleted in all of these chromosomes and in each case the phenotype is α^0 thalassaemia; some patients have α^0-thalassaemia trait ($\alpha\alpha/(\alpha\alpha)$), others have HbH disease ($-\alpha/(\alpha\alpha)$).

Interspecific hybrids, each containing an abnormal copy of chromosome 16 from these patients, have been made by fusing Epstein–Barr (EB) virus cell lines with mouse erythroleukaemia (MEL) cells. In contrast to normal copies of chromosome 16, the abnormal chromosomes produce less than one per cent of human α-globin mRNA, indicating that deletions which remove HS –40 severely downregulate expression of the α-globin genes and are responsible for the associated α^0 thalassaemia. More recently a specific 'knockout' of HS –40 (Bernet *et al.* 1994) from such a chromosome, together with many experiments in transgenic mice (Higgs *et al.* 1998), have con-

firmed that HS –40 is the major element deleted by these arrangements.

The mechanisms by which these mutations have arisen are quite diverse. In the $(\alpha\alpha)^{RA}$ chromosome the deletion resulted from recombination between partially homologous *Alu* repeats that are normally 62 kb apart (Hatton *et al.* 1990). The $(\alpha\alpha)^{MB}$ chromosome (Flint *et al.* 1996) resulted from a subtelomeric rearrangement; the breakpoint was found in an *Alu* element located ~105 kb from the 16p subtelomeric region. The broken chromosome was stabilized with a new telomere acquired by recombination between this *Alu* element and a subtelomeric *Alu* repeat associated with the newly acquired chromosome end.

In five cases ($(\alpha\alpha)^{CMO}$ $(\alpha\alpha)^{IdF}$ $(\alpha\alpha)^{TAT}$ $(\alpha\alpha)^{IC}$ and $(\alpha\alpha)^{TI}$) (Fig. 4.8) the chromosomes appear to have been broken and then stabilized by the direct addition of telomeric repeats to non-telomeric DNA (Flint *et al.* 1994). Sequence analysis suggests that these chromosomes are 'healed' by the action of telomerase, an enzyme that is normally involved in maintaining the integrity of telomeres (Blackburn 1992; Flint *et al.* 1994).

In the three remaining examples ($(\alpha\alpha)^{IJ}$ $(\alpha\alpha)^{MCK}$ and $(\alpha\alpha)^{SN}$ (Fig. 4.8), the mechanism has not yet been established. However, it is interesting that in both

$(\alpha\alpha)^{IJ}$ and $(\alpha\alpha)^{MCK}$ the deletions appear to have arisen *de novo*, since neither parent has the abnormal chromosome.

A deletion extending downstream of the α-gene cluster

During a study to identify thalassaemia in families from the Czech Republic, Indrák *et al.* (1993) reported a new deletion (>18 kb) involving the α1 and θ1 gene, α–^{ZF} (Fig. 4.6). Heterozygotes have a mild hypochromic, microcytic anaemia (Hb 12.6 g/dl, MCH 22 pg, MCV 68 fl) with a reduced α/β-globin synthesis ratio (0.62–0.66) and HbH inclusions. These findings suggest that, although the α2 gene appears to be intact, it has been inactivated by the deletion.

Further analysis of this deletion (Higgs *et al.* 1998; Barbour *et al.* 2000) has confirmed that the remaining α2 gene on the α–^{ZF} chromosome is structurally intact, including all its critical *cis*-acting sequences, and has no inactivating point mutations. Nevertheless, functional studies in which the abnormal chromosome was isolated as an interspecific hybrid with MEL cells, confirmed that the α2 gene has been inactivated by the deletion; such hybrids produce no human α mRNA.

Detailed *in vivo* analyses of this mutation have shown that the α gene and its promoter have been made inaccessible to DNase1 and other endonucleases. Furthermore, the CpG island associated with the gene, which spans the α-gene promoter, has become fully methylated whereas normally this region is unmethylated. At present the mechanism by which this occurred is not clear but it is of interest that the region of the chromosome abutted to the α2 gene by the deletion corresponds to an *Alu*-dense, methylated region that contains no DNase1-hypersensitive sites (Flint *et al.* 1997). Perhaps the simplest explanation is that the juxtaposition of the α2 gene next to a piece of relatively inert chromatin has induced a chromosomal position effect. In such situations it is thought that a repressive chromatin structure spreads over a gene that is normally active and prevents its expression (Shaffer *et al.* 1993). Further studies will be needed to test this hypothesis.

It is not clear whether this mutation has simply identified an unimportant block of 'heterochromatin', or if this region normally plays an important role in regulating the α-gene cluster. Studies in transgenic mice have shown that, although this region contains no positive regulatory sequences, α-globin mRNA expression from a large construct containing it occurs at higher levels than those which do not span this area, and in a more stable manner (Higgs *et al.* 1998). Further studies are under way to assess the role of this fascinating area of the α-gene cluster.

Non-deletional types of α thalassaemia

In all surveys reported so far, α thalassaemia is much more frequently due to deletions, as described in previous sections, than to single-point mutations or oligonucleotide insertions and deletions involving the canonical sequences that control gene expression, the so-called 'non-deletion variants', in which the affected gene is denoted α^T.

Non-deletional types of α thalassaemia were first described in 1977 (Kan *et al.* 1977a) and shown to result from a variety of mechanisms (Higgs *et al.* 1981). At present we know of 41 well defined types of non-deletion α⁺ thalassaemia (Table 4.2); 25 occur in the α2 gene, seven in the α1 gene, and six on a –α chromosome. In three cases the mutation has not yet been assigned to the α1 or α2 genes. As a group, they appear to have a more severe effect on α-globin gene expression and the haematological phenotype than simple deletions that remove one or other of the α genes (–α) (see Chapter 11). This may be because the majority of mutations affect the α2 gene, the expression of which may predominate over the α1 gene; this may also lead to a bias in ascertainment. In addition, unlike the situation in which one α-globin gene is deleted, there does not appear to be a compensatory increase in expression of the remaining functional α-globin gene when its partner is inactivated by a point mutation. Furthermore, some highly unstable variants may have multiple secondary effects on red-cell structure and function, producing a more severe phenotype than would be predicted from the decrease in α-gene expression. At present these ideas are based on a small number of observations and further evaluation of the pathophysiology of each mutation is needed.

Mutations that affect RNA splicing

Three mutations affect RNA splicing. One ($\alpha^{IVS1; \, 5bp \, del}\alpha$) results from a pentanucleotide deletion at the 5′ donor site of IVS1 of the α2-globin gene (Orkin *et al.* 1981a; Felbar *et al.* 1982). This involves the invariant GT sequence and eliminates splicing from the normal donor site, while activating a cryptic donor consensus in exon 1. Aberrantly spliced mRNA can be detected in a transient expression system and in bone marrow. In contrast, in peripheral blood very little, if any, mRNA from the altered $\alpha 2$-globin gene can be detected, suggesting that the aberrantly spliced RNA is unstable. Heterozygotes for this mutation have the phenotype of α-thalassaemia trait and homozygotes have a correspondingly more severe form of α^+ thalassaemia.

A mutation of the acceptor site of IVS1 of the $\alpha 2$ gene ($^{IVS1-116(A \rightarrow G)}\alpha$) was described by Harteveld *et al.* (1996c). Abnormal splicing leads to the retention of IVS1 which introduces a premature stop at codon 31. The low levels of abnormal mRNA found in reticulocytes are thought to be due to post-transcriptional instability. Although all 11 carriers for this mutation have reduced α/β-globin synthesis ratios (0.78–0.85) their haematological findings are remarkably normal (Harteveld *et al.* 1996c). It remains to be seen if this applies in further cases.

A third splicing defect is caused by a mutation at IVS1-117 of the $\alpha 1$-globin gene ($\alpha^{IVS1-117(G \rightarrow A)}\alpha$) (Çürük *et al.* 1993a). In this case, the nature of the abnormal splicing has not been established. Furthermore, the evidence that this mutation causes α thalassaemia is based solely on its consistent effect of lowering the level of HbS in sickle-cell heterozygotes; it will be interesting to document the haematological effect of this mutation.

Mutations affecting the poly(A) addition signal

The highly conserved sequence motif AATAAA is present 10–30 bp upstream of most poly(A) addition sites and forms part of the signal for mRNA cleavage and polyadenylation of primary transcripts (see Chapter 2). This sequence is required for transcriptional termination; when mutated, transcription may proceed into neighbouring genes and 'interfere' with their expression.

Four mutations of the $\alpha 2$-gene polyadenylation signal (PA) have been described (Table 4.2). The first to be identified (AATAAA$\rightarrow$AATAAG, or $\alpha^{PA6:A \rightarrow G}$) was found in the Saudi Arabian population. Heterozygotes have the haematological phenotype of the more severe forms of α-thalassaemia trait, while homozygotes have HbH disease, with 5–15% HbH in their peripheral blood (Pressley *et al.* 1980b; Dr J. Zhao, personal communication).

Homozygotes for other non-deletion mutations that inactivate the $\alpha 2$ gene do not always have HbH disease and, even when they do, it is often mild with low levels of HbH. In contrast, homozygotes for the $\alpha^{PA6:A \rightarrow G}\alpha$ chromosome always have HbH disease with high levels of HbH. It is interesting that $\alpha 2$ mRNA is reduced but not absent and therefore, if the $\alpha 1$ gene were fully active, a severe form of α-thalassaemia trait rather than HbH disease might be expected. The implication of these findings is that the poly(A) site mutation downregulates both $\alpha 2$ and $\alpha 1$ genes on the same chromosome. Occasionally, the $\alpha^{PA6:A \rightarrow G}$ mutation is duplicated, producing a chromosome with three α genes, $\alpha^{PA6:A \rightarrow G}\alpha^{PA6:A \rightarrow G}\alpha$, which still interacts with the $\alpha^{PA6:A \rightarrow G}\alpha$ chromosome to produce HbH disease (Thein *et al.* 1988b).

Further analysis of the $\alpha^{PA6:A \rightarrow G}$ mutation has shown that it has at least two effects. It reduces the amount of $\alpha 2$ mRNA and, in a transient assay, read-through transcripts extending beyond the mutated poly(A) addition site are detected. Extended transcripts were also detected in reticulocytes of patients with this defect using RT-PCR (Molchanova *et al.* 1995). It is possible that transcription extending through the normal termination point could run on and interfere with expression of the linked $\alpha 1$ gene.

Given the reduction in α-chain synthesis associated with the $\alpha^{PA6:A \rightarrow G}\alpha$ chromosome it is surprising that compound heterozygotes for this mutation and a common α^0-thalassaemia determinant are not more severely affected (Dr J. Zhao, personal communication).

Since the original description of the $\alpha^{PA6:A \rightarrow G}$ allele, three other poly(A) signal mutations have been described (Table 4.2). At present there are insufficient data to know whether these mutations downregulate α-globin gene expression in a similar way. In particular no homozygotes have been identified. Compound heterozygotes for these mutations and α^0 thalassaemia have HbH disease, as expected (Fei *et al.* 1992; Yüregir *et al.* 1992).

Mutations affecting initiation of mRNA translation

Several non-deletion mutations affect mRNA translation, five of which disrupt the initiation consensus sequence CCRCCATG (Table 4.2). Two mutations, which involve the initiation (IN) codon, occur on chromosomes with a single α gene. In one ($-\alpha^{IN:A \rightarrow G}$),

Table 4.2 Non-deletion mutants that cause α thalassaemia.

Affected gene	Affected sequence	Location§	Mutation	Alternative notation	Identification	Distribution	Reference
mRNA processing							
α2	IVS1 (donor)	163008–163012	IVS1;5-bp del	$\alpha^{Hph}\alpha$	– Hph 1	Mediterranean	Orkin et al. (1981a)
α2	IVS1-116 (acceptor)	163122	IVS1;116 A→G		+ Sac 2	Dutch Caucasian	Harteveld et al. (1996c)
α1	IVS1-117 (acceptor)	166927	IVS1;117 G→A		– Fok 1	Asian Indian	Çürük et al. (1993a)
α2	Poly(A) signal	163673–163688	PA;16-bp del		– Hae III	Arab	Tamary et al. (1997)
α2*	Poly(A) signal	163693	PA;6 A→G	$\alpha^{TSaudi}\alpha$		Middle East; Mediterranean	Higgs et al. (1983a)
α2	Poly(A) signal	163691	PA;4 A→G			Mediterranean	Yüregir et al. (1992)
α2	Poly(A) signal	163692–163693	PA;2-bp del			Asian Indian	Hall et al. (1994); Harteveld et al. (1994)
mRNA translation†							
–α	Initiation codon	163912	IN;→G		– Nco 1	Black	Olivieri et al. (1987)
$-\alpha^{3.7II}$	Initiation codon	162909–162910	IN;2-bp del			North African; Mediterranean	Morlé et al. (1985, 1986)
α2	Initiation codon	162913	IN;T→C		– Nco 1	Mediterranean	Pirastu et al. (1984b)
α1	Initiation codon	166716	IN;A→G		– Nco 1	Mediterranean	Paglietti et al. (1986); Moi et al. (1987)†
α2	Initiation codon	162913	IN;1-bp del		– Nco 1	Vietnam	Waye et al. (1996)†
–α	Exon I	163005–163006	CD30/31;2-bp del			Black	Safaya & Rieder (1988)†
α2	Exon II	163146–163154	CD39/41;del/ins			Yemenite-Jewish	Oron-Karni et al. (1997)†
α1	Exon II	166986–167000	CD51–55;13-bp del		– Bst NI	Spain	Ayala et al. (1997)†
α2	Exon III	163509–163520	CD113–116;12-bp del			Spanish	Ayala et al. (1996)
α2	Exon III	163519	CD116;G→T		+ Bfa 1	Black	Liebhaber et al. (1987)
α2	Termination codon	163597	TER;T→C (Constant Spring)	$\alpha^{CS}\alpha$	– Mse 1	South-east Asian	Clegg et al. (1971b)
α2	Termination codon	164597	TER;T→A (Icaria)	$\alpha^{Ic}\alpha$	– Mse 1	Mediterranean	Clegg et al. (1974); Efremov et al. (1990)
α2	Termination codon	163598	TER;A→C (Koya Dora)	$\alpha^{KD}\alpha$	– Mse 1	Indian	de Jong et al. (1975)
α2	Termination codon	163597	TER;T→G (Seal Rock)	$\alpha^{SR}\alpha$	– Mse 1	Black	Bradley et al. (1975); Merritt et al. (1997)
α2	Termination codon	163599	TER;A→T (Paksé)		– Mse 1	Laotian	Waye et al. (1994e)

Post-translational

Gene	Exon	Codon/mutation	Number§	Variant	Enzyme	Population	Reference
−α	Exon I	CD14;T→G (Evanston){W→R}	162954			Black	Honig et al. (1984)
α2	Exon I	CD29;T→C (Agrinio){L→P}	163000			Mediterranean	Hall et al. (1993b)
α2	Exon I	CD30;3-bp del {ΔE}	163002–163004			China	Chan et al. (1997)
α1	Exon II	CD38/39;3-bp del; (Taybe){ΔT}	163143–163145			Arabia	Pobedimskaya et al. (1994)
α1	Exon II	CD59;G→A (Adana){G→D}	167011			Turkey	Çürük et al. (1993b)
α2	Exon II	CD59;G→A (Adana){G→D}	163207			China	Chan et al. (1997)
α1	Exon II	CD60/61;3-bp del (Clinic){ΔK}	167013–167018		+ Dde 1	Spain	Ayala et al. (1998)
α2	Exon II	CD62;3-bp del	163215–163217			Greece	Harteveld (1998)
α2	Exon II	CD66;T→C (Dartmouth)				Cambodia	Fairweather et al. (1999)
α2	Exon III	CD104;G→A (Sallanches){C→Y}	163484		+ Bsp M1	French	Morlé et al. (1995)
α2	Exon III	CD109;T→G (Suan Dok){L→R}	163499	$\alpha^{SD}\alpha$	+ Sma 1	South-east Asia	Sanguansermsri et al. (1979)
α	Exon III	CD110;C→A (Petah Tikva){A→D}	(163502)	$\alpha^{PT}\alpha$		Middle East	Honig et al. (1981)
α2	Exon III	CD125;T→C (Quong Sze){L→P}	163547	$\alpha^{QS}\alpha$	+ Msp 1	South-east Asia	Goossens et al. (1982)
$-\alpha^{3.7}$	Exon III	CD125;T→A {L→Q}	163547			Israel	Oran Kani (personal communication)
α1	Exon III	CD129;T→C (Tunis-Bizerte){L→P}	167370		+ Nci 1	Tunisia	Darbellay et al. (1995)
α2	Exon III	CD129;T→C (Utrecht){L→P}	163559		+ Hpa II	Netherlands	Harteveld et al. (1996a)
α2	Exon III	CD130;G→C (Sun Prairie){A→P}	163561			Asian Indian	Harkness et al. (1990)
α2	Exon III	CD131;T→C (Questembert){S→P}	163564			Yugoslavia	Rochette et al. (1995)
α2	Exon III	CD 136;T→C (Hb Bibba){L→P}	163580			Caucasian	Prchal et al. (1995)

Uncharacterized

Gene	Exon	Codon/mutation	Number§	Variant	Enzyme	Population	Reference
α	Unknown	Not determined	Unknown			Black	Mathew et al. (1983)
α	Unknown	Not determined	Unknown			Greek‡	Trent et al. (1986c)
α	Unknown	Not determined	Unknown			Pacific	Hill et al. (1987b)

* This mutation has been found in both α2-like genes on an $\alpha\alpha\alpha^{3.7}$ chromosome present in Saudi Arabian individuals.

† The elongated α chains associated with Hb Wayne, which results from a frameshift (deletion of either C at α138 or A at α139 of the α2-globin gene), and Hb Grady, which results from a crossover in phase (with insertion of three residues at α118), are not known to be associated with α thalassaemia although the critical interactions that would clearly reveal this have not been described.

‡ Its interaction with α^{0}-thalassaemia determinants to produce the Hb Bart's hydrops fetalis syndrome suggests that both α-globin genes may be affected.

§ These numbers refer to the sequence published in Flint et al. (1997); location in brackets assumes α2 defect.

'−', removes; '+', creates restriction enzyme site.

the mutation abolishes translation of mRNA. It was identified through its interaction with a second α-thalassaemia chromosome ($-\alpha^{IN:A\rightarrow G}/-\alpha$); affected persons had the typical haematological features of HbH disease, with 2.4 and 7.2% HbH (Olivieri *et al.* 1987). In the other case ($-\alpha^{IN:2bp\ del}$) a 2-bp deletion from the consensus sequence reduced the level of mRNA translation by 30–50% (Morlé *et al.* 1985, 1986). This mutation produces HbH disease in homozygotes ($-\alpha^{IN:2bp\ del}/-\alpha^{IN:2bp\ del}$), who have a mild hypochromic microcytic anaemia (Hb 9.7–9.9, MCV 63, MCH 18–20) with 4.5–5.6% HbH (Tabone *et al.* 1981).

Two mutations ($\alpha^{IN:T\rightarrow C}\alpha$ and $\alpha^{IN:1bp\ del}\alpha$) abolish translation of mRNA from the α2 gene. Six of seven homozygotes for the $\alpha^{IN:T\rightarrow C}\alpha$ haplotype have a severe form of α-thalassaemia trait, but one had a mild form of HbH disease, with 2.6% HbH (Cao *et al.* 1991; Galanello *et al.* 1992). Compound heterozygotes for this mutation with common α^0 thalassaemias have HbH disease with substantial amounts of HbH (~8–24%) in the peripheral blood.

One mutation, $\alpha\alpha^{IN:A\rightarrow G}$, abolishes translation of mRNA from the α1-globin gene (Moi *et al.* 1987). In the single family reported, compound heterozygotes ($--/\alpha\alpha^{IN:A\rightarrow G}$) had relatively low levels of HbH (1.5% and 3%), suggesting that the mutation of the α1 gene causes a less severe degree of α-chain deficit than a similar mutation of the α2 gene. The finding of this mutation adds weight to the argument that the α2 gene is expressed at a higher level than the α1 gene.

In-frame deletions, frameshifts and nonsense mutations

In 1988 Safaya and Rieder described an Afro-American with HbH disease and HbG Philadelphia ($-\alpha^{68\ Asn\rightarrow Lys}$) who synthesized only α^G and no α^A chains. The patient was shown to have the genotype $-\alpha/-\alpha^G$, and it was concluded that the $-\alpha$ chromosome was inactivated by a further mutation. Sequence analysis showed that the remaining α gene has a dinucleotide deletion from one or other of the Glu (GAG) or Arg (AGG) codons (30 and 31). The loss of two nucleotides leads to a frameshift and a new sequence in exon II from codons 31–54, followed by a new, in-phase termination codon (TAA) at position 55. Hence the $-\alpha^{Cd30/31:2bp\ del}$ chromosome is an inactive α^0-thalassaemia determinant.

Mutations affecting the α-globin gene translational reading frame have also been found on chromosomes with two α genes (αα); three affect the α2-globin gene. In one ($\alpha^{Cd39/41\ del/ins}\alpha$) there is a deletion of 9 bp (codons 39–41) replaced by an 8-nucleotide insertion which duplicates the adjacent downstream sequence. The mutation changes the mRNA reading frame, introducing a new termination signal (TGA) 10 codons downstream. In another case a 12-bp deletion of the α2 gene results in the loss of four amino acids (codons 113–116) from the α chain, which is reduced from its normal length of 141 amino acids to 137. It is thought that this results in an unstable α chain which is rapidly broken down and unable to form a haemoglobin tetramer, like some variants described later. In a heterozygote this mutation produced the phenotype of α-thalassaemia trait. The third mutation in this group has a single base change ($\alpha^{Cd116:G\rightarrow T}\alpha$) which results in a premature termination codon and inactivation of the α2 gene. Again, carriers have α-thalassaemia trait.

A single Spanish family with a frameshift mutation in the α1-globin gene has been described by Ayala *et al.* (1997). Direct sequence analysis of the α1 gene revealed a 13-bp deletion, between codons 51 and 55 ($\alpha\alpha^{Cd51-55:13bpdel}/\alpha\alpha$). This mutation results in an mRNA reading frameshift which introduces a new stop signal at codon 62. Two affected persons have α-thalassaemia trait.

Chain-termination mutations

There are potentially nine single nucleotide variants of the natural termination codon (TAA) of the α2-globin gene; two (TGA and TAG) generate new stop (nonsense) mutations and the others encode amino acids (Fig. 4.9). When mutations change the stop codon to one that encodes an amino acid it allows mRNA translation to continue to the next in-phase termination codon (UAA) located within the polyadenylation signal (AAUAAA), in each case extending the α chain by 31 amino acids from the natural C-terminal arginine (codon 141). Of the six predicted α2 variants, five have been described, each with a unique amino acid at α142: Hb Constant Spring (α142 Gln), Hb Icaria (α142 Lys), Hb Koya Dora (α142 Ser), Hb Seal Rock (α142 Glu) and Hb Paksé (α142 Tyr). An extended α-globin chain variant with leucine at position 142 is predicted but has not yet been described.

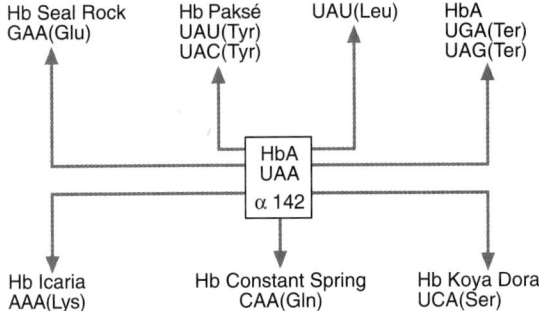

Fig. 4.9 The potential and actual α-chain-termination mutant haemoglobins that can be produced by a single base change in the α-globin mRNA termination codon, α142 UAA. Redrawn from Weatherall and Clegg (1975).

The mechanism by which chain-termination mutations cause α thalassaemia has been difficult to elucidate although there are now sufficient observations to provide a plausible explanation. Nevertheless, we still do not fully understand how the unusual haematological phenotype associated with these mutations arises (see Chapters 5 and 11 for further discussion). Heterozygotes clearly have α thalassaemia, but the MCV is higher than normally seen in this condition (for examples see Weatherall & Clegg 1975; Schrier *et al.* 1997). Homozygotes have an unexpectedly severe form of thalassaemia, considering that only two of the four α genes are inactive (Lie-Injo *et al.* 1974; Pootrakul *et al.* 1981c), and compound heterozygotes ($\alpha^{TER:T\rightarrow C}\alpha/--$) have an unusually severe form of HbH disease (for example, see Fucharoen *et al.* 1988a).

Hb Constant Spring (CS) is the most extensively studied of this group. Heterozygotes for this mutation ($\alpha^{TER:T\rightarrow C}\alpha/\alpha\alpha$) have ~1% HbCS in their red cells rather than the ~25% usually found in carriers of α-chain variants (Weatherall & Clegg 1975). It seems likely that the α2 gene containing this mutation is transcribed normally, although this has not been formally demonstrated. Substantial amounts of the abnormal α^{CS} mRNA are found in erythroid precursors from the bone marrow but the level decreases during erythroid maturation and is virtually absent from reticulocytes (Liebhaber & Kan 1981; Hunt *et al.* 1982). The synthesis of α^{CS} globin follows the same pattern, decreasing from bone marrow to reticulocytes (Kan *et al.* 1974c; Weatherall & Clegg 1975).

From these findings it was suggested that α^{CS} mRNA is unstable, possibly due to disruption of a sequence(s) in the 3′ non-coding region that is translated inappropriately as a result of the chain-termination mutation (Hunt *et al.* 1982). Recent experimental data support this interpretation. Weiss & Liebhaber (1994) showed that translational readthrough disrupts a putative RNA/protein complex associated with the α2-globin 3′ UTR which is required for mRNA stability in erythroid cells.

Recent studies on the pathophysiology of the forms of α thalassaemia associated with Hb Constant Spring, and the reasons that they may differ from other forms of α thalassaemia, are summarized in Chapter 5.

Unstable α-chain variants associated with α thalassaemia

It is well established that some globin variants alter the tertiary structure of the haemoglobin molecule, making the dimer (αβ) or tetramer ($\alpha_2\beta_2$) unstable. Such molecules may precipitate within the red cell, forming insoluble inclusions (Heinz bodies) which damage the red-cell membrane. As outlined in Chapters 2 and 11, this results in a chronic haemolytic anaemia with equal loss of α- and β-like globin chains from the red cell.

Some α-globin variants are so unstable that they undergo very rapid, postsynthetic degradation. In this case, since they do not form dimers or tetramers, there is no associated loss of normal β chains, which remain, in excess, within the red cell. These patients, by definition, have α thalassaemia. Many of these variants are so unstable that they cannot be detected by conventional protein analysis. Therefore patients often present with non-deletional α thalassaemia that can only be explained when the mutation is identified by DNA sequence analysis.

The haematological findings are complex because the mutations may involve the α1 or α2 gene, cause different degrees of globin instability and be influenced by interacting alleles. For example, some variant α chains may be fully or temporarily stabilized when incorporated into a dimer or tetramer; the co-inheritance of α thalassaemia will reduce the normal pool of free α chains and drive abnormal α chains into dimers or tetramers. In this case, subsequent instability may cause loss of both α-like and β-like chains, changing the clinical picture from α tha-

Table 4.3 Phenotypes of unstable α-chain variants.

Variant	Base change	Residue/substitution	Phenotype
Hb Agrino	CD29 CTG→CCG	α29 (B10) Leu→Pro	α⁺-thalassaemia trait
Hb Taybee	CD38/39 –'ACC	α38/39 (C3/4) Thr→O	α⁺-thalassaemia trait
Hb Torino	—	α43 (CE1) Phe→Val	Heinz-body haemolytic anaemia
Hb Hirosaki	CD43 TTC→TTG	α43 (CE1) Phe→Leu	Haemolytic anaemia
Hb Adana	CD59 GGC→GAC	α59 (E8) Gly→Asp	α⁺-thalassaemia trait
Hb Sallanches	CD104 TGC→TAC	α104 (G11) Cys→Tyr	α⁺-thalassaemia trait
Hb Suan Dok	CD109 CTG→CGG	α109 (G16) Leu→Arg	α⁺-thalassaemia trait
Hb Pehah Tikva	—	α110 (G17) Ala→Asp	α⁺-thalassaemia trait
Hb Quong Sze	CD125 CTG→CCG	α125 (H8) Leu→Pro	α⁺-thalassaemia trait
Hb Tunis-Bizerte (Hb Utrecht)	CD129 CTG→CCG	α129 (H12) Leu→Pro	α⁺-thalassaemia trait
Hb Sun Prairie	CD130 GCT→CCT	α130 (H13) Ala→Pro	α⁺-thalassaemia trait
Hb Questembert	—	α131 (H14) Ser→Pro	α⁺-thalassaemia trait
Hb Bibba	—	α131 (H19) Leu→Pro	Heinz-body haemolytic anaemia
Hb Toyama	—	α136 (H19) Leu→Arg	Heinz-body haemolytic anaemia

lassaemia to a haemolytic anaemia. The easiest way to appreciate the effect of these mutations is to observe their effects in simple heterozygotes; they usually have the phenotype of α-thalassaemia trait with low or undetectable amounts of the α-globin-chain variant.

To date, 17 unstable α-globin-chain variants have been shown to produce this phenotype to a greater or lesser extent (Table 4.3). The mutations most frequently affect the haem pocket, internal hydrophobic regions of the molecule that normally maintain its conformation, or hydrophobic residues involved in the formation of $\alpha_1\beta_1$ contacts.

The patterns of precipitation and association of these highly unstable α-globin chains with β chains are extremely variable and produce a series of complex phenotypes (Table 4.3). Indeed, studies of haemoglobin synthesis in some of these conditions have led to them being characterized as disorders of β-globin-chain production (Ho *et al.* 1996b). We shall return to the problem of the phenotypic distinctions between disorders due to unstable α-globin-chain variants in Chapter 11.

The β thalassaemias

In the previous chapter we described how the β thalassaemias are classified into β^0 and β^+ varieties, reflecting an absence or reduction of β-globin synthesis, respectively. We also discussed how the latter may be further divided into β^+ and β^{++}, reflecting variabil-

ity in the degree of severity of the defect in β-globin production. As shown in Table 3.1, the β thalassaemias are further subdivided into several categories, depending on the clinical manifestations and levels of Hbs F and A_2 in heterozygotes. Here we shall describe the different kinds of mutations that underlie these conditions.

Almost 200 β-thalassaemia alleles have now been characterized. Unlike the α thalassaemias, the vast majority of β thalassaemias are caused by point mutations within the β-globin genes or their immediate flanking sequences. A few β-thalassaemia mutations which segregate independently of the β-globin gene cluster have been described, presumably involving *trans*-acting regulatory factors. The main classes of mutations that underlie β thalassaemia, together with their level of function, are summarized in Table 4.4.

Gene deletions or insertions which cause β thalassaemia

In contrast to the α thalassaemias, the β thalassaemias are rarely caused by major gene deletions. There are two notable exceptions: a family of upstream deletions, which downregulate the β-globin LCR (see Chapter 2); and another which involve only the β-globin genes themselves. Since the upstream deletions involve the whole β-globin gene complex and cause $(\varepsilon^G\gamma^A\gamma\delta\beta)^0$ thalassaemia, they are described in a later section.

Table 4.4 Main classes of mutations that cause β-thalassaemias.

Transcription
  Deletions
  Insertions
  Promoter
  5′ UTR

Processing of mRNA
  Junctional
  Consensus sequence
  Cryptic splice sites in introns
  Cryptic splice sites in exons
  Poly(A) addition site
  Other 3′ UTR sites

Translation
  Initiation site
  Nonsense
  Frameshift

Post-translational stability
  Highly unstable β-chain variants

Determinants unlinked to β-globin-gene cluster

Determinants of unknown molecular pathology

Deletions restricted to the β-globin genes

Fourteen deletions affecting only the β-globin gene have been described (Fig. 4.10). They range in size from 290 bp to >60 kb. Of these, only the 619-bp deletion at the 3′ end of the β gene is common, and even that is restricted to the Sind and Punjabi populations of India and Pakistan, in whom it accounts for ~20% of β-thalassaemia alleles (Thein *et al.* 1984b; Varawalla *et al.* 1991a). The other deletions, although extremely rare, are of particular functional and phenotypic interest because they are associated with an unusually high level of HbA$_2$ in heterozygotes.

These deletions differ widely in size, but remove in common a region from positions −125 to +78 relative to the mRNA CAP site in the β promoter, which includes the CACCC, CCAAT and TATA elements. The mechanism underlying the unusually high levels of HbA$_2$ and the variable increases in HbF in heterozygotes for these deletions appear to involve the removal of the 5′ promoter region of the β-globin gene. This may release competition for the upstream LCR, leading to its increased interaction with the γ

and δ genes in *cis*, so enhancing their expression. Indeed, studies of an individual heterozygous for the 1.39 kb β-thalassaemia deletion and a δ-chain variant showed that there is a disproportionate increase of HbA$_2$ (δ chain) derived from the δ-globin gene *cis* to the β-globin gene deletion (Codrington *et al.* 1990). This mechanism may also explain the moderate increases in HbF which characterizes this group of deletional β thalassaemias and those due to point mutations affecting the promoter regions. Although the increases in HbF are variable, and modest in heterozygotes, they are adequate to compensate for the absence of β-globin production in homozygotes; two homozygotes for different deletions of this kind are not transfusion dependent and have a mild form of β thalassaemia intermedia (Schokker *et al.* 1966; Craig *et al.* 1992).

An insertion involving the β-globin genes

Earlier in this chapter we described how transposable elements may occasionally disrupt human genes and result in their inactivation. There is one example of the insertion of such an element, a retrotransposon of the family called L1, associated with the phenotype of β thalassaemia. This resulted in a chromosomal rearrangement involving the insertion of 6–7-kb DNA into IVS2. Sequence analysis of the inserted fragment showed that it is similar to an L1 transposon and the L1 element is in reverse orientation with respect to the β-globin gene. The insertion breakpoint is located at the 3′ end of IVS2 within a recombinational region previously identified to be part of an ancestral L1 element. The affected gene expresses full length β-globin transcripts at a level corresponding to about 15% of normal β-globin mRNA (Divoky *et al.* 1996). A similar insert has been found in the factor VIII gene in a patient with haemophilia.

The non-deletional forms of β thalassaemia

These conditions account for the vast majority of β-thalassaemia alleles. They result from single base substitutions, small insertions, and deletions within the β-globin gene or its immediate flanking sequences. They may affect any level of gene expression (Table 4.5). Their sites are summarized in Fig. 4.11.

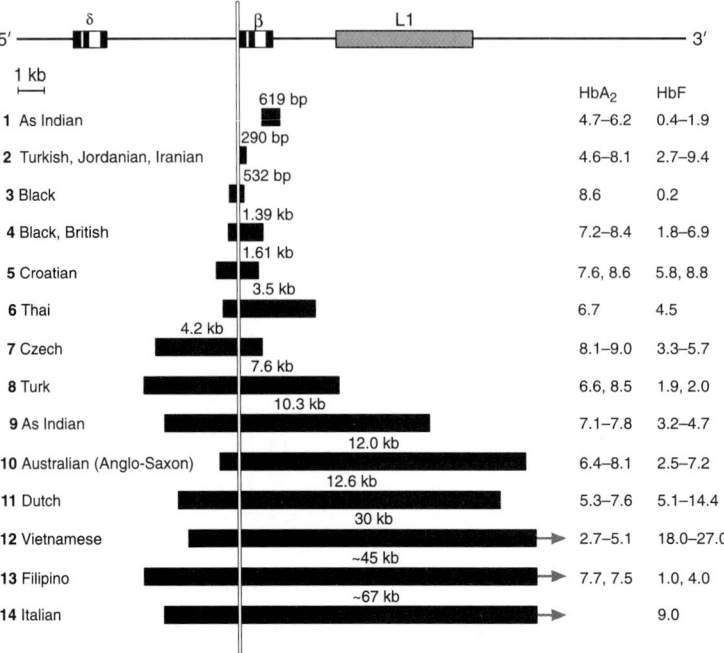

Fig. 4.10 Deletions restricted to the β-globin gene. The hatched box represents the 6.4 kb *Kpn* repeat 3′ of the β gene. Deletions are represented by the horizontal shaded boxes below. The vertical shaded box represents the region (from position −175 to +28 relative to the β mRNA CAP site) lost in all the deletions, with the exception of the 619 bp variety. The corresponding levels of HbA_2 (%) and HbF (%) observed in heterozygotes for the different deletions are shown on the right.
References to the deletions are: 1 Orkin *et al.* 1980; 2. Diaz-Chico *et al.* 1987; Spiegelberg *et al.* 1989; Thein *et al.* 1992; 3. Waye *et al.* 1991; 4. Padanilam *et al.* 1984; Thein *et al.* 1989; 5. Dimovski *et al.* 1993; 6. Lynch *et al.* 1991; 7. Popovich *et al.* 1986; 8. Öner *et al.* 1995 (the mutation includes a 7.6-kb upstream deletion extending 1.5 kb 5′ of the β gene to ~4.5 kb 3′ of the β gene); 9. Craig *et al.* 1992; 10. Motum *et al.* 1992; 11. Gilman, 1987a; 12. Motum *et al.* 1993a (the deletion of ~27 kb noted by Dimovski *et al.* 1994 is probably similar); 13. Motum *et al.* 1993b; 14. Lacerra *et al.* 1997.

Mutations affecting β-globin gene transcription

Promoter mutations

This group of mutations are single base substitutions in the conserved DNA sequences that form the β-globin promoter (Fig. 4.11). Transient expression systems show that they result in an output of β-globin mRNA ranging from 10 to 25% of normal, a level compatible with the relatively mild phenotype of these $β^+$ thalassaemias (Treisman *et al.* 1983). They emphasize the role of the conserved promoter sequences in the binding of transcription factors involved in expression of the β-globin genes. For example, binding of EKLF, a zinc-finger transcription factor, to the CACCC element is critical for normal expression (see Chapter 2). It has been found that the mutation at position −87 specifically ablates EKLF binding (Feng *et al.* 1994). To date, no mutations have been observed within the conserved CCAAT box at position −70.

These lesions have been described in diverse ethnic groups and variation in phenotype has been observed. Africans homozygous for the −29 A→G mutation have an extremely mild disease (Antonarakis *et al.* 1984; Safaya *et al.* 1989), while Chinese homozygous for the same mutation have thalassaemia major (Huang *et al.* 1986). A modulating factor appears to be the presence or absence of the C→T polymorphism at position −158 upstream of the $^Gγ$-globin gene (*Xmn*-I $^Gγ$ site), which is associated with increased fetal haemoglobin production

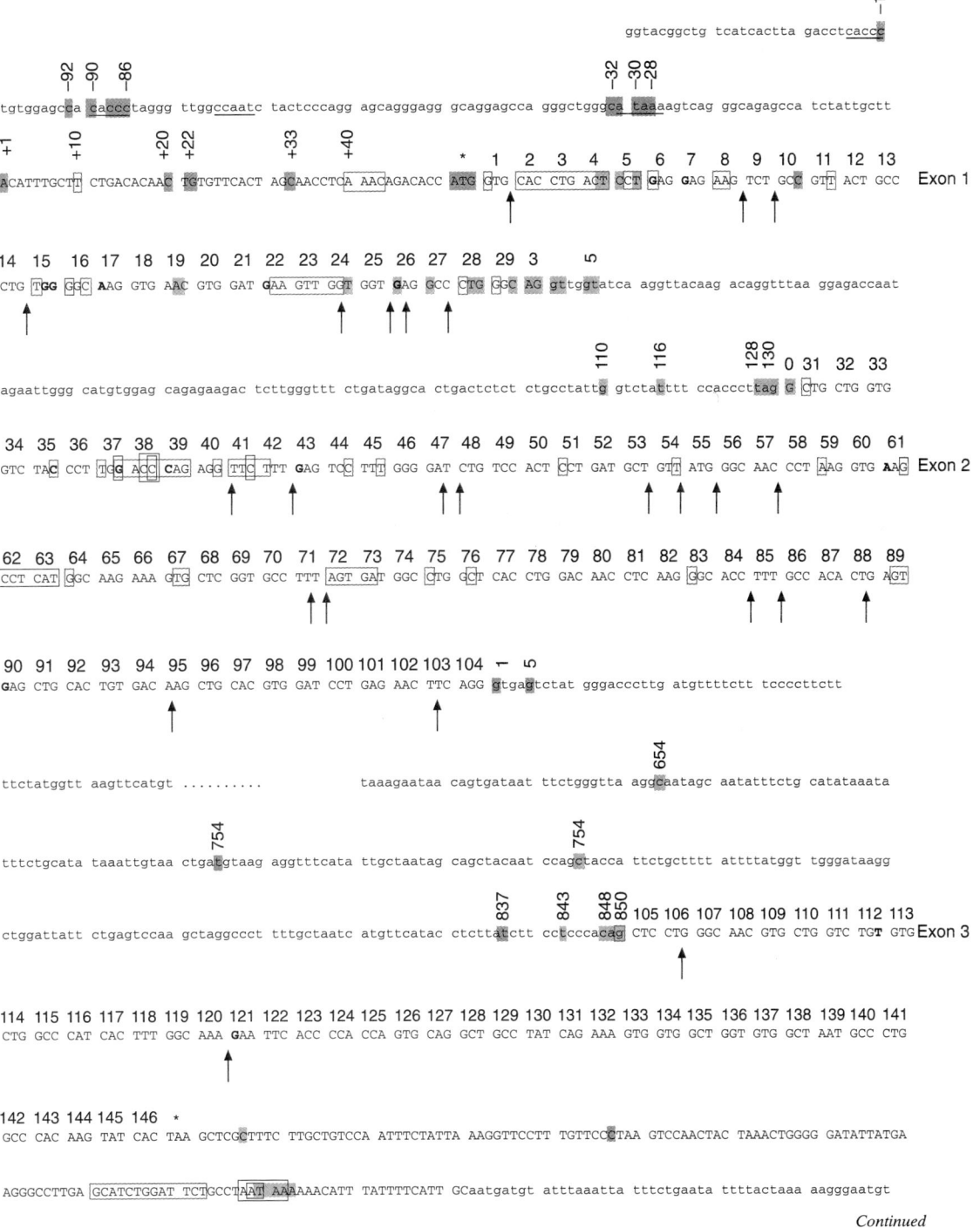

Fig. 4.11 Sequence of the β-globin gene with sites of recessively inherited mutations. Sequences in the 5′ and 3′ UTRs and coding regions are shown in upper case. The regulatory elements in the promoter region (ATAAA, CCAAT, proximal and distal CACCC) and the poly(A) site (AATAAA) in the 3′ UTR are underlined. Boxed sites represent minor deletions, upward arrows indicate the sites of insertions, shaded bases indicate sites of base substitutions, and bases in bold indicate the sites of substitutions leading to stop codons. For details of the changes refer to Table 4.5.

gacctcaccc tgtggagcca cacccctaggg ttggccaatc tactcccagg agcagggagg gcaggagcca gggctgggca taaaagtcag ggcagagcca

```
                    ⊤                                          *  1   2   3   4   5   6   7   8   9   10
                    ⊥                                            Val His Leu Thr Pro Glu Glu Lys Ser Ala     Exon 1
tctattgcttÂCATTGCTT CTGACACAAC TGTGTTCACT AGCAACCTCA AACAGACACC ATG GTG CAC CTG ACT CCT GAG GAG AAG TCT GCC
```

```
11  13  14  14  15  16   17  18  19  20  21  22  23  24  25  26  27  28  29  3
Val Thr Ala Leu Trp Gly Lys Val Asn Val Asp Glu Val Gly Gly Glu Ala Leu Gly Ar
GTT ACT GCC CTG TGG GGC AAG GTG AAC GTG GAT GAA GTT GGT GGT GAG GCC CTG GGC AG gttggtatca aggttacaag acaggtttaa
```

```
                                                                                                    0
                                                                                                    g
ggagaccaat agaaattggg catgtggag cagagaagac tctttgggttt ctgataggca ctgactctct ctgcctattg gtctatttt ccacccttag G
                                                                                                    ↑
```

```
31  32  33  34  35  36   37  38  39  40  41  42  43  44  45  46  47  48  49  50  51  52  53  54  55  56  57  58
Leu Leu Val Val Tyr Pro Trp Thr Glu Arg Phe Phe Glu Ser Phe Gly Asp Leu Ser Thr Pro Asp Ala Val Met Gly Asn Pro
CTG CTG GTG GTC TAC CCT TGG ACC CAG AGG TTC TTT GAG TCC TTT GGG GAT CTG TCC ACT CCT GAT GCT GTT ATG GGC AAC CCT    Exon 2
```

```
59  60  61  62  63  64  65  66  67  68  69  70  71  72  73  74  75  76  77  78  79  80  81  82  83  84  85  86
Lys Val Lys Ala His Gly Lys Lys Val Leu Gly Ala Phe Ser Asp Gly Leu Ala His Leu Asp Asn Leu Lys Gly Thr Phe Ala
AAG GTG AAG GCT CAT GGC AAG AAA GTG CTC GGT GCC TTT AGT GAT GGC CTG GCT CAC CTG GAC AAC CTC AAG GGC ACC TTT GCC
```

```
87  88  89  90  91  92  93  94  95  96  97  98  99  100 101 102 103 104
Thr Leu Ser Glu Leu His Cys Asp Lys Leu His Val Asp Pro Glu Asn Phe Arg ∩
ACA CTG AGT GAG CTG CAC TGT GAC AAG CTG CAC GTG GAT CCT GAG AAC TTC AGG gtgagtcttat gggacccttg atgtttttctt
                                ↑                      ↑                  ↑
```

tcccctctt ttctatggtt aagttcatgt ....   taaagaataa cagtgataat ttctgggtta aggcaatagc aatatttctg

catataaatatttctgcata taaattgtaa ctgatgtaag aggtttcata ttgctaatag cagctacaat ccagctacca ttctgctttt attttatggt

```
                                                                            105 106 107 108 109 110
                                                                            Leu Leu Gly Asn Val Leu      Exon 3
tgggataagg ctggattatt ctgagtccaa gctaggccct tttgctaatc atgttcatac ctcttatctt cctcccacag CTC CTG GGC AAC GTG CTG
```

```
111 112 113 114 115 116 117 118 119 120 121 122 123 124 125 126 127 128 129 130 131 132 133 134 135 136 137 138
Val Cys Val Leu Ala His His Phe Gly Lys Glu Phe Thr Pro Pro Val Gln Ala Ala Thr Gln Lys Val Val Ala Gly Val Ala
GTC TGT GTG CTG GCC CAT CAC TTT GGC AAA GAA TTC ACC CCA CCA GTG CAG GCT GCC TAT CAG AAA GTG GTG GCT GGT GTG GCT
            ↑                            ↑                        ↑                              ↑
```

```
139 140 141 142 143 144 145 146  *
Asn Ala Leu Ala His Lys Tyr His
AAT GCC CTGGCC CAC AAG TAT CAC TAA GCTCGCTTTC TTGCTGTCCA ATTTCTATTA AAGGTTCCTT TGTTCCCTAA GTCCAACTAC TAAACTGGGG
```

GATATTATGA AGGGCCTTGA GCATCTGGGAT TCTGCCTAAT AAAAAACATT TATTTTCATT GCaatgatgt atttaaatta tttctgaata ttttctaaa

Fig. 4.11 *Continued.*

under conditions of erythropoietic stress (see Chapters 2 and 10); this site is occupied by T on the chromosome carrying the −29 A→G mutation in Africans, and C in the Chinese.

The C→T mutation at position −101 to the β-globin gene appears to cause an extremely mild deficit of β-globin. The allele is so mild that it is 'silent' in heterozygotes, who have normal HbA₂ levels and normal red-cell indices. We shall consider it further, together with its interactions, in Chapter 13.

Table 4.5 Point mutations causing β thalassaemia. (Identification refers to particular restriction enzymes that identify mutation or allele-specific oligonucleotide (ASO) probe.)

Mutation	Type	Identification	Distribution	References
I–Transcriptional mutations				
Promoter regulatory elements				
1 −101 (C→T)	β++(silent)	ASO	Mediterranean	Gonzalez-Redondo et al. (1989a)
2 −92 (C→T)	β+(silent)	ASO	Mediterranean	Kazazian (1990); Divoky et al. (1993a); Kimberland et al. (1995); Rosatelli et al. (1995)
3 −90 (C→T)	β+		Portuguese	Faustino et al. (1992)
4 −88 (C→T)	β++	+Fok I	US Blacks, Asian Indians	Orkin et al. (1984a);Thein et al. (1988a)
5 −88 (C→A)	β+	ASO	Kurds	Rund et al. (1991)
6 −87 (C→G)	β++	−Avr II	Mediterranean	Treisman et al. (1983); Meloni et al. (1992)
7 −87 (C→T)	β++	−Avr II	German, Italian	Kulozik et al. (1991b); Meloni et al. (1992)
8 −87 (C→A)	β++	−Avr II	US Blacks	Coleman et al. (1992)
9 −86 (C→G)	β+	−Avr II	Thai, Lebanese	Kazazian (1990);Thein et al. (1990b)
10 −86 (C→A)	β++	−Avr II	Italian	Meloni et al. (1992)
11 −32 (C→A)	β+		Taiwanese	Lin et al. (1992b)
12 −31 (A→G)	β+		Japanese	Takihara et al. (1986)
13 −31 (A→C)	β+		Italian	Huisman et al. (1997)
14 −30 (T→A)	β+		Mediterranean, Bulgarian	Fei et al. (1988b)
15 −30 (T→C)	β+		Chinese	Cai et al. (1989)
16 −29 (A→G)	β+	+Nla III	US Blacks, Chinese	Antonarakis et al. (1984); Huang et al. (1986)
17 −28 (A→C)	β+		Kurds	Poncz et al. (1983)
18 −28 (A→G)	β+		Blacks, south-east Asians	Orkin et al. (1983b);Antonarakis et al. (1984); Huang et al. (1986)
19 −27 (A→T)	β+		Corsican	Badens et al. (1999)
5′ UTR				
20 CAP +1 (A→C)	β++(silent)		Asian Indian	Wong et al. (1987)
21 CAP +8 (C→T)	β++(silent)		Chinese	Ma et al. (1999)
22 CAP +10 (−T)	β++(silent)		Greeks	Athanassiadou et al. (1994)
23 CAP +20 (C→T)‡	?		Bulgarian	Gonzalez-Redondo et al. (1989a)
24 CAP +22 (G→A)	β++		Mediterranean, Bulgarian	Öner et al. (1991a); Cai et al. (1992)
25 CAP +33 (C→G)	β++(silent)	+Nla IV	Greek Cypriot	Ho et al. (1996c)
26 CAP +40 to +43 (−AAAC)	β+	+Dde I	Chinese	Huang et al. (1991)

Continued

Table 4.5 *Continued.*

II–RNA processing

Splice junction

Mutation	Type	Identification	Distribution	References
1 IVS1-(−2) CD30 (AGG→GGG)	β^0		Sephardic Jews	Waye *et al.* (1998)
2 IVS1-(−1) CD30 (AGG→ACG) (Arg→Thr)	β^0	−*Bsp* MI	Mediterranean, US Blacks, N. African, Kurds, UAE	Chibani *et al.* (1988);Gonzalez-Redondo *et al.* (1989c); Vidaud *et al.* (1989); Rund *et al.* (1991); El-Kalla & Mathews (1997)
3 IVS1-(−1) CD30 (AGG→AAG)	β^0		Bulgaria, UAE	Kalaydjieva *et al.* (1989); El-Kalla & Mathews (1997)
4 IVS1-1 (G→A)	β^0	−*Bsp* MI	Mediterranean	Orkin *et al.* (1982a)
5 IVS1-1 (G→T)	β^0	−*Bsp* MI	Asian Indian, south-east Asian, Chinese	Kazazian *et al.* (1984)
6 IVS1-2 (T→G)	β^0	−*Bsp* MI	Tunisian	Chibani *et al.* (1988)
7 IVS1-2 (T→C)	β^0	−*Bsp* MI	US Blacks	Gonzalez-Redondo *et al.* (1989d)
8 IVS1-2 (T→A)	β^0	−*Bsp* MI	Algerian, Italian	Bouhass *et al.* (1990);Murru *et al.* (1991)
9 IVS2-1 (G→A)	β^0	−*Hph* I	Mediterranean, US Blacks	Baird *et al.* (1981a);Treisman *et al.* (1982)
10 IVS2-1 (G→C)	β^0		Iranian	Nozari *et al.* (1995)
11 IVS2-2 (−T)	β^0		Chinese	Ma *et al.* (1999)
12 IVS1-3′ end del 17bp	β^0		Kuwaiti	Kazazian & Boehm (1988)
13 IVS1-3′ end del 25bp	β^0		Asian Indian, UAE	Orkin *et al.* (1983c)
14 IVS1-3′ end del 44bp	β^0		Mediterranean	Gonzalez-Redondo *et al.* (1989b)
15 IVS1-130 (G→C)	β^0	−*Del* I/*Sau* I	Italian, Japanese, UAE	Renda *et al.* (1992a); Yamamoto *et al.* (1992); El-Kalla & Mathews (1997)
16 IVS1-130 G→A	β^0	−*Dde* I	Egyptian	Deidda *et al.* (1990); Öner *et al.* (1990)
17 IVS1-130 (+1) CD30 (AGG→AGC) (Arg→Ser)	β^0		Middle East	El-Kalla & Mathews (1997)
18 IVS2-849 (A→G)	β^0		US Blacks	Antonarakis *et al.* (1984);Atweh *et al.* (1985)
19 IVS2-849 (A→C)	β^0		US Blacks	Padanilam & Huisman (1986)
20 IVS2-850 (G→C)	β^0		Yugoslavian	Jankovic *et al.* (1992)
21 IVS2-850 (G→A)	β^0		N. European	Çürük *et al.* (1995)
22 IVS2-850 (G→T)	β^0		Japanese	Ohba *et al.* (1997)
23 IVS2-850 (−G)	β^0		Italian	Rosatelli *et al.* (1992c)
Consensus splice sites				
24 IVS1-5 (G→C)	β^0		Asian Indian, south-east Asian, Melanesian	Treisman *et al.* (1983); Hill *et al.* (1988)
25 IVS1-5 (G→T)	β^+		Mediterranean, N. European	Atweh *et al.* (1987a); Eigel *et al.* (1989)
26 IVS1-5 (G→A)	β^+	+*EcoR* V	Mediterranean, Algerian	Lapoumeroulie *et al.* (1986)

27 IVS1-6 (T→C)	+*Sfa* NI	β+	Mediterranean	Orkin *et al.* (1982a); Tamagnini *et al.* (1983)
28 IVS1-(-3) CD29 (GGC→GG**T**)	-*Bsp* MI	β++	Lebanese	Chehab *et al.* (1987)
29 IVS1-128 (T→G)		β+	Saudi Arabian	Wong *et al.* (1989a)
30 IVS1-129 (A→G)			German	Vetter *et al.* (1997)
31 IVS2-5 (G→C)		β+	Chinese	Jiang *et al.* (1993)
32 IVS2-843 (T→G)		β+	Algerian	Beldjord *et al.* (1988)
33 IVS2-844 (C→G)		β++ (silent)	Italian	Murru *et al.* (1991); Rosatelli *et al.* (1994)
34 IVS2-848 (C→A)		β+	US Blacks, Egyptian, Iranian	Gonzalez-Redondo *et al.* (1988a); Wong *et al.* (1989a)
35 IVS2-848 (C→G)		β+	Japanese	Hattori *et al.* (1992)
Cryptic splice sites in introns				
36 IVS1-110 (G→A)		β+	Mediterranean	Spritz *et al.* (1981); Westaway & Williamson (1981)
37 IVS1-116 (T→G)	+*Mae* I	β0	Mediterranean	Metherall *et al.* (1986)
38 IVS2-654 (C→T)		β0/β+	Chinese, south-east Asians, Japanese	Cheng *et al.* (1984); Takihara *et al.* (1984)
39 IVS2-705 (T→G)		β+	Mediterranean	Dobkin *et al.* (1983)
40 IVS2-745 (C→G)	+*Rsa* I	β+	Mediterranean	Orkin *et al.* (1982a)
41 IVS2-837 (T→G)		?	Asian Indian	Varawalla *et al.* (1991b)
Cryptic splice sites in exons				
42 CD10 (GCC→GC**A**)		β++	Asian Indian	Pawar *et al.* (1997)
43 CD19 (AAC→A**G**C) Hb Malay (Asn→Ser)		β++	South-east Asian	Yang *et al.* (1989); Thein *et al.* (1990b)
44 CD24 (GGT→GG**A**)		β++	US Black, Japanese	Goldsmith *et al.* (1983); Hattori *et al.* (1989)
45 CD26 (GAG→AAG) (Glu→Lys, HbE)	-*Mnl* I	β+	South-east Asian, European	Flatz *et al.* (1965a); Fairbanks *et al.* (1980); Orkin *et al.* (1982b)
46 CD27 (GCC→TCC) (Ala→Ser, Hb Knossos)	-*Sau* 96 I or -*Hae* III	β+	Mediterranean	Arous *et al.* (1983); Orkin *et al.* (1984b); Baklouti *et al.* (1986); Olds *et al.* (1991)
3' UTR				
RNA Cleavage—Poly(A) signal				
47 AATAAA→AACAAA		β++	US Blacks	Orkin *et al.* (1985)
48 AATAAA→AATGAA		β++	Mediterranean	Jankovic *et al.* (1990b)
49 AATAAA→AATAGA		β++	Malay	Jankovic *et al.* (1990b)
50 AATAAA→AATAA**G**		β++	Kurd	Rund *et al.* (1991)
51 AATAAA→AA—AA		β+	French, US Blacks	Ghanem *et al.* (1992); Kimberland *et al.* (1995)
52 AATAAA→A——		β+	Kurd, UAE	Rund *et al.* (1992); El-Kalla & Mathews (1997)
Others				
53 Term CD+6, C→G		β++ (silent)	Greek	Jankovic *et al.* (1991); Maragoudaki *et al.* (1998)
54 Term CD+90, del 13 bp	-*Hinf* I	β+	Turkish	Basak *et al.* (1993)
55 Term CD+47 (C→G)	-*Dde* I	β+	Armenian	Author's laboratory

Continued

Table 4.5 Continued.

Mutation	Type	Identification	Distribution	References
III—RNA translation				
Initiation codon				
1 ATG→GTG	β^0		Japanese	Hattori et al. (1991)
2 ATG→ACG	β^0	–Nco I	Yugoslavian	Jankovic et al. (1990a)
3 ATG→AGG	β^0	–Nco I	Chinese	Lam et al. (1990)
4 ATG→AAG**	β^0	–Nco I	N.European	Waye et al. (1997a)
5 ATG→ATC	β^0		Japanese	Ohba et al. (1997)
6 ATG→ATA	β^0		Italian, Swedish	Saba et al. (1992); Landin et al. (1995)
7 ATG→ATT	β^0		Iranian	Nozari et al. (1995)
Nonsense codons				
1 CD6 GAG→TAG, CD4 ACT→ACA, CD5 CCA→TCA	β^0		Italian	Dr. C. Rosatelli (personal communication)
2 CD7 GAG→TAG	β^0		English	Author's laboratory
3 CD15 TGG→TAG	β^0		Asian Indian, Japanese	Kazazian et al. (1984); Ohba et al. (1997)
4 CD15 TGG→TGA	β^0		Portuguese, Japanese	Ribeiro et al. (1992); Ohba et al. (1997)
5 CD17 AAG→TAG	β^0	+Mae I	Chinese, Japanese	Chang & Kan (1979); Ohba et al. (1997)
6 CD22 GAA→TAA	β^0		Reunion Island	Ghanem et al. (1992)
7 CD26 GAG→TAG	β^0	–Mnl I	Thai	Fucharoen et al. (1990a)
8 CD35 TAC→TAA	β^0	–Acc I	Thai	Fucharoen et al. (1989a); Thein et al. (1990b)
9 CD37 TGG→TGA	β^0	–Ava II	Saudi Arabian	Boehm et al. (1986)
10 CD39 CAG→TAG	β^0	+Mae I/+Bfa I	Mediterranean	Orkin & Goff (1981b); Trecartin et al. (1981); Fiori & Mach (1982)
11 CD43 GAG→TAG	β^0	–Hinf I	Chinese, Thai	Atweh et al. (1988)
12 CD61 AAG→TAG	β^0	–Hph I	Black	Gonzalez-Redondo et al. (1988a)
13 CD90 GAG→TAG	β^0		Japanese	Fucharoen et al. (1990d)
14 CD112 TGT→TGA	β^0		Slovenian	Divoky et al. (1993b)
15 CD121 GAA→TAA*	β^0	–EcoR I	Czechoslovakian	Indrák et al. (1992); Yamamoto et al. (1992)
Frameshift				
1 CD1 –G	β^0		Mediterranean	Rosatelli et al. (1992b)
2 CD2/3/4 (–9 bp,+31 bp)	β^0		Algerian	Badens et al. (1996)
3 CD5 –CT	β^0	–Dde I	Mediterranean	Kollia et al. (1989)
4 CD6 –A	β^0	–Dde I/–Mst II	Mediterranean, US Blacks	Chang et al. (1983); Kazazian et al. (1983)

	Mutation	Restriction site	Type	Population	Reference
5	CD8 –AA		β⁰	Mediterranean	Orkin & Goff (1981b); Filon et al. (1995)
6	CD8/9 +G		β⁰	Asian Indian, Japanese	Kazazian et al. (1984); Ohba et al. (1997)
7	CD9/10 +T		β⁰	Greek, Arab	Waye et al. (1994c)
8	CD11 –T		β⁰	Mexican	Economou et al. (1991)
9	CD14 +T			Azerbajian	
10	CD14/15 +G		β⁰	Chinese	Chan et al. (1988)
11	CD15 –T		β⁰	Malay	Fucharoen et al. (1990b)
12	CD15/16 –G			German	Vetter et al. (1997)
13	CD16 –C		β⁰	Asian Indian	Kazazian et al. (1984)
14	CD22/23/24 –7 bp (–AAGTTGG)		β⁰	Turkish	Özçelik et al. (1993)
15	CD24 –G; +CAC		β⁰	Egyptian	Deidda et al. (1991)
16	CD25/26 +T		β⁰	Tunisian	Fattoum et al. (1991)
17	CD26 +T		β⁰	Japanese	Hattori et al. (1998)
18	CD27/28 +C		β⁰	Chinese, Thai	Cai et al. (1991); Lin et al. (1991)
19	CD28 –C		β⁰	Egyptian	El-Hashemite et al. (1997)
20	CD11 –C		β⁰	Portuguese	Cabeda et al. (1999)
21	CD28/29 –G		β⁰	Japanese, Egyptian	El-Hashemite et al. (1997); Ohba et al. (1997)
22	CD31 –C		β⁰	Chinese	Ko et al. (1997a)
23	CD35 –C	–Acc I	β⁰	Malay	Yang et al. (1989)
24	CD36/37 –T		β⁰	Kurd, Iranian	Rund et al. (1991); Nozari et al. (1995)
25	CD37 –G		β⁰	Kurdish	
26	CD37/38/39 del 7 bp (–GACCCAG)		β⁰	Turkish	Schnee et al. (1989)
27	CD38/39 –C	–Ava II	β⁰	Czechoslovkian	Indrak et al. (1991)
28	CD38/39 –CC	–Ava II	β⁰	Belgian	Heusterspreute et al. (1996)
29	CD40 –G	–Ava II	β⁰	Japanese	Ohba et al. (1997)
30	CD40 +86 bp		β⁰	Portuguese	Cabeda et al. (1999)
31	CD40/41 +T		β⁰	Chinese	Ko et al. (1997a)
32	CD41 –C		β⁰	Thai	Fucharoen et al. (1991b)
33	CD41/42 –TTCT		β⁰	Chinese, south-east Asian, Indian	Kimura et al. (1983); Kazazian et al. (1984)
34	CD42/43 +T		β⁰	Japanese	Oshima et al. (1996)
35	CD42/43 +G		β⁰	Japanese	Ohba et al. (1997)
36	CD44 –C		β⁰	Kurdish	Kinniburgh et al. (1982); Rund et al. (1991)
37	CD45 –T		β⁰	Pakistani	El-Kalla & Mathews (1997)
38	CD47 +A	–Xho I	β⁰	Surinamese	Codrington et al. (1990)
39	CD47/48 +ATCT		β⁰	Asian Indian	Garewal et al. (1994); El-Kalla & Mathews (1995)
40	CD51 –C		β⁰	Hungarian	Ringelhann et al. (1993)

Continued

Table 4.5 *Continued.*

Mutation	Type	Identification	Distribution	References
41 CD53/54 +G	β^0		Japanese	Fucharoen *et al.* (1990d)
42 CD54 −T	β^0		Swedish	Landin & Berglund (1996)
43 CD54/55 +A	β^0		Asian Indian	Garewal *et al.* (1994)
44 CD56−60 +14 bp	β^0		Iranian	Ghaffari *et al.* (1997)
45 CD57/58 +C	β^0		Asian Indian	El-Kalla & Mathews (1995)
46 CD59 −A	β^0		Italian	Meloni *et al.* (1994)
47 CD61/63 del 7 bp (−GGCTCAT)	β^0		Italian	Dr. C. Rosatelli (personal communication)
48 CD64 −G**	β^0		Swiss	Chehab *et al.* (1989)
49 CD67 −TG	β^0		Filipino	Eng *et al.* (1993)
50 CD71/72 +T	β^0		Chinese	Chan *et al.* (1989)
51 CD71/72 +A	β^0	+*Mse* I	Chinese	Cheng *et al.* (1984)
52 CD72/73 −AGTGA, +T	β^0	−*Hae* II	British	Waye *et al.* (1997b)
53 CD74/75 −C	β^0		Turkish	Basak *et al.* (1992a)
54 CD76 −C	β^0		Italian	Di Marzo *et al.* (1988); Giambona *et al.* (1995)
55 CD82/83 −G	β^0		Czech, Azerbaijan	Schwartz *et al.* (1989); Çürük *et al.* (1992b)
56 CD83−86 del 8 bp (−CACCTTTG)**	β^0		Japanese	Hattori *et al.* (1998)
57 CD84/85 +C	β^0		Japanese	Ohba *et al.* (1997)
58 CD84/85/86 +T	β^0		Japanese	Ohba *et al.* (1997)
59 CD88 +T	β^0		Asian Indian	Varawalla *et al.* (1991b)
60 CD88 −TG	β^0		Japanese	Hattori *et al.* (1998)
61 CD89/90 −GT	β^0		Japanese	Ohba *et al.* (1997)
62 CD95 +A	β^0		South-east Asian	Winichagoon *et al.* (1992b); Cai & Chehab (1996)
63 CD106/107 +G	β^0		US Black, Egyptian	Wong *et al.* (1987); Hussein *et al.* (1993)
64 CD120/121 +A†	β^0		Philippino	Hopmeier *et al.* (1996)

* Unlike the majority, some heterozygotes for the CD121 G→T mutation do not have an unusually severe phenotype.
† This frameshift leads to predicted truncated variant of 13 amino-acid residues with an abnormal carboxy terminal. Heterozygotes do not appear to have an unusually severe phenotype.
‡ Occurs in *cis* to the IVS2-745 C→G mutation.
β^+ Also occurs in *cis* to 7201-bp deletion involving delta gene.
β^{++} Occurs in *cis* to 59 −A.
** Probably *de novo*.

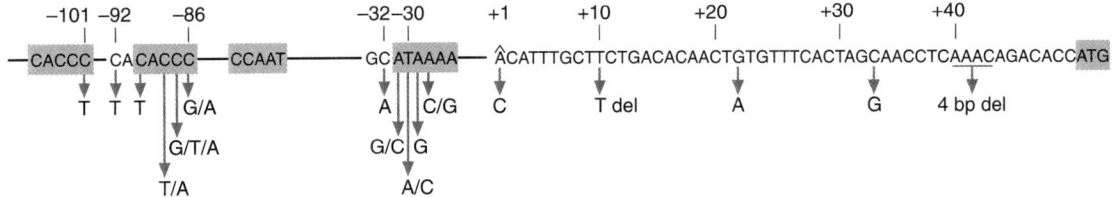

Fig. 4.12 Mutations in the promoter and 5′ untranslated region (UTR) of the β-globin gene. Positions of the four conserved motifs and the initiation codon are indicated. Single base substitutions and minor deletions at the positions indicated result in β⁺ thalassaemias, the majority of which are very mild.

Mutations of the 5′ UTR

Several mutations in the 5′ UTR have been characterized since the original description of the CAP +1 A→C allele (Wong *et al.* 1987). They include single base substitutions and minor deletions distributed along this stretch of 50 nucleotides. As in the case of the −101 C→T mutation, this class of mutations is 'silent'; the extremely mild phenotype is exemplified by a homozygote for the CAP +1 A→C mutation who has the haematological picture of β-thalassaemia trait (Wong *et al.* 1987). *In vivo* and *in vitro* studies show that the +33 C→G mutation leads to a reduction of β-globin mRNA of about 33% of normal, more than is associated with mutations involving the promoter elements (Ho *et al.* 1996c). Compound heterozygotes for mutations in the 5′ UTR and the more severe β-thalassaemia alleles tend to have a mild disease (see Chapter 13).

Mutations affecting mRNA processing

Intervening sequences (IVS) must be removed from the precursor mRNA and the coding regions joined to produce a functional template. As described in Chapter 2, sequences critical in this process include the invariant dinucleotides, GT at the 5′ (donor) and AG at the 3′ (acceptor) splice junctions between exons and introns (Breathnach & Chambon 1981; Mount 1982). The regions flanking these invariant dinucleotides are fairly well conserved and hence consensus sequences can be recognized at exon–intron boundaries (see Table 2.5). They encompass the last three nucleotides of the exon and the first six nucleotides of the intron for the 5′ donor site, and the last 10 nucleotides of the intron and the first nucleotide of the exon for the 3′ acceptor site. Both

exons and introns also contain 'cryptic' splice sites, sequences which mimic the consensus sequence for a splice site but which are not normally used. Mutations can occur in these sites, however, creating a sequence that resembles more closely the normal splice site. During RNA processing the newly created site is utilized preferentially, leading to aberrant splicing.

Junctional mutations

Mutations that affect either of the invariant dinucleotides in the splice junction completely abolish normal splicing and produce the phenotype of β⁰ thalassaemia. Genes with these mutations appear to transcribe normally, but, although some alternative splicing occurs at 'cryptic' donor or acceptor sites, the mis-spliced mRNA does not allow the translation of functional β globin.

Consensus-sequence mutations

Mutations within the consensus sequences at the splice junctions reduce the efficiency of normal splicing to varying degrees and produce a β-thalassaemia phenotype that ranges from mild to severe. For example, mutations at position 5 of IVS1 G→C, T or A, considerably reduce splicing at the mutated donor site. They appear to activate three 'cryptic' donor sites, two in exon 1 and one in IVS1, which are utilized preferentially to the normal donor site (Treisman *et al.* 1983). On the other hand, the substitution of C for T in the adjacent nucleotide, IVS1 position 6, only mildly affects RNA splicing even though it activates the same three cryptic donor sites as the IVS1-5 mutations (Treisman *et al.* 1983). The IVS1-6 T→C mutation, often referred to as the Portuguese form of β thalassaemia, is particularly common in the Mediterranean and accounts for the majority of the mild β thalassaemias in this region (Tamagnini *et al.* 1983).

Cryptic splice-site mutations in introns

Several splice mutations involve base substitutions within introns rather than consensus splice sites. The first to be characterized was a G→A substitution at position 110 of IVS1 (Spritz *et al.* 1981; Westaway & Williamson 1981). This region contains a sequence similar to a 3′ acceptor site although it lacks the invariant AG dinucleotide. The change at position 110 creates an AG with the result that 90% of the RNA is spliced to the newly created site (Busslinger *et al.* 1981). The mis-spliced mRNA retains 19 nucleotides from IVS1 and introduces a premature termination codon at position 36. Due to the early in-phase termination, it is likely that the aberrantly spliced mRNA is subjected to nonsense-mediated decay (see Maquat 1996 for review). Hence, the majority of the low level of β-globin mRNA present in erythroid cells is of the normal type. Since only a small amount of normal β mRNA is produced, the phenotype is a severe β⁺ thalassaemia. Another β-thalassaemia gene, with a T→G substitution in position 116 of IVS1 leading to a new 3′ acceptor site, has been characterized. In this case, little or no normal

β-globin mRNA is produced, resulting in a β^0-thalassaemia phenotype (Metherall *et al.* 1986).

Three β-thalassaemia alleles have substitutions within IVS2 that generate new donor sites (Orkin *et al.* 1982a; Dobkin *et al.* 1983; Cheng *et al.* 1984). In each case, an upstream acceptor site at position 579 is activated such that the normal 5′ donor site at exon 2/IVS2 is spliced to the activated site at position 579, while the newly created donor site is spliced to the normal 3′ acceptor site at IVS2/exon 3. This results in the retention of part of IVS2 in the mis-spliced β mRNA. Variable amounts of splicing from the normal donor to the normal acceptor also occur, resulting in phenotypes that range from β^+ to β^0 thalassaemia.

Several heterozygotes for the IVS2-654 C→T mutation (Fig. 4.13) with an unusually severe phenotype have been described (Naritomi *et al.* 1990; Zeng *et al.* 1995; Ho *et al.* 1996a, 1998b). In a father and son, the ratio of aberrant to normal β mRNA was 10-fold that in asymptomatic heterozygotes for the same mutation (Ho *et al.* 1996a). It was suggested that the unusually severe disease in these heterozygotes results from the accumulation of the mis-spliced mRNA, which, presumably, translates into a highly unstable β-chain variant with a dominant-negative effect (see later section). However, it was not possible to demonstrate translation of the aberrant mRNA. Further *in vivo* and *in vitro* studies (Ho *et al.* 1998b,

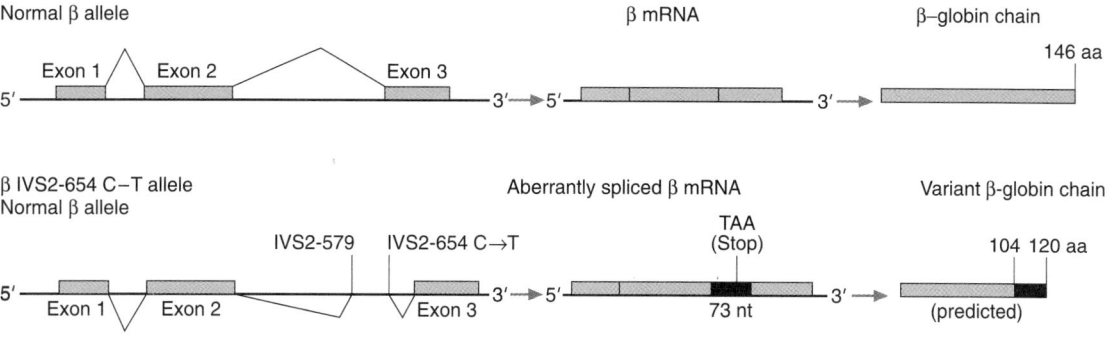

Fig. 4.13 The IVS2-654 C→T mutation is an example of a mutation within an intron that creates a new splice site. In this case, the mutation creates a donor splice site which is spliced to the normal 3′ acceptor site, while an acceptor site is activated upstream at position 579 of intron 2 and spliced to the normal donor site at the exon 2/intron 2 junction. This results in the incorporation of 73 nucleotides of intron 2 into the aberrantly spliced mRNA. A shift in the reading frame results in the generation of a premature termination codon at position 121 and the predicted synthesis of a truncated variant β chain with an abnormal carboxy-terminal end from codon 105.

1999) showed that the β^{654T} mRNA is very unstable. The discrepancy between the reticulocyte α/β mRNA ratios, which were within the range observed in asymptomatic heterozygotes, and the considerably imbalanced α/β-chain synthesis implies that the unusually severe phenotype is due to a second defect that acts at the translational or post-translational level. It appears that the higher levels of β^{654T} mRNA in the thalassaemia intermedia cases were simply a reflection of the higher levels of reticulocytes and younger donor population of red cells in these cases (Ho *et al.* 1998b).

Cryptic splice sites in exons One of the cryptic splice sites used in alternative splicing in mutations

inactivating the IVS1 donor site contains the sequence GT GGT GAG G, spanning codons 24 to 27 in exon 1 (Treisman *et al.* 1983). Three mutations within this region activate this cryptic site, which then acts as an alternative donor site in RNA processing (Fig. 4.14). The codon 24 GGT→GGA substitution is translationally silent (Goldsmith *et al.* 1983), while the codon 26 GAG→AAG and codon 27 GCC→TCC changes result in the variants, HbE and Hb Knossos, respectively (Orkin *et al.* 1982b, 1984b). The mutations in codons 26 and 27 are associated with only a minor activation of the alternative splicing pathway. Hence there is only a moderate reduction of the normally spliced β-globin mRNA which

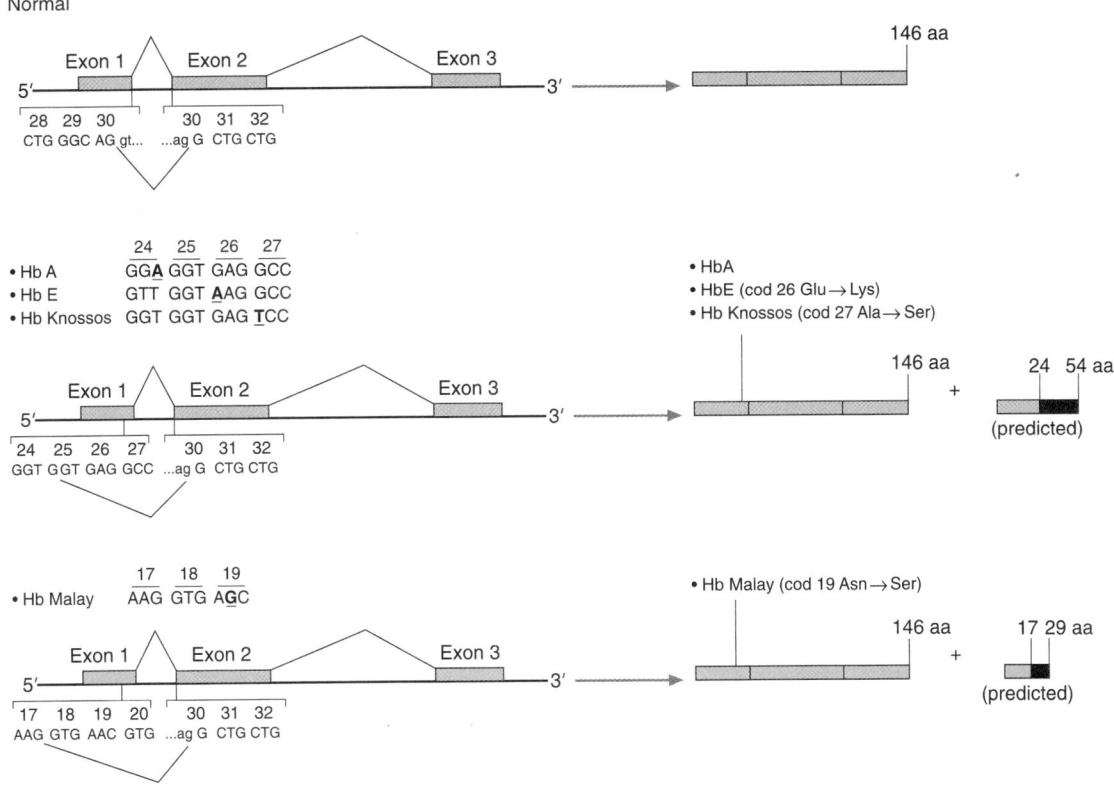

Fig. 4.14 Examples of aberrant splicing due to mutations that create an alternate donor splice in the first exon. Three mutations (CD24 GG**T**→GG**A**, CD26 **G**AG→**A**AG, CD27 **G**CC→**T**CC) activate an alternate splice site at CD25 generating a truncated variant haemoglobin (predicted) but the majority of the β-globin mRNA is correctly spliced and leads to haemoglobins incorporating the different amino acid substitutions (HbE and Hb Knossos). The mutation in CD24 does not lead to a change of amino acid. Similarly, Hb Malay (CD19 A**A**C→A**G**C) activates an alternate donor splice site at CD17/CD 18.

encodes for the particular β-globin variants; the associated phenotype is a very mild form of β thalassaemia.

Abnormal splicing into the codon 24–27 region does not produce any recognizable β globin. Similarly, an A→G mutation in codon 19 activates another cryptic donor site in this region, resulting in a reduced level of the normally spliced β-globin mRNA which encodes for Hb Malay (Yang *et al.* 1989) (Fig. 4.14).

The reduction in normal splicing is therefore the molecular basis for the mild β$^+$-thalassaemic phenotype associated with all these structural variants. The β^E gene is particularly prevalent in south-east Asia, reaching a frequency of 75% in north-east Thailand. Its interaction with β thalassaemia accounts for a large proportion of severe β thalassaemia in south-east Asia (see Chapter 9).

Poly(A) addition-site mutations

Four nucleotide substitutions and two minor deletions affecting the conserved AATAAA sequence in the 3′ UTR have been described. Transient expression studies in two cases showed that only 10–20% of the RNA transcript is cleaved appropriately; the majority is not processed until transcription proceeds beyond the next AATAAA signal, which lies 1 to 3 kb 3′ from the β-globin gene (Orkin *et al.* 1985). These elongated transcripts are unstable, although some normal ones are also produced. These mutations generally lead to a phenotype of mild β$^+$ thalassaemia. Functional analysis of RNA derived from peripheral blood of patients with two different mutations affecting the poly(A) site indicates that an intact AATAAA signal is not an absolute requirement for correct cleavage of the transcript (Rund *et al.* 1992). Furthermore, the extended mRNAs are translatable *in vivo*.

Other mutations in the 3′ UTR

Mutations affecting other sites in the 3′ UTR, a C→G substitution at nucleotide 6 and a 13-bp deletion at nucleotide 90 downstream of the termination codon, also result in β$^+$ thalassaemia.

Mutations affecting mRNA translation

Mutations which are expressed at the level of mRNA translation involve either the initiation or elongation phases of globin synthesis. Unlike the α thalassaemias, no chain-termination mutations have been found.

Initiation

Five mutations affecting the initiation codon have been described, all of which produce β^0 thalassaemia. They are single base substitutions, one affecting the first (A), two the second (T) and two the third (G) nucleotide of ATG (Jankovic *et al.* 1990a; Lam *et al.* 1990; Hattori *et al.* 1991; Saba *et al.* 1992; Ohba *et al.* 1997).

Elongation

Approximately half the β-thalassaemia alleles are characterized by premature β-chain termination, reflecting frameshift or nonsense mutations. They nearly all result in premature termination in exons 1 or 2, with two exceptions which terminate in exon 3 (Fig. 4.15). The preponderance of these in-phase termination mutations in exon 1 and 2 is probably related to their 'positional' effect on nonsense-mediated decay of the abnormal β-globin mRNA (for review see Maquat 1995). Mutations that result in premature termination in exons 1 and 2 are associated with very low levels of the mutant β-globin mRNA in erythroid progenitors (Takeshita *et al.* 1984; Baserga & Benz 1988; Gonzalez-Redondo *et al.* 1989d). In heterozygotes, about half the normal amount of β globin is produced, the product of the normal allele, resulting in a mild hypochromic anaemia. In contrast, mutations that produce in-phase termination later in the β sequence, in exon 3, are associated with substantial levels of abnormal β-globin mRNA comparable to that from the normal β allele. The mutant β mRNA, presumably, is translated to produce variant β globin (Hall & Thein 1994), which, as we shall see later, precipitates in the red-cell precursors, resulting in the more severe phenotype of dominantly inherited β thalassaemia (Ho *et al.* 1997). The position effect of these premature termination codons (PTCs) on the accumulation of mRNA is referred to as nonsense-mediated decay (NMD), which could be an mRNA surveillance mechanism to eliminate mRNAs encoding truncated polypeptides. It is not clear how this is achieved, but it could be related to coupling between transcription and translation at the nuclear membrane (Sachs 1993). This

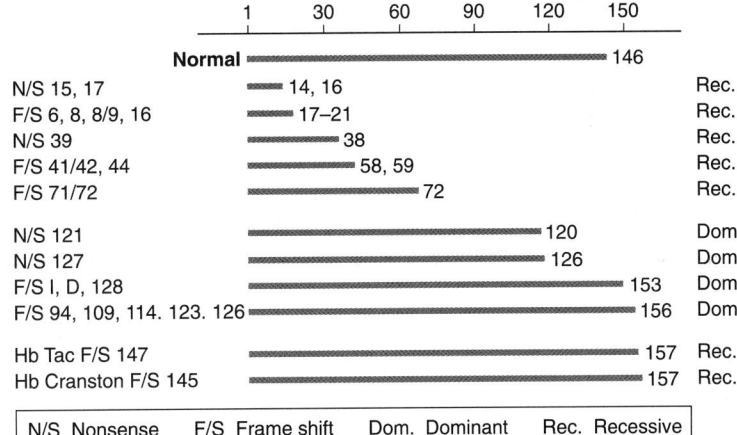

Fig. 4.15 Mutations that underlie dominant β thalassaemia. The mechanisms are described in the text. The amino acid residues are numbered at the top. Below is the normal β chain.

question has been addressed in detail by Thermann *et al.* (1998) and Zhang *et al.* (1998a), who propose that only those termination codons located >50–55 nucleotides upstream of the 3′-most exon–exon junction (after splicing) cause a reduction in the quantity of mRNA. Nonsense codons that reside 54 bp or more upstream of the 3′-most intron of the β-globin gene, intron 2, reduce the abundance of nuclear mRNA to 10–15% of normal. The level of cytoplasmic mRNA is also reduced to 10–15% of normal, indicating that decay occurs in the nucleus. The mechanisms by which this is executed are still not clear but are thought to involve the interaction of a 'tag' marking the 3′-most exon–exon border and the cytoplasmic translation-termination complex.

The milder phenotypes associated with exon 1 or 2 mutations may have come under intense selection; the more severe disorders due to exon 3 mutations would not have been expanded in this way. This may explain the preponderance of exon 1 and 2 mutations in thalassaemic populations today.

Trans-acting determinants

Population studies have shown that ~1% of the β-thalassaemia genes remain uncharacterized despite extensive sequence analysis including the flanking regions. It has been postulated that the mutations might be found in the upstream β LCR or in the enhancer region, 700–1100 bp 3′ of the β gene. However, in several families, linkage studies demonstrate that the β-thalassaemia phenotype segregates independently of the β-globin gene cluster, suggesting that the genetic determinant is *trans*-acting (Murru *et al.* 1992; Thein *et al.* 1993; Pacheco *et al.* 1995; Gasperini *et al.* 1998). Two large families from Sardinia have recently been reported (Gasperini *et al.* 1998) in which heterozygotes for the β codon 39 C→T thalassaemia allele have the phenotype of thalassaemia intermedia. Family studies suggested that the second putative mutation was not linked to the β-globin gene cluster.

Variants of β thalassaemia

'Silent' β thalassaemia

Rarely, the phenotype of β-thalassaemia trait results from homozygosity or compound heterozygosity for very mild or 'silent' β-thalassaemia alleles (Wong *et al.* 1987; Gonzalez-Redondo *et al.* 1988a). The 'silent' β thalassaemias cause only a minimal deficit of β-globin production and do not produce a detectable haematological phenotype when present in a single copy; the only abnormality is a very mild imbalance of globin synthesis. It is not surprising therefore that these mutations are usually identified in the compound heterozygous states with a severe β-thalassaemia allele, where they cause thalassaemia intermedia, or in homozygotes, who have a typical β-thalassaemia trait phenotype. 'Silent' β-thalassaemia alleles include the C→T mutation at position −101 to the β gene (Gonzalez-Redondo *et al.* 1989a), some of the promoter mutations (Rosatelli *et al.* 1995) and

Table 4.6 'Silent' β-thalassaemia alleles.

Position	Mutation	Hb (g/dl)	MCV (fl)	MCH (pg)	HbA₂ (%)	HbF (%)	Distribution	Reference
−101	C→T	11–17	70–92	23–33	3.0–4.4	0.1–3.4	Mediterraneans	Gonzalez-Redondo *et al.* (1989a); Maragoudaki *et al.* (1999)
−92	C→T	12–16	79–86	25–30	3.4–4.0	<1	Mediterraneans	Divoky *et al.* (1993a)
CAP +1	A→C	12–14	76–81	25–27	3.4–3.6	<1	Asian Indians	Wong *et al.* (1987
CAP +8	C→T	51.1	98	33.7	3.0	1.8	Chinese	Ma *et al.* (1999)
CAP +10	(−T)	14–16	94–102	30–33	2.5–2.7	<1	Greeks	Athanassiadou *et al.* (1994)
CAP +33	C→G	12–14	85–86	28–29	2.8–3.0	1.6–2.0	Greeks	Ho *et al.* (1996c)
IVS2-844	C→G	13–16	73–90	26–31	3.0–3.8	<1	Italians	Rosatelli *et al.* (1994)
Terminal CD +6	C→G	12–17	79–95	20–31	1.9–3.4	0.3–3.0	Greeks	Maragoudaki *et al.* (1998)

those affecting the 5′ and 3′ UTR (Wong *et al.* 1987; Gonzalez-Redondo *et al.* 1989a; Jankovic *et al.* 1990b; Athanassiadou *et al.* 1994; Ho *et al.* 1996c). They are summarized in Table 4.6.

It has been suggested that $(TA)_X (T)_Y$ sequence variation at position −530 to the β gene may also be responsible for some 'silent' forms of β thalassaemia (Semenza *et al.* 1984). The reduced β-globin gene expression has been related to the increased binding of a repressor protein (BP1) isolated from K562 cells (Berg *et al.* 1991). However, population surveys and clinical studies do not show a consistent correlation between the sequence variation (+ ATA, −T) and a β-thalassaemia phenotype, suggesting that it is a neutral polymorphism (Wong *et al.* 1989b).

We shall take up the story of these extremely mild forms of β thalassaemia again in Chapter 13 when we consider their interactions with more severe β-thalassaemia alleles as the basis for different clinical grades of thalassaemia intermedia.

β-Thalassaemia trait with unusually high HbA₂ levels

Despite the vast heterogeneity of mutations, the increased levels of HbA₂ observed in β-thalassaemia heterozygotes in different ethnic groups are remarkably uniform, usually 3.5–5.5% and rarely exceeding 6%. The little that is known of the relationship between the level of HbA₂ and particular mutations is described in Chapter 7.

Unusually high levels of HbA₂, over 6.5%, seem to be the hallmark of a subgroup of β thalassaemias caused by deletions that remove the TATA box and other regulatory elements in the β promoter (Fig. 4.11). As discussed earlier, the increase in HbA₂, accompanied by a variable but sometimes marked elevation of HbF, may be related to the removal of competition for the upstream LCR and hence its greater availability to interact with the δ and γ genes in *cis*.

β-Thalassaemia trait with normal HbA₂ levels

It has been customary to classify this form of β thalassaemia into type 1, or the 'silent carrier' state, in which there are minimal or no haematological abnormalities, and type 2, in which the blood picture is typical of heterozygous β thalassaemia except for the normal level of HbA₂. This phenotypic classification is now of limited use following the characterization of the truly 'silent' β-thalassaemia alleles (see above) and the realization that most forms of β-thalassaemia trait with normal HbA₂ levels result from the co-inheritance of δ thalassaemia.

β Thalassaemia with δ thalassaemia in **cis** *or* **trans**

One relatively common form of normal HbA₂ β thalassaemia is that associated with Hb Knossos. This β-chain variant, which results from a **GCC→TCC** mutation at codon 27, is not detectable by electrophoresis under standard conditions. Like HbE, the mutation activates an alternative splicing site in exon

1, giving rise to a reduced amount of β-globin gene transcript containing the amino acid substitution (Orkin *et al.* 1984b). Unlike HbE, the HbA$_2$ level is not elevated in heterozygotes (Baklouti *et al.* 1986; Olds *et al.* 1991). The molecular basis for the normal HbA$_2$ level is a δ^0-thalassaemia mutation (CD59 (−A)) *cis* to the β gene (Loudianos *et al.* 1991a; Olds *et al.* 1991). Beta-globin gene haplotype analysis suggests that the δ^{0}CD59 (−A)/β^{Knossos} allele is a relatively common cause of normal HbA$_2$ β thalassaemia in the Middle East and Mediterranean.

Other cases of normal A$_2$ β thalassaemia are also due to the co-inheritance of a defective δ gene, either in *cis* or in *trans* to a β-thalassaemia gene, which can be of the β$^+$ or β^0 type. Examples include: δ 3′ UTR (+69 G→A) in *cis* to βIVS2-745 C→G (Moi *et al.* 1992); and the δ+27 G→T in *cis* or *trans* to βIVS2-745 C→G (Oggiano *et al.* 1987; Loudianos *et al.* 1990); and the δ$^+$26 G→T in *cis* to the β^{0}39 C→T mutation (Oggiano *et al.* 1994). The δ-thalassaemia mutations are discussed in a later section.

Other causes of the normal HbA$_2$ β-thalassaemia phenotype

Another fairly common cause of the normal HbA$_2$ β-thalassaemia phenotype in the Greek population is the Corfu form of δβ thalassaemia, which removes 720-bp DNA from the 3′ end of the ψβ gene to IVS1 of the δ gene (Wainscoat *et al.* 1985; Traeger-Synodinos *et al.* 1991). The β gene in *cis* is down-regulated by a G→A mutation in position 5 of IVS1 (Kulozik *et al.* 1988b). Heterozygotes for the Corfu δβ thalassaemia have a δβ-thalassaemia phenotype characterized by a variable increase in HbF and low-normal levels of HbA$_2$, while homozygotes have almost 100% HbF, no HbA$_2$, trace amounts of HbA, and a β-thalassaemia intermedia phenotype. The two lesions in Corfu δβ thalassaemia have also been described as separate mutations in two different populations. The normal β gene in *cis* to the 7.2-kb deletion in an Italian is expressed at normal levels (Galanello *et al.* 1990a), while Algerian homozygotes for the βIVS1-5 G→A mutation have a severe transfusion-dependent anaemia (Lapoumeroulie *et al.* 1986).

The clinical picture of normal HbA$_2$ β thalassaemia is also seen in individuals with deletions of the entire β-globin complex (the εγδβ thalassaemias) as well as the upstream deletions which involve the LCR (see later section).

Dominantly inherited β thalassaemia

In some forms of β thalassaemia the inheritance of a single β-thalassaemia allele, in the presence of a normal complement of α genes, results in a clinically detectable phenotype. This unusual form of β thalassaemia was first recognized in an Irish family in 1973; moderately severe anaemia, jaundice, enlargement of the spleen, gross abnormalities of the erythrocytes and inclusion bodies in red-cell precursors were transmitted through three generations as a single allele in an autosomal dominant fashion (Weatherall *et al.* 1973).

Apart from the usual features of heterozygous β thalassaemia, such as increased levels of HbA$_2$ and increased α/β-globin biosynthesis ratios, this group of disorders is also characterized by dyserythropoiesis associated with large intraerythroblastic inclusions. Hence the term 'inclusion-body β thalassaemia' was proposed by Stamatoyannopoulos *et al.* (1974). However, since similar intraerythroblastic inclusions are found in all severe forms of β thalassaemia this term does not seem appropriate.

Molecular pathology

The molecular lesion in the original Irish family was a complex rearrangement involving two minor deletions of 4 and 11 bp interrupted by an insertion of 5 bp in exon 3 of the β gene, giving rise to a frameshift and the predicted synthesis of an elongated β-chain variant with an abnormal carboxy terminus (Thein *et al.* 1990a). Since its first description, numerous families with dominantly inherited β thalassaemia have been described, arising from a heterogeneous group of lesions which include mis-sense mutations, minor deletions leading to the loss of intact codons, frameshifts arising from minor insertions and deletions, all of which result in elongated β chains with abnormal carboxy-terminal ends or truncated β chains (see Table 4.7 and Fig. 4.15).

Unlike the more common recessively inherited varieties, which lead to a quantitative reduction in normal β globin, they result in the synthesis of β-chain variants which are so unstable that, in many cases, the dominantly inherited β-thalassaemia alleles are not detectable and are only implicated from the DNA sequence. The predicted synthesis is supported by the presence of substantial amounts of abnormal β-globin mRNA in reticulocytes, compara-

Table 4.7 Dominantly inherited β thalassaemias.

	β Variant	Identification§	Distribution	References
I–Mis-sense mutations				
1	CD28 (**CTG**→**CGG**) Leu→Arg	Hb Chesterfield*	–*Bst* NI	English	Thein *et al.* (1991)
2	CD32 (**CTG**→**CAG**) Leu→Glu in *cis* with CD98 (**GTG**→**ATG**) Val to Met, Hb Köln	Hb Medicine Lake*	ASO	US Caucasian	Coleman *et al.* (1995)
3	CD60 (**GTG**→**GAG**) Val to Glu	Hb Cagliari*	ASO	Italian	Podda *et al.* (1991)
4	CD110 (**CTG**→**CCG**) Leu to Pro	Hb Showa-Yakushiji	+*Msp* I	Japanese	Kobayashi *et al.* (1987)
5	CD114 (**CTG**→**CCG**) Leu to Pro	Hb Durham/Hb Brescia	+*Msp* I	US Irish, Italian	Çürük *et al.* (1994); de Castro *et al.* (1994)
6	CD115 (**GCC**→**GAC**) Ala to Asp	Hb Hradec Kralove	ASO	Czech	Divoky *et al.* (1993c)
7	CD127 (**CAG**→**CCG**) Gln to Pro	Hb Houston	ASO	US English	Kazazian *et al.* (1992)
8	CD127 (**CAG**→**CGG**) Gln→Arg	Hb Dieppe	ASO	French	Girodon *et al.* (1992)
II–Deletion or insertion of intact codons→Destabilization				
1	CD30–31 (+CGG) +Arg		ASO	Spanish	Arjona *et al.* (1996)
2	CD32–34 (–GGT) –Val	Hb Korea*	ASO	Korean	Park *et al.* (1991)
3	CD33–35 (–6'bp) Val-Val-Try→Asp	Hb Dresden	–*Mae* II	German	Vetter *et al.* (2000)
4	CD108–112 (–12'bp) Asn-Val-Leu-Val-Cys to Ser‡		ASO	Swedish	Landin & Rudolphi (1996)
5	CD124–126 (CCA) +Pro		ASO	Armenian	Çürük *et al.* (1994)
6	CD127–128 (–AGG) Glu-Ala to Pro	Hb Gunma	ASO	Japanese	Fucharoen *et al.* (1990c)
7	CD134–137 (–12, +6) Val-Ala-Gly-Val to Gly-Arg		ASO	Portuguese	Öner *et al.* (1991c)
III–Premature termination→Truncated β variant				
1	CD121 (**GAA**→**T**AA) Glu to Term (120aa)		–*EcoR* I	Caucasian, N. Europeans	Kazazian *et al.* (1986); Fei *et al.* (1989b); Thein *et al.* (1990a)
2	CD127 (**CAG**→**T**AG) Gln to Term (127aa)		–*Bsg* I	English	Hall *et al.* (1991)

IV – Frameshift or aberrant splicing →Elongated or truncated variants with abnormal carboxy terminal

1	IVS2: 2,3 (+11, −2)		−HinfI	Iranian	Kaeda et al. (1992)
2	IVS2: 4,5 (−AG)→aberrant splicing		ASO	Portuguese	Faustino et al. (1992)
3	CD94 (+TG)→156aa	Hb Agnana*	ASO	S. Italian	Ristaldi et al. (1990b)
4	CD100 (−CTT, +TCTGAGAACTT)→158aa		ASO	S. African	Williamson et al. (1997)
5	CD109 (−G)→156aa	Hb Manhattan	ASO	Lithuanian	Kazazian et al. (1992)
6	CD114 (−CT, +G)→156aa	Hb Geneva	+ApaI	Swiss-French	Beris et al. (1988)
7	CD123 (−A)→156aa	Hb Makabe	−HphI	Japanese	Fucharoen et al. (1990e)
8	CD1232−125 (−ACCCCACC)→135aa	Hb Khon Kaen	−HphI	Thai	Fucharoen et al. (1991a)
9	CD124 (−A)→156aa		ASO	Russian	Çürük et al. (1994)
10	CD125 (−A)→156aa		ASO	Japanese	Ohba et al. (1997)
11	CD126 (−T)→156aa	Hb Vercelli*	ASO	N. Italian	Murru et al. (1991)
12	CD126−131 (−17bp)→132aa	Hb Westdale¶	ASO	Trinidad, Pakistan	Waye et al. (1995); Ahmed et al. (1996)
13	CD128−129 (−4,+5,−11)→153aa		ASO	Irish	Thein et al. (1990a)
14	CD131−132 (−GA)→138aa		ASO	Swiss	Deutsch et al. (1998)

* Spontaneous mutations.

† Several families reported, including one spontaneous mutation.

‡ Heterozygotes do not have a particularly severe phenotype.

§ Identification: (+) indicates creation, and (−) removal of restriction enzyme sites. Otherwise, mutations are detectable by allele-specific oligonucleotide (ASO) hybridization.

¶ Difficult to evaluate phenotypes of heterozygotes as only homozygote and compound heterozygotes, both with thalassaemia major, reported.

ble in amounts to that produced from the normal β-globin allele (Hall & Thein 1994; Ho *et al.* 1997). In a few cases, the β-chain variant can be detected when newly synthesized, as in Hb Houston (β127 Gln→Pro) (Kazazian *et al.* 1992). In the case of the β121 GAA→TAA mutation, the truncated β variant was detected indirectly by studies of haemoglobin synthesis (Ho *et al.* 1997). In a similar study of a patient with the same mutation, the truncated β121 chain comprised 0.05–0.1% of the total non-α chains (Adams *et al.* 1990). The abnormal β variant that is truncated to β120 should bind haem and have some secondary structure and, presumably, is not as unstable as those in which no abnormal globin can be demonstrated, such as Hb Showa-Yakushiji (β110 Leu→Pro) and Hb Durham NC (β114 Leu→Pro) (Kobayashi *et al.* 1987; de Castro *et al.* 1994).

Phenotype–genotype relationships

All of the in-phase chain-termination mutations associated with dominantly inherited β thalassaemia are in exon 3 or beyond, while the vast majority (71/75) of the in-phase mutations that are recessively inherited lead to termination in exon 1 or 2 (see Figs 4.12 and 4.15). The latter are associated with minimal amounts of abnormal β-globin mRNA and hence the quantitative reduction of β-globin typical of recessive β thalassaemia (Hall & Thein 1994) (see p. 164). In contrast, mutations which cause termination later in the β-globin sequence, in exon 3, result in the production of substantial amounts of mRNA, leading to the synthesis of unstable β-chain variants. In short, in-phase termination mutants exemplify how shifting the position of a nonsense codon can alter the phenotype of recessive inheritance characterized by haplo-insufficiency, to a dominant negative effect due to the synthesis of an abnormal and deleterious protein.

Analysis of tryptic peptides prepared from inclusion bodies from the red cells of patients with mutations of this kind showed that they contain precipitated α- and β-globin chains (Weatherall *et al.* 1973). This was recently confirmed in two heterozygous cases of the β121 GAA→TAA mutation by immunoelectron microscopy using mouse monoclonal antibodies against human α- and β-globin chains (Ho *et al.* 1997). In contrast, the intraerythroblastic inclusions found in homozygous β thalassaemia consisted only of precipitated α globin. It is quite clear that the cellular pathology underlying this

group of β thalassaemias is related to the synthesis of highly unstable β globin, which fails to form functional tetramers and precipitates intracellularly, the concomitant excess of α chains accentuating the ineffective erythropoiesis. In addition, there is also a haemolytic component, as shown by an increased level of reticulocytes.

Clearly, the dominantly inherited β thalassaemias belong to a phenotypic class of their own. Unlike the other β-thalassaemia haemoglobinopathies, the synthesis of β-chain variants is usually implicated but they are undetectable due to their hyper-instability. But they share the other hallmarks of heterozygous β thalassaemia, i.e. raised HbA$_2$ levels, varying degrees of hypochromic microcytosis and α/β-globin imbalance. The factors which determine the pathophysiology of mutations involving the β-globin gene in the heterozygous state thus appear to include: whether a β-chain variant is synthesized; the stability of the product; its ability to bind haem and to form αβ dimers and tetramers; and the stability of the tetramers. At one end of the spectrum are typical β-thalassaemia traits due to a 'pure' quantitative defect characterized by a very mild anaemia and hypochromic microcytic red cells, while at the other there are predominantly haemolytic anaemias due to instability of haemoglobin tetramers. The dominantly inherited β thalassaemias, characterized by the synthesis of highly unstable β-chain variants, fall in between the two extremes. They resemble the intermediate forms of β thalassaemia by virtue of the ineffective erythropoiesis, but also have elements of congenital haemolytic anaemias in that there is a variable degree of haemolysis.

Distribution

Unlike recessive β thalassaemia, which is prevalent in malaria-endemic regions, dominant β thalassaemias are rare, occurring in dispersed geographical regions including Northern and Eastern Europe, Japan and Korea, where the gene frequency for β thalassaemia is very low (Thein 1993). Except for the codon 121 GAA→TAA mutation and codon 114 CTG→CCG mutations, all the dominant β-thalassaemia alleles have been described in single families, many as *de novo* mutations (Table 4.7). As mentioned earlier, it is likely that their low frequency reflects the lack of positive selection that occurs in the recessive forms.

δ Thalassaemia

Mutations affecting the δ-globin gene cause either a reduction (δ^+ thalassaemia) or absence (δ^0 thalassaemia) of δ-globin synthesis (Table 4.8). Although these conditions are clinically silent they are of importance in that, when co-inherited with β thalassaemia, they prevent an increase in the level of HbA_2, which can confuse the diagnosis of the β-thalassaemia carrier state. The co-inheritance of a mutation in the δ gene in *cis* or *trans* is the most common cause of normal HbA_2 β thalassaemia (see earlier section).

A fairly common condition that resembles δ^0 thalassaemia in the Mediterranean population, Corfu δβ thalassaemia, is caused by a deletion of 7201 bp (see p. 167) (Traeger-Synodinos *et al.* 1991). As discussed earlier, the *cis* β gene contains a G→A mutation at IVS1-5, but subsequent to the initial report both the 7.2-kb deletion and the β IVS1-5 G→A mutation have been identified as separate lesions. Presumably Corfu δβ thalassaemia has arisen from a recombination event between two different chromosomes, each carrying the separate lesions.

The other mutations causing δ thalassaemia resemble those found in β thalassaemia. They include insertions and deletions causing frameshifts, nonsense codons and base changes that lead to abnormal splicing. Several lead to the production of δ-globin variants similar to the β-thalassaemic haemoglobinopathies. Although some of the mutations in δ thalassaemia have their equivalents in the β-globin sequence in β thalassaemia, far fewer mutations causing δ thalassaemia and δ-globin variants have been described. This may be related to ascertainment bias from the lack of clinical and haematological abnormalities, or a lack of selective pressure from malaria. The identical nucleotide changes in the same positions in the β and δ genes have presumably arisen as either independent mutations or gene conversions. Some of the δ-thalassaemia mutations have been observed both *cis* and *trans* to β thalassaemia, e.g. δ27 C→T and β^+ IVS2-745 thalassaemias (Loudianos *et al.* 1990; Pirastu *et al.* 1990). Again, this presumably has arisen from either recombination or gene conversion. Other δ thalassaemias reported *cis* to β-thalassaemia genes include the δ poly(A) +69 G→A/βIVS2-745 C→G (Moi *et al.* 1992), δCD59 (−A)/β Knossos (Olds *et al.* 1991). The δCD27 (C→T) has also been reported in *cis* to the β^0CD39 (C→T)

(Oggiano *et al.* 1994) and β Knossos (Loudianos *et al.* 1991a).

δβ Thalassaemia and hereditary persistence of fetal haemoglobin

As outlined in the previous chapter, almost all the β thalassaemias are associated with increased levels of fetal haemoglobin production which persist after the neonatal period. In most cases the output is insufficient to compensate for the primary deficit of β-globin chain production. However, there is a rarer group of conditions, including δβ thalassaemia and hereditary persistence of fetal haemoglobin (HPFH), in which persistent HbF synthesis occurs at a much higher level and hence is able to compensate much more effectively for the reduction or absence of β-globin production. As we shall see in Chapters 8 and 10, on clinical and haematological criteria there is some degree of overlap between the δβ thalassaemias and HPFH.

The first gene-mapping studies of these conditions, described in Chapter 1, demonstrated that both are often associated with deletions of the δ- and β-globin genes, underlining their similarity at the molecular level. As outlined in Chapter 3, analyses of the structure of the HbF that is produced, together with their further definition at the molecular level, have led to their classification along the lines of the other forms of thalassaemia. Thus the δβ thalassaemias can be subdivided into $(\delta\beta)^+$ and $(\delta\beta)^0$ varieties, and the latter can be further divided into $^{G}\gamma^{A}\gamma(\delta\beta)^0$ and $^{G}\gamma(^{A}\gamma\delta\beta)^0$ thalassaemias; they are more logically described as $(\delta\beta)^0$ and $(^{A}\gamma\delta\beta)^0$ thalassaemia. Similarly, HPFH can be subclassified based on the same principles; that is, on the presence or absence of β-globin production and on the structure of the associated HbF. Broadly, therefore, HPFH can be subdivided into $^{G}\gamma^{A}\gamma(\delta\beta)^0$, $^{G}\gamma^+$ and $^{A}\gamma^+$ varieties; in line with the δβ thalassaemias, $^{G}\gamma^{A}\gamma(\delta\beta)^0$ HPFH is now usually called $(\delta\beta)^0$ HPFH. In addition, there is a heterogeneous group in which there is hereditary persistence of low levels of HbF for which some of the genetic determinants may be in the β-globin gene cluster, while others are probably on other chromosomes. A classification of these conditions along these lines was outlined in Chapter 3 and a more detailed breakdown in shown in Table 4.9.

Deletions are responsible for most forms of δβ thalassaemia and for most of the varieties of HPFH in

Table 4.8 Mutations causing δ thalassaemia.

	Type	Identification*	Distribution	Reference
Deletions				
1 Corfu deletion 7.2 kb† (3′ of ψβ to δ-IVS2)	δ^0	*Eco*R V	Greek/Italian	Kulozik *et al.* (1988b); Galanello *et al.* (1990a); Traeger-Synodinos *et al.* (1991)
Point mutations				
I–TRANSCRIPTION				
1 −77 T→C	δ^0	ASO	Japanese	Matsuda *et al.* (1992)
2 −65 A→C	δ^+	ASO	Greek	Papadakis *et al.* (1997)
3 −55 T→C	δ^+	ASO	Greek	Papadakis *et al.* (1997)
4 −36 C→A	δ^+	ASO	Greek	Papadakis *et al.* (1997)
II–RNA PROCESSING				
Splice junction				
1 CD30 AGG→ACG	δ^0	ASO	Italian	Loudianos *et al.* (1992)
2 IVS1-2 T→C	δ^0	ASO	Italian	Moi *et al.* (1988)
3 IVS2 −1 AG→GC	δ^0	+*Sac* II	Greek	Trifillis *et al.* (1991)
Cryptic splice sites				
4 CD4 ACT→ATT (Thr→Ile)	δ^+	−*Ple* I	Greek	Trifillis *et al.* (1993)
5 CD27 GCC→TCC (Ala→Ser, HbA₂-Yialousa)	δ^+	+*Hae* III or −*Eco* O 109 I	Mediterranean	Moi *et al.* (1988); Trifillis *et al.* (1991); Renda *et al.* (1992b)
RNA cleavage + polyadenylation				
6 Term CD +69 bp G→A‡	δ^+	ASO	Italian	Moi *et al.* (1992)
III–RNA TRANSLATION				
Nonsense codons				
1 CD37 TGG→TAG	δ^0	ASO	Italian	Gasperini *et al.* (1994)
Frameshift				
2 CD59 −A§	δ^0	−*Sau* I	Egyptian, Mediterranean	Olds *et al.* (1991)
3 CD91 +T	δ^0	ASO	Belgium	Losekoot *et al.* (1989)
IV–POST-TRANSLATIONAL				
1 CD11 GTC→GGC (HbA₂-Pylos)	δ^+	+*Cac* 81	Greek	Drakoulakou *et al.* (1997)
2 CD85 TTT→TCT (HbA₂-Etolia)	δ^+	ASO	Greek	Drakoulakou *et al.* (1997)
3 CD98 GTG→ATG (Val→Met)	δ^+	ASO	US Black	Codrington *et al.* (1989)
4) CD116 CGC→TGC (Arg→Cys)	δ^+	+*Sau* 96 I	Greek Cypriot	Loudianos *et al.* (1991b); Trifillis *et al.* (1991)
5 CD141 CTG→CCC (Leu→Pro, HbA₂-Pelendri)	δ^0	+*Hpa* II	Greek Cypriot	Trifillis *et al.* (1991)

* Restriction enzyme sites affected are noted: (+) indicates creations of site and (−) indicates removal. Otherwise point mutations are detectable by ASO (allele-specific oligoprobe) hybridization.

† Originally described in *cis* to β IVS1-5 G→A mutation.

‡ In *cis* to β IVS2-745 C→G thalassaemia mutation.

§ In *cis* to β^Knossos (β27 GCC→TCC).

which levels of HbF of 20% or more are found in heterozygotes. Over 20 different deletions of this type have now been characterized and the endpoints of many of them have been cloned and sequenced. Their positions relative to the β-globin gene cluster are shown in Fig. 4.16 and Table 4.9, in which the larger deletions that result in the phenotype of β thalassaemia are included, for comparison.

Table 4.9 The molecular pathology of the δβ thalassaemias and deletional forms of hereditary persistence of fetal haemoglobin. The deletions that underlie the deletional forms of β thalassaemia are shown for comparison.

Condition	Type	5′ Breakpoint	3′ Breakpoint	Deletion size (kb)
β Thalassaemia	Turkish	~43	~50.6	7.6
	Turkish	~58	~65.6	7.6
	Filipino	57876	(~103)>165	(45)>108
	US Asian	59145	69474	10.329
	Dutch	59711	72333	12.622
	Australian	61354	73377	12.023
	South Italian	58523	~125	~67
δβ Fusion	Hb Lepore	54874–55238	62483–63572	7.4
δ Thalassaemia	Corfu	48.841	56051	7.201
γβ Fusion	Hb Kenya	39846–39869	62521–62534	22.5
(δβ)^0 Thalassaemia	Mediterranean	55961	69321	13.4
	South-east Asian	56007	68591	12.6
	East European	53230	62352	9.1
	Black	50725	64052 or 64776	12.5
	Macedonian/Turkish	54704	66169	11.465
	Macedonian/Turkish	73813	75406	1.593
	Indian	42151	74772	32.621
	Spanish	51976	~165	114
	Japanese	43120	>70	>130
$^G\gamma(^A\gamma\delta\beta)^0$ Thalassaemia	Black	40701	76508	35.807
	Chinese	40471	~140	~100
	Belgian	40730	~94	50
	Indian	40073	40903	0.830
	Indian	56192	63651	7.459
	Yunnanese	~39.3	~130	~90
	Malay 2	~40	>80	>40
	German	~38	~90	52
	Turkish	37075	73286	36.234
	Thai	37252	~138	~101
	Malay 1	~35	>65	>30
	Cantonese	~35	>67	>30
	Italian	39768	92	52
(δβ)^0 HPFH	Black	51086	~154	~106
	Ghanaian	46495	~148.5	~105
	Indian	45026	~94	~48.5
	Italian	~50.5	~91	40
	Sicilian	51504	64414	12.910
	South-east Asian	60202	~88	~28

The δβ thalassaemias

(δβ)⁺ Thalassaemias

Haemoglobin Lepore was defined by Gerald & Diamond (1958) as a structural haemoglobin variant associated with a thalassaemia-like disorder. In 1962 Baglioni showed that the non-α chain of haemoglobin Lepore is a hybrid of δ and β chains. It was shown subsequently that the δβ-fusion chain of haemoglobin Lepore is synthesized inefficiently and gives rise to a form of thalassaemia in which both β- and δ-chain production are affected, i.e. a δβ thalassaemia. Because some δβ-chain fusion product

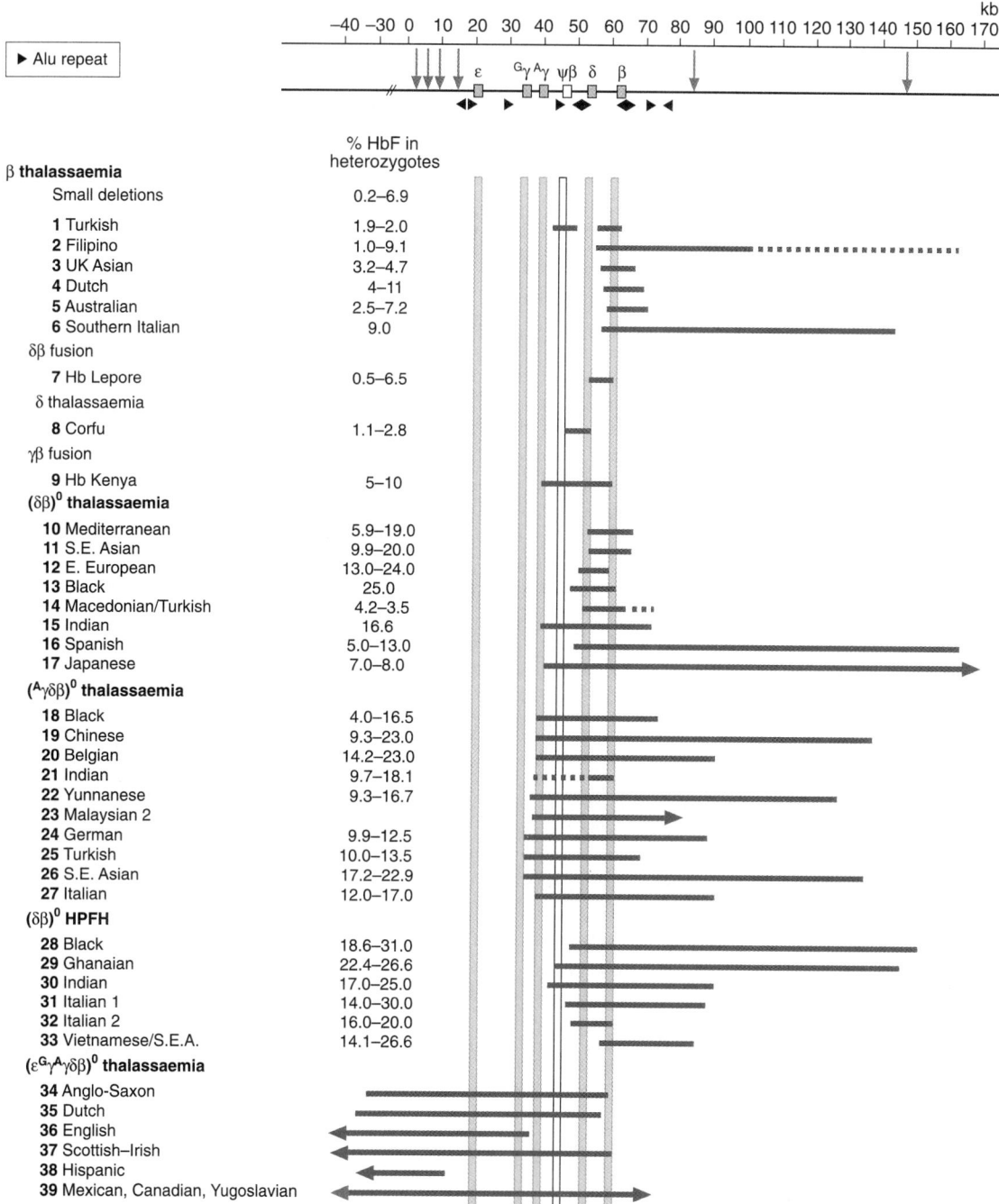

Fig. 4.16 The deletions that generate δβ thalassaemia and the deletional forms of hereditary persistence of fetal haemoglobin. The upper set of arrows indicate DNase1-sensitive sites.

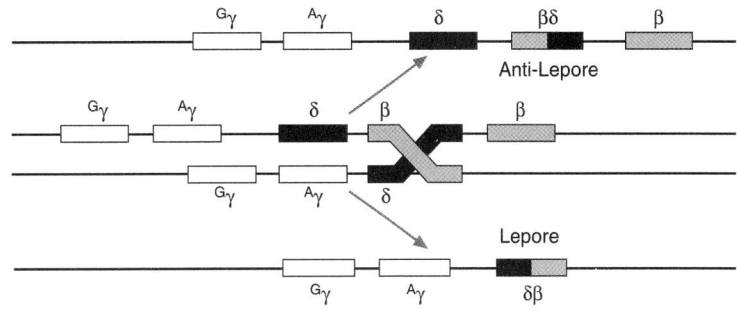

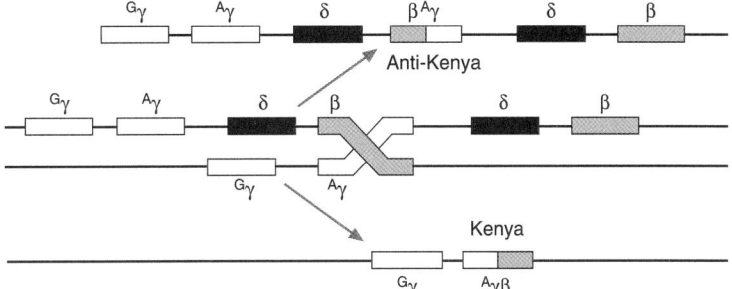

Fig. 4.17 The generation of the Lepore and anti-Lepore haemoglobins and haemoglobin Kenya.

is synthesized, it is designated a form of $(\delta\beta)^+$ thalassaemia.

Baglioni suggested that the δβ-fusion gene was formed by unequal crossing over between the δ- and β-chain genes (Fig. 4.17). This was later confirmed by gene mapping (Flavell *et al*. 1978; Mears *et al*. 1978a). Three different forms of Hb Lepore have been described, containing different relative amounts of the δ and β chains; Hb Lepore Hollandia has a breakpoint between amino acids 22 and 50, Hb Lepore Baltimore between amino acids 50 and 86 and Hb Lepore Boston/Washington between amino acids 87 and 116.

Later, it was possible to confirm these protein structural studies by direct analysis of the globin genes of patients with different forms of haemoglobin Lepore. Southern blotting, and later direct sequence analysis, defined the crossover region in Lepore Boston/Washington as being between δ^{87} and β^{IVS2-8} (Baird *et al*. 1981b; Mavilio *et al*. 1983; Fioretti *et al*. 1992; Ribeiro *et al*. 1997). The breakpoints for Hbs Lepore Baltimore and Hollandia have been defined as being between codons δ^{68} and β^{84} and δ^{22}

and nucleotide 16 of β IVS1, respectively (Miranda *et al*. 1994; Waye *et al*. 1994d; Huisman *et al*. 1997; Ribeiro *et al*. 1997). In the case of Hb Lepore Boston–Washington the unequal recombination event generating the deletion must have taken place in a segment of only 125 bp. Despite this relatively short segment, which makes repeated crossover events unlikely, evidence which is cited in Chapter 8 suggests that Hb Lepore Boston–Washington has, in fact, arisen on a number of different occasions.

We shall consider the structure of the δ-globin gene promoter, which is probably responsible for the reduced rate of production of the Lepore haemoglobins, when we consider their pathophysiology in Chapter 8.

Misaligned crossing over between the β and δ genes can also result in the production of a βδ-fusion gene lying between normal copies of the two genes (Fig. 4.17). A number of examples of these so-called anti-Lepore haemoglobins have been reported, such as Hb Miyada (Ohta *et al*. 1971a) and HbP Nilotic (Badr *et al*. 1973). They are described in Chapter 8.

Phenocopies of (δβ)⁺ thalassaemia

The combination of independently inherited δ- and β-thalassaemia genes may occasionally give rise to the phenotypic picture of (δβ)⁺ thalassaemia.

Corfu δβ thalassaemia

The original description of the Corfu type of δβ thalassaemia identified a 7.2-kb deletion involving the δ gene (see Fig. 4.16), which was believed to inactivate the β-globin gene and to be responsible for the high level of HbF in the homozygote (Wainscoat *et al.* 1985). Subsequently, it was shown that, in this patient, the β-globin gene carried the IVS1-5 (G→A) mutation, accounting for the reduced β-chain production (Kulozik *et al.* 1988b). When the deletion was discovered in Italian patients without the β-thalassaemia mutation (Galanello *et al.* 1990a) it became clear that it acts only on the δ-globin gene, with normal β-chain production and no increase in HbF in heterozygotes, i.e. it is a deletional form of δ thalassaemia (see earlier section).

Homozygotes with the combined deletion and β-thalassaemia mutation have the clinical picture of thalassaemia intermedia. Whether the deletion plays any role in producing relatively high levels of HbF in homozygotes remains to be established (Traeger-Synodinos *et al.* 1991).

Sardinian δβ thalassaemia

In this disorder there is no deletion and the HbF contains predominately ᴬγ chains. Analysis of the ᴬγ and β genes (Ottolenghi *et al.* 1987) demonstrated two separate mutations in *cis*; the common β⁰CD39 (C→T) premature stop codon in the β gene and a point mutation at position –196 in the ᴬγ gene, an established non-deletion HPFH mutation (see below).

Other δβ-thalassaemia phenocopies

Two Chinese families with the phenotype of δβ thalassaemia/HPFH with an intact β-globin gene cluster have also been described (Zeng *et al.* 1985a; Atweh *et al.* 1986). The HbF in these patients contains both ᴳγ and ᴬγ chains. Sequencing of the β-globin gene in one of these cases identified a point mutation in the TATA box at position –29 that leads to β⁺ thalas-

saemia (Atweh *et al.* 1987b). The same mutation does not lead to high HbF levels in African or in other Chinese families. No non-deletion HPFH mutations were observed in the γ-gene promoters but a non-polymorphic base substitution was found in the regulatory element 3′ to the ᴬγ gene (Balta *et al.* 1994). If this element plays a role in γ-gene silencing it is possible that such a mutation may be involved in the high HbF levels in these patients, but this has yet to be demonstrated.

(δβ)⁰ Thalassaemia

At least nine different deletions have been described that underlie the phenotype of (δβ)⁰ thalassaemia (Fig. 4.16, Table 4.9). Several have been found in single families while others are more common. The Mediterranean (or Sicilian) type occurs throughout the Mediterranean region, where it is by far the most common form of δβ thalassaemia. Several families with the Spanish type have been described, including 10 homozygotes, suggesting that it is the most common form in Spain, while the Turkish/Macedonian inversion–deletion types have been found in Greece and Italy as well as Turkey and Macedonia.

Sicilian (δβ)⁰ thalassaemia (Mediterranean/Southern Italian δβ thalassaemia)

Delta beta thalassaemia is frequently encountered among the populations of the Mediterranean. Gene mapping studies demonstrated a deletion that gave abnormal-sized bands with a probe from IVS2 of the δ gene (Bernards *et al.* 1979a; Fritsch *et al.* 1979; Ottolenghi *et al.* 1982a; Tuan *et al.* 1983). It extended beyond the β-globin gene and encompassed ~13 kb in total. Cloning and sequencing of the breakpoint showed that the deletion begins within δ IVS2, 188 bp upstream of exon 3, and ends within an L1 repeat (Henthorn *et al.* 1990).

Laotian (δβ)⁰ thalassaemia (South-East Asian δβ thalassaemia)

Three independent reports of (δβ)⁰ thalassaemia from south-east Asia describe a 12.5-kb deletion that is similar to, but clearly different from, Mediterranean δβ thalassaemia. It starts in IVS2 of the δ gene and ends in the same L1 repeat. Restriction-enzyme analysis of the Laotian (Zhang *et al.* 1988a) and Thai

(Trent *et al.* 1988) cases are indistinguishable at that level of resolution, but sequence analysis was not reported. Craig *et al.* (1994) sequenced the breakpoints of a deletion found in a Vietnamese patient and showed that it lies within that of the Sicilian type, but is truncated by 47–48 bp at the 5′ end, and 747–748 bp at the 3′ end. It is not entirely clear whether this is identical to the Laotian case, in which fine mapping suggested that the 5′ breakpoint lay 18–24 bp downstream of that sequenced in the Vietnamese case. It is possible that closely related but subtly different recombinations between the δ IVS2 and L1 regions have produced very similar deletions and, not surprisingly, similar phenotypes.

Eastern European (δβ)⁰ thalassaemia

A 9.1-kb deletion resulting in δβ thalassaemia was characterized in a single family of east European origin. The breakpoint was cloned and sequenced and shown to extend from 1.6 kb 5′ to the δ-gene CAP site into IVS1 of the β-globin gene (Palena *et al.* 1992).

Black (δβ)⁰ thalassaemia

A deletion of ~12.5 kb that removed the δ and β genes was found in an Afro-American woman who had a βˢ gene on the other chromosome (Anagnou *et al.* 1985). No simple heterozygotes for this condition were found but the normal MCH, balanced globin synthesis and a pancellular distribution of the HbF pointed to an HPFH phenotype. Restriction mapping of the 5′ and 3′ breakpoints indicated that this deletion is very similar to, but differs from, HPFH 5 (see later section). A similar deletion was described in a second Afro-American family (Waye *et al.* 1994a) in which, in the absence of βˢ, a phenotype of δβ thalassaemia was observed. Sequencing of the breakpoints showed that these two deletions were identical and differed slightly in position from those of HPFH 5 (Dr NP Anagnou, personal communication).

Turkish/Macedonian (δβ)⁰ thalassaemia

Delta beta thalassaemia was described in two families from Macedonia by Efremov *et al.* (1975). Gene mapping demonstrated a deletion extending 18–23 kb from 5′ to the δ-globin gene to 3′ to the β gene (Efremov *et al.* 1986b). However, some inconsistencies in expected band sizes were observed. Subse-

quently, Kulozik *et al.* (1992) described a Turkish family with δβ thalassaemia in which there were two deletions, with inversion of the sequences between them. The 5′ deletion begins 53 bp 5′ to the δ gene CAP site and ends 11.5 kb downstream, beyond the β gene and just 5′ to the L1 repeat. The second deletion, of 1.6 kb, begins beyond the inverted L1 repeat. The restriction map of this complex rearrangement is similar to that described for the Macedonian cases, suggesting that the two may be the same. Craig *et al.* (1994), using PCR to identify deletion mutants, described further cases of this inversion–deletion in one Greek and two Italian families. Using the same technique to re-analyse the original Macedonian cases, they found that the Macedonian and Turkish cases had identical deletions (Craig *et al.* 1995).

Indian (δβ)⁰ thalassaemia

A unique deletion causing δβ thalassaemia was found in a single individual of Indian origin. Cloning and sequencing of the breakpoints demonstrated that the deletion begins about 1 kb 3′ of the ᴬγ gene and terminates in an L1 repeat, about 11 kb 3′ to the β gene, encompassing 32.6 kb in total (Mishima *et al.* 1989; Gilman *et al.* 1992).

Spanish (δβ)⁰ thalassaemia

Cases of δβ thalassaemia, including homozygotes, were first reported from Spain in 1979 (Gimferrer *et al.* 1979). The 5′ end of the deletion was mapped to an *Alu* repeat upstream of the δ-globin gene (Ottolenghi *et al.* 1982a,b). The 3′ breakpoint was shown to lie 8.5–9.0 kb beyond the HPFH 1 deletion (Camaschella *et al.* 1987b) (see later section) and it has been cloned and sequenced (Feingold & Forget 1989).

Japanese (δβ)⁰ thalassaemia

A Japanese δβ-thalassaemia homozygote, from a consanguineous marriage, was shown to have a deletion that starts ~2 kb 3′ to the ᴬγ gene and extends beyond the β gene (Matsunaga *et al.* 1985). Cloning and sequencing of the breakpoint demonstrated that the 3′ end of the deletion is further 3′ than any of the other characterized deletions, including the Spanish δβ-thalassaemia deletion (Shiokawa *et al.* 1988).

Turkish-2 $(\delta\beta)^0$ thalassaemia

A second deletion causing $(\delta\beta)^0$ thalassaemia was reported from Turkey by Öner *et al.* (1996). The deletion begins downstream of the $^A\gamma$ gene, at a position close to the 5′ ends of the Indian and Japanese types. It extends for ~30 kb, ending in an L1 repeat 3′ to the β gene.

$(^A\gamma\delta\beta)^0$ Thalassaemia

Deletions that remove not only the δ- and β-globin genes but also the $^A\gamma$ gene result in δβ thalassaemia in which the HbF contains only $^G\gamma$ chains. At least nine different varieties have been reported (Fig. 4.16). The Black, Chinese and Indian types have been found in many families within their respective populations.

Black $(^A\gamma\delta\beta)^0$ thalassaemia

Numerous examples of patients with high HbF containing only $^G\gamma$ chains have been reported in Afro-American populations, some originally described as $^G\gamma$ HPFH, others as $^G\gamma$ δβ thalassaemia (Altay *et al.* 1977b). Molecular analyses of 10 families demonstrated that they all had the same deletion, ~34 kb beginning within the 3′ end of the $^A\gamma$ gene (Henthorn *et al.* 1985). Cloning and sequencing of the junction showed that its 5′ end was within IVS2 of the $^A\gamma$ gene, 87 bp from exon 3, while the 3′ end was located within the L1 repeat 3′ of the β-globin gene.

Chinese $(^A\gamma\delta\beta)^0$ thalassaemia

The first Chinese family with $(^A\gamma\delta\beta)^0$ thalassaemia was reported by Mann *et al.* (1972). Genomic mapping demonstrated that the 5′ breakpoint of the deletion lay within the $^A\gamma$ gene (Jones *et al.* 1981b). When the junction was cloned and sequenced, the 5′ end was shown to be in IVS2 of the $^A\gamma$ gene, while the 3′ end was ~100 kb away, approximately 11 kb on the 5′ side of the HPFH 2 deletion (Mager *et al.* 1985). An insert of 36–41 bp from an L1 repeat lay between the two junctions. Additional families with the same deletion were described by Trent *et al.* (1984b) and Craig *et al.* (1994).

Belgian $(^A\gamma\delta\beta)^0$ thalassaemia

A third deletion that starts within the $^A\gamma$ gene was

described in a single Belgian family (Losekoot *et al.* 1991a), 30 bp downstream from that of the Black $(^A\gamma\delta\beta)^0$-thalassaemia breakpoint. It extends for ~50 kb, terminating just 4 bp upstream from the 3′ end of the HPFH 3 deletion (see later section) and 1 bp from the midpoint of the 160-bp palindrome that lies in this region (Fodde *et al.* 1990).

Italian $(^A\gamma\delta\beta)^0$ thalassaemia

An Italian patient with $(^A\gamma\delta\beta)^0$ thalassaemia, originally described in 1989, has recently been characterized and shown to have a deletion beginning in exon 2 of the $^A\gamma$ gene and extending for ~52 kb. The 3′ breakpoint of this deletion is close to those of Indian HPFH (HPFH 3) and Belgian $(^A\gamma\delta\beta)^0$ thalassaemia, in the region of the L1 repeat and 160 bp palindrome (De Angioletti *et al.* 1997).

Indian $(^A\gamma\delta\beta)^0$ thalassaemia

A complex double-deletion/inversion rearrangement has been reported in several Indian families with $(^A\gamma\delta\beta)$ thalassaemia (Jones *et al.* 1981a) with similarities to that found in the Macedonian/Turkish $(\delta\beta)^0$ thalassaemia described above. There is a loss of 834 bp from IVS2 and exon 3 of the $^A\gamma$ gene and deletion of 7.46 kb between exon 3 of δ and the 3′ untranslated region of the β gene (Jennings *et al.* 1985). Additional families with this deletion have been described from India (Matthews *et al.* 1981; Trent *et al.* 1984b), Kuwait (Amin *et al.* 1979) and Iran (Craig *et al.* 1994), suggesting that it may be widespread in the Middle East and across the Indian subcontinent.

Yunnanese $(^A\gamma\delta\beta)^0$ thalassaemia

A single family from Yunnan province of China was described in which there were several heterozygotes and a homozygote from a consanguineous mating with a large deletion starting just upstream of the $^A\gamma$ gene (Zhang *et al.* 1993). The 5′ breakpoint was close to an *Nco* I site 0.14 kb upstream of the $^A\gamma$ CAP site and the deletion extended ~66 kb, terminating ~13 kb upstream of the 3′ breakpoint of the Chinese $(^A\gamma\delta\beta)^0$ thalassaemia.

Malaysian-2 $(^A\gamma\delta\beta)^0$ thalassaemia

George *et al.* (1986) described an $(^A\gamma\delta\beta)^0$-

thalassaemia homozygote who had been adopted and whose relatives were therefore not available. The deletion in this patient also began close (~200-400 bp) to the $^A\gamma$-gene CAP site and extended beyond the β gene to an undetermined extent. The size of the abnormal fragments hybridizing with a γ-gene probe demonstrates that this deletion is clearly different from the Yunnanese type, even though the two have very close 5′ breakpoints.

German $(^A\gamma\delta\beta)^0$ thalassaemia

A three-generation German family with $(^A\gamma\delta\beta)^0$ thalassaemia was described by Anagnou *et al.* (1988). The deletion starts ~2 kb 3′ to the $^G\gamma$ gene and ends ~27 kb 3′ to the β gene, close to the 3′ breakpoints of the HPFH 3 and HPFH 4 deletions and the Belgian $(^A\gamma\delta\beta)^0$-thalassaemia deletion (Kosteas *et al.* 1996). Sequence data demonstrated that the 3′ end of the deletion lies 120 bp downstream of the breakpoint in HPFH 4 (Dr NP Anagnou, personal communication).

Turkish $(^A\gamma\delta\beta)^0$ thalassaemia

A Turkish family with $(^A\gamma\delta\beta)^0$ thalassaemia, including a homozygote, was reported by Reyes *et al.* (1978) and Dinçol *et al.* (1981). Gene mapping demonstrated a large deletion beginning between the $^G\gamma$ and $^A\gamma$ genes (Fritsch *et al.* 1979; Orkin *et al.* 1979a). Sequencing of the breakpoints showed that the 5′ site lay 1 kb 3′ to the $^G\gamma$ gene and extended for 36 kb, terminating 48 bp beyond the L1 repeat 3′ to the β gene (Henthorn *et al.* 1990).

South-east Asian (Malay-1, Thai, Cantonese) $(^A\gamma\delta\beta)^0$ thalassaemia

A deletion with a 5′ breakpoint close to that of the Turkish case was described in a Malaysian family by Trent *et al.* (1984b). Direct comparison of the two samples demonstrated that the deletions were different but the 3′ extent of the deletion was not determined. A second family with the same 5′ restriction map was described by Fucharoen *et al.* (1987).

Another deletion beginning close to the 3′ end of the $^G\gamma$ gene was described in a family from Canton (family C (Zeng *et al.* 1985a)); the extent was not ascertained. There were similarities in several abnormal restriction-fragment sizes between the Cantonese and Malay-1 deletions, with some apparent differences in weaker bands. Sequencing of the

breakpoint junctions will be necessary to confirm the reasonable assumption that the Malay and Cantonese deletions are identical.

Winichagoon *et al.* (1990b) described a Thai family in which there was a large deletion starting close to the 3′ end of the $^G\gamma$ gene, extending for ~100 kb and ending just short of the Chinese $(^A\gamma\delta\beta)^0$-thalassaemia deletion. The abnormal restriction fragments identified with a γ-globin gene probe were similar to those of the Malay-1 deletion. The identity of the Malay and Thai cases was demonstrated by direct comparison with the Malay sample by Fucharoen *et al.* (1987).

Haemoglobin F levels are higher in the Malay, Cantonese and Thai deletion families than in the other forms of $(^A\gamma\delta\beta)^0$ thalassaemia, again consistent with them being identical. There is a pancellular distribution of HbF (Trent *et al.* 1984b; Winichagoon *et al.* 1990b), leading to some descriptions of this condition as HPFH 6 (Kosteas *et al.* 1997). An enhancer-like sequence has been identified in the region between the endpoint of the south-east Asian and Chinese $(^A\gamma\delta\beta)^0$ thalassaemias; the retention of this element could be responsible for the higher HbF levels in the former condition (Dr NP Anagnou, personal communication).

Hereditary persistence of fetal haemoglobin (HPFH)

$(\delta\beta)^0$ HPFH

Early studies using solution hybridization suggested that some forms of African HPFH were due to a deletion of the δ- and β-globin genes (Kan *et al.* 1975d; Ottolenghi *et al.* 1976; Ramirez *et al.* 1976) and this was confirmed when restriction-enzyme mapping was introduced (Fritsch *et al.* 1979; Ottolenghi *et al.* 1979; Bernards & Flavell 1980; Tuan *et al.* 1980). Furthermore, although the cases studied by Fritsch *et al.*, on the one hand, and Tuan *et al.* and Bernards and Flavell, on the other, appeared to be phenotypically identical, there was clearly heterogeneity at the molecular level, with one deletion extending about 5 kb further at the 5′ end than the other. The extent of the deletion at the 3′ end remained unknown at that time. Since then, conditions resembling HPFH have been recognized and analysed in other populations and four additional deletions have been characterized, one from India, two from Italy and one that is found in south-east Asia (Fig. 4.16).

Black HPFH (HPFH 1)

The deletion in this condition begins about 3.75 kb upstream of the δ-globin gene (Fritsch *et al.* 1979; Tuan *et al.* 1979, 1983) in an *Alu* repetitive sequence (Jagadeeswaran *et al.* 1982) and extends for approximately 105 kb (Collins *et al.* 1987). The breakpoint has been cloned and the newly juxtaposed sequence from the 3′ end characterized (Feingold & Forget 1989). There is no sequence homology between the 5′ and 3′ ends; an additional five 'orphan' nucleotides have been inserted at the breakpoints.

The sequence situated 1 kb beyond the 3′ breakpoint contains an erythroid-specific DNase1-hypersensitive site (Elder *et al.* 1990). This region contains a CpG dinucleotide that is specifically hypomethylated in erythroid cells, as well as a number of sequence elements previously described in enhancers, including a 14/18 match to a motif found in the $^A\gamma$ enhancer and 3′ to the chicken β-globin gene. This element functions as an enhancer in transient transfection assays using a γ-promoter-CAT reporter assay (Feingold & Forget 1989) and in transgenic mice in the presence of the β LCR, where it is necessary to produce an HPFH phenotype (Arcasoy *et al.* 1997) (see below).

Ghanaian HPFH (or HPFH 2)

The deletion begins ~5 kb upstream of that which causes HPFH 1 deletion (Bernards & Flavell 1980; Tuan *et al.* 1980). The 3′ end is also shifted ~ 5 kb to the 5′ side of the HPFH 1 3′ breakpoint (Vanin *et al.* 1983) such that the overall size of these deletions is almost the same. From pulsed-field gel electrophoresis, the HPFH 1 and 2 deletions have been estimated to be ~106 and 105 kb, respectively (Collins *et al.* 1987).

The breakpoint of the HPFH 2 deletion has been cloned and sequenced (Mager *et al.* 1985; Henthorn *et al.* 1990). It starts within IVS2 of the ψβ gene and ends in an L1 repeat element, with three homologous base pairs at the junction itself and no orphan nucleotides.

Indian HPFH (or HPFH 3)

Six Indian families with HPFH (Schroeder *et al.* 1973b; Wainscoat *et al.* 1984b) have been studied at the molecular level and shown to have the same deletion (Kutlar *et al.* 1984; Wainscoat *et al.* 1984b). The 5′ end lies just upstream of the ψβ gene in an *Alu* repeat. It extends for 48.5 kb, much shorter than the HPFH 1 and HPFH 2 deletions, and ends within a perfect 160-bp palindrome that lies between an L1 repeat and a set of 41-bp repeats (Henthorn *et al.* 1986).

Italian HPFH (or HPFH 4)

Analysis of three families with HPFH from southern Italy showed that they all had the same deletion that removed the δ and β genes (Saglio *et al.* 1986). The 5′ breakpoint lies between the ψβ and δ genes, close to that of the HPFH 1 deletion. The deletion extends for 40 kb, with the 3′ end lying ~2 kb upstream of the HPFH 3 deletion. Sequence analysis of the breakpoint region has not been reported.

Sicilian HPFH (or HPFH 5)

Two brothers with an HPFH phenotype from a Sicilian family were shown to have a much smaller deletion, only ~13 kb (Camaschella *et al.* 1990c). The 5′ end lies within an *Alu* repeat while the 3′ breakpoint is located 692–695 bp downstream of the β-globin gene poly(A) site. The breakpoints share a 4-bp homology, and there are five 'orphan' nucleotides inserted. The deletion ends within the enhancer 3′ to the β gene, removing one of the four GATA-1 sites (Camaschella *et al.* 1990c). The functional significance of this observation remains unclear.

South-east Asian HPFH

Motum *et al.* (1993a) described two unrelated Vietnamese persons with HPFH in whom there was a 30-kb deletion that differed from any previously described. An apparently identical deletion was subsequently described in families from Vietnam, Cambodia and China (Dimovski *et al.* 1994), suggesting that this condition may occur throughout south-east Asia and may be responsible for cases of HPFH previously reported from this region (Wasi *et al.* 1968b; Winichagoon *et al.* 1994).

This form of HPFH is the only one described in which the δ gene remains intact. The deletion starts 2 kb upstream of the β-globin gene and extends for ~30 kb, with its 3′ terminus within 5 kb of those of the HPFH 3 and 4 deletions.

$(^A\gamma\beta)^+$ HPFH Hb Kenya

Structural analysis of the abnormal β-like chain of Hb Kenya demonstrated that it was a hybrid γβ chain, analogous to the hybrid δβ chain of Hb Lepore (Huisman *et al.* 1972; Kendall *et al.* 1973). The amino acids from position 1 to 80 were those of a γ chain while those from 87 to 145 were β-like in sequence. As the persistent HbF in this condition was virtually all of the $^G\gamma$ type, it was suggested that a non-homologous crossover between the $^A\gamma$ and β genes had given rise to the $^A\gamma\beta$ Kenya chain. This interpretation has been confirmed by analysis of DNA from the propositus in the original report; restriction-enzyme analysis was consistent with a deletion of ~22.5 kb and the loss of sequences stretching from exon 2 of the $^A\gamma$ gene to exon 2 of the β gene (Ojwang *et al.* 1983).

No examples of the hypothetical anti-Kenya (Fig. 4.17) globin gene have yet been described.

$^G\gamma\beta^+$ and $^A\gamma\beta^+$ non-deletional forms of HPFH

Background

When it became possible to analyse the β-globin gene cluster at the molecular level, it soon became clear that not all types of HPFH were due to gene deletions. In 1975, Huisman *et al.* (1975b) and colleagues described a family in which the propositus had a haemoglobin pattern of approximately 50% HbS, 25% HbA and 25% HbF, with a low level of HbA$_2$. The β^S gene was inherited from a parent with normal HbF levels while the other parent had HbA and a high level of HbF. This implies that β^A and γ chains were being produced from the same chromosome. Furthermore, the γ chains were almost entirely $^G\gamma$. The condition was therefore characterized as $^G\gamma\beta^+$ HPFH.

Reports on a number of other forms of HPFH that were not due to gene deletions, and in which the HbF contained only $^G\gamma$ or $^A\gamma$ chains, soon followed. Greek HPFH, first characterized in 1964 (Fessas & Stamatoyannopoulos 1964), was shown to have mostly $^A\gamma$ chains (Clegg *et al.* 1979) and to have an intact β-globin cluster (Bernards & Flavell 1980; Tuan *et al.* 1980; Jones *et al.* 1982). Homozygotes for Greek HPFH, with HbA and 24% HbF, were subsequently discovered (Camaschella *et al.* 1989a). A British family with an $^A\gamma$ form of HPFH included

homozygotes with ~20% HbF, normal levels of HbA$_2$ and the remainder HbA, pointed to there being active γ, δ and β genes on the same chromosome (Weatherall *et al.* 1975). In this case, too, there was no deletion within the β-globin cluster (Jones *et al.* 1982).

Molecular studies

The molecular basis of the first of these conditions was reported by Collins *et al.* (1984), who showed that the $^G\gamma$ gene from a $^G\gamma\beta^+$ HPFH chromosome carried a C→G mutation at position –202 to the $^G\gamma$ gene. At that stage there was no direct evidence that this base substitution was itself responsible for the condition, but similar reports rapidly followed. Giglioni *et al.* (1984) demonstrated a C→T substitution at –196 in the $^A\gamma$ gene of an Italian HPFH patient; Greek HPFH was shown to have a G→A substitution at $^A\gamma$-117 (Collins *et al.* 1985; Gelinas *et al.* 1985); and the British form of HPFH was found to have a T→C substitution at –198 in the $^A\gamma$ gene (Tate *et al.* 1986).

It was soon shown that these changes were not simple polymorphisms but were always associated with high levels of HbF (Waber *et al.* 1986; Metherall *et al.* 1988). Furthermore, the same rare mutation turned up in different population groups in individuals with similar phenotypes, suggesting independent origins (Gelinas *et al.* 1986). Finally, direct evidence that the point substitutions were responsible for persistent γ-gene expression was provided in transgenic mice. Whereas a normal LCR-γβ-gene construct showed suppression of the γ locus in adults, the same construct carrying the $^A\gamma$-117 HPFH mutation showed high levels of γ mRNA in adult life (Berry *et al.* 1992; Ronchi *et al.* 1996).

Heterogeneity

To date, 13 mutations in the promoters of the $^G\gamma$ or $^A\gamma$ genes have been described (Fig. 4.18, Table 4.10). Haemoglobin F levels range from marginal increases (2 to 5%) to values that equal or exceed those found in deletional forms of HPFH. The lesions cluster in three regions. One, around positions –114 to –117, involves the distal CCAAT box, while a second, at –175, may involve an overlapping Oct1/GATA-1 site. A third group, from –195 to –202, does not directly involve a known protein binding site but may disrupt binding to a neighbouring G-rich box.

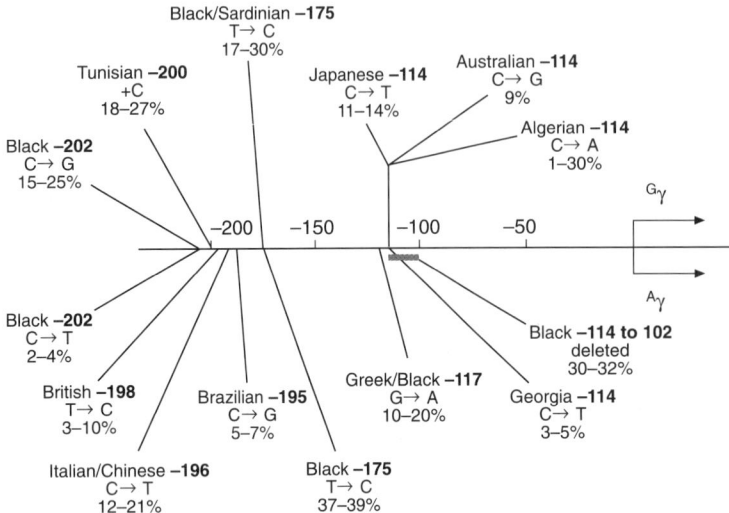

Fig. 4.18 The point mutations in the γ-globin genes that generate non-deletional forms of hereditary persistence of fetal haemoglobin.

Table 4.10 Non-deletional forms of hereditary persistence of fetal haemoglobin.

Type	Position	Substitution	% HbF in heterozygotes	% $^G\gamma$ or $^A\gamma$	*Xmn* I at −158 in *cis*
$^G\gamma$ *mutations*					
Black	−202	C→G	15–25	88–97	−
Tunisian	−200	+C	18–27	100	+
Black/Sardinian	−175	T→C	17–30	90–100	−
Japanese	−114	C→T	11–14	86–92	+
Australian	−114	C→G	8.6	90	−
$^A\gamma$ *mutations*					
Black	−202	C→T	2–4	86–96	−
British	−198	T→C	3–10	90–96	−
Italian/Chinese	−196	C→T	12–21	81–95	−
Brazilian	−195	C→G	5–7	86–91	?
Black	−175	T→C	37–39	62–82	+
Greek/Black	−117	G→A	10–20	85	−
Black	−114 to −102	Deleted	30–32	81–90	−
Georgia	−114	C→T	3–5	87–91	?

Two mutations have been found in both the $^G\gamma$ and $^A\gamma$ genes. A C→T change at −114 produces higher HbF levels when it occurs in the $^G\gamma$ gene than in the $^A\gamma$ gene (and slightly higher levels than a C→G mutation in the same position of the $^G\gamma$ gene). In contrast, a T→C mutation at −175 produces high HbF levels whether the $^G\gamma$ or $^A\gamma$ genes are affected. A 13-bp deletion of −102 to −114 also results in HbF levels of about 30%, while an additional base inserted at position −200 of the $^G\gamma$ gene produces HbF levels of up to 28% in heterozygotes and 48% in homozygotes (Table 4.10).

Phenotype/genotype relationships

Individuals with γ-promoter mutations have balanced globin synthesis and a normal MCH (see Chapter 10). This tells us that the combined output from the genes on the affected chromosome is approximately normal and therefore that the increased γ-chain production is matched by a decrease in β-chain output. This reciprocity only occurs in *cis*; when a non-deletion HPFH gene is inherited together with HbS or HbC on the opposite chromosome, the abnormal haemoglobin comprises about 50% of the total. A *cis*-active reciprocal relationship between one of the γ genes and the β gene could be explained if there were competition between the two genes for access to an element in *cis*, the most likely candidate being the LCR.

Mechanisms of increased haemoglobin F production

It seems probable that the non-deletion HPFH mutations alter the binding of various transcription factors to the γ-gene promoter. For instance, if adult red-cell precursors contain factors which bind to the γ-gene promoter to repress expression, a mutation might decrease the avidity of the factor for its recognition sequence, hence partially relieving the repression. Alternatively, the change may allow the binding of a positively acting factor present in adult red-cell precursors which normally would not be able to bind. Attempts have been made to analyse the proteins that bind to this region and to document the changes that occur with the mutant sequences. They have demonstrated the complexity of the region, in which

binding sites for different proteins frequently overlap (Fig. 4.19).

Altered binding of Sp1 (see Chapter 2) to the G-rich area upstream of the −195 to −202 region has been reported in gel-shift assays comparing normal and mutant oligonucleotides. However, binding increased in the ^{G}γ-202 (G→C) (Sykes & Kaufman 1990) and ^{A}γ-198 mutations (Ronchi *et al.* 1989; Fischer & Nowock 1990; Gumucio *et al.* 1991) but decreased in the ^{A}γ-202 (C→T) (Sykes & Kaufman 1990) and ^{A}γ-196 mutations (Ronchi *et al.* 1989; Gumucio *et al.* 1991). The ^{G}γ-202 (G→C) mutation also creates a new binding site for the stage-selector protein (Jane *et al.* 1993). It has also been suggested that mutations in this region disrupt an intramolecular triplex which may be the binding site for a repressor (Ulrich *et al.* 1992).

The −175 mutation abolishes the binding of the Oct1 protein and alters the binding of GATA-1, which also includes this residue in its binding site. However, different reports suggest that this binding is either slightly increased (Mantovani *et al.* 1988), decreased (Martin *et al.* 1989), or unaffected (Gumucio *et al.* 1988).

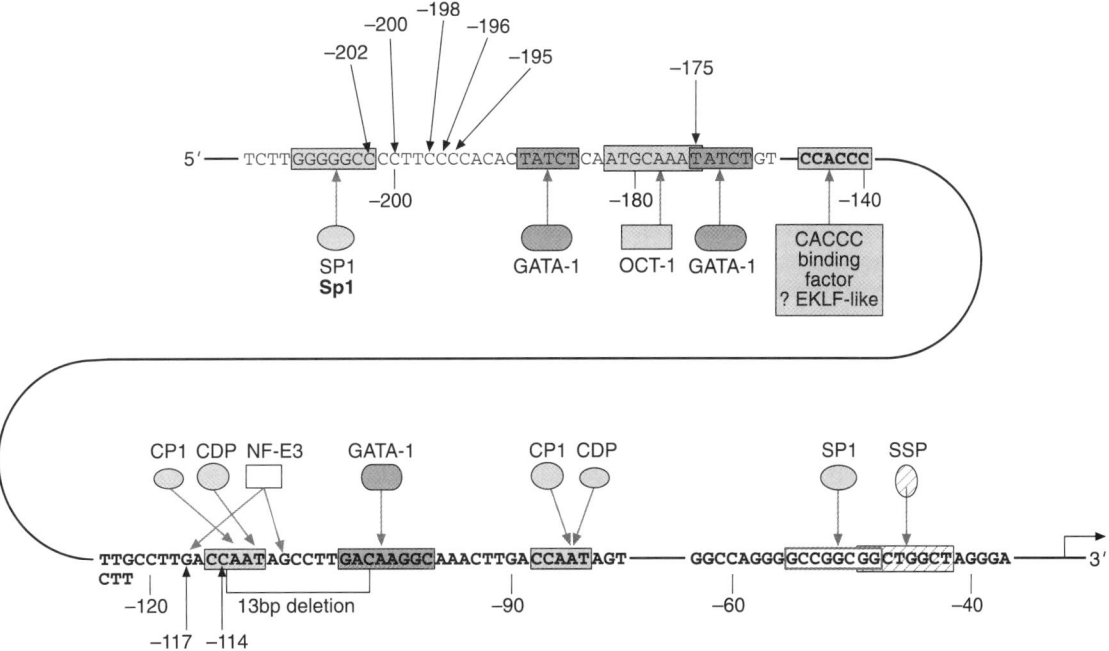

Fig. 4.19 Relationship of some mutations that generate non-deletional forms of hereditary persistence of fetal haemoglobin to γ-gene promoters. The function of the DNA binding regulatory proteins are described in the text.

The distal CCAAT box can bind at least two CCAAT binding proteins, CP1 and CDP; binding of both proteins is increased by the $^A\gamma$-117 mutation (Gumucio *et al.* 1988; Mantovani *et al.* 1988; Superti-Furga *et al.* 1988). This mutation also decreases the binding of GATA-1 to the 3′ side of the CCAAT box as well as the binding of NF-E3, an uncharacterized protein (Mantovani *et al.* 1988; Superti-Furga *et al.* 1988). CP1 binding is abolished in the $^G\gamma$-114 (C→T) mutation (Fucharoen *et al*, 1990f) while CP1, CDP, and NF-E3, but not GATA-1, binding is lost in the 13-bp deletion of this region.

Clearly, no consistent themes run through these binding studies and, as with the deletional forms of HPFH, different mechanisms may operate for each mutation. Furthermore, the results of these *in vitro* studies may not truly reflect the pattern of binding *in vivo*, when the DNA is in chromatin. The results are not always reproducible, reflecting the use of different oligonucleotide probes and differences in nuclear protein extraction procedures.

Several of these mutations have also been studied in transient-transfection assays or *in vitro* transcription assays, usually involving a comparison of the normal and abnormal promoter to drive transcription of a reporter gene such as chloramphenicol acetyl transferase (CAT). The results have been variable, with either little or no difference seen or a three- to eightfold increase in expression (Rixon & Gelinas 1988; Lanclos *et al.* 1989; Nicolis *et al.* 1989; Fischer & Nowock 1990; Gumucio *et al.* 1990; Ulrich & Ley 1990; Lloyd *et al.* 1992). The increased expression of 50–100-fold seen *in vivo* has not been reproduced, again reflecting the inadequacies of these expression systems.

Direct evidence that the base substitution is directly responsible for the HPFH phenotype comes from studies in transgenic mice. High levels of $^A\gamma$-gene expression in adults was seen in mice carrying the $^A\gamma$-117 mutation, either as an LCR-$^A\gamma$-117 construct (Berry *et al.* 1992; Ronchi *et al.* 1996) or as an intact β cluster (Peterson *et al.* 1995). No adult γ expression was observed in the same constructs lacking the HPFH lesion. No adult expression was seen in the absence of any LCR element (Starck *et al.* 1994) and reduced levels were obtained when only HS2 was present (Roberts *et al.* 1997b), suggesting that an intact LCR is necessary to obtain maximum effect.

Other sequence changes in the β-globin-gene cluster affecting haemoglobin F production

Point mutations

Other sequences within the β-globin cluster may affect HbF levels to a minor degree in normal individuals, but have a greater effect in patients with sickle-cell anaemia or β thalassaemia. The best characterized is the C→T change at position −158 in the promoter of the $^G\gamma$ gene, which creates an *Xmn* I cleavage site (Gilman *et al.* 1984; Labie *et al.* 1985a). The most consistent change caused by this substitution in normal persons is a high proportion of $^G\gamma$ chains in the HbF. A similar effect is seen with a G→A substitution at $^G\gamma$ −161 (Gilman *et al.* 1987). The change at $^G\gamma$ −158 does not usually raise the HbF level in otherwise normal individuals. However, using the more sensitive F-cell assay it has been shown that HbF levels are related to the status of the *Xmn*-I site, with *Xmn*-I+/+ individuals having the highest levels (Sampietro *et al.* 1992). Analysis of Yugoslav patients with 'Swiss'-type HPFH, in which slightly raised HbF levels of 1–5% are found, showed seven families in which the increased HbF was associated with *Xmn*-I+/+ or ± genotypes (Efremov *et al.* 1987). However, nearly half of the normal members of this population had these genotypes with no increase in HbF level, suggesting that the presence of this substitution may be necessary but not sufficient to increase the level of HbF.

Rearrangements

A gene conversion which has created a $^G\gamma^G\gamma$ arrangement instead of $^G\gamma^A\gamma$ (Gilman & Huisman 1984) occurs frequently among Afro-Americans (~5%), who have a high proportion of $^G\gamma$ chains but normal levels of HbF (Kutlar *et al.* 1990). Most of these persons are *Xmn*-I negative. However, two families originally described as having the Atlanta type of HPFH (Altay *et al.* 1976–77; Huisman *et al.* 1985) were subsequently shown to have the $^G\gamma^G\gamma$ arrangement on one chromosome in which both $^G\gamma$ genes were *Xmn*-I positive (Efremov *et al.* 1994b). Members of these families have HbF levels of 2–6% as adults, and much higher levels in early childhood.

Restriction-fragment length polymorphisms (RFLPs)

The different RFLP haplotype of the β-gene cluster are described in Chapter 2. Patients with sickle-cell anaemia with haplotypes containing the *Xmn* I site tend, as a group, to have higher HbF levels. In Africa, those with the 'Senegal' haplotype, which contains this site, have ~12% HbF on average, compared with those with the Benin and Bantu (CAR) haplotypes, who have 8–10% HbF. Much higher levels of HbF (20–35%) are found in this disorder in eastern Saudi Arabia and India, where the β^S gene also occurs on a chromosome that *is Xmn* I positive (Kulozik *et al.* 1987a; Miller *et al.* 1987). Thus, while the $^G\gamma$-158 site may contribute towards increasing HbF levels, other factors must be acting in the Arabian and Indian populations.

Among β-thalassaemics, those with the same 5′ haplotype as the Senegal and Arab–Indian sicklers, which are *Xmn* I positive, have a high proportion of $^G\gamma$ chains (Labie *et al.* 1985b). Homozygotes for haplotype IX (++−+++ ++), where the bold + is the $^G\gamma$ *Xmn* I site, have very high levels of HbF and tend to have a milder disease (Labie *et al.* 1985b; Thein *et al.* 1987b). Again, the $^G\gamma$-158 site cannot be the only determinant; haplotype III (++−+++ +−) is also positive for this site and has a high proportion of $^G\gamma$ chains but is not associated with high levels of HbF (Labie *et al.* 1985b).

Given the proximity of the $^G\gamma$-158 site to other substitutions within the γ-gene promoters that cause an HPFH phenotype, the C→T substitution may be directly responsible for the minor increases in HbF in normal individuals and the more marked effects in those with sickle-cell anaemia and β thalassaemia. However, this has not been verified experimentally. A small increase in promoter activity was observed with −158T in a transient assay in one study (Lanclos *et al.* 1989) but not in another (Motum *et al.* 1993c). It is also possible that the −158T residue is in linkage disequilibrium with other, so far unidentified, sequence changes within the β-globin gene cluster.

Other structural changes

The problem of linkage disequilibrium also applies to other sequence polymorphisms that tend to associate with increased HbF levels. Sequence variations are common throughout the β-globin gene cluster, many of which reach polymorphic frequencies. As discussed earlier in this chapter, the region 520–540 bp upstream of the β-globin gene has a variable sequence that can be written as $(AT)_x(T)_y$, where $x=7$ to 9 and $y=4$ to 9 (Elion *et al.* 1992). It has been proposed that this region binds a putative repressor protein, BP1 (Berg *et al.* 1989), and that binding is increased in the $(AT)_9(T)_5$ variant characteristic of the Indian β^S chromosome. It has therefore been suggested that decreased β^S output may predispose to increased γ-chain output from these chromosomes (Elion *et al.* 1992). However, as noted earlier, there is no consistent correlation between sequence variation at this ATA motif and a β-thalassaemia phenotype, and evidence that this is any more than a neutral polymorphism is unconvincing.

Numerous single base substitutions have been described upstream of the $^G\gamma$ gene and in γ IVS2. Different combinations are found among the various β^S haplotypes found in sickle-cell anaemia. Chromosomes associated with increased HbF have similar combinations that differ from those found on those associated with low HbF (Lanclos *et al.* 1991). Polymorphisms also occur in the region between 1.15 and 1.65 kb upstream of the Gγ gene, which contains binding sites for GATA-1, Sp1 and a cyclic AMP response element (CRE). They are closely linked to four different β^S haplotypes and also show altered affinities in factor-binding assays and different activities in an enhancer-dependent reporter-gene assay (Pissard & Beuzard 1994). This suggests that they may be of functional significance and hence could affect HbF levels in patients with sickle-cell anaemia.

Polymorphic sequence changes have also been observed within the HS2 element of the β-globin LCR (see Chapter 2), including an $(AT)_xN_{12}(AT)_y$ motif, where $x=8$ to 10 and $y=10$ to 12 (Beris *et al.* 1992; Öner *et al.* 1992; Merghoub *et al.* 1996). One pattern has been associated with higher levels of HbF in sickle-cell anaemia and β thalassaemia (Öner *et al.* 1992) as well as with increased HbF and F-cell levels in those with the sickle-cell trait who share the same β^S haplotype (Merghoub *et al.* 1996). There are no functional data to suggest that this is a direct effect rather than a reflection of linkage disequilibrium.

HPFH due to determinants which are not linked to the β-globin gene cluster

Several families have been reported in which increased levels of HbF, usually demonstrated in an interaction with β thalassaemia or sickle-cell disease, apparently segregate independently of the β-globin gene cluster (Gianni *et al.* 1983; Giampaolo *et al.* 1984b; Martinez *et al.* 1989; Thein & Weatherall 1989; Oppenheim *et al.* 1990; Seltzer *et al.* 1992). Analysis of these families is difficult because of the potential genetic heterogeneity and incomplete penetrance. Furthermore, the distribution of HbF levels in these families may be continuous, rendering phenotypic identification of normal and affected individuals extremely difficult. Thus the pattern of inheritance is rarely clear; examples of autosomal or sex-linked, dominant, or co-dominant, and recessive varieties have all been reported.

Analysis of HbF levels in healthy Japanese adults led Miyoshi *et al.* (1988) to suggest that an X-linked gene was involved in increasing HbF levels, with a frequency of 11% affected males and 21% of female carriers. Support for this notion came from analyses of the levels of reticulocytes in which HbF can be demonstrated, called F reticulocytes, in males and females with the sickle-cell trait, and from sib-pair studies in the same population. Dover *et al.* (1992) suggested that a co-dominant, bi-allelic F-cell production locus with high and low alleles resides on the X chromosome and is linked to markers at Xp22.2–22.3. Furthermore, it was proposed that this locus accounts for 40% of the variability in HbF levels in those with the β^S gene, an effect of much greater magnitude than β-globin haplotype, age, sex or α-gene status, which, together, could only account for ~10% of the variability (Chang *et al.* 1995b).

The value of a single large family in the study of unlinked HPFH was underlined by Thein and Weatherall (1989). Starting from a patient homozygous for β^0 thalassaemia who had an extremely mild course, with 10–12 g/dl HbF, a family study was carried out that showed clear-cut evidence for an HPFH-like gene unlinked to the globin cluster. The family study was extended (across four continents!) until nearly 200 members were accumulated. Initially, the pattern of inheritance was unclear and assignments of phenotypes were difficult, not only reflecting the large number of β-thalassaemia carriers but also because α thalassaemia was found in the family.

Nevertheless, by using statistical analysis to take account of the influence of α and β thalassaemia, $^G\gamma$ −158 status, age and sex, it was possible, by multiple regression analysis, to demonstrate a major gene affecting F-cell levels (Thein *et al.* 1994). By using polymorphic markers covering the whole genome it proved possible to localize this gene to a small area of chromosome 6, 6q22.3–q24 (Craig *et al.* 1996; Garner *et al.* 1998).

Other families with a form of HPFH unlinked to the β-globin cluster do not show linkage to chromosome 6 or the X chromosome, suggesting that other autosomal loci exist (Craig *et al.* 1997).

The mechanism by which either the chromosome 6 or X-chromosome-linked genes affect HbF and F-cell levels remains unknown. It is possible that these loci code for *trans*-acting factors that bind within the β-globin gene cluster and directly affect γ-gene transcription. It is equally plausible that there are genes that act much more indirectly, perhaps by altering the kinetics of erythropoiesis and mimicking the increased HbF seen in stress erythropoiesis.

Lessons from the molecular pathology of hereditary persistence of fetal haemoglobin and δβ thalassaemia

Mechanisms producing gene deletions in the β-globin cluster

The nature of the breakpoints

The deletions responsible for Hbs Lepore and Kenya are believed to arise by crossing over between misaligned, partially homologous genes (Fig. 4.17). The same process produces the anti-Lepore haemoglobins, Hbs Miyada and P Nilotic and, potentially, anti-Kenya haemoglobins, although the latter have not been described. This mechanism is similar to that responsible for generating −α and ααα and −γ and γγγ gene arrangements. As there is less homology between γ and β and δ and β genes, these events are likely to be less common than rearrangements among the nearly identical, duplicated α and γ genes.

The deletions responsible for $(\delta\beta)^0$ thalassaemia $(^A\gamma\delta\beta)^0$ thalassaemia and HPFH (as well as those for β and δ thalassaemias) do not involve homologous regions at their 5′ and 3′ breakpoints, and result from illegitimate recombinations. It is not clear whether the latter simply reflect chance breakage and rejoining or whether there may be a common underlying mechanism. Small regions of homology consisting of only a few nucleotides are common at the breakpoints, while in many cases the two sequences are joined directly. In others, however, there are several 'orphan' nucleotides inserted that are usually of unknown origin, although in one case they appear to have originated from an L1 repeat sequence.

Several of the deletions involve repetitive sequence elements, such as the inverted *Alu* repeats between ψβ and δ, and the L1 and truncated L1 repeats that lie downstream of the β-globin gene. However, their involvement does not appear to occur more frequently than would be expected by chance for sequences occupying ~20% of the region (Henthorn *et al.* 1990). Furthermore, although breakpoints within the genes occur more frequently than expected, in this case there is potential for ascertainment bias.

Length of the deletions

The staggered ends of the breakpoints of HPFH 1 and HPFH 2, as well as those of $\varepsilon^G\gamma^A\gamma\delta\beta$ thalassaemias 1 and 2 (see later section), suggested to Vanin *et al.* (1983) that these deletions may have resulted from the loss of a complete chromosomal loop. The variation in the positions of the deletions indicates either that the anchorage points of the loops are not fixed or that DNA is moved through them, perhaps during replication. Breakage and rejoining at the base of the loops would then generate deletions of similar overall lengths, but with different and staggered breakpoints at their 5 and 3′ ends. This idea was further supported when the sizes of the $\varepsilon^A\gamma^G\gamma\delta\beta$ thalassaemia (Taramelli *et al.* 1986), HPFH (Collins *et al.* 1987) and Chinese $(\delta\beta)^0$ thalassaemia (Mager *et al.* 1985) deletions were determined and shown to range from 95 to 105 kb. Three other deletions, Filipino β thalassaemia, Spanish $(\delta\beta)^0$ thalassaemia and Thai $(^A\gamma\delta\beta)^0$ thalassaemia, are also of a similar overall size.

However, when further deletions were characterized, it became less clear that there are discrete size classes (Fig. 4.16). There are four deletions of ~50 kb, six are evenly spread between 20 and 40 kb, a cluster of seven between 11.5 and 13.5 kb, and seven between 7 and 10 kb. There is no obvious correlation between their size and the resulting phenotype.

The mechanisms for increased haemoglobin F production

It was always hoped that the characterization of the deletions in the various disorders with increased HbF production in adult life would provide insights into the mechanisms underlying the increase and, at the same time, provide insights into how haemoglobin switching is regulated. However, an appraisal of Fig. 4.16 quickly demonstrates that there is unlikely to be a simple explanation for how the loss of different downstream sequences results in the continued activation of the γ genes. Several hypotheses have been proposed, including loss of specific regulatory regions, movement of enhancer sequences into the proximity of the γ genes, and removal of competition from the δ- and β-gene promoters.

Loss of regulatory regions

Huisman *et al.* (1974) first proposed that a regulatory region responsible for the repression of the γ genes in adult life might lie between the $^A\gamma$ and δ genes. This was based on the assumption, subsequently shown to be correct, that the δβ and γ fusion proteins of Hbs Lepore and Kenya reflected a gene order $^G\gamma^A\gamma\delta\beta$, and that the fusion proteins result from deletions of the missing sequences. Thus, since Hb Kenya has an HPFH phenotype but Hb Lepore is a form of β thalassaemia, the negative regulator of γ-gene expression would lie in the $^A\gamma$-δ region. As more deletions were characterized, this idea became less tenable. Bernards and Flavell (1980) modified it to suggest that there are two mutually exclusive domains within the cluster, one fetal and one adult, marked by 'domain' boundaries; loss of parts of the adult domain would make it defective and shift the equilibrium toward γ-gene expression.

Even with the large number of deletions now characterized, it is still not possible to delineate any single area which, when deleted, results in β thalassaemia, δβ thalassaemia or HPFH phenotypes. Overlapping deletions in Turkish deletion β thalassaemia, Corfu δ thalassaemia, Hb Lepore and Indian β^0 thalassaemia, all of which show only minimal increases in HbF in adults, demonstrate that the loss of no single element within the region from 2 kb downstream of the $^A\gamma$ gene to 5 kb downstream of the β gene can result in persistent HbF production. The Australian and Dutch β-thalassaemia deletions extend further in the

3′ direction; some (but not all) of these cases have slightly higher levels of HbF. Furthermore, these conditions have only been described in single families and the influence of other factors such as the sequence at $^G\gamma$ −158 (see below) or unlinked genes modifying the HbF response, has not been excluded.

Other comparisons of deletions with the level of HbF in heterozygotes are equally uninformative. The east European $(\delta\beta)^0$-thalassaemia deletion (~18% HbF) differs from Hb Lepore (~3% HbF) only by the removal of 1.5 kb immediately upstream of the δ gene, including its promoter. In contrast, the Mediterranean (~10% HbF) and south-east Asian (~10% HbF) $(\delta\beta)^0$-thalassaemia deletions differ from Hb Lepore only by the deletion of sequences 3′ to the β gene. When sequences both 5′ to δ and 3′ to β are deleted, much higher levels of HbF are found in adults (Italian 2 HPFH with ~20% HbF and black $(\delta\beta)^0$ thalassaemia with 22% HbF). It is possible therefore that there are two or more regions around the δ- and β-globin genes that act in combination and are involved in keeping the γ genes switched off in adult life.

Effect of enhancer sequences

An alternative explanation for increased HbF production associated with some of these deletions is that newly opposed sequences at the 3′ end contain enhancer-type elements that are brought close to the γ genes and influence their expression (Tuan *et al.* 1983; Feingold & Forget 1989). In the Hb Kenya deletion, for example, fusion of the $^A\gamma$ and β genes might allow the β IVS2 and 3′ enhancers to activate the promoter of the $^A\gamma\beta$ gene and the $^G\gamma$ gene. Support for this suggestion came from analysis of the sequences immediately 3′ to the large HPFH 1 deletion. This region is marked by an erythroid-specific DNase1-hypersensitive site extending from 1.1 to 1.4 kb 3′ to the HPFH 1 breakpoint (Elder *et al.* 1990); this sequence has enhancer activity in a classical transient-transcription assay (Feingold & Forget 1989). Furthermore, this site is no longer hypersensitive on a chromosome from which the LCR has been deleted, suggesting that it is influenced by this regulatory element even though it lies > 150 kb away (Forrester *et al.* 1990). As a result of the HPFH 1 and 2 deletions, this sequence is brought to within 10–15 kb of the γ genes.

A 0.7-kb region with similar enhancer activity in transiently transfected erythroid cells has been identified immediately 3′ to the HPFH 3 3′ breakpoint (Kosteas *et al.* 1996). This element has sequences homologous to the simian virus 40 enhancer as well as to the human $^A\gamma$ and chick β enhancers. Its activity was restricted to the γ and ε promoters, having no effect on the δ- or β-gene enhancers. The HPFH 3 deletion moves this sequence to within ~5 kb of the $^A\gamma$ gene; a similar degree of proximity occurs in the Italian 2 and SEA HPFHs as well as the Belgian and Turkish, and Italian $(^A\gamma\delta\beta)^0$-thalassaemia deletions.

A third region with enhancer activity in transient-expression systems lies between the breakpoints of the Thai and Chinese $(^A\gamma\delta\beta)^0$-thalassaemia deletions, and is deleted in the latter (Kosteas *et al.* 1997). In 10 Chinese $(^A\gamma\delta\beta)^0$-thalassaemia cases from five families, HbF ranged from 9% to 23% (mean 13% HbF). HbF levels in the three members of the Thai family ranged from 17% to 23% (mean 20%) and this condition has also been referred to as HPFH 6 (see earlier section). While the difference in HbF levels between the two conditions is consistent with a positive effect of this enhancer element, additional families with the Thai defect are needed to confirm that high HbF levels are always associated with this deletion. An open reading frame in the enhancer sequence shares 36% homology with the open reading frame in the HPFH 1 enhancer, and both appear to be related to an olfactory receptor gene. Furthermore, this element appears to enhance only γ genes and not ε or β genes in these transient-transfection assays.

Indirect evidence that sequences within the human β-cluster region are necessary to produce the HPFH phenotype was produced in transgenic mice. Rearrangements of a YAC containing the whole of the β-globin cluster on insertion into transgenic mice have mimicked the deletional forms of HPFH. The LCR, $^G\gamma$ and $^A\gamma$ sequences remain intact, but the truncated inserts lack any of the human 3′ sequences that would normally be opposed by the deletion. Instead, at the 3′ end of the transgene there are mouse sequences from the random site of integration. These transgenes are expressed in embryonic and fetal life but are switched off in adult life: that is, they do not contain any of the putative 3′ enhancers and do not show an HPFH phenotype (Peterson *et al.* 1995).

As enhancers detected in transient-transfection assays do not always show the same activity when they are incorporated into a chromosome, particularly if they come under the influence of strong regulatory elements such as the LCR (Ryan *et al.* 1989; Collis *et al.* 1990; Roberts *et al.* 1997b), it was important to test this element *in vivo*. Arcasoy *et al.* (1997) produced transgenic mice involving various constructs containing the β LCR core elements, the two γ genes and the enhancer from 3′ to the HPFH 1 and 2 deletions (Fig. 4.16). Only mice containing the construct with all three elements produced significant amounts of γ-gene expression in adult life. This demonstrates unequivocally that this enhancer element is essential for activating the γ genes in this experimental model and provides strong evidence that it is likely to function in the same way in individuals with HPFH. Similar experiments with the other two enhancer elements are required to confirm their functional importance.

If these enhancers are active *in vivo* and increase γ-gene expression when they are close to the genes, could similar elements be responsible for the increased HbF in all the other deletion conditions? Figure 4.20 shows the 3′ extent of the deletions, with the three enhancer-like sequences marked with arrows. It is not possible to estimate how many such sequences would be necessary to cover all the deletions because the distance over which an enhancer is effective is unknown. However, a number of deletions that result in a β-thalassaemia phenotype without raised levels of HbF terminate in the region between 50 and 75 kb in this diagram, as well as several δβ-thalassaemia deletions. So, if there were further active enhancer-like elements in this area, additional factors must be responsible for their differential phenotypic effects.

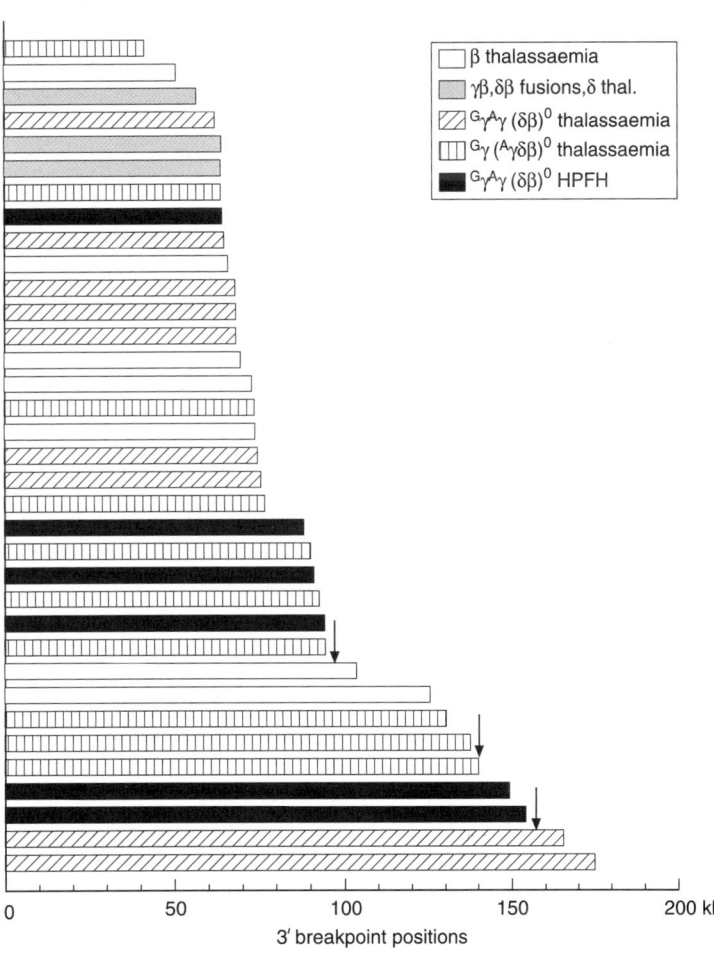

Fig. 4.20 3′ breakpoints of some deletions of the β-globin gene cluster. Positions of downstream enhancers are marked with arrows.

Competition between promoters

It has been suggested that, since globin-gene expression appears to involve interaction of the LCR with gene promoters, the γ genes may be in competition with the δ and β genes during adult life. In normal circumstances, this competition would favour the δ and β genes as a result of chromatin conformation or the action of *trans*-acting factors, or both. However, when both the δ- and β-gene promoters are deleted, the γ promoters may be free to interact with the LCR, albeit at submaximal levels, resulting in persistent HbF production (Wood 1989; Townes & Behringer 1990). This suggestion is supported by analyses of non-deletion HPFH in which there seems to be clear evidence for competition between the β and γ genes. As there are several β-thalassaemia mutations in which the β-globin promoter is deleted and which do not have HbF levels as high as those seen in δβ thalassaemia and HPFH, but which do have very high levels of HbA$_2$, it is necessary to postulate that both δ and β promoters would have to be deleted for such an effect to be seen. For most of the HPFH and δβ-thalassaemia deletions this is the case. The southeast Asian form of HPFH is a clear exception, however; the δ gene is intact and yet HbF levels of > 20% are found in heterozygotes. Furthermore, in three of the (δβ)^0 thalassaemias (Mediterranean, south-east Asian, Macedonian/Turkish), the 5′ end of the deletion lies within the body of the δ gene, leaving the promoter intact.

Competition between β- and γ-gene production could not, on its own, explain the phenotypic differences between (δβ)^0 thalassaemia and HPFH. Neither is it compatible with the data from transgenic mice that show autonomous regulation and switching off of γ-gene expression during development in constructs that lack the β-globin gene (Dillon & Grosveld 1991; Peterson *et al.* 1995). However, in that the mouse does not have a fetal haemoglobin and the human γ gene is expressed largely in embryos in mice, it is not clear whether this model system faithfully reflects all aspects of human globin gene regulation.

Conclusions

It is clear therefore that there is no simple explanation for persistent γ-gene expression in the deletional forms of HPFH and δβ thalassaemia. While there may be a unifying mechanism linking them all which has so

far escaped us, it is equally possible that all of them play a role, the relative importance of each varying from deletion to deletion. Given the large number of elements within the β-globin cluster that affect the regulation of its genes, both positively and negatively, it is not surprising that other elements capable of these functions lie in the region downstream of the genes. The precise balance between regulatory sequences which tend to increase the interaction of the LCR with the γ-gene promoters compared with those that might disrupt this function may ultimately determine the amount of HbF in red cells and hence the degree of compensation for the lack of β-globin production. If these interactions are probabilistic, they may also explain the heterocellular distribution of HbF in the δβ thalassaemias. The lower probability of LCR and γ-gene interaction in this condition may result in some cells not producing any HbF while others contain relatively large amounts. If the probability is higher, then most if not all cells will produce HbF, resulting in higher HbF levels and the pancellular (but still heterogeneous) distribution in HPFH.

(ε^{G}γ^{A}γδβ)^0 Thalassaemia

Several deletions have been described which appear to remove either the whole of the β-globin cluster or large parts of it, and inactivate any remaining genes (Fig. 4.16). Total deletions have been found in those of Mexican (Fearon *et al.* 1983), Canadian and Yugoslavian (Diaz-Chico *et al.* 1988a) and Scottish–Irish (Pirastu *et al.* 1983b) ancestry, clearly explaining the lack of globin production. Similarly, no globins were produced in an Anglo-Saxon patient in whom a large deletion terminated within the β-globin gene itself (Orkin *et al.* 1981b).

An English patient was reported to have a deletion of the 5′ end of the complex, terminating in the ^{G}γ gene, also with an inactive β gene (Curtin *et al.* 1985). In a Dutch patient with (ε^{G}γ^{A}γδβ)^0 thalassaemia there was an extensive deletion which spared the β-globin gene, but nevertheless led to its inactivation (Taramelli *et al.* 1986). It was later work on this deletion that led to the identification of the β-globin LCR (see Chapter 2). The critical importance of this region *in vivo* was confirmed by the discovery of the Hispanic forms of (ε^{G}γ^{A}γδβ)^0 thalassaemia, in which the deletion removed HS2, HS3 and HS4 of the β LCR, sparing all of the globin genes, but inactivating them (Driscoll *et al.* 1989).

It is presumed that the homozygous inheritance of these long deletions would be lethal. In the heterozygous state they produce the clinical phenotype of β-thalassaemia trait with a normal HbA$_2$ level. We shall consider their pathophysiology and clinical features in Chapter 8.

When we wrote the last edition of this book we could not have anticipated the extraordinary numbers and diversity of the mutations that would be found to underlie the thalassaemias. In the chapters which follow we shall summarize how the conse-quences of these mutations are manifested at the level of cells and organs, and their frequency and distribution among different populations. The remainder of the book will describe how they interact to produce the diverse phenotypes that make up the thalassaemia syndromes. The remarkable heterogeneity of mutations at the different globin loci that we have described in this chapter, and the fact that many patients will have inherited more than one of them, should be ample warning to readers that relating phenotype to genotype in these diseases will not be easy.

Chapter 5
The pathophysiology of the thalassaemias

Introduction

The New Shorter Oxford English Dictionary defines the rather clumsy word 'pathophysiology' as 'the branch of medicine that deals with the disordered physiological processes associated with disease or injury'. Its increasing usage reflects the importance ascribed to trying to understand disease in terms of the breakdown of normal homeostatic function. In the thalassaemia field this entails an explanation of how the many different mutations of the α- and β-globin genes, described in the previous chapter, give rise to an extraordinarily diverse family of clinical phenotypes. And, as is the case for any monogenic disease, it must ultimately take us one step further, and try to account for the wide diversity of clinical manifestations that can arise from the *same* mutations.

It follows, therefore, that the exploration of the pathophysiology of a single-gene disorder has to evolve through several stages. First, the consequences of abnormal gene action at the affected locus have to be understood, and other genes, which may modify the action of the primary genetic defect, must be identified. Next, the functional consequences of damage acquired by cells, tissues and organs as the result of the primary genetic lesions have to be characterized. Finally, the effects of the environment on the disease must be considered. This not only involves an understanding of how their habitats and social backgrounds can alter patients' responses to their illness but, in the case of diseases like thalassaemia which have come under strong selection, also includes an appreciation of their evolutionary history and of how the genotypes of affected ethnic groups may differ one from another as a consequence of selective pressures, and how this too may modify patients' responses to the disease and its complications. The main factors to be considered in the pathophysiology of thalassaemia are summarized in Table 5.1.

In this chapter we shall describe and contrast the pathophysiology of the two main classes of thalassaemia and outline their interactions one with another. We hope this will help the reader to appreciate the complex interplay between genotypes and phenotypes that underlies the conditions that are described in later chapters, where particular aspects of their pathophysiology are discussed in more detail. Although there are differences in detail, the principles described in this chapter apply to every form of thalassaemia.

The β thalassaemias

The pathophysiology of β thalassaemia is reasonably well understood, at least in outline (Fig. 5.1). The basic defect, as described in the previous chapter, is a reduction in the output of β chains. This leads to imbalanced globin synthesis and to the production of an excess of α chains. Although HbF synthesis persists after birth to a varying degree in all the severe forms of β thalassaemia, its overall output is insufficient to compensate for the deficiency of HbA. In other words the output of β and γ chains is never sufficient to match that of α chains; unbalanced globin production and an excess of α chains is therefore the hallmark of β thalassaemia. Unbound α chains precipitate in the red-cell precursors in the marrow and in their progeny in the peripheral blood, leading to defective erythroid precursor maturation and ineffective erythropoiesis, and a shortened red-cell survival. The resulting anaemia causes an intense proliferative drive in the ineffective bone marrow, which leads to its expansion. This results in skeletal deformities and a variety of growth and metabolic abnormalities. The anaemia may be further exacerbated by haemodilution caused by shunting of blood through the vastly expanded marrow, and also by splenomegaly due to entrapment of abnormal red cells in the spleen. The hyperplasia of the bone marrow leads to increased iron absorption and iron loading, often exacerbated by the need for regular blood transfusion. This leads to progressive iron deposition in the tissues, organ failure and, if the iron is not removed, death.

In the sections which follow we shall examine each

Table 5.1 Pathophysiology of thalassaemia.

Effect of primary mutation on globin output
  Imbalanced globin synthesis
Consequences of excess globin on red-cell metabolism and
    survival
  Anaemia
Consequences of abnormal red cells on organ function
  Anaemia, splenomegaly, hepatomegaly, hypercoagulable
    state
Consequences of profound anaemia
  Erythropoietin production and marrow expansion
  Skeletal deformity. Metabolic abnormalities
  Adaptivity changes in cardiovascular function
Consequences of abnormal iron metabolism
  Iron loading. Damage to liver, endocrine organs and
    myocardium
  Susceptibility to specific infections
Effects of cell selection
  Raised levels of HbF. Heterogeneity of red-cell
    populations
Effects of secondary genetic modifiers
  Variation in phenotype, particularly through HbF
    response
  Variations in bilirubin, iron and bone metabolism
Effects of therapy
  Iron overload, bone disease, blood-borne infection, drug
    toxicity
Effects of evolutionary history
  Variation in genetic background, response to infection
Ecological and ethnological factors

of these mechanisms in more detail and try to relate them to the overall clinical picture and heterogeneity of the β thalassaemias.

Imbalanced globin synthesis

Although early studies of the thalassaemias that analysed their interactions with the structural haemoglobin variants suggested that they might be the result of defective α- or β-globin synthesis, it was not until methods for the quantitative measurement of α- and β-chain production became available that it was possible to put these ideas on to a solid experimental footing. The methods for *in vitro* radioactive labelling and separation of the α and β chains of human haemoglobin that were devised in the mid-1960s (Clegg *et al.* 1965; Weatherall *et al.* 1965; Clegg *et al.* 1966) have been used widely to study haemoglobin synthesis in reticulocytes and their precursors in patients with different forms of β thalassaemia major (Weatherall *et*

al. 1965; Bank & Marks 1966; Bargellesi *et al.* 1967; Modell *et al.* 1969; Weatherall *et al.* 1969b) and minor (Vigi *et al.* 1969; Schwartz 1970; Clegg & Weatherall 1972; Kan *et al.* 1972c; Shchory & Ramot 1972; Knox-Macaulay *et al.* 1973; Chalevelakis *et al.* 1975, 1976).

How is globin synthesis assessed?

Before we outline what was learnt from these studies it is important that readers coming to this field for the first time appreciate the principles (and pitfalls) of analysing haemoglobin synthesis in the test-tube. After newly made globins have been labelled by incubating bone marrow or peripheral blood with radiotagged amino acids, and separating them chromatographically, two types of measurement can be made. First, the *total amount of radioactivity* that cochromatographs with each globin can be determined. This gives an approximate assessment of the amount of each type of globin synthesized during the period of the incubation. However, if any of the globins are degraded during this period, it may give a false impression of the overall rates of globin production. It is also possible to determine the *specific activity* of each type of globin, that is, the counts incorporated/mg protein/min. Since, during a short period of *in vitro* incubation, relatively few newly synthesized, and hence labelled, globin molecules are added to a large pre-existing pool, this measurement tells us something about the stability and rate of turnover of globin chains. If, for example, two different types of globin are synthesized at the same rate, neither of which is being destroyed and turning over more rapidly than its partner, they will have the *same* specific activity; if, on the other hand, a particular globin type is preferentially destroyed it will have a *higher* specific activity than its partner. In the former case the newly labelled globin is added to a large pool of previously synthesized and unlabelled globin molecules that reflects their overall rate of production; in the latter, the more rapidly turning over labelled molecules are added to a smaller pool of unlabelled globin, reflecting their instability, and hence they will have relatively higher counts/mg protein.

We can take these analyses one step further. Instead of studying globin synthesis at a single time-point we can plot the rate of incorporation of radioactivity into different globins over a period of time. If

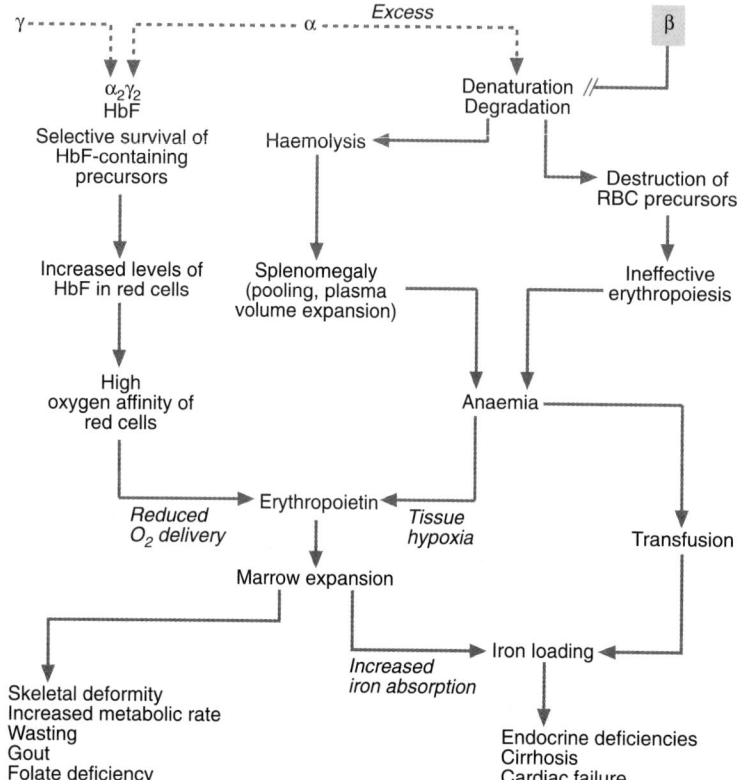

Fig. 5.1 An outline summary of the pathophysiology of β thalassaemia.

they are stable there will be a linear pattern of synthesis, whereas if they are turning over rapidly their incorporation curves will tend to reach a plateau at the point at which their rate of synthesis is balanced by their rate of destruction. When assessing the literature on globin synthesis in thalassaemia, all these points must be taken into consideration.

Globin synthesis in β thalassaemia

In normal red-cell precursors and reticulocytes, α- and β-globin synthesis is almost synchronous; there is a very small pool of free α chains, indicating a slight excess of α-chain production (Weatherall *et al.* 1965) (Fig. 5.2). In red-cell precursors from patients with different forms of β thalassaemia major there is always more radioactivity incorporated into the α chains than into the combined β- and γ-chain fractions (Fig. 5.3); the ratio of α/β + γ radioactivity varies considerably, with a published range of 1.5–30; in β⁰ thalassaemia no β chains are synthesized. Furthermore,

the specific activities of the α chains are greater than those of the β chains, indicating that there must be a relatively faster turnover and destruction of α chains during the period of the experiment.

The finding of excess α-chain synthesis implies that there should be a substantial amount of free α chains in the red cells, a prediction that was confirmed by both gel filtration (Modell *et al.* 1969) and DEAE-cellulose chromatography (Weatherall *et al.* 1969b) (Fig. 5.4). It appears from the gel-filtration studies that soluble α chains exist as both monomers and dimers. Furthermore, α chains from this pool can combine with β and γ chains to produce HbA and HbF (Modell *et al.* 1969). The free α chains are also unstable and become associated with the red-cell membrane, even after short periods of red-cell incubation (Bargellesi *et al.* 1968; Weatherall *et al.* 1969b). It is not certain how much of this denatured material is removed by proteolysis during the red cell's lifespan; degradation of free α chains occurs *in vitro* in thalassaemic reticulocytes, but whether this reflects the *in vivo* rate of

Fig. 5.2 Globin synthesis in non-thalassaemic reticulocytes. The reticulocytes were incubated with radioactive leucine for 1 h, after which the globins were separated by CM-cellulose chromatography. The amount of radioactivity incorporated into the α and β chains is approximately equal, indicating that during the period of the experiment almost equal numbers of α and β chains were synthesized.

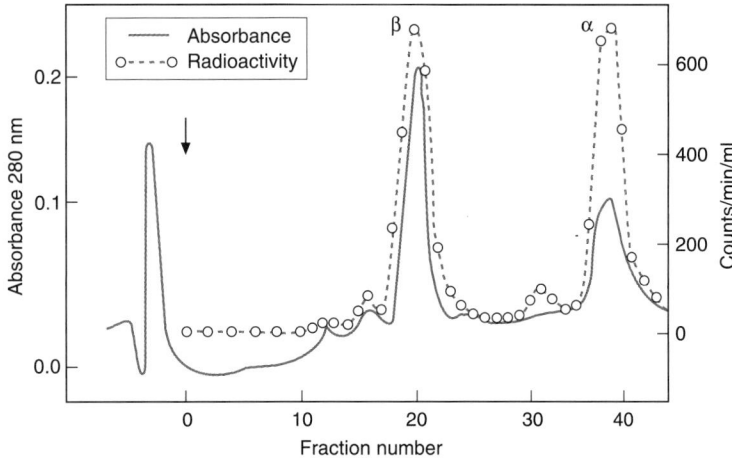

Fig. 5.3 Haemoglobin synthesis in homozygous β thalassaemia. An identical experiment to that shown in Fig. 5.2 was carried out using reticulocytes of a patient homozygous for β thalassaemia. Clearly there is marked imbalance of globin synthesis with an excess of α chains over non-α chains produced during the 1-h incubation period.

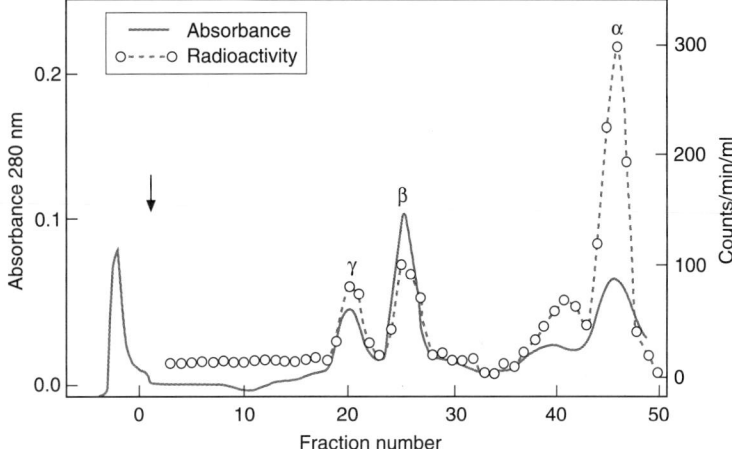

chain removal is uncertain (Bank & O'Donnell 1969; Weatherall & Clegg 1972).

Early studies of globin synthesis in β thalassaemia described apparent discrepancies between the relative rates of production of globins in the peripheral blood and bone marrow. In some reports they were similar (Bargellesi *et al.* 1967; Shchory & Ramot 1972; Nienhuis *et al.* 1973), in others α/β+γ synthesis ratios were higher in the blood than in the marrow, while in β⁰ thalassaemia α/γ ratios were higher in the marrow (Braverman & Bank 1969; Friedman *et al.* 1972). On the other hand, Nathan and Benz (1976) found less imbalance in the blood than in the marrow; in β⁰ thalassaemia α/γ ratios were very much higher in the

blood than in the marrow. Similar findings were reported by Weatherall *et al.* (1974a), who also observed that the α/β+γ, β/γ and α/γ ratios changed quite markedly depending on the period of incubation. These discrepancies between the apparent rates of globin synthesis between the marrow and blood appeared at first to be even more marked in heterozygous β thalassaemia. Schwartz (1970) reported that there was balanced globin synthesis in heterozygous β-thalassaemic marrow, while in the peripheral blood synthesis appeared to be imbalanced, a finding later noted by several other groups (Kan *et al.* 1972c; Shchory & Ramot 1972; Gallo *et al.* 1975).

However, these apparent inconsistencies were

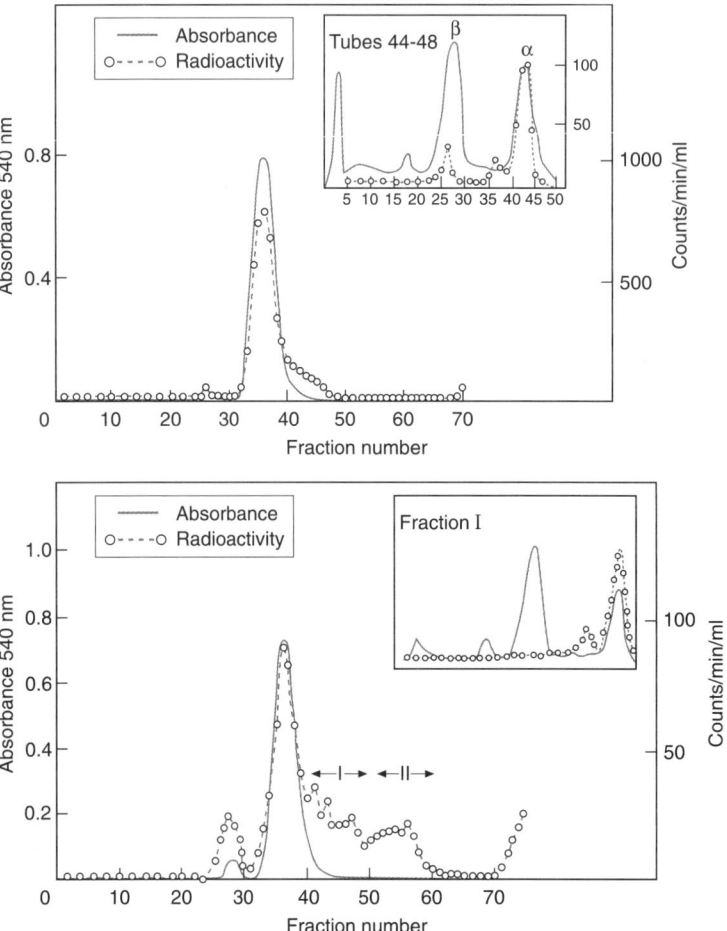

Fig. 5.4 The demonstration of free α chains in homozygous β-thalassaemic reticulocytes. Red cells were incubated with radioactive leucine for 20 min, washed and lysed and the lysate applied to a Sephadex G75 column. The main haemoglobin protein peak is shown by the continuous line. The experiment at the top shows the pattern obtained from a non-thalassaemic patient. In addition to a major radioactive peak with the same molecular weight as haemoglobin, there is a small tail. This material was added to unlabelled haemoglobin and the globins separated by CM-cellulose chromatography as shown in the insert. Most of this radioactive 'tail' consists of free α chains but there is only a very small pool in normal reticulocytes. The experiment shown below is identical except that in this case the red cells were obtained from an individual homozygous for β thalassaemia. In this case there is a relatively large amount of low molecular weight radioactivity, and again this consists almost entirely of free α chains. This experiment demonstrates a large pool of free α chains in the red cells of the thalassaemic patient.

eventually reconciled to provide a fairly clear picture of disordered globin synthesis in β thalassaemia. Most haemoglobin synthesis occurs in red-cell precursors in the bone marrow, and in reticulocytes represents only about 1% of the total output. As we shall see later, precursors which synthesize relatively greater amounts of HbF preferentially survive their passage through the bone marrow and peripheral blood of patients with β thalassaemia. Thus the peripheral-blood reticulocytes represent a highly selected population which have survived *because* they are synthesizing more HbF. Hence it might be expected that there would be relatively more γ-chain than β-chain synthesis in the peripheral blood than in bone marrow (Weatherall *et al.* 1974a; Nathan & Benz 1976) (Fig. 5.5).

It must also be remembered that haemoglobin synthesis is a dynamic process and that the results of *in vitro* radioactive labelling experiments reflect an equilibrium between production and destruction of globin molecules; if some of the excess of α chain is lost by proteolysis during the course of an experiment the apparent ratios of production may give quite erroneous results (Weatherall *et al.* 1974a). As we shall see later, proteolysis is much more active in red-cell precursors than in reticulocytes. Hence it is likely that the rate of proteolytic degradation of excess α chains is greater in the bone marrow than in the peripheral blood. Indeed, when time-course experiments were carried out on the rates of incorporation of radioactive amino acids into α, β and γ chains it was found that this was linear in the peripheral blood, while in the

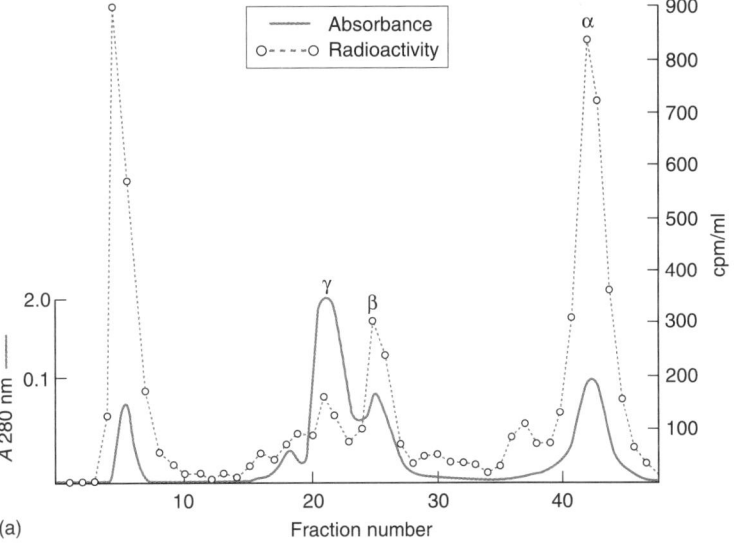

(a)

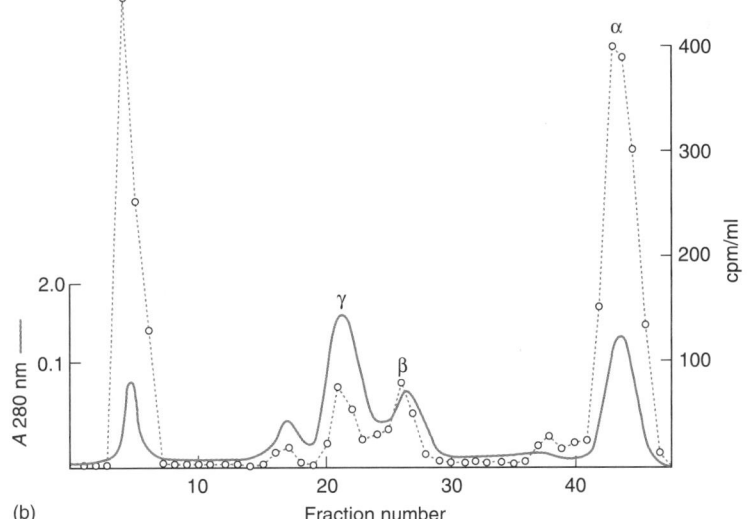

(b)

Fig. 5.5 A comparison of haemoglobin synthesis in the bone marrow and peripheral blood of an individual homozygous for β thalassaemia. The experimental conditions were identical to those described in Figs 5.2 and 5.3. (a) The results of a bone-marrow incubation; (b) results of peripheral blood incubation. Clearly the relative amount of radioactivity incorporated into the β chains is greater in the bone marrow than in the peripheral blood. These findings suggest that the cell populations synthesizing relatively more HbF survive their passage through the bone marrow and therefore that there are relatively more HbF-producing reticulocytes in the peripheral blood.

bone marrow, although incorporation into β and γ chains was linear, incorporation into α chains tended to plateau early over a 1-h incubation period (Weatherall *et al*. 1974a; Chalevelakis *et al*. 1975), findings that were later substantiated (Hanash & Rucknagel 1978).

Finally, there is an important technical artefact that has to be taken into account when assessing the relative rates of globin synthesis in the bone marrow; there are other proteins synthesized that co-chromatograph with the β chains and which, if not removed, may alter the apparent synthesis ratios (Clegg & Weatherall 1972; Chalevelakis *et al*. 1975, 1976; Hanash & Rucknagel 1978; Cividalli *et al*. 1979). When these observations are taken into account it is clear that there is always marked imbalance between α- and β-chain production in both homozygotes and heterozygotes, regardless of whether bone marrow or blood is studied.

What have these experiments told us about globin

synthesis in β thalassaemia? First, it is imbalanced, in both β thalassaemia major and minor. The excess of α chains that are produced enter an unstable pool from which they either combine with β or γ chains, become associated with the red-cell membrane or are subjected to proteolytic attack, a process which is more active in the bone marrow than in the peripheral blood. It is also apparent that red-cell precursors that synthesize more HbF survive preferentially and hence there is relatively more γ- than β-chain synthesis in reticulocytes than in their nucleated precursors; at every stage of erythroid maturation there is likely to be a marked heterogeneity of cell populations with respect to the relative amount of β- and γ-chain synthesis.

While these studies have given us a reasonably clear picture of the dynamics of globin-chain production in β thalassaemia, they provide only an approximation of the *absolute* amount of globin synthesis. To obtain a more accurate measure of the rate of production of globin and degree of imbalance it would be necessary to isolate early red-cell precursors from the marrow and to carry out a time-course experiment, measuring α/β+γ ratios at varying times over, say, 30 min, and then to extrapolate the ratios back to zero time. As far as we know this difficult experiment has never been done and therefore it seems likely that most of the published data have, if anything, underestimated the degree of globin imbalance in β thalassaemia. Overall, however, these studies have left us with a fairly clear picture of the degree of globin imbalance in the different varieties of β thalassaemia and related disorders, as well as the α thalassaemias, and have clarified other important issues, notably the turnover and initial fate of globin that is produced in excess.

The fate of the excess of α chains in β thalassaemia

Morphological studies

Fessas (1963) reported that there are inclusion bodies in the erythroblasts of the bone marrow and peripheral blood of patients with β thalassaemia, and suggested that they might result from precipitation of excess α chains. He went on to show that they consist of haemoglobin-like material consisting mainly, but perhaps not exclusively, of precipitated α chains (Fessas *et al.* 1966). Later work by Rachmilewitz and

Thorell (1972) demonstrated that each inclusion consists of a focus of precipitated haemichromes, haemoglobin subunits in which both the fifth and sixth coordination positions of the haem iron are liganded to nitrogenous bases. Much later Yuan *et al.* (1993) and Wickramasinghe *et al.* (1996), using an immunoelectromicroscopic technique, confirmed that the inclusion bodies in β thalassaemia consist entirely of precipitated α globin.

In an analysis of marrow aspirated from patients with thalassaemia major, Yataganas and Fessas (1969) found that the proportion of erythroblasts containing intracellular precipitates and the average quantity of precipitation per cell increased with increasing nuclear diameter. They concluded that α-chain precipitation commences early during erythroid maturation, increases as these cells mature, and that a proportion of the late red-cell precursors do not contain detectable precipitates, observations which were confirmed using different methods by Wickramasinghe *et al.* (1973). Yataganas *et al.* (1972) found an inverse correlation between the amount of α-chain precipitate and soluble haemoglobin in individual red cells, and in a further study showed that the α-chain precipitates are not confined to the cytoplasm but are sometimes present in the nucleus (Yataganas *et al.* 1974).

These early descriptions of α-chain inclusions were augmented by ultrastructural studies of erythroblasts from thalassaemic patients (Polliack & Rachmilewitz 1973; Polliack *et al.* 1974a; Yataganas *et al.* 1974; Wickramasinghe & Bush 1975; Wickramasinghe 1976). The α-chain precipitates appear as foci of amorphous material, the electron density of which is higher than that of the cell cytoplasm (Fig. 5.6). They vary in size, are usually multiple and tend to become confluent. They are rarely seen in basophilic erythroid precursors but are found in about 3% of early polychromatophilic cells, in 20% of late polychromatophilic cells, and in virtually all circulating late polychromatophilic erythroblasts. They differ in several ways from the Heinz bodies that can be produced experimentally by phenylhydrazine treatment of red cells. In particular, in thalassaemic red-cell precursors there are no large marginated inclusions attached to the red-cell membrane. In addition, many of the early erythroid precursors show vacuoles that contain little or no electron-dense material, or membrane-bound vesicles. Wickramasinghe and Bush (1975) suggested that the latter represent small autophagic vacuoles.

In addition to these cytoplasmic changes there are nuclear abnormalities, confined largely to late polychromatic erythroblasts (Polliack *et al.* 1974a,b; Wickramasinghe 1976). They include loss or reduplication of parts of the nuclear membrane and α-chain precipitates or particles containing iron. Wickramasinghe (1976) suggested that the intranuclear precipitates represent intracytoplasmic α-chain precipitates which are trapped in the nuclear territory during mitosis, or, alternatively, precipitates which enter the interphase nucleus through a defect in the nuclear membrane.

Loss of α chains by proteolysis

As mentioned earlier, studies of globin synthesis suggest that excess α chains precipitate and become associated with the membrane, and that some of them are rapidly lost by proteolytic destruction (Bank & O'Donnell 1969; Weatherall *et al.* 1969b; Wood *et al.* 1975).

The proteolytic systems of human red cells and their precursors have received only limited attention. In rabbit reticulocytes there is a proteolytic pathway that is dependent on adenosine triphosphate (ATP); during the transformation of reticulocytes to mature erythrocytes this activity is gradually lost, a finding which has been also noted in human red cells and their precursors (Etlinger & Goldberg 1977; Speiser & Etlinger 1982; Rieder *et al.* 1988). With respect to β-thalassaemic reticulocytes it has been observed that degradation of newly synthesized α chains is not only ATP dependent but also requires the presence of ubiquitin (Shaeffer 1983, 1988). In this degradative pathway the C terminus of ubiquitin is activated in an ATP-dependent reaction, and, through a series of enzymatic steps, activated ubiquitin molecules are covalently linked to the ε-amino groups of lysine residues of the protein destined for proteolysis. These conjugates are then recognized through their ubiquitin tag by the 26S proteasome, a multisubunit protease complex. The protein substrate is then degraded in a further ATP-dependent process. Interestingly, Shaeffer and Cohen (1997) have shown how, by the use of ubiquitin aldehyde, a synthetic inhibitor of isopeptidases, it is possible to increase the rate of ATP-dependent proteolysis of α-globin subunits in β-thalassaemic cells. The ubiquitin–proteasome pathway has been reviewed in detail recently (Ciechanover 1998).

Individual variation in the rate of α-chain proteolysis

Presumably the size of the α-chain precipitates reflects a balance between their rates of proteolytic digestion and the speed with which they form insoluble aggregates which are no longer susceptible to attack in this way. Since, as we shall see, damage to the red-cell precursors and red cells by these precipitates is the major factor in causing the anaemia of β thalassaemia, an increased capacity for their proteolytic removal might be beneficial. Very little is known about individual variation in the rate of proteolysis as a potential basis for the phenotypic heterogeneity of the β thalassaemias, and the few reported experiments that have addressed this important question have given rather equivocal results (Braverman *et al.* 1982). In one study there appeared to be a correlation between proteolytic activity and the steady-state haemoglobin level in patients with HbE thalassaemia (Promboon *et al.* 1988). Clearly these potentially important observations need to be followed up and the activities of other proteolytic systems of red cells, which could also have a role in modifying the anaemia of β thalassaemia, must be dissected further. Possible candidates include the cytosolic calcium-dependent proteases and calpains, their inhibitors (Murachi *et al.* 1981; Melloni *et al.* 1982; Macotpet *et al.* 1988) and the ubiquitin system (Ciechanover 1998).

α-Globin precipitation and the anaemia of β thalassaemia

Defective red-cell maturation and survival in β thalassaemia

Ineffective erythropoiesis

Although there is a shortened red-cell survival, the most important factor in the anaemia of β thalassaemia is ineffective erythropoiesis, with large-scale destruction of red-cell precursors in the bone marrow (Crosby & Akeroyd 1952; Sturgeon & Finch 1957; Erlandson *et al.* 1958; Larizza *et al.* 1958; Malamos *et al.* 1961; Finch *et al.* 1970; Murachi *et al.* 1981). This conclusion is based largely on ferrokinetic and erythrokinetic studies, although the destruction of erythroblasts is also reflected in the pattern of bilirubin metabolism (Grinstein *et al.* 1960). The remarkable

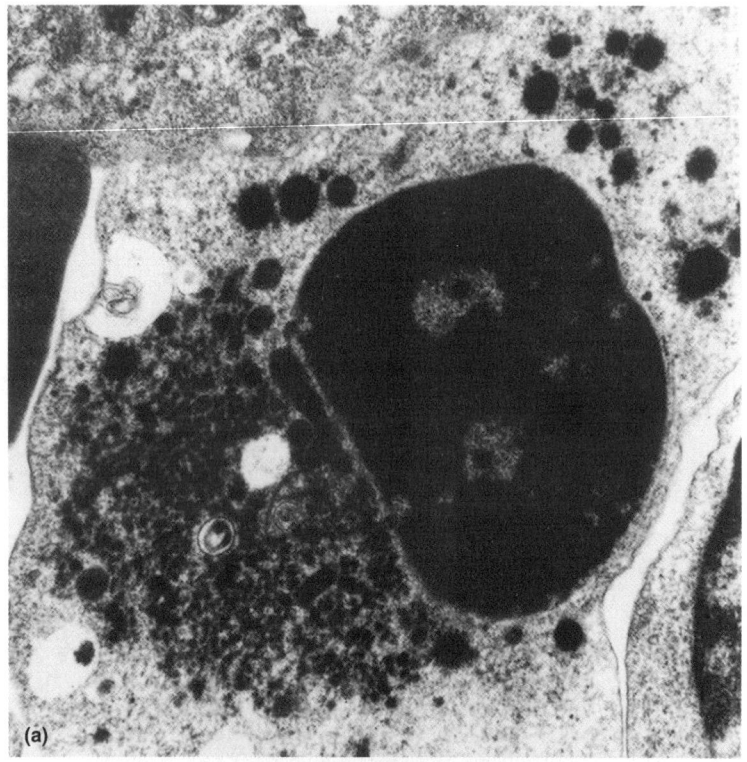

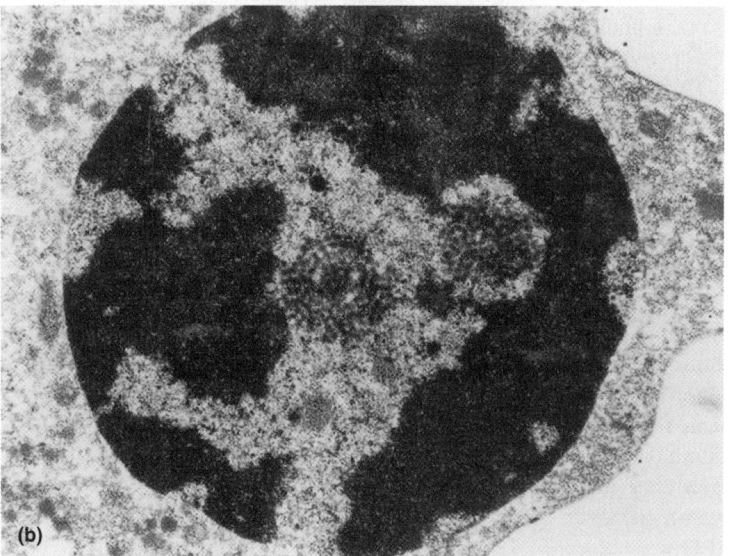

Fig. 5.6 Electron-microscopic appearance of the bone marrow in homozygous β thalassaemia. (a) Inclusion bodies in the cytoplasm and nucleus (× 1550). (b) Similar to (a) at a magnification of × 13 600. *Continued.*

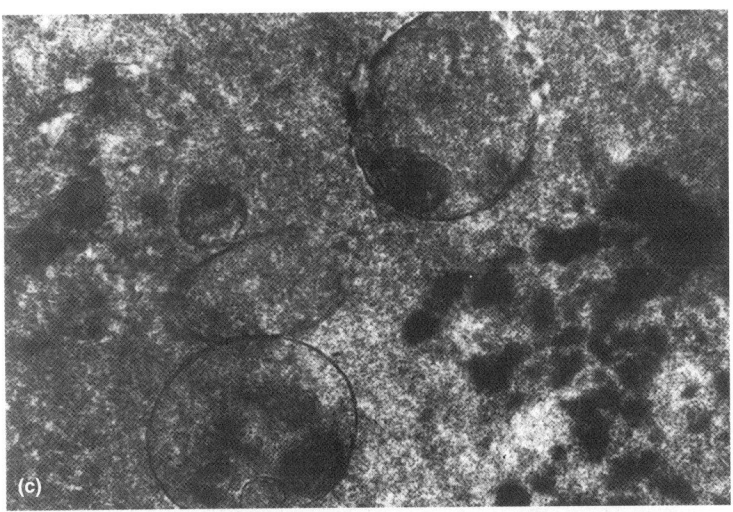

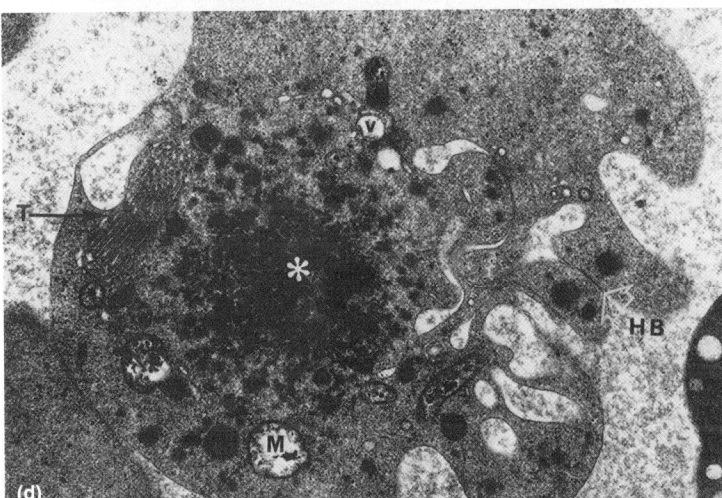

Fig. 5.6 *Continued.* (c) Inclusion bodies and myelin figures in the cell cytoplasm (×15 000). (d) A reticulocyte with irregular indentations of the membrane and cytoplasmic projections containing Heinz (inclusion) bodies (HB). Note the amorphous, partially confluent Heinz body (star), mitochondria (M) with degenerative changes containing haemosiderin, small vacuoles (V) and parallel arrays of tubules (T) (×10 875). From Polliack and Rachmilewitz (1973), with permission.

degree of ineffective erythropoiesis, the only other disease reaching comparable levels being pernicious anaemia, is well exemplified by the study of Finch *et al.* (1970). In 10 severe β thalassaemics the plasma iron turnover (PIT) and erythrocyte iron turnover (EIT) showed a wide discrepancy; the PIT was higher than in any other disease, reaching a level of 10 times greater than normal, while the EIT was only slightly elevated. These findings reflect major destruction of developing red cells in the marrow, together with extensive hypertrophy of the erythron. The latter has been confirmed in more recent studies that estimated

the level of circulating transferrin receptor as a measure of erythropoiesis (Huebers *et al.* 1990; Beguin 1992; Olivieri & Brittenham 1997). Erythrokinetic studies have also demonstrated suppression of erythropoiesis after blood transfusion (Cavill *et al.* 1978).

Haemolysis

There is also a reduced red-cell survival in β thalassaemia, although this is less important than ineffective erythropoiesis in determining the severity of the anaemia. Using either the Ashby or ^{51}Cr-labelling methods, survival times have ranged from 7 to 22 days (Kaplan & Zuelzer 1950; Sturgeon & Finch 1957; Erlandson *et al.* 1958; Vullo & Tunioli 1958; Blendis *et al.* 1974; Cavill *et al.* 1978). There are two populations of red cells, one which is very rapidly destroyed (Kaplan & Zuelzer 1950; Bailey & Prankerd 1958; Hillcoat & Waters 1962). There is evidence, discussed later in this chapter, that the short-lived population contains mainly HbA or α-chain precipitates, while the longer-lived cells are richer in HbF. External counting indicates that some, but by no means all, of the premature red-cell destruction occurs in the spleen (Prankerd 1963; Blendis *et al.* 1974).

Is excess α-chain production the main cause of the anaemia of β thalassaemia?

In a study which examined both *in vitro* chain synthesis and *in vivo* red-cell survival, Vigi *et al.* (1969) found a good correlation between the magnitude of excess α-chain synthesis in the peripheral blood of β thalassaemics and the degree of shortened red-cell survival. Earlier, in their seminal analysis of the red cells of splenectomized patients with severe β thalassaemia, Nathan and Gunn (1966) observed that the largest inclusions were found in the most lightly stained cells, i.e. those which contain relatively less HbF. These findings, taken in conjunction with haemoglobin synthesis studies described earlier, showing that there is relatively more γ-chain synthesis in the peripheral blood than in the bone marrow, suggest that α-chain precipitation is the major cause of the intramedullary destruction of red-cell precursors, and that those which synthesize relatively more γ chains are protected, presumably because excess α chains combine with γ chains to form fetal haemoglobin. This interpretation is entirely consistent with the *in vivo* observation that cells containing relatively more HbF turn over more slowly than those containing mainly HbA (Gabuzda *et al.* 1963), and with differential centrifugation experiments on red cells of patients with β thalassaemia intermedia, which show that the older populations are richer in HbF while the lighter cells contain predominantly HbA and HbA$_2$ and α-chain precipitates (Loukopoulos & Fessas 1965; Weatherall *et al.* 1979).

How does α-chain precipitation interfere with erythroid maturation?

Knowledge of the cellular events that lead to the intramedullary destruction of red-cell precursors in β thalassaemia has come from several sources. Early studies focused on the patterns of erythroid maturation. More recently, with the availability of large numbers of erythroid precursors obtained at the time of bone-marrow transplantation, it has been possible to analyse the structure and function of their membranes.

Kinetics of red-cell maturation

The complex abnormalities of red-cell maturation that have been demonstrated by *in vitro* labelling experiments using red-cell precursors from the bone marrows of β thalassaemics were summarized by Wickramasinghe (1976). There is a major accumulation of early polychromatophilic cells in the G1 phase of the cell cycle which may be caused by substantial prolongation of G1 and/or failure of G1 cells to enter S. Wickramasinghe *et al.* (1973) investigated the possibility that α-chain precipitates might be responsible for this abnormality by examining the relationship between the number of intracytoplasmic precipitates and the DNA synthetic activity of individual early polychromatic erythroblasts. They found that there is a reduced incorporation of ^{3}H-thymidine into polychromatic erythroblasts which contain moderate or large quantities of α-chain precipitates. An unexpected finding was that even in precursors that did not contain precipitates there was a marked reduction in DNA synthesis. In other words it appeared that many cells without detectable inclusions were also arrested in G1. This could reflect the loss of inclusions from the cell after they had caused the arrest or, as seems more likely, this type of maturational arrest may be produced by an expanded pool of soluble α chains. The suggestion of Yataganas *et al.* (1974) that the abnormality of proliferation might be related to the presence of nuclear rather than cytoplasmic precipitation was not borne out by the later studies of Wickramasinghe and Bush (1975), who observed that intranuclear α-chain precipitates rarely occur in dividing early polychromatophilic erythroblasts. Whether intranuclear iron deposition plays a role in the defect in cell division is also unclear (Polliack *et al.* 1974a,b). In normal marrow the non-dividing late polychromatophilic erythroblasts appear to be formed solely as a consequence of division of earlier chromatophilic precursors (Wickramasinghe 1976). On the other hand, in patients with β thalassaemia a significant proportion of late erythroblasts must be the progeny of early polychromatophilic erythroblasts which have been arrested in G1, without an intervening cell division. Autoradiographic studies have shown that there is a gross defect in protein synthesis in late erythroblasts containing the largest quantities of precipitate, though approximately 20% of cells without detectable precipitates also fail to incorporate labelled amino acids. Interestingly, even very early red-cell precursors, in which there is minimal haemoglobin synthesis, seem to have a reduced proliferative capacity (Dörmer & Betke 1978).

It appears therefore that at least part of the ineffective erythropoiesis of β thalassaemia is the result of intramedullary death of late polychromatophilic erythroblasts which are grossly defective in protein synthesis, and from the loss of earlier precursors which are arrested in G1. It is probable that both these effects are due to excess α chains, although whether they reflect precipitation in the nucleus or cytoplasm or whether the damage results from a more subtle mechanism is still not clear.

Mechanisms of damage to red-cell precursors

More recently, research in this field has focused on abnormalities of the membrane of red-cell precursors and on the mechanisms whereby these changes lead to their premature removal by the cells of the reticulo-endothelial system. Much of this work has followed increased knowledge about the structure and function of normal red-cell membranes (Platt 1994; Lux & Palek 1995).

In health, the red-cell membrane is a mixture of phospholipids, esterified cholesterol and glycolipids, arranged in a bilayer and traversed randomly by transmembrane protein channels and receptors. The membrane contains 10–15 major proteins that fall into two classes. First, there are integral membrane proteins, which traverse the bilayer, interact with the hydrophobic lipid core and are tightly bound; they include band 3, the anion-exchange protein, and glycoprotein surface antigens. Second, there are peripheral membrane proteins, which are confined to the cytoplasmic membrane surface; they include spectrin and actin, and some red-cell enzymes.

It appears that there are a number of simultaneous processes underlying the premature destruction of red-cell precursors in β thalassaemia. It has been found that there is an accelerated rate of apoptosis, that is, programmed cell death (Yuan *et al.* 1993). How might this be mediated? Excess α chains accumulate at the membrane and its skeleton where they probably cause alterations in membrane deformability, stability and cellular hydration (Shinar *et al.* 1987; Schrier *et al.* 1989). These abnormalities are associated with changes in the membrane characterized by a reduced spectrin/band 3 ratio, and partial oxidation and defective function of band 4.1 (Advani *et al.* 1992b). They seem to reflect the early accumulation of α globin and its colocalization with band 4.1 and spectrin at sites of membrane discontinuity. It seems likely that these changes reflect the fact that haem, haemichromes and iron components of α globin serve as foci for generation of reactive oxygen species that result in the partial oxidation of band 4.1 and the decrease in spectrin/band 3 ratio. The deficiency of band 3 in the youngest erythroid precursors occurs without any evidence of interaction with α globin, nor is there membrane discontinuity of band 3. It has been suggested therefore that α globin interferes at an earlier stage, in the complex processes of synthesis, trafficking and membrane insertion of band 3 (Aljurf *et al.* 1996). Interestingly, it appears that the protein 3 defect tends to disappear at the intermediate or late normoblast stage, suggesting either that it is temporary or, as seems more likely, that red-cell precursors that are most deficient in band 3 are destroyed during early erythroid maturation.

It has also been observed that aggregates of red-cell membrane proteins, including spectrin and proteins 3 and 4.1, occur in erythroid progenitors of patients with β thalassaemia and in late erythroblasts isolated from the bone marrow of β-thalassaemic mice (Shinar & Rachmilewitz 1993). It is presumed that they result from abnormal cytoskeleton assembly and it is suggested that they might result in IgG and complement binding, in the same way that has been observed in erythrocytes of patients with β thalassaemia (see later section).

Red-cell precursor damage is multifactorial

Although many questions remain therefore, the intramedullary loss of red-cell precursors in β thalassaemia appears to be an extremely complex process involving precipitation of α globin with subsequent effects on red-cell plasticity, maturation and membrane structure and metabolism, together with accelerated apoptosis, all of which combine to render the precursor both unable to mature and susceptible to premature destruction.

Removal of damaged red-cell precursors

The marrow shows intense phagocytic activity, with many large foamy cells resembling Gaucher's cells, which are also found in the spleen. Ultrastructural studies (Zaino *et al.* 1971; Zaino & Rossi 1974) demonstrate that they contain intracytoplasmic tubules and phagocytosed mature and immature red cells (Fig. 5.7). Further details of the fine structure of the macrophages in thalassaemic marrow are given by Wickramasinghe and Hughes (1978).

How does α-chain precipitation result in a shortened red-cell survival?

As we have seen, free α chains tend to oxidize, first to methaemoglobin and later to irreversible haemichromes which precipitate in the red cells as inclusion bodies (Rachmilewitz 1974). There is a good correlation between the magnitude of excess α-chain synthesis in the peripheral blood of β thalassaemics and the degree of shortened red-cell survival (Vigi *et al.* 1969). Red cells containing inclusions are only seen in the blood after splenectomy and it is therefore clear that either they must be trapped in the spleen, or the inclusion bodies must be removed in the spleen and the damaged cells returned to the circulation (Rifkind 1966; Jacob 1970). Electron-microscopic studies have shown rigid inclusion-containing parts of cells being retarded during their passage from splenic cords to sinusoids in thalassaemic spleens (Slater *et al.* 1968).

While these early studies focused on the mechanical consequences of globin precipitation, more recently interest has shifted to the functional effects of globin imbalance on red-cell membrane metabolism. As mentioned earlier, much of this work has stemmed from a rapid increase in knowledge about the structure and function of the normal and abnormal red-cell membrane (Rachmilewitz *et al.* 1985; Rouyer-Fessard *et al.* 1989; Shinar & Rachmilewitz 1990a,b, 1993; Schrier 1994; Rund & Rachmilewitz 1995; Schrier 1997). It appears that, as well as mechanical factors, premature destruction of the red cells

results from two major mechanisms, the generation of haemichromes from excess α chains with subsequent structural changes to the red-cell membrane, and damage to the membrane mediated through the degradation products of α chains.

Haemichrome

The formation of membrane-bound haemichrome creates a copolymer of macromolecular dimensions which promotes clustering of band 3 in the membrane, first shown in sickle-cell erythrocytes (Waugh *et al.* 1987) and later observed in the red cells of β thalassaemics (Yuan *et al.* 1992a; Turrini *et al.* 1994). It seems likely that these clusters are opsonized with autologous IgG and complement and hence removed by macrophages (Turrini *et al.* 1991; Yuan *et al.* 1992b; Mannu *et al.* 1995).

α-Chain degradation products

The products of degradation of free α chains, i.e. α-globin protein, haem, haemin (the oxidized form of haem) and free iron, may also play a role in damaging red-cell membranes.

Excess globin binds to different membrane proteins and probably alters both their structure and function. The pattern is different in α and β thalassaemia, an observation which may explain some of their phenotypic differences (Shinar *et al.* 1989; Yuan *et al.* 1995) (see p. 231). Although binding to spectrin does not seem to cause major alterations in function, protein 4.1 shows a decreased ability to enhance the binding of spectrin to actin in β-thalassaemic red cells, an important function for maintenance of the normal stability of the cytoskeleton (Shinar *et al.* 1989). Band 4.1 is also partially oxidized (Advani *et al.* 1992b). These mechanisms may also be responsible for the increased susceptibility to fragmentation under sheer stress, observed in β- but not in α-thalassaemic red cells (Schrier *et al.* 1989).

Normally the red cell is protected from *iron* by chelation of free iron via its carrier, transferrin, and its storage protein, ferritin, a vital function in order to prevent iron from catalysing lipid and protein peroxidation. The mechanisms of iron toxicity are summarized by Hershko (1989) and are discussed further in a later section. By generating oxygen free radicals it has

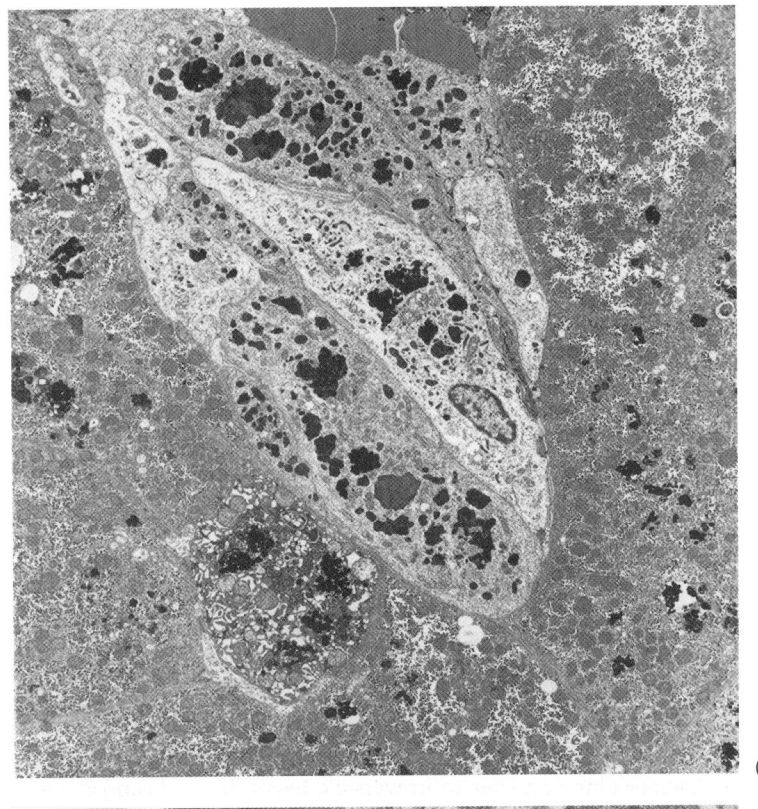

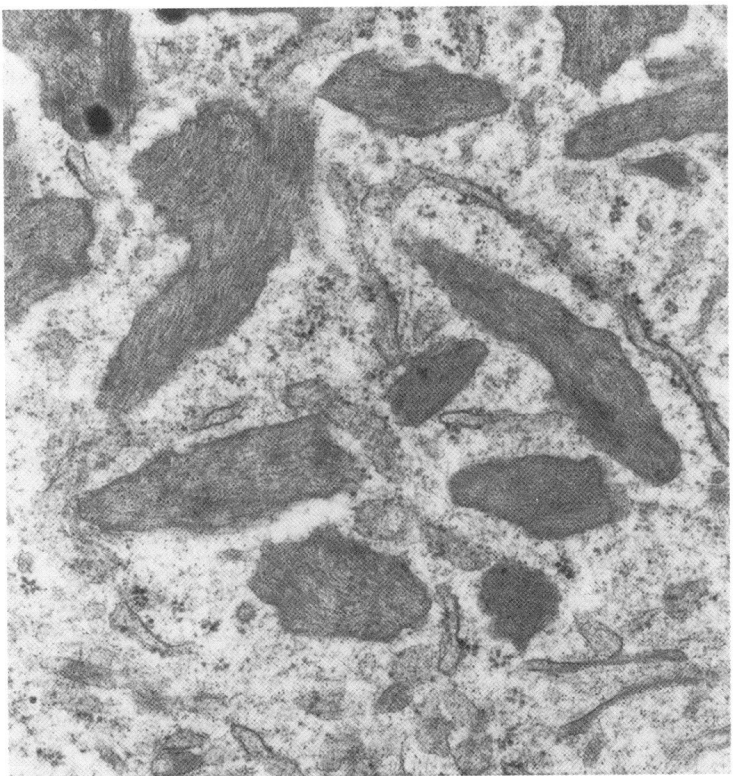

Fig. 5.7 Gaucher-like cells in thalassaemia. (a) Kupffer cells with Gaucher-like structure within hepatic sinusoids (centre). The surrounding hepatocytes contain haemosiderin pigment (dark staining) (×2678). (b) A Gaucher-like cell in the spleen showing membrane-bound fusiform saccules filled with microtubules in the cytoplasm (×18 600). Figures kindly prepared by Professor David Ferguson.

the potential to damage several membrane components including lipids and protein, as well as intracellular organelles such as mitochondria and lysosomes. Abnormally high levels of iron are present in the cytosol and in the membrane of the red cells of β thalassaemics (Repka *et al.* 1993; Shinar & Rachmilewitz 1993). Early studies showed that, as judged by serum α-tocopherol levels, many β thalassaemics are vitamin E deficient, this suggesting that it may be consumed in neutralizing oxidative damage to the red cell (Rachmilewitz *et al.* 1979). Recent experimental studies have confirmed that excess iron accumulation is catalytically active in propagating free-radical reactions (Grinberg & Rachmilewitz 1995; Grinberg *et al.* 1995). These findings correlate with those of others (Hebbel 1985) on the generation of free radicals in the red cells of patients with sickle-cell anaemia, thus indicating a similar pattern of oxidative damage in these two haemoglobin disorders.

More direct evidence for the deleterious effects of iron on red-cell membrane function in β thalassaemia has been obtained by Browne *et al.* (1997). Mice with β thalassaemia were treated with intraperitoneal injections of the iron chelator deferiprone for 4 weeks. This resulted in an improvement in red-cell survival, a reduction in oxidation of membrane proteins and an improvement in the metabolic activities of the red cells and, as measured by osmotic-gradient ektacytometry, there was a trend towards improved hydration of the red cells.

The potentially toxic effects of *haem* and its products on the red-cell membrane are summarized by Vincent (1989) and Jarolim *et al.* (1990). These agents can catalyse the formation of a variety of reactive oxygen species and they are potent photosensitizers, able to transfer the energy of their excited states to oxygen, forming superoxide radicals. Haem can damage membrane lipids and protein, in the free state or complexed with haem proteins. It may react with hydrogen peroxide to form oxygen intermediates; oxidized haem gives rise to protoporphyrin cation radicals while ferrous haem catalyses the formation of hydroxyl radicals. All these agents are capable of causing major oxidative damage to various components of the membrane.

Haemin is of particular importance in membrane damage because it combines directly with skeletal proteins to produce local oxidative damage to surrounding lipids and protein. It can also induce potassium leak, decreased osmotic fragility, alterations in the conformation of band 4.1 and its oxidative state and association with spectrin, and weakening of spectrin dimer–dimer associations; all these changes have been observed in thalassaemic red cells (Avissar *et al.* 1984; Liu *et al.* 1985; Rachmilewitz *et al.* 1985; Shinar *et al.* 1989).

These observations have been supported by *in vitro* experiments in which haem-containing α globin has been inserted into normal red cells. After 20 h of incubation, these cells show considerable cytosolic and membrane changes indicative of oxidative damage, including increased levels of methaemoglobin, excess hydrogen peroxide generation and reduced glutathione stability, which correlates with the rate of α-chain oxidation and the amount of membrane-bound globin (Scott *et al.* 1990, 1993). In keeping with observations on thalassaemic cells, this model also demonstrates elevated levels of haem and non-haem iron, and increased lipid peroxidation. These findings provide additional support for the role of oxidative stress in the pathophysiology of the β-thalassaemic red cell.

It appears therefore that, at least as judged by studies of membrane structure and function, oxidative denaturation plays an important role in the premature destruction of red cells in β thalassaemia (Shinar & Rachmilewitz 1990a). These changes are also mirrored by an abnormal distribution of membrane phospholipids, with most of the phosphatidyl-choline (PC) on the inner bilayer leaflet, and phosphatidyl-ethanolamine (PE) on the outer leaflet. Furthermore, there is a reduction in the percentage of PE together with an increase in the amount of polyunsaturated fatty acids (PUFAs). Both PE and PUFAs are known to be particularly susceptible to peroxidation and their relative decrease in thalassaemic red-cell membranes suggests that they may have been damaged in this way.

We shall return to the question of oxidative damage to the red-cell membrane later in this chapter when we discuss the differences in the patterns of membrane changes between α and β thalassaemia.

In vitro *evidence of membrane damage*

As well as the reduction in their survival the red cells of β thalassaemics show in vitro evidence of red-cell membrane damage. Cividalli *et al.* (1971) demonstrated a marked increase of sodium permeability, and similar findings, together with an increased leakage of potassium, elevated levels of calcium, a higher rate of glycolysis and lactate formation, and low and unstable levels of ATP, were reported by Nathan *et al.* (1969), Shalev *et al.* (1984) and Bookchin *et al.* (1988). Overall, the β-thalassaemic red cell is dehydrated compared with normal or α-thalassaemic erythrocytes (Bunyaratvej *et al.* 1994). Several workers have found that many of these changes are more marked in the upper, younger cells obtained after centrifugation, which contain more inclusion bodies than those from the lower layers (Loukopoulos & Fessas 1965; Nathan & Gunn 1966; Nathan *et al.* 1969). This provides further evidence that these abnormalities are due directly to damage caused by α-chain precipitation as the cells traverse the microcirculation (Nathan *et al.* 1969). The complex relationship between haemichrome formation and the activity of the hexose monophosphate shunt and antioxidant enzymes is discussed by Cappellini *et al.* (1999).

Membrane function in the red cells of β-thalassaemia heterozygotes

These changes are mirrored by similar though milder abnormalities of membrane function in β-thalassaemia heterozygotes (Gunn *et al.* 1972; Chapman *et al.* 1973; Knox-Macaulay & Weatherall 1974; Vettore *et al.* 1974). There is an increased flux of K^+, an effect which is accentuated when the red cells are incubated for 24 h at 37°C, but minimal increase in intracellular Na^+. Adenosine triphosphate (ATP) levels are normal or slightly reduced, but on incubation the cells lose ATP more rapidly than normal, an effect which can be reversed by the addition of glucose. It appears therefore that the cells can compensate for their increased cation pumping by increasing the transport-regulated component of glycolysis and hence can maintain normal ATP levels except under conditions of stress. Interestingly, in the studies of Chapman *et al.* (1973), Knox-Macaulay and Weatherall (1974), Falezza *et al.* (1977) and Vettore *et al.* (1977a,b,c) similar functional abnormalities were found in other hypochromic anaemias such as iron-deficiency and sideroblastic anaemia. It is likely therefore that some of these changes reflect under-haemoglobinized red cells rather than globin imbal-

ance. In favour of this concept is the observation that similar changes were found in the cells of individuals who had inherited both α and β thalassaemia, in which there was minimal globin imbalance (Knox-Macaulay *et al.* 1972).

These findings also explain the increased osmotic resistance of thalassaemic red cells and how this further increases after incubation for 24 h. With excessive loss of K^+ and water, and cellular dehydration, there is a decrease in red-cell volume and hence in osmotic activity. This phenomenon is accentuated after incubation, but if glucose is added it provides adequate energy for ATP regeneration and hence for maintaining the Na^+–K^+ pump to counteract excess loss of K^+ and water from the cells. The observation that increased osmotic resistance can be demonstrated even in the presence of glucose by inhibition of the Na^+–K^+ membrane pumps by ouabain or ethrynic acid is further evidence in favour of this mechanism (Knox-Macaulay & Weatherall 1974).

The red cells of β thalassaemics have therefore a shortened survival that reflects both excess α-chain production and under-haemoglobinization. In the severe forms of the disease damage is also mediated by mechanical trauma and complex interactions which combine to overcome the red cells' defence mechanisms which, except in the case of senescent cells, normally protect haemoglobin and the red-cell membrane components from oxidative damage. The end result is a dehydrated, rigid cell. Some of the complex interactions that lead to red-cell damage of this kind are summarized in Fig. 5.8 and Table 5.2. We shall return to the practical implications of these issues when we describe the potential role of antioxidants in the management of β thalassaemia in Chapter 15.

Secondary effects of ineffective erythropoiesis and anaemia

Response to anaemia

Because methods for estimating erythropoietin (Epo) levels in blood and urine were, until recently, extremely tedious and difficult to standardize, evidence about the physiological response to the anaemia of β thalassaemia has been slow in coming. The pioneering studies of Hammond *et al.* (1962) suggested that there are significantly elevated levels of Epo in the blood and urine of patients with haemo-

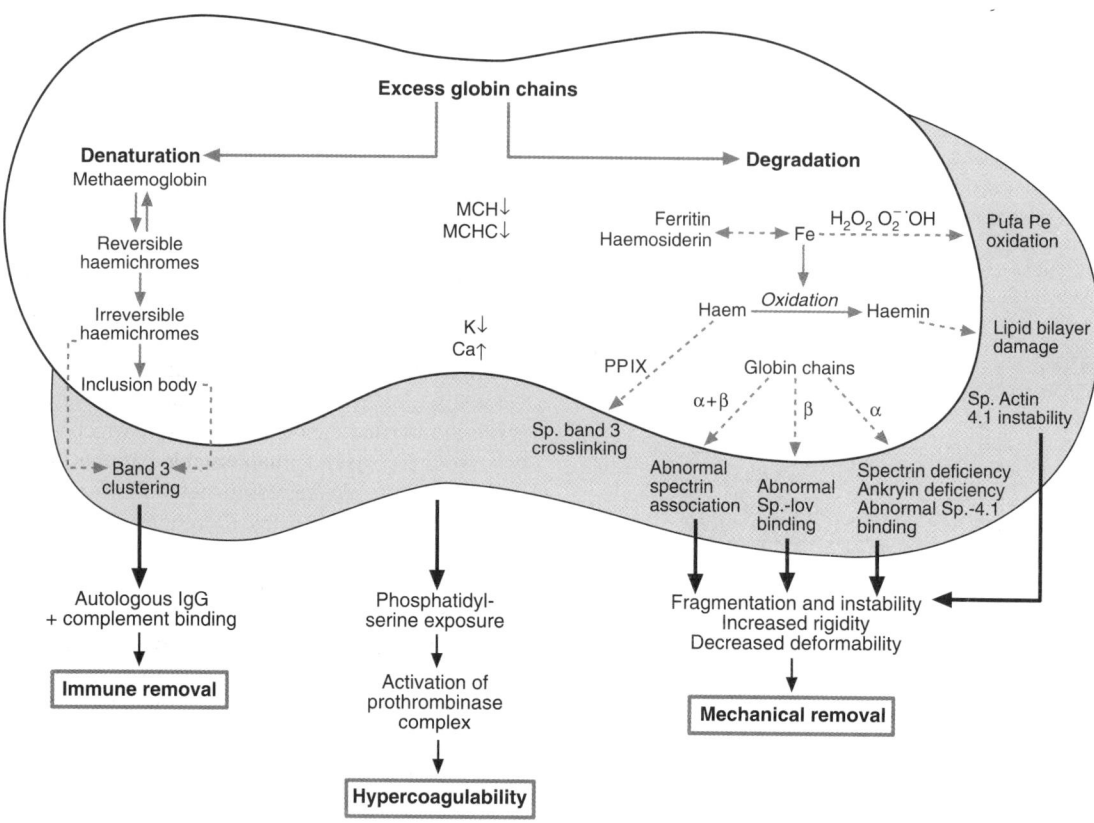

Fig. 5.8 A representation of the main pathways that are involved in membrane damage and shortened red-cell survival in the α and β thalassaemias. The figure also shows one of the proposed mechanisms for generating a hypercoagulable state. Iov, inside-out vesicles; MCH, mean cell haemoglobin; MCHC, mean cell haemoglobin concentration; Pe, phosphatidyl ethanolamine; Pufa, polyunsaturated fatty acid; Sp, spectrin. From Weatherall (1998).

globin values of 7.0 g/dl or less. Interestingly, the level of Epo in plasma and urine was higher in patients with hypoplastic anaemia than thalassaemics with comparable haemoglobin levels.

More recently published data on Epo levels in β thalassaemia, though often difficult to interpret because of the different transfusion status of the patients, have given similar results although there are some puzzling inconsistencies (Manor *et al.* 1986; Andre *et al.*1991; Kalmanti *et al.*1991; Dore *et al.*1993; Sergiacomi *et al.* 1993; Galanello *et al.* 1994; Cazzola *et al.* 1995). Some of these studies included patients with thalassaemia intermedia and hence the results were not confused by transfusion. In many, though not all, there was a reasonable correlation between the steady-state haemoglobin and serum Epo levels

and there was an appropriate response to transfusion reflected by a marked reduction in the level of Epo production. However, the same discrepancy that had been noted by Hammond and colleagues with respect to different Epo responses at the same haemoglobin level in patients with aplastic anaemia and those with β thalassaemia has been confirmed. In one study the Epo response was different in children and older patients, suggesting that it is less effective with increasing age (Manor *et al.* 1986). Another, which attempted to assess the relationship between Epo production and both haemoglobin and HbF levels, reported that these two variables were independently correlated (Galanello *et al.* 1994); patients with thalassaemia intermedia with particularly high HbF levels showed an expansion of erythropoiesis to as

Table 5.2 Summary of mechanisms of damage to red cells and precursors in β thalassaemia.

Red-cell precursors; infective erythropoiesis
Imbalanced globin synthesis. α-Chain precipitation
Inclusion-body formation
Haemichrome formation
Oxidative damage to membrane components by haem, haemin and iron
Defective maturation of erythroid precursors
Accelerated apoptosis
Enhanced phagocyte activity

Red cells; haemolysis
α-Chain precipitation
Inclusion-body formation—mechanical trauma
Haemichrome formation. Band 3 clusters. IgG binding
Oxidative damage to membrane by haem, haemin and iron. Band 4.1 oxidation
Low ATP and potassium; increased calcium
Dehydration and rigidity
Metabolic consequences of hypersplenism

---

much as 4–9 times normal at the same haemoglobin level as patients with much lower levels of HbF. It was concluded that HbF exerts an independent regulatory effect on Epo production. The possibility that some patients have a suboptimal erythropoietin response received further credence when it was found that there is a modest increase in haemoglobin level following the long-term administration of recombinant Epo (Rachmilewitz *et al.* 1995).

It is difficult to reconcile all these findings. While it seems certain that there is a marked Epo response to the anaemia of β thalassaemia, and that this is the main factor involved in erythroid expansion, whether this is always optimal, and whether it persists over the lifespan of a thalassaemic patient, remains to be determined. And further work is needed to define its relationship to HbF production and to other factors that may determine the position of the oxygen dissociation curve of the complex heterogeneous red-cell populations of β thalassaemics, a problem which we shall return to later in this chapter.

Erythroid expansion

The expansion of the ineffective erythroid mass that occurs in β thalassaemia, estimated to range between 10 and 30 times normal in some cases (Finch *et al.* 1970; Fessas & Loukopoulos 1974), is of profound importance in the generation of many of the more distressing clinical features of the disease, particularly bone deformity and, occasionally, the production of extramedullary tumour masses (see Chapter 13). It also imposes an excessive metabolic burden, particularly on young children, with the result that they fail to grow, muscular development is poor, and body fat and weight are reduced. Shunting of blood through this massively expanded marrow may be partly responsible for the increase in plasma volume (Blendis *et al.* 1974), which, together with splenomegaly, is undoubtedly responsible for exacerbating the anaemia. Anaemia and hypervolaemia combine to produce cardiomegaly and the high-output state which is seen in profoundly anaemic thalassaemic patients. It also seems likely that the increased metabolic burden and cell turnover are responsible for other features of the disease such as temperature elevation, anorexia and other non-specific symptoms. A poor nutritional state, together with an increased rate of cell turnover, probably explains the occurrence of folate deficiency, another factor which may worsen the anaemia (Jandl & Greenberg 1959; Luhby & Cooperman 1961; Luhby *et al.* 1961; Vatanavicharn *et al.* 1978). The increased rate of destruction of red-cell precursors is mirrored by an elevated level of urates in the urine, and serum uric acid levels that are higher than in control subjects; clinical features of gout are uncommon, however (Paik *et al.* 1970; Fessas & Loukopoulos 1974).

Splenomegaly and hypersplenism

Mechanisms

One of the functions of the spleen is to act as a filter, retaining defective blood cells and foreign particles in a bed of phagocytes (Weiss 1995). Approximately 5–10% of splenic blood is diverted into the red pulp and slowly percolates through a non-endothelialized mesh containing macrophages, after which it re-enters the circulation through narrow slits, measuring 1–3 μm, in the endothelial sinuses. Sometimes called 'work hypertrophy', a term which at least hides our total ignorance of the mechanisms involved, the exposure of the reticuloendothelial elements of the spleen to abnormal red cells like those of β thalassaemics leads to its progressive enlargement. This concept is supported by the observation that children who have received regular blood transfusions from early in life, and hence who do not have many abnormal red cells in their circulation, do not develop significant splenomegaly. The early observations of Fessas (1963) that blood cells carrying inclusions only appear in the peripheral blood after splenectomy also pointed to the central importance of the spleen in the pathophysiology of the anaemia. Extramedullary haemopoiesis may also contribute to splenomegaly, and hepatomegaly.

Morphological and metabolic studies of red cells from patients who have undergone splenectomy, when separated into young and old populations by centrifugation, also provide valuable evidence about the role of the spleen in the anaemia of β thalassaemia. Cells from the upper layer contain more inclusion bodies than the older populations from the lower layers; the former have a lower haemoglobin content and more crateral distortions, and show abnormalities of membrane function, higher rates of glycolysis and lactate formation, and low, unstable levels of ATP. It is presumably these younger, inclusion-containing populations that are trapped in the spleen (Loukopoulos & Fessas 1965; Nathan & Gunn 1966; Nathan *et al.* 1969).

Consequence of splenomegaly

All the formed elements of the blood may be trapped in the spleen, producing anaemia, thrombocytopenia and neutropenia. The anaemia has a complicated basis, with shortening of the red-cell survival, a dilutional element caused by pooling of a proportion of the red-cell mass in the spleen, and the ill-understood effect of increasing the plasma volume. Several studies have reported red-cell mass and survival data in thalassaemic children with large spleens (Lichtman *et al.* 1953; Smith *et al.* 1955; Reemsta & Elliot 1956; Blendis *et al.* 1974). There is shortening of the homologous red-cell survival, evidence of entrapment of red cells in the splenic pool and a marked expansion of the total blood volume. Cells trapped in the splenic pool accounted for between 9 and 40% of the total red-cell mass in the study of Blendis *et al.* (1974). The spleen is also the site of extensive extramedullary haematopoiesis in patients with severe forms of β thalassaemia.

Interestingly, Blendis *et al.* (1974) noted that splenectomy may be associated with a growth spurt, suggesting that an enlarged spleen might have a deleterious effect on development. Whether this follows the beneficial effect of removing a large mass of ineffective erythropoietic tissue, with its associated metabolic demands, or a more subtle effect of hypersplenism remains to be determined.

Many children with severe β thalassaemia that are inadequately transfused, or those with thalassaemia intermedia, have palpable hepatomegaly. Experienced clinicians have noted that this may tend to become more marked after splenectomy, particularly if the patient is not receiving adequate blood transfusion. There are no convincing explanations for either of these findings. They could reflect the effects of hepatic extramedullary erythropoiesis (see Fig. 7.13, Chapter 7) or sequestration of abnormal red cells in the liver. Recent studies by the authors of children with this clinical picture in Sri Lanka suggest that the former explanation is more likely.

Plasma volume expansion

As mentioned earlier, plasma volume expansion is a common finding in severe β thalassaemia, particularly if patients are inadequately transfused. This has the effect of worsening the anaemia and posing a greater load on the myocardium. It is not due entirely to splenomegaly; the plasma volume does not always return to normal after splenectomy (Blendis *et al.* 1974). It has been suggested that it results from the expanded bone marrow acting as a vascular shunt, a mechanism that is thought to result in plasma volume expansion in other diseases.

Iron overload

Generalized iron loading of the organs has been recognized as a complication of thalassaemia for many years (Whipple & Bradford 1936; Howell & Wyatt 1953; Ellis *et al.* 1954; Erlandson *et al.* 1964b; Fink 1964). The excess iron is derived both from intestinal absorption and from transfusion; in adequately transfused children the latter mechanism predominates, while in patients who have been inadequately transfused and in those with intermediate forms of β thalassaemia increased absorption from the gut is the major route.

Mechanisms and rate of iron loading

Current views on iron metabolism in thalassaemia are based on knowledge about normal iron homeostasis

(Brittenham 1994; Kühn 1994). The main pathway of internal iron flux is from transferrin, the iron transport protein, to the erythron and thence to the monocyte/macrophage system, which ingests effete red cells, and back to plasma transferrin. Approximately 0.5% of the total body iron is acquired or lost each day. Because humans cannot increase the rate of excretion of iron, balance is regulated by the control of absorption. The two major factors that influence the rate of absorption from the intestine are the amount of iron in the body stores and the level of erythropoietic activity. A normal adult has a total body iron of about 5 g, of which approximately 3.5 g are in the erythron, 1 g in the storage compartments and 0.5 g in the tissues.

From these physiological considerations it is easy to see why iron loading occurs in β thalassaemia. A unit of blood contains approximately 200 mg of iron and, since there is no way of excreting excess iron, a regular transfusion regimen rapidly increases the body iron load. At the same time, iron absorption increases dramatically in the presence of ineffective erythropoiesis and erythroid expansion; the drive to increased iron absorption overcomes the physiological mechanisms whereby it is normally reduced in the presence of increased body stores.

The degree of iron load derived from transfusion depends on the type of regimen. Modell (1976) estimated that by the time children maintained asymptomatic on a high transfusion programme reach the age of 11 years they will have accumulated approximately 28 g of iron. Although it is only at about this level of loading that patients begin to show signs of hepatic, cardiac and endocrine disturbances similar to those seen in adults with primary haemochromatosis, organ damage starts much earlier. In a group of babies and children studied by serial liver biopsies it was found that tissue damage occurs soon after transfusions are initiated (Iancu *et al.* 1977a,b; Iancu & Neustein 1977). For example, in three babies aged 5, 6 and 13 months, although the hepatic architecture was normal, most of the hepatocytes contained a number of round or oval structures, single and membrane bound, which were identified as secondary lysosomes; two of these biopsies already showed increased total iron content. To what extent this early iron loading reflects increased absorption associated with anaemia before the beginning of regular transfusion or the effect of the first transfusions is not clear. The pathology of hepatic iron loading is considered further in Chapter 7.

Though iron absorption studies in patients with transfusion-dependent thalassaemia give variable results, presumably depending on the transfusion regimen that is being followed, overall there is an increased rate of absorption in children who are anaemic, which is corrected after adequate transfusion (Smith *et al.* 1955; Larizza *et al.* 1958; Erlandson *et al.* 1962; Bannerman 1964; Necheles *et al.* 1969; Heinrich *et al.* 1973). For example, Heinrich *et al.* (1973) found that inorganic iron absorption was markedly increased 64–300 days after transfusion, whereas it fell into the normal range when measured 3–17 days afterwards.

In intermediate forms of β thalassaemia, in which the picture is not complicated by the effects of blood transfusion, there is increased iron absorption and subsequent iron overload, although this occurs at a slower rate than in transfusion-dependent patients (Pippard *et al.* 1979). Combined measurements of iron absorption and ferrokinetics have demonstrated a consistent relationship between the magnitude of the increase in erythropoiesis and radioactive iron absorption in patients of this kind (Pootrakul *et al.* 1988).

Mechanisms of tissue damage in iron loading

Although vital for living processes iron can, under certain circumstances, generate extremely toxic free radicals, which cause widespread tissue damage. In health, it is tightly bound to storage or transport proteins; binding of plasma iron to transferrin, for example, prevents its catalytic effect in free-radical production (Hershko & Peto 1987). However, with increasing iron loading transferrin becomes saturated and a potentially toxic, non-transferrin-bound fraction of plasma iron (NTPI) becomes detectable in plasma (Hershko *et al.* 1978; Gutteridge *et al.* 1985; Wagstaff *et al.* 1985). The rate of low molecular weight iron uptake from this source by cultured rat heart cells is over 300 times that of transferrin iron (Link & Pinson 1985). Furthermore, transferrin iron uptake is inhibited by high tissue iron concentration due to the downregulation of transferrin receptor production, whereas NTPI uptake is actually increased in high tissue iron concentrations (Randell *et al.* 1994).

The advances in free-radical chemistry which have clarified the toxic properties of iron are summarized by Gutteridge and Halliwell (1989) and the effects of free-radical damage mediated by iron are reviewed by Hershko and Weatherall (1988), Hershko *et al.*

(1998b) and Grinberg and Rachmilewitz (1995). Activation of the respiratory burst in macrophages and granulocytes is associated with a marked increase in the production of superoxide (O_2^-) and peroxide (O_2^{2-}). At physiological pH, peroxide is rapidly protonated to hydrogen peroxide (H_2O_2). The superoxide radical and hydrogen peroxide are poorly reactive in aqueous solution, but the hydroxyl radical ($^{\cdot}OH$) is highly reactive and toxic. Hydrogen peroxide readily crosses biological membranes and can propagate oxygen-related damage. Free hydroxyl radicals are produced from O_2 and H_2O_2 as follows:

$$Fe^{+++} + O_2 \rightarrow Fe^{++} + O_2^-$$
$$Fe^{++} + H_2O_2 \rightarrow Fe^{+++} + {}^{\cdot}OH + OH^-$$

Hydroxyl radicals, and possibly other oxygen-derived species, may cause considerable damage by degrading DNA and hyaluronic acid, and by membrane peroxidation (Slater 1984; Hershko & Weatherall 1988). The end result of the lipid damage is loss of fluidity, a fall in membrane potential, increased permeability to H^+ and other ions, and eventual rupture leading to release of cell and organelle contents including lysosomal hydrolytic enzymes. The damaging effects of lipid peroxidation are discussed in detail by Gutteridge and Halliwell (1989).

It has been found that the low molecular mass iron that is present in the serum of patients with iron overload (Hershko et al. 1978) is also present in many other tissues. Although iron is usually tightly associated with haem and non-haem proteins such as ferritin, transferrin and haemoglobin, imposing an oxidant stress on iron-containing proteins can cause them to release some 'free' iron. It thus seems likely that oxidant damage itself generates at least some of the iron necessary to complete the toxic sequences of the reactions outlined above (Gutteridge & Halliwell 1989). Although there are several defence mechanisms against free-radical damage (Table 5.3), including such first-line antioxidant systems as superoxide dismutase, catalase and glutathione peroxidase, it appears that in heavily iron-loaded patients they are inadequate to prevent oxidative damage.

Autopsies of patients who have died of β thalassaemia have shown widespread iron deposition (Whipple & Bradford 1936; Astaldi et al. 1951; Ellis et al. 1954; Sansone et al. 1955; Fink 1964; Putignano et al. 1973; Modell & Matthews 1976). Although iron is deposited throughout many organs, the most important pathological consequences result from its involvement of the liver, heart and endocrine glands.

Table 5.3 Some important antioxidant systems. Modified from Gutteridge and Halliwell (1989).

Antioxidant	Mode of action
Intracellular	
Superoxide dismutases	Removal of superoxide radical (O_2^-)
Catalase	Removal of hydrogen peroxide (H_2O_2)
Glutathione peroxidase	Removal of hydrogen peroxide and organic hydroperoxides
Membrane	
Vitamin E	Lipid-soluble, lipid-radical, chain-breaking antioxidant
β-Carotene	Singlet oxygen and $^{\cdot}OH$ scavenger
Extracellular	
Transferrin	Iron binding
Lactoferrin	Iron binding at low pH
Ceruloplasmin	Oxidation of ferrous ions to ferric state
Haptoglobin/haemopexin	Bind free haemoglobin/haem
Albumin	Binds copper tightly and iron weakly
Superoxide dismutases	As above
Urate; uric acid	Inhibitors of radical reactions
Glucose	High rate constant for reaction with $^{\cdot}OH$ radicals

Liver

As mentioned earlier, Iancu and colleagues have carried out serial liver and other tissue biopsies from thalassaemic children from very early in life and described both the light- and electron-microscopic appearances of the tissue damage mediated by iron deposition (Iancu & Neustein 1977; Iancu *et al.* 1977a,b; Masera *et al.* 1980; Iancu 1989). In the first year, liver biopsies show ferritin particles in the cytocell and siderosomes of hepatocytes. With progressive transfusion therapy there is increasing siderocytosis of both parenchymal and reticuloendothelial cells (Fig. 5.9a). Fibrosis, initially interhepatocytic, progresses to capillarization of sinusoids and cirrhosis (Fig. 5.9b). Finally, hepatocytes disappear within connective-tissue scars containing clumps of haemosiderin.

There are extensive autopsy data, collected over many years, which indicate that in children who have not had adequate iron chelation therapy, severe hepatic fibrosis and siderosis are common accompaniments of iron loading (Frumin *et al.* 1952; Howell & Wyatt 1953; Ellis *et al.* 1954; Witzleben & Wyatt 1961). Furthermore, it is clear, both from the sequential studies described above and from autopsy data, that serious hepatic damage may be mediated very early in life (Wollstein & Kreidel 1930; Panizon & Vullo 1952) (see Chapter 7).

Parkes *et al.* (1995) have shown that human liver cells in culture upregulate the transport of non-transferrin-bound iron in response to iron loading, a factor that may be of considerable importance in generating liver damage in diseases like thalassaemia.

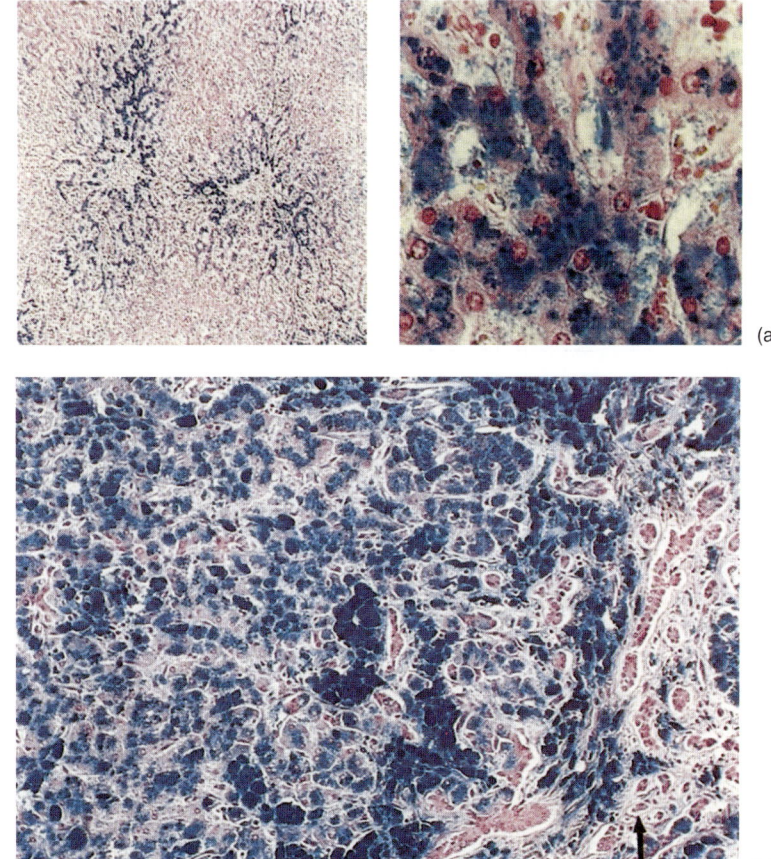

Fig. 5.9 Liver pathology in β thalassaemia. (a) Early iron deposition in a 2-year-old child, showing liver cells at the periphery of lobules. The left-hand section is magnified × 100 and the right-hand section × 450. (b) Severe iron loading with early cirrhosis in HbE β thalassaemia; Prussian blue stain, × 100. From Sonakul (1989), with permission.

Heart

While for obvious reasons there have been no sequential biopsy studies of the heart in thalassaemic patients there are extensive autopsy data on the distribution and patterns of iron loading. Detailed descriptions of the myocardium and conducting tissues of the heart have been reported by Engle (1964), Buja and Roberts (1971), Modell and Matthews (1976) and Sonakul *et al.* (1988a). Although the dry weight of iron is less than in the liver it is widely distributed together with lipofuscein in small granules which may represent lysosomes (Fig. 5.10). Curiously, the iron is not distributed uniformly in the myocardium but is found at a much greater concentration in the epicardial region. Hence assessment of cardiac iron loading by endomyocardial biopsy may give falsely low values. Additional changes observed at autopsy have included extensive myocardial fibre disruption and variable fibrosis (Howell & Wyatt 1953; Witzleben & Wyatt 1961; Schellhammer *et al.* 1967).

There have been several studies of heart cells maintained in culture to examine the kinetics of cardiac iron loading and the likely effects of iron chelation (Link & Pinson 1985; Parkes *et al.* 1993). Parkes and colleagues found that previous iron loading of rat myocardiocytes promoted a dose- and time-dependent increase in the rate of uptake of non-transferrin-bound iron, an effect which, interestingly, resulted in a reduction in spontaneous beating of the cells by over 50%. The rate of uptake of non-transferrin-bound iron reverted to control levels after treatment with therapeutic concentrations of iron chelators. These results suggest that a vicious circle may be created whereby iron loading exacerbates the uptake of toxic, non-transferrin-bound iron leading to cardiac damage and further iron loading, in a similar fashion to that described for liver cells earlier in this section. It seems likely that the generation of free hydroxyl radicals results in the damage to the lysosomal membrane of myocytes and leads to the disruption of the sarcolemmal membrane and inhibition of the mitochondrial respiratory chain (Link *et al.* 1994, 1996; Hershko *et al.* 1998b).

While it is clear that iron loading of the myocardium is the major factor in the pathophysiology of cardiac disease in thalassaemic patients, there are a number of other mechanisms which may be involved. There is increasing evidence that right-heart strain

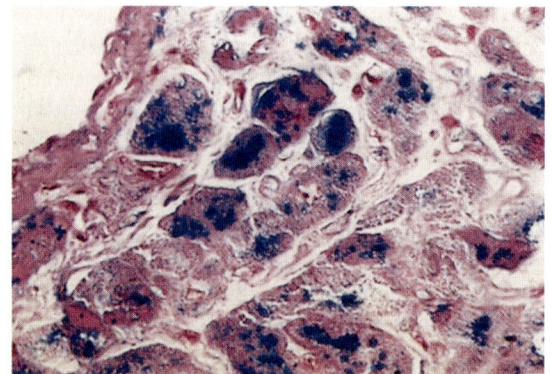
(a)

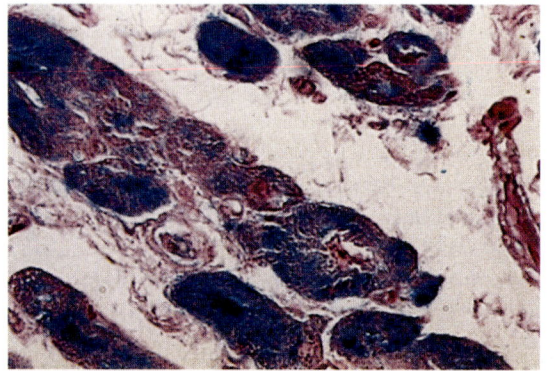
(b)

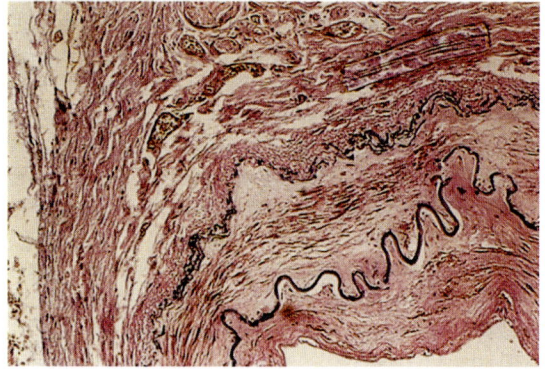
(c)

Fig. 5.10 Iron deposition in the myocardium. (a) Paranuclear deposition of iron in the early stages of iron loading. (b) Distribution of iron throughout the myocardial fibres which occurs with heavy iron loading. (c) Iron encrusting of the elastic lamina of a small coronary artery. Prussian blue stain; (a,b) × 450, (c) × 100. From Sonakul (1989), with permission.

may be provoked by pulmonary hypertension resulting from either structural damage to the lungs or multiple pulmonary emboli (see later section). Furthermore, as we shall see in Chapter 7, in the past recurrent pericarditis was a fairly frequent complication, although it has been seen less frequently over recent years. However, recent studies have suggested that myocarditis, not necessarily associated with iron overload, may be a fairly frequent complication; in a study of 1000 patients, approximately 5% developed serious cardiac disease secondary to myocarditis with no evidence of iron overload (Kremastinos et al. 1996). These infective complications which involve the heart may vary in different populations. For example Wasi (1972) found an elevated level of antistreptolysin O titres in thalassaemic patients with pericarditis in Thailand, and suggested that at least some of them might represent rheumatic pericarditis. As far as we know, this suggestion has not been followed up and there have not been reports of similar serological changes from other populations.

Endocrine glands

There is widespread haemosiderosis involving most of the endocrine organs in iron-loaded thalassaemics (Ellis et al. 1954; Erlandson et al. 1964b; Fink 1964). This early work focused on the high frequency of pancreatic involvement and subsequent diabetes as a complication of severe thalassaemia (Ellis et al. 1954; Erlandson et al. 1964b; Bannerman et al. 1967); more recently these studies have been confirmed and detailed analyses of carbohydrate homeostasis in thalassaemic patients have been reported (Toccafondi et al. 1970b; Lassman et al. 1974a; Flynn et al. 1976; Saudek et al. 1977; De Sanctis et al. 1988a,b,c; Merkel et al. 1988).

Later, it was found that iron-loaded patients with β thalassaemia may suffer from a variety of other hormone deficiencies involving any endocrine organ, including the gonads (Kuo et al. 1968; Canale et al. 1974; Lassman et al. 1974b; Flynn et al. 1976; McIntosh 1976a,b; Tuchinda et al. 1978; Masala et al. 1984; De Sanctis et al. 1989; Vullo et al. 1990; Perignon et al. 1993; Jensen et al. 1997; Low 1997).

More detailed studies of individual endocrine gland function have confirmed that there may be variable hormone deficiencies of the pituitary (Zaino et al. 1969; Toccafondi et al. 1970a; Canale et al. 1974; Costin et al. 1979; Saenger et al. 1980; Pintor et al. 1986;

Sklar et al. 1987; De Sanctis et al. 1988a, 1989; Chatterjee et al. 1993b; Roth et al. 1997), adrenal (Kuo et al. 1968; Canale et al. 1974; McIntosh 1976b; Sklar et al. 1987), thyroid (Gabrielle 1971; Lassman et al. 1974b; Oberklaid & Seshadri 1975; Flynn et al. 1976; Spitz et al. 1984), parathyroid (Flynn et al. 1976; Aloia et al. 1982; Spitz et al. 1984; De Sanctis et al. 1992) and gonads (Canale et al. 1974; Lassman et al. 1974b; Flynn et al. 1976; Modell 1976; De Sanctis et al. 1988b; Wang et al. 1989).

Several authors have suggested that, in very severely iron-loaded patients, end-organ fibrosis may be an important factor in producing endocrine insufficiency (Canale et al. 1974; Flynn et al. 1976). Autopsies have revealed varying degrees of testicular interstitial fibrosis with small, heavily pigmented undifferentiated seminiferous tubules, hyalinized slings and an absence of Leidig cells (Canale et al. 1974).

As we shall see when we discuss the clinical manifestations of endocrine deficiency in β thalassaemia in Chapter 7, it is now clear that growth failure, delayed sexual maturation and bone disease, all in part reflecting hypogonadotrophic hypogonadism, due to the extreme sensitivity of the hypothalamic/pituitary axis to iron excess, are the most important manifestations of iron loading of the endocrine system. Diabetes remains a problem, while hypothyroidism and hypoparathyroidism are encountered less frequently.

While this type of pathology undoubtedly explains the definable endocrine deficiencies in β thalassaemia it does not explain the remarkable pigmentation which was observed by Cooley in his first description of the disease. Like other iron-loading diseases, darkening of the skin is due to increased melanin rather than iron. The skin rapidly lightens on treatment with chelating agents and it has been suggested (Graziano 1976) that the increased melanin deposition results from a free-radical mechanism similar to that responsible for sunlight-induced melanin synthesis; this reaction may be catalysed in thalassaemic children by the slight increase of iron in their skin.

Iron involvement of other organs

While the most serious effects of iron overload are manifest in the liver, heart and endocrine system, there is increasing evidence that it may be of importance in other ways. In Chapter 7 we shall discuss the increasing evidence that it may cause pulmonary pathology, and in the next section we shall mention briefly its possible role in growth retardation and bone disease. It is also clear that it affects the exocrine pancreas, although whether this is of functional importance is not yet clear (see Chapter 7).

Bone disease

The characteristic deformities of the skull and face, and other skeletal features of severe thalassaemia, were emphasized in many of the early descriptions of the disease by workers in the USA and Europe. It has been clear for many years that they can be prevented by adequate blood transfusion (Johnston & Roseman 1967; Piomelli *et al.* 1969). It seems likely therefore that these changes are largely due to expansion of the bone-marrow mass, a process that can lead to a variety of distressing complications. Spontaneous fractures, or fractures following minor trauma, are relatively common in poorly transfused children (Wolman 1964; Herrick & Davis 1975; Novikova & Abrakhanova 1975; Michelson & Cohen 1988). Uncontrolled maxillary overgrowth can lead to a grotesque appearance (Logothetis *et al.* 1971a) and can also result in severe dental deformities, particularly malocclusion (Asbell 1964).

While most of these skeletal deformities are largely prevented by regular transfusion, bone disease, as manifested by a varying degree of osteoporosis and its complications, remains an important problem for β-thalassaemia patients (Jensen *et al.* 1998).

Mechanisms

The pathophysiological mechanisms whereby expanded marrow causes bone deformity and osteoporosis are not known. There is a paucity of information about the histological features of the bones of thalassaemic patients. Pootrakul *et al.* (1981a) studied two patients with serial biopsies, metabolic measurements and ferrokinetic analyses. Limited histological data are reported, but there was evidence of healing as bone-marrow activity was reduced by transfusions. Rioja *et al.* (1990) examined iliac crest biopsies from 70 transfusion-dependent children. In each case radiological examination had revealed typical skeletal changes, including expansion of the medullary spaces and widespread osteoporosis; ricket-like lesions were not observed. Iron deposits were detected histochemically in the bone marrow, at

the marrow/bone interface, along cement lines and in mineralizing perimeters. Minor changes only were present in trabecular bone; osteomalacia was not observed. In contrast, the cortical bone exhibited severe osteoporotic changes, including fissures and focal defects in mineralization.

Virtually nothing is known about the mechanisms that underlie the relationship between hyperplasia of the bone marrow and skeletal pathology. The regulation of bone formation, a 'coupled' interaction between osteoblasts and osteocytes, is extremely complex and not fully understood. The stimulus for local remodelling appears to be a product, or products, of bone resorption and there is increasing evidence that cytokine release may be involved. Osteoblasts are responsive to many different cytokines (Smith 1996; Rodan 1998). Osteoclast activity, on the other hand, although regulated directly by hormones such as calcitonin, appears to be more passive and is controlled to a considerable degree by osteoblast activity, though the way these interactions are coupled is not clear. The recent discovery of osteoprotegerin and its ligand, which may play a major role in regulating bone mass, should enable rapid progress to be made in determining the mechanisms of this process (Simonet *et al.* 1997; Lacey *et al.* 1998). It is possible therefore that at least some of the stimuli to the remodelling and associated osteoporotic changes that occur in response to marrow expansion in β thalassaemia are mediated by locally produced cytokines, possibly the products of marrow cells. Whether the marked increase in vascularization associated with marrow hypertrophy also plays a role is equally uncertain.

To what extent is the bone disease of β thalassaemia related to additional metabolic disturbances? There is no evidence for a major abnormality of vitamin D metabolism in this disease (Dandona *et al.* 1987; Rioja *et al.* 1990). Clinical hypoparathyroidism with metabolic bone disease has been reported (Gabrielle 1971; Oberklaid & Seshadri 1975; Flynn *et al.* 1976) but is unlikely to be a factor in the large majority of cases. It has also been suggested that ascorbate deficiency secondary to iron overload plays a role in osteoporosis (Charlton & Bothwell 1976; Michelson & Cohen 1988); in Bantu populations with dietetic iron loading severe osteoporosis is a frequent complication. It is not clear, however, whether ascorbate deficiency plays a major part in the bone disease of β thalassaemia. Recently it has become clear that hypogonadism plays an important role in the genesis of the osteoporosis that is observed in patients with severe forms of β thalassaemia, particularly in those in whom there is evidence of severe iron loading (Fabbri *et al.* 1991; Anapliotou *et al.* 1995; Jensen *et al.* 1998). In two extensive series of patients with primary or secondary hypogonadism there was a reasonable correlation between gonadal function and the degree of osteoporosis. There is also some preliminary evidence that polymorphisms of the COLIAI and vitamin D receptor genes may play a role in modifying the likelihood of developing osteoporosis (see Chapter 7).

Clearly, therefore, much remains to be learnt about the pathophysiology of the skeletal deformities and thinning of the bones that occur in β thalassaemia. However, until more is known about the regulation of osteoblast and osteoclast activity, and the relationship between marrow hypertrophy and skeletal pathology, it may be very difficult to make further progress. What is becoming clear, however, is that hormonal deficiency secondary to iron loading, particularly if it involves the gonads via the hypothalamic/pituitary axis or, less commonly, the parathyroids, may contribute significantly (Wonke 1998). Whether variability at gene loci involved with bone or hormone metabolism is also important requires further study. Finally, as we shall discuss in Chapter 15, there is increasing evidence that long-term chelation therapy may also have important effects on growth and bone metabolism.

Bleeding, thrombosis and coagulation defects

Bleeding

The earlier literature on thalassaemia suggested that a bleeding tendency occurs occasionally in severely affected patients, particularly if they have not been adequately transfused. The most common problem is recurrent epistaxis (Hilgartner & Smith 1964; Esposito *et al.* 1976; Bertorello *et al.* 1977; Caocci *et al.* 1978). It has also been suggested that there is an increased incidence of intraocular haemorrhage (Toselli *et al.* 1969). In the study of Hilgartner and Smith no specific coagulation factor deficiencies could be demonstrated, despite poor liver function due to iron loading in some of their cases. Hypersplenism may be associated with severe thrombocytopenia and bleeding. In older, iron-loaded patients defective liver function with a prolonged prothrombin time may be responsi-

ble. Abnormal platelet function was observed in some of these early reports (Eldor 1978a,b).

Thrombotic complications

While recent reviews of coagulation in thalassaemia have stressed the importance of thrombotic complications, it is not clear how commonly they are encountered in practice. There were early reports of an increased frequency of transient ischaemic attacks and cerebrovascular accidents (Logothetis *et al.* 1972a; Sinniah *et al.* 1977; Paolini *et al.* 1983). However, many of these incidents occurred in severely anaemic children. Later, it was reported that both peripheral arterial and venous thromboses and an increase in pulmonary emboli found at autopsy are found quite frequently in splenectomized patients with HbE thalassaemia (Sonakul *et al.* 1980; Sumiyoshi *et al.* 1992). In a review of 735 Italian patients, 32 were reported to have experienced one or more important thromboembolic events (Borgna-Pignatti *et al.* 1998a).

Thrombotic mechanisms

It has been known for many years that after splenectomy there is an inverse relationship between the steady-state haemoglobin level and the platelet count; patients who remain anaemic tend to have a persistently high count and Hirsh and Dacie (1966) reported that they are at high risk for thromboembolism. A number of studies have examined the role of spontaneous platelet activation and aggregation, particularly after splenectomy (Winichagoon *et al.* 1981; Eldor *et al.* 1991; Laosombat *et al.* 1992; Opartkiattikul *et al.* 1992a; Del Principe *et al.* 1993). There appears to be a significant shortening of platelet lifespan in thalassaemic patients (Eldor *et al.* 1989). The notion that this might reflect increased activation and turnover was strengthened by the finding of significantly increased levels of urinary metabolites of thromboxane A2 and prostacyclin (Eldor *et al.* 1991).

It has also been observed that there is an increased interaction between thalassaemic red cells and endothelial cells (Butthep *et al.* 1992; Hovav *et al.* 1999) and evidence for an increased rate of activation of the coagulation system (Caocci *et al.* 1978; Mazzone *et al.* 1984; Cappellini *et al.* 1996; Ruf *et al.* 1997). Using thalassaemic red cells as a source of phospholipids, enhanced thrombin generation has been demonstrated in a prothrombinase assay (Borenstein-Ben Yashar *et al.* 1993; Cappellini *et al.* 1996). This procoagulant effect of thalassaemic red cells appears to be due to an increased expression of anionic phospholipids such as phosphatidylethanolamine and phosphatidylserine. This effect was also observed in studies using annexin V, a protein with a high affinity and specificity for these phospholipids which blocks the procoagulant effect of isolated thalassaemic red cells (Helley *et al.* 1996). It appears therefore that the procoagulant surface of thalassaemic red cells may accelerate thrombin generation *in vivo*, which, in turn, triggers platelet activation. Recent experimental studies have confirmed that this may be an important mechanism in the hypercoagulable state of β thalassaemia (Ruf *et al.* 1997).

Other coagulation changes have been observed in β thalassaemia. Some but not all studies have shown a reduction in antithrombin III, protein C and protein S (Musumeci *et al.* 1987; Leonardi *et al.* 1990; Shirahata *et al.* 1992). More recently it has been found that there are low levels of heparin cofactor II, a protein with similar properties to antithrombin III, a finding that can be reversed by blood transfusion (O'Driscoll *et al.* 1995). The mechanism for this change is also not clear; it could result from binding of the heparin cofactor to abnormal erythrocytes.

Recently, Eldor *et al.* (1999) have obtained evidence which suggests that the features of a chronic hypercoagulable state is present from early life in patients with β thalassaemia, and may contribute to later cardiac and pulmonary complications.

Is the hypercoagulable state important?

Although there seems little doubt that thalassaemic red cells have potential procoagulant properties, the frequency of clinical manifestations based on these laboratory abnormalities is still not clear. The recent Italian study of Borgna-Pignatti *et al.* (1998a), mentioned earlier, suggests that they may be commoner than hitherto realized. The case of splenectomized patients with HbE β thalassaemia in Thailand is also of particular interest in this context (see Chapter 9). In this setting there appears to be a definite increase in the frequency of pulmonary thromboembolic disease (Sonakul *et al.* 1988b). This study and the beautifully illustrated atlas produced by Sonakul (1989) reveal a complex pathology with pulmonary arterial obstructive lesions and evidence of thromboembolism (Fig. 5.11). These findings are associated with rather non-specific cardiopulmonary abnormalities (Israngkura *et al.* 1987) together with arterial hypoxia, which may or may not be reversed by aspirin, an observation which might implicate platelet aggregation in the genesis of the pulmonary artery lesions. Clearly the whole question of thrombotic vascular disease of the lungs and its cardiac consequences requires a great deal more study, not just in this group of patients but in other forms of β thalassaemia.

Infection

The risk of infection

Though an increased risk of infection in thalassaemia has been questioned (Valassi-Adam *et al.* 1976), and it has been the impression of clinicians that the incidence in early childhood is reduced by blood transfusion (Modell 1976), children still die from infection. In an attempt to assess its importance, Modell *et al.* (1980) reported on 48 episodes of serious infections among 129 patients with thalassaemia major and intermedia. The incidence of pneumonia was one for every 54 patient years, and for other serious infections was one for every 63 years. Severe infection was believed to be the primary cause of death in 10 of 55 patients who died with thalassaemia major.

The role of splenectomy

Undoubtedly, thalassaemic children are at increased risk of infection from iatrogenic causes; as we shall see later, infections derived from blood products, particularly viral hepatitis, are common in some populations. Carl Smith was the first to point out that splenectomy in young thalassaemic children may be followed by an increased incidence of severe and often overwhelming infection (Smith *et al.* 1962, 1964). The highest incidence is in the first 2 years after splenectomy and the greatest period of risk is in the first few years of life. The hazard of overwhelming infection after splenectomy, or in children with sickle-cell anaemia in whom splenic function is defective, has been confirmed in many studies (Eraklis *et al.* 1967; Erikson *et al.* 1968; Ein *et al.* 1977). Several organisms may be involved, although the encapsulated bacteria *S. pneumoniae*, *H. influenzae* and *N. meningitidis* are by far the most important. Very little is known about the pathogenesis. In a recent review

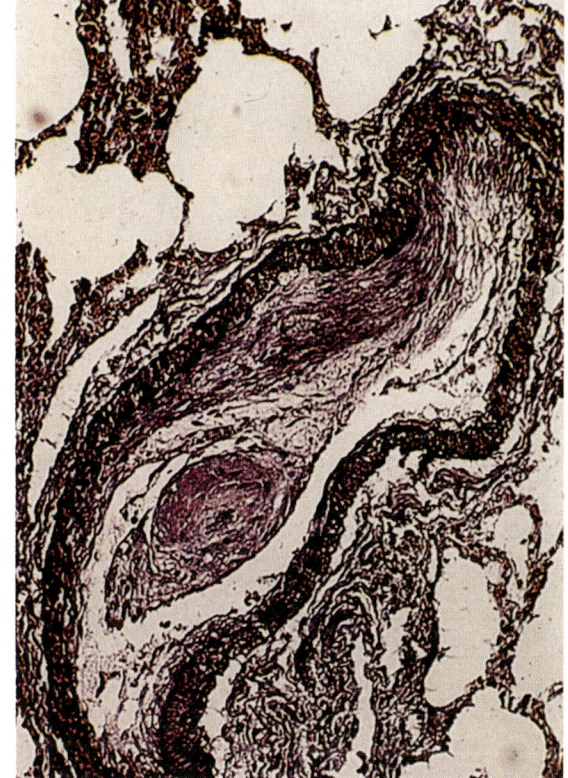

(a)

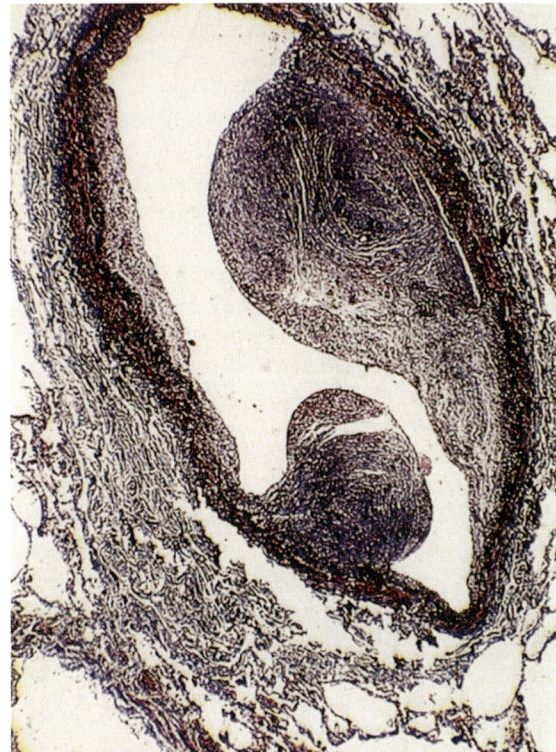

(b)

Cohen (1996) suggests that the two most important factors are the role of the spleen in generating an antibody response to polysaccharide antigens and its ability to act as a phagocytic filter, especially for the removal of damaged or senescent erythrocytes, an observation which may explain the association of increased rates of infection with babesia and malaria in certain populations. Other factors may play a role; there is evidence of complement dysfunction, and of defective production of tuftsin, a small peptide that has opsonic properties for bacteria. With the exception of work in Thailand (Wasi *et al.* 1971), studies that have examined immunoglobulin levels in splenectomized and non-splenectomized β thalassaemics have shown no significant difference (Caroline *et al.* 1969; Valassi-Adam *et al.* 1976; Constantoulakis *et al.* 1978).

The role of iron in infection

This is a difficult and contentious subject. In two critical reviews (Hershko & Weatherall 1988; Hershko *et al.* 1988) the evidence for this association was analysed in detail. It was concluded that iron overload is not associated with an impressive increase in the incidence or severity of bacterial infections. The one exception is infection with *Yersinia enterocolitica*, a normally non-virulent pathogen which is unable to produce its own siderophore but which has receptors for ferrioxamine and hence which may be pathogenic in the presence of iron bound to desferrioxamine (Robins-Browne & Prpic 1985).

Cellular and humoral immunity

Cell-mediated immunity has been examined by following skin responses to a variety of antigens; no differences between thalassaemic and normal children were observed (Suvatte *et al.* 1978). The same group demonstrated normal transforming properties of peripheral blood lymphocytes, both pre- and post-splenectomy. Neutrophil function tests have also

Fig. 5.11 Pulmonary arterial occlusion in HbE β thalassaemia. (a) Old thrombi forming a polypoid structure in a small artery. (b) Old thromboemboli forming 'cushions' attached to the walls of small arteries. Elastic-Masson stain, × 100. From Sonakul (1989), with permission.

been carried out before and after splenectomy, and found to be normal (Caroline *et al.* 1969; Genova *et al.* 1975; Tovo *et al.* 1977; Tuchinda *et al.* 1978). The distribution of circulating B and T lymphocytes is the same in thalassaemic patients as in controls of the same age (Kulapongs *et al.* 1978). These authors also noted a modest reduction in serum opsonic activity. Similar non-specific changes have been reported, including defects in the alternative pathway for complement (De Ciutiis *et al.* 1978), and increased levels of immune complexes (Casali *et al.* 1978) and inhibitors of granulopoiesis (Luban & Miller 1978).

Recently, more sophisticated approaches have been applied to study neutrophil and monocyte function and the modulation of natural killer cell activity, and to relate these activities to iron loading. There appears to be defective phagocytic and lytic activity of peripheral blood monocytes in β thalassaemics which is broadly correlated with the degree of iron loading (Ballart *et al.* 1986); the same association has been found for neutrophil dysfunction (Cantinieaux *et al.* 1987). Pittis *et al.* (1994) have noted defective phagolysosomal fusion in peripheral blood monocytes from thalassaemic patients, which can be partially corrected by iron chelation. Iron-loaded patients may also exhibit impaired neutrophil chemotaxis and migration (Matzner *et al.* 1993). Iron loading has also been related to defects in natural killer activity together with a subnormal cellular release of α interferon.

It is difficult to draw many firm conclusions about the pathophysiology of infection in β thalassaemia. Research in this field has been carried out in populations with widely differing states of nutrition and exposure to pathogens, and on very heterogeneous groups of patients. It is clear that splenectomy is an important risk factor and that iron-loaded patients who are treated with desferrioxamine are susceptible to infection with *Yersinia enterocolitica*; the relationship of this complication to chelation therapy is described in more detail in Chapter 15. Blood-borne infections, particularly viral, are also common in some populations (see Chapter 7). Beyond this we know very little. Indeed, it is not clear whether, with these exceptions, thalassaemic children are more prone to infection than any child with a chronic, debilitating disease.

Fetal haemoglobin production and other 'adaptive' factors

Fetal haemoglobin

Why is there persistent fetal haemoglobin production in β thalassaemia?

Although as we learn more about the mechanisms of fetal haemoglobin production in β thalassaemia it becomes increasingly difficult to regard it as an 'adaptive' process, nevertheless HbF makes up the bulk of such haemoglobin as is produced by many patients with the disease. Furthermore, the amount that is made plays a major role in determining its phenotypic severity. But why does fetal haemoglobin production persist after birth in the β thalassaemias to a greater extent than in almost any other disease?

In Chapter 2 we discussed what is known about the regulation of the switch from fetal to adult haemoglobin during normal human development. We saw how it is never quite complete; normal adults have small amounts of fetal haemoglobin in their blood, apparently confined to a subset of red cells which have been called 'F cells'. An 'F cell' is simply a red cell in which HbF can be demonstrated by chemical or immunological means. There is no evidence that it is derived from a separate stem-cell population and it is possible that most adult red cells contain some HbF but that it is only in F cells that it reaches detectable levels. What is clear is that the mechanism of suppression of γ-chain synthesis in adult life is, in effect, slightly 'leaky', and that the amount produced after the first year of life varies widely between different red-cell precursors, even though the level of HbF and the number of F cells is remarkably constant in each of us.

The relative numbers of F cells in the blood may increase in response to some types of acute erythroid hyperplasia and increased red-cell turnover, or 'stress erythropoiesis' as it is sometimes called. For example, there is an increase in the middle of pregnancy at the time when the red-cell mass is rapidly expanding (Boyer *et al.* 1975; Popat *et al.* 1977), in patients recovering after myelotoxic treatment for leukaemia (Sheridan *et al.* 1976) or after bone-marrow transplantation (Alter *et al.* 1976c), and in babies following transient erythroblastopenias (Alter *et al.* 1979b), or after infection (Boyer & Dover 1979). A more dramatic response is observed in baboons made anaemic by venesection (De Simone *et al.* 1978, 1979). On the other hand, it does not usually rise in patients with chronic, well compensated haemolytic anaemias, although modest increases have been reported in patients with severe megaloblastic anaemia (Beaven *et al.* 1960).

These observations suggest therefore that in certain conditions of 'erythroid stress', reflecting regeneration or hyperplasia, and in some forms of dyserythropoiesis with maturational arrest, the propensity to produce HbF may be increased (Beaven *et al.* 1960). Stamatoyannopoulos *et al.* (1987) have suggested that F cells represent the progeny of progenitor cells which have undergone an 'accelerated' pathway of erythroid differentiation. Normally, very few cells follow this route, but under conditions of increased erythroid demand a higher proportion do so, leading to an increased number of F cells and higher levels of HbF.

The other observation that is particularly relevant to the problem of HbF production in β thalassaemia is that red-cell precursors and their progeny that synthesize relatively more γ chains enjoy preferential survival, in both the marrow and peripheral blood. Evidence that this is the case has been outlined in earlier sections of this chapter. In short, the *in vivo* turnover of HbF is much slower than that of HbA (Gabuzda *et al.* 1963). Globin synthesis studies indicate that there is a selective survival of cells that are synthesizing HbF, in both the blood and marrow (Weatherall *et al.* 1974b), and differential centrifugation studies show that the older, longer-surviving cell populations in the blood of β thalassaemics contain significantly more HbF than younger cell populations (Loukopoulos & Fessas 1965; Nathan & Gunn 1966; Weatherall *et al.* 1979) (Fig. 5.12).

In severe β thalassaemia, therefore, those cells which synthesize relatively more γ chains, and hence in which there is less globin imbalance, are selected, both in the bone marrow and in the blood. Because there is wide variation in the amount of γ-chain synthesis between different red-cell precursors there is a marked heterogeneity of cell populations in the peripheral blood with respect to the amount of HbF that they contain; the higher the concentration, the greater chance they have of surviving. The reason for the differences in the level of γ-chain production between different red-cell precursors is not clear. Perhaps it is simply a reflection of the heterogeneity of the cellular distribution of HbF that occurs in normal people after the first year of life.

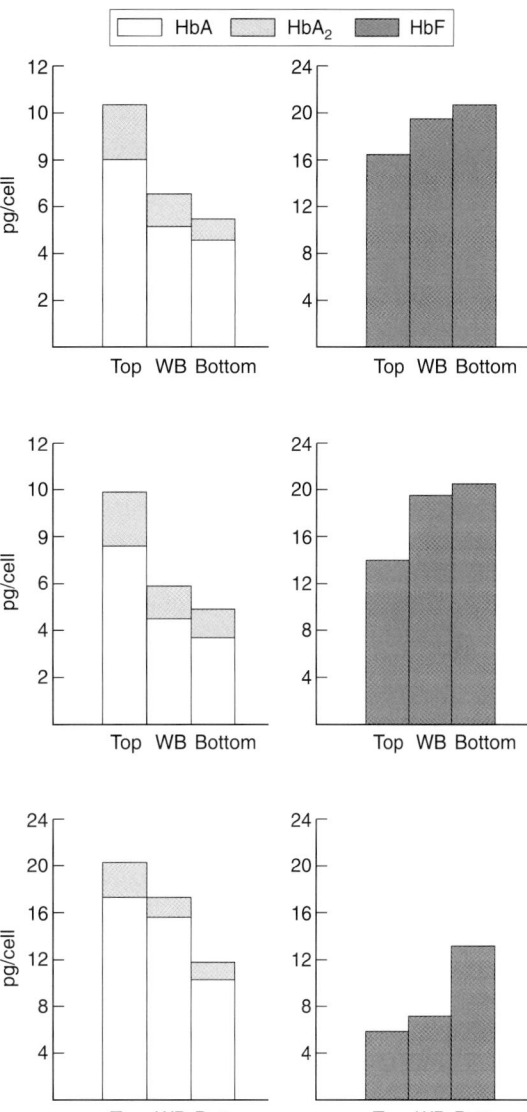

Fig. 5.12 Differential centrifugation experiments showing the heterogeneous distribution of haemoglobins F and A$_2$ among the red cells of three patients with severe β$^+$ thalassaemia intermedia. WB, whole blood uncentrifuged. Clearly the denser cell population contains relatively more HbF while the lighter population contains relatively more HbA$_2$. From Weatherall *et al.* (1979).

Based on these observations, in previous editions of this book and elsewhere we set out a theoretical model to account for the production of fetal haemoglobin in β thalassaemia (Weatherall 1976; Weatherall *et al.* 1977). As mentioned earlier, the small amount of fetal haemoglobin in normal adults, found in approximately 5% of the peripheral blood cells, constitutes approximately 150 mg HbF/dl of whole blood. If a patient with severe β thalassaemia synthesizes no more fetal haemoglobin than normal, but simply expands their total erythroid mass by 10–30-fold they would be capable of producing up to 4.5 g/dl of HbF. Within this expanded bone marrow, many of the red-cell precursors do not survive. But those that synthesize relatively more γ chains come under intense selection. Combining these mechanisms it is undoubtedly possible to account for the production of 2–4 g/dl of HbF, particularly if the increased drive to erythropoiesis also makes γ-chain synthesis more likely, as occurs in other conditions of erythroid 'stress'. In short, the red cells in severe β thalassaemia represent the tip of the erythropoietic iceberg, a highly selected population, many of which only survive to reach the circulation because of their relatively high content of HbF. These considerations can account for the elevation of HbF in severe β thalassaemics without the need to invoke even more complicated mechanisms.

The concept that the red cells of the profoundly anaemic, untransfused β-thalassaemic patient are the end product of intense selection in a stressed, dyserythropoietic marrow is supported by globin synthesis studies on the blood of patients with HbE thalassaemia who have received transfusions to maintain their haemoglobins at a near-normal level. They synthesize α, γ and βᴱ chains; the relative amount of γ-chain production is markedly reduced after transfusion (Rees *et al.* 1998b). Thus it appears that the relatively high levels of HbF which are nearly always found in this condition require both erythroid expansion and the selective survival of precursors that are synthesizing relatively more HbF; if these conditions are reversed by transfusion the red-cell precursors show a more typical pattern of adult globin-chain synthesis.

Why does the output of fetal haemoglobin vary so much?

While providing an explanation for the baseline output of HbF in β thalassaemia, these mechanisms do not explain the wide variation in the amount produced. There is growing evidence that much of this is genetically determined. This should not surprise us; the level of fetal haemoglobin and the percentage of F cells in healthy people is under genetic control (Popat *et al.* 1977; Garner *et al.* 2000). In addition, there are other genetic factors that can modify fetal haemoglobin production in patients with β thalassaemia (Table 5.4), all of which are described in greater detail in other parts of this book. Particular β-thalassaemia mutations, notably those that involve small deletions of the 5′ end of the β-globin gene, are associated with higher levels of fetal haemoglobin production than single-point mutations of the β-globin gene. There are a variety of different *cis*-acting forms of hereditary persistence of fetal haemoglobin (HPFH), other forms of HPFH that are not encoded in the β-globin-gene cluster, and many different deletions that give rise to δβ thalassaemia or HPFH, all of which are associated with much higher levels of γ-chain production and, incidentally, much milder phenotypes. There is also some modest post-translational tuning of the level of HbF; α chains have a greater affinity for β than γ chains and if they are in short supply, due to co-existent α thalassaemia for example, the relative amounts of HbA and HbF may be modified in β thalassaemia.

The picture that is emerging, therefore, is that the remarkably variable levels of HbF in β thalassaemia are the result of erythroid hyperplasia and cell selec-

Table 5.4 Some mechanisms of haemoglobin F production in β thalassaemia.

Basic mechanisms
Erythroid hyperplasia and expansion of marrow
?Ineffective erythropoiesis
Selective survival of F cells

Individual variability
Genetic
   Variability in F cells
   Particular β-thalassaemia mutations*
   Co-inheritance of hereditary persistence of fetal
      haemoglobin†
Acquired
   Cytotoxic agents. Butyrate analogues‡

* See Chapter 7.
† See Chapter 10.
‡ See Chapter 15.

tion set in a background of many different genetic (and possibly environmental) factors that can modify γ-chain production after the neonatal period. This problem, which is central to current thalassaemia research because of its therapeutic implications, is discussed in greater detail in Chapters 4, 10, 13 and 15.

Compensation for the anaemia of β thalassaemia

A complex battery of compensatory mechanisms are normally brought into play in response to anaemia (Weatherall 1996). Lowering the haemoglobin concentration reduces proportionally the oxygen-carrying capacity of the blood. In response, there is an increase in the production of erythrocyte 2,3-diphosphoglycerate (2,3-DPG), which shifts the dissociation curve to the right, so enhancing tissue oxygen delivery. With increasing severity of anaemia there is a progressive increase in 2,3-DPG, which may facilitate oxygen delivery by as much as 40% for the same haemoglobin concentration. A price is paid for this adaptive function, however. In effect, it results in a lower venous oxygen content and hence a lower reserve of oxygen available for further increase in oxygen demand, as might occur on exercise for example.

It seems likely that moderate anaemia is compensated for mainly by a shift in the oxygen dissociation curve. However, when the haemoglobin level falls below 7–8 g/dl there is an increase in cardiac output, both at rest and after exercise. There is an associated increase in stroke rate; a hyperkinetic circulation develops, characterized by tachycardia, arterial and capillary pulsation, a wide pulse pressure and haemic (flow) murmurs. Studies involving orthostatic stress or the administration of pressor amines suggest that redistribution of blood volume and vasodilatation with reduced afterload play a dominant role in the hyperkinetic response to chronic anaemia.

These compensatory mechanisms may be impaired in β thalassaemia. Red cells containing relatively large amounts of HbF have a reduced p50, i.e. a higher oxygen affinity, than cells containing HbA. This is because HbF interacts with 2,3-DPG much less readily than with HbA. Some information about HbF and 2,3-DPG values in a small series of patients with β thalassaemia intermedia that were studied in the author's laboratory is summarized in Table 5.5. Clearly, they are at a distinct disadvantage because they are unable to compensate for their anaemia by a

Table 5.5 Oxygen dissociation analysis (pH 7.4, P_{CO_2} 40 mmHg, 37°C) on blood samples from four untransfused homozygous β thalassaemics.

Hb (g/dl)	HbF (%)	p50
5.7	61.6	23.0
10.5	70.0	22.0
8.3	79.0	23.0
4.1	96.8*	18.5

* Patient homozygous for β^0 thalassaemia. (The normal p50 range is 27–32 mmHg.)

right shift in their oxygen dissociation curve; all of them have high levels of HbF and p50 values which are *lower* than normal.

Gallo *et al.* (1970) and de Furia *et al.* (1974) have studied the oxygen dissociation curves and 2,3-DPG concentrations in a series of transfused thalassaemics. They also found inappropriately low p50 values and 2,3-DPG concentrations for the diminished red-cell mass. They suggest that these abnormalities are due to increased levels of HbF and postulate that there might also be decreased 2,3-DPG synthesis due to abnormal glucose metabolism in thalassaemic cells. Correra *et al.* (1984) found inappropriately low red-cell 2,3-DPG and p50 values in transfused β thalassaemics and suggested that the red cells of chronically transfused patients may be unable to adapt to the decline in haemoglobin that occurs during the inter-transfusion interval.

Thus anaemic patients with β thalassaemia cannot compensate to the same degree as those with other forms of anaemia. For example, a patient with sickle-cell anaemia, because of the low oxygen affinity of HbS, is able to compensate for anaemia by a right shift in the oxygen dissociation curve; i.e., they can oxygenate their tissues more readily at a given haemoglobin level. Although it is not absolutely clear how important these adaptive mechanisms are in practice, and they may be less so in well-transfused patients, they undoubtedly are of importance in patients with thalassaemia intermedia with particularly high levels of HbF and in those whose cardiac function is compromised by iron loading.

The α thalassaemias

The pathophysiology of the α thalassaemias has much in common with the β thalassaemias. In this section we shall focus on the main differences between the two, which stem largely from the properties of the globin that is produced in excess. As is the case for the β thalassaemias, the broad principles of the pathophysiology of the α thalassaemias are quite well understood, though a number of problems remain to be worked out.

The clinical phenotypes of α thalassaemia reflect the degree of defective α-chain synthesis and are best understood in terms of gene dosage effects. As we saw in the previous chapter, there are two major classes, α^+ and α^0 thalassaemia, in which either one or both of the linked α-globin genes are inactivated, either by a deletion (–) or by a mutation (T). Loss of a single α-globin gene, $-\alpha/\alpha\alpha$ or $\alpha^T\alpha/\alpha\alpha$, has virtually no effect on the phenotype. The heterozygous state for α^0 thalassaemia, $--/\alpha\alpha$, or the homozygous state for α^+ thalassaemia, $-\alpha/-\alpha$ or $\alpha^T\alpha/\alpha^T\alpha$, results in a very similar phenotype to the carrier state for β thalassaemia. Loss of three of the four α-globin genes, $-\alpha/--$ or $\alpha^T\alpha/--$, results in a disorder of moderate severity, HbH disease. Finally, the homozygous state for α^0 thalassaemia, $--/--$, is incompatible with survival, the Hb Bart's hydrops syndrome.

The fundamental defect in α thalassaemia is, like β thalassaemia, imbalanced globin synthesis. However, there are two major pathophysiological differences between the conditions. First, since α chains are shared by both fetal and adult haemoglobin the α thalassaemias, unlike the β thalassaemias, are manifest in fetal life, and cells that synthesize HbF do not come under selection. Second, the properties of the excess γ and β chains that are synthesized consequent on defective α-chain production are quite different from the excess α chains that are produced in β thalassaemia (Fig. 5.13). Rather than precipitating in the red-cell precursors they form the soluble tetramers, γ_4, Hb Bart's, and β_4, HbH. Finally, because the α-globin genes are duplicated and the α thalassaemias reflect a broad spectrum of gene dosage effects, as outlined above, we can expect a wider range of phenotypes as a direct reflection of the underlying molecular pathology.

Globin-chain imbalance

The relative rates of α- and β-chain production have been studied in reticulocytes and bone marrow obtained from patients with each of the clinical phenotypes of α thalassaemia as outlined above

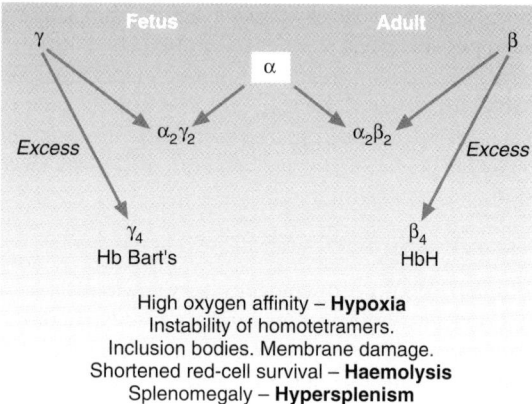

Fig. 5.13 An outline of the pathophysiology of α thalassaemia.

(Weatherall *et al.* 1965; Clegg & Weatherall 1967; Kan *et al.* 1968; Schwartz *et al.* 1969; Weatherall & Clegg 1969; Clegg *et al.* 1971b; Knox-Macaulay *et al.* 1972; Shchory & Ramot 1972; Ramot *et al.* 1973; Russo *et al.* 1973b; Wood & Stamatoyannopoulos 1976–77; Hunt *et al.* 1980). In all these studies there was marked imbalance of globin synthesis, with an excess of non-α chains compatible with the degree of severity of the clinical phenotype.

In a study of globin synthesis in the peripheral blood reticulocytes and nucleated red cells of a liveborn baby with the Hb Bart's hydrops syndrome, i.e. homozygous for α^0 thalassaemia, it was found that only γ- and β-chain production could be demonstrated; there was no α-chain synthesis (Weatherall *et al.* 1970). Similar findings were reported by Sophocleous *et al.* (1981). Surprisingly, although these infants had approximately 20% of the embryonic haemoglobin, Hb Portland ($\zeta_2\gamma_2$), in the peripheral blood, no radioactively labelled ζ chains could be demonstrated. This may reflect the particular method used for separation of the globins, or it may indicate that there is heterogeneity among the red-cell populations of these babies and that those with relatively large amounts of embryonic haemoglobin survive longer than those with lower levels.

In the first studies of globin synthesis in HbH disease, it was also possible to examine the kinetics of globin production in the face of β-chain excess (Weatherall *et al.* 1965; Clegg & Weatherall 1967). Overall, it was found that there is a marked imbalance, with α-/β-chain synthesis ratios of 0.2–0.5, with a mean of about 0.4. However, if, after incubation of reticulocytes with radioactive amino acids, HbA and HbH were first separated, there was much more radioactive labelling of the α chains than the β chains of HbA. This indicated that there is a relatively large intracellular pool of β chains and that these combine with newly synthesized α chains as they become available. It was also observed that the specific activities of the β chains were very much greater than those of the α chains. This suggested that labelled HbH, or the total intracellular pool of β chains, were not present in the amounts that would be expected from their levels in the peripheral blood, thus providing unequivocal evidence of intracellular destruction of HbH during the lifespan of the red cells (Fig. 5.14).

In a subsequent study, in which globin synthesis was examined both in bone-marrow cells of different ages separated by centrifugation and in peripheral blood reticulocytes, Wood and Stamatoyannopoulos (1976–77) found that the α-/β-chain production ratio is constant at all stages of erythroid maturation in HbH disease.

These findings provided a fairly clear picture of the synthesis of HbA and HbH in HbH disease. In short, there is imbalanced globin synthesis and the resulting excess of β chains exist in two forms: the majority form β₄ tetramers but there is also an intracellular pool of β chains which are capable of combining with newly made α chains as they become available. In addition, there is clear-cut evidence that HbH must be lost from red cells during their time in the circulation.

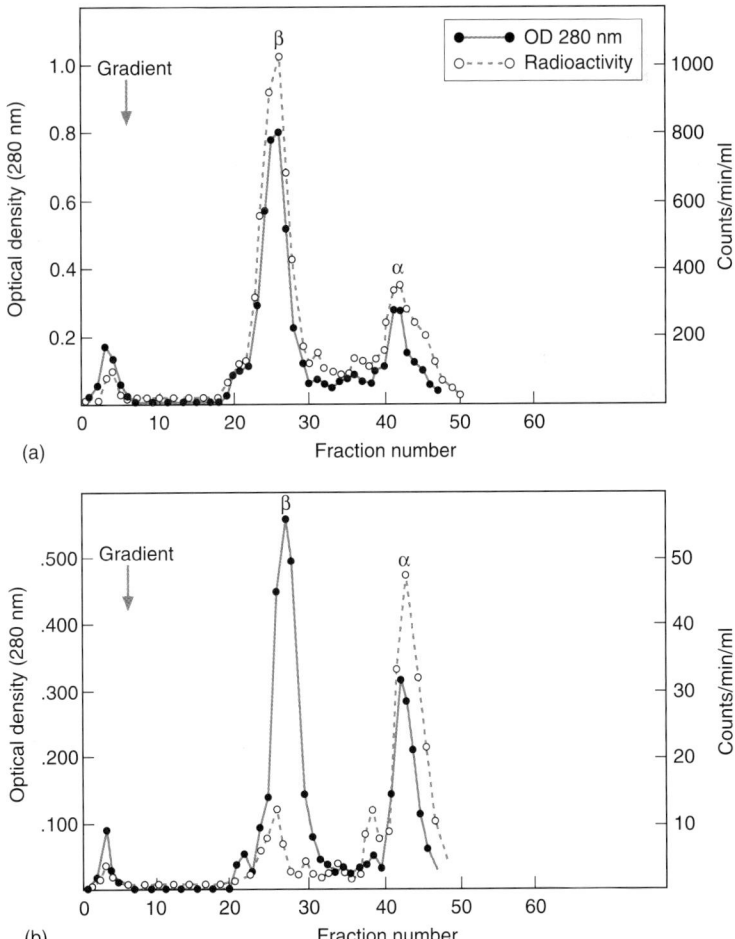

Fig. 5.14 Globin synthesis in HbH disease. (a) Red cells were incubated for 60 min together with radioactive leucine and the globins separated by CM-cellulose chromatography (see Fig. 5.2). The elution profiles are shown; clearly there is a marked deficiency of α-chain synthesis. (b) A similar experiment to that described in (a) except that, after incubating the reticulocytes, Hbs A and H were separated by column chromatography and then the globin subunits of HbA were separated under the same conditions as described above. There is now very much more radioactive labelling of the α chains than the β chains. This result indicates that newly synthesized α chains combine with unlabelled β chains from a large intracellular pool of the latter to synthesize HbA. Thus the excess β chains in the red cells of patients with HbH disease exist both as HbH (β₄) and as a small pool capable of combining with newly made α chains.

Globin synthesis in what we now know must have been heterozygotes for α^0 or α^+ thalassaemia was reported by Kan *et al.* (1968), Schwartz *et al.* (1969), Pootrakul *et al.* (1975a) and Hunt *et al.* (1980). All these studies showed some degree of globin imbalance, although there was overlap between α^0 and α^+ thalassaemia heterozygotes with respect to the α-/β-chain synthesis ratios (see Chapter 11).

The consequences of defective α-globin synthesis

Homotetramer formation

As we saw in Chapter 1, it was appreciated early during the development of knowledge about the heterogeneity of the thalassaemias that the excess β and γ chains that result from defective α-chain production are able to form homotetramers rather than precipitate like the excess α chains in β thalassaemia. Haemoglobin H was first described in 1955 (Gouttas *et al.* 1955; Rigas *et al.* 1955) and shown to be a tetramer of normal β chains, β_4, by Jones *et al.* (1959). Haemoglobin Bart's was first identified by Ager and Lehmann (1958) and later shown to be a tetramer of normal γ chains, γ_4, by Hunt and Lehmann (1959) and Kekwick and Lehmann (1960).

The notion that HbH and Hb Bart's might reflect defective α-chain synthesis in adult and fetal life was formally set out by Ingram and Stretton (1959) and Ramot *et al.* (1959). While this hypothesis was attractive, subsequent studies disclosed a puzzling dilemma: several workers observed that babies who had increased levels of Hb Bart's in their cord blood, in the 2–10% range, if followed into later life did not produce detectable amounts of HbH (Minnich *et al.* 1962; Weatherall & Boyer 1962; Weatherall 1963; Pootrakul *et al.* 1967b, 1970). It was suggested that perhaps these babies might be carriers for milder forms of α thalassaemia, and an argument to explain the non-appearance of HbH was developed along the following lines. During the neonatal period, at the time of the switch from fetal to adult haemoglobin production, both γ and β chains are competing for available α chains. Hence a mild deficiency of α chains will become evident during this stage of development and be reflected by a small excess of γ chains, particularly as α chains bind β chains in preference to γ chains. Indeed, using sensitive electrophoretic methods, traces of Hb Bart's can be found in many

normal babies at the time of birth (Fessas & Mastrokalos 1959; Weatherall 1963; Huehns *et al.* 1964a). Once the switch from γ- to β-chain production is complete, the deficiency of α chains may be too small to produce detectable amounts of HbH (Weatherall 1963). This concept was useful in that it led to the notion that the neonatal period might be the most useful time to demonstrate the α-thalassaemia carrier state. Later studies, in which it was possible to analyse the α-globin genes directly, confirmed that this concept is correct, though showed that not all babies heterozygous for α^+ thalassaemia, the mildest form of the condition, have levels of Hb Bart's at birth which are detectable by standard electrophoretic methods.

The properties of haemoglobin homotetramers

Haemoglobin H shows no haem/haem interaction or Bohr effect and has an oxygen affinity 10 times that of HbA. The oxygen dissociation curve of purified HbH resembles a rectangular hyperbola (Benesch *et al.* 1961). The curve of whole blood from patients with HbH disease may show two components due to the combined presence of HbA and HbH. Consequently, patients carrying large amounts of HbH have a whole-blood oxygen dissociation curve which is shifted to the left; less oxygen is given up at physiological tensions, a factor which causes a reduced capacity to compensate for the anaemia associated with HbH disease. 2,3-Diphosphoglycerate binds equally to the oxy and deoxy forms of HbH (Benesch *et al.* 1968a,b). In other words the interaction of 2,3-DPG with HbH is not oxygen linked. This is because HbH does not change its quaternary conformation on oxygenation.

Haemoglobin H is unstable and thermolabile (Scott *et al.* 1970). It contains two reactive SH groups per β chain; the β chains in HbA have only one reactive SH group, in the oxy form. Gabuzda (1966) suggested that the relative susceptibility of HbH to oxidation might result from the presence of the eight free thiols, which could confer a lower net reduction–oxidation potential on the molecule.

The temporal pattern of the precipitation of HbH in red cells was studied in detail by Rigas and Koler (1961) and by Nathan and Gunn (1966). The former workers pointed out that single preformed inclusions of HbH are only seen in the peripheral blood after splenectomy (Fig. 5.15). Furthermore, when they and, later, Nathan and Gunn separated the red cells of patients with HbH disease into different age popula-

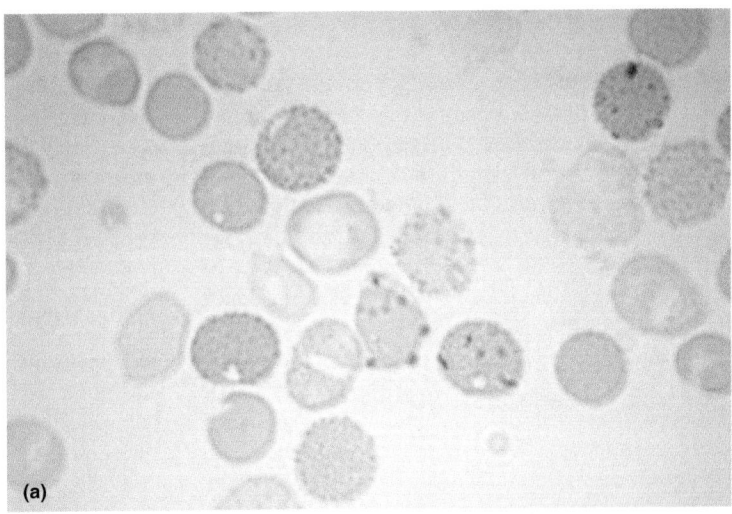

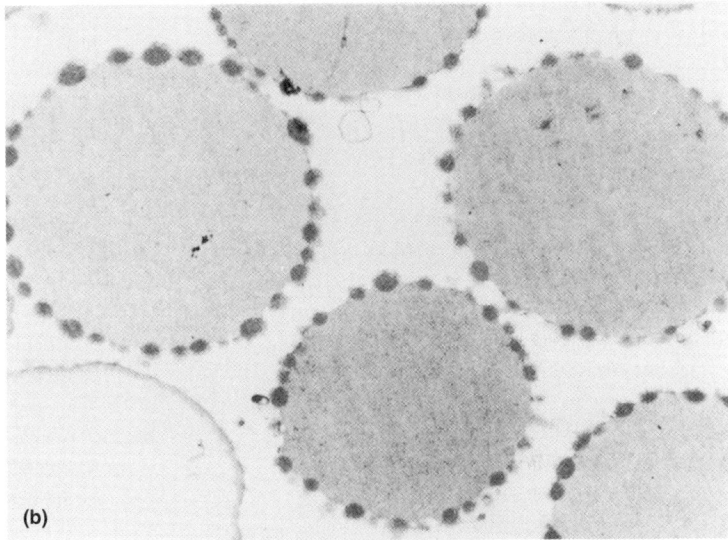

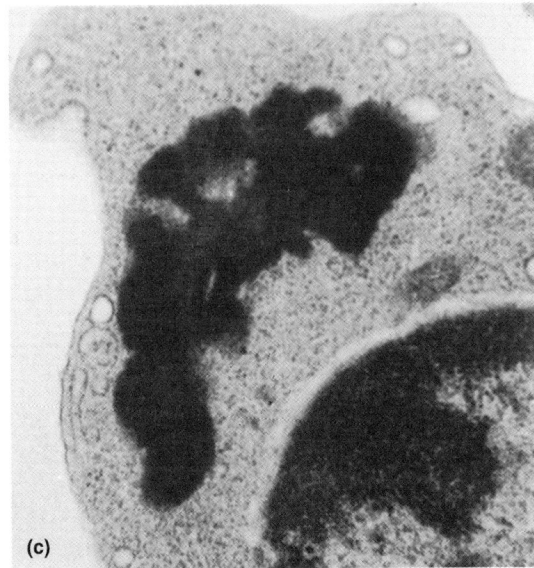

Fig. 5.15 HbH inclusions. (a) Multiple inclusions generated by incubation of red cells with brilliant cresyl blue. A few large inclusions, which are most easily seen after staining with methyl violet and which only appear in large numbers in the peripheral blood after splenectomy, are also present. (b) An electron micrograph of the inclusion bodies generated by brilliant cresyl blue in the cells of a patient with HbH disease ($\times 6425$). (c) Precipitation of HbH in erythroblasts from the bone marrow of a patient with HbH disease ($\times 14\,300$). The electron-microscopy preparations were kindly supplied by Professor Sunitha Wickramasinghe.

tions by centrifugation, it was found that the pre-formed inclusions are mainly in the older, denser cell populations, while soluble HbH is much more abundant in the younger, lighter cells and is absent or considerably reduced in the older cells. Rigas and Koler demonstrated that the rate of inclusion-body formation was greatly accelerated in the presence of agents such as amyl or sodium nitrite which produce methaemoglobin; this effect was counteracted by the addition of reduced glutathione or sodium ascorbate. It was discovered later that, as in the case of excess α-globin chains in β thalassaemia, the generation of HbH is associated with haemichrome formation (Rachmilewitz 1969; Rachmilewitz *et al.* 1969). The notion that HbH precipitates during the lifespan of red cells is compatible with *in vivo* labelling experiments in which it has been found that it has a much faster turnover and disappears from the circulation much more rapidly than HbA (Gabuzda *et al.* 1965).

As we shall discuss later, the precipitation of HbH is not confined to the older erythrocytes in the peripheral blood. It seems likely that once a HbH tetramer is formed it survives its passage through the bone marrow and into the peripheral blood, where it tends to precipitate in older red cells. On the other hand, some of the excess of β chains that are synthesized in the marrow become associated with the red-cell precursor membrane. We shall see how these processes contribute to the pattern of anaemia of α thalassaemia in the next section.

Less is known about the properties of Hb Bart's. It has an extremely high oxygen affinity and no haem/haem interaction or Bohr effect (Horton *et al.* 1962), findings very similar to those for HbH. In the red cell it oxygenates independently from HbA (Bellingham & Huehns 1968). However, it is thought not to be as unstable as HbH. Newborn infants with relatively high levels of Hb Bart's do not have HbH-like inclusions and differential centrifugation experiments have not shown a major loss in older cell populations (unpublished data). A possible explanation for its greater stability was offered by Rachmilewitz and Harari (1972), who demonstrated that the rate of haemichrome formation of Hb Bart's is considerably slower than for HbH.

These abnormal properties of the haemoglobin homotetramers of α thalassaemia are of profound importance in determining its pathophysiology. Particularly in the Hb Bart's hydrops syndrome, and to a lesser degree in HbH disease, patients may have a considerable proportion of their haemoglobin in this form. Hence the oxygen-carrying capacity of their blood may be seriously compromised; while their haemoglobin levels may appear to be relatively high, a considerable proportion of what is being measured is physiologically useless.

Globin imbalance and mechanisms of anaemia

The mechanisms of the anaemia of α thalassaemia are fundamentally different from those in β thalassaemia. As we saw earlier in this chapter, the latter is characterized by major intramedullary destruction of red-cell precursors with ineffective erythropoiesis, while the haemolytic component is probably less important. It appears that in α thalassaemia the ability to produce soluble tetramers from excess γ or β chains results in more effective erythropoiesis and hence haemolysis plays a more important role.

From the limited erythrokinetic studies that have been reported in patients with HbH disease it is apparent that red-cell production is considerably more effective than in severe β thalassaemia, although there is still a significant degree of ineffective erythropoiesis (Pearson & McFarland 1962). Red-cell survival, as judged by ^{51}Cr studies, is shortened, reported figures ranging from 8 to 17 days for the ^{51}Cr half-life (Rigas & Koler 1961; Pearson & McFarland 1962; Woodrow *et al.* 1964; Knox-Macaulay *et al.* 1972; Tso *et al.* 1982). Initially there were concerns about the validity of these data because of uncertainty about the rate of elution of ^{51}Cr from HbH, but later studies did not suggest that there is a significant loss of the isotope from the red cells (Tso *et al.* 1982). The pattern of red-cell survival curves is much more uniform than that found in β thalassaemia, reflecting the more homogeneous nature of the cell populations that are being destroyed (Malamos *et al.* 1962; Nathan & Gunn 1966). External scanning studies have shown that the spleen is the site of much of the red-cell destruction (Rigas & Koler 1961; Woodrow *et al.* 1964).

These observations, while they suggest that haemolysis is the predominant mechanism of the anaemia of α thalassaemia, at least in HbH disease, raise questions about the pattern of erythropoiesis in this condition. Earlier studies using light microscopy showed that there are a few inclusion bodies even in the red-cell precursors (Fessas & Yataganis 1968). On electron microscopy they appear to be highly condensed, branching intracytoplasmic bodies, which can be seen in early and late polychromatic erythroblasts and reticulocytes (Fig. 5.15). Autoradiographic analysis has also demonstrated the addition of newly synthesized protein, possibly β chains, into these inclusions (Wickramasinghe *et al.* 1980). In mature erythrocytes the pattern of the inclusions is different from that observed in β thalassaemia.

Clearly the precipitation of HbH during the lifespan of the red cell is a dynamic and complex process. The biosynthetic studies of Weatherall *et al.* (1965) showed that both free β chains and β_4 tetramers are present in the red cells of patients with HbH disease. It seems likely that once soluble tetramers have formed they are relatively stable until later in the lifespan of the red cell. On the other hand, it is clear that some free β chains precipitate early in the red-cell precursors and may be responsible for the element of ineffective erythropoiesis that has been described in this condition. The pattern of anaemia, haemolytic rather than dyserythropoietic, may reflect the relative rate of stable homotetramer formation compared with loss of excess β chains on the membranes of red-cell precursors.

Mechanisms of red-cell damage

Mechanical destruction

We have seen how HbH precipitates during the ageing of the red cells to form large single Heinz bodies. Early ultrastructural studies focused on the mechanisms of removal of these cells by the spleen (Wennberg & Weiss 1968). Two major mechanisms were demonstrated. First, the intracellular precipitates are removed and, second and more commonly, the red cells appear to be split into two or more fragments during their passage from splenic cords to sinuses. These elegant studies describe how relatively large hypochromic cells can be divided into two small, dense cells, leaving behind fragments which may be phagocytosed by splenic macrophages. In short, they provide a mechanical basis for how the spleen removes preformed inclusions and for the poikilocytosis which is seen after splenectomy.

Metabolic changes

Damage to the red-cell membranes in HbH disease is reflected by a variety of metabolic abnormalities

(Gabuzda 1966; Nathan *et al.* 1969; Scott *et al.* 1970; Knox-Macaulay *et al.* 1972). The rates of glucose utilization and lactate formation are increased and both young and old cells have increased cation permeability, the most marked changes being in the older populations which contain single inclusion bodies in splenectomized individuals. Red-cell ATP levels are normal or slightly reduced but fall more rapidly than normal after sterile incubation. These cells also have an increased rate of methaemoglobin production. Reduced glutathione (GSH) levels are also lower in the old cell populations as is hexose monophosphate shunt (HMPS) activity. It has been suggested that, since HbH is particularly sensitive to oxidative precipitation, its reactive thiols may participate in cellular reduction reactions and thus substitute for glutathione. Thus HMPS activity would be reduced in a situation in which glutathione is spared, i.e. in the younger cell population, but be increased with cell ageing as HbH precipitates and becomes less available. The totally unexpected finding of elevated glutathione peroxidase levels (Beutler *et al.* 1977) has never been adequately explained.

Membrane damage

More recent studies have focused on the mechanisms of red-cell membrane damage in α thalassaemia, how these differ from β thalassaemia, and their consequences (Schrier *et al.* 1989; Shinar *et al.* 1989; Advani *et al.* 1992a; Schrier 1994, 1997).

The mechanisms of membrane damage by excess α chains in β thalassaemia were reviewed earlier in this chapter. They include the formation of haemichromes with direct damage to the red-cell membrane and the action of haemoglobin degradation products in causing oxidative damage to a variety of membrane structures. It turns out that, while the red-cell membranes in β thalassaemia are more mechanically unstable, possibly due to oxidation of protein (band) 4.1, in α thalassaemia the membranes are hyperstable and there is no evidence of oxidation or any dysfunction of this protein. Furthermore, the state of cellular hydration is different in the two forms of thalassaemia. Accumulation of excess α chains in β thalassaemia leads to cellular dehydration, whereas accumulation of β chains in α thalassaemia appears to result in increased hydration (Schrier *et al.* 1989; Olivieri *et al.* 1992e; Bunyaratvej *et al.* 1994). It has been suggested that these findings reflect the results of the action of different kinds of oxidized globin chains on the K^+–Cl^- cotransporter, and possibly on other transport pathways.

The mechanical properties of red cells induced by free α or β chains have been studied in normal red cells loaded with haem-containing globin (Scott *et al.* 1990; Shalev *et al.* 1996). It was found that entrapment of α chains causes a significant decrease in cellular and membrane deformability, associated with reduced amounts of spectrin and ankyrin, and a decrease in membrane-reactive thiol groups. On the other hand, the entrapment of β chains does not result in any significant changes in membrane protein function or thiol concentrations, but causes changes in cellular deformability, similar to those described in the red cells of patients with HbH disease by Schrier *et al.* (1989).

Because the cytoplasmic domain of band 3 of the red-cell membrane is the high-affinity binding site for native haemoglobin, as well as for its denatured metabolites, its interaction with β globin in α thalassaemia is of particular interest. It has been found to be abnormal in red cells of patients with HbH disease, with a similar pattern to that found in other unstable haemoglobin disorders (Shinar *et al.* 1989). These observations have been augmented by *in vitro* studies which examined the same spectrin–ankyrin band 3 interactions using entrapped α or β globin in normal red-cell membranes (Shalev *et al.* 1995). It was shown that inside-out vesicles (IOVs) derived from membranes incubated with β globin bound only 4% as much spectrin as IOVs from unincubated control membranes. On the hand, IOVs from membranes incubated with α chains were almost normal, that is, they bound between 83 and 86% of control values.

Shinar and Rachmilewitz (1993) have offered a possible explanation for the differences in behaviour between α and β subunits in the thalassaemias and related disorders. They suggest that the larger β subunits, which precipitate in α thalassaemia and in unstable β-chain haemoglobinopathies, tend to bind more tightly to protein band 3, the 'native' binding site on the membrane. On the other hand, the small α subunits, which precipitate early in the lifespan of red cells in β thalassaemia, are more widely dispersed over the cytoplasm before reacting with specific sites on the membrane. These observations are in keeping with the different electron-microscopic appearances of α- and β-chain binding to thalassaemic red cells (Rachmilewitz *et al.* 1985).

In a further series of experiments using the red-cell IOV loading model Shalev *et al.* (1996) confirmed that β chains produce defective spectrin binding that may result in damage to ankyrin, similar to that observed with unstable haemoglobins (Platt & Falcone 1988). They suggest that this results from structural changes in the 62-kDa domain of ankyrin, the spectrin binding site, mediated by β chains.

It is also likely that the membranes of α-thalassaemic cells undergo oxidative damage by broadly similar mechanisms to those described earlier in this chapter for β thalassaemia. The nature of the haem carrier protein plays an important role in this process (Shinar & Rachmilewitz 1993). For example, it has been shown that β-globin chains lose haem eight times faster than α-globin chains, but that α chains are more likely to auto-oxidize. Hence pathological haem loss may be a feature of both globin chains and participate in red-cell damage in α as well as β thalassaemia.

Clearly, these experiments provide strong evidence for a fundamental difference in the mechanisms of membrane damage between α and β thalassaemia. However, more work is required before the precise details of how this injury is mediated are understood.

There is one form of α thalassaemia which causes particularly characteristic red-cell changes. As described in the previous chapter, there is a family of haemoglobin variants, of which Hb Constant Spring was the first to be discovered, which are caused by mutations in the stop codon of the $\alpha 2$ gene. They result in the very low output of an α chain with 31 additional amino acid residues at the C-terminal end. Homozygotes are anaemic, with evidence of haemolysis, and their red cells are large and quite different from those seen in any other form of thalassaemia (reviewed by Weatherall & Clegg 1975). Recent studies suggest that these cells are markedly overhydrated relative to those of the deletional forms of α thalassaemia. Furthermore, the derangement of volume regulation and cellular hydration seems to occur early in erythroid maturation and is fully expressed at the reticulocyte stage. The membrane rigidity and mechanical stability of these cells is increased compared with those of patients with HbH disease and other forms of α thalassaemia. It has been found that their membranes are associated with oxidized β and α^{CS} chains (Schrier 1997). At first sight this is a surprising observation, particularly as detailed studies of the synthesis of Hb Constant Spring have shown that, although it is produced at a very low rate, it is relatively stable throughout the lifespan of the erythrocyte (Derry *et al.* 1984). Yet it has been suggested that it is the binding of oxidized α^{CS} chains to the membrane that is responsible for the associated abnormalities in membrane function (Schrier 1997). These observations may not be incompatible, however. If, because of their steric properties, α^{CS} chains associate more slowly with β chains than is the case for normal α chains, but once they have combined the resulting molecule is stable, some α^{CS} chains, together with β chains, may also become associated with the membranes of early red-cell precursors. In other words, in early erythroid progenitors, in which the level of α^{CS} chains is highest, they may either slowly combine with β chains to form a stable tetramer, or become associated with the red-cell membrane.

It appears therefore that damage to the red-cell membrane occurs in both α and β thalassaemia, but that because of the particular properties of free α and β chains in their interactions with its different components there are considerable differences in the end results. However, despite some overlap, the fundamental distinction between the two major forms of thalassaemia lies in the degree of ineffective erythropoiesis as compared with haemolysis, which is considerably greater in β than in α thalassaemia.

Consequences of the anaemia of α thalassaemia compared with β thalassaemia

Although there are similarities in the clinical pictures of α and β thalassaemia there are also some fundamental differences (Table 5.6). As already described, this in part reflects the properties of the abnormal homotetramers of γ or β chains that are produced in α thalassaemia. These effects are seen at their most extreme in the homozygous state for α^0 thalassaemia, the Hb Bart's hydrops syndrome. Thus, although these stillborn babies are usually not grossly anaemic compared with those with hydrops fetalis due to other causes, the clinical picture, described in detail in Chapter 11, is one of profound intrauterine hypoxia. This reflects the fact that Hb Bart's, with its extremely high oxygen affinity, constitutes approximately 80% of the haemoglobin.

In HbH disease, which results from a deficit of approximately three of the four α-globin genes, there is a variable haemolytic anaemia, which, in some cases, is associated with sufficient erythroid expansion to produce skeletal changes similar to those observed in β thalassaemia (Wasi *et al.* 1969). Patients with high levels of HbH, because of its high oxygen affinity, may not be able to compensate for their anaemia as well as those with similar haemoglobin levels due to other causes. The bombardment of the spleen with abnormal erythrocytes invariably causes splenomegaly, which may be progressive and result in the features of hypersplenism, similar to those that occur in β thalassaemia.

Because the degree of ineffective erythropoiesis is less in the α thalassaemias than in β thalassaemia it appears that the rate of iron loading in untransfused patients is also slower. Indeed, early observations

Table 5.6 Some important differences between α and β thalassaemia.

	α Thalassaemia	β Thalassaemia
Mutations	Gene deletions common	Gene deletions rare
Properties of excess globin	Soluble γ_4 or β_4 tetramers Slow rate of haemichrome formation Band 4.1 not oxidized Binds to band 3	Insoluble α-chain aggregates Rapid rate of haemichrome formation Oxidation of band 4.1 Less interaction with band 3
Red cells	Overhydrated Rigid Membranes hyperstable p50↓	Dehydrated Rigid Membranes unstable p50↓
Anaemia	Mainly haemolytic	Mainly dyserythropoietic
Bone changes	Rare	Common
Iron loading	Rare	Common

suggested that iron loading of the tissues was unusual in HbH disease (Wasi *et al.* 1969) and that there is much less tissue haemosiderosis than in autopsy material obtained from patients with homozygous β thalassaemia or HbE thalassaemia (Sonakul *et al.* 1978). However, later studies described a steady rise with age in the serum ferritin levels in patients with HbH disease (Tso *et al.* 1984), indicating that the erythroid hyperplasia is associated with some increase in the rate of iron loading. However, with the exception of patients who are maintained on regular transfusion, the widespread effects of iron loading on the pancreas, endocrine organs, liver and myocardium, characteristic of β thalassaemia, have not been observed.

The erythroid hyperplasia is also reflected by increased requirements for folate; although there have been few reports of clinical folate deficiency, subclinical deficiency has been documented (Vatanavicharn *et al.* 1978).

As mentioned earlier, some forms of β thalassaemia may be associated with an increased risk of thromboembolic disease. In the last edition of this book we discussed a curious condition which we had observed in a patient with HbH disease who, following splenectomy, developed the combination of superficial migrating thrombophlebitis with deep venous disease (see Chapter 11). A further group of similarly affected patients with HbH disease was reported by Tso *et al.* (1982) and, subsequently, we have observed several other patients with this disorder, who, in addition, have had recurrent pulmonary emboli. All these patients have been splenectomized and have relatively high platelet counts, although not in excess of those often observed after this operation. Whether the removal of the spleen results in the persistence in the circulation of red cells with membrane damage similar to that which may generate the prethrombotic element of β thalassaemia is not clear. Indeed, very little attention has been paid to the study of haemostasis and coagulation in the α thalassaemias.

Secondary changes in haemoglobin constitution

As we saw earlier, one of the cardinal features of the β thalassaemias is persistent fetal haemoglobin production. Does anything like this happen in α thalassaemia? Babies homozygous for α^0 thalassaemia, with the Hb Bart's hydrops syndrome, undoubtedly have persistent ζ-chain production, and their cord bloods, when they are stillborn late in pregnancy, contain from 10 to 20% of Hb Portland ($\zeta_2\gamma_2$) (Todd *et al.* 1970; Weatherall *et al.* 1970). Since in our original radiolabelling experiments we were not able to demonstrate labelling of Hb Portland in the blood of these babies, we do not know for sure whether this represents the true level of synthesis late in pregnancy or whether it may be lower and the levels observed reflect selective survival of cells that synthesize relatively larger amounts of this type of embryonic haemoglobin. However, there seems little doubt that embryonic ζ-globin synthesis does persist at a very low level in α^0 thalassaemia; trace amounts of ζ globin can be identified in the blood of heterozygotes of all ages (Chung *et al.* 1984; Chui *et al.* 1986).

Unlike the case of β thalassaemia, in which there is marked dyserythropoiesis and erythroid expansion, and in which red-cell precursors that synthesize γ chains come under intense selection, there seems no a priori reason why there should be persistence of HbF in the α thalassaemias; HbF and HbA both have α chains and hence their synthesis will be equally affected. Curiously, however, there is increased γ-chain synthesis in some of the α thalassaemias, though not to the same level as is observed in the β thalassaemias. Many patients with HbH disease have Hb Bart's as well as HbH, even in later childhood and adult life (Ramot *et al.* 1959; Huehns *et al.* 1960; Sturgeon *et al.* 1961; Fessas *et al.* 1966). Indeed, occasionally the level of Bart's may exceed that of HbH (Ramot *et al.* 1959). It should be remembered, however, that the level of Hb Bart's may be partly determined at the post-translational stage of globin synthesis during the combination of subunits one with another to form dimers and tetramers. In the face of a deficiency of α chains, and if the γ-chain loci remain active, both β and γ chains will be competing for a depleted pool of α chains. Since α chains associate with β chains in preference to γ chains the overall result may be a greater excess of γ_4 than β_4 molecules; since the latter are more unstable the final level of Hb Bart's in the blood of patients with HbH disease may not be a direct reflection of the rate of γ-chain production.

These complex issues are highlighted in the interactions between α thalassaemia and β-globin chain variants like HbE, which are extremely common in south-east Asia and which are described in detail in Chapter 11. Individuals who have the genotype of HbH disease and who also are carriers of HbE produce only Hbs A, E and Bart's; the latter may constitute up to 10% of the total haemoglobin. Why do they produce Hb Bart's rather than HbH? Clearly, the γ-chain genes must remain active and thus γ, $β^A$ and $β^E$ chains are competing for a limited number of α chains. It seems likely that $β^A$ chains compete better than $β^E$ chains for the relatively few α chains, so leaving an excess of γ and $β^E$ chains. The $γ_4$ tetramer is stable but the $β_4^E$ tetramer is probably not (Tuchinda *et al.* 1967). Hence these patients have only Hbs Bart's, A and E. Similarly, the rare occurrence of the homozygous state for sickle-cell disease in association with the genotype for HbH disease is characterized by the production of Hbs S, F and Bart's (Weatherall *et al.* 1969a). Although early studies suggested that individuals who have defective α-chain synthesis with the sickle-cell gene might produce trace amounts of a molecule with the structure $β_4^S$, Hb Augusta 1 (Huisman 1960a,b), more recent studies have not confirmed these findings. Indeed, it seems likely that the variant β-globin chains of Hbs S, E and C are unable to form stable $β_4$ tetramers.

Clearly, therefore, there is a persistent γ-chain production in the more severe forms of α thalassaemia, although whether this reflects a higher level than that seen in many conditions with erythroid hyperplasia and some degree of ineffective erythropoiesis is difficult to be sure. While the relatively high levels of Hb Bart's in some of the interactions with HbE suggest that this may be the case, the complex post-translational events relating to the relative affinities of different globin subunits that we have just considered suggest that factors other than the rates of γ-chain production are involved in the final level of both HbF and $γ_4$ tetramers in the peripheral blood.

Finally, another characteristic feature of β thalassaemia is the absolute increase in δ-chain production, both *cis* and *trans* to the β-thalassaemia determinant. As might be expected, since HbA_2 shares α chains with HbA, the HbA_2 level tends to be normal or reduced in the more severe forms of α thalassaemia such as HbH disease. In truth, very little is known about the overall level of δ-chain production in α thalassaemia. Using a combined chromatographic and electrophoretic approach, a haemoglobin was isolated from the blood of a patient with HbH disease which consisted entirely of the δ chains of HbA_2 (Dance *et al.* 1963). It is not known how commonly this variant is produced in α thalassaemia, or whether it has the molecular formula $δ_4$; no molecular weight

determinations have been reported. Again, this may be a post-translational phenomenon; δ chains are known to have a lower affinity for α chains than β chains and hence, in the face of a deficiency of α chains, β chains will be bound in preference to δ chains, a phenomenon which may explain the presence of free δ chains in the blood of patients with α thalassaemia. There is no reason to suppose that δ-chain production is increased.

In summary, the final haemoglobin constitution of patients with α thalassaemia reflects a primary deficiency of α chains, the production of homotetramers of γ and β chains, and a complex series of alterations in the levels of both fetal haemoglobin and associated β-chain variants, which reflect, at least in part, the different affinities of globin subunits one for another.

Genotype/phenotype relationships

As we have seen, the principles that underlie the pathophysiology of α thalassaemia are in many ways similar to those for β thalassaemia. The major pathological process is imbalanced globin synthesis, the clinical consequences of which hang largely on the deleterious effects of the particular globin subunit that is produced in excess. Based on these observations, and a knowledge of the molecular pathology of the α thalassaemias as described in the previous chapter, it is possible to make some sense of the pathophysiology and genetic heterogeneity of these diseases. They are described in detail in Chapter 11; here we shall outline the principles involved.

As we have seen, the α thalassaemias are, overall, elegant examples of gene dosage effects, reflecting the clinical consequences of the loss of between one and four α-globin genes. Much of their clinical heterogeneity is explicable in this way, but there are also further subtleties that depend on the fact that the output of the two linked α-globin genes is not equal, and that they may be inactivated either by deletions or by point mutations.

The most marked heterogeneity is observed among the α thalassaemias of intermediate severity, that is, the various forms of HbH disease. This disorder has a remarkably variable clinical phenotype, ranging from a transfusion-dependent disorder to one which is symptom free and associated with very little clinical disability (Minnich *et al.* 1958; Na-Nakorn 1959; Na-Nakorn *et al.* 1965; Wasi *et al.* 1969). In large series of patients reported from Thailand the steady-state haemoglobin values ranged from 3 to 12 g/dl (Wasi *et al.* 1969; Piankijagum *et al.* 1978). Similar heterogeneity has been observed in more recent reports (Styles *et al.* 1997). Furthermore, although HbH is unstable and some of the variability in its reported levels may reflect technical problems in its estimation, there is no doubt that its level varies enormously in patients with HbH disease, published figures showing anything between 2 and 40% of the total haemoglobin (Na-Nakorn *et al.* 1965; Wasi *et al.* 1969).

Studies which have related the molecular pathology of HbH disease to its clinical phenotype typify some of the successes and frustrations of the thalassaemia field over recent years. For while it has been possible to relate some of this clinical heterogeneity to underlying mutations of the α-globin genes, many questions remain unanswered. Overall, the forms that result from the coinheritance of α^0 with α^+ thalassaemia of the deletional varieties ($--/\alpha-$) are milder than those which result from the interactions of α^0 with α^+ thalassaemia of the non-deletional forms ($--/\alpha^T\alpha$) (Galanello *et al.* 1983b; Fucharoen *et al.* 1988a; Kattamis *et al.* 1988; Styles *et al.* 1997). These differences probably reflect two major pathophysiological processes. First, the α-chain output is different depending on whether the α^+-thalassaemia mutation that is inherited together with α^0 thalassaemia is of the deletion or non-deletion variety. If the upstream ($\alpha2$) gene is deleted, its downstream partner can increase its output; if it is inactivated by a mutation, this does not seem to be possible. Hence, in compound heterozygotes for α^0 and α^+ thalassaemia of the non-deletion variety, there is a greater degree of globin imbalance, compatible with the higher levels of HbH that are found in this condition. These differences are also reflected in the homozygous states for the deletional and non-deletional forms of α^+ thalassaemia. In the former case the clinical phenotype is α-thalassaemia trait, while in the latter it may be HbH disease (Pressley *et al.* 1980b).

The second possibility for heterogeneity reflects the nature of the mutation that inactivates the α-globin gene in the non-deletional forms of α thalassaemia. As we have already seen, the production of elongated α-globin chains in the case of the chain-termination mutants such as Hb Constant Spring may have a particularly deleterious effect on red-cell membrane function. This, together with the fact that Hb Constant Spring is due to a point mutation which

leaves the $\alpha2$ gene intact, may explain the more severe clinical phenotype associated with HbH disease due to the interaction of α^0 thalassaemia with α^+ thalassaemia due to the inheritance of this variant (Fucharoen *et al.* 1988a; Styles *et al.* 1997).

HbH disease also provides a good example of how environmental factors may combine with a genetic disease to modify the phenotype. Because of the instability and sensitivity to oxidants of HbH it tends to precipitate after the administration of drugs such as sulphonamides (Rigas & Koler 1961). It is not clear how often its marked heat lability causes the same phenomenon in the presence of the types of fevers encountered with infections in tropical countries (see Chapter 11).

Many questions about the pathophysiology of HbH disease and other forms of α thalassaemia remain unanswered, however. It is not known why the degree of anaemia or level of HbH varies so much within a particular genotype. Similarly, it is not clear whether the degree of anaemia is related to the level of HbH. We do not understand why only a small proportion of patients with the condition develop serious thromboembolic complications after splenectomy. We shall return to these and the many other unanswered questions about the pathophysiology of the α thalassaemias in Chapter 11.

The relationship between pathophysiology and clinical diversity

A greater knowledge of the pathophysiology of the main forms of thalassaemia has been the major factor in helping us better to understand the remarkable clinical diversity of its different forms. We shall discuss the various interactions and genetic and environmental modifiers that are responsible for the different intermediate forms of thalassaemia in Chapter 13. Although there are many gaps in our knowledge about why this disease is so variable in its presentation and course, at least some principles have been established.

Throughout this chapter we have seen that the cardinal feature of all the thalassaemias is imbalanced globin synthesis. Thus anything that lessens the degree of imbalance will have a beneficial effect on the clinical phenotype. These principles have been established for the β thalassaemias, at least to some extent (Table 5.7). It turns out that patients with severe forms of β thalassaemia who have also been

Table 5.7 Some factors which modify the β-thalassaemia phenotype. From Weatherall (2001).

Genetic
  Primary
    Severity of the β-globin-gene mutation
  Secondary
    Co-inheritance of α thalassaemia
    Increased level of HbF; several determinants
  Tertiary
    Iron, bilirubin or bone metabolism
    Genetic background based on evolutionary
      adaptation

Acquired
  Splenomegaly and hypersplenism
  Consequences of organ damage due to iron loading
  Nutritional factors

Ecological and ethnological factors

---

fortunate enough to inherit α thalassaemia have, in general, a milder disease. This is because the α-thalassaemia determinant has the effect of reducing the overall degree of globin imbalance. Similarly, patients with different forms of β thalassaemia who have also inherited genes that encourage more effective HbF production are also protected. Again this is an elegant example of how a reduction in globin imbalance, in this case by γ chains making up for β chains, can transform the clinical picture of severe thalassaemia.

It is also becoming apparent that, as well as modification of the β-thalassaemic phenotype by heterogeneity at the loci that regulate the α- or γ-globin genes, other, more subtle, genetic polymorphisms may play a role in determining the phenotype. As we shall see in later chapters these include polymorphisms at loci which are involved in the regulation of iron, bilirubin and bone metabolism. There seems little doubt that, as the complications of older patients with thalassaemia are explored in more detail, more of these secondary modifiers will be discovered.

Finally, as outlined in the next section, it is becoming increasingly clear that the remarkable genetic differences between populations in which thalassaemia is common which have resulted from their evolutionary history, particularly with respect to the presence of infective agents such as malaria, may also have had an important effect on a thalassaemia patient's ability to cope with infection and other environmental factors. The way in which these complex interactions modify the genotype of β thalassaemia are summarized in Table 5.7.

The heterogeneity of thalassaemia: genes, environment and evolution

In this chapter we have outlined and contrasted the major features of the pathophysiology of the α and β thalassaemias. We have seen how the fundamental disease process, that is, imbalanced globin synthesis, is the same in the two conditions but how, because of the different properties of the particular globins that are produced in excess, their pathophysiology differs. We have also seen how their clinical phenotypes may be modified according to the different underlying molecular lesions together with a number of other genetic and environmental factors.

These principles of the pathophysiology of the two main forms of thalassaemia provide the basis for a clearer understanding of the remarkable heterogeneity of the disease. The central issue is always imbalanced globin production. It follows that milder defects in α- or β-chain production, because they result in less imbalance, will be associated with milder clinical phenotypes. But we can take this argument one step further. Since the cardinal feature of severe thalassaemia is the production of an excess of one type of globin over another, it follows that the *co-inheritance* of *both* α and β thalassaemia should tend to cause them to cancel each other out. That is, patients with severe forms of β thalassaemia who co-inherit α thalassaemia might be expected to have a milder clinical condition, and vice versa. As we shall see in later chapters this is indeed the case; an important part of the heterogeneity of the β thalassaemias can be ascribed to variation in the severity of the underlying β-globin-gene mutation together with the interaction of α thalassaemia. Furthermore, as pointed out earlier, there is remarkable variability in the level of HbF production in β thalassaemia. This again plays a major role in determining the phenotype.

In the chapters which follow we shall describe the bewilderingly complex series of interactions between the α and β thalassaemias, either with themselves or with structural haemoglobin variants, which comprise the thalassaemia syndromes. However, we should not delude ourselves into thinking that even this sophisticated knowledge of events at the molecular and cellular level can, in itself, provide anything like a complete picture of the remarkable clinical diversity of these diseases. Many other genetic, acquired and environmental factors must be involved.

Table 5.8 Genetic polymorphisms associated with variation in susceptibility to malaria.

Haemoglobin
   Structural variants
   Thalassaemia
Red-cell membrane
   Band 3 deletion; ovalocytosis
   Blood groups; Duffy, ABO(H), Le(a), Kidd
   Glycophorins
Red-cell metabolism
   Glucose-6-phosphatase deficiency
HLA/DR
Iron transport
TNFα
ICAM 1

ICAM, intercellular adhesion molecule; TNFα, tumour necrosis factor α.

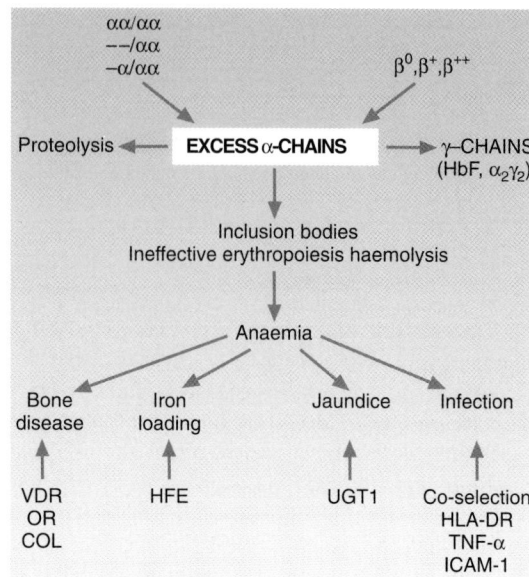

Fig. 5.16 A summary of the factors which may modify the pathophysiology and clinical phenotype of the β thalassaemias. The magnitude of the excess of α chains may be modified by the degree of β-chain deficiency, the number of α-globin genes and the ability to synthesize γ chains after birth. It could also be affected by the degree of proteolysis. There are a number of other genetic factors which may also modify the phenotype to some degree. COL, heterozygosity of the loci directing collagen synthesis; HFE, hereditary haemochromatosis locus; ICAM, intercellular adhesion molecule; OR, oestrogen receptor; TNF, tumour necrosis factor; UGT-1, UDP-glucuronosyltransferase 1; VDR, vitamin D receptor.

It is becoming clear that there is a remarkable diversity in the genetic backgrounds of patients with the different forms of thalassaemia. A good example is their response to infection. As we shall see in the next chapter, one of the major factors which has maintained the thalassaemias at their high frequency is heterozygote resistance to severe forms of malaria. But thalassaemia is not the only polymorphism which has been maintained in this way: there is increasing evidence that many others, involving not just the red cell and its contents but also many of the arms of the immune system and its effectors, have also arisen (Table 5.8). Because of our relatively short (at least in evolutionary terms) exposure to malaria, these polymorphisms tend to be different in each population, just as thalassaemia mutations differ in the same way (Weatherall *et al.* 1997). Thus thalassaemic children from various parts of the world may vary profoundly in their response to infection. No doubt genetic heterogeneity involving other responses to the disease will have been mediated in the same way.

The environmental and cultural backgrounds of thalassaemic patients may also differ widely and play a major role in modifying the severity of the illness and the reaction of patients and their family to these diseases. Exposure to infection or malnutrition may result in a completely different course of the disease in children in poorer countries from those in richer, Western societies. And different cultural and religious attitudes to the disease may have a profound effect on an individual patient's response to their condition. It is against this highly complex background of events at the molecular and cellular level, overlaid with broader aspects of genetic and environmental heterogeneity (Fig. 5.16), that we must examine the clinical disorders that comprise the thalassaemia syndromes.

Chapter 6
Distribution and population genetics of the thalassaemias

Introduction

The idea that thalassaemia reached high frequencies in many parts of the world as a result of malarial selection is now generally accepted. But in 1981, when the last edition of this book was published, there was still much scepticism about the 'malaria hypothesis', as it was known. Although this was first mooted in 1948 by J.B.S. Haldane, really convincing experimental or epidemiological evidence, certainly as it applied to the thalassaemias, was sparse. And even what seemed to some the best circumstantial evidence—the geographical overlap between endemic malaria and thalassaemia—did not survive close inspection. Central and South America have malaria but the indigenous populations are remarkably free of haemoglobinopathies. In contrast, parts of the central and eastern Pacific, which have always been malaria free, have relatively high frequencies of thalassaemia.

That important observation, made in the early 1980s, proved a turning-point for the malaria hypothesis. For the first time the newly emerged DNA technologies were brought to bear on a population genetics problem. While previously only phenotypes could be identified, now genotypes could be characterized with base-pair precision. And haplotypes, clusters of DNA polymorphisms that enabled different chromosomal types to be identified, could be used to provide information about the origins of mutations and about population relationships.

The upshot of this new approach was to show decisively that the variety of thalassaemia in the central and eastern Pacific was a single, extremely unusual, molecular variant of α^+ thalassaemia (the $-\alpha^{3.7\mathrm{III}}$ deletion), identical to that which had arisen in Melanesia, where malaria *was* common. Canoes, not malaria, were responsible for the arrival of thalassaemia in Tahiti, and the malaria hypothesis survived a crucial challenge.

We shall discuss the detailed evidence for the hypothesis later in this chapter. Suffice it to say here that the new methods have provided a much clearer insight into the world distribution of the various haemoglobinopathies. Paradoxically, however, they appear to have left one important aspect somewhat overshadowed. In the previous edition we remarked on the rather unsatisfactory state of much of the gene frequency data for α and β thalassaemia. Sadly, despite, or perhaps because of, the new technology we are—with a few notable exceptions—still in the dark about the true gene frequencies of the thalassaemias in many parts of the world, although a detailed repertoire of molecular variants is often available!

The reasons for this are many and varied. Accurate prevalence data usually need large-scale surveys, preferably not hospital based, and involving a lot of hard work and expense. In many countries, local variations in geography and climate mean that malarial endemicity, and therefore thalassaemia frequencies, may vary widely. Population movements and malaria eradication programmes will often have broken the link between the two, so that pockets of thalassaemia, or its absence, cannot always be readily predicted.

Furthermore, because thalassaemia was one of the first common genetic diseases to be recognized, many surveys were carried out with less than ideal methods, with little incentive to repeat all the hard work as better methods later became available. So it is rarely the case that full diagnostic criteria have been used for the different forms of thalassaemia being surveyed. Add to this variations in technique, and even in definitions of 'normal', and it becomes obvious why prevalence data are so imprecise, and perhaps why the relatively straightforward determination of genotypes has largely replaced assessment of the nature and extent of phenotypic variation.

In this chapter we shall discuss what is known about the distribution and frequency of the common forms of α and β thalassaemia. The distribution of the $\delta\beta$ thalassaemias is considered in Chapter 8, the interactions of structural haemoglobin variants with the β thalassaemias in Chapter 9, hereditary persistence of fetal haemoglobin in Chapter 10, and the dominant β thalassaemias in Chapter 13.

Overall distribution

Thalassaemia has a high incidence in a broad region extending from the Mediterranean basin and parts of Africa, through the Middle East, the Indian subcontinent, south-east Asia and Melanesia and out into the Pacific (Fig. 6.1). These are the regions where most of the public health problems occur (together with some countries in Central and South America that had substantial immigration from Europe, mainly Italy, in the last century). But it is also evident that thalassaemia occurs, albeit at very low frequencies, in many other parts of the world. Indeed, wherever serious attempts have been made to find it, they have usually been successful. We now know that this follows to some extent from the molecular basis of the disease. Unlike sickle-cell anaemia, for example, which results from a unique single-base mutation in the β-globin gene, any mutation that leads to a reduced output of globin will be a thalassaemia mutation. Not surprisingly, therefore, there are many of them, because there are so many 'targets' in the α and β genes for such mutations. In effect, the mutation

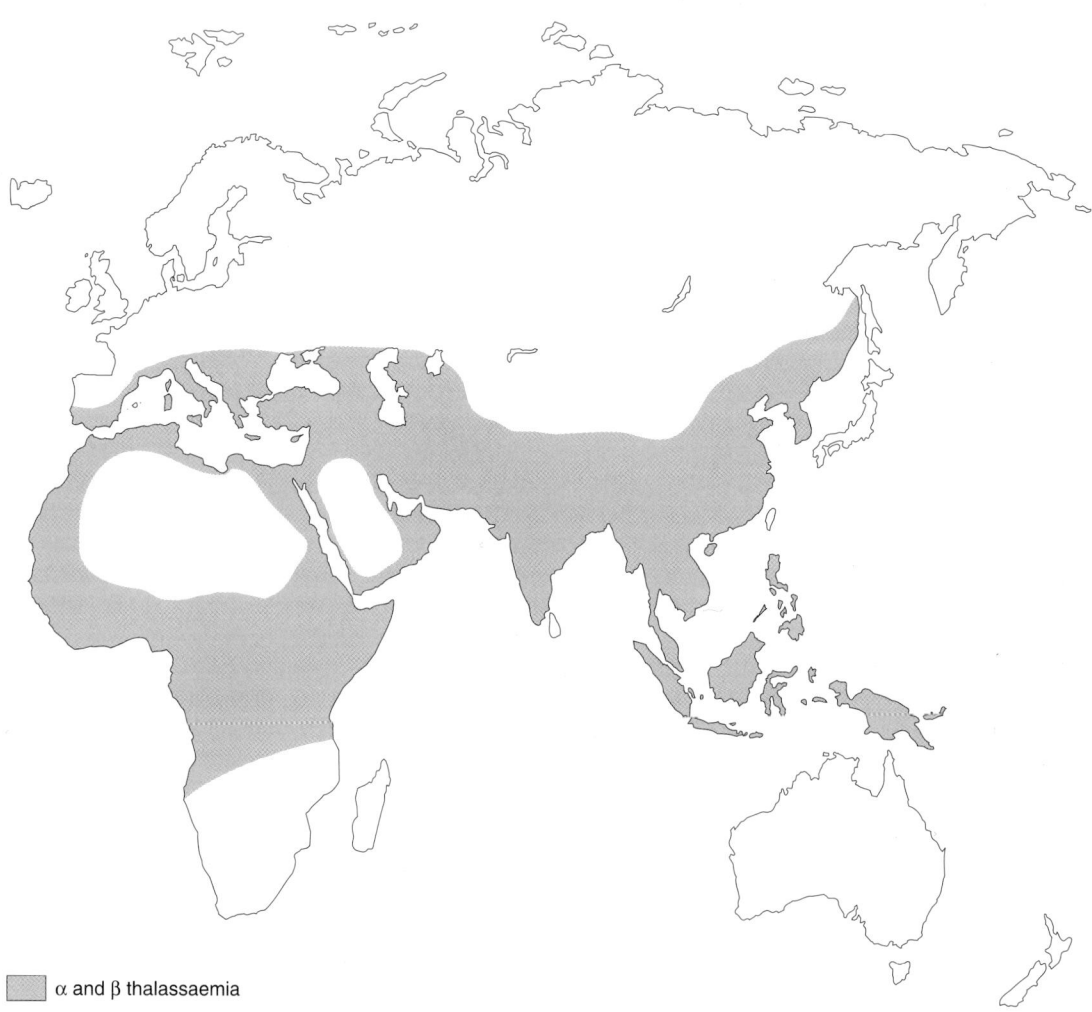

☐ α and β thalassaemia

Fig. 6.1 World distribution of α and β thalassaemia.

rate for 'thalassaemia' is quite high, and the consequence, helped along by population movements, is the sporadic occurrence of thalassaemia in most populations that have been looked at. These mutations are, of course, the raw material for malarial selection to act upon in the endemic regions of the world.

Early descriptions of the distribution of thalassaemia genes appear in the reviews by Chernoff (1959) and Bannerman (1961). An excellent account of data published before DNA technologies appeared can be found in the monograph by Livingstone (1967) together with an updated tabular survey covering almost 150 countries or areas and with over 2000 references (Livingstone 1985). The topic is also reviewed in several WHO publications (WHO 1983, 1985, 1989b, 1994) and by Angastiniotis and Modell (1998).

In a series of annual workshops, held under the auspices of the WHO, an attempt has been made to estimate the frequency of the α and β thalassaemias and the common haemoglobin variants throughout the world. These data are summarized in the latest of these publications (WHO 1994) and in a review of the work of this programme by Angastiniotis and Modell (1998). These publications, in which the sources of the gene frequency data are not referenced, are not designed to provide absolutely accurate information about the frequency of different forms of thalassaemia and haemoglobin disorders in each population, but rather to give an overall view of the global problem of the disease together with advice for its control and management. The data are based on a certain amount of published work

together with personal figures supplied by local clinicians (Dr Bernadette Modell, personal communication). As we shall see throughout this chapter, where it has been studied in detail, the distribution of the haemoglobin disorders is always patchy, and hence the WHO figures may be inaccurate, at least for some populations. However, they provide a useful guideline to an approximation of the clinical problems that these diseases will pose in the future. An overall assessment of the numbers of patients with the important haemoglobin disorders derived from the WHO Working Party is shown in Table 6.1.

β Thalassaemia

Distribution and frequency

In the sections that follow we shall largely confine ourselves to the high-incidence areas where thalassaemia poses serious health issues. Since haemoglobin E is associated with a mild thalassaemic phenotype, and can interact with β-thalassaemic alleles to cause a severe form of β thalassaemia (see Chapter 9), we include a description of its distribution and frequency in this account.

Europe

Italy

Some of the earliest and largest surveys were those carried out in Italy by Silvestroni, Bianco and their

Table 6.1 Global summary of approximate numbers of annual births of babies with severe haemoglobin disorders. Modified from WHO (1994).

WHO region	Population (millions)	Births (millions)	Births of homozygotes or compound heterozygotes (thousands)*
Africa	650	30.0	230
Americas	730	17.5	5.0
Asia	3150	84.0	120.0
Europe	780	11.0	1.6
Oceania	30	0.5	0.2
Total	5340	143.0	356.8†

* The disorders vary according to the region. In Africa sickle-cell anaemia accounts for most of the cases, while in Asia β thalassaemia, HbE β thalassaemia and α^0 thalassaemia are the most important disorders. In Europe β thalassaemia is the predominant haemoglobin disorder.
† These figures may be an underestimate; accurate gene frequencies for many populations are not available, and birth rates are based on current figures rather than World Bank projections.

colleagues between 1944 and 1981 (Silvestroni & Bianco 1947, 1959, 1963, 1966, 1968, 1975; Silvestroni *et al.* 1978, 1981a,b). Because methods in use changed during the course of these surveys, they are not strictly comparable; nevertheless they reveal considerable variation in β-thalassaemia frequencies in Italy, with the highest incidences found in the Po delta in the north and in the southern regions of Campania, Calabria, Puglia, Lucania and Sardinia. In the Po delta the incidence ranges from 7 to 19%. Barrai *et al.* (1984) estimated frequencies for the Po provinces of Rovigo and Ferrara as ~8%, and also included a comparison between the osmotic-fragility method extensively employed in the early surveys and quantitative HbA$_2$ methods. They concluded that estimates of heterozygote frequencies by the former method may have been inflated by at least 8%. Elsewhere in northern and central Italy β-thalassaemia frequencies are in the range of 0.5–2%.

In addition to the extensive surveys of Silvestroni and Bianco, other large surveys have been carried out in Italy. Brancati (1961) studied 33 000 people in 121 areas of Calabria. There was remarkable variation in the frequency of the disease (from less than 4% to over 9%, reaching just under 20% in a few places), which was commoner in low-lying areas and particularly on the coast of the Ionian Sea. A similar high incidence has been recorded in Calabria by Quattrin *et al.* (1970, 1973). Six per cent of over 25 000 individuals studied were found to be carriers for some form of thalassaemia, almost 90% of which was β thalassaemia, the remainder being a mixture of other haemoglobinopathies including Hb Lepore and δβ thalassaemia.

Sicily and Sardinia

There are limited data available for Sicily, with the frequency of β thalassaemia ranging from ~3 to 9% in five studies (Schiliro 1987; Pepe *et al.* 1992). Schiliro (1978) makes the point that Sicily is something of a Mediterranean halfway house, with a fair selection of most of the haemoglobinopathies found in the region: of 7143 haematological patients, almost 30% had some haemoglobin disorder with the majority being heterozygotes for β thalassaemia. The high incidence of β thalassaemia in Sardinia, first reported by Carcassi *et al.* (1957b), was confirmed in later studies by Cao *et al.* (1978, 1981) using modern quantitative methods. They found that one in eight of the popula-

tion were carriers for β thalassaemia. Only a handful of other β-cluster disorders, like δβ thalassaemia, Hb Lepore and HbS, were recorded.

Greece

Beta thalassaemia is also common in Greece, but as in Italy there is an uneven distribution. Malamos *et al.* (1962) studied 1600 Greek Air Force personnel drawn from all over the country and found ~5% with the β-thalassaemia trait. Stamatoyannopoulos and Fessas (1964) looked at four mainland areas (Korditsa, Elasson, Petromagoula and Arta) and two islands (Corfu and Serifos); the incidence of β thalassaemia ranged from 6 to 19%. Barnicot *et al.* (1963) found an incidence of 3.9% for the Chalkdiki peninsula, and somewhat higher values for Atalanta (7.6%) and Korditsa (9.8%). Schizas *et al.* (1977) estimated an average Greek mainland figure of ~7%. In general, low-altitude fertile areas have the highest incidence, while in the mountains and the north frequencies rarely exceed 2% (Tegos *et al.* 1987).

Mediterranean islands

Beta thalassaemia is also widespread throughout the islands of the Mediterranean. We have already noted its impact in Sardinia. On *Crete*, frequencies of between 4 and 9% were reported, and on *Rhodes* it reaches 25% in the Massori and Laerma regions (Barnicot *et al.* 1963). In *Cyprus*, β thalassaemia presents a public health problem as serious as that in Sardinia (Plato *et al.* 1964; Ashiotis *et al.* 1973; Bate 1975). Ashiotis *et al.* (1973) found an overall incidence in Greek Cypriots of 15%, and a similar figure is reported for the Turkish Cypriot population (Ashiotis *et al.* 1973; Cin *et al.* 1984). Angastiniotis and Hadjiminas (1981) give an overall figure of 17.2% based on a survey of 14 624 people in the Cyprus Thalassaemia Centre in Nicosia. On *Malta* 3.5% of 1500 individuals surveyed were found to be β-thalassaemia carriers (Cauchi 1970).

Western Mediterranean

Thalassaemia is less common at the western end of the Mediterranean. There appears to be little in southern *France* except in individuals of Italian or Spanish origin (Orsini *et al.* 1974). Surveys in *Spain* have revealed a patchy distribution throughout the country apart from the Basque region, where it is absent. Elsewhere it occurs at frequencies of 1–2%, reaching a high of 3.4% in Murcia (Pellicer & Casado 1970). It is also quite common in the Barcelona region and on the island of Minorca (Gimferrer & Baiget 1979). These authors (Baiget & Gimferrer 1986) also make the point that the distribution of β thalassaemia in Spain largely fits with areas previously known to be occupied by the Moors, or in areas where malaria was endemic (except Galicia in the north-west). In *Portugal*, thalassaemia frequencies vary from about 1% in the south of the country to less than 0.5% in the north (Faustino *et al*. 1992).

East Europe

Early reports (Fraser *et al*. 1966) that there might be a significant incidence of β thalassaemia in what was then Yugoslavia have been borne out by later studies. Sadikario *et al*. (1969) looked at 2861 children from *Macedonia* and found that 4.7% were β-thalassaemia carriers. More localized surveys within Macedonia revealed frequencies varying from 1.6 to 5.0% (Efremov *et al*. 1982). Further north, in *Croatia*, the frequency falls to about 1%, with intermediate values in *Serbia* and *Bosnia Herzegovina* (Efremov 1992).

At the time we wrote the previous edition, it was only just becoming apparent to haematologists in the West that thalassaemia was a serious problem in countries bordering on the Black Sea. Most reports were found in local journals and we were fortunate in getting the help of Dr K.N. Kantchev of Burgas to translate the Bulgarian literature for us. β Thalassaemia is most common in the south-west of the country with frequencies of about 2%, declining to 0.05% in the north-east. It reaches 3.4% in a few isolated pockets (Rashkov 1978), with an average overall of between 2 and 3% (Tasheva *et al*. 1987).

Central Europe

Moving further north into central Europe it is clear that thalassaemia is found at low levels in many countries, *Romania* (Predescu *et al*. 1968), *Czechoslovakia* (Efremov & Huisman 1983; Indrák *et al*. 1992), *Hungary* (Efremov & Huisman 1983; Szelényi *et al*. 1983), *Germany* (Laig *et al*. 1990b) and the *UK* (Knox-Macaulay *et al*. 1973), although no large-scale systematic surveys have been carried out in these regions. A summary of much of the European data

can be found in Efremov and Huisman (1983). These authors reiterate the point made earlier, that many of the data can only be regarded as a rough guide to the true frequency because some surveys were conducted with limited methodology, which also often failed to differentiate between the different forms of thalassaemia. In general, though, it is clear that β thalassaemia is found at the highest frequencies in and around the Mediterranean. As we shall see in a later section, the molecular characterization of variants has enabled us to get a much clearer picture of the origins and movements of these different thalassaemia genes around Europe during the past few thousand years.

The Middle East and west Asia

Beta thalassaemia is widespread throughout the Middle East. In *Turkey* the average frequency is about 1.7% (Çavdar & Arcasoy 1971) ranging from 0.8% in Erzurum to 10.8% in western Thrace (Aksoy 1991) although higher incidences, particularly in western parts of the country, are known (Aksoy *et al*. 1985). The disorder is found throughout *Lebanon* at frequencies ranging from 0.5% to 2.5%, with the highest prevalence in the mountainous areas. It has also been reported in *Jordan* where it averages ~3.5% (Saba *et al*. 1992) and in the Arabian peninsula. The oasis populations of *Saudi Arabia*, where the sickle-cell gene is the predominant β haemoglobinopathy, have a low frequency of β thalassaemia. It is, however, clear that β thalassaemia occurs in significant proportions in other parts of the country because of the regular occurrence of patients with HbS β thalassaemia. Perrine *et al*. (1981) screened 2341 infants from the oases of eastern Saudi Arabia and found six cases of HbS $β^0$ thalassaemia compared with 43 cases of sickle-cell disease. Elsewhere in the Arabian peninsula, β thalassaemia has been reported at frequencies of ~2% in *Oman*, the *United Arab Emirates* and the *Yemen* (White *et al*. 1986). Much lower frequencies (<1%) have been reported in a large series from *Kuwait* (Ghosh *et al*. 1993).

In Yemenite Jews now residing in *Israel* low frequencies have been reported, and this is also the case with Iranian and north African Jews. On the other hand, much higher frequencies (15–20%) have been reported in Kurdish Jews, and in Bnei Israel and Cochin Jews from India (Ramot *et al*. 1964). It seems likely that the differences in thalassaemia prevalence in these Jewish groups have arisen since their exile from ancient Israel in 721 BC after the destruction of the first Temple, probably because they moved to areas where malarial selection pressures were so different. The disorder is virtually absent in Ashkenazi Jews. In the Arab communities of Israel, frequencies >10% have been reported in some areas. Overall carrier frequencies for β thalassaemia are ~1–2%, but this covers considerable extremes.

There is evidence that β thalassaemia is a serious public health problem in *Iran* (Pouya 1959; Nasab 1979) and *Iraq* (Taj-Eldin *et al.* 1968). We have already noted its occurrence in Jews from Kurdistan, a region straddling eastern Turkey, western Iran and northern Iraq. Nozari *et al.* (1990) reported that β thalassaemia is widespread in the north and north-western parts of Iran with frequencies reaching 4–5%, and there is clinical evidence of a high incidence of the disease in the Fars region in the south.

Moving north we encounter the various republics of the former *Soviet Union*. In the previous edition we gained some insight into the distribution of β thalassaemia in various parts of the country from Professor Y.N. Tokarev and colleagues at the Central Institute of Haematology and Blood Transfusion in Moscow. The major foci of the disorders are found in the Transcaucasian region and central Asia. Particularly high frequencies were noted in Armenia (0–2%), Georgia (3%), Azerbaijan (6%), Uzbekistan (3%), Tadjikistan (5%) and Dagestan (3.5%) (summarized in Tokarev & Spivak 1982). Since the break-up of the USSR it has become easier for researchers in Western countries to establish links with clinical centres in the various republics. Some of the fruits of these collaborations can be seen later in this chapter when we discuss the distribution of the molecular variants of thalassaemia.

The Indian subcontinent

Beta thalassaemia is probably the commonest inherited haemoglobin disorder on the Indian subcontinent, with an uneven distribution among the different endogenous populations (Sukumaran 1975). In addition, Hbs S and E are common among some tribal groups. HbS was probably originally present in the Indus valley and was dispersed into India following invasions from the north (Labie *et al.* 1990). It reaches its highest frequencies in the Nilgiri district of Madras (up to 20%), parts of Andhra Pradesh (up to

17%), Madhya Pradesh (up to 20%), Maharashba (10%), Gujerat (up to 30%) and Orissa (up to 25%) (Livingstone 1985). It seems likely that the HbE in India reflects ancient population movements from the high-prevalence regions (Burma, Thailand, Cambodia) to the west. Chatterjea (1966) summarized the early literature on thalassaemia in India. More recent reviews can be found in Saha and Banerjee (1973), Sukumaran and Master (1974) and Sukumaran (1975). The average incidence is 3.3% (Modell & Petrou 1983), although there are considerable individual variations.

In early surveys of Bengalis, Chatterjea (1959) found a carrier frequency of 3.7% for β-thalassaemia trait, and a high preponderance of HbE β thalassaemia (Chatterjea 1966). Ajmani *et al.* (1976) in a survey of 205 West Bengalis found 8.8% with β-thalassaemia trait and ~3.5% with HbE trait. Further north, in Assam, β thalassaemia is found at carrier frequencies that range from 0.3% in the Khasi population to 5.5% in Assamese (Flatz *et al.* 1972). HbE frequencies in these two populations are 45% and 20%, respectively. Similarly, Das and Deka (1975) and Das *et al.* (1980) found that HbE reached gene frequencies of over 50% among the mongoloid Bodo tribes living in the Brahmaputra valley. HbE has also been reported in Bhutan (Glasgow *et al.* 1968) and in Nepal at carrier frequencies of between 0.5 and 4% (Adams 1974; Gupta *et al.* 1977, 1979). Beta thalassaemia was also more common in the south-east of the country with frequencies varying from 0 to 8% among different population groups (Adams 1974). In north-western India carrier frequencies of 4.4% were recorded in Chitrapur Saraswats and 13.6% in Lohnas (Sharma *et al.* 1971). In a similar type of study of the Banushali community of Bombay, β thalassaemia was reported in 14.9% of 599 screened (Mehta *et al.* 1972). A high incidence was also noted in the Bohra Muslim community of Udaipur, Rajasthan.

The incidence of β thalassaemia in the tribal populations has not been extensively studied. It has been reported in the populations of Dadra and Bagar Haveli region (Joshi *et al.* 1978). Jain *et al.* (1983) recorded 3% in the Bhils of southern Rajasthan and 7.9% in the Damar tribe (who had no HbS). In Madhya Pradesh, which has the largest tribal population in India, 50 individuals were identified with β-thalassaemia trait out of 2781 screened (~2%). In this same group the carrier frequencies for Hbs S and E were 16.8 and 0.6%, respectively. In the Santal and Bhumji tribal populations of West Bengal β thalassaemia was found in about 6% of 197 individuals, with only one example of HbE trait (Giri *et al.* 1982).

There is less information available from Pakistan. Studies on over 1000 people in Karachi suggested that the incidence of β-thalassaemia trait is about 1.4% (Farzana *et al.* 1975; Hashmi & Farzana 1976). In a survey of 500 healthy adults from the northern parts of Punjab and North-West Frontier Province, Khattak and Saleem (1992) reported an incidence of 3.3% in Punjabis rising to almost 8% in the 201 Pathans studied. There are no data available for Afghanistan.

Early reports from Sri Lanka revealed a considerable amount of HbE (~20%) in the Veddahs (Wickremasinghe *et al.* 1963). In a recent survey of school children from different parts of the island it was found that, even though in the small population the distribution is patchy, the incidence of β-thalassaemia trait is about 2%, while that for HbE is 0.5–1% (De Silva *et al.* 2000).

There are few frequency data available for Bangladesh, although it is clear from the many cases of β thalassaemia and HbE β thalassaemia seen during a visit by one of the authors many years ago and in the Bangladeshi community in the UK that both HbE and β thalassaemia must be quite common.

Africa

The haemoglobinopathies in much of Africa, particularly south of the Sahara desert, are dominated by sickle-cell anaemia. Nevertheless, β thalassaemia occurs sporadically throughout the continent. In a later section we shall discuss some of the reasons for this uneven distribution.

North Africa

Beta thalassaemia is found throughout the populations of north Africa. In parts of *Algeria* it reaches frequencies of 3% (Belhani *et al.* 1977; Godet *et al.* 1977; Labie *et al.* 1990) with an average of 1–2%. Cabannes *et al.* (1969a) reported similar frequencies in a number of sedentary northern Saharan populations (Berbers, Arabs, Harratin) and the disease is also seen in *Morocco* (Grozdea *et al.* 1966) and *Libya*, where frequencies of ~7% have been recorded (Jain

1985). Beta thalassaemia has been reported in *Tunisia* (Chibani *et al.* 1988; Fattoum *et al.* 1991) though no prevalence data are given. In *Egypt* incidences of between 2.6% and 4% have been reported (Habib & Böök 1982; Novelletto *et al.* 1989; Novelletto *et al.* 1990) and the disease is a serious public health problem with a predicted 1000 live births annually (Hussein *et al.* 1993). Similar high frequencies have been suggested by small surveys in *Sudan*. Vella (1965) reported 6% of hospital patients to be likely β-thalassaemia heterozygotes. Ibrahim *et al.* (1970), studying members of the Beni Amer tribe (by 'persuasive techniques'!), recorded about 5% with β thalassaemia; a similar frequency was reported by Saha *et al.* (1978) for residents of Khartoum. Similarly, Mourant *et al.* (1974) reported ~5% β thalassaemia in the Kunama and Baria tribes of north-west *Eritrea*. Further south, there are few studies of east African populations that have frequency data for β thalassaemia. An exception is that of Nowicki *et al.* (1975), who reported an incidence of ~3.5% in the Chuabo and Macua groups of *Mozambique*.

West Africa

There are numerous reports of β thalassaemia in West Africa, though few substantive surveys. One of the most systematic is that of Coquelet *et al.* (1978), who screened 10 000 students arriving in France from sub-Saharan Africa. In general, gene frequencies were low in central and eastern Africa. The highest incidences were recorded in the Baoule of *Ivory Coast* (4.6%), the Mossi of *Upper Volta* (2.6%) and the Djerma of *Niger* (2.6%), a similar frequency being reported by Cabannes *et al.* (1967a). Beta thalassaemia was also seen in individuals from *Dahomey*, *Togo*, *Mali*, *Senegal* and *Chad*. In similar studies on West Africans in France by Labie *et al.* (1978), an average frequency of 3.1% was reported for 540 immigrants from *Mali*, *Mauritania* and *Senegal*. Hiernaux (1976) reported a frequency of ~5% in the Sara Majingay of southern *Chad*. Beta thalassaemia has been well documented in *Liberia*. Early surveys were carried out by Olesen *et al.* (1959) and Neel *et al.* (1961). Willcox (1975) found an incidence of 9% in a northern population, and even higher frequencies in the southern Kru-speaking peoples. Bienzle *et al.* (1983b) studied 1578 individuals from four Liberian populations. The incidence of β thalassaemia ranged from 1.6% in the Kissi west Atlantic group to 12.9% in the Sapo Kru, with an overall average of 8.9%, only slightly lower than the 9.8% for HbS. Ringelhann *et al.* (1968) recorded an average incidence of 4% for four populations in *Ghana*, with the highest frequency in the Kassena tribe close to the northern border with Upper Volta. Weatherall *et al.* (1971) recorded lower frequencies of 1.7% for the north and 1.3% for a southern Ghanaian population. The gene frequency is lower in *Nigeria*. Folayan Esan (1970) screened 3002 blood donors in Ibadan and found 23 (0.8%) with β-thalassaemia trait. There have been a number of studies from the *Ivory Coast* in addition to that of Coquelet *et al.* (1978) mentioned earlier. Cabannes *et al.* (1967b, 1969b, 1974) found frequencies ranging from 2% to a high of nearly 5% in a large survey of the Akan. Lower frequencies were noted in the Koulango, who are of Upper Voltaic origin.

South-east Asia

The haemoglobinopathies are widespread throughout south-east Asia, although gene frequency data for many countries are sparse. Large parts of the mainland, from Burma in the west to Vietnam in the east are dominated by HbE; consequently as well as homozygous β thalassaemia, HbE β thalassaemia is a serious public health problem throughout the region (Fig. 6.2).

Burma

Beta thalassaemia has been recognized in Burma for many years (Perabo 1954) and is found at a frequency of about 0.5% (Aung-Than-Batu *et al.* 1968). In contrast HbE reaches a carrier frequency of ~26% in Burmese, 24% in Shans and Mons and 4–10% in Karens and Kachins (Aung-Than-Batu & Hla-Pe 1971).

Thailand, Cambodia and Vietnam

Much more is known about thalassaemia in Thailand as a result of the work of Na-Nakorn, Wasi and Flatz and their colleagues. The overall incidence of β thalassaemia is 4.8%, with the highest incidence of ~11% in northern Thailand and the lowest in Khmer-speakers of the north-east (Flatz *et al.* 1965b), where, in contrast, HbE frequencies reach 50%. Similarly, east of Thailand in Laos the frequency of β thalassaemia averages about 6% (Sicard *et al.* 1979) and HbE

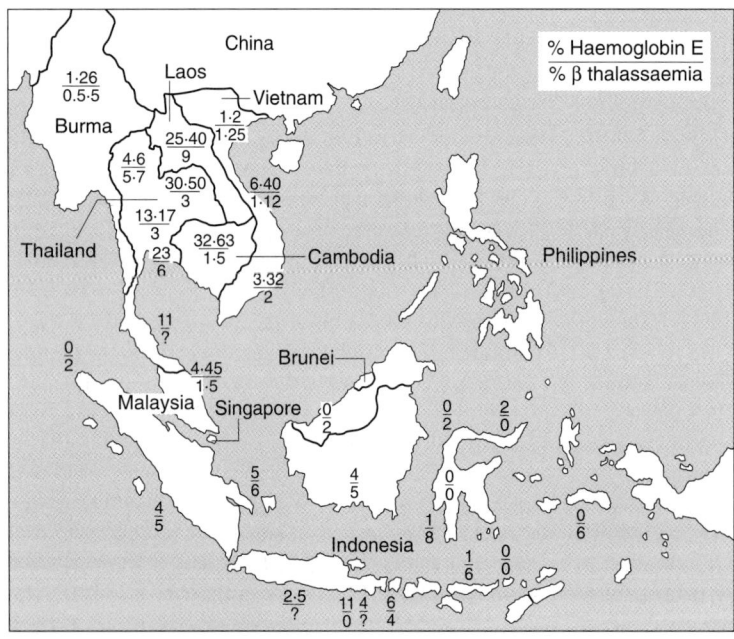

Fig. 6.2 Distribution of β thalassaemia and HbE in south-east Asia. Data obtained from references in text and from unpublished studies by the authors.

carrier frequencies vary from 20% in the north of Laos, to 50% in the south bordering Cambodia (Sicard *et al*. 1979). The frequency of HbE in Cambodia itself varies from 30 to 60% (Goueffon & du Saussay 1967; Sanguansermsri *et al*. 1987; Bashir *et al*. 1992a), averaging ~33% (Satta *et al*. 1970). Beta thalassaemia is much less common: in a study of 264 rural Cambodians, Sanguansermsri *et al*. (1987) found 3.4% with raised HbA$_2$ levels. In Vietnam, β thalassaemia occurs at an average frequency of ~2% (de Traverse *et al*. 1959; Pornpatkul *et al*. 1980). HbE frequencies vary markedly, with the highest (72%) in the Stieng group located close to the border with central Cambodia, and the lowest in Vietnamese from the south.

China

Few data were available from China when the previous edition of this book was written. Much of the information, which had come from Chinese in Hong Kong and Singapore, was summarized in the paper of McFadzean and Todd (1971). It has since become clear that β thalassaemia is a major public health problem, particularly in the south of the country. Zeng and Huang (1987) surveyed over 360 000 people from 12 provinces and found an average incidence of 0.66% with the highest frequencies in Guizhou (2.21%), Sichuan (2.18%), Guangxi (1.52%) and Guangdong (1.08%). A similar overall figure of 0.67% was reported by Yang *et al*. (1985). The incidences for most of the regions studied were similar to those reported by Zeng *et al*. except for Yunnan, where a much higher frequency of 5% is given in the earlier study. A recent summary given to the authors by Professor B. Liu of the West China University of Medical Sciences also reports an incidence of ~2% in the southern provinces of Sichuan, Yunnan and Guizhou, which collectively have a population of over 200 million. A crude estimate would therefore suggest that there are 4 million heterozygotes, and 20 000 homozygous live births per annum in this part of China. In contrast to the countries to the west, HbE is almost unknown in China and, when seen, can usually be traced to an origin in the high-frequency areas of Thailand, Laos and Cambodia. In Taiwan a survey of 4100 women showed that 1.1% of them were β-thalassaemia heterozygotes (Ko *et al*. 1989), a reflection of the mainland ethnic background of most Taiwanese.

Malaysia

Thalassaemia is encountered frequently amongst the Chinese and Malays of the Malay peninsula (Vella 1958b, 1959; Lie-Injo & Chin 1964; Wong 1966). Remarkably, considering the public health problems encountered, there appear to be no reliable gene frequency data available. The incidence of HbE is, however, well documented. Lie-Injo and Chin (1964) reported frequencies of 26 and 45% in the Semai and Temiar aboriginal Malays. Much lower frequencies of 3–10% were seen in the non-aboriginal population (Vella 1962a; Lie-Injo 1970; Lie-Injo & Duraisamy 1972; Ganesan *et al*. 1976). In a study of hospital patients with thalassaemia major, George *et al*. (1992a) reported that HbE β thalassaemics outnumbered β-thalassaemia homozygotes by about 4 to 1 (whereas in Chinese the ratio was 1 to 3). Assuming that fewer HbE β thalassaemics are ascertained than homozygous β thalassaemias, this might imply that the frequency of β thalassaemia in Malays is probably less than 1%.

Indonesia

Thalassaemia is widespread throughout island southeast Asia, though there are few prevalence data available in the literature except for HbE (Lie-Injo 1959b; Vella & Tavaria 1961; Lie-Injo *et al*. 1968). A series of studies in Indonesia by Wahidiyat *et al*. (1987), Sofro *et al*. (1985), Untario *et al*. (1986), Untario (1988) and Sofro (1995) revealed that the incidence of β thalassaemia varied between 4.5 and 7.8%. More recently the authors have had the opportunity to collaborate with Dr A.S.M. Sofro on another detailed survey of several regions of Indonesia. There are remarkable variations of the frequencies of both β thalassaemia and HbE. The highest incidences (10%) of β thalassaemia were seen in central and south Sumatra, with the lowest (0%) in parts of central and north Sulawesi. Intermediate levels were found in south Sulawesi, Kalimantan on the island of Borneo, Lombok, Ambon and Flores. HbE was equally patchily distributed. The highest frequencies are the islands of Savu (25%), Sumbawa (8%) and Madura and in eastern Java (10%) in the south of the archipelago. Elsewhere, frequencies vary between 0 and 5%. The overall average frequencies for β thalassaemia and HbE are 3.7% and 2.7%, respectively. Given that the population of Indonesia is at present approaching 200 million and is projected to reach 265 million by 2025 it is obvious that homozygous β thalassaemia and HbE β thalassaemia present massive public health problems in this region.

Philippines

Beta thalassaemia was found in the Philippines at low frequency (<1%) in a survey of 403 residents of Manilla (Motulsky *et al.* 1964).

Melanesia

Beta thalassaemia was first recognized in Melanesians from New Guinea in 1961 (Ryan 1961). Since then numerous surveys have been carried out and some quite high frequency pockets have been identified. In general β thalassaemia is rare in the malaria-free highland populations, averaging 0.2% in a survey of almost 1000 individuals from four regions. On the coast, where malaria prevalences can be very high, the frequency averaged 5% in surveys of 2600 individuals from 11 regions (summarized in Hill *et al.* 1988). Elsewhere in Melanesia β thalassaemia is uncommon, except for the island of Maewo in Vanuatu, where carrier rates of 13% have been reported (Bowden *et al.* 1987b). There are no reports of β thalassaemia in the indigenous island populations of the central and eastern Pacific.

The Americas

The indigenous populations of the Americas are remarkably free of haemoglobinopathies. Wherever they are found in any significant frequency, there is usually evidence of admixture from immigrant populations from Africa or Europe. But, because of the scale of immigration in some countries, thalassaemia, HbE and sickle-cell disease contribute to a substantial public health problem. Beta thalassaemia occurs in several populations in the Americas. In North America it is found mainly in the immigrant populations of Greeks and Italians and more recently southeast Asians, while in American blacks its incidence reflects that of West Africa. In a 1977 survey, Pierce *et al.* (1977) reported that 1.4% of healthy adults were β-thalassaemia heterozygotes.

In reviewing the data available for Mexico, Ruiz Reyes (1983) concluded that β thalassaemia is extremely rare in the Mayan and Amerindian groups

of Mexico. Lisker (1981) (summarized in Ruiz Reyes 1983) surveyed 3311 'pure' Indians belonging to 20 linguistic groups and found only three HbS heterozygotes. Similar qualitative findings were noted by Matson *et al.* (1963). There are few other frequency data for Central America. In contrast there have been substantial studies for some regions of South America, notably in Venezuela and Brazil. Arends (1984) reviewed a large number of studies on 26 000 Venezuelans, comprising Indian, black and mixed populations. Three β-thalassaemia heterozygotes were seen in 722 members of the Waros tribe of the Orinoco delta, and one individual in 170 Sharapu from Tukoko. Otherwise in over 4500 individuals from 20 tribes, β thalassaemia was absent. In contrast, β thalassaemia was often seen, at frequencies up to 1.4%, in mixed and black populations. For Venezuela as a whole Arends (1984) estimated that there would be over 30 000 β-thalassaemia heterozygotes and over 100 homozygotes in the population of 14.5 million. Sickle-cell anaemia represents a more serious problem, with over 2000 cases estimated.

Beta thalassaemia is not recognized in surveys of Brazilian Indian populations (Salzano & Tondo 1982). The frequencies in non-Indian Brazilians range from 0.8% to 1.1% in southern mixed populations. Most carriers are of Italian descent (Zago & Costa 1985).

The pattern of β thalassaemia in individuals of European descent is also seen in Argentina. Abreu de Miani and Peñalver (1983) found that 0.8% of 4000 blood donors screened in Buenos Aires were heterozygotes and that 97% of these individuals had identified Mediterranean ancestry, mostly Italian. In Surinam, on the other hand, it seems likely that β thalassaemia was introduced from Africa via the slave trade. Pik *et al.* (1965) studied 70 negroid individuals from four regions and found carrier frequencies of between 0.9 and 2.3%. HbS frequencies in these groups varied between 10 and 20%. Native Indians now make up only ~2% of the population of Bolivia. Restrepo (1971) found no abnormal HbS or thalassaemia in 766 people from five tribes. In the black population the frequency of β thalassaemia was about 0.5%, while mulattos and mestizos, who constitute the bulk of the population, had ~0.1%. Haemoglobinopathies in the Caribbean are dominated by HbS and HbC. Frequencies of β thalassaemia are generally low, for example 0.3% in Guadeloupe and Martinique (Gentilini *et al.* 1975).

Finally, we shall end this section with one of the few data sets that cover much of the world. Coquelet *et al.* (1983) studied abnormal haemoglobins and thalassaemia in 35 000 individuals from 99 countries who were examined at the Centres Eurafricain, Euraméricain, Eurasiatique de Biologie Humaine (CEABH) in Paris. Whatever one may say about the limitations of particular studies, at least in this one we assume any there were were consistent across nations! Briefly, their findings were as follows. Among 9417 black Africans the average β-thalassaemia frequency was 0.58% (range for three regions 0.2–1.1%); for 7370 individuals from north Africa and the Mediterranean 'orientale' (Lebanon, Syria, Turkey, Cyprus, Greece), 1.18% (range for 10 countries 0.3–7.1%); for 1793 individuals from Arabia, the Middle East and India, 1.56% (range for 11 countries 0–3.3%); for 2277 individuals from north and south Asia, 1.36% (range for 10 countries 0–3.4%); for 4738 from the Americas, 0.2%; and for Europe (7383 individuals), 0.18%.

Molecular variation of β thalassaemia

When the previous edition of this book was written the impact of the recombinant DNA revolution was only just beginning to make itself felt in the thalassaemia field. Classification of $β^0$ and $β^+$ thalassaemia was about as much as prevailing methods would allow, and even this was difficult in heterozygotes. Indeed, the most reliable approach was the old established one of studying interaction of β-thalassaemia determinants with β structural variants like HbS and HbE.

In the intervening period, characterization of mutations at the molecular level has become commonplace. As we somewhat despondently noted in the introduction to this chapter, we often now have an extremely detailed picture of the different molecular variants that make up the spectrum of the thalassaemia syndromes in a particular country, while remaining in almost complete ignorance about the true scale of the problem.

But the new molecular information has enabled us to tackle questions that were virtually unanswerable previously. We can now make sensible inferences about the origins and movements of particular variants, and as we shall show later we have been able to use this information to address the old issue of the relationship between thalassaemia and malaria.

Distribution of β-thalassaemia alleles

Almost 200 mutations that cause β thalassaemia have been described. Many of them are rare, often encountered only once, but a substantial proportion are extremely common, albeit sometimes with a limited geographical distribution.

In Table 6.2 and Fig. 6.3 we have listed the most frequently reported variants, with a crude geographical breakdown of their distribution. Two features stand out: variants are not uniformly distributed, but have obvious geographical specificity; and, although most populations have a fair number of different variants, two or three usually account for most of the thalassaemia; 20 alleles constitute more than 80% of β-thalassaemia determinants (Table 6.3). Each region has one, or at most two, mild alleles (see Chapter 13).

So in Europe and the Middle East four variants, codon 39 C→T (28%), IVS110 G→A (25%), IVS1-1 G→A (10%) and IVS1-6 T→C (10%), account for almost three-quarters of the β thalassaemia in the region, the first two, in fact, for over 50%. Two of the four are $β^0$ thalassaemias (CD39, IVS1-1 G→A) and the other two are $β^+$. A similar situation is seen in India and south-east Asia. There, three variants, IVS1-5 G→C (33%), CD41/42 (27%) and IVS1-1 G→C (9%), account for over two-thirds of the β thalassaemias in the combined region. In addition a further set of three variants, CD8/9 +G (9%), CD15 G→A (2%) and the 619-bp 3′ deletion (16%), comprise most of the remainder in India, and three different variants, −29 A→G (7%), CD16 −C (10%) and IVS2-654 C→T (14%), bring up the total in the rest of south-east Asia. As in Europe, they comprise a mix of $β^0$ and $β^+$ types. In Africa, the distribution is even more restricted with just two variants, −29 A→G (60%) and −88 C→T (21%), accounting for over three-quarters of the β thalassaemia. It is interesting to note that both these variants are $β^+$ types, largely accounting for the relative mildness of β thalassaemia in black Africans. In addition, compound heterozygotes of these mild β thalassaemias and HbS are likely to have a less severe phenotype than HbS $β^0$-thalassaemia interactions. It is intriguing that in India, where most of the β-thalassaemia variants are $β^0$, the HbS mutation occurs on a haplotype that allows higher levels of HbF production in

Table 6.2 World distribution of β thalassaemia mutations: **(a)** Africa.

Mutation	Type	Egypt 26, 41	Algeria 6, 32	Tunisia 11, 17	US Blacks 23
−101 C→T	+				
−90 C→T	+				
−88 C→A	+				
−88 C→T	+				21.4
−87 C→A	+	0.8			
−87 C→G	+				
−87 C→T	+				
−86 C→G	+				
−30 T→A	+		0.3	2.7	
−29 A→G	+		3.0		60.3
−28 A→G	+				
−28 A→C	+				
−28 A→T	+				
−31 A→G	+				
CAP +1 A→C	+				
CAP +22 G→A	+				
In codon T→C	0				
In codon T→G	0				
In codon A→G	0				
In codon G→A	0				
CD5 −CT	0	1.7		1.8	
CD6 −A	0	1.7	17.7	10.7	0.8
CD8 −AA	0	1.7		0.9	
CD8/9 +G	0				
CD9/10 +C	0				
CD14 +T	0				
CD14/15 +G	0				
CD15 G→A	0				
CD16 −C	0				
CD17 A→T	0				
CD19 A→G	+				
CD22/23/24 (−7)	0				
CD24 T→A	+				2.4
CD25/26 +T	0			0.9	
CD27 G→T	+	0.8	0.3		
CD27/28 +C	0				
CD28 T→G	0				
CD29 C→T	+				
CD30 G→C	0		0.7	1.8	0.8
CD30 A→G	0				
IVS1-1 G→C	0				
IVS1-1 G→T	0				
IVS1-1 G→A	0	11.8	10.5	0.9	
IVS1-2 T→G	0			0.9	
IVS1-2 T→C	0		2.6		0.8
IVS1-2 T→A	0		1.0		
IVS1-5 G→C	+		0.3		
IVS1-5 G→T	+				1.6
IVS1-5 G→A	+		0.7	0.9	
IVS1-6 T→C	+	15.1	3.3	6.3	
IVS1-110 G→A	+	35.3	24.9	12.5	
IVS1-116 T→G	0				

Continued

Table 6.2(a) Africa *Continued.*

References Mutation	Type	Egypt 26, 41	Algeria 6, 32	Tunisia 11, 17	US Blacks 23
IVS1-128 T→G	+				
IVS1-130 G→C	0				
IVS1 –25 bp (+252 to +276)	0				
CD35 C→A	0		3.0		
CD35 –C	0				
CD36/37 –T	0				
CD37 –G	0	1.7			
CD37 G→A	0				
CD38/39 –C	0				
CD39 C→T	0	1.7	21.6	27.7	
CD41 –C	0				
CD41/42 –TCTT	0				
CD43 G→T	0				
CD44 –C	0			3.6	
CD47/48 +4	0				
CD51 –C	0				
CD55 +A	0				
CD61 A→T	0				0.8
CD71/72 +A	0				
CD76 –C	0				
CD82/83 –G	0				
CD90 G→T	0				
IVS2-1 G→A	0	3.4			0.8
IVS2-4/5 –AG	+				
IVS2-654 C→T	+				
IVS2-705 T→G	+				
IVS2-745 C→G	+	5.0	0.7	4.5	
IVS2-843 T→G	+		0.3		
IVS2-848 C→A	+	6.7	0.3	0.9	0.8
IVS2-849 A→C	+				1.6
IVS2-849 A→G	0				2.4
IVS2-850 G→C	0				
IVS2-850 –G	0				
CD106/107 +G	0	1.7			1.6
CD121 G→A	0				
CD121 G→T	0				
CD123–125 (–8)	0				
CD127 C→T	0				
CD127/128 (–3)	0				
Poly(A) (AAA→AAG)	+				
Poly(A) (AAA→GAA)	+				
Poly(A) (AAT→AAC)	+				0.8
Poly(A) (AAA→AGA)	+				
290-bp deletion (–124 to +167)	0				
619-bp deletion (+1065 to 1683)	0				
1393-bp deletion (–485 to +908)	0				1.6
1605-bp deletion (–984 to +620)	0				
Unknown/others		10.9	8.8	23.2	
Chromosomes		119	305	112	126

Table 6.2(b) Southeast and northeast Asia.

Mutation	Type	Burma	China	Malaysia Malays	Malaysia Chinese	Indonesia	Thailand	Taiwan	Japan/Korea
References		7	8, 25, 29 35, 38, 57	22		36	19, 20, 34, 52	9, 37	60
−101 C→T	+								
−90 C→T	+								
−88 C→A	+								
−88 C→T	+								
−87 C→A	+								
−87 C→G	+								
−87 C→T	+								
−86 C→G	+						0.2		
−30 T→A	+								
−29 A→G	+		2.3		1.4			0.3	
−28 A→G	+	4.2	12.4	3.1	11.3		5.8		
−28 A→C	+			2.0	1.4				
−28 A→T	+							6.7	
−31 A→G	+								16.1
CAP +1 A→C	+								
CAP +22 G→A	+								
In codon T→C	0							1.7	
In codon T→G	0								4.3
In codon A→G	0								7.5
In codon G→A	0								0.2
CD5 –CT	0								
CD6 –A	0								
CD8 –AA	0								
CD8/9 +G	0						0.2		
CD9/10 +G	0								
CD14 +T	0								
CD14/15 +G	0		0.1				0.2		
CD15 G→A	0					6.8			1.0
CD16 –C	0								
CD17 A→T	0	7.4	16.6	7.1	2.8	1.7	21.2	10.0	0.2
CD19 A→G	+			10.2	4.2		5.4		
CD22/23/24 (−7)	0								
CD24 T→A	+								
CD25/26 +T	0								
CD27 G→T	+								
CD27/28 +C	0							2.7	
CD28 T→G	0								
CD29 C→T	+								
CD30 G→C	0					1.7			
CD30 A→G	0								
IVS1-1 G→C	0								
IVS1-1 G→T	0	35.8	1.3	9.2	1.4	10.2	3.8	0.3	1.0
IVS1-1 G→A	0					1.7			
IVS1-2 T→G	0								
IVS1-2 T→C	0			1.0					
IVS1-2 T→A	0								
IVS1-5 G→C	+	28.4	1.8	45.9	1.4	54.2	9.6		
IVS1-5 G→T	+								
IVS1-5 G→A	+								
IVS1-6 T→C	+								

Continued

Table 6.2(b) Southeast and northeast Asia *Continued.*

		Burma	China	Malaysia		Indonesia	Thailand	Taiwan	Japan/Korea
				Malays	Chinese				
References		7	8, 25, 29 35, 38, 57	22		36	19, 20, 34, 52	9, 37	60
Mutation	Type								
IVS1-110 G→A	+								
IVS1-116 T→G	0								
IVS1-128 T→G	+							0.3	
IVS1-130 G→C	0								
IVS1-25 (+252 to +276)	0								
CD35 C→A	0						0.8		
CD35 –C	0			4.1		1.7			
CD36/37 –T	0								
CD37 –G	0								
CD37 G→A	0								
CD38/39 –C	0								
CD39 C→T	0								
CD41 –C	0						0.2		
CD41/42 –TCTT	0	22.1	42.3	7.1	53.5	1.7	40.2	38.2	7.2
CD43 G→T	0		0.4					0.3	
CD44 –C	0								
CD47/48 +4	0								
CD51 –C	0								
CD55 +A	0								
CD61 A→T	0								
CD71/72 +A	0		5.8		2.8		2.4	0.3	
CD76 –C	0								
CD82/83 –G	0								
CD90 G→T	0								15.7
IVS2-1 G→A	0								10.8
IVS2-4/5 –AG	+								
IVS2-654 C→T	+	2.1	12.1	4.1	19.7	11.9	6.0	39.2	13.6
IVS2-705 T→G	+								
IVS2-745 C→G	+								
IVS2-843 T→G	+								
IVS2-848 C→A	+								
IVS2-849 A→C	+								
IVS2-849 A→G	0								
IVS2-850 G→C	0								
IVS2-850 –G	0								
CD106/107 +G	0								
CD121 G→A	0								2.9
CD121 G→T	0								
CD123–125 (–8)	0						0.2		
CD127 C→T	0								
CD127/128 (–3)	0								3.9
Poly(A) (AAA→AAG)	+								
Poly(A) (AAA→GAA)	+								
Poly(A) (AAT→AAC)	+								
Poly(A) (AAA→AGA)	+		1.0						
290-bp deletion	0								
619-bp deletion	0								
1392-bp deletion	0								
1605-bp deletion	0								
Unknown/others				5.1		8.5	3.8		15.7
Chromosomes		95	710	98	71	59	533	301	279

Table 6.2(c) West Asia and the Middle East.

Mutation	Type	Turkey 2,3,4,42	Lebanon 10,56	Israel 63	UAE 16,44	Jordan 59	Iran 58	Kurdistan 48	Azerbaijan 13,31,49,50
−101 C→T	+	0.5			1.4				
−90 C→T	+			0.2					
−88 C→A	+						0.9		0.5
−88 C→T	+		0.6	0.2					
−87 C→A	+								
−87 C→G	+	1.2	0.6			2.2			
−87 C→T	+								
−86 C→G	+								
−30 T→A	+	3.5	0.6	0.7					1.1
−29 A→G	+								
−28 A→G	+								
−28 A→C	+	0.4		6.0				28.8	0.5
−28 A→T	+								
−31 A→G	+					3.3			
CAP +1 A→C	+								
CAP +22 G→A	+								0.8
In codon T→C	0								
In codon T→G	0								
In codon A→G	0								
In codon G→A	0								
CD5 −CT	0	2.4	3.1	1.7	4.7	3.3			0.3
CD6 −A	0	0.6		0.2					
CD8 −AA	0	5.9	5.0	2.5	3.4		3.7		30.4
CD8/9 +G	0	2.0			8.5		4.6		6.4
CD9/10 +G	0	0.1							
CD14 +T	0								0.3
CD14/15 +G	0								
CD15 G→A	0	0.2		0.7	2.1				1.6
CD16 −C	0								0.5
CD17 A→T	0								
CD19 A→G	+						0.9		
CD22/23/24 (−7)	0								0.3
CD24 T→A	+								
CD25/26 +T	0								
CD27 G→T	+	0.1		0.2		3.3			
CD27/28 +C	0								
CD28 T→G	0								
CD29 C→T	+		5.0			1.1			0.8
CD30 G→C	0				0.9				0.8
CD30 A→G	0		1.2						
IVS1-1 G→C	0				0.4	3.0	0.9		
IVS1-1 G→T	0								1.3
IVS1-1 G→A	0	3.7	11.8	5.5			3.7		1.9
IVS1-2 T→G	0								
IVS1-2 T→C	0								
IVS1-2 T→A	0								
IVS1-5 G→C	+	1.0	3.1	1.4	56.6	5.5	7.4		1.6
IVS1-5 G→T	+	0.5							0.3
IVS1-5 G→A	+	0.1							
IVS1-6 T→C	+	13.3	6.2	12.1	3.0	6.6	4.6		4.5
IVS1-110 G→A	+	40.6	46.6	23.7	1.3	22.0	6.5	13.6	11.9
IVS1-116 T→G	0	0.1							

Continued

Table 6.2(c) West Asia and the Middle East *Continued.*

References Mutation	Type	Turkey 2,3,4,42	Lebanon 10,56	Israel 63	UAE 16,44	Jordan 59	Iran 58	Kurdistan 48	Azerbaijan 13,31,49,50
IVS1-128 T→G	+								0.3
IVS1-130 G→C	0	0.2							
IVS1 –25 (+252 to +276)	0		0.6		6.8		3.7		
CD35 C→A	0								
CD35 –C	0								
CD36/37 –T	0			1.1			1.9		1.3
CD37 –G	0				0.9				
CD37 G→A	0			5.5		8.8			
CD38/39 –C	0								
CD39 C→T	0	3.8	1.2	11.6	4.3	2.2	5.5	1.7	2.1
CD41 –C	0								
CD41/42 –TCTT	0								
CD43 G→T	0								
CD44 –C	0		1.2	9.4	0.9		3.7	38.9	2.4
CD47/48 +4	0								
CD51 –C	0								
CD55 +A	0								
CD61 A→T	0								
CD71/72 +A	0								
CD76 –C	0								
CD82/83 –G	0								3.7
CD90 G→T	0								
IVS2-1 G→A	0	6.9	6.8	7.7	3.8	20.0	13.8		15.9
IVS2-4/5 –AG	+								
IVS2-654 C→T	+								
IVS2-705 T→G	+								
IVS2-745 C→G	+	2.7	3.7	2.5		12.1	3.7		0.8
IVS2-843 T→G	+								
IVS2-848 C→A	+					2.2			
IVS2-849 A→C	+								
IVS2-849 A→G	0								
IVS2-850 G→C	0								
IVS2I-850 –G	0								
CD106/107 +G	0			0.2					
CD121 G→A	0								
CD121 G→T	0								
CD123–125 (–8)	0								
CD127 C→T	0								
CD127/128 (–3)	0								
Poly(A) (AAA→AAG)	+			2.8				15.3	
Poly(A) (AAA→GAA)	+								
Poly(A) (AAT→AAC)	+								
Poly(A) (AAA→AGA)	+								
290-bp deletion	0		1.9						
619-bp deletion	0								
1392-bp deletion	0								
1605-bp deletion	0								
Unknown/others		10.0	0.6	2.3		4.4	36.1	1.7	7.7
Chromosomes		817	161	446	235	91	108	59	377

Table 6. 2(d) Europe.

References Mutation	Type	Portugal 12, 18, 51	Spain 1,40	France 39	UK 24	Germany 33	Italy 47
−101 C→T	+						0.4
−90 C→T	+	1.2					
−88 C→A	+						
−88 C→T	+						
−87 C→A	+						
−87 C→G	+						1.5
−87 C→T	+						0.1
−86 C→G	+						
−30 T→A	+						
−29 A→G	+						
−28 A→G	+						
−28 A→C	+						
−28 A→T	+						
CAP +1 A→C	+						
CAP +22 (G→A)	+						
In codon T→C	0						
In codon T→G	0						
In codon A→G	0						
In codon G→A	0						
CD5 −CT	0				8.7		
CD6 −A	0		2.9				1.2
CD8 −AA	0		1.0				
CD8/9 +G	0						
CD9/10 +C	0						
CD14 +T	0						
CD14/15 +G	0						
CD15 G→A	0	7.9					
CD16 −C	0						
CD17 A→T	0						
CD19 A→G	+						
CD22/23/24 (−7)	0						
CD24 T→A	+						
CD25/26 +T	0						
CD27 G→T	+						
CD27/28 +C	0						
CD28 T→G	0				4.3		
CD29 C→T	+						
CD30 G→C	0						0.1
CD30 A→G	0						
IVS1-1 G→C	0						
IVS1-1 G→T	0						
IVS1-1 G→A	0	21.0	11.5	10.5	8.7	2.6	10.4
IVS1-2 T→G	0						
IVS1-2 T→C	0						
IVS1-2 T→A	0						
IVS1-5 G→C	+						0.2
IVS1-5 G→T	+						
IVS1-5 G→A	+						0.1
IVS1-6 T→C	+	19.0	12.6	8.6	4.3		10.1
IVS1-110 G→A	+	11.5	16.5	25.7	4.3	7.7	23.5
IVS1-116 T→G	0						
IVS1-128 T→G	+						

Yugoslavia 15	Czechoslovakia 27	Hungary 45	Bulgaria 28, 43	Greece 30	Sardinia 46	Sicily 14	Cyprus 5
			0.5	0.5			
0.4							
0.8			2.6	2.0	0.2	1.0	
0.8							
0.4							
		13.8					
2.1			3.1	0.3			
1.2			6.2	2.8	2.1		0.1
4.2			3.6	1.1			0.2
			3.6				
1.2							
10.3	45.2	31.0	4.1	13.9	< 0.1	3.1	6.0
21.5		6.9	9.8	8.8	0.1	28.9	6.4
38.8	5.4		27.3	43.1	0.5	26.8	78.4

Continued

Table 6. 2(d) Europe *Continued.*

References Mutation	Type	Portugal 12, 18, 51	Spain 1, 40	France 39	UK 24	Germany 33	Italy 47
IVS1-130 G→C	0	0.8					0.4
IVS1 –25 bp (+252 to +276)	0						
CD35 C→A	0						
CD35 –C	0						
CD36/37 –T	0						
CD37 –G	0						
CD38/39 –C	0						
CD39 C→T	0	37.3	50.0	41.9	34.8	51.3	41.0
CD41 –C	0						
CD41/42 –TCTT	0				4.3		
CD43 G→T	0						
CD44 –C	0						0.7
CD47/48 +4	0						
CD51 –C	0						
CD55 +A	0						
CD61 A→T	0						
CD71/72 +A	0						
CD76 –C	0						0.4
CD82/83 –G	0						
IVS2-1 G→A	0			1.0		5.1	3.9
IVS2-4/5 –AG	+						
IVS2-654 C→T	+						
IVS2-705 T→G	+		1.0				
IVS2-745 C→G	+		1.0	2.8			5.2
IVS2-843 T→G	+						
IVS2-848 C→A	+						
IVS2-849 A→C	+						
IVS2-849 A→G	0						
IVS2-850 G→C	0						
IVS2-850 (–G)	0						0.1
CD106/107 +G	0						
CD121 G→A	0				13.0		
CD121 G→T	0	0.4					
CD123–125 –8	0						
CD127 C→T	0				4.3		
Poly(A) (AAA→AAG)	+						
Poly(A) (AAA→GAA)	+						
Poly(A) (AAT→AAC)	+						
Poly(A) AATAAA→AATAGA	+						
290-bp deletion (–124 to +167)	0						0.1
619-bp deletion (+1065 to 1683)	0						
1393-bp deletion (–485 to +908)	0						
1605-bp deletion (–984 to +620)	0						
Unknown/others		0.4	3.9	9.5	13.0	33.3	0.4
Chromosomes		252	103	105	23	39	893

Yugoslavia 15	Czechoslovakia 27	Hungary 45	Bulgaria 28, 43	Greece 30	Sardinia 46	Sicily 14	Cyprus 5
3.7	7.5 / 2.2	34.5	19.6	20.9	95.7	36.1	2.5
		3.4					
					0.7	1.0	
0.1	7.5 / 14.0	6.9	2.1	2.0	< 0.1		
1.7	4.3	3.4	8.2	3.0	0.4	3.1	5.7
1.7							
0.4							
	11.8						
3.7			0.5				
0.4 / 5.4	2.2		8.8	1.6			1.9
242	93	29	194	642	3000	97	937

Table 6.2(e) Indian subcontinent.

Reference Mutation	Type	Gujerat 53	Punjab 21, 53, 55	Maharastra 21, 53	Tamil Nadu 53, 54
−101 C→T	+				
−90 C→T	+				
−88 C→A	+				
−88 C→T	+		1.6		
−87 C→A	+				
−87 C→G	+				
−87 C→T	+				
−86 C→G	+				
−30 T→A	+				
−29 A→G	+				
−28 A→G	+				
−28 A→C	+				
−28 A→T	+				
−31 A→G	+				
CAP+1 A→C	+		3.7		
CAP +22 G→A	+				
In codon T→C	0				
In codon T→G	0				
In codon A→G	0				
In codon G→A	0				
CD5 −CT	0		0.5	1.8	
CD6 −A	0				
CD8 −AA	0				
CD8/9 +G	0	4.0	12.5	1.8	2.9
CD9/10 +G	0				
CD14 +T	0				
CD14/15 +G	0				
CD15 G→A	0	1.5	0.3	14.0	
CD16 −C	0		1.9		
CD17 A→T	0				
CD19 A→G	+				
CD22/23/24 (−7)	0				
CD24 T→A	+				
CD25/26 +T	0				
CD27 G→T	+				
CD27/28 +C	0				
CD28 T→G	0				
CD29 C→T	+				
CD30 G→C	0	2.0	0.3	1.8	
CD30 A→G	0				
IVS1-1 G→C	0				
IVS1-1 G→T	0	16.8	14.9	1.8	
IVS1-1 G→A	0			1.8	
IVS1-2 T→G	0				
IVS1-2 T→C	0				
IVS1-2 T→A	0				
IVS1-5 G→C	+	41.1	34.1	59.6	85.9
IVS1-5 G→T	+				
IVS1-5 G→A	+				
IVS1-6 T→C	+				
IVS1-110 G→A	+				
IVS1-116 T→G	0				
IVS1-128 T→G	+		0.3		
IVS1-130 G→C	0				
IVS1 −25 (+252 to +276)	0				
CD35 C→A	0				

Haryana 55	Uttar Pradesh 55	Rajasthan 55	Bihar 55	Bengal 55	Pakistan 53,55, 61,62
1.7	4.9				0.2
1.7	3.3				1.2
					2.1
1.7	11.5	10.0	15.2	3.2	24.1
	4.9				3.3
1.7	4.9	4.0	3.0		1.8
	1.6	2.0		0.8	2.3
			6.1		0.5
10.2		2.0			10.4
					0.5
57.6	49.2	66.0	66.7	76.0	32.4

Continued

Table 6.2(e) Indian subcontinent *Continued.*

Reference Mutation	Type	Gujerat 53	Punjab 21,53,55	Maharastra 21,53	Tamil Nadu 53,54
CD35 –C	0				
CD36/37 –T	0				
CD37 –G	0				
CD37 G→A	0				
CD38/39 –C	0				
CD39 C→T	0				
CD41 –C	0				
CD41/42 –TCTT	0	8.6	12.8	1.8	9.3
CD43 G→T	0				
CD44 –C	0				
CD47/48 +4	0		0.3		
CD51 –C	0				
CD55 +A	0			1.8	
CD61 A→T	0				
CD71/72 +A	0				
CD76 –C	0				
CD82/83 –G	0				
CD90 G→T	0				
IVS2-1 G→A	0		0.3	1.8	
IVS2-4/5 –AG	+				
IVS2-654 C→T	+				
IVS2-705 T→G	+				
IVS2-745 C→G	+				
IVS2-843 T→G	+				
IVS2-848 C→A	+				
IVS2-849 A→C	+				
IVS2-849 A→G	0				
IVS2-850 G→C	0				
IVS2-850 –G	0				
CD106/107 +G	0				
CD121 G→A	0				
CD121 G→T	0				
CD123–125 (–8)	0				
CD127 C→T	0				
CD127/128 (–3)	0				
Poly(A) (AAA→AAG)	+				
Poly(A) (AAA→GAA)	+				
Poly(A) (AAT→AAC)	+				
Poly(A) (AAA→AGA)	+				
290-bp deletion	0				
619-bp deletion	0	25.9	15.7	5.3	1.0
1392-bp deletion	0				
1605-bp deletion	0				
Unknown/others			0.8	7.0	1.0
Chromosomes		197	375	57	205

The percentage gene frequencies of each mutation identified are given for the total number of thalassaemic chromosomes examined. This table is compiled from studies attempting to establish the prevalence of different mutations in populations. Therefore the table should not be taken as a guide to whether or not a mutation is present in a population. We have presented only quantitative data, where available, for mutation frequencies. References: 1. Amselem *et al.* (1988); 2. Atalay *et al.* (1993); 3. Aulehla-Scholz *et al.* (1990); 4. Basak *et al.* (1992); 5. Baysal *et al.* (1992); 6. Bennani *et al.* (1994); 7. Brown *et al.* (1989); 8. Chan *et al.* (1987a); 9. Chang *et al.* (1994); 10. Chehab *et al.* (1987); 11. Chibani *et al.* (1988); 12. Coutinho Gomes *et al.* (1988); 13. Çürük *et al.* (1992b); 14. Di Marzo *et al.* (1988); 15. Efremov *et al.* (1982); 16. El-Kalla and Mathews (1993); 17. Fattoum *et al.* (1991); 18. Faustino *et al.* (1992); 19. Fucharoen *et al.* (1989b); 20. Fukumaki *et al.* (1992); 21. Garewal *et al.* (1994); 22.

Haryana 55	Uttar Pradesh 55	Rajasthan 55	Bihar 55	Bengal 55	Pakistan 53,55, 61,62
					0.1
8.5	13.1	12.0	3.0	9.6	6.3
					0.4
					0.6
16.9	3.3	4.0		0.8	13.1
	3.3		6.1	9.6	0.7
59	61	50	33	125	2490

George *et al.* (1992a); 23. Gonzalez-Redondo *et al.* (1991); 24. Hall *et al.* (1992); 25. Huang *et al.* (1990); 26. Hussein *et al.* (1993); 27. Indrák *et al.* (1992); 28. Kalaydjieva *et al.* (1989); 29. Kazazian *et al.* (1986a); 30. Kollia *et al.* (1992); 31. Kuliev *et al.* (1994); 32. Labie *et al.* (1990); 33. Laig *et al.* (1990b); 34. Laig *et al.* (1989); 35. Liang *et al.* (1994); 36. Lie-Injo *et al.* (1989); 37. Lin *et al.* (1991); 38. Liu *et al.* (1989); 39. Milland *et al.* (1987); 40. Molina *et al.* (1994); 41. Novelletto *et al.* (1990); 42. Öner *et al.* (1990); 43. Petkov *et al.* (1990); 44. Quaife *et al.* (1994); 45. Ringelhann *et al.* (1993); 46. Rosatelli *et al.* (1992b); 47. Rosatelli *et al.* (1992c); 48. Rund *et al.* (1991); 49. Tagiev *et al.* (1993); 50. Tagiev *et al.* (1994); 51. Tamagnini *et al.* (1993); 52. Thein *et al.* (1990b); 53. Varawalla *et al.* (1991a); 54. Venkatesan *et al.* (1992); 55. Verma *et al.* (1997); 56. Zahed *et al.* (1997); 57. Zhang *et al.* (1988b); 58. Nozari *et al.* (1995); 59. Sadiq *et al.* (1994); 60. Ohba *et al.* (1997); 61. Ahmed *et al.* (1996); 62. Khan and Riazuddin (1998); 63. Filon *et al.* (1994).

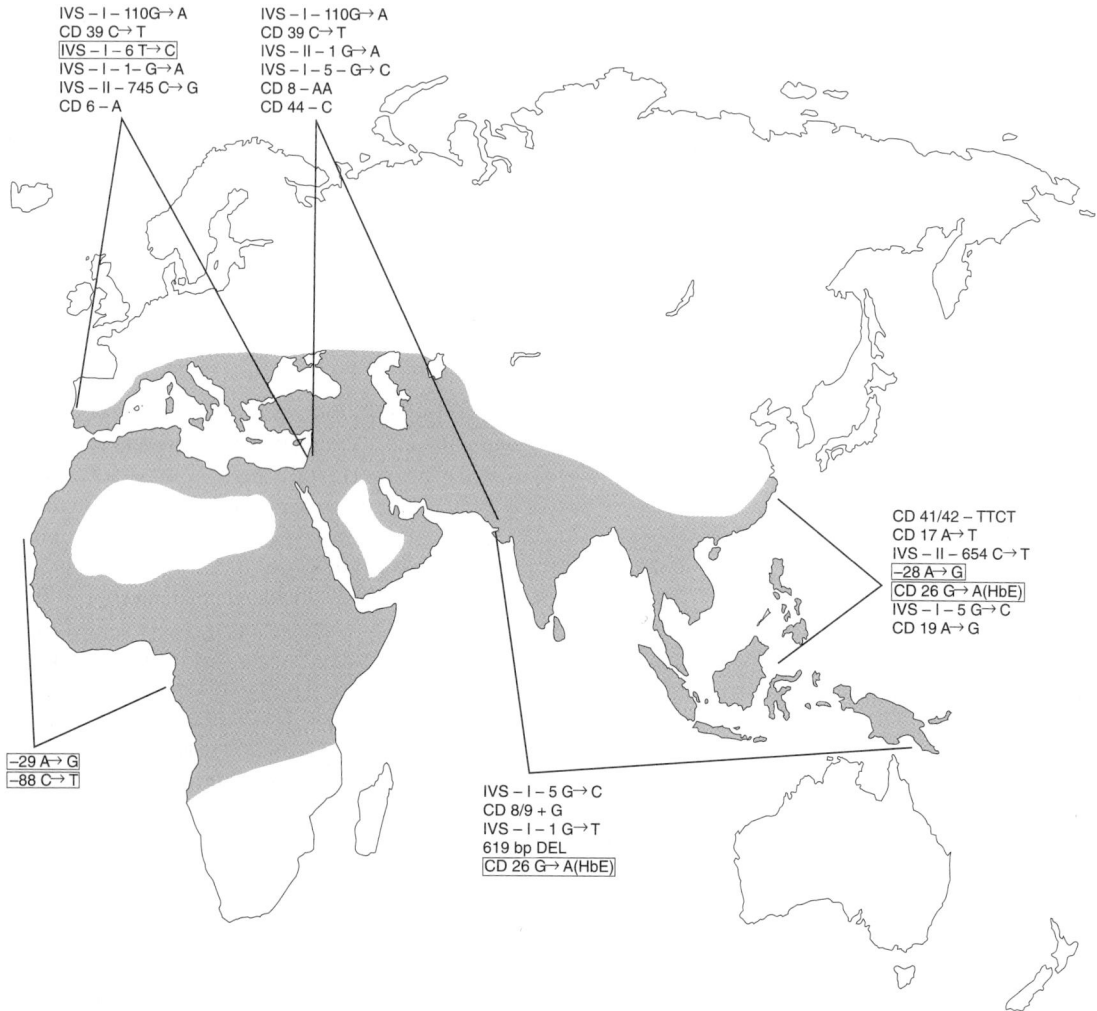

IVS – I – 110G→ A
CD 39 C→ T
IVS – I – 6 T→ C
IVS – I – 1 – G→ A
IVS – II – 745 C→ G
CD 6 – A

IVS – I – 110G→ A
CD 39 C→ T
IVS – II – 1 G→ A
IVS – I – 5 – G→ C
CD 8 – AA
CD 44 – C

CD 41/42 – TTCT
CD 17 A→ T
IVS – II – 654 C→ T
–28 A→ G
CD 26 G→ A(HbE)
IVS – I – 5 G→ C
CD 19 A→ G

–29 A→ G
–88 C→ T

IVS – I – 5 G→ C
CD 8/9 + G
IVS – I – 1 G→ T
619 bp DEL
CD 26 G→ A(HbE)

Fig. 6.3 Distribution of the common β-thalassaemia alleles. The boxed mutations are mild alleles.

homozygotes or compound heterozygotes with β tha-lassaemia. In India and Africa, therefore, the particu-lar combinations of β-thalassaemia mutations and HbS haplotype are those that minimize the severity of the compound heterozygous state. Nevertheless, it seems likely that the co-existence of β thalassaemia in India and Africa with HbS, and in south-east Asia with HbE, is (or was until the intervention of modern medicine) a transient affair. As Livingstone (1967, 1985) has argued, a higher relative fitness of β^S and β^E genes in malarial regions would ultimately result in the replacement of β-thalassaemia genes by the struc-tural variants.

α Thalassaemia

Prior to the introduction of DNA analysis, popula-tion surveys for α thalassaemia were based entirely on measurement of Hb Bart's levels in cord bloods. Although relatively straightforward, this assay has certain drawbacks, which only became apparent when the molecular basis of the α thalassaemias was established. The most important is that single-gene-deletion heterozygotes do not always have detectable Hb Bart's in the neonatal period (Higgs *et al.* 1980b), unlike homozygotes (−α/−α) and α^0-thalassaemia heterozygotes (−−/αα), which usually have Hb Bart's

Table 6.3 The common β-thalassaemia alleles which comprise over 80% of all β-thalassaemia determinants. Modified from Huisman *et al.* (1997).

Allele	Main ethnic groups
–88 C→T	African
–31 A→G	Japanese
–29 A→G	African
–28 A→G	Chinese, Thai, Israeli
CD6 –A	North African
CD8 –AA	Arab
CD8/9 +G	Indian, Arab
CD17 A→T	Chinese, Thai
CD19 A→G	Thai
IVS1-1 G→T	Indian, Thai
IVS1-5 G→C	Indian, Thai, Indonesian, Malay, Arab
IVS1-6 T→C	Mediterranean
IVS1-110 G→A	Mediterranean
CD39 C→T	Mediterranean, Arab
CD41/42 –TTCT	Chinese, Thai, Indian, Malay
CD44 –C	Arab
CD90 G→T	Japanese
IVS2-1 G→A	Arab, Turkish
IVS2-654 C→T	Chinese, Thai
IVS2-745 C→G	Mediterranean
619-bp deletion	North Indian

levels in the 3–6% range. In practice, this meant that the gene frequency of –α could not be reliably determined, especially in low-incidence regions where –α/–α homozygotes were rare. In addition, where α thalassaemia was common—south-east Asia for example—and where, as we now know, both –α (α⁺) and α⁰ determinants are present, a raised Hb Bart's, say, 5%, could represent either the –α/–α or ––/αα genotypes.

The introduction of Southern blotting clarified some of these issues, but highlighted others, particularly that of non-deletion α thalassaemia. Moreover, Southern blotting is an expensive technique, so it has by no means replaced Hb Bart's screening in population surveys.

Thus, for a number of reasons, reliable data on population frequencies for the various forms of α thalassaemia are not always available. But it is clear that α thalassaemia is common throughout the malarial (and even parts of the non-malarial) world (Fig. 6.4 and Table 6.4). Indeed it seems likely that it is probably the most common of all single-gene disorders, as a result of selection by malaria. This is a topic we shall return to later in the chapter.

Because of the difficulties in screening for α thalassaemia phenotypically, we shall describe what is known of its distribution and frequency, combining the information from the level of Hb Bart's in neonates with the limited amount of data that are available from studies at the DNA level.

Distribution and frequencies

Europe

Italy

Although some of the earliest surveys (Silvestroni & Bianco 1962) suggested that α thalassaemia was relatively uncommon in Italy, this has not been borne out by more recent work. Iolascon *et al.* (1982) found that 25 of 1147 (2.17%) consecutive newborns from the Naples area had Hb Bart's levels exceeding 1%. Izzo *et al.* (1979) noted 1.63% of 550 newborns from Apulia had Hb Bart's levels >2% (with a further 6.18% having detectable but 'non-measurable' levels). In Naples, Pepe *et al.* (1982) recorded somewhat lower figures of 1.6% with traces of Hb Bart's, with a further 0.2% having levels >1%. This compares with an early study of Pinto *et al.* (1978), who found 2.7% of 319 cord bloods from Campania had Hb Bart's levels >1%. Further north, Velati *et al.* (1983) found that ~3.1% of 3037 cord bloods collected in Milan had detectable Hb Bart's; in Turin the figure was 1.5% and for Genoa ~6.1%. Velati *et al.* make the point that each of these three cities has a very heterogeneous population mix, Genoa in particular having many individuals of Sardinian origin, where α thalassaemia is common (see below). Despite this, Pinto *et al.* (1978) noted that only two of 40 cases of HbH disease recorded in Italy up to the end of 1977 had been seen in the north, the remainder being evenly divided between the south, Sicily and Sardinia.

Sicily

In Sicily, Maggio *et al.* (1982) reported 3.5% of over 1000 cord bloods collected from five western hospitals had Hb Bart's levels >1%, while a further 1.5% had levels of less than 1%. The heterogeneity of molecular defects underlying these figures has recently been elucidated in a study of over 1000 adults by Fichera *et al.* (1997). Their data reveal a gene fre-

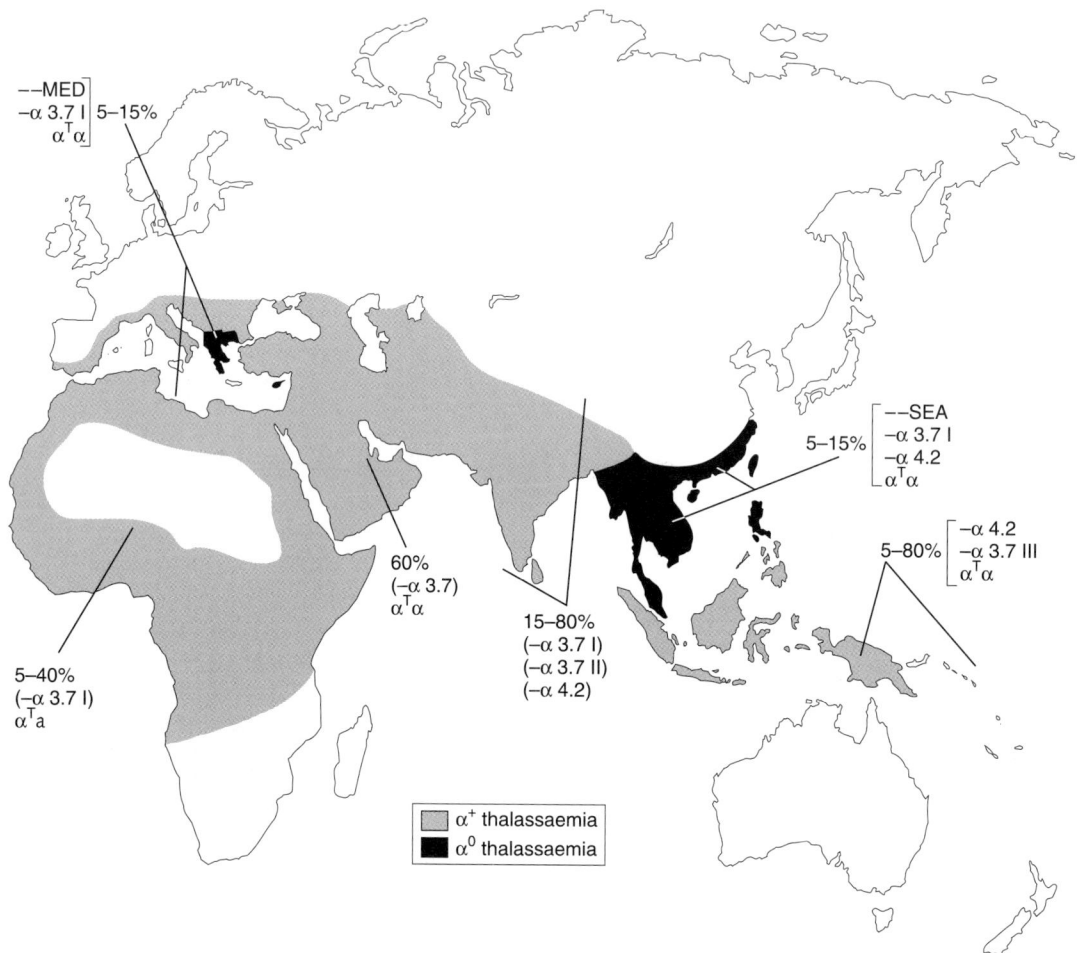

Fig. 6.4 World distribution of α^+ and α^0 thalassaemia.

quency for α^+ thalassaemia of 4.1%. The $\alpha^{3.7I}$ deletion was the most frequently seen (87%) variant but $-\alpha^{4.2}$, $-\alpha^{3.7II}$, $\alpha 2$ IVS1 5 bp deletion (also known as $\alpha^{Hph1}\alpha$) and $\alpha 2$ initiation codon T→C (also known as $\alpha^{Nco1}\alpha$), were also seen at low frequency. Two defects, $--^{MED}$ and $--^{CAL}$, accounted for the α^0 variants present. Three α-thalassaemia determinants that were specifically sought: $-\alpha^{(20.5)}$ and two poly(A) mutations (AATAAA→G; AATA→G) were not found.

Sardinia

Early studies in Sardinia (Bianco *et al.* 1972) suggested that α thalassaemia might be quite common

on the island. Detectable Hb Bart's was noted in 4.3% of a series of 465 cord bloods. A similar incidence of 4.79% was noted in a survey of 11 160 cord bloods in northern Sardinia (Meloni *et al.* 1981). Extensive surveys by Professor Cao's group (Galanello *et al.* 1980) revealed an even higher incidence in southern Sardinia: 12.6% of 2291 cord bloods had Hb Bart's levels exceeding 1%, most falling into two groups with either 1–2% or ~5% Hb Bart's, and four individuals had ~25% (indicative of HbH disease). Professor Cao and colleagues have explored the molecular basis of α thalassaemia in Sardinia in some detail (Pirastu *et al.* 1982; Cao *et al.* 1991; Galanello *et al.* 1992), mainly by characterizing

Table 6.4 World distribution of α^+-thalassaemia.

Country	$-\alpha^{3.7}$	$-\alpha^{4.2}$	$-\alpha^{3.7I}$	$-\alpha^{3.7II}$	$-\alpha^{3.7III}$	Number of chromosomes	Reference
Africa (Bantu-speaking)		0	29			76	Dodé *et al.* (1988)
Africa (Beninian Gulf)		0	40			20	Dodé *et al.* (1988)
Africa (Gambia)	8	0				106	Abdalla *et al.* (1989); present authors (unpublished)
Africa (Kenya)	19	0					Present authors (unpublished)
Africa (San)	6	0				202	Ramsay & Jenkins (1987)
Africa (southern)	9	0				306	Ramsay & Jenkins (1987)
Africa (west Atlantic)		0	17			41	Dodé *et al.* (1988)
Africa (Zambia)	27					218	Muklwala *et al.* (1989)
Australia (Aboriginal)	3	0				238	Roberts-Thomson *et al.* (1996)
China (south)	<1	<1				202	Chan *et al.* (1986b)
Cyprus (Greek)	7	0				100	Pirastu *et al.* (1982)
Egypt	8	<1				124	Novelletto *et al.* (1989)
Greece	7	0				454	Kanavakis *et al.* (1988)
India	18	8				282	Kulozik *et al.* (1988a)
India, Andhra Pradesh (Konda Doya)		32	26	1		50	Fodde *et al.* (1988)
India, Andhra Pradesh (Konda Reddi)		0	53			32	Fodde *et al.* (1988)
Indonesia	4	1				979	A.S.M. Sofro and present authors (unpublished) (various islands)
Italy	5	0				100	Velati *et al.* (1986)
Melanesia	0–28	2–60				3000	O'Shaughnessy *et al.* (1990)
Micronesia		<1	<1		2	844	O'Shaughnessy *et al.* (1990)
Nepal (non-Tharu)		0	6			68	Modiano *et al.* (1991)
Nepal (Tharu)		0	75	5		72	Modiano *et al.* (1991)
Polynesia		<1	<2		2–9	662	O'Shaughnessy *et al.* (1990)
Portugal	4	<1				200	Peres *et al.* (1995)
Sardinia		0	18			96	Di Rienzo *et al.* (1986)
Saudi Arabia	9	<1				152	D.R. Higgs (unpublished)
Sicily	4	<1				2000	Fichera *et al.* (1987)
Spain	1					800	Villegas *et al.* (1992)
Taiwan	2	≤1				2418	Ko *et al.* (1993a)
Thailand (north-east)		2	15			128	Hundreiser *et al.* (1990)
Thailand (northern)	9	<1				212	Hundreiser *et al.* (1988)
Turkey	3	0				138	Fei *et al.* (1989a)

cases of HbH disease. The most prevalent genotype is $--/-\alpha^{3.7}$, accounting for nearly 84% of cases; $--/\alpha^{Ncol}\alpha$ (9.8%) is the next commonest. The $--/-\alpha^{4.2}$ combination is relatively rare (1.4%) as is the $--/\alpha^{Hph1}\alpha$.

This is a similar spectrum of α-thalassaemia mutations to that seen in Sicily and, although there are few published data (Velati *et al.* 1986), one assumes, Italy.

Greece

The first description of HbH disease in Greece was reported by Gouttas *et al.* (1960) and some of the early work on the genetics of the disease was carried out by Fessas (1959). Despite these early beginnings, information about the prevalence of α thalassaemia in Greece has been limited. A survey of 500 cord bloods by Fessas (1961) showed that 0.3% had elevated Hb Bart's levels. One survey, relying on haematological changes in a population from the lowland region of Arta (Fraser *et al.* 1964), suggested that the prevalence of α thalassaemia might be as high as 5%. In a much later study, Kanavakis *et al.* (1986) compared the incidence of α thalassaemia determined by Hb Bart's analysis of 227 cord bloods from Athens with analyses of DNA from the same samples. Five out of the 227 (2.2%) had raised Hb Bart's levels >1%, whereas there were 19 clear-cut carriers of an α-thalassaemia determinant (mostly $-\alpha/\alpha\alpha$), an overall carrier frequency of 8.3%. This clearly emphasizes the problem that reliance on Hb Bart's levels may well lead to a substantial underestimation of the prevalence of α thalassaemia, especially when the overall frequency is quite low (and therefore few $-\alpha/-\alpha$ homozygotes or $--/$ heterozygotes are present).

As in other parts of the Mediterranean, several genotypes interact to produce HbH disease in Greece. Tzotzos *et al.* (1986) examined DNA from 16 individuals with HbH disease: eight had the genotype $--^{\text{MED}}/-\alpha^{3.7}$, four the genotype $-(\alpha)^{20.5}/-\alpha^{3.7}$ and three the genotype $--^{\text{MED}}/\alpha\alpha^{\text{T}}$. Subsequent work by the same group (Traeger-Synodinos *et al.* 1993) looked at a number of $\alpha\alpha^{\text{T}}$ variants in detail. Nine (out of 16) turned out to have the $\alpha^{\text{Poly(A)(AATAA}\rightarrow\text{G})}\alpha$ mutation, two the α2 IVS1 pentanucleotide deletion (GA**GGTGA**GG→GAGG) ($\alpha^{\text{Hph1}}\alpha$), two the chain-termination variant Hb Icaria ($\alpha^{\text{Ic}}\alpha$), one the initiation-codon variant ATG-ACG ($\alpha^{\text{Nco1}}\alpha$), and two were uncharacterized. In the former Yugoslavia a survey of 1100 cord bloods revealed detectable Hb Bart's in 3.2% (Efremov *et al.* 1982).

Cyprus

Alpha thalassaemia is common on the island of Cyprus. Ashiotis *et al.* (1973) found that 21 of 176 (12%) newborn infants had raised Hb Bart's levels and a similar finding was made by Hadjiminas *et al.* (1979). They looked at 1200 Greek Cypriots and 132 Turkish Cypriots and found raised Hb Bart's levels in 12.4% and 6.8%, respectively. In a study using DNA analysis Pirastu *et al.* (1982) found that the carrier rate for the $-\alpha^{3.7}$ deletion was 14%.

Spain and Portugal

There are fewer data available for the western end of the Mediterranean. Villegas *et al.* (1989) found that less than 0.5% of Spanish newborns had increased levels of Hb Bart's. Similar data were reported by Baiget and Gimferrer (1986). Other studies by direct gene analysis suggested that the carrier frequency of α thalassaemia was about 2% (Fei *et al.* 1989a; de las Nieves *et al.* 1990). Villegas *et al.* (1992) analysed the DNA of 400 cord bloods and found nine were heterozygotes for the $-\alpha^{3.7}$ deletion and one was heterozygous for the $--^{\text{MED}}\alpha^0$ deletion. Significantly, only five out of the 10 individuals with α-thalassaemia deletions had raised Hb Bart's levels. Peres *et al.* (1995) studied a series of 100 consecutive cord bloods from the greater Lisbon region of Portugal. They found seven heterozygotes for the $-\alpha^{3.7}$ deletion and three examples of $-\alpha^{4.2}$, an overall carrier frequency of 10%. In a subsequent analysis of 342 selected subjects, examples of the $--^{\text{MED}} \alpha^0$ deletions and $\alpha^{\text{Nco1}}\alpha$ variant were also observed.

The Middle East and west Asia

Alpha thalassaemia has been reported in many populations, though with one or two exceptions prevalence data are limited.

Jewish populations

One of the earliest papers on α thalassaemia was that of Ramot *et al.* (1959), who described a case of HbH disease in an Oriental Jewess. Subsequent surveys revealed that the disorder is largely confined to the Yemeni and Iraqi communities. Halbrech and Ben-Pora (1971) surveyed 3218 cord bloods from various Jewish and Arab ethnic groups and recorded a high incidence of a 'fast-moving' Hb component on electrophoresis. The highest incidence was recorded in Yemeni newborns, in whom it was found in 17.3%. Ashkenazi Jews and north Africans had the lowest frequency (0.7% and 0.8%, respectively), with intermediate values of 2–5% in Sephardic Jews, Iraqi/Iranians and Arabs. Similar results were obtained by Zaizov and Matoth (1972) in a survey of 286 newborns. The underlying molecular defects in a number of Yemeni HbH disease cases was studied by Shalmon *et al.* (1994). They found a new α^0 defect ($-–^{\text{YEM}}$), involving a deletion of at least 39 kb in the α complex, interacting with either $-\alpha^{3.7}$ or $\alpha\alpha^{\text{T}}$ mutations. Although not characterized, the latter is probably the $\alpha2^{\text{Poly(A) AATAAA}\rightarrow\text{G}}$ mutation first characterized in Saudi Arabs (Higgs *et al.* 1983a; Thein *et al.* 1988b).

Saudi Arabia

A number of studies have shown that α thalassaemia is extremely common among populations of the Arabian peninsula. We have already noted its occurrence in Yemeni Jews (who only arrived in Israel after 1948). If anything, α thalassaemia is even more common in the oasis populations of the eastern peninsula. Pembrey *et al.* (1975) studied cord bloods from 345 Shiite Saudi Arab infants and identified Hb Bart's in 52%, at levels ranging from 0.5 to 16% of the total haemoglobin. Somewhat lower frequencies were noted in the north-western and south-western provinces of Saudi Arabia (El-Hazmi 1987; El-Hazmi *et al.* 1991).

In re-analysing cases of α thalassaemia from eastern Saudi Arabia Pressley *et al.* (1980) found that 45% of the population carried the single-gene-deletion variant $-\alpha^{3.7}$, while 15% had a hitherto unrecognized non-deletion variant $(\alpha\alpha^T)$ (now known to be the poly(A) mutation AATAAA→G on the α2 gene (Higgs *et al.* 1983a; Thein *et al.* 1988b)), which gave rise to HbH disease in the homozygous state. This is a form of inheritance for HbH disease that is quite different from the usual interaction of α^0 and α^+ variants.

Other Arabian populations

Elsewhere on the Arabian peninsula α-thalassaemia frequencies ranging from 1 to 60% have been reported (Adekile 1997). White *et al.* (1986) studied 800 cord bloods of newborns of Omani, Yemeni and United Arab Emirates origin. Hb Bart's levels were elevated in 17.5% of Yemenis in accord with analysis of Yemeni Jews residing in Israel, in 15.2% of individuals from the UAE and in 54% of Omanis. White *et al.* (1993) subsequently estimated that 45% of Omanis are homozygotes for the $-\alpha^{3.7}$ deletion (a gene frequency of ~0.67). In Kuwait about a third of the population have α thalassaemia, mostly (70%) the $-\alpha^{3.7}$ variant with the remainder being the α2Poly(A) AATAAA→G mutation and the α2 IVS1 5-bp deletion $(\alpha^{Hph1}\alpha)$ (Adekile & Haider 1996).

Turkey

Although HbH disease has been recognized in Turkey since 1968 (Aksoy & Erdem 1968c) there are few prevalence data. Arcasoy and Çavdar (1978) screened 700 cord bloods and found one with an elevated Hb Bart's level. Fei *et al.* (1989a), using DNA methods to analyse cord bloods, found that 3% carried the $-\alpha^{3.7}$ deletion variant. It seems likely that this is an underestimate of the true prevalence. In an investigation of 25 Turkish patients with HbH disease, Öner *et al.* (1997) found that the $-\alpha^{3.7}$ deletion was present in only half the cases. The $-\alpha^{4.2}$ deletion and the two common non-deletion defects α2 IVS1 5-bp deletion $(\alpha^{Hph1}\alpha)$ and α2 poly(A) AATAAA→G made up the remainder. The most common α^0 determinants were the $-(\alpha)^{20.5\,kb}$ and the $--^{17.5\,kb}$ ($--^{MED}$) deletions. Three examples of the $--^{26.5\,kb}$ deletion were also seen.

There is some evidence that α thalassaemia occurs in Jordan, probably at a frequency of less than 3% (Bashir *et al.* 1992b). Frequencies of 9% have been recorded in a survey of three regions of Azerbaijan (Gaziev 1983).

The Indian subcontinent

The limited information available at the time the previous edition of this book was published suggested that α thalassaemia was not very common in India. Chouhan *et al.* (1970) found nine newborns with elevated Hb Bart's levels in a survey of 438 cord bloods in Bombay. Equally low frequencies (~1%) were seen in a survey of 720 (mostly) Bengali Hindus from Calcutta (Das *et al.* 1973). Earlier studies of Indians born in Singapore (Vella 1959) or Malaysia (Lie-Injo & Ti 1961) had also found Hb Bart's frequencies of ~1%. In part, these low frequencies may be due to technical limitations. Desai *et al.* (1997) compared four electrophoretic methods—paper, cellulose acetate and starch gel electrophoresis, and isoelectric focusing, and found that Hb Bart's detection was very insensitive using paper electrophoresis. With cellulose acetate they found that ~15% of 798 cord bloods from Bombay had detectable Hb Bart's.

A quite different picture of α thalassaemia in India emerges when tribal groups are included in the surveys and DNA analysis is used for screening. Kulozik *et al.* (1988a) studied 282 individuals with sickle-cell trait from Orissa and found a gene frequency of $-\alpha$ deletions of 0.29 (i.e. a prevalence of ~50%). The predominant form was $-\alpha^{3.7}$, although $-\alpha^{4.2}$ accounted for about 30% of the total. Two examples of a rare variant involving a 3.5-kb deletion that removed the entire α1 gene ($-\alpha^{3.5}$) were also seen. Hb Bart's screening in the Orissa population in contrast revealed 12.6% of cord bloods with raised Hb Bart's levels (Misra *et al.* 1991). In another study of Indian tribals, Brittenham *et al.* (1980) determined $-\alpha$ frequencies in a group of Valmiki, Khonda Reddi and Koya Dora, revealing a remarkably high gene frequency, 0.58, in this group, implying that over 80% of individuals are either $-\alpha$ heterozygotes or homozygotes. Similar data were obtained by Fodde *et al.* (1991) in studies of tribals from the same Andhra Pradesh region of east central India. Gene frequencies ranged from 0.35 in the Khonda Reddi to 0.92 in the Kolam. Non-tribals from the same region had a $-\alpha$ frequency of 0.12. Another interesting feature of the data is the variety of $-\alpha$-thalassaemia mutations in these groups. Four $-\alpha$ deletion variants were noted, $-\alpha^{3.7I}$, $-\alpha^{3.7II}$, $-\alpha^{4.2}$ and $-\alpha^{3.7\,Rampa}$, in addition to the α2 chain-termination variant Hb Koya Dora, which has a similar phenotype to Hb Constant Spring. These variants, moreover, are found on an extremely diverse set of α haplotypes. In studies of another central India tribe, the Baiga, Reddy *et al.* (1995) screened the entire population of 17 villages (3115 individuals) and obtained circumstantial evidence that α thalassaemia was extremely common. Ten individuals chosen at random were studied for $-\alpha$ deletions. Of their 20 chromosomes-16, six had $-\alpha^{3.7}$ and seven $-\alpha^{4.2}$ deletions, an overall $-\alpha$ gene frequency of 0.65. Similar high frequencies were observed in the Gond tribe from the Maudla and Jabalpur districts of central India (Gupta *et al.* 1991). Again $-\alpha^{3.7}$ and $-\alpha^{4.2}$ deletions were common and the overall $-\alpha$ allele frequency was ~0.52. A few examples of Hb Koya Dora ($\alpha^{KD}\alpha$) were also noted. As in Andhra Pradesh the allele frequency of $-\alpha$ was low (0.07) in non-tribals from the same area.

Further north, in the Tharu people of the Terai region of southern Nepal, an even higher frequency for $-\alpha$ of 0.8 has been reported (Modiano *et al.* 1991). There are few data available for Pakistan. Rehman *et al.* (1991) screened 500 cord bloods from the northern population of Rawalpindi and found 12 (2.4%) with raised Hb Bart's levels. This may be an underestimate: Hassall *et al.* (1998) noted a carrier frequency of 15% in British Asians of Pakistani origin. Similar figures were seen in Gujeratis (11%) and Punjabis (13%). Bengalis had a much lower incidence. Approximately 80% of these mutations were $-\alpha^{3.7}$ and the rest (with one unidentified exception) $-\alpha^{4.2}$.

Although no formal population studies have been carried out, the α-globin genes of over 400 patients from Sri Lanka with β thalassaemia have been analysed in our laboratory. Both the $-\alpha^{3.7}$ and $-\alpha^{4.2}$ deletions were encountered, with an overall gene frequency of about 14% for $-\alpha^{3.7}$ and 2% for $-\alpha^{4.2}$ (De Silva *et al.* 2000).

Thus it appears that α thalassaemia is extremely common in the tribal groups of the Indian subcontinent, and indeed reaches some of the highest frequencies recorded anywhere in the world. Although isolated cases of HbH disease have been recorded in India, none of the surveys published so far have reported finding evidence for an α^0-thalassaemia determinant, although they are known to exist (Drysdale & Higgs 1988).

South-east Asia

Alpha thalassaemia is widespread throughout south-east Asia. Because both α^0 and α^+ determinants are relatively common in these populations HbH disease and the Hb Bart's hydrops syndrome are seen frequently. Despite having a lower overall incidence than the tribal groups of central India and the island populations of Melanesia, α thalassaemia is thus a much more serious public health problem in mainland south-east Asia than elsewhere.

Alpha thalassaemia was first described in Burma by Aung-Than-Batu *et al.* (1968). These authors later described 20 cases of HbH disease (Aung-Than-Batu *et al.* 1971) and recorded 10.5% of cord bloods with raised Hb Bart's in a survey of newborns from Rangoon (Aung-Than-Batu & Hla-Pe 1971).

Thailand

The most extensive surveys for α thalassaemia have been carried out over a number of years in Thailand, many by groups in the Siriraj Hospital, Bangkok. In early surveys for Thai infants with raised Hb Bart's levels, Tuchinda *et al.* (1959) and Pootrakul *et al.* (1967b) suggested that ~5% might be carriers of α thalassaemia. Later surveys produced much higher incidences. Pootrakul *et al.* (1970) recorded an incidence of over 20% in a survey of 1408 infants from Bangkok, and 15% in a separate survey of 2404 newborns. Tanphaichitr *et al.* (1985) studied 406 cord bloods and reported raised Hb Bart's in 25%. This same series was also studied by DNA analysis: eight individuals with no detectable Hb Bart's had the $-\alpha/\alpha\alpha$ genotype.

Elsewhere in Thailand, α thalassaemia occurs just as frequently. Na-Nakorn and Wasi (1970) noted 16.3% of cord bloods from Chiangmai Province in the north had raised Hb Bart's levels. Hundreiser *et al.* (1988, 1990) determined the frequency of α thalassaemia in northern and north-east Thailand using DNA methods. Twenty-five per cent of adults from the Chiangmai region had some form of the disorder, mostly the $-\alpha^{3.7I}$ variant. Only five (4%) heterozygotes for the $--^{SEA}$ α^0 mutation were observed, a considerably lower frequency than that previously estimated (Na-Nakorn & Wasi 1970) on the basis of Hb Bart's determinations. Hundreiser *et al.* (1988) suggest that the discrepancy arose because of previously unrecognized causes of α thalassaemia like Hb Constant Spring or other non-deletion variants making a substantial contribution to the intermediate Hb Bart's category in cord blood analyses. Higher frequencies were seen in the Khonkaen and Ubal areas of north-east Thailand. Hundreiser *et al.* (1990) found that 40% of adults had some form of α thalassaemia: $-\alpha$ deletions (mainly $-\alpha^{3.7}$) accounted for almost 70% of affected chromosomes with $\alpha^{CS}\alpha$ (20%) and $--^{SEA}$ (10%) making up the balance.

In the So tribal group α thalassaemia reaches its highest frequency ($\sim$75%) in any Thai population group (Hundreiser *et al.* 1990). Lemmens-Zygulska *et al.* (1996) studied 215 adults from the same region and found 74 (34.4%) had some form of α thalassaemia ($-\alpha^{3.7}/\alpha\alpha$ in 36; $-\alpha^{3.7}/-\alpha^{3.7}$ in 3; $--^{SEA}/\alpha\alpha$ in 30; $\alpha^{CS}\alpha/\alpha\alpha$ in 5). These figures imply that as many as 2% of children born in northern Thailand will have HbH disease or the Hb Bart's hydrops syndrome. In southern Thailand (Songkla Province) 16.3% of newborns have elevated Hb Bart's levels (Laosombat *et al.* 1979). Only in the north-east of the country (Khon Kaen Province) are frequencies for raised Hb Bart's levels in the 5% range as recorded in the very early surveys (Saichua *et al.* 1983). Winichagoon *et al.* (1992a) suggest, on the basis of DNA analyses, that the prevalence of α thalassaemia is highest in northern Thailand (4.7% α^0, 26.4% α^+) compared with the central region (3.45% and 16.25%) with the lowest incidence in the south. The distribution of Hb Constant Spring follows a similar pattern, with 1.5% in the south and centre, and 6–11% in the north (Laig *et al.* 1990a).

Laos

Alpha thalassaemia is extremely common in Laos. Sicard *et al.* (1979) studied cord bloods from 147 infants, and found 63 (43%) with raised Hb Bart's levels. Thirteen of the cord bloods with increased Hb Bart's had Hb Constant Spring; of the remaining 50, 37 were consistent with a $-\alpha/\alpha\alpha$ genotype, 11 with $-\alpha/-\alpha$, $--/\alpha\alpha$ or $-\alpha/\alpha^{CS}\alpha$ and 3 with HbH disease.

Vietnam

There seems to be less α thalassaemia in Vietnam. Pornpatkul *et al.* (1980) estimated an incidence of 6.3% in 810 refugees in a camp in southern Thailand, although this was based solely on haematological criteria, and the authors accepted that their figure was probably an underestimate.

China

Until the mid-1980s α thalassaemia in Chinese had been documented almost exclusively in immigrant populations elsewhere in the world. These studies, conducted in Hong Kong (Todd *et al.* 1969; Li *et al.* 1982), Singapore (Vella 1959; Wong 1971), Malaysia (Lopez & Lie-Injo 1971; Lie-Injo *et al.* 1982) and Canada (Gray & Marion 1971), revealed incidences of raised Hb Bart's in cord bloods ranging from 3.0 to 7.4%.

Beginning in 1980 some extremely large surveys of residents of the People's Republic of China have enabled us to get a better idea of the distribution of α thalassaemia within China itself. Zeng (1981) summarized the results of a survey of over 123 000 individuals in 14 provinces. Although gene frequencies for α thalassaemia were not given, over 300 cases of HbH disease were recorded, mainly in Guangxi and Guangdong provinces. Similar data were obtained by Zaino and Yang (1981). Yang *et al.* (1985) surveyed over 400 000 individuals from 22 provinces and identified 223 cases of HbH disease, again mainly from Guangxi and Guangdong provinces. A survey of 11 000 cord bloods from six provinces by the same authors revealed an incidence of 2.93% with elevated Hb Bart's levels. The highest incidence (14.95%) occurred in Guangxi, followed by Guangdong (4.11%), Jiangxi (2.60%), Sichuan (1.92%), Xinjiang (0.47%) and Shanghai (0.34%).

An even larger survey was carried out by Zeng and

Huang (1987). They looked at 900 000 people from 28 provinces, including cord bloods from over 13 000 infants. The average incidence of α thalassaemia was calculated to be 2.64%, with the highest at 14.95% in the Guangxi region bordering Vietnam, where HbH disease and the Hb Bart's hydrops syndrome are serious problems. Zeng and Huang (1987) looked at 60 cases of HbH disease and many of their parents; $-\alpha^{3.7}$, $-\alpha^{4.2}$, $\alpha^{CS}\alpha$ and an uncharacterized non-deletion α^{+} defect were identified in addition to the α^{0} determinants. Wen *et al.* (1992) studied 50 cases of HbH disease from Guangxi province and found that $--/-\alpha$ genotypes accounted for just over half the total. Of the remainder, 33% were $--/\alpha^{CS}\alpha$. Besides HbCS, one case of HbH disease involving Hb Quong Sze, a highly unstable α-chain variant with an α-thalassaemia phenotype, was seen. Similar findings were seen by Zhao *et al.* (1992). They looked at 57 newborns from Nanning with α thalassaemia. Roughly equal numbers of $-\alpha^{3.7}/\alpha\alpha$, $-\alpha^{4.2}/\alpha\alpha$ and $\alpha^{CS}\alpha/\alpha\alpha$ heterozygotes (30 in all) were seen, along with 19 α^{0} heterozygotes ($--^{SEA}/\alpha\alpha$), one HbH disease ($--^{SEA}/-\alpha^{3.7}$) and one Hb Quong Sze homozygote. The remaining six samples could not be characterized.

Taiwan

Most of the people now living in Taiwan are the descendants of Chinese immigrants from the mainland. Lin *et al.* (1977) studied 3013 Chinese newborns in Taiwan and found 1.42% with raised Hb Bart's levels. The molecular variants present have been characterized by Liu *et al.* (1994) for 67 cases of HbH disease. All involved the $--^{SEA}$ α^{0} determinant in combination with α^{+} determinants, which were evenly divided between $-\alpha$ and Hb Constant Spring. Of the $-\alpha$ deletions 80% were $-\alpha^{3.7I}$, 10% $-\alpha^{3.7II}$ and 10% $-\alpha^{4.2}$. Ko *et al.* (1991) also concluded that the majority of α^{0} variants in Taiwan Chinese were $--^{SEA}$, although five of 87 cases of the Hb Bart's hydrops syndrome were compound heterozygotes for $--^{SEA}$ and $--^{THAI}$. The aboriginal inhabitants of Taiwan now number only about 300 000 and live in the mountainous regions and on the east coast. Ko *et al.* (1993a) studied 1309 individuals from the four major aboriginal groups. In the Ami 8% of adults had some form of α thalassaemia as revealed by DNA analysis, divided almost exactly into α^{0} (mostly $--^{THAI}$, but with some $--^{SEA}$ and $--^{FIL}$) and α^{+} types (almost all $-\alpha^{3.7}$). The other three tribal groups had

much less α thalassaemia (an incidence of 0.2–1.6%). It seems likely therefore that the $--^{SEA}$ α^{0} determinant is a Chinese introduction to Taiwan, with the aboriginal groups contributing the $--^{THAI}$ variant.

Japan

Alpha thalassaemia is uncommon in Japan. In a survey of over 3000 cord bloods, Imamura *et al.* (1980) found three with raised Hb Bart's levels.

Malaysia

Alpha thalassaemia is well documented on the Malay peninsula. Cases of the Hb Bart's hydrops were reported as early as 1960 (Lie-Injo & Jo 1960b) and cord blood surveys of indigenous Malays, as well as individuals of Chinese or Indian ancestry revealed that as many as 7% of those studied had elevated Hb Bart's levels. Lopez and Lie-Injo (1971) found Hb Bart's in 7% of 568 Chinese, 4.9% of 205 Malay and 1.8% of 226 Indian newborns. A later survey in 1431 Malays, Chinese and Indians (Lie-Injo 1973) found 6.9% of cord bloods with raised Hb Bart's levels. In surveys of Chinese in Singapore, Vella (1959) and Wong (1971) found 4.0% and 3.4% of cord bloods with raised Hb Bart's levels. Hb Constant Spring is seen frequently on the Malay peninsula, especially in Malays, in which it occurs in 2.2% of individuals studied. An even higher incidence (3.2%) was seen in Temuan aboriginals but it was not found in either of the two groups of Senoi aboriginals (Lie-Injo *et al.* 1975).

Indonesia

Early surveys of Indonesia by Lie-Injo (1959b) suggested that α thalassaemia was much less common than on the mainland of south-east Asia. Few data have been published since, but we have recently gathered some preliminary data through a collaboration with Dr A.S.M. Sofro of Gadjah Madah University in Yogyakarta. The incidence of α thalassaemia varies considerably from island to island, with the lowest (<1%) on Bangka, south Sumatra and the highest (>13%) on Lombok. Both $-\alpha^{3.7}$ and $-\alpha^{4.2}$ deletions are present, with the former predominating. Lie-Injo (1959b) described a number of well documented cases of HbH disease in families of Chinese/Indonesian extraction but the disease appears to be much less common in eastern Indonesia, suggesting that the frequency of α^0 determinants there is very low. Occasional examples of Hb Constant Spring have been reported in regions closest to the south-east Asian mainland (Lie-Injo *et al.* 1975).

Philippines

Alpha thalassaemia is not uncommon in the Philippines. One survey reported 5.4% of 313 cord bloods had raised Hb Bart's levels (Koenig & Vedvick 1975) and HbH disease and the Hb Bart's hydrops fetalis syndrome have been well documented (Dozy *et al.* 1977).

Papua New Guinea and island Melanesia

Further east, in New Guinea and the islands to the south and east, α thalassaemia reaches much higher frequencies, indeed the highest in the world with the exception of one or two Indian tribal groups. The first evidence for α thalassaemia in Melanesia came from the observation of Ryan *et al.* (1961) of a case of HbH disease. Others were later described by Booth (1966) and Russell *et al.* (1971). Early surveys for Hb Bart's in cord bloods suggested a moderate incidence of α thalassaemia in New Guinea. Beaven *et al.* (1974) reported that 36 out of 86 samples had some Hb Bart's; a similar figure (36%) was noted by Booth (1981) in a survey of 50 cord bloods from the Papuan Gulf. An even higher incidence was observed by Oppenheimer *et al.* (1984): Hb Bart's was detected in 81% of cord blood samples from infants born in Madang on the north coast of Papua New Guinea. Subsequent studies (Flint *et al.* 1986; Yenchitsomanus *et al.* 1986) using DNA techniques confirmed these high frequencies on the coast. Flint *et al.* also showed that the mountainous regions of New Guinea are largely devoid of α thalassaemia. Alpha thalassaemia is also common in the island archipelagos to the south and east of New Guinea. Bowden *et al.* (1985) surveyed 17 islands in Vanuatu (formerly the New Hebrides) and found incidences of α thalassaemia of 9–60%.

None of these studies identified any forms of α^0 thalassaemia, consistent with the absence of any recorded cases of the Hb Bart's hydrops fetalis syndrome. In New Guinea, the predominant form of α thalassaemia is the $-\alpha^{4.2}$ deletion with a smaller contribution from the $-\alpha^{3.7I}$ and $-\alpha^{3.7III}$ deletion variants.

In Vanuatu, in contrast, the $-\alpha^{3.7III}$ is the major α^+-thalassaemia determinant, with only a small proportion of $-\alpha^{3.7I}$ and $-\alpha^{4.2}$. Throughout the south-west Pacific there is good evidence for the presence of a non-deletion α-thalassaemia variant which occurs at frequencies of 1–5% (Bowden *et al.* 1985; Allen 1997). Although not yet characterized, this variant, in the homozygous state, is responsible for the cases of HbH disease seen in the region (Hill *et al.* 1987b; unpublished observations of D.K. Bowden and D.R. Higgs).

Micronesia and Polynesia

Alpha thalassaemia is found throughout Micronesia and Polynesia (O'Shaughnessy *et al.* 1990) in the central and eastern Pacific, at incidences ranging from an average 2% in Micronesia to 16% in Polynesia, and reaching a maximum of ~30% in some of the Society Islands. Both $-\alpha^{3.7}$ and $-\alpha^{4.2}$ variants are found in Micronesia, whereas the α^+ thalassaemia in Polynesia is almost exclusively $-\alpha^{3.7III}$. By determining the α haplotypes and spectrum of 5' and 3' HVR alleles associated with the $-\alpha$ deletions in the Pacific, O'Shaughnessy *et al.* (1990), Martinson (1991) and Martinson *et al.* (1994) showed that they originated in the islands of the south-west Pacific and so were probably carried into the central and eastern Pacific during the early Polynesian colonizing voyages.

Similarly, it appears that the α^+ thalassaemia found in north coastal aboriginal Australians at low frequencies probably reached Australia in migrants from island Melanesia and Indonesia (Roberts-Thomson *et al.* 1996).

Africa

Alpha thalassaemia is found throughout sub-Saharan Africa. Many of the early data were derived from studies of the descendants of (mostly) West Africans resident in the USA. Surveys in various cities (Horton *et al.* 1962; Minnich *et al.* 1962; Weatherall 1963; Schmaier *et al.* 1973; Friedman *et al.* 1974a) showed raised Hb Bart's levels in cord bloods varying from 2 to 30%. It seems likely that much of this variation resulted from different definitions of 'normal' levels of Hb Bart's, and from the differential sensitivities of the techniques used. Thus Higgs *et al.* (1980b) in a prospective study of over 200 infants in Jamaica (whose antecedents probably came from the same parts of Africa as the infants studied in the USA) showed that 7% had detectable Hb Bart's in the neonatal period. The Hb Bart's levels fell within two modes at 0.5% and 4.5%. Infants with Hb Bart's levels in the 3–8% range were shown by DNA analysis to be $-\alpha/-\alpha$ homozygotes, while those in the 0.1–2% range were $-\alpha$ heterozygotes. However, Higgs et al. concluded that a significant proportion of infants without detectable Hb Bart's must be $-\alpha$ heterozygotes, since the estimated frequency for $-\alpha$ carriers, based on the number of homozygotes, was 25% (see Chapter 11). This study clearly showed that α-thalassaemia frequencies can be grossly underestimated by Hb Bart's analysis, particularly when, as in Africans, there is a predominance of the less severe single-gene-deletion ($-\alpha$) forms of α^{+}-thalassaemia determinants. Hendrickse et al. (1960) studied 100 infants born in Ibadan, Nigeria, and noted that 11 of the cord bloods had a 'fast-moving' component (= Hb Bart's). A later survey in Nigeria (Folayan Esan 1970) revealed a lower incidence of 4.5%. In contrast to these two surveys, Falusi et al. (1987) showed that almost 50% of Nigerians were carriers of the $-\alpha$ deletion. Two surveys in the Congo produced somewhat lower incidences. Van Baelen et al. (1969) found almost 18% of cord bloods had elevated levels of Hb Bart's and Lallemant et al. (1986) recorded over 23%. On the east coast of Africa in Tanzania, Nhonoli et al. (1979) found 11.1% of a sample of 325 cord bloods had detectable Hb Bart's. Further studies in eastern Africa revealed considerably higher incidences for α thalassaemia. Ojwang et al. (1987) showed that approximately 50% of Kenyans (with sickle-cell disease, compared with 40% in our unpublished survey on normal Kenyans) had the $-\alpha^{3.7}$ deletion variant (with both subtypes I and II present) and a similar incidence was seen in Zambia (Muklwala et al. 1989). Further south, the prevalence of α thalassaemia is somewhat lower. Ramsay and Jenkins (1987) looked at a number of groups including the Bantu-speaking Venda, the Nguni-speaking Zulu, Ndebele, Swazi and Zhosa, and four tribes from the Sotho-Tswana group. Alpha-thalassaemia prevalences ranged from 12% in the Nguni and Sotho-Tswana to 35% in the Venda. Ramsay and Jenkins (1987) also studied a group of San bushmen from north-east Namibia and found that 12% had α thalassaemia. Without exception, the α^{+}-thalassaemia determinant in these southern African populations

was the $-\alpha^{3.7}$ deletion. Other surveys using DNA analysis have reinforced this observation. In Senegal where the incidence of α thalassaemia is 20% and Benin/Upper Volta (40%), Pagnier et al. (1984) and Dodé et al. (1988) found only the $-\alpha^{3.7I}$ variant. Similarly Abdalla et al. (1989) in their survey of Gambians found all 13% of individuals with α thalassaemia had the $-\alpha^{3.7}$ deletion. However, this is not the case in black Americans or Jamaicans, where, in addition to $-\alpha^{3.7}$, occasional $-\alpha^{4.2}$ deletions have been noted (Embury et al. 1985b; D.R. Higgs, unpublished), although there is always a preponderance of the $-\alpha^{3.7}$ variant (Dozy et al. 1979b; Goossens et al. 1980; Serjeant et al. 1986). This suggests some element of admixture from other ethnic groups (e.g. Chinese in Jamaicans) in these populations.

There is limited information on α thalassaemia in north Africa, although it is clear that in some regions it may be quite common. In Algeria, for example, Trabuchet et al. (1977a) reported 12 cases of HbH disease. Cord blood surveys (Henni et al. 1981) suggested a prevalence of at least 10%. It appears that at least two single-deletion forms of α thalassaemia are present in that population: the $-\alpha^{3.7I}$ and a variant $-\alpha^{3.7II}$ which has a deletion of two nucleotides preceding the initiation codon ($\alpha^{Nco1}\alpha$). It is this variant which, in the homozygous state, is responsible for the HbH disease in Algeria. There are no reports of this variant being found further east. Thein et al. (1984a) found that 16% of Egyptians were heterozygous for the single-gene-deletion form ($-\alpha$) of α thalassaemia, mostly the $-\alpha^{3.7I}$ type. A similar incidence was noted by Novelletto et al. (1989). One example of the $-\alpha^{4.2}$ deletion was seen in 23 $-\alpha$ deletions characterized, the remainder being $-\alpha^{3.7}$.

South America and the Caribbean

There are only a few reports of α thalassaemia in south and central America, and few, if any, of well defined examples in the indigenous populations. It seems likely that Europe and Africa are the major sources of the disorder. For example Pereira et al. (1973) described a case of HbH disease in a Greek immigrant family in Brazil and Zago and Costa (1985) report three families in which the α-thalassaemia genes were probably of Italian or African origin. Zago et al. (1983) found four newborns, out of a mixed population of 606 (0.7%), with high levels of Hb Bart's. In a survey of 190 black newborns in Brazil, Motta *et al.* (1983) found 6.8% with raised Hb Bart's. These findings suggest that α thalassaemia is not uncommon in Brazil, but largely confined to individuals of immigrant descent. Other studies, such as those of Daiber *et al.* (1976) in *Chile* and Arends (1984) in *Venezuela* mention the occurrence of α thalassaemia in these populations, but do not give any information about prevalence. There are a few reports of haemoglobin H disease in *Mexico* (Angles-Cano *et al.* 1977). Cord blood surveys of 5100 newborns from Puebla and Guadalajara failed to detect any with increased Hb Bart's levels, and only one example of α thalassaemia was identified in a survey of over 1600 individuals from Jalisco state.

Occasional cases of HbH disease have been reported in *Jamaica*, usually in Chinese families or individuals of mixed Chinese/black ancestry (Went & MacIver 1961), and HbH disease in association with Hb Constant Spring was first reported in a Chinese family in Jamaica (Milner *et al.* 1971). Alpha thalassaemia in the black population is similar to that seen in the USA. Higgs *et al.* (1980b) reported 7% of 2000 cord bloods with detectable Hb Bart's, an underestimate of the true α-thalassaemia frequency which was nearer 30% (all $-\alpha^{3.7}$) when assessed by DNA analysis. Cord blood surveys in *Cuba* (Martinez & Colombo 1976) suggest that α thalassaemia is probably as common as in Jamaica.

Population genetics of thalassaemia and the malaria hypothesis

As discussed in Chapter 1, it was J.B.S. Haldane (1949b) who suggested that the high frequencies of haemoglobinopathies might be due to selection by malaria.

At the end of World War II in 1945, sickle-cell anaemia and thalassaemia were reasonably well understood clinical disorders. Although both had been described before 1925 their genetic basis was, for reasons that we summarized in Chapter 1, not properly understood until the late 1940s. By then it was clear that both thalassaemia major (in fact β thalassaemia) and sickle-cell disease were the homozygous states for recessive genes, and information on gene frequencies was beginning to accumulate. To quantitative geneticists, used to thinking of mutation rates for human genetic disorders in the order of 10^{-5}, the thalassaemia and sickle-gene figures were incredible.

On the assumption that the fitness of the homozygote is zero, and the heterozygote is selectively neutral, Neel and Valentine (1947) calculated a mutation rate for β thalassaemia of 1 in 2500. An even higher rate was proposed by Silvestroni *et al.* (1949). But the sickle gene provided the most extreme case, and the general unease was summed up by Neel (1950):

> If sickle-cell disease is in Africa the same disease that it is in [the USA], then some very thorny problems in gene dynamics are raised.
>
> Thus [for] a 20% incidence of sickling, the mutation rate necessary to maintain this frequency, assuming the heterozygote to be neutral . . . , would be approximately 1×10^{-2} — a truly staggering figure.
>
> Just as in the case of thalassaemia, the most logical alternative to the assumption of so high a mutation rate is positive selection in favour of the heterozygote.
>
> . . . is it a matter of chance that we find in such geographical proximity two anaemias presenting us with similar problems in population dynamics?

Silvestroni *et al.* (1949) had also suggested some sort of positive selection for the β-thalassaemia heterozygote, but, as described in Chapter 1, it was Haldane who, at the 8th International Congress of Genetics in Stockholm in 1948, proposed the specific example of malaria and how it might operate (Fig. 6.5). Although the malaria hypothesis was originally addressed to β thalassaemia, it soon became apparent that the problems posed applied equally to sickle-cell anaemia (Fig. 6.6). Largely for practical reasons, the most convincing early evidence for it came from a series of studies on sickle-cell anaemia carried out in Africa (mostly) during the 1950s and 1960s (reviewed extensively by Allison 1954; Rucknagel & Neel 1961; Allison 1964; Motulsky *et al.* 1964; Allison 1965; Livingstone 1967, 1971).

Allison obtained three different kinds of evidence regarding interaction between the sickle gene and malaria. First, he demonstrated that children with the sickle-cell trait have a lower parasitaemia; second, he showed that adult sickle-cell heterozygotes inoculated with *P. falciparum* did not show infections as frequently as normal individuals; and, third, he showed that the frequency of the sickle-cell gene in east Africa is correlated with endemicity of malaria. Although some of this work proved difficult to repeat in detail, later studies confirmed the protective effect

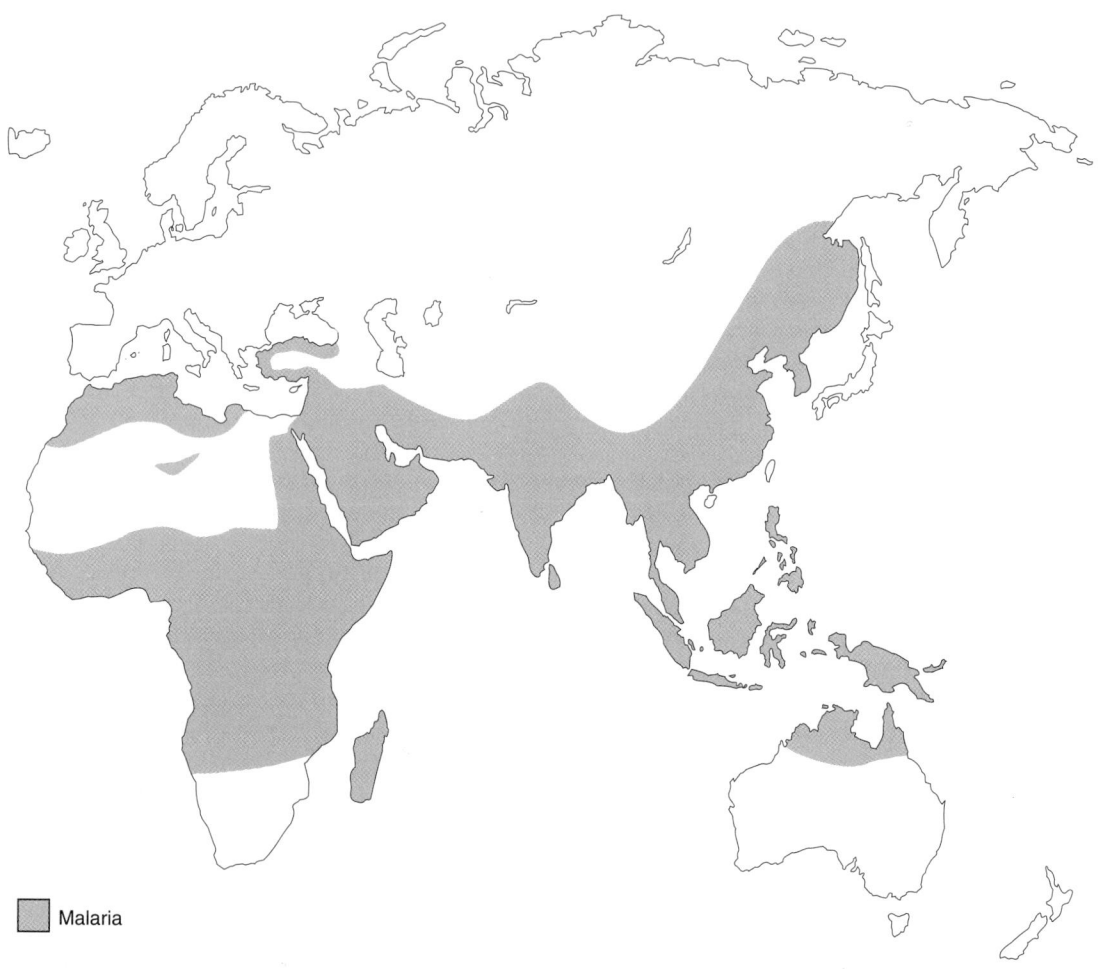

Fig. 6.5 Old-World distribution of malaria. This figure outlines the distribution of malaria before control programmes were established.

of HbS against *P. falciparum*. In particular it was found that deaths from cerebral malaria in early childhood were much less common in sickle-cell heterozygotes than in normal children.

Given that the fitness of sickle-cell homozygotes in their natural environment is zero, the most convincing evidence in favour of heterozygote advantage (protection) ought to be seen in relative mortality/ morbidity rates between sickle heterozygotes and normal individuals. Recently, in a convincing case–control study, this was very nicely demonstrated by Hill *et al*. (1991), who showed that carriers of the sickle gene were 90% protected against hospitalization from severe *P. falciparum* malaria.

There has been a great deal of interest in the possible cellular mechanism for this protective effect. Luzzatto *et al*. (1970) suggested that, when the malarial parasite enters an HbS-containing red cell, by utilizing oxygen it may cause the cell to sickle and that the sickled red cell is trapped in the spleen or other parts of the reticulo-endothelial system, so preventing the parasite completing its life cycle. More recent work using *in vitro* culture systems for the malarial parasite has provided clear evidence that the parasite cannot develop in HbS-containing cells maintained at reduced oxygen tension similar to that encountered in venous blood or the deep tissues. Indeed, growth of the parasite is almost completely prevented under

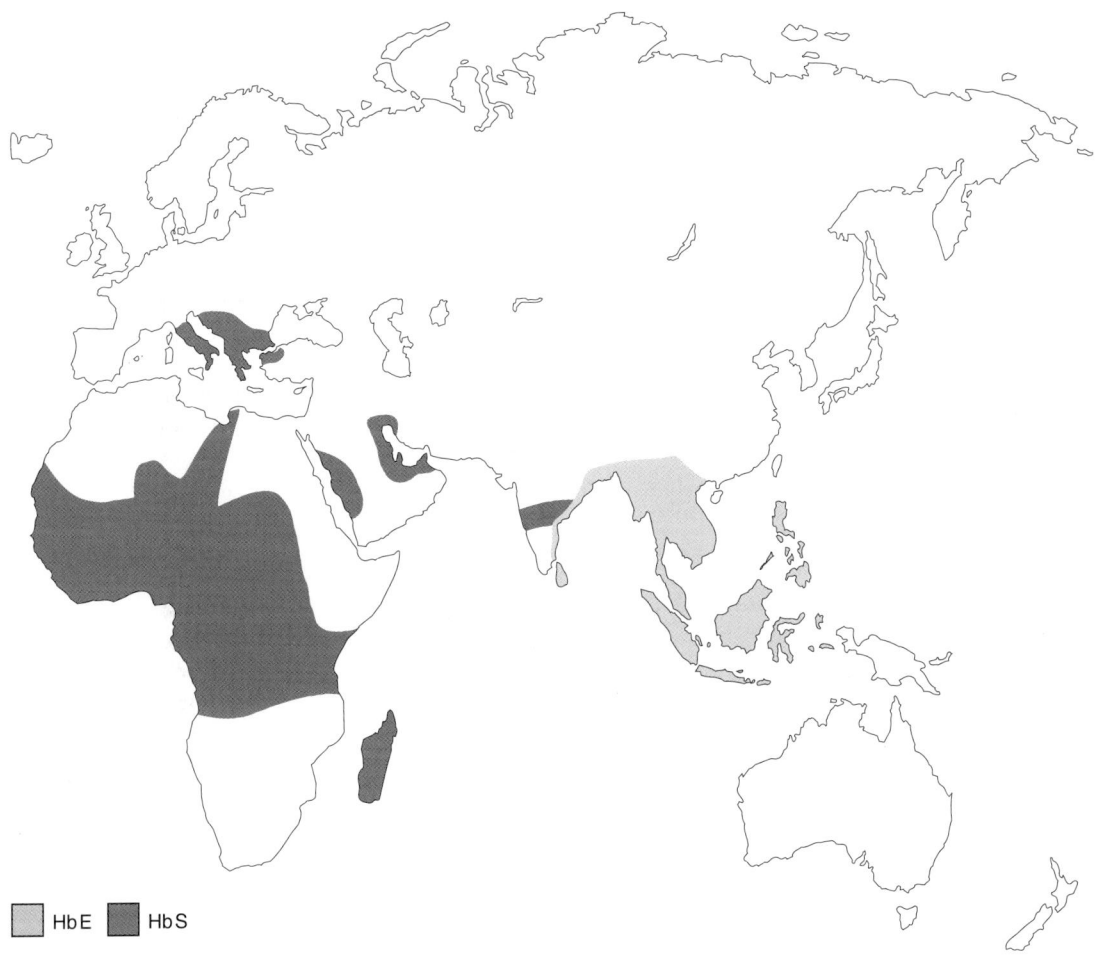

HbE   HbS

Fig. 6.6 World distribution of haemoglobins S and E.

these conditions (Friedman 1978; Pasvol. *et al.* 1978; Friedman *et al.* 1979).

These observations provide a possible explanation for the protection against *P. falciparum* malaria afforded to sickle-cell heterozygotes. The malarial parasite spends the first half of its maturation cycle mainly in the well oxygenated peripheral blood and the later part of the cycle in the capillaries of the deep tissues, where it will be exposed to lower oxygen tensions than in the peripheral blood. Because of the reduced rate of development of the parasite at reduced oxygen tensions it seems likely that the later part of the parasite life cycle will be inhibited and hence some degree of protection afforded sickle-cell

carriers. Whether the defective parasite maturation in red cells containing HbS is due to the direct properties of the haemoglobin molecule altering the environment of the cells as they sickle, the potassium concentrations for example (Friedman 1978; Friedman *et al.* 1979), or whether it results from more subtle metabolic changes which occur consequent upon sickling and the presence of the parasite in the cell remains to be determined.

The malaria hypothesis and thalassaemia

It is perhaps at first sight surprising that work on β

thalassaemia and sickle-cell disease proceeded independently throughout the 1950s. Indeed, as far as we can tell, the first reference to Haldane's paper did not appear in the sickle-cell literature until 1964. But, to early medical workers in the field, sickle-cell anaemia was an 'African' problem, and thalassaemia a 'Mediterranean' one, with little in common between them. All sorts of possible links with environmental, infectious and dietary factors (among many others) were considered and rejected, many of these studies starting well before Haldane's seminal paper was published (for example Beet 1946). The presence at very high frequencies of such serious diseases was both puzzling and worrying to clinicians. The population geneticists, on the other hand, approached the problem from a completely different angle. One serious red-cell disease with an apparently anomalously high mutation rate was one thing, but two, in proximity, was asking too much of coincidence. Some common factor linking them seemed the obvious way out of the dilemma, and malaria, with its intimate involvement with the red cell, was the obvious candidate.

In fact, well before Haldane's paper, Vezzoso (1946), investigating the notion that malaria in parents causes thalassaemia in their offspring, had noted that the distribution of thalassaemia in Italy appeared to correlate with that of malaria. But despite this and Haldane's specific proposal for a possible mechanism, the first studies on parasite–host interaction in β thalassaemia were not undertaken until the 1970s in Thailand (Kruatrachue *et al.* 1969, 1970), and then with inconclusive results. Further epidemiological studies were equally ambiguous. The positive findings in the classical studies of Carcassi *et al.* (1957b) and Siniscalco *et al.* (1966) in Sardinia were not seen in other studies in the Mediterranean —Greece (Fraser *et al.* 1964; Stamatoyannopoulos & Fessas 1964); Malta (Gilles *et al.* 1967; Livingstone 1967); Cyprus (Plato *et al.* 1964)—or in Sudan and New Guinea. Indeed, the Siniscalco study itself was subsequently criticized (Brown 1981) for using secondary evidence for malarial endemicity. Two small series in Liberia by Willcox *et al.* (1983a,b) did provide evidence for lower parasitaemias in β-thalassaemia trait, consistent with relative resistance of carriers to *P. falciparum* malaria.

The picture drawn from the early epidemiological studies on the relationship of thalassaemia to malaria was suggestive but inconclusive, and might have

remained so had not the techniques of molecular genetics intervened. Their application to epidemiological investigations has brought substantial benefits. The problem with the malaria hypothesis is an old one in practical population genetics. Theory describes many processes—mutation, selection, genetic drift, migration, for example—that can affect gene frequencies for a particular variant, but in practice it has rarely been possible to disentangle these effects. The molecular techniques have provided a new approach to tackling these difficult questions by enabling direct determination of genotypes. Characterization of variants by DNA sequencing can distinguish between apparently identical phenotypes, and conversely confirm the genetic identity of apparently variable phenotypes. Haplotype analysis provides information on genetic variation within and between populations, and can be a powerful indication of genetic affiliations.

Perhaps by way of illustration we can pose some (now rhetorical) questions that were unanswerable (but highly relevant) at the time the previous edition of this book was written: is β thalassaemia in Italy the same molecular disease as that seen in Thailand? were there independent mutations or are we witnessing the effects of ancient population movements? why do some haemoglobinopathies have such a patchy distribution in contrast to others? This last question has to address several issues: the continuum of β thalassaemia spread from the western Mediterranean through to the Far East; HbC confined almost exclusively to West Africa and HbE to south-east Asia, with a focus in northern Thailand, Laos and Cambodia; and HbS largely in Africa but with outcrops in Arabia, India, the Mediterranean basin and the Caribbean. Why do some of these disorders occur where there has never been malaria? The molecular evidence provides plausible, and often convincing, answers and in doing so narrows the options of population genetics-related factors that can be invoked to explain the epidemiological observations.

The molecular characterization of variants has obvious applications to population genetics. Indeed, it was the development of methods for prenatal diagnosis of haemoglobinopathies by DNA analysis that stimulated much of the research that subsequently proved so useful for population studies. To date, over 180 different molecular variants of β thalassaemia have been described, and we now know that the deletions (previously unidentifiable by classical biochemical methods) responsible for α^+ thalassaemia are probably the commonest of all single-gene disorders. The haplotype associations of many of these variants have been determined over the years, often as part of the early prenatal diagnostic programmes using DNA analysis. In most populations only a few (typically less than 10) of the possible repertoire of haplotypes are present at polymorphic frequencies (Flint *et al.* 1993a,b). Probably as a result of genetic drift, population movements, etc., there can be major variations in the (normal) haplotype make-up of different populations. For example, three α haplotypes that comprise 90% of those present in Melanesia rarely account for more than 10% in most other populations. West Africans have two β haplotypes that are almost unknown elsewhere. These features help in distinguishing one population from another. New mutations will be inherited by future generations on the same haplotype background as that on which the mutation arose (barring rare recombination events), and so the haplotype 'signature' can be used to trace the mutation's subsequent migrations, and to distinguish it from other identical mutations that arose independently (but on other haplotypes). Together these mutation–haplotype associations can often be used to infer population origins of a particular mutation. This information has helped to build up a remarkable picture of the world-wide distribution of thalassaemia. Moreover it has provided some important clues to the history of thalassaemia in human populations.

Selection not migration: α thalassaemia in Melanesia

Prior to 1975 the molecular basis of α thalassaemia was unknown and the true geographical distribution could only be guessed at from foci of severe conditions like HbH disease and the Hb Bart's hydrops fetalis syndrome, and from cord blood surveys for Hb Bart's. It was not until the gene deletions responsible for the commonest form of the disorder, α^+ thalassaemia, could be easily detected by Southern blotting that it was realized that this form of α thalassaemia is probably the world's commonest genetic disorder, reaching, as we have seen earlier, gene frequencies of 90% in some places and with a distribution from the Mediterranean to the eastern Pacific.

The frequency of α^+ thalassaemia in the south-west Pacific (Flint *et al.* 1986) follows a clinal distribution from north-west to south-east, at its highest on the north coast of New Guinea and gradually falling to <5% in New Caledonia (and in the high mountains of New Guinea) (Fig. 6.7). Malarial endemicity, as recorded in pre-eradication surveys, revealed a

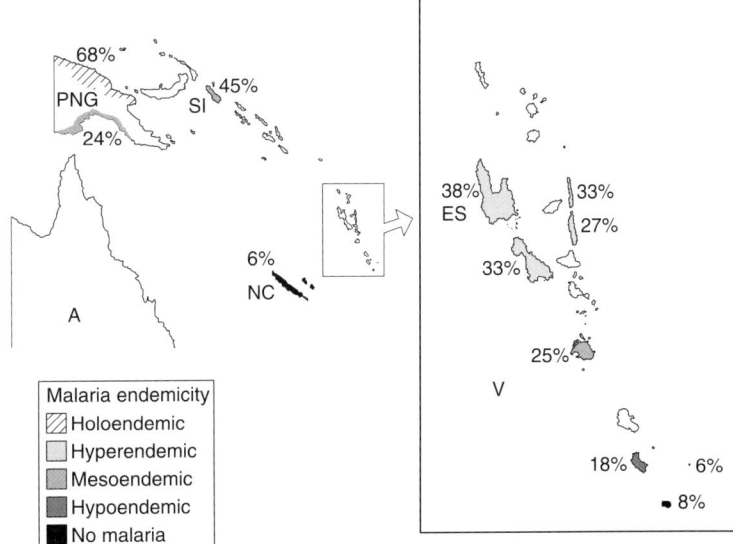

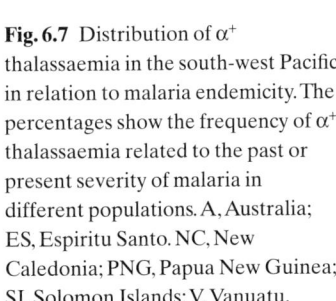

Fig. 6.7 Distribution of α^+ thalassaemia in the south-west Pacific in relation to malaria endemicity. The percentages show the frequency of α^+ thalassaemia related to the past or present severity of malaria in different populations. A, Australia; ES, Espiritu Santo. NC, New Caledonia; PNG, Papua New Guinea; SI, Solomon Islands; V, Vanuatu.

Malaria endemicity
Holoendemic
Hyperendemic
Mesoendemic
Hypoendemic
No malaria

highly significant correlation with α-thalassaemia distribution. There was no correlation of malarial endemicity with other ('neutral') genetic markers tested (Fig. 6.8). Three different deletions ($-\alpha^{3.7I}$, $-\alpha^{3.7III}$, $-\alpha^{4.2}$) are found in the south-west Pacific, and these three types can be further subdivided on the basis of their associated α haplotypes: three $-\alpha^{3.7I}$ chromosomes, six different $-\alpha^{4.2}$s and a single $-\alpha^{3.7III}$ chromosome. The deletions are not uniformly distributed throughout the frequency cline: $-\alpha^{4.2}$ is predominantly a north-coast New Guinea variant, though it occurs elsewhere as a minor component; $-\alpha^{3.7III}$ occurs mainly in Vanuatu, though it too is found sporadically elsewhere; $-\alpha^{3.7I}$ has a focus in southern New Guinea. Most striking of all, each of these α^+-thalassaemia mutations is found on α haplotypes that are very common in Melanesia (types IIIa, IVa, Vc) and rare, often almost unknown, elsewhere. The presumption is that these are all mutations that have arisen in Melanesia and been amplified to high frequencies by some locally acting mechanism (Flint *et al*. 1986). And this must have happened quickly, because the islands of Vanuatu were only occupied 4000 years ago (Bellwood 1989).

Had one only the information that the α^+-thalassaemia frequency is strongly correlated with malarial endemicity, then the picture in Melanesia would still be a good piece of circumstantial evidence in favour of the malaria hypothesis. But it is greatly enriched by the molecular data. A frequency cline is not characteristic of other neutral DNA polymorphisms common in the region (Flint *et al*. 1986). A number of independent mutations with virtually the same phenotype have reached high frequencies where there is endemic malaria, implying that the process responsible is acting on the phenotype and not the genotype. The mutations were not imported from south-east Asia (where there is also malaria and thalassaemia) and they are of relatively recent origin (the different molecular subtypes have not yet been evenly distributed by population movements and, in any case, the islands have only recently been occupied). Together, these findings, while supporting selection, also argue against some of the confounding forces that could otherwise be invoked to explain some of the gene frequency data—migration, or genetic drift, for example.

Population migrations and founder effects: α thalassaemia in Polynesia

Despite the convincing evidence that high frequencies of α thalassaemia in the south-west Pacific are the result of malarial selection, elsewhere in the Pacific—from Fiji in the west to Tahiti and beyond in the east, and from the great arc of Micronesian atolls in the north to New Zealand in the south—the disorder occurs at gene frequencies varying from 1 to 15% (O'Shaughnessy *et al*. 1990), yet malaria has never been recorded anywhere in this vast region (Lambert 1949). Detailed molecular analysis has resolved this paradox and, in the process, provided new insights into Pacific prehistory.

It turns out that in Polynesia almost all (>99%) of the α^+ thalassaemia can be accounted for by the $-\alpha^{3.7III}$ mutation previously seen mainly in northern Vanuatu (O'Shaughnessy *et al*. 1990). Moreover, the deletion is found on the IIIa haplotype, as in Vanuatu, and carries a very restricted subset of the 3′ HVR alleles seen in Vanuatu (Martinson 1991). (The 3′ HVR is a region near the α genes (see Fig. 2.13, Chapter 2) that consists of tandemly repetitive DNA. Its high mutation rate generates new alleles so quickly that differences between populations separated by a few thousand years are apparent.) In Micronesia, examples of the $-\alpha^{4.2}$ variant are found in addition to the $-\alpha^{3.7III}$; these $-\alpha^{4.2}$s are also found

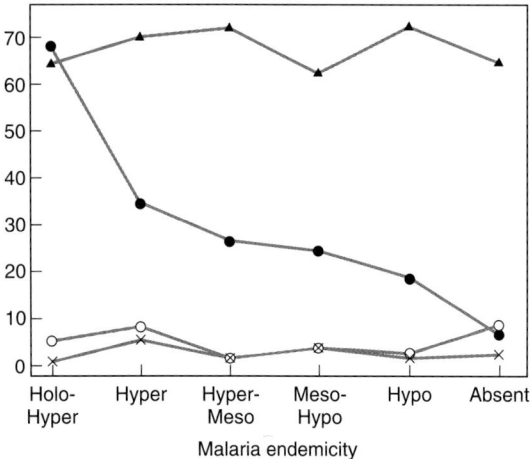

Fig. 6.8 Diagrammatic representation of the distribution of α thalassaemia in the south-west Pacific shown in Fig. 6.7. The percentage frequencies of the following polymorphisms are shown: $-\alpha$ (●), Hp1 (▲), γγγ (x) and $-\gamma$ (○).

on the IIIa haplotype backgrounds common in Melanesia.

Seen in isolation, the finding of $-\alpha^{3.7III}$ in Polynesia and Melanesia might be explained by independent mutations, but there are strong molecular genetic grounds for the view that this mutation was a unique event, and that all extant examples derive from it (Hill *et al.* 1989). Archaeological and linguistic versions of the colonization history of the Pacific provide a more convincing explanation for its distribution (Bellwood 1989). Although the islands of New Guinea and the Bismarck archipelago were first occupied over 30 000 years ago, the more southerly parts of island Melanesia, Micronesia and Polynesia only received their first humans within the past 4000 years. This wave of occupation began in south-east Asia, with seafaring peoples speaking Austronesian languages (in contrast to the Papuan of the old established New Guinea populations) moving south into coastal parts of New Guinea about 4000 years ago. Subsequently they spread rapidly through island Melanesia south to New Caledonia and, by about 1500 BC, east to Fiji and thence to Tonga and Samoa. Expansion eastward into all parts of Polynesia began ~2000 years ago, culminating in the colonization of New Zealand in AD 900. Less is known about the colonization of Micronesia, but it seems that these archipelagos, too, were settled by people of south-east Asian origins within the past 3000–4000 years.

The $-\alpha^{3.7III}$ deletion occurs at high frequency in northern Vanuatu and almost certainly originated there. Knowing this, we can surmise that the proto-Polynesians acquired the $-\alpha^{3.7III}$ variant during their passage through island Melanesia *en route* to the central Pacific. Thereafter, the $-\alpha^{3.7III}$ chromosomes were deposited, like calling cards, across the Pacific as islands were colonized. The colonizing parties were probably small, a situation known to disturb gene frequencies by genetic drift, so, by chance, some islands would have much higher, or lower, frequencies than others. And lacking any selective forces to drive up or maintain gene frequencies, they can further fluctuate by genetic drift. Deleterious mutations, in the absence of *positive* selection, ought to be removed by *negative* selection, but the $-\alpha^{3.7}$ mutations are relatively benign in the heterozygous state. In the 2000 years since occupation, there probably has been insufficient time for the forces of natural selection to eradicate these fairly harmless genes from the island populations of Polynesia.

In Micronesia, the $-\alpha^{3.7III}$ mutation probably arrived with Polynesian voyagers; whether by accident or intent is unknown. Major 'outlier' islands like Kapingimerangi are probably examples of the latter. The $-\alpha^{4.2}$ variants, on the other hand, are all represented in New Guinea (O'Shaughnessy *et al.* 1990). There is ample evidence of drift voyages between Micronesia and New Guinea, and linguistic evidence suggests strong contacts between the two.

Malarial selection may have been recent: the example of β thalassaemia

Despite the β-thalassaemic antecedents of the malaria hypothesis, convincing epidemiological evidence for a relationship between the two diseases has been hard to come by. As we mentioned earlier, the countries of the Mediterranean basin were an early focus for epidemiological studies. But population migration and malaria control programmes had probably disturbed any equilibrium that had previously existed in most areas, and the same may be true of parts of Thailand, where similar studies were undertaken. Whatever the reason, the epidemiological evidence for a causal relationship between β thalassaemia and malaria is not very convincing. Do the molecular data add anything?

The first striking finding, which stems from the efforts made to establish prenatal diagnosis programmes, is the sheer number of β-thalassaemia mutations — now nearly 180. Secondly, the majority of them are regionally specific (Table 6.2 and Fig. 6.3). Thirdly, particular mutations are closely associated with specific β-globin haplotypes; most strongly with the 3′ subhaplotype (which contains the β gene) but with substantial linkage to the 5′ subhaplotype, despite the fact that 5′ and 3′ subhaplotypes are separated by a recombination hotspot (Flint *et al.* 1993a,b). In contrast to the extreme patchiness of the world-wide distribution of β-thalassaemia mutations, the background of normal β-globin haplotypes is much more homogeneous. Together these observations point towards the following conclusions. The regional specificity of mutations suggests local processes for their elevation to high frequencies. The close association with specific haplotypes suggests a recent cause — migration has not had sufficient time to disperse most mutations (unlike the normal background haplotypes), nor has recombination yet disrupted that linkage. At the sequence level some of these features are even more striking. In Vanuatu, the sequences of a 3-kb region around the β gene from 60 normal chromosomes revealed 17 different alleles involving 19 polymorphic sites. In contrast 12 β-thalassaemia chromosomes carrying the IVS1-5 G→C mutation were totally monomorphic over the same 3 kb (Fullerton *et al.* 1994).

The inferences seem clear: β-thalassaemia genes throughout the malarial regions of the world have been amplified to high frequency so recently that none of the equilibrating forces—migration, recombination, genetic drift—has had sufficient time or opportunity to bring them into spatial or genetic equilibrium with their background.

The structural variants: haemoglobins S, C and E

We have seen how the relatively smooth geographical distribution of β thalassaemia as a disease belies its extreme heterogeneity at the molecular level. What can be said of the structural variants, each of which, in complete contrast to β thalassaemia, owes its existence to a single nucleotide substitution in the β gene? How can we account for HbS in Africa, Arabia, Sicily, the Caribbean and India; and within India (for example) how can one explain its uneven distribution?

Haemoglobin S in Africa

Haplotype analysis of HbS can explain many of the features of the distribution of the disease in Africa (and elsewhere); but it also raises some new questions, which, ironically, hark back to the old problem of mutation rates (p. 273).

The current distribution of HbS is shown in Fig. 6.6. The most interesting feature is that, although for the most part the disease is found from the Atlantic west coast almost to the borders of South Africa, it is, at the molecular level, compartmentalized. The mutation is found predominantly on four β-globin-gene-cluster haplotypes, and each of these is regionally specific. It has been argued that this implies independent mutations (Chebloune *et al.* 1988; Nagel & Ranney 1990; Lapouméroulie *et al.* 1992), but it is not so simple. There is tight linkage between the 5′ and 3′ subhaplotypes: as for β thalassaemia, this suggests recency, as does the circumscribed distribution of the haplotypes. The fact that HbE in south-east Asia has similar population genetics features (localized distri-

bution, multiple haplotypes) (see Figs 6.2 & 6.6) raises the obvious question: if recurrent mutation can provide multiple examples of these same mutations in the same locale, why are they not found throughout the malarial world? But put the question another way and ask if a single mutation could find its way on to numerous haplotypes, and there is a way out of this dilemma. There are molecular processes—localized recombination and gene conversion—that could account for the molecular genetics of HbS, especially as the HbS (and HbE) mutation site is known to lie in a highly recombinogenic part of the β-globin-gene cluster (Fullerton *et al.* 1994). This seems a more plausible explanation of the molecular observations than recurrent mutation at a single nucleotide site in the β gene.

Haemoglobin S in India

HbS is a common haemoglobinopathy in India, but it is found predominantly in a few high-frequency pockets (Livingstone 1985) with the intervening regions having mostly α and β thalassaemia. The general picture is thus of a patchwork distribution of haemoglobin disorders throughout the malarial regions of the subcontinent. Haplotype analysis reveals that almost all β^S chromosomes have the same haplotype (Kulozik *et al.* 1986; Labie *et al.* 1989); moreover this haplotype only accounts for ~2% of normal β^A haplotypes in India. It is unlikely that a β^S mutation has arisen independently in three separate locations on the same minor haplotype background; moreover, the tight linkage between the 5′ and 3′ parts of the haplotype implies that all mutations would have to have been recent events. Fortunately, there is a more plausible interpretation. Anthropological and archaeological evidence points to a single ancestral population, possibly living in the Indus valley, as the forerunners of today's HbS-carrying ethnic groups. Invasions from the north by peoples whose descendants now comprise most of the Indian population probably led to the dispersal of the original HbS-carrying population (Labie *et al.* 1989). The distribution of HbS in India is thus probably a consequence of warfare and migrations that occurred over 5000 years ago.

Migrations can similarly account for the HbS present in the eastern oases of Saudi Arabia. Haplotype analysis suggests that the eastern Saudi and Indian mutations share a common origin (Kulozik *et al.*

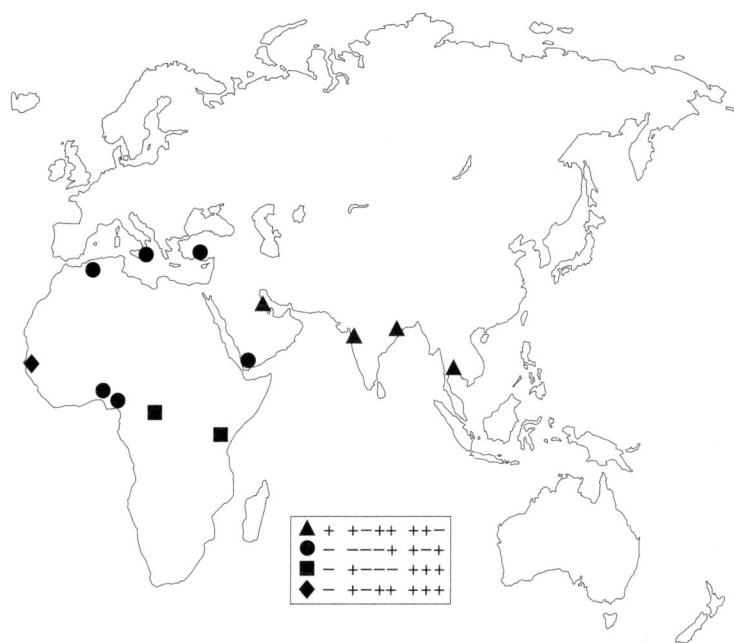

Fig. 6.9 The different β-globin-gene-cluster restriction-fragment length polymorphisms associated with the sickle-cell gene in Africa, the Middle East and India. The polymorphic sites, + or –, are described in Fig. 2.15, Chapter 2.

1986) (Fig. 6.9), and there is ample evidence of ancient trade routes between the two countries. Precisely where the mutation arose is, however, unknown.

Population migrations

Apart from the major foci of HbS in Africa and India, the variant is found at significant frequencies in many parts of the world. We have seen that the Indian and eastern Saudi Arabia clusters are related, but what of the Mediterranean and Caribbean countries? Leaving the India–Arabia region aside, haplotype analysis shows that most of the HbS outside equatorial Africa almost certainly originated there. HbS in Algeria is found on the same β haplotype that characterizes HbS from the Benin region of Nigeria (Flint *et al.* 1993a). This haplotype accounts for over half of all normal $β^A$ chromosomes in West Africa but less than 5% in north Africa, making it unlikely that the HbS mutation arose there and then migrated to equatorial Africa, rather than vice versa. Using similar arguments it can be shown that HbS in Greece and Sicily is also derived from the Benin area (Ragusa *et al.* 1988; Schiliro *et al.* 1990).

In the New World, haplotypes can be used not only to confirm the African provenance of HbS genes but also to pinpoint their regions of origin. Seventeenth-century shipping records of slave consignments correlate remarkably with the haplotype compositions of HbS carriers in the Caribbean (Nagel 1984; Nagel & Ranney 1990). The slave trade is also implicated in the HbS found on the Iberian peninsula (Monteiro *et al.* 1989).

A malarial region without haemoglobinopathies

In south and central America where malaria is a major problem from Mexico to Brazil, we have seen that there is little evidence for haemoglobinopathies in the native populations. At first sight this contradicts our previous inferences, and the conventional answer, that malaria—or *P. falciparum*—was a post-Columbian introduction, for which the evidence is not very strong (Bruce-Chwatt 1965), begs the question because it assumes that *if* there had been sufficient time for selection to operate, haemoglobin variants would be as common now as they are elsewhere in the malarial world.

Lacking mutations to study, molecular genetics cannot contribute, except indirectly, but recent work on DNA polymorphisms in *P. falciparum* in Brazil hints of restricted variation (Shi *et al.* 1992) suggestive of a population bottleneck (and consistent with a recent introduction). Clearly, this is not conclusive evidence, but is at least compatible with the overall picture.

In this short section we have tried to show how the new molecular data affect the 'malaria hypothesis'. By their nature, the evidence they provide is circumstantial; only experiments that show a direct protective effect of phenotype on malaria mortality or morbidity, as we describe below, can do otherwise. But they can, and do, address many of the issues that have eluded and confused the epidemiological approaches, especially the apparent contradictions to the hypothesis. It is now possible to at least begin to tease out some of the previously unfathomable population genetics influences on gene frequency that have always been invoked as alternatives to selection. Although any one of these bits of evidence might be regarded as anecdotal, collectively they are all telling the same story—the one consistent factor that accounts for the high frequencies of such lethal diseases as thalassaemia and sickle-cell anaemia is selection by malaria.

Finally, and perhaps unexpectedly, we may also be learning new insights into malaria from this new source of information. It seems inescapable that the mutations we are considering have only reached high frequencies in recent historical times—perhaps within the past 5000 years. Although malaria is probably an old parasite of humans, it may be that it has only become a serious scourge within the past 10 000 years as a result of increased population densities made possible by agriculture.

The mechanism of protection against malaria by thalassaemia

The population data described above provide convincing evidence for a causal relationship between thalassaemia and malaria. In the case of α thalassaemia at least, we now have good direct evidence for protection against malaria. The first hints of this came from studies in Papua New Guinea by Oppenheimer *et al.* (1987) and in Nepal by Professor Luzzatto and colleagues (Terrenato *et al.* 1988). The latter workers found from a retrospective analysis of health records that the incidence of both *P. falciparum* and *P. vivax* malaria was nearly seven times lower amongst Tharus compared with sympatric non-Tharus living in the highly malarial Terrai region. Subsequently,

Modiano *et al.* (1991) showed that Tharus have an extremely high frequency of α thalassaemia, with the majority (90%) being homozygous for the single-gene-deletion (–α) variant. It was estimated that there is a 10-fold reduction in morbidity from malaria in (–α/–α) homozygotes. Yates (1995) analysed the relationship between severe malaria and α thalassaemia in two large African case–control studies. Individually, neither study gave a clear-cut result. When combined, however, there was a significant protective effect in α[+]-thalassaemia homozygotes. More recently, Allen *et al.* (1997) carried out a prospective case–control study of nearly 250 children with severe malaria admitted to Madang hospital on the north coast of Papua New Guinea, where malaria transmission is intense. Compared with normal children, the risk of contracting severe malaria was 0.4 in α[+]-thalassaemia homozygotes (and as low as 0.2 for cases defined by the strictest WHO guidelines), and 0.66 for α[+]-thalassaemia heterozygotes. As we noted earlier, α[+] thalassaemia affects approximately 90% of the indigenous population. Thus α thalassaemia has a profound beneficial effect on the population in this highly malarial environment.

Unfortunately, none of the epidemiological experiments indicate how the protective effect might be mediated at the cellular level. Suggestions made following Haldane's paper, and summarized in the previous edition, all followed the notion that thalassaemic cells might, in some way, be an unfavourable environment for parasite growth and development, through lack of key metabolites, small cell size, susceptibility to oxidant stress and so on. With this mechanism in mind a number of studies have been conducted to examine the efficacy of invasion and re-invasion of thalassaemic red blood cells. Almost all have found that invasion is reduced in the more severe forms of thalassaemia, such as homozygous HbE (Nagel *et al.* 1981; Bunyaratvej *et al.* 1992) or HbH disease (Ifediba *et al.* 1985; Brockelman *et al.* 1987; Bunyaratvej *et al.* 1992), and in complex haemoglobinopathies such as α and β thalassaemia in conjunction with Hbs Constant Spring or E (Brockelman *et al.* 1987; Yuthavong *et al.* 1987; Udomsangpetch *et al.* 1993). However, since it is unlikely that the severe forms of thalassaemia would have come under selection, the relevance of these findings is not clear. In contrast, the majority of studies have found that invasion of cells from individuals with clinically 'silent' forms of thalassaemia, such as the heterozygous states for α thalassaemia and β thalassaemia or HbE, show normal rates of invasion and subsequent growth over a single red-cell cycle (Nagel *et al*. 1981; Yuthavong *et al*. 1988; Luzzi *et al*. 1990; Bunyaratvej *et al*. 1992). There have been several attempts to monitor parasite growth in cells from heterozygous α- or β-thalassaemics over a number of cycles, but the results have been inconsistent. Thus, while Ifediba *et al*. (1985) found no reproducible decrease in re-invasion or growth rates in minor forms of α thalassaemia even after prolonged culture, others have found a reduced rate of re-invasion (Senok *et al*. 1997).

Other workers have attempted to demonstrate abnormal biological properties of parasite-infected thalassaemic red cells. For example, two groups have presented data suggesting that rosette formation, a phenomenon which has been found to be correlated with an adverse outcome in some studies, may be reduced, at least *in vitro*, in infected heterozygous α- and β-thalassaemic red cells (Udomsangpetch *et al*. 1993; Carlson *et al*. 1994). Others have studied the cytoadherence potential of infected α-thalassaemic cells. For example, Luzzi and Pasvol (1990) found no reduction in cytoadherence to C32 amelanotic melanoma cells in heterozygous α⁰-thalassaemic red cells infected with *P. falciparum*, while Udomsangpetch *et al*. (1993) found some reduction of *in situ* adherence to human umbilical-vein endothelial cells by heterozygous α- and β-thalassaemic cells treated in the same way. Two groups have analysed the binding of malaria hyperimmune serum to the surface of *P. falciparum*-infected thalassaemic red blood cells. Luzzi *et al*. (1991) found that infected α- and β-thalassaemic red cells bound significantly more antibody per unit area from immune serum than control cells. Udomsangpetch *et al*. (1993), on the other hand, found no significant difference in binding to either variant cell type. However, this apparent conflict may reflect methodological differences: the former group used a radiometric method to assess binding to live cells while the latter used a flow-cytometric method to quantify binding to fixed cells.

Given the complexities and difficulties in repro-ducing *in vitro* culture systems for malarial parasites, and the fact that the red cells in more severe forms of thalassaemia show many metabolic and structural abnormalities (see Chapter 5), it is not surprising that these *in vitro* studies have given variable results and that no definitive answers have emerged. However, what is clear is that the rates of invasion and develop-ment, at least through one cycle, of malarial parasites introduced into red cells obtained from α⁺-thalas-saemia heterozygotes or homozygotes, or β-thalas-saemia heterozygotes, appear to be normal.

It is likely that the key period of susceptibility to *P. falciparum* malaria in holoendemic areas is in the first 18 months of life. During the first few months there may be a measure of passive protection from mater-nal antibodies, but this effect may be relatively short-lived. After this period infants subjected to infection will either die or become increasingly immune during the first or second year. Thus the critical phase is probably the period between the ages of 4 and 18 months. The issue that concerns us, then, is in what way are the red cells of thalassaemia heterozygotes different from those of a normal infant during this period?

There is good evidence that the rate of decline of HbF production in heterozygous β-thalassaemic infants is retarded as compared with normal individ-uals (see Chapter 7). There is some limited evidence from short-term culture experiments that HbF affects the growth and development of malaria parasites in red cells *in vitro* (Pasvol *et al*. 1977). However, even if this were shown to be effective *in vivo*, it would only be applicable to β thalassaemia. Recently, another more intriguing possibility has emerged. Williams *et al*. (1996a) studied a large cohort of children with and without α thalassaemia on an island with holoendemic malaria in Vanuatu in the south-west Pacific. Surprisingly, they found that the incidence of uncomplicated malaria and the prevalence of splenomegaly, an index of malaria infection, were significantly *higher* in young children with α thalassaemia than in normal children. More-over, the effect was most marked in the youngest children and with the non-lethal parasite *P. vivax*. Williams *et al*. suggest that the early susceptibility to *P. vivax* may be acting as a natural vaccine by induc-ing cross-species protection against *P. falciparum*. It seems likely that α⁺ thalassaemia, like other mild forms of the disorder, is probably associated with a degree of ineffective erythropoiesis and reduced red-cell survival (Chapter 11), resulting in a higher pro-portion of circulating young red cells. Infection with both *P. falciparum*, which preferentially invades young metabolically active cells, and *P. vivax*, which only invades reticulocytes (Pasvol. *et al*. 1980), would thus be more efficient. An increased susceptibility to malaria during the neonatal period may thus lead to improved immunity to later severe disease. If this is indeed the basis of the protective mechanism, one would expect that it would be equally applicable to β-thalassaemia heterozygotes and HbE homozygotes, both of which have comparable haematological characteristics to homozygous α^+ thalassaemia, and even possibly to G6PD-deficient individuals.

There are other hints that protection by thalassaemia may have at least some degree of immunological involvement. As mentioned earlier, Luzzi *et al.* (1991) observed that surface antigen expression in *P. falciparum*-infected α-thalassaemic red cells is almost twice that of normal cells, a phenomenon that may lead to better presentation of parasite antigens to the immune system. Furthermore, rosette formation, which has been associated with cerebral malaria, appears to be hindered in thalassaemic red cells (Carlson *et al.* 1994). Perhaps the most important piece of indirect evidence comes from the case–control study of Allen *et al.* (1997). This revealed that α thalassaemia protects not only against severe malaria, but equally against hospitalization from other (mainly) infectious disease. This striking finding suggests that acquired antidisease immunity against malaria has a more general basis, possibly by inducing tolerance to important mediators of the systemic inflammatory response, like tumour necrosis factor (TNFα).

Postscript

These successes in establishing a clear relationship between α thalassaemia and resistance to malaria are encouraging and suggest that it should be possible to test these relationships for other forms of thalassaemia in the near future. Over recent years it has become clear that other red-cell polymorphisms, including glucose-6-phosphate dehydrogenase deficiency and variation in membrane structure and blood groups, have been shaped by malaria (Weatherall *et al.* 1997). However, it has also become apparent that genetic variability due to selection by malaria is not confined to red cells. It is now known that certain polymorphisms of the HLA-DR system are associated with substantial protection against both cerebral malaria and severe malarial anaemia. Another polymorphic system which has been uncovered, and which is clearly related to malaria, involves the gene encoding TNFα. For example, a single-base change in the promoter is associated with a markedly increased risk of cerebral malaria and death. Thus it seems likely that some polymorphisms may have been selected by other infectious illnesses which alter malaria susceptibility in a deleterious way.

These are examples of how malaria, quite probably over a relatively short period, has dramatically changed the genetic make-up of populations. As mentioned in Chapter 5, these new observations have important implications for a better understanding of the complex pathophysiology of the thalassaemias. Just as every population has a different series of thalassaemia alleles, so there is wide variability in a variety of other polymorphisms which, like the thalassaemias, have come under intense selection in malarious regions. Thus individual responses to intercurrent infection or iron loading may vary widely between different thalassaemic populations and have an important effect on the pattern of infectious illnesses and on other complications of the disease. In the thalassaemia field, like many other branches of medicine, we are just beginning to see the importance of the role of evolutionary biology in helping us to better understand the remarkable variability of individual response to both genetic and acquired disease.

Part 3
Clinical features of the thalassaemias

Contributors:
R. Gibbons
D.R. Higgs
Nancy F. Olivieri
W.G. Wood

Chapter 7
The β thalassaemias

Introduction

The β thalassaemias are a diverse group of disorders of haemoglobin synthesis, all of which result from a reduced output of the β chains of adult haemoglobin. Clinically, either alone or through their interactions with β-globin structural haemoglobin variants, they are by far the most important forms of thalassaemia. Their control and management will pose an increasing drain on health-care resources, particularly in developing countries, in which improvements in sanitation and public health measures have dramatically reduced the number of deaths from malnutrition and infection early in life, and hence in which babies with thalassaemia are now surviving long enough to present for diagnosis and treatment.

In this chapter we describe the clinical and laboratory features of the severe, transfusion-dependent forms of β thalassaemia and their carrier states. The diverse disorders which fall between these extremes, the β thalassaemia intermedias, are described, together with the other forms of thalassaemia that cause a similar clinical picture, in Chapter 13.

Classification and genotype/phenotype relationships

As we saw in Chapter 1, the different clinical conditions that were later realized to be forms of β thalassaemia attracted a variety of different names. However, with the exception of some current Italian literature (see, for example, Bianco Silvestroni 1992), it is now customary to call the severe, transfusion-dependent forms of β thalassaemia thalassaemia major, or Cooley's anaemia, and the symptomless carrier states thalassaemia minor, or trait. Because of the wide variability of the haemoglobin constitution in all the severe forms of β thalassaemia, it has been necessary to resort to describing the different phenotypic subtypes by the more consistent findings in carriers, particularly the level of HbA_2. Most of the common forms of β thalassaemia are associated with increased levels of HbA_2 in heterozygotes. There are, however, varieties in which it is in the normal range. These 'normal HbA_2' types of β thalassaemia are further subdivided into those in which carriers have a typical thalassaemic morphology of their red cells, and those in which there are no haematological changes, the 'silent' β thalassaemias. Other forms of β thalassaemia have been identified in which carriers have unusually high levels of Hbs F or A_2. Finally, there is a group characterized by a dominant rather than the usual recessive form of inheritance. A summary of the different varieties of β thalassaemia based on their heterozygous phenotypes is given in Table 7.1.

Beta thalassaemia major usually results from the compound heterozygous state for two different β-globin-gene mutations or, less commonly and mainly in populations with a high frequency of consanguineous marriages, from the homozygous state for the same mutation. As we saw in Chapters 3 and 4, the majority of the β thalassaemias are caused by mutations at the β-globin gene loci, which result in either no output of β globin, $β^0$ thalassaemia, or a reduced output, $β^+$ thalassaemia. Hence compound heterozygotes may be heterozygous for both $β^+$ and $β^0$ thalassaemia or for two different forms of either $β^0$ or $β^+$ thalassaemia. The term $β^{++}$ thalassaemia, which was introduced to describe the β thalassaemias with a mild reduction in β-globin synthesis, is used less now that these diseases can be defined at the molecular level.

Because many different mutations underlie the β thalassaemias, and those that cause $β^+$ thalassaemia vary in their overall effect on β-chain synthesis, it is not surprising that, either alone or through their interactions with structural haemoglobin variants or with α thalassaemia, they generate the wide variety of different phenotypes that are described in this and subsequent chapters. As mentioned in Chapter 4, and discussed in more detail in Chapter 13, although it is clear that some β-thalassaemia mutations are usually

Table 7.1 The different forms of β thalassaemia.

β thalassaemia major
   β⁰ thalassaemia
   β⁺ thalassaemia
   (β⁺⁺ thalassaemia)*
β thalassaemia intermedia†
β thalassaemia minor (trait)
   With raised level of HbA_2
      Normal or slightly elevated levels of HbF
      Unusually high levels of HbF
      Unusually high levels of HbA_2
   Normal levels of HbA_2
      β thalassaemia and δ thalassaemia
      Mild β thalassaemia‡
      Silent β thalassaemia
   Dominant β thalassaemia
   β thalassaemia with genetic determinant unlinked to
      β-globin-gene locus

* Term to describe very mild alleles; not in common usage.
† Classified in full in Chapter 13.
‡ HbA_2 may be slightly elevated.

associated with a mild disease, and hence are some-times called 'mild' or 'silent' mutations, these relationships are not yet consistent enough to make it possible to develop a diagnostic classification of β thalassaemia that relates genotype to phenotype with any degree of accuracy.

In the sections which follow, the main clinical, laboratory and diagnostic features of the different forms of β thalassaemia are described. The pathophysiology of β thalassaemia is considered in detail in Chapter 5 and the mechanisms that underlie its remarkable heterogeneity and its intermediate forms are considered in Chapter 13.

β Thalassaemia major

The major forms of β thalassaemia, still sometimes called Cooley's anaemia, are defined as genetic disorders of β-globin synthesis in which life can only be sustained by regular blood transfusion.

The early descriptions of severe thalassaemia by Cooley and colleagues present a picture of the disease as it was, and unfortunately still is, seen in children who have either not been transfused at all or not been given adequate transfusion. If children are adequately treated in this way many of the 'typical' features of thalassaemia do not appear in early child-hood and most of the clinical problems, which occur after the first decade, are the result of iron accumulation. For this reason it is necessary to consider this disease in two settings, that is, the inadequately treated child and the child who has been transfused from early in life.

General clinical features and course

Age and symptoms at presentation

Since β-chain synthesis replaces γ-chain synthesis during the first months of life it might be expected that β thalassaemia would become manifest at about that time. This is usually the case. Severe forms of β thalassaemia commonly present during the first year. For example, Kattamis *et al.* (1975) noted that the mean age at presentation was 13.1 months (±8.1 months), with a range from 2 to 36 months. In reviewing 121 patients, Modell and Berdoukas (1984) found that 60% presented within the first year; the mean age at presentation was 6 months. Similarly, Cao (1988) found that, comparing a group of transfusion-dependent with non-transfusion-dependent β-thalassaemics, the mean age of presentation of the former was 8.4±9.1 months while in the latter it was 17.4±11.8 months. The mean haemoglobin level at presentation in the transfusion-dependent group was 8.28 g/dl as compared with 9.16±1.2 g/dl in the group with the milder disease.

Some infants with severe β thalassaemia present later than the first year. Their haemoglobin values are in the 6–9 g/dl range and after presentation it is not clear whether they are going to fall into the major or intermediate category. However, after observation for several months it is apparent that they are failing to thrive or not growing adequately, and it is clear that they require regular transfusion. The same reasoning applies to even older children who have been categorized as having thalassaemia intermedia but in whom poor growth or the development of other complications indicates that they fall into the transfusion-dependent category. The age spectrum of presentation of severe and milder forms of β thalassaemia is summarized in Table 7.2.

A wide variety of symptoms may alert the parents to the fact that the child has a serious illness. Frequently, affected infants fail to thrive and gain weight normally and become progressively pale. Feeding problems, diarrhoea, irritability, recurrent bouts of infection, progressive enlargement of the abdomen due to splenomegaly and failure to recover from an infective episode are common presenting symptoms. Less usual presentations include the incidental finding of an enlarged spleen, a fever of unknown origin or the mother noticing that the infant's urine stains the napkin (diaper) pink or brown (Modell & Berdoukas 1984). At this stage of the illness the infant may look pale but otherwise there may be no abnormal signs. On the other hand, splenomegaly may already be present. Thus an accurate diagnosis at this stage depends on the haematological findings described later in this chapter, together with the demonstration of the β-thalassaemia trait in both parents.

If a firm diagnosis is made at this stage and the infant is started on a regular blood transfusion regimen, subsequent growth and development may be relatively normal over the next decade. However, if the child is not adequately transfused the typical clinical picture of β thalassaemia major develops over the next few years.

Diagnostic difficulties at presentation

When babies with β thalassaemia major present with failure to thrive and anaemia, whether or not splenomegaly is already present, the diagnosis is easily made from the appearances of the peripheral blood film, the finding of an unusually high level of fetal haemoglobin and the demonstration of a carrier state in both parents. However, infants often present with an acute infective episode and the extent to which their anaemia reflects infection rather than severe thalassaemia is not clear. Although the blood picture can be examined it is often necessary to transfuse these infants to tide them over this acute episode. All too often the infant is then assumed to be transfusion dependent and labelled as having the major form of the illness. However, it is very important to stop transfusions, either immediately or after a period, to allow the child to fully recover, and to observe the steady-state haemoglobin off transfusion. Only in this way is it possible to identify the milder, intermediate forms of the disease which have been exacerbated by acute infection. The problems of distinguishing between the major and intermediate forms of the disease are discussed further in Chapter 13.

Although the diagnosis of β thalassaemia major is usually fairly straightforward the authors have observed a number of cases, particularly in the developing countries, in which difficulties arose. For example, the disease may present with an acute illness, and there are certain infections that can mimic β thalassaemia. Malaria causes anaemia and splenomegaly, and although the peripheral blood findings are quite different it may be necessary to treat the infant with antimalarial agents and carefully re-examine the child to see if the spleen has regressed, and to assess the haematological findings, before the diagnosis of β thalassaemia is confirmed. Occasionally, the anaemia and splenomegaly associated with leukaemia may superficially resemble β thalassaemia; juvenile chronic myeloid leukaemia, particularly because of the associated high level of fetal haemoglobin production, may sometimes cause confusion. Severe iron deficiency can usually be diagnosed from the haematological picture together with

Table 7.2(a) Age at presentation of infants with thalassaemia major or intermedia (from Modell & Berdoukas 1984).

Age (years)	Thalassaemia major	Thalassaemia intermedia
<1	75 (62%)	4 (11%)
1–2	35 (29%)	11 (30%)
>2	11 (9%)	22 (59%)
Total	121	37

Table 7.2(b) Further data on the age of presentation of different β-thalassaemia phenotypes.

	Number of patients	Age at diagnosis (months)	
Thalassaemia major	52	10.8 ± 6.4	Kattamis *et al.* (1975)
Thalassaemia intermedia	23	34.6 ± 22.3	
Thalassaemia major	19	8.4 ± 9.1	Cao (1988)
Thalassaemia intermedia	15	17.5 ± 11.8	

the low serum iron and ferritin values, while the blood pictures associated with other congenital haemolytic anaemias are sufficiently different to make them unlikely to be confused with β thalassaemia. We have seen several patients with congenital dyserythropoietic anaemia that have been thought to have β thalassaemia; although the blood pictures are quite different, the associated splenomegaly and dyserythropoiesis may cause confusion.

Course through childhood in inadequately transfused patients

The under-transfused thalassaemic child is often growth retarded; many are noticeably smaller than their normal siblings, although, in some, slowing of growth is more marked as puberty approaches. There is pallor of the mucous membranes and skin, a variable degree of icterus, and the dirty brown pigmentation first noticed by Cooley in his early descriptions of the disease may develop. These children fail to thrive and show features of a hypermetabolic state, including poor musculature, reduction in body fat, recurrent fever, poor appetite and lethargy; the neglected β thalassaemic, with characteristic protuberant abdomen, poor musculoskeletal development and spindly legs, looks very much like a child with malignant disease (Fig. 7.1). There is a variable degree of hepatosplenomegaly together with skeletal changes which produce a characteristic facial appearance, with bossing of the skull (Fig. 7.2a), hypertrophy of the maxilla, which tends to expose the upper teeth, prominent malar eminences with depression of the bridge of the nose, puffiness of the eyelids and a tendency to a mongoloid slant of the eyes (Fig. 7.2b). There may also be proximal muscle weakness and a genu valgum. Recurrent ulceration of the legs may occur at any time throughout childhood.

The skeletal changes are mirrored by characteristic radiological changes of the skull, long bones and hands. The skull shows dilatation of the diploic space, and the subperiosteal bone grows in a series of radiating striations, giving a typical 'hair on end' appearance (Fig. 7.3). There is cortical thinning of the long bones with porous rarefaction; similar changes are found in the small bones of the hands and feet (Fig. 7.4). These radiological changes, noted as early as 1930 by Voght and Diamond, have been the subject of many reviews (Moseley 1962; Baker 1964; Capelli

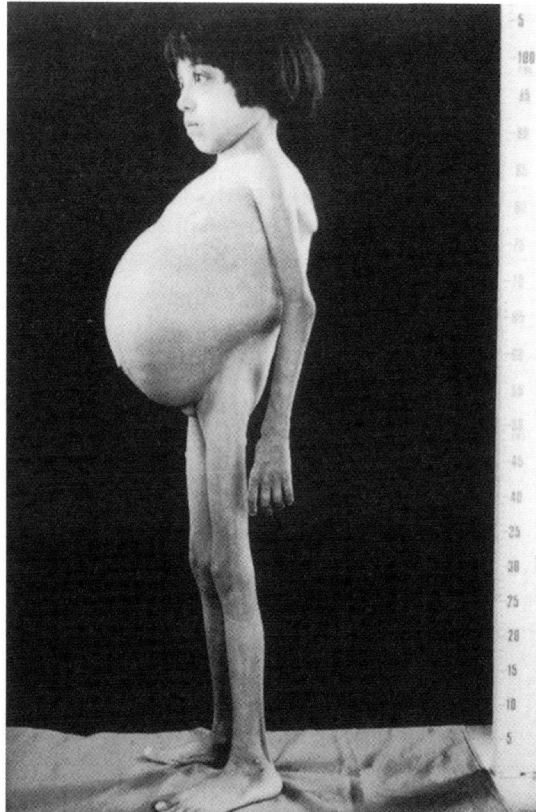

Fig. 7.1 Some clinical features of severe β thalassaemia. This child has massive hepatosplenomegaly and wasting of the limbs. The stance, with arching of the back, is characteristic.

1966; Middlemis & Raper 1966; Cammisa & Sabella 1967; Roy *et al.* 1971; Aksoy *et al.* 1973; Moseley 1974; Ribio Perez *et al.* 1976 ; Orzincolo *et al.* 1994). Pathological fractures are also a major feature of inadequately transfused β thalassaemics (Michelson & Cohen 1988) (Fig. 7.5).

The early childhood of these patients is interspersed with numerous complications. These include recurrent infections associated with worsening of the anaemia, spontaneous fractures and a variety of other complications due to progressive bone deformity, folate deficiency, a bleeding tendency, increasing hypersplenism, gallstones, leg ulcers, and a variety of syndromes due to tumour masses resulting from extramedullary haemopoiesis. If they survive to puberty they often develop similar complications to children who, because they have been adequately

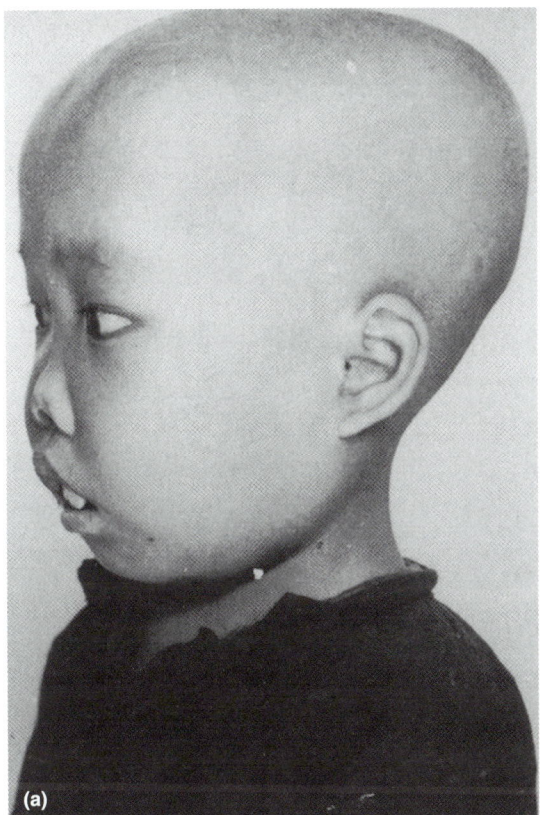 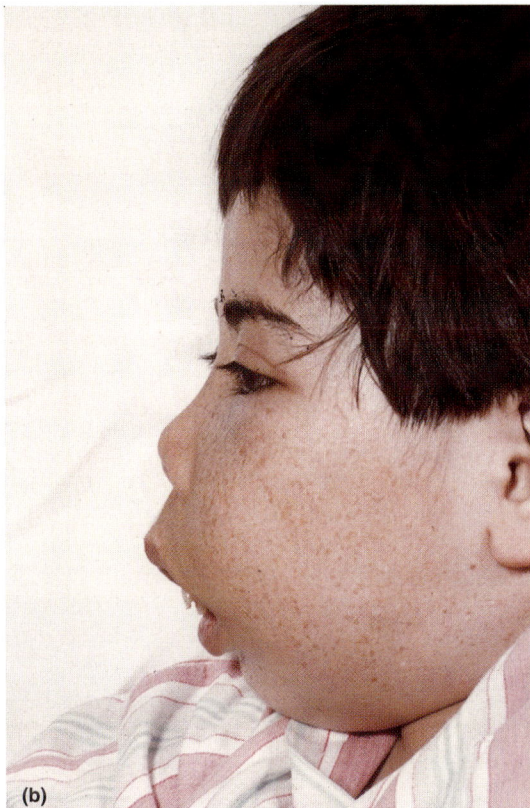

Fig. 7.2 Facial appearances in severe β thalassaemia. (a) Bossing of the skull. (b) Typical dental deformity.

transfused, have had a relatively trouble-free childhood.

The well transfused thalassaemic child

Well transfused thalassaemic children often remain asymptomatic until the age of 10–11 years. Their future course then depends on whether they have received adequate iron chelation. If not, they begin to show signs of hepatic, endocrine and cardiac disturbances resembling those seen in adults with familial haemochromatosis. The first observable changes are often a failure or reduction of the pubertal growth spurt, sometimes associated with delayed sexual maturation. Throughout their teenage life these children suffer from a variety of complications due to different endocrine deficiencies and they nearly all develop cardiac symptoms in the latter half of the second decade.

Many children who are adequately transfused and are fully compliant with respect to iron chelation grow and develop normally, enter puberty and become sexually mature. Though in some cases they may suffer from the side-effects of long-term chelation therapy, this type of treatment has revolutionized the management of the disease and many of these patients are now reaching adult life in good health.

This subdivision of the course of severe β thalassaemia is, of course, rather artificial; many patients are encountered who fall between the two groups. In the sections that follow we shall consider the major complications which underlie the clinical manifestations of this condition. Readers coming to the field for the first time will find it helpful to read them in conjunction with Chapter 5, which outlines the major pathophysiological mechanisms involved.

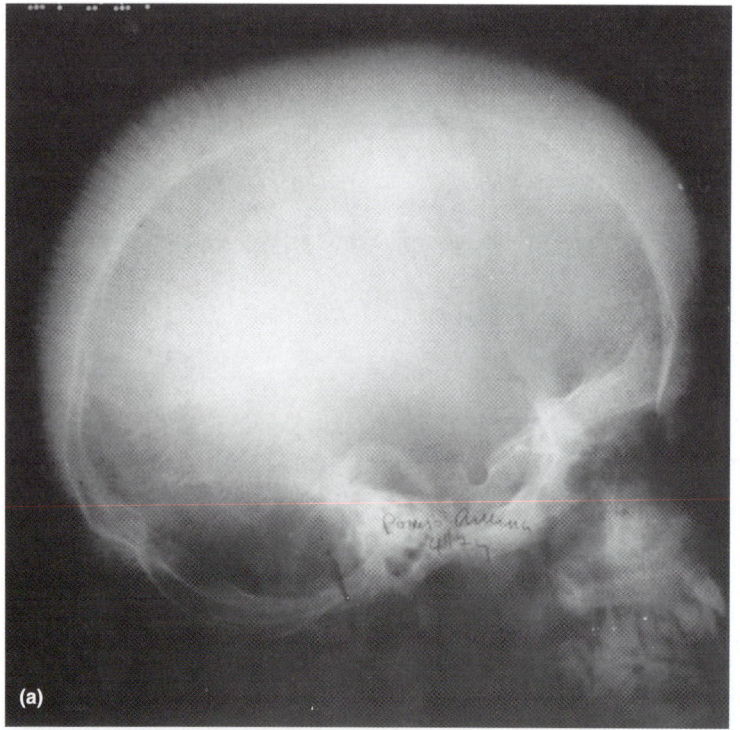

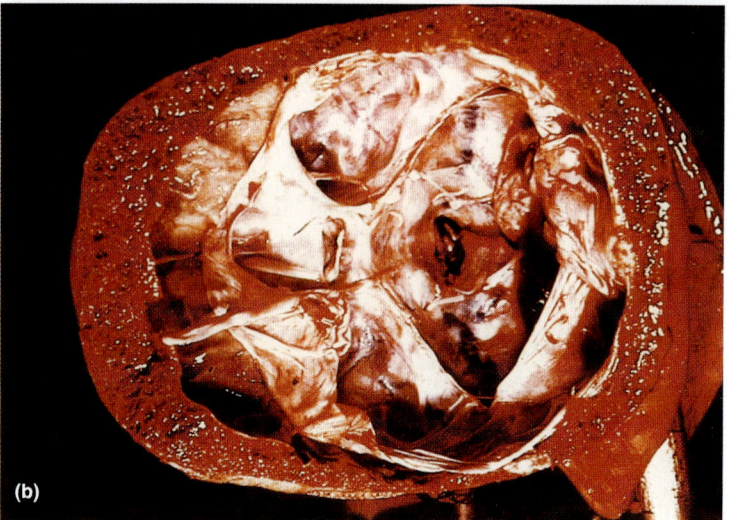

Fig. 7.3 Skull changes in severe β thalassaemia. (a) An X-ray showing the typical 'hair on end' appearance. (b) A skull at autopsy, showing massive hypertrophy of the marrow. From Sonakul (1989), with permission.

Complications

The frequency and severity of many of the complications of β thalassaemia depend to a large extent on the way that patients are managed, particularly with respect to their steady-state haemoglobin level and effectiveness of chelation therapy. In this section we shall group all the complications under particular headings and try, in each case, to relate the particular patterns of management to the severity of each complication.

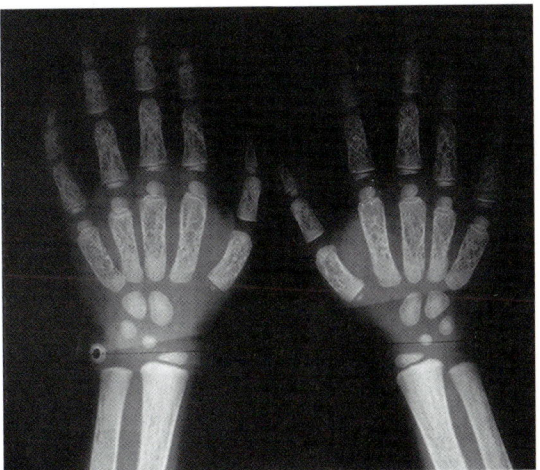

Fig. 7.4 X-ray changes in the bones of the hand in severe β thalassaemia.

Hypersplenism and plasma volume expansion

All the early literature on thalassaemia stresses the occurrence of progressive splenomegaly in the major form of the illness. Splenectomy for the treatment of thalassaemia has also been practised from the time that the disease was first identified. The pathophysiology and mechanisms of hypersplenism are considered in Chapter 5, and its diagnosis and management are discussed in Chapter 15.

As soon as there was sufficient experience of children who had been maintained at relatively high haemoglobin levels it became apparent that marked splenomegaly and hypersplenism were being seen much less frequently (O'Brien *et al.* 1972; Modell 1976). In a series of careful measurements of the annual blood requirements of her patients Modell demonstrated how it was possible to calculate an average annual transfusion requirement to maintain a mean haemoglobin level of approximately 10 g/dl (Fig. 7.6). She found that patients who exceeded this figure by 50% or more almost invariably returned to their 'ideal' transfusion requirements after splenectomy (Modell 1976, 1977; Modell & Berdoukas 1984). These observations were confirmed by others, who found that children who need more than 200 ml of packed cells/kg body weight/year to maintain average haemoglobins at about 10 g/dl have significant hypersplenism, and that splenectomy significantly reduces these blood requirements (Cohen

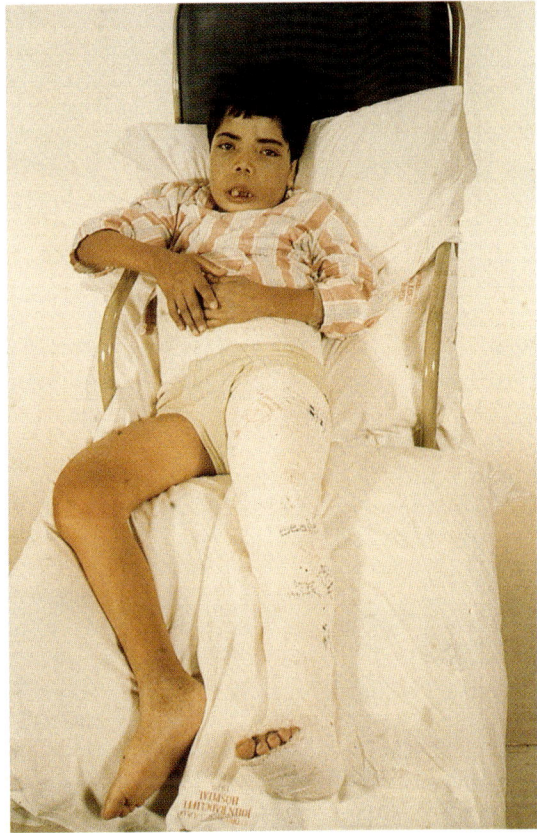

Fig. 7.5 Recurrent fractures in a patient with β thalassaemia. This child had been inadequately transfused for many years and at the time of this photograph had suffered from over 20 fractures after minor trauma.

et al. 1989a). More recent experience suggests that hypersplenism may usually be avoided by early and regular transfusion, and that many patients reaching adolescence after following a regimen of this type do not require splenectomy (Olivieri & Brittenham 1997).

As discussed in Chapter 5, the mechanisms of splenic enlargement are complex and ill-understood. Among several factors that may be involved, the constant bombardment of the reticulo-endothelial elements of the spleen with abnormal red cells, and the development of extensive extramedullary erythropoiesis are of particular importance. Both of these would undoubtedly be modified by maintaining patients at a relatively high haemoglobin level with transfusions of normal red cells.

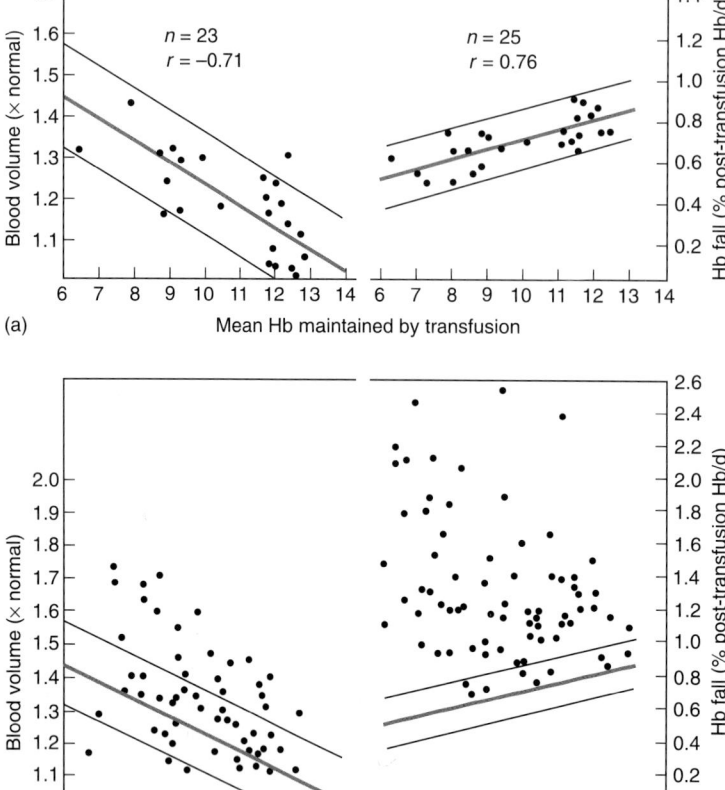

Fig. 7.6 Changes in transfusion requirements related to hypersplenism. (a) The relationship between the mean haemoglobin maintained by transfusion and apparent blood volume (left), and the rate of haemoglobin fall in splenectomized thalassaemic patients (right). (b) Blood volume expansion and the rate of haemoglobin fall in hypersplenic patients in the year before splenectomy, plotted on the standard curves in (a). The rate of haemoglobin fall is expressed as a transfusion quotient, as described in the text. From Modell and Berdoukas (1984), with permission.

Splenic enlargement may cause a variety of complications. Occasionally, there is physical discomfort simply due to the size of the spleen. The formed elements of the blood may be trapped in the splenic pool, producing anaemia, thrombocytopenia and some degree of neutropenia. The anaemia of hypersplenism has a complex pathophysiology, which was discussed in detail in Chapter 5. Several studies have reported red-cell mass and survival data in thalassaemic children with large spleens (Lichtman *et al.* 1953; Smith *et al.* 1955; Reemsta & Elliot 1956; Blendis *et al.* 1974). There is invariably some shortening of the autologous red-cell survival, trapping of a proportion of the red cells in the splenic red-cell pool, and a marked expansion of the total blood volume. In the study of Blendis *et al.* (1974) the trapped cells in the splenic pool accounted for between 9 and 40% of the total red-cell mass. These workers also showed that there is marked expansion of the plasma volume,

which has the effect of worsening the anaemia and, incidentally, producing a greater load on the myocardium. The reasons for the changes in plasma volume, which occur in patients with splenomegaly associated with other diseases, is not entirely clear. It is not due entirely to splenomegaly or hepatosplenomegaly; the plasma volume may remain significantly expanded after splenectomy for many months (Blendis *et al.* 1974). One factor which has been incriminated is the expanded bone marrow, which may act as a vascular shunt; the latter is thought to result in plasma volume expansion in a number of other settings.

Finally, it should be remembered that a very large spleen constitutes an extensive mass of ineffective haemopoietic tissue as well as a potential pool for the trapping of the formed elements of the blood. Thus, as it enlarges, it increases the metabolic demands of the growing child while, at the same time, causing haemodilution and plasma volume expansion. The improved feeling of well-being, which is often reflected by a growth spurt, both of which often follow splenectomy, is probably the best evidence we have that a large spleen may be deleterious to a child with thalassaemia in many different ways.

Iron overload

Iron overload has been a recognized feature of severe forms of thalassaemia since the first autopsy reports (Whipple & Bradford 1932, 1936). The history of how this puzzled workers in the thalassaemia field for many years, and of the gradual realization that it resulted from both increased intestinal absorption and from blood transfusion, is outlined in Chapter 1. The mechanisms of iron toxicity, its tissue distribution and way that it causes organ failure are discussed in Chapter 5. The methods by which the total body iron burden can be assessed are discussed later in this chapter. Here, we shall outline the main features of iron accumulation as a background to the description of its effects on individual organs that follow.

It was quite apparent from the results of the first iron absorption studies, and the transfusion histories of thalassaemic children in the days before high transfusion regimes were instituted, that iron loading was the result of increased absorption and transfusion, however inadequate. When assessing the results of higher transfusion regimens Modell (1976) estimated that by the time children maintained asymptomatic at a relatively high haemoglobin level reached the age of 11 years they would have accumulated approximately 28 g of iron. She suggested that it was only at about this level of iron loading that patients begin to show signs of hepatic, cardiac and endocrine disturbance, similar to those seen in adults with hereditary haemochromatosis.

Since iron overload was to become the major cause of death in thalassaemia it was clearly important to attempt to derive more accurate approaches to assessing the level of iron accumulation which would render patients at risk from life-threatening complications. Letsky *et al.* (1974) found that there was a good correlation between the serum ferritin and liver iron concentration in β thalassaemics maintained on high transfusion regimens. The values in most of their older patients were extremely high and well within the range seen in untreated hereditary haemochro-

matosis. However, these workers noticed that during the period over which the first 50–100 units of blood were transfused there was a steep rise in ferritin levels, after which the rate of increase was less marked. Later studies also indicated that the correlation between transfusion load and serum ferritin may not be so clear-cut (Pippard *et al.* 1978b). Indeed, Worwood *et al.* (1980) found that a maximum plasma ferritin concentration of about 4000 μg/l probably reflects the upper physiological limit of the rate of its synthesis; higher concentrations are now thought to be caused by the release of intracellular ferritin from damaged cells. Several other factors probably determine the level of circulating ferritin including ascorbate deficiency, infection, hepatic damage, haemolysis and ineffective erythropoiesis (Roeser *et al.* 1980; Baynes *et al.* 1986).

But the most clear-cut data that showed that the serum ferritin level cannot be relied on as an accurate assessment of total body iron burden were reported by Olivieri *et al.* (1995b). These workers found that over a wide range of serum ferritin levels and hepatic iron values, there was quite a broad scatter and, indeed, that the 95% prediction intervals in hepatic iron concentrations for a given plasma ferritin were so broad as to make determination of plasma ferritin a poor predictor of body iron stores (Fig. 7.7).

More recent work, reviewed by Olivieri and

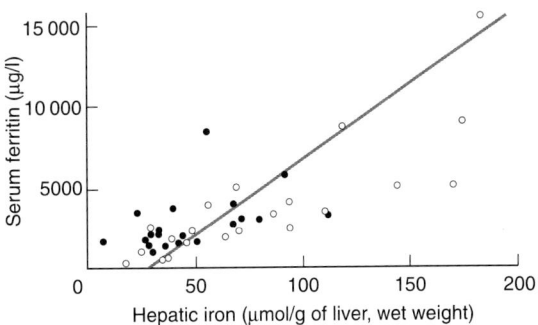

Fig. 7.7 Comparison of hepatic iron and serum ferritin concentrations in patients with thalassaemia major. In this study patients were assessed before treatment with oral iron chelation therapy (open circles) and after therapy extending from 1 or 5 years (solid circles). The diagonal line denotes the simple linear least-squares regression between two variables. By permission of the *New England Journal of Medicine*, Olivieri *et al.* (1995b). Copyright 1995 Massachusetts Medical Society, all rights reserved.

Brittenham (1997) and described in more detail later in this chapter and in Chapter 15, has provided much more accurate information about the levels of hepatic iron at which patients are at risk of serious complications of iron overload. These studies, which extrapolate from data obtained from patients with genetic haemochromatosis, show that patients with hepatic iron levels of approximately 40–80 μmol iron/g liver, wet weight, which is about 7–15 mg iron/g liver, dry weight, are at an increased risk of hepatic disease and endocrine organ damage. Patients with higher body iron burdens are at particular risk of cardiac disease and early death (Fig. 7.8). Later in this chapter we shall consider how these hepatic iron values can be determined by non-invasive means.

Although in the following sections we shall focus our attention on the consequence of iron loading of the heart, endocrine glands and liver, it is likely that excess body iron has other, less dramatic pathological consequences. It is certainly responsible for the curious grey pigmentation which has been a well recognized feature of the severe forms of thalassaemia ever since they were first described. What is known of the pathophysiology that underlies this complication is described in Chapter 5. The complex relationship between iron loading and increased susceptibility to infection was also touched on briefly in Chapter 5 and will be considered further later in this chapter.

Cardiac complications

The cardiac complications of β thalassaemia are the most important factors in determining the survival in both transfused and untransfused patients. While they have been recognized for decades, many aspects of cardiac disease in this condition are still poorly understood. It is clear that it is multifactorial, reflecting as it does chronic anaemia, iron overload, the consequences of pulmonary disease, myocarditis, pericarditis, and probably many other mechanisms.

Mechanisms

As discussed in Chapter 5, many of the cardiological changes observed in under-transfused children with severe thalassaemia are part of the adaptive changes to hypoxia which occur in all forms of anaemia. They include enhanced left ventricular contractility, an elevated cardiac output, left ventricular hypertrophy and, ultimately, dilatation, and, in cases of profound anaemia, all the manifestations of congestive cardiac failure.

As described in Chapter 1, the advent of more effective transfusion regimens rescued many thalassaemic children from the distressing complications of early life but, until the development of effective chelation regimens, only bought time until they died

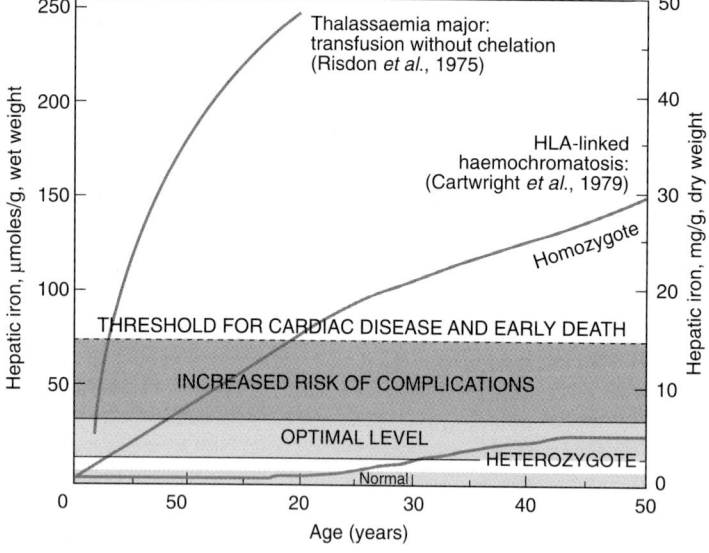

Fig. 7.8 The relationship of hepatic iron concentration to complications in transfusion-dependent patients with β thalassaemia major. Hepatic iron concentrations shown are those in normal individuals, those in heterozygotes for hereditary haemochromatosis associated with normal survival free of complications of iron load, those associated with an increased risk of iron-induced complications including hepatic fibrosis and diabetes, and those associated with a greatly increased risk for iron-induced cardiac disease and early death. Modified from Olivieri and Brittenham (1997).

from a cardiac death or other complications of iron loading towards the end of the second decade of life (Engle 1964). As we shall see in Chapter 15, there is now good evidence that effective chelation may protect transfusion-dependent patients from developing cardiac disease. However, because many patients do not adhere sufficiently strictly to their chelation programmes, and because their expense precludes their use in many developing countries, cardiac disease still remains a major challenge in the management of patients with severe forms of thalassaemia. The mechanisms of cardiac damage due to iron loading are discussed in Chapter 5 and later in this chapter.

It should be emphasized that the cardiological complications of thalassaemia are not restricted to the effects of anaemia and iron loading, though they are by far the most important factor (Table 7.3). More recently it has been recognized that, at least in some countries, patients with thalassaemia major may be unusually prone to myocarditis (Kremastinos *et al.* 1996). In addition, it has been observed that some patients with severe forms of thalassaemia may have an additional burden of right-heart strain due to chronic pulmonary hypertension (Grisaru *et al.* 1990). It has been suggested that this too may be related to iron overload (see later section), but it may also follow recurrent, small pulmonary emboli. Unfortunately, except for the data from Thailand on the frequent occurrence of this type of complication in patients with HbE β thalassaemia, reviewed in detail in Chapter 9, there have been few studies which have pursued this possibility. Recently, Hoeper *et al.* (1999) have suggested that there is an increased risk of pulmonary hypertension in patients who have

undergone splenectomy for any cause; autopsy data showed abundant pulmonary thrombotic lesions. The relationship of these changes to persistent thrombocytosis and an increased propensity to thromboembolic disease is discussed in Chapters 5 and 9, and later in this chapter.

Children with severe β thalassaemia were also prone to recurrent attacks of pericarditis. Smith *et al.* (1955, 1960) first reported that a benign, transient pericarditis often develops in thalassaemic children after splenectomy. This complication was later well documented by others (Orsini *et al.* 1970; Wasi 1972). Engle (1964) had also observed this complication but could find no causal or temporal relationship with splenectomy and suggested that these events may coincide towards the end of the first decade of life. Several workers, notably Orsini *et al.* (1970) examined the relationship between pericarditis and iron loading but could find no convincing evidence that the two are related. Over recent years this complication has been seen less frequently.

Pathology

Most of the information that is available on the pathology of the myocardium in β thalassaemia comes from autopsy studies, many of which were published in the era prior to the introduction of iron chelation therapy. In most cases a diffuse, rust-brown staining of the myocardium was observed, together with right and left ventricular hypertrophy, dilatation and a greatly increased cardiac weight (see Engle 1964). In most of the early series evidence of pericarditis was found (Engle 1964; Arnett *et al.* 1975). Interestingly, an autopsy report of 19 patients with cardiac iron loading and anaemia due to causes other than thalassaemia did not describe pericarditis (Buja & Roberts 1971).

Estimations of the iron content of the myocardium have shown gross elevations, to as much as 20 times normal. However, they also have underlined the marked variation in cardiac iron content, for example from 0.9 to 9.2 mg/iron/g of heart, dry weight (Schellhammer *et al.* 1967; Buja & Roberts 1971). In an extensive examination of iron-loaded hearts in patients who had received transfusions for conditions other than thalassaemia, iron was present in myocardial fibres as well as in the connective tissue (Fig. 7.9). The endocardium was reported to have an iron concentration equal to less than 50% of that in the peri-

Table 7.3 Cardiac complications of β thalassaemia.

Iron loading of the myocardium
  Cardiac failure with or without dysrhythmias

Right-sided failure
  Recurrent pulmonary emboli
  ?Obliterative pulmonary artery disease*
  Structural damage to lung tissue due to iron loading

Pericarditis

Myocarditis

*Thought to be due to platelet aggregation, particularly postsplenectomy in intermediate forms of thalassaemia. Some due to pulmonary emboli.

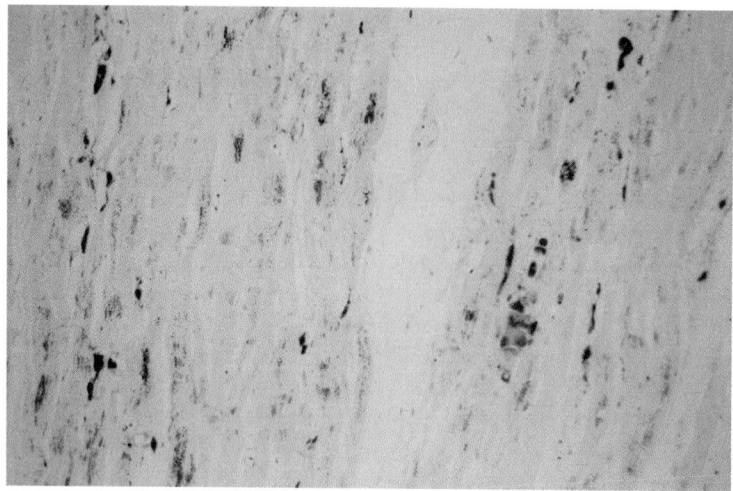

Fig. 7.9 A biopsy of the myocardium from a patient with β thalassaemia major showing iron-containing granules (Perl's stain×280).

cardium; iron was concentrated in the left ventricular septum and free wall, with maximal concentration in the left ventricular epicardium (Buja & Roberts 1971). The preferential deposition of iron in the epicardium, only later involving the remainder of the myocardium, may explain the preservation of systolic ventricular function early in the course of the disease. Attempts to study the relationship between cardiac function and the degree of iron overload suggest that high concentrations of iron correlate reasonably well with the degree of dysfunction, though, surprisingly, in many patients iron deposition in the conduction system appears to be relatively mild, even in those who die of cardiac dysrhythmias (Schellhammer *et al.* 1967; Buja & Roberts 1971).

Other changes that have been observed at autopsy include extensive myocardial fibre disruption and variable fibrosis (Howell & Wyatt 1953; Witzleben & Wyatt 1961; Schellhammer *et al.* 1967). Witzleben and Wyatt reported findings in two children aged 8 and 10 years, respectively. There was prominent right ventricular hypertrophy and pericarditis, but cardiac fibrosis was absent or minimal, despite the presence of hepatic cirrhosis. Although these studies suggested that iron deposition alone might not be enough to produce a fibrotic reaction, later work showed that iron loading is probably a major factor in generating these changes (Lombardo *et al.* 1995). Endomyocardial biopsies have demonstrated that interstitial fibrosis correlates reasonably well with persistent electrophysiological disturbances, at least in primary haemochromatosis (Short *et al.* 1981).

Pathophysiology

The mechanisms of iron-mediated tissue damage were discussed in detail in Chapter 5. It is clear from the iron concentrations observed in autopsy studies that the heart can accommodate a lower iron load than the liver, possibly because cardiac cells have a relatively small amount of storage protein and may be more sensitive to free iron-induced oxygen radicals. There is some evidence that very low levels of myocardial iron may interfere directly with diastolic function (Spirito *et al.* 1990), a process which resembles the effect of hypercalcaemia, and which is characterized by inadequate relaxation, spontaneous early depolarization and subsequent failure of contractility (Liu & Olivieri 1994). As discussed in Chapter 5, the generation of free hydroxyl radicals may result in damage to the lysosomal membrane of cardiac cells and lead to the disruption of the sarcolemmal membrane and inhibition of the mitochondrial respiratory chain (Link *et al.* 1994, 1996; Hershko *et al.* 1998b). The effects of iron may be augmented by a number of variables, including the reduction of ferric iron to ferrous iron and the addition of low concentrations of ascorbic acid; conversely, the effects of iron may be inhibited by high concentrations of ascorbic acid, alpha tocopherol and desferrioxamine (Hershko *et al.* 1998b).

In inadequately transfused patients, the magnitude of the body iron burden appears to be the chief factor in the development of cardiac disease (Olivieri & Brittenham 1997). This appears to be true even though lung disease and myocarditis may aggravate iron-induced cardiac disease, as shown in a 5-year study of more than 1000 thalassaemic patients, of whom approximately 5% developed serious cardiac disease secondary to myocarditis with no evidence of iron overload (Aessopos *et al.* 1995). While the low incidence of iron-induced cardiac disease in this young and well treated population is not surprising, it should be emphasized that infectious myocarditis may play a role in the development of cardiac disease and, conversely, that iron-promoted free-radical formation may contribute to the pathogenesis of infectious myocarditis (Hiraoka *et al.* 1993; Suzuki *et al.* 1993).

Clinical presentations

Considering this complex pathology it is not surprising that the clinical presentation of cardiac disease in thalassaemia is extremely variable. It should be expected in any patient over the age of 15 years who has been inadequately transfused and chelated, has been maintained at a high haemoglobin level with inadequate chelation and, in particular, has a hepatic iron concentration in excess of 15 mg/g liver, dry weight (Olivieri & Brittenham 1997). As mentioned in the previous section, the serum ferritin level is an unreliable guide but the liver iron level shows a strong correlation with the likelihood of the onset of cardiac complications.

The clinical descriptions over recent years have never bettered those of Engle (1964). She described a progressive staging for cardiac disease in irregularly transfused patients with thalassaemia. In the first stage, observed at about the age of 10 years, asymptomatic but progressive cardiac enlargement was noted. This was often followed by attacks of pericarditis at a mean age of approximately 11 years, sometimes associated with large pericardial effusions. This complication was observed in nearly half the patients; no infective cause could be found. The third stage was characterized by the appearance of first-degree heart block, occasional atrial premature beats and abnormal T waves. Finally, the typical signs of congestive cardiac failure appeared, with features of both right and left ventricular failure in parallel with serious disturbances of rhythm and conduction. The peak incidence of the final stage was between 10 and 15 years. The duration of life after the onset of failure was less than 3 months in over half the

patients, and one-third died within a month of the appearance of cardiac failure.

This general pattern of progression of cardiac disease is still observed although, as mentioned earlier, pericarditis is seen much less frequently. Very occasionally the picture may be predominantly of right-heart failure (Engle 1964; Ehlers *et al.* 1980; Zurlo *et al.* 1989). As pointed out by Jessup and Manno (1998), in older, adequately chelated patients, who are often asymptomatic, there may be much more subtle abnormalities of both systolic and diastolic function that are multifactorial in origin.

The clinical diagnosis of iron-induced cardiomyopathy is extremely difficult. The symptoms parallel those of left ventricular failure, but there may be no abnormalities until the rapid onset of overt cardiac failure. Palpitations may simply be related to anaemia or other cardiac abnormalities. Similarly, a poor exercise tolerance may also be related to anaemia.

Detection of cardiac dysfunction

Despite all the technological might of modern cardiology the investigation of cardiac function in thalassaemia remains problematic. Conduction/rhythm abnormalities correlate poorly with conduction tissue infiltration in autopsy sections of patients who have died of cardiac dysrhythmias. Moreover, the subendocardial iron concentration is much less than that found in the epicardial region, so that endomyocardial biopsy may underestimate the degree of iron deposition (Fitchett *et al.* 1980). As pointed out by Jessup and Manno (1998) there is no particular electrocardiographic finding that is indicative of iron-induced cardiac dysfunction, although they suggest that serial tracings may be useful in that a significant change is often indicative of a process other than increased iron deposition. There is a large literature on the value of echocardiography in the diagnosis of iron loading of the myocardium (Henry *et al.* 1978; Hussain *et al.* 1979; Bahl *et al.* 1992; Lattanzi *et al.* 1993; Kremastinos *et al.* 1996). In general, systolic function, cardiac dimensions and myocardial wall thickness are normal until there are unequivocal symptoms of cardiac failure. A standardized quantification of diastolic function is helpful but more difficult to obtain. The measurement of the ventricular end-systolic pressure dimension ($LVPD_{ES}$) assesses contractility dependent on ventricular loading. This approach has shown some abnormalities of function in a proportion of patients with advanced thalassaemia (Borow *et al.* 1982) but does not seem to have been widely studied or applied.

Probably the most experience has been gained with radionuclide studies of the left and right ventricular ejection fraction (EF) by first-pass or gated techniques, or with low-dose dobutamine stimulation (Spirito *et al.* 1990), although they seem to have met with little more success than resting echocardiography. Leon *et al.* (1979) described the estimation of the left ventricular EF during exercise in 24 patients; the number of transfusions seemed to predict an abnormal exercise LVEF by first pass.

The assessment of the risk of cardiac disease by various methods used for imaging of tissue iron is reviewed by Olivieri and Brittenham (1997). Reasonable correlations with magnetic resonance imaging (MRI) have been observed in a thalassaemic mouse model (Liu *et al.* 1996), and MRI changes consistent with a reduction of cardiac iron, paralleled by improvement in cardiac function, have been reported in individual patients (Olivieri *et al.* 1992d). But, although it is clear that this technique has the potential to detect iron in the heart, it is uncertain whether it will be possible to apply it to quantify the concentrations of cardiac iron. Other approaches, such as magnetic susceptometry, which provides a direct measurement of hepatic storage iron, have not yet been applied for the evaluation of cardiac iron. And although some abnormalities have been detected by ultrasonic analysis (Lattanzi *et al.* 1993) this approach has not been widely used or calibrated for the evaluation of cardiac disease in thalassaemia.

The measurement of serum atrial natriuretic peptide has been reported to be of value in the identification of preclinical cardiac involvement (Derchi *et al.* 1992), though further experience of this approach is required. Recently, decreased antioxidant activity of apolipoprotein E, related to the frequency of the apolipoprotein E4 allele, has been proposed as a genetic risk for left ventricular failure in thalassaemia (Economou-Petersen *et al.* 1998).

In a critical review of the current state of assessing cardiac function in iron-loaded patients Jessup and Manno (1998) emphasize that none of the methods that have been used to assess early myocardial impairment have been rigorously tested in a prospective manner. Indeed, they point out that the combined information obtained from the patient's transfusion record, serial serum ferritin levels, details of their adherence to a chelation regime and, most importantly, hepatic iron concentration, provides as much predictive power as any of the non-invasive tests just described. Thus, while future research should be directed at a full assessment of these different techniques in patients with well defined body iron loads, best obtained from hepatic biopsy, for day-to-day practice these simple approaches to the assessment of a patient with cardiac disease are probably as good as any.

Changing pattern of cardiac disease

With the advent of adequate chelation therapy there has been a major change in the frequency of cardiac disease over recent years (Olivieri & Brittenham 1997). Two trials have shown quite unequivocally that the effective, sustained use of desferrioxamine results in long-term survival and the absence of cardiological complications. In one, which used the serum ferritin as a measure of iron loading, those who maintained concentrations of less than 2500 μg/l had an estimated cardiac disease-free survival of 91% after 15 years; patients in whom most of the serum ferritin concentrations had exceeded this figure had an estimated cardiac disease-free survival after 15 years of less than 20% (Olivieri *et al.* 1994b). The other study assessed successful chelation therapy in terms of hepatic iron storage; values of 80 μmol of iron/g liver weight (15 mg iron/g liver, dry weight) were used as a cut-off point above and below which patients were classified as having received ineffective or effective chelation therapy, respectively. The probability of survival to at least 25 years was only 32% among patients above the threshold (Brittenham 1994). We shall return to this important topic when we discuss the management of iron chelation agents in Chapter 15.

Lung disease

Over the last two decades there has been an increasing recognition of the possible role of chronic lung disease in thalassaemia, which may aggravate cardiac disease. It has been suggested that iron deposition in the lungs may provoke pulmonary hypertension and right ventricular strain, dilatation and failure (Koren *et al.* 1987).

A variety of functional abnormalities have been

reported, including small-airway obstruction, hyper-inflation and hypoxaemia, possibly as the result of several different pathological processes (Keens *et al.* 1980; Hoyt *et al.* 1986; Grisaru *et al.* 1990; Santamaria *et al.* 1994). Other studies have described a primarily restrictive pattern of lung disease, with abnormalities consistent with obstructive airways disease (Cooper *et al.* 1980; Grisaru *et al.* 1990; Bacalo *et al.* 1992; Factor *et al.* 1994). Studies of total lung capacity have given inconsistent results, as have the effects of trans-fusion on pulmonary function (Santamaria *et al.* 1994).

These abnormalities of pulmonary function have been related to autopsy findings of the lungs, which have shown massive accumulation of haemosiderin in alveolar phagocytes in the perivascular and sup-porting framework (Witzleben & Wyatt 1961; Cooper *et al.* 1980). In some but not all series fibrosis was noted in the majority of cases (Landing *et al.* 1987). In addition, and as discussed in more detail in Chapter 9, sclerotic vascular lesions and thromboemboli have been observed in some series, and have been at-tributed to platelet thrombi.

A variety of mechanisms have been proposed to account for this pathology. They include tissue damage due to the generation of free hydroxyl radi-cals secondary to iron deposition, ferrugination of connective tissue resulting in reduced capillary com-pliance (Landing *et al.* 1987), and other less well defined abnormalities of the alveolar capillary mem-brane (Tai *et al.* 1996). Abnormal growth and devel-opment of the alveolus, either secondary to intrinsic disease or due to frequent transfusions, have also been proposed as a contributing factor (Tai *et al.* 1996). The additional possibility of pulmonary dis-ease due to recurrent pulmonary thromboembolic episodes resulting from platelet aggregates is dis-cussed in more detail in Chapters 5 and 9. Because a progressive acute pulmonary syndrome has been described in patients receiving high-dose desferriox-amine (Freedman *et al.* 1990), it has been suggested that drug toxicity may also play a role.

In summary, although our knowledge of the evolu-tion and importance of pulmonary disease in β thalassaemia is still limited, it seems likely that restrictive lung dysfunction resulting from parenchy-mal disease may lead to a reduced arterial oxygen saturation. It is possible that this may, in some cases, lead to pulmonary hypertension and right ventricular strain and failure. However, until the pathophysiol-ogy of this condition is worked out, and the complex interactions between damage to lung tissue and the effects of pulmonary embolic disease are understood, it will be difficult to determine the overall importance of these mechanisms in the generation of cardiac disease in thalassaemia.

Thromboembolic disease

As discussed in Chapter 5, because of a variety of abnormalities of platelets and coagulation factors and their antagonists, and the properties of the red-cell membrane, it might be expected that patients with β thalassaemia would be at increased risk of thromboembolic disease. In a study which examined the causes of death in thalassaemia major carried out in Italy in 1989 it was found that thromboembolism was the primary cause in four of 159 thalassaemic patients (Zurlo *et al.* 1989). In Israel, Michaeli *et al.* (1992) reported thromboembolic events, either recurrent arterial occlusion or, more commonly, pul-monary thromboembolism, in 4% of patients with thalassaemia major. More recently, Borgna-Pignatti *et al.* (1998a) identified 32 patients with thromboem-bolic episodes out of a total of 735 patients with β tha-lassaemia, 683 with thalassaemia major and 52 with thalassaemia intermedia. The commonest variety was stroke, which made up half of their cases. Other manifestations included pulmonary embolism, mesenteric or portal thrombosis and deep venous thrombosis in either the upper or lower limbs. Two cases of intracardiac thrombosis were observed. In this survey the frequency of thromboembolic events was significantly higher in association with cardiac disease, diabetes, non-specific liver function abnor-malities and hypothyroidism.

The complex relationship between an increased propensity to thrombosis in patients with inherited haemolytic anaemias has been reviewed recently (Barker & Wandersee 1999). As well as abnormalities of platelet function and the potential prethrombotic properties of the abnormal red-cell membranes of patients with β thalassaemia, it appears that other factors, both genetic and acquired, may contribute towards an increased likelihood of thromboembolic disease. For example, as mentioned earlier, thalas-saemic patients with heart failure have a higher risk of thrombosis if they carry the apolipoprotein E4 allele (Economou-Petersen *et al.* 1998). Recently, it has been observed that thalassaemic patients with hepatitis C may have an increased frequency of anti-cardiolipin antibodies and lupus anticoagulant, and that this may also be associated with an increased risk of thromboembolic events (Giordano *et al.* 1998).

It appears therefore that there is a genuine increased risk of thromboembolic disease in patients with β thalassaemia. This may be more common in those with β thalassaemia intermedia and in those who have undergone splenectomy. The problems of recurrent pulmonary embolus and pulmonary artery occlusion associated with thrombocytosis were discussed earlier in this chapter and are considered in detail in relationship to HbE β thalassaemia in Chapter 9.

Endocrine dysfunction

It was recognized many years ago that the iron loading of the tissues which occurs in severe forms of β thalassaemia has a particular predilection for the endocrine organs (Ellis *et al.* 1954; Erlandson *et al.* 1964b; Fink 1964; Bannerman *et al.* 1967). Over the years there have been many analyses of endocrine function in thalassaemic children over a wide range of ages and body iron burden (Kuo *et al.* 1968; Toccafondi *et al.* 1970a,b; Canale *et al.* 1974; Lassman *et al.* 1974a,b; Flynn *et al.* 1976; McIntosh 1976a,b; Anoussakis *et al.* 1977; Costin *et al.* 1977; Landau *et al.* 1978; Tuchinda *et al.* 1978; Costin *et al.* 1979; Kletsky *et al.* 1979; De Sanctis *et al.* 1989; Vullo *et al.* 1990; Perignon *et al.* 1993; El-Hazmi *et al.* 1994; Grundy *et al.* 1994; Italian working Group on Endocrine Complications in Non-endocrine Diseases 1995; Kwan *et al.* 1995; Jensen *et al.* 1997; Low 1997). Although these studies have been carried out in very heterogeneous populations of patients it has become apparent that the most common endocrine abnormalities in the present era are hypogonadotrophic hypogonadism, growth hormone deficiency and diabetes mellitus; the frequencies of hypothyroidism, hypoparathyroidism and adrenal insufficiency seem to be much lower.

Retarded growth and development

Although the all too common problems of growth and development in thalassaemic children are multi-factorial, and not all related to endocrine deficiency, because recent work has emphasized the importance of hypogonadism in many of these cases, we shall consider this topic here.

The early literature on thalassaemia major frequently emphasized defective growth and development. This was highlighted in several series which were reported just before or during the period when adequate transfusion regimens were first introduced (Erlandson *et al.* 1964a; Logothetis *et al.* 1972b; Constantoulakis *et al.* 1975). These workers noted a particular tendency for retarded growth at about the age of 8–10 years and pointed out that many affected children attained a very short final height. They also reported that, although the estimated bone age may be normal in early life, it was frequently delayed after the age of 6–7 years (Erlandson *et al.* 1964a). With the introduction of high transfusion regimens many workers reported improvements in the rates of growth (Beard *et al.* 1969; Modell 1976) although others were less impressed (Johnsen *et al.* 1966; Brook *et al.* 1969; Wolff & Luke 1969).

In 1984 Modell and Berdoukas also reported that early growth failure can often be corrected by raising the haemoglobin level by adequate transfusion or by splenectomy. More recent studies have generally confirmed these observations and suggested that linear growth rates and final heights are related to the haemoglobin levels that have been maintained throughout early life (De Sanctis *et al.* 1994).

Growth disturbances associated with low transfusion regimens are characterized by lack of weight gain and, in particular, a reduced muscle mass, which often gives the limbs a characteristic stick-like appearance and limits exercise tolerance through weakness (Fig. 7.1). Modell and Berdoukas (1984) noted that under-transfused patients have a much lower level of creatinine excretion in their urine than those maintained on higher transfusion regimens. Since approximately 2% of muscle creatine is broken down to creatinine each day, and this provides the only source of urinary creatinine, these studies were compatible with the concept that a low transfusion regime is associated with a reduced muscle mass and development.

The introduction of high transfusion regimens for thalassaemic children did not entirely solve the problem of growth retardation, however. Indeed, as pointed out by Modell and Beck (1974) and Modell (1976), one of the first indications of tissue damage due to iron overload is a failure of the normal pubertal growth spurt. However, this is not the whole story because even children who are well transfused and adequately chelated, and who have apparently normal sexual development, may still show some degree of growth retardation and a reduced final height (Modell & Berdoukas 1984; Borgna-Pignatti *et al.* 1985; Kattamis *et al.* 1990).

The reasons for growth retardation in well transfused children are extremely complex, multifactorial and not entirely understood (Table 7.4). Undoubtedly iron accumulation due to variability in the effectiveness of chelation therapy plays a major role. Here again, several mechanisms may be involved. Delayed pubertal growth has been attributed to iron-induced selective central hypogonadism (Costin *et al.* 1979; Kletsky *et al.* 1979; Wang *et al.* 1989; Landau *et al.* 1993), or interference by iron with the production of insulin-like growth factor (IGF-1) (Saenger *et al.* 1980; Herington *et al.* 1981; Werther *et al.* 1981). Other mechanisms which have been proposed include impaired growth hormone (GH) response to growth-hormone-releasing hormone (GHRH) (Pintor *et al.* 1986), abnormalities in growth-hormone secretion (Shehadeh *et al.* 1990) and, because growth-hormone reserves appear to be normal in many patients (Masala *et al.* 1984; Tolis *et al.* 1988; Leger *et al.* 1989), a defect in its receptor, although it has not been possible to demonstrate a lesion of this kind in hepatic tissues.

Several studies underline the complexities of these issues. In one, nearly half of a group of patients, most of whom had received regular transfusions and chelation therapy from an early age, had evidence of reduced growth-hormone reserve and low IGF-1 levels, with a substantial proportion also demonstrat-

Table 7.4 Some possible causes of defective growth in β thalassaemia.

Inadequate transfusion

Iron overload
  Selective central hypogonadism
  Defective production of insulin-like growth factor 1
  Impaired growth-hormone response to growth-
    hormone-releasing hormone
  Abnormal growth-hormone secretion
  Abnormality of growth-hormone receptor
  Reduced secretion of adrenal androgen

Zinc deficiency

Free-haemoglobin-induced inhibition of cartilage growth

Desferrioxamine toxicity

---

ing reduced levels of IGF-BP3, the predominant IGF-1 binding protein which results in prolongation of the serum half-life of IGF peptides, and which is growth-hormone dependent. However, the reduction in growth-hormone reserve was not shown to be correlated with short height or delay in bone age (Cavallo *et al.* 1997).

In a similar analysis of 32 patients with thalassaemia major, 14 of whom were short in stature, Roth *et al.* (1997) investigated 13 of the group who exhibited a particularly short stature or reduced growth rate. The stimulated GH secretion in 10 lay in the normal range. However, studies of their spontaneous GH secretion during the night revealed that they had markedly reduced amplitudes of their GH peaks (see next section). Low IGF-1 levels were also seen in growth-retarded patients. Stimulation tests showed a marked increase in both IGF-1 and insulin-like growth factor binding protein 3 (IGF-BP-3) levels, indicating intact IGF-1 generation by the liver. After priming with gonadotroplin-releasing hormone (GnRH), no change in either oestradiol or testosterone levels or in luteinizing hormone (LH) or follicle-stimulating hormone (FSH) response to GnRH was observed, suggesting a severe degree of pituitary gonadotrophin insufficiency. These results indicate that low GH secretion and low levels of IGF-1 in thalassaemic patients are related to severe neurosecretory dysfunction rather than liver damage. In short, it was apparent that hypogonadotrophic hypogonadism was a major factor, particularly in the growth-retarded patients who had impaired sexual development.

Evidence has also been presented for the existence of a state of partial growth-hormone insensitivity due to a postreceptor defect in growth-hormone action, which can be overcome with supraphysiological doses of exogenous growth hormone (Scacchi *et al.* 1991; Low *et al.* 1995; Wonke *et al.* 1998b). Other contributing factors include a reduced level of secretion of adrenal androgen (McIntosh 1976b; Sklar *et al.* 1987), zinc deficiency (Arcasoy *et al.* 1987) and free haemoglobin-induced inhibition of cartilage growth (Vassilopoulou-Sellin *et al.* 1989). Over recent years it has been recognized that short stature, related primarily to disproportionate truncal growth and loss of sitting height, may be related to the direct effect of desferrioxamine on spinal cartilage (De Sanctis *et al.* 1994; Hatori *et al.* 1995; Olivieri *et al.* 1995b; Rodda *et al.* 1995; De Sanctis *et al.* 1996). We shall return to a consideration of desferrioxamine toxicity in Chapter 15.

It is clear therefore that growth retardation in thalassaemia is both multifactorial and extremely common, an observation which will be further emphasized when we discuss the effects of treatment in Chapter 15. In inadequately transfused patients it seems likely that hypoxia plays a role, while in those who are well transfused but inadequately chelated iron-mediated damage to the hypothalamic/pituitary axis is the main factor.

It follows that, because of the extreme sensitivity of some of the endocrine organs to iron excess, and the fact that chelating agents like desferrioxamine in therapeutic doses can inhibit fibroblast proliferation and collagen formation and chelate other metals, even for thalassaemic children who have, by all other criteria, received ideal treatment, the potential for growth retardation is still considerable.

Delayed puberty and defective function of the hypothalamic/pituitary axis

Arrest or failure of puberty occurs in approximately 50% of both male and female patients. In one large series secondary amenorrhoea was documented in 23% of females, arrested puberty in 16% of males and 13% of females, and oligomenorrhoea or irregular menstrual cycles in 13% of females (Italian Working Group on Endocrine Complications in Non-endocrine Diseases 1995). While a conflicting literature has accumulated regarding the overall effects of iron chelation on sexual maturation, most recent studies have observed an improvement, with significantly reduced serum ferritin concentrations in those who achieve a normal puberty (Italian Working Group on Endocrine Complications in Non-endocrine Diseases 1995; Jensen *et al.* 1997). However, there have been no studies of this type involving adequate follow-up of patients whose body iron loads have been assessed by hepatic biopsy.

While in inadequately treated patients hypogonadism may be a reflection of chronic anaemia, deficiency of IGF-1 secondary to liver dysfunction, cirrhosis, diabetes and low adrenal androgen production, there is now abundant evidence that, in those who are more adequately managed, the major mechanism involved in failure of sexual maturation is selective central hypogonadism; rarely, it may result

from end-organ unresponsiveness (Kletsky *et al.* 1979; De Sanctis *et al.* 1988b; Maurer *et al.* 1988; Wang *et al.* 1989; Chatterjee *et al.* 1993b; Landau *et al.* 1993). Some males tend to have a low baseline testosterone level but their response to human chorionic gonadotrophin is usually normal. Although defective ovarian function has been reported in some cases (De Sanctis *et al.* 1988b), patients who show retarded sexual development usually demonstrate blunted responses to GnRH rather than to FSH.

The hypothalamic/pituitary axis appears to be particularly vulnerable to the effects of iron loading. This is supported by histological studies showing selective deposition in pituitary gonadotropes (Bergeron & Kovacs 1978) and the observation of loss of anterior pituitary volume in iron-loaded patients, demonstrated by MRI scanning (Chatterjee *et al.* 1998) (Fig. 7.10).

Over recent years the importance of the linkage of the function of endocrine organs to circadian cycles has been emphasized. One of the most carefully studied is the pulsatile secretion of LH and FSH, which reflects the intermittent release of GnRH from the hypothalamus. In a long-term prospective study of thalassaemic women with secondary amenorrhoea it was found that all of them developed gonadotrophin pulse abnormalities together with evidence of GnRH secretory insufficiency (Chatterjee *et al.* 1993b); over the 10-year period there was a progressive deterioration of hypothalamic/pituitary function, and 66% of the patients became apulsatile with marked reduction in the levels of gonadotrophin.

These studies emphasize the importance of studying the hypothalamic/pituitary axis in patients with amenorrhoea or other evidence of failure of sexual development. Although there were early reports of heavy testicular and ovarian involvement with iron (Canale *et al.* 1974) it seems likely that, with improvements in the management of β thalassaemia, end-organ unresponsiveness will play a relatively small role in problems of sexual maturation and function in the future.

Thus, although there has been an increase in fertility in men and women with thalassaemia over the last decade, it is disappointing that secondary amenorrhoea may eventually develop in approximately a quarter of thalassaemic women. This suggests that the anterior pituitary may be particularly susceptible

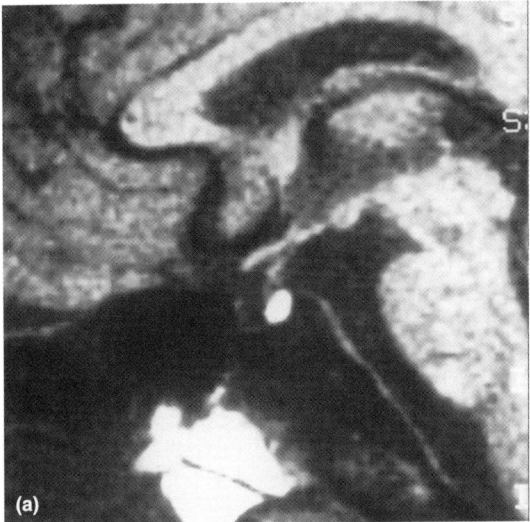

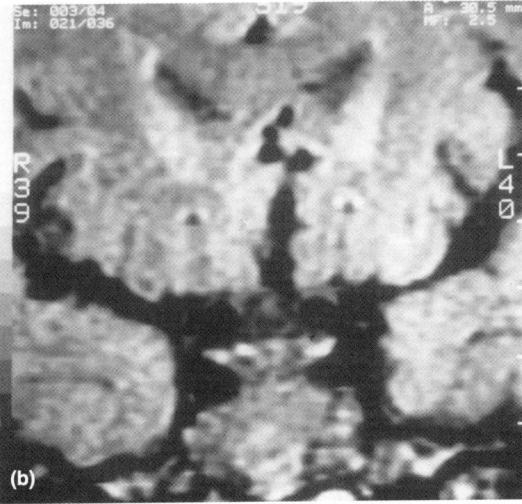

Fig. 7.10 Iron loading of the pituitary gland. (a) Sagittal T_1 spin-echo image showing heavy iron loading of the pituitary gland. The normal high signal from the posterior pituitary is shown; the low signal from the enhancer pituitary is consistent with iron loading. (b). Coronal T_1-weighted MRI showing a lower signal than normal from the pituitary. These images were kindly reviewed by Drs Niall Moore and David Lindsell.

over time to iron-induced damage (see next section) and that, unlike the heart and liver, the consequences of iron deposition may be irreversible. There are no reports in the literature describing improvement in potency, fertility or normalization of testosterone levels and sperm counts after reduction of iron load in thalassaemia major, though this may occur in primary haemochromatosis. Recent studies have suggested that body iron burdens corresponding to a hepatic iron concentration of between 9 and 30 mg/g liver, dry weight, may be associated with a high risk of development of pituitary failure (Olivieri 2000). Further studies to quantify body iron and anterior pituitary function in patients from early in life should provide more secure conclusions with respect to the threshold of risk.

Diabetes mellitus

Diabetes is a relatively common complication in children who have been inadequately iron chelated and is also observed in those who have been well transfused and chelated. In an extensive study of transfused and chelated patients it occurred in 4–6% of cases (Italian Working Group on Endocrine Complications in Non-endocrine Diseases 1995). It has been attributed to impaired secretion of insulin secondary to chronic pancreatic iron overload (Ellis *et al.* 1954; Lassman *et al.* 1974a; Costin *et al.* 1977; Saudek *et al.* 1977; Zuppinger *et al.* 1979; De Sanctis *et al.* 1988c). There have also been a number of reports of insulin resistance in diabetes (Dandona *et al.* 1983; Merkel *et al.* 1988; Dmochowski *et al.* 1993; Cavello-Perin *et al.* 1995), although the mechanism is not absolutely clear. It has also been linked temporally to episodes of acute viral hepatitis (De Sanctis *et al.* 1986, 1988c).

However, it appears that iron-mediated damage to the pancreas is the major factor in producing diabetes in iron-loaded children; there is a good relationship between the development of diabetes and the severity and duration of iron overload (De Sanctis *et al.* 1988c; Olivieri *et al.* 1990b). This conclusion is strengthened by consecutive studies over a long period which have shown early and progressive loss of pancreatic β-cell mass, manifested by decreased insulin release in response to secretagogues before the development of significant insulin resistance or diabetes (Karahanyan *et al.* 1994; Soliman *et al.* 1996). In addition, there appears to be a reduction in the frequency of diabetes in patients who have been more adequately chelated (Brittenham 1994).

Hypothyroidism

Mild abnormalities of thyroid function were described in some iron-loaded patients with β thalassaemia by Lassman *et al.* (1974b) and Flynn *et al.* (1976). These findings have been substantiated in later studies (Sabato *et al.* 1983; Magro *et al.* 1990) including patients who had been well managed by transfusion and iron chelation. Grundy *et al.* (1994) described two adolescents with moderately reduced levels of plasma thyroxine and marked elevations in thyroid-stimulating hormone (TSH); both had clinical features of hypothyroidism. In the study of Jensen *et al.* (1997) there was a strong correlation between serum ferritin concentrations and the presence of thyroid dysfunction. Although it appears that hypothyroidism is relatively uncommon in transfusion-dependent thalassaemia (Vullo *et al.* 1990), because its clinical features are so insidious it is very important to bear this complication in mind.

Hypoparathyroidism

Defective parathyroid function has been well documented for many years (Flynn *et al.* 1976; Costin *et al.* 1979; Gertner *et al.* 1979; De Sanctis *et al.* 1992) and florid, clinical hypoparathyroidism has been described in a few cases (Gabrielle 1971; Oberklaid & Seshadri 1975; Flynn *et al.* 1976; McIntosh 1976b). The symptoms and signs are all attributable to hypocalcaemia and hyperphosphataemia. The early signs are quite non-specific and include neuromuscular irritability, paraesthesiae involving the face, fingers and toes, and abdominal cramps. The full clinical picture of acute irritability, emotional lability, memory impairment, lethargy and convulsions has been rarely reported in thalassaemia. The diagnosis is easily made by the finding of hypocalcaemia and hyperphosphataemia, together with a reduction in the level of plasma parathyroid hormone (PTH). In a recent study of 113 transfusion-dependent cases, 12.4% showed subnormal PTH levels, suggesting that subclinical hypoparathyroidism is relatively common (Pratico *et al.* 1998).

Adrenal insufficiency

There is much less information about functional adrenal insufficiency in thalassaemic patients. Such as there is suggests that it is uncommon and that, although there may be measurable abnormalities of adrenal function (Lassman *et al.* 1974b), they are rarely associated with the clinical picture of adrenal failure (Kuo *et al.* 1968; Canale *et al.* 1974; McIntosh 1976b; Vullo *et al.* 1990). Interestingly, there seems to be some dissociation of the different adrenal hormone functions in cases in which defects have been observed. For example, Sklar *et al.* (1987) observed low levels of adrenal androgen secretion with a normal glucocorticoid reserve. Early suggestions that part of the skin pigmentation in thalassaemia might be due to the melanophore-stimulating effect of raised plasma ACTH levels were not confirmed by Costin *et al.* (1979).

Conclusions

It is clear therefore that one of the relative failures of the high transfusion/adequate chelation programme that has otherwise changed the lives of thalassaemic patients has been the persistence of endocrine dysfunction, particularly involving the hypothalamic/pituitary axis. Although the reasons are not clear, it may well be that the pituitary is particularly sensitive to even mild degrees of iron overload and that even chelation regimens that are adequate to retain the function of other organs may simply not be good enough to protect it.

Bone disease

The bone changes in inadequately transfused thalassaemic children were described earlier in this chapter. As soon as the high transfusion regimens were instituted in the mid-1960s it became apparent that the gross skeletal deformities that had been seen earlier could be prevented (Johnston & Roseman 1967; Piomelli *et al.* 1969). It seems likely therefore that they reflect expansion of the bone-marrow mass, a process which can lead to a variety of other distressing symptoms, particularly spontaneous fracture or fracture following minor trauma (Wolman 1964; Herrick & Davis 1975; Novikova & Abrakhanova 1975). Similarly, poor dentition (Poynton & Davey 1968; Catena 1975; Tas *et al.* 1976) and attacks of recurrent sinusitis due to inadequate drainage (Hazell & Modell 1976) appear to be much less common.

What little is known of the histology and pathophysiology of bone disease in thalassaemia is discussed in Chapter 5. While it is clear that marrow expansion plays a major role in inadequately treated patients, the osteoporosis which occurs in many patients who have been reasonably well transfused, but in whom there is severe iron loading, may be related to hypogonadism (Fabbri *et al.* 1991; Anapliotou *et al.* 1995). Indeed, it has been apparent that even in well transfused patients with thalassaemia major there may be a relatively high frequency of osteoporosis (Giardina *et al.* 1995; Goni *et al.* 1995; Vichinsky 1998; Wonke 1998).

Jensen *et al.* (1998) investigated 82 transfusion-dependent patients of both sexes, with a mean age of 27 years. The incidence of osteoporosis was 51%. Multivariant analysis showed that hypogonadotrophic hypogonadism, sex and diabetes were significant risk factors. There was no association with ethnic group, smoking, exercise, calcium supplementation or age at starting chelation therapy or, indeed, the serum ferritin concentration. This study also highlighted some features of osteoporosis in thalassaemia which are different from those in the post-menopausal variety. In thalassaemia, men are more commonly and more severely affected and their lumbar vertebrae and femoral necks are involved, whilst in women osteoporosis mainly involves the spine. This is surprising because most of the women in this study were receiving hormone replacement therapy. Many of these patients were symptomatic with varying degrees of bone pain.

This study, which in parts confirms and extends the earlier findings of Fabbri *et al.* (1991) and Anapliotou *et al.* (1995) in incriminating hypogonadism as an important factor in the development of osteoporosis in thalassaemia, further underlines the importance of pituitary failure, even in patients who have been treated adequately.

Some of the other factors which have been suggested as contributing towards bone disease in β thalassaemia are outlined in Chapter 5. Recently, there has been considerable interest in the possibility that there may be subsets of individuals who are genetically susceptible to developing osteoporosis (Eisman 1996). So far very few studies along these lines have been reported in patients with thalassaemia. Rees *et al.* (1998c) showed that there was a modest correlation between homozygosity for the SS polymorphism of vitamin D receptor and the likelihood of developing osteoporosis of the femoral neck but not the lumbar spine. Jensen *et al.* (1998) could find no rela-

tionship between osteoporosis and polymorphisms of the gene for the oestrogen receptor. Hanslip *et al.* (1998) found a correlation between osteoporosis and a promoter polymorphism of the COLIAI gene in males but not in females. Clearly, this important question needs further study.

Suggestions that β thalassaemia minor might be a risk factor for osteoporosis (Giuzio *et al.* 1991; Greep *et al.* 1992) have not been confirmed in further studies (Kalef-Exra *et al.* 1995).

Infection

The notion that thalassaemic children are particularly prone to infection has been an accepted part of the thalassaemia literature for many years. As symptomatic management improved, this concept was questioned (Valassi-Adam *et al.* 1976) and it was suggested that the incidence of infection in early childhood had been markedly reduced in children maintained at an adequate haemoglobin level (Modell 1976).

In recent years, although there is still an awareness of the dangers of infection, particularly after splenectomy, there has been a major change in emphasis towards concerns about blood-borne infection, notably hepatitis B and C and human immunodeficiency virus (HIV).

In Chapter 5 we reviewed the large and not very informative literature about the mechanisms which might render thalassaemic children more prone to infection, particularly after splenectomy, and the vexed question of the relationship of infections such as pericarditis to iron loading. Here we shall briefly review the pattern of infections in thalassaemic children with particular respect to those that are blood borne. One of the difficulties that faces anybody who approaches this complex field is that, with the possible exception of a single study of patients with HbE β thalassaemia, which is summarized in Chapter 9, there have been no well controlled studies comparing the frequency of infection in thalassaemic and non-thalassaemic children in the same environment.

General patterns of infection with changing management

In an extensive retrospective study of the patterns of infection in thalassaemic children maintained at different haemoglobin levels Modell and Berdoukas

(1984) concluded that the most serious infections were pneumonia, pericarditis, the sequelae of streptococcal infections, meningitis, peritonitis and osteomyelitis. Further analysis suggested that pneumonia and septicaemia are significantly associated with splenectomy and a low transfusion regimen, and that in patients who had been maintained at a satisfactory mean haemoglobin level these infections had almost disappeared. They also observed that other serious infections, including meningitis, peritonitis and osteomyelitis, are only seen in splenectomized patients and that they have no obvious relationship to anaemia. Finally, they noted that pericarditis is also unrelated to anaemia and splenectomy but is very clearly related to age, occurring in childhood or later. They suggested that the latter observation may reflect a relationship between iron overload and pericarditis. Modell and Berdoukas also provided some comparative information from other countries indicating that this overall pattern of infection is common in most thalassaemic populations. These observations were in keeping with the earlier studies of the dangers of infection in splenectomized thalassaemic children (Smith *et al.* 1962, 1964) and, indeed, in any child who has had the spleen removed early in life (Eraklis *et al.* 1967; Erikson *et al.* 1968). In this case the most important organisms are *Streptococcus pneumoniae*, *Haemophilus influenzae* and *Neisseria meningitidis*.

The widespread use of prophylactic penicillin and appropriate immunization after splenectomy has undoubtedly reduced the frequency of severe infections in splenectomized thalassaemic children (see Chapter 15).

Organisms that attack iron-loaded patients

Although, as discussed in Chapter 5, there has been a great deal of controversy as to whether the frequent attacks of pericarditis in thalassaemic children are related to iron loading, no organism has ever been implicated. The only pathogens that have been shown quite unequivocally to occur with an increased frequency in iron-loaded patients are those of the *Yersinia* genus, which normally have a low pathogenicity and an unusually high requirement for iron. They do not secrete siderophores but have receptors for ferrioxamine and become pathogenic in the presence of iron bound to desferrioxamine (Green 1992). There are numerous reports of severe infections in thalassaemic patients due to infections with *Yersinia*

spp. (Robins-Browne & Prpic 1985; Gallant *et al.* 1986; Kelly *et al.* 1987; de Mazzoleni *et al.* 1991; Green 1992). They are usually characterized by severe abdominal pain, diarrhoea, vomiting, fever and sore throat. They may also be associated, on occasion, with rupture of the bowel.

Hepatitis B virus (HBV)

It is estimated that about 350 million individuals world-wide are persistent carriers of hepatitis B. The virus persists in about 10% of infected immunocompetent adults. Approximately 25% of all patients with chronic hepatitis progress to cirrhosis, about 20% of whom develop hepatocellular carcinoma. During the first phase of chronicity, virus replication continues in the liver; markers of this stage include HBV DNA and a soluble antigen, hepatitis Be antigen (HBeAg). In most persons there is an immune clearance of infected hepatocytes, associated with seroconversion from HBeAg to anti-HBe.

Because HBV is primarily a blood-borne infection, transfusion-dependent thalassaemic children are at particular risk, depending on its prevalence in their community and the effectiveness of donor screening programmes. The early experience in Europe was summarized by Schanfield *et al.* (1975) and by Modell and Berdoukas (1984). At that time, in British, Cypriot, Sardinian and Greek populations the frequency of antibody positivity ranged from 30 to 90%, with an appropriately low level of those with persistent antigen positivity. Mela *et al.* (1988) found that about 60% of transfused thalassaemic patients in Thailand showed evidence of previous HBV infection. Studies from Greece have shown how the application of adequate screening and vaccination programmes results in a major fall in the frequency of HBV infection (Politis 1989).

Although the frequency of HBV infection is now very low in countries in which screening and immunization programmes have been established, HBV-related hepatitis is still seen frequently in parts of the world where these precautions are not taken. The diagnosis of chronic active hepatitis depends on the presence of abnormal liver function tests, particularly elevated transaminases, the appearances on liver biopsy and, in the early stages, the presence of Hbe antigen and, later, the presence of anti-HBe. In the early phase there is an Hbe-positive viraemia which usually becomes negative as the disease progresses.

Hepatitis C virus (HCV)

Following the identification of HCV it soon became clear that this infection is widespread and presents a serious risk to patients with transfusion-dependent thalassaemia. The prevalence of anti-HCV in patients with thalassaemia major varies in different parts of the world, ranging from 11.7% in Turkish Cypriots, through 30% in Malaysians and Chinese to nearly 75% in Italians (Wonke *et al.* 1990; Bozkurt *et al.* 1993; Cancado *et al.* 1993; Lau *et al.* 1993; Kaur & Kaur 1995; Cao *et al.* 1996; Wonke *et al.* 1998b).

An initial HCV infection is almost invariably anicteric and can only be diagnosed by screening for elevated serum transaminases; jaundice is rare. Until recently it was believed that only 50% of patients recover, and the remainder develop persistent viraemia with hepatitis. Of these about one in five develop cirrhosis and run the risk of hepatocellular carcinoma. Recently, however, long-term follow-up of children who had contracted HCV during the first few years of life during cardiac surgery showed that, after 19 years, 50% had demonstrable HCV-RNA, but of these very few had progressive liver damage (Vogt *et al.* 1999). Clearly we need to know more about the natural history of this disease, particularly when contracted in childhood and in the setting of an associated iron-loading condition.

Antibodies to structural and non-structural proteins of the virus can be found at various times after infection. Viraemia is detected by the polymerase chain reaction (PCR), which can identify HCV-RNA. Patients with chronic active hepatitis are invariably HCV-RNA positive and also have IgG anti-HCV, which is also present after recovery. There is some evidence that the liver damage associated with persistent HCV infection, or response to therapy, may be modified by the presence of excess iron (Clemente *et al.* 1994; Olynyk & Bacon 1995; Rubin *et al.* 1995).

Clearly, therefore, any patient with persistently raised serum transaminases must be screened for HCV using PCR to identify HCV-RNA. If this test is positive it is important to proceed to a liver biopsy to identify those patients who have histological changes of chronic active hepatitis. The liver histology shows predominantly chronic persistent hepatitis with a low incidence of periportal piecemeal necrosis and lobular hepatitis. The further investigation and management of these patients is discussed in Chapter 15.

Other forms of viral hepatitis

Hepatitis D virus (HDV) only replicates in patients already infected with HBV. Infection is common among HBV carriers in the Mediterranean region and may occur at the same time as HBV. The clinical course is that outlined earlier for HBV infection.

Hepatitis E virus (HEV) is enterically transmitted and, like hepatitis A virus, although it may produce acute hepatitis, is not associated with persistent infection. Evidence of infection with HEV was obtained in 2.4% of transfusion-dependent thalassaemic patients in Athens (Psichogiou *et al.* 1996) and in 10.7% of a similar population in Saudi Arabia (al-Fawaz *et al.* 1996).

Hepatitis G virus (HGV) was discovered in 1995 (reviewed by Stransky 1996). It produces a mild form of hepatitis and there is evidence that some patients may go on to develop chronic hepatitis. It can be identified by assessment of HGV-RNA by PCR in a similar way to HCV. Its prevalence in USA blood donors is approximately 1.5%. In a study of 40 Italian transfusion-dependent β thalassaemics HGV-RNA was detected in 22% of cases. In patients who were also viraemic for HCV the clinical manifestations of the coinfection were no different from those of patients with HCV alone. The authors concluded that although HGV is highly prevalent among Italian polytransfused individuals there is no evidence for a clinically significant role in liver disease (Sampietro *et al.* 1997). Similar conclusions came from a study of Chung *et al.* (1997) in Taiwan, where the prevalence of HGV-RNA positivity was 14%; again the presence of the virus did not seem to be associated with significant hepatitis. In a further follow-up of Italian patients with HGV it was concluded that in over 25% of cases the infection resolved within 6 years (Prati *et al.* 1998). Similar conclusions were reported by Zemel *et al.* (1998), who found an incidence of HGV infection of 19.4% in a population in Tel Aviv; follow-up studies suggested that there is persistent viraemia but no significant biochemical evidence of liver damage. The frequency of HGV infections in southeast Asia seems to be even higher, with reports of frequencies in transfusion-dependent thalassaemic children of 32% (Poovorawan *et al.* 1998).

All these studies suggest that HGV infection, while very common, does not often seem to be associated

310 *Chapter 7*

with a serious form of hepatitis or long-term liver damage. Although preliminary studies suggested that it might have an ameliorating effect on HCV infections, the question needs much further study. Indeed, more careful, long-term follow-up data on HGV-infected patients are required.

Human immunodeficiency viruses (HIVs)

The human immunodeficiency viruses HIV-1 and HIV-2 belong to the lentivirus subfamily of retroviruses. They can both give rise to the acquired immunodeficiency syndrome (AIDS). Globally, HIV-1 is responsible for the world-wide pandemic of AIDS, while HIV-2, though mainly confined to western Africa, is starting to spread rapidly, notably in India. It is currently estimated by the WHO that by the year 2000 approximately 40 million people world-wide will be infected. More than 90% of them will live in the developing countries in sub-Saharan Africa, south and south-west Asia, Latin America and the Caribbean. Since these viruses can be transmitted by blood transfusion or perinatally it is clear that thalassaemic patients form a high-risk subgroup in any population in which this infection is common.

It should be remembered that most people in the world with HIV infections are asymptomatic. Prospective studies of cohorts of infected people with known dates of seroconversion have suggested that 50–60% of them will develop symptoms and signs of disease within 10 years of infection. During the asymptomatic phase many individuals show abnormal laboratory tests such as low CD4 lymphocyte counts and hypergammaglobulinaemia. It is beyond our scope to deal with the various symptom complexes of AIDS, which have been classified by the Centers for Disease Control (CDC) into several subgroups (Table 7.5).

It is not surprising therefore that HIV infection has become a major concern for multitransfused patients with thalassaemia (Manconi *et al.* 1998). In the mid-1980s, when it was becoming apparent that HIV infection was going to pose a serious problem for children who had received regular blood products, a European–Mediterranean WHO Working Group on Haemoglobinopathies together with the Cooleycare Group established a programme to coordinate data collection. Work from this group and colleagues has provided valuable information about the change in prevalence of HIV infection after donor screening

Table 7.5 Centers for Disease Control (CDC) classification for HIV infection.

Group I	Acute infection
Group II	Asymptomatic infection
Group III	Persistent, generalized lymphadenopathy
Group IV	Other disease

Subgroup A Constitutional disease (one or more of: fever for more than 1 month; weight loss >10% baseline; diarrhoea for more than 1 month)
Subgroup B Neurological disease
Subgroup C Secondary infection
   C1   As specified by CDC surveillance definition
   C2   Others
Subgroup D Secondary cancers
Subgroup E Other conditions

was established and about the course of the illness in those who were affected (Girot *et al.* 1991). Early prevalence figures from Italy and Greece ranged from 2.3 to 11% (De Martino *et al.* 1985; Politis *et al.* 1986; Zanella *et al.* 1986), while the infection rate in transfused thalassaemic patients in the USA was reported to be about 12% (Robert-Guroff *et al.* 1987). The European–Mediterranean WHO Working Group carried out a further study of 3633 patients in 36 centres from 13 countries and found an overall frequency of HIV positivity of 1.56%. Further data collected after establishment of screening (reviewed by Girot *et al.* 1991) revealed a sharp fall in the number of HIV-positive patients although there is still a very low level of transmission from HIV blood obtained from seronegative donors (Jullien *et al.* 1988). However, in the period after 1988 an analysis of nearly 3000 patients in 13 European centres found no HIV-1-positive patients.

The same WHO Working Group started a follow-up study of 79 seropositive thalassaemic patients to observe the natural history of HIV infection in thalassaemic children (Costagliola *et al.* 1992). The median follow-up period was 4 years 11 months. At the end of the study, 43 patients were CDC stage II, 23 in CDC stage III, and 13 in CDC stage IV, including seven patients with AIDS, of whom three had died. The rate of progression to AIDS was not associated with intercurrent infection, splenectomy, age or sex. For the group, an accumulative AIDS incidence rate of 1.4% was observed at 3 years, and of 9% at 5 years.

The situation in other parts of the world, where screening started later or has not yet been established, is much less encouraging. Khan (1992) reported a frequency of 8.4% HIV positivity in 203 thalassaemic children in New Delhi; in a further study of 203 children in the same city Sen *et al.* (1993) reported a frequency of 8.9%. Kumar *et al.* (1994) found a frequency of 8.9% in a transfusion clinic in Manapur, India. These data provide some indication of the magnitude of the problem that will be posed by HIV infection in thalassaemic children in many parts of the world unless urgent steps are taken to institute donor screening. This problem is highlighted by Kumar and Khuranna (1998), who have recently reported on a prospective analysis of the outcome of pregnancies in 123 women with transfusion-dependent β thalassaemia, of whom 81 were HIV positive; using the CDC classification 39 were stage C2 and 42 stage A2 (see Table 7.5). All 22 preterm babies of mothers with stage C2 had positive viral cultures for HIV-1 within 1 week of birth; 10 of these neonates died of AIDS by 8 weeks, and the remaining 12 by 15 months of age. Of 39 C2-stage pregnancies, five died undelivered at 32 weeks' gestation due to fulminating *Pneumocystis carinii* pneumonia. Although there may be a successful outcome of pregnancies in thalassaemic women with asymptomatic HIV disease, the presence of AIDS indicator conditions is associated with an appreciable perinatal and maternal morbidity and mortality.

Malaria

Following early hopes on the part of the WHO that malaria was being contained in many parts of the world, events of the last few years have proved just how unpredictable the control of an important infection can be. The disease has returned to many countries from which it seemed to have disappeared and, even more frighteningly, drug resistance is now widespread. Children with severe forms of thalassaemia are subject to attacks of acute malaria like any other child. The protective effect of thalassaemia against malaria, described in Chapter 6, is statistical; no form of thalassaemia protects any individual completely against the infection. Chronic malaria, as well as exacerbating the anaemia of thalassaemia, may also increase the degree of splenomegaly.

Thalassaemic children are particularly at risk from blood-borne infection. In a study from India of the

blood of children immediately after transfusion Choudhury *et al.* (1990) found that in 6.4% of cases there was evidence of transfusion-transmitted malaria infection. Thus it is clear that there must be a high frequency of chronic malaria in blood donors in endemic regions. We shall return to the prevention of this complication in Chapter 15.

Another important question regarding malarial infection in thalassaemic children is the effect of splenectomy on the course of the disease. This complex issue was reviewed by Looareesuwan *et al.* (1993). Although there have been anecdotal reports suggesting that malaria may be particularly severe in those who have been splenectomized, there is no convincing evidence that this is the case, but this question requires further study.

Severe malaria is not always associated with high parasitaemias, however. Therefore in any thalassaemic child in a malarious area who presents with fever, drowsiness progressing to coma, renal failure, haemoglobinuria, hypoglycaemia or simply a rapidly worsening anaemia, a diagnosis of malaria must be considered, regardless of the number of parasites in the peripheral blood.

Liver disease

In young adults with thalassaemia major, liver disease remains a common cause of morbidity and mortality. For many years the major factor in the generation of liver damage was iron overload, acquired through transfusion and increased gastrointestinal absorption. More recently, with the increasing recognition of viral hepatitis contracted from blood products, it has become clear that the pathogenesis of liver damage is extremely complex.

Mechanisms of liver damage

The mechanisms of organ damage resulting from excess iron were discussed in Chapter 5. In short, iron produces cellular injury with progression to fibrosis and cirrhosis. This may be mediated in several ways. Iron promotes free-radical-mediated lipid peroxidation and mitochondrial dysfunction (Tsukamoto *et al.* 1995; Hershko *et al.* 1998a). The deposition of haemosiderin in lysosomes may lead to fragility and subsequent rupture of their membranes. Early studies also suggested that another important mechanism may be excess collagen deposition induced by iron-promoted catalysis of collagen synthesis, or decreased collagen breakdown due to lysosomal blockade following iron overload; a similar mechanism has been observed in other storage diseases (Iancu *et al.* 1977a). Furthermore, iron overload may potentiate further iron loading; upregulation of the transport of non-transferrin-bound iron has been observed in cultured hepatocytes (see Chapter 5).

As mentioned in earlier sections in this chapter, the high frequency of blood-borne viral infections is another major factor in the generation of liver disease in thalassaemic patients. As we also saw earlier, iron may potentiate the action of viral hepatitis, and other factors such as alcohol may act synergistically in accelerating the development of liver damage. Clearly, therefore, the hepatic pathology is extremely complex and many questions about the mechanisms of tissue damage and its pattern of progression remain to be worked out.

Assessment of iron loading and liver damage

The methods for assessing body iron burden in general, and the level of liver iron in particular, are discussed later in this chapter and in Chapter 15. Hepatic biopsy provides definitive information with respect to quantitative body iron stores (Brittenham 1994). In addition, it offers the only direct approach for determining both the pattern and extent of liver damage.

Early studies of inadequately treated patients

In the period before children were treated adequately, severe hepatic fibrosis and siderosis were regular findings at autopsy (Frumin *et al.* 1952; Howell & Wyatt 1953; Ellis *et al.* 1954; Witzleben & Wyatt 1961). Indeed, in the absence of adequate chelation therapy, hepatic fibrosis was an inevitable consequence of iron overload; in most patients, it developed during childhood and progressed to frank cirrhosis during the second decade of life.

How soon does liver damage begin in patients with thalassaemia? In several early investigations the relationship between liver iron content and liver disease was examined in babies of less than 2 years of age (Wollstein & Kreidel 1930; Koch & Shapiro 1932; Panizon & Vullo 1952; Iancu & Neustein 1977). Hepatic fibrosis of varying degree was reported in five of these 16 babies but unfortunately the hepatic

iron concentration was not determined. Importantly however, screening tests were of limited clinical value and there was no biochemical evidence of hepatic damage (Panizon & Vullo 1952). The histological and electron-microscopic changes in liver pathology in early childhood, as described in the consecutive studies of Iancu and Neustein (1977), are discussed in detail in Chapter 5.

Early studies in older children with thalassaemia (Cooley *et al.* 1927; Baty *et al.* 1932; Whipple & Bradford 1936; Frumin *et al.* 1952; Panizon & Vullo 1952; Ellis *et al.* 1954; Witzleben & Wyatt 1961) suggested that fibrosis and cirrhosis were common in transfused, non-chelated children after the age of 3 years. The age and iron content at which significant fibrosis and cirrhosis were likely to develop is unclear. A relationship between liver iron concentration and transfusional iron overload was best expressed as an exponential, not linear, function of the transfused load (Barry *et al.* 1974). Higher liver iron concentrations relative to transfusion load might have been expected in patients who had undergone splenectomy, but this was not always observed (see below). The imperfect correlation in these earlier reports between the amount of iron administered by transfusion and the development of fibrosis may be accounted for, in part, by the fact that many children were maintained on a low haemoglobin level, which would not have substantially reduced gastrointestinal iron loading.

Factors influencing the development of liver disease

Of the many factors which appear to be involved in the rate of development of cirrhosis, age, the iron content of the liver (Fig. 7.11), associated hepatitis and, possibly, splenectomy may all play a role.

Risdon *et al.* (1975) suggested that the severity of fibrosis is related to age in a normal linear fashion, but that, even when iron accumulation is rapid, severe fibrosis may not be expected before 10 years of age. However, this pattern of the evolution of fibrosis does not seem to have been consistent between series of transfused, poorly chelated children with thalassaemia. One study reported fibrosis as early as 3 years of age, and cirrhosis as early as 8 years; by the age of 16 years, almost all children showed cirrhosis (Jean *et al.* 1984). Liver biopsies, obtained in 51 regularly transfused patients aged 5–36 years (mean, 18 years), showed that only six did not have some degree of

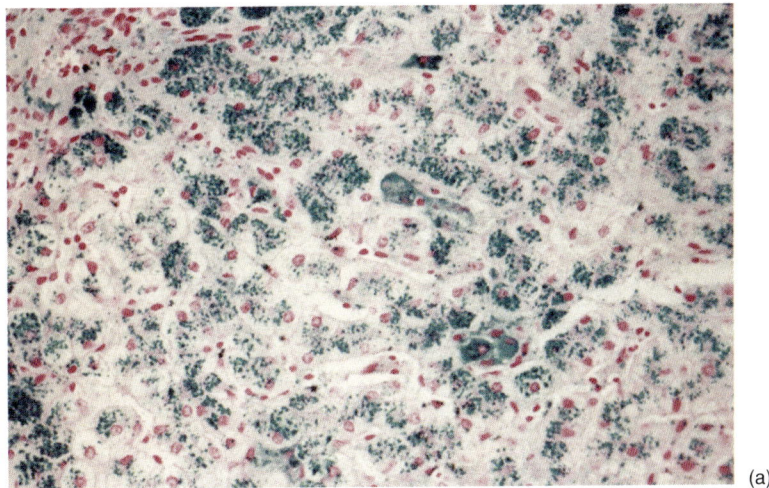

(a)

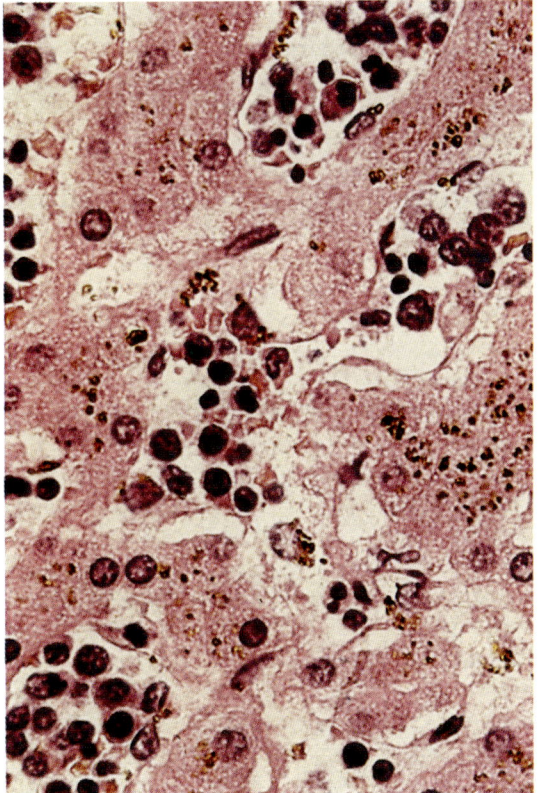

(b)

Fig. 7.11 Liver histology in homozygous β thalassaemia. (a) Perl's stain showing periportal iron deposition and iron-loaded macrophages together with some distended Kupffer cells (×200). (b) Extramedullary erythropoiesis in the hepatic sinusoids of a child with β thalassaemia major (H and E stain×450); from Sonakul (1989), with permission.

fibrosis; in five, cirrhosis was fully developed (Aldouri *et al.* 1987). In another study, involving 16 patients aged 3–17 years, it was observed that all but two, both aged 3 years at the time of the biopsy, had moderate to massive fibrosis or cirrhosis; three older patients, aged 4 and 5 years, already demonstrated a severe degree of hepatic fibrosis (Maurer *et al.* 1988). A further report suggested that fibrosis is observed in about 50% of transfused, irregularly chelated patients under the age of 6 years, and in 90% of similarly treated children over the age of 5 years (Angelucci *et al.* 1993), an observation which has been confirmed in more recent analyses of poorly chelated patients (Thakerngpol *et al.* 1996).

It has been suggested that, following splenectomy, the iron content of the liver may increase and fibrosis may be accelerated (Witzleben & Wyatt 1961). A possible mechanism was proposed, based on the observation that, in some studies, extremely high concentrations of iron were found in the spleens of patients with iron-loading anaemias, suggesting that the spleen is a major site of iron deposition (Lukens & Neuman 1971). On the other hand, others found that the iron content of the spleen was low (Borgna-Pignatti *et al.* 1984a), and that there is a rapid redistribution of iron from the initial site of deposition to the parenchymal tissues. Furthermore, Risdon *et al.* (1975) could demonstrate no increase in fibrosis in splenectomized patients. Thus, although the question of the relationship between splenectomy and iron loading remains open, the balance of evidence is against this being an important mechanism for potentiating liver damage.

There is extensive evidence that the major factor in the development of fibrosis is the concentration of iron in the liver. Risdon *et al.* (1975) noted an exponential relationship between iron content and fibrosis in a series of 52 liver biopsies in 19 patients studied over 13 years. The relationship between tissue iron concentration and hepatic cirrhosis was also explored by the same group (Barry *et al.* 1974) in children maintained on a high transfusion regimen who did, or did not, receive intramuscular desferrioxamine, and demonstrated a clear reduction in the degree of fibrosis in the former. In early attempts to establish a threshold of hepatic iron associated with the development of hepatic damage it was observed that fibrosis was only present in patients whose iron levels exceeded 7.6 mg/g, dry weight (Witzleben & Wyatt 1961). Later, De Virgiliis *et al.* (1980) reported findings of chronic persistent hepatitis, or chronic active hepatitis with periportal lesions, but only in patients with liver iron concentrations exceeding 10 mg/g, dry weight. Aldouri *et al.* (1987) reported a mean hepatic iron concentration of approximately 12.5 mg/g, dry weight, in patients with moderate or severe fibrosis, although fibrosis was observed in the presence of lower concentrations of hepatic iron.

As already mentioned, the first clear evidence that fibrosis can be arrested by iron chelation therapy was

obtained by Barry *et al.* (1974). This is a particularly interesting study because this effect was obtained at a dose which would now be considered inadequate, and the benefit was observed at a liver iron concentration in excess of 20 mg/g, dry weight, a level which was subsequently shown to be associated with a heightened risk of cardiac disease and early death (Brittenham *et al.* 1994). Arrest of fibrosis was observed in several other small studies (Aldouri *et al.* 1987; Maurer *et al.* 1988).

In the absence of prospective clinical trials to evaluate lifelong therapy for the prevention of tissue damage in thalassaemia, guidance about the risk of hepatic fibrosis has had to be derived from the clinical experience with hereditary haemochromatosis. Minor iron loading develops in about a quarter of heterozygotes for this condition, though their body iron stores do not seem to increase beyond two to four times the upper limit of normal, that is, up to approximately 7 mg/g, dry weight. In contrast, homozygotes who have iron burdens exceeding 7 mg/g, dry weight, have a definite increased risk of hepatic fibrosis. We shall take up this question again later in this chapter and in Chapter 15.

It is clear, however, that the toxic manifestations of iron overload do not depend entirely on the amount of iron in the liver. They are also modified by the rate of iron accumulation, the duration of exposure to increased iron, the partition of the iron load between relatively harmless sites in macrophages and more hazardous deposits in parenchymal cells, ascorbate status, which probably helps to determine this partition effect, the extent of internal redistribution of iron between macrophages and parenchymal sites, and factors unrelated to iron. Indeed, as we saw when we discussed hepatitis C, it is clear that liver damage associated with persistent infection, or response to therapy, may be considerably modified by the presence of excess iron (Clemente *et al.* 1994; Olynyk & Bacon 1995; Rubin *et al.* 1995). Furthermore, it has been reported recently that the use of the oral chelating agent deferiprone may result in the progression of hepatic fibrosis (Olivieri *et al.* 1998a; Berdoukas *et al.* 2000). We shall return to this important question in Chapter 15.

Assessment of liver function

Given the extremely complex and multifactorial nature of liver disease in β thalassaemia, the assessment of liver function and determination of the reasons for abnormalities of liver function tests may be extremely difficult. As mentioned earlier, there may be significant liver damage due to iron excess without any changes in standard liver function tests. Most patients with β thalassaemia, unless their bone marrow is suppressed by transfusion, have elevated serum bilirubin levels, reflecting both ineffective erythropoiesis and a shortened red-cell survival. The level of bilirubin is extremely variable and, as mentioned later in this chapter, it is becoming apparent that some patients who remain deeply jaundiced may have an additional genetic defect in bilirubin conjugation. Hepatocellular damage is reflected by a rise in the activity of serum aspartate aminotransferase (AST) and alanine aminotransferase (ALT). Since these enzymes are not specific for the liver, elevated levels must be assessed with caution. Since gallstones occur quite frequently in patients with β thalassaemia, particularly of the intermediate variety, a typical picture of obstructive jaundice may occur with raised levels of serum alkaline phosphatase, 5′ nucleotidase and γ-glutamyl transferase.

In assessing patients with suspected liver disease an estimation of the size of the liver may be helpful. A moderate degree of hepatomegaly is quite common in patients who have been maintained at a relatively low haemoglobin level. It has been the impression of clinicians for many years that in some patients the liver may enlarge dramatically after splenectomy, a condition sometimes referred to as the 'large liver syndrome'. This does not seem to be a feature of those maintained at an adequate haemoglobin level. We have observed a number of patients like this with HbE β thalassaemia in Sri Lanka. The liver biopsies show a complex picture, with iron loading and early fibrosis in many cases, and widespread extramedullary haemopoiesis (Fig. 7.11), nearly all of the erythroid lineage as demonstrated by a variety of staining techniques. Hence the typical picture of extramedullary haemopoiesis involving all the cell lines may not be observed in patients with thalassaemia. A large, tender liver should raise the suspicion of underlying hepatitis or, in grossly iron-loaded patients, associated cardiac failure.

An elevation of the liver enzymes should always be investigated, particularly if the level is rising with time. It is essential to screen for the different forms of hepatitis, as discussed earlier in this chapter. A liver biopsy should be performed and, where possible, the hepatic iron level estimated chemically. The liver should be examined histologically using standard stains, together with special stains to demonstrate iron, collagen and, where appropriate, hepatitis antigen.

Exocrine pancreas

As well as diabetes, described earlier in this chapter, there is increasing evidence that iron may also cause damage to the exocrine pancreas (Gullo *et al.* 1993). In a combined ultrasonographic and pancreatic enzyme study, the frequency of exocrine pancreatic damage was assessed in 39 consecutive patients with β thalassaemia and iron overload. Most of them had markedly increased echogenicity of the pancreas, with decreased size of the gland, as compared with controls. These changes showed a significant correlation with age and the duration of transfusion. Serum concentrations of trypsin and lipase was significantly lower in patients than in controls. The lowest values were found in older patients with a longer duration of transfusion therapy, who also had the most marked sonographic changes. Although the functional significance of these findings is not clear it is possible that, in cases of extreme damage to the exocrine pancreas, malabsorption may occur.

Folic acid and vitamin B$_{12}$ deficiency

The early literature on thalassaemia offered clear evidence that in inadequately treated patients folate deficiency is relatively common (Jandl & Greenberg 1959; Luhby & Cooperman 1961; Luhby *et al.* 1961). These findings were confirmed in studies carried out in Thailand (Vatanavicharn *et al.* 1978, 1979). Interestingly, Chanarin in his monograph, written in 1980, pointed out that the bone marrow may not show features which are absolutely typical of a megaloblastic anaemia in patients with thalassaemia and co-existent folate deficiency. In several of these early reports it was noted that severe bone pain may follow the administration of folic acid to folate-deficient patients. Folate deficiency is seen less commonly in well transfused patients although it is still an important problem in those with the intermediate forms of thalassaemia (see Chapter 13).

Vitamin B$_{12}$ levels are usually normal or elevated (Luhby *et al.* 1969) and only one, probably incidental, report of vitamin B$_{12}$-related neuropathy in a thalassaemic patient has been described (Robinson 1976).

Other vitamin and trace metal deficiencies

In addition to folic acid deficiency, described earlier, there are several other vitamin deficiency states which occur relatively commonly in patients with severe β thalassaemia, though their clinical significance is less clear.

Ascorbic acid

Early studies suggested that leucocyte ascorbic acid concentrations are significantly reduced in patients with severe forms of β thalassaemia (Wapnick *et al.* 1969; Modell & Beck 1974). It was suggested by Charlton and Bothwell (1976) that this is due mainly to iron overload. Subsequent studies confirmed that low ascorbic acid levels are found in iron-loaded thalassaemic patients (O'Brien 1974; Cohen *et al.* 1981; Chapman *et al.* 1982). It seems likely that ascorbic acid, because of its role as a biological reducing agent, may well be utilized in combating some of the complex free-radical damage that may be mediated by excess iron in the tissues. Its role in this process, and how this may differ at varying tissue concentrations of ascorbate, is reviewed by Gutteridge and Halliwell (1989). Although clinical scurvy must be unusual in iron-loaded patients (Cohen *et al.* 1981), ascorbate deficiency is of great importance in determining the response to chelating agents like desferrioxamine. Although the mechanism is uncertain it seems likely that this effect is mediated by expansion of the chelatable iron pool to which desferrioxamine has access (O'Brien 1974; Nienhuis 1981; Bridges & Hoffman 1986). We shall return to this question, and the potential dangers of the administration of high doses of ascorbic acid to iron-loaded patients, when we discuss the management of iron loading in Chapter 15.

Vitamin E deficiency

It has long been established that severe β thalassaemics may be vitamin E depleted (Hyman *et al.* 1974; Modell & Beck 1974). Hyman and colleagues found that baseline serum DL-α-tocopherol levels and vitamin E stores were low, and that serial biopsies of skin, liver, thyroid and testes showed increased deposits of lipofuscin, which are associated with vitamin E deficiency. These findings were corroborated by Rachmilewitz (1976), who suggested that, because of the continual process of peroxidation of thalassaemic red-cell membranes, the low serum vitamin E levels reflect its consumption as an antioxidant rather than a primary defect in vitamin E absorption or metabolism. This explanation seems likely to be correct; the antioxidant properties of vitamin E are discussed by Gutteridge and Halliwell (1989).

In their studies of the effects of vitamin E supplementation, Rachmilewitz *et al.* (1979) showed that it was possible to produce a fourfold increase in both serum and red-cell vitamin E levels, that the serum vitamin E level dropped rapidly after discontinuation of therapy, that there was a reduction in oxidant stress in red cells due to reduced peroxidative damage, and that in three of seven patients treated there was a significant increase in red-cell survival. These findings confirmed the role of vitamin E as an antioxidant in thalassaemic red cells although, unfortunately, as we shall discuss in Chapter 15, vitamin E seems to have no place in the treatment of β thalassaemia. The role of vitamin E as an antioxidant and the mechanisms of red-cell damage relating to peroxidation of the lipid portion of red-cell membranes are discussed further in Chapter 5.

Trace metal deficiencies

There have been conflicting reports about the levels of certain trace metals in the blood of thalassaemic patients, and even less is known about their significance. Erlandson *et al.* (1964b, 1965) found an increased serum copper and decreased serum magnesium levels. Prasad *et al.* (1965) also reported increased serum copper levels and Hyman *et al.* (1980) confirmed that at least some patients have decreased serum magnesium levels. The significance of these observations is not clear although Hyman and colleagues suggested that markedly reduced magnesium levels might have a deleterious effect on cardiac function.

Prasad *et al.* (1965) also reported a reduction in serum zinc levels, at least in some patients. Again the mechanism is not clear although this appears to be a general feature of other haemolytic states, including sickle-cell anaemia. Low levels of serum zinc were also found in a study in Thailand by Silprasert *et al.*

(1998). Incidentally, this study also confirmed the earlier findings of elevated levels of serum copper, although there was no correlation between copper and zinc levels. These authors point out that, at least in experimental animals with zinc and vitamin A deficiency, there is lack of response to vitamin A which can be corrected by zinc supplementation. Zinc deficiency has also been incriminated in growth retardation, although this has not been documented in thalassaemia.

Overall, we know very little about the significance of these changes in the levels of trace elements. Since many chelating agents remove metals other than iron, and even desferrioxamine is not entirely specific for iron, trace metal deficiency may also be exacerbated by treatment (see Chapter 15).

Gallstones

Gallstone formation is common in under-transfused β thalassaemics and in thalassaemia intermedia (Mazzone & Distefano 1969; Dewey *et al.* 1970). This problem is discussed further in Chapter 13.

Secondary gout

Because of the rapid turnover of red cells in their bone marrow, many patients with β thalassaemia who are maintained on a low transfusion regime are hyperuricaemic (Rosmino *et al.* 1968). Secondary gout has been well documented (Fessas & Loukopoulos 1974) and gouty arthropathy has been reported (Paik *et al.* 1970). These complications are rarely seen in well transfused patients. This topic is discussed further in Chapter 13.

Neuromuscular abnormalities

Neuromuscular complications of thalassaemia are not common. Logothetis *et al.* (1972a) summarized their studies on 138 consecutive patients with thalassaemia major who had been maintained on only a moderate transfusion regimen. They noted that walking was delayed beyond 18 months in about one-third of the patients, while speech and intellectual development appeared to proceed normally. Twenty-six of their patients developed a curious myopathic syndrome with proximal weakness, mostly in the lower extremities, and a myopathic electromyographic pattern. This complication was associated with severe skeletal stigmata, suggesting that it occurred in inadequately transfused patients. Certainly it does not seem to be a feature of adequately transfused thalassaemic children.

In the series of Logothetis *et al.* 27 patients had histories of episodes suggesting cerebral ischaemia, with focal neurological episodes. Similar episodes were described by Sinniah *et al.* (1977). Neurosensory deafness has been noted by McIntosh (1976a), who described improvement in hearing after commencement of regular blood transfusion and, in the same paper, noted that deafness was relatively common in inadequately transfused young thalassaemics. This complication was also reported by Hazell and Modell (1976). There is no doubt that severe cranial deformities resulting from massive expansion of the bone marrow can result in symptoms of this kind, or involvement of the optic nerve, but these complications are only seen in patients who have been maintained at extremely low haemoglobin levels.

We shall discuss the various neurological syndromes that can follow compression by haemopoietic cell tumour masses when we describe the complications of thalassaemia intermedia in Chapter 13. There are also several neurological and sensory complications of desferrioxamine therapy; these are described in Chapter 15.

Intelligence and behavioural patterns

Logothetis *et al.* (1971b) evaluated the mental status of 138 consecutive cases of thalassaemia major in Greece. Intelligence testing revealed no difference from normal children of the same age and social group. A trend to lower IQ scores was found in those subjected to less vigorous transfusion regimes. Abnormalities of behaviour and character were noted in 96 cases and abnormal emotional responses, mainly depression and anxiety, were observed in 67 of the children. In summarizing their experience these workers concluded that their findings were similar to those in any group of children with chronic disease.

More recent studies have attempted to use some of the modern techniques of psychology and psychiatry to assess the behavioural and emotional problems of young children with thalassaemia. For example, Tsiantis (1990) assessed a group of Greek children using the methods that were pioneered by Michael Rutter and colleagues (Rutter & Graham 1968) for studying the reliability and validity of psychiatric assessment of children. Using these strict criteria it was found that approximately 40% of the thalassaemic children, compared with about 30% of a control group of chronically sick children, were defined as having an emotional or behavioural disorder which would be classified as requiring some kind of psychiatric help. Problems relating to denial and displacement, which are considered to be maladaptive mechanisms, seem to be particularly common. In a further study of group interactions with the parents of thalassaemia children a number of factors were disclosed which may have contributed to the children's problems: death anxiety, denial, overprotective behaviour and, surprisingly, excessive pressure on the sick child to achieve.

These brief examples of studies of the behavioural problems of thalassaemic children and their families, while making it absolutely clear that it is not a topic that can be neglected, underline the difficulties that will be encountered when we try to learn more about this important subject. We shall return in more detail to the practical implications of these studies and to other social aspects of the disease when we discuss the management of thalassaemia in Chapter 15.

Pregnancy

Until the era of adequate transfusion and chelation, pregnancy in patients with severe forms of β thalassaemia was not observed. Pregnancies had occurred occasionally in patients with the intermediate forms of β thalassaemia (see Chapter 13). However, many patients are now passing through a relatively normal puberty and most centres that look after large numbers of thalassaemic patients have had some experience of managing pregnancy in those who are on regular transfusion and chelation therapy.

A number of reports have appeared over recent years of series of successful pregnancies in transfusion-dependent β-thalassaemic patients. These have included spontaneous pregnancies, twin pregnancies and pregnancies following *in vitro* fertilization (Seracchioli *et al.* 1994; Tampakoudis *et al.* 1997). Presumably because pregnancy would only be likely to occur in women who had been adequately chelated, and therefore in whom it is unlikely that there would be serious hepatic, cardiac or endocrine complications, most of these pregnancies seem to have gone to term and there have been no major problems. The

patients have maintained their usual haemoglobin levels by regular transfusion but have usually avoided chelating drugs during pregnancy. We shall return to the question of the management of pregnancy in thalassaemia in Chapter 15.

Complications not covered in this chapter

Iatrogenic disease

Like all branches of medicine, the natural course of thalassaemia may be modified by the complications of treatment. We shall consider these, and the way in which problems such as iron loading and infection are modified by bone-marrow transplantation, in Chapter 15.

Renal disease

There are no renal complications directly attributable to thalassaemia. Chronic renal failure due to other causes may modify the clinical course, particularly with respect to anaemia and blood requirements. We shall discuss briefly our experience of renal transplantation in thalassaemia in Chapter 15.

The effects of complications on prognosis

The prognosis relating to different forms of treatment and the occurrence of complications is discussed in Chapter 15.

Autopsy findings

With one notable exception the recent literature of the thalassaemia field has, like that of the rest of medicine, completely neglected the value of the autopsy. The one exception is the beautifully illustrated atlas produced by Sonakul (1989).

There are, however, many excellent descriptions of the morbid anatomy of thalassaemia in its earlier literature (Whipple & Bradford 1936; Astaldi *et al.* 1951; Ellis *et al.* 1954; Sansone *et al.* 1955; Fink 1964; Chaptal *et al.* 1967; Putignano *et al.* 1973; Modell & Matthews 1976). Perhaps the most valuable information to come from these reports is the distribution of iron among the different organs. The weight of iron per organ in the series of autopsies reported by Modell and Matthews (1976) is shown in Table 7.6. Most of the findings at autopsy reflect the various

Table 7.6 Tissue iron concentration (% dry weight) in patients dying from thalassaemia major. The iron loading quotient is derived from the observed iron load/expected load from standard weight curves. Data from Modell and Matthews (1976).

Patient	Age	Fe (g)	Iron loading quotient	Liver	Heart	Pancreas	Kidney	Thyroid	Para-thyroid	Adrenal	Testis
1	3 months	0.0	—	0.38	0.06	—	0.12	—	—	—	—
2	22 months	0.8	0.23	0.44	0.09	—	0.88	—	—	—	—
3	3–6 months	2.2	0.5	—	0.12	—	0.13	—	—	—	0.1
4	4–6 months	1.5	0.2	0.6	0.06	—	0.15	—	—	—	—
5	2–3 months	0.05	0.14	1.17		1.38	0.22	—	—	—	—
6	7 yrs	4.2	0.3	7.2	0.2	3.18	0.16	0.24	—	—	—
7	10 yrs	21.0	0.9	3.7	0.14	1.69	0.24	—	—	0.16	—
8	11 yrs	44.0	1.8	5.7	1.32	1.49	0.58	3.3	7.3	—	—
9	18 yrs	48.0	1.0	4.9	0.6	—	0.42	—	—	—	—
10	21 yrs	74.0	1.3	3.7	0.95	3.9	0.49	2.7	—	1.4	0.4
11	5 yrs	8.5	1.0	1.5	0.41	0.86	—	—	—	0.34	0.12

pathologies that have been described in different sections of this chapter. The most striking finding in all these reports is the widespread deposition of iron with varying degrees of organ fibrosis. As might be expected the organs most affected include the liver, spleen, endocrine glands, pancreas, heart and kidneys. The degree of fibrosis varies between most marked in the liver and least noticeable in the thyroid gland. The spleen, if present, is enlarged and congested with thickened reticulum. It may contain Gaucher-like cells similar to those seen in the marrow (Resegotti *et al.* 1974, 1975). Data on the levels of gangliosides and glucocerebrosides are given by Fabris *et al.* (1978). Detailed studies of the myocardium and conductive tissues are reported by Buja and Roberts (1971) and Modell and Matthews (1976). Iron may constitute up to 1% of the dry weight. It is laid down with lipofucin, in small granules which are probably lysosomes. Muscle fibres show early degeneration with swelling of the granules. As shown most elegantly in the atlas of Sonakul (1989) there may be extensive extramedullary haematopoiesis. This work is also notable for the elegant pictures of obliterative changes in the small vessels of the lungs seen in some Thai patients with HbE β thalassaemia and pulmonary hypertension.

The blood and bone marrow

Red cells

There is always a severe degree of anaemia, which is typically hypochromic and microcytic with a low mean cell haemoglobin (MCH) and mean cell volume (MCV). The mean cell haemoglobin concentration (MCHC) is inconsistent. The red-cell indices derived from electronic cell counters do not always reflect the degree of haemoglobinization of the red cells judged from inspection of the peripheral blood film. This is particularly noticeable after splenectomy and in patients with thalassaemia intermedia (see Chapter 13). Many factors may be involved in this discrepancy, particularly heterogeneity of cell populations (see below), with large numbers of extremely small cells which may not be 'seen' by the electronic cell counter, and artefacts produced by the large numbers of nucleated red cells, white cells and platelets which are nearly always present after splenectomy.

The most striking and consistent haematological finding is the marked abnormality of the morphological appearances of the red cells (Fig. 7.12). These changes include anisocytosis, poikilocytosis, misshapen microcytes, occasional macrocytes and a variable number of target cells. In addition, there may be some well haemoglobinized normocytes or macrocytes, almost transparent hypochromic elliptocytes, small spherocytes and spiculated cells together with variable numbers of tear-drop and elongated forms and a great assortment of bizarre poikilocytes and distorted cell remnants. Erythroblasts are almost always present and their number seems to be related to the degree of anaemia. Some of these changes are illustrated in Fig. 7.13.

The red-cell morphology in β thalassaemia tends to change after splenectomy (Nathan & Gunn 1966).

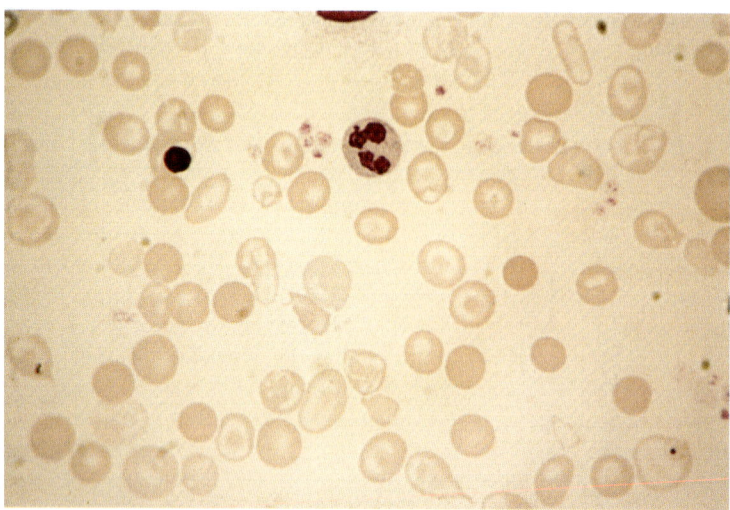

Fig. 7.12 The peripheral blood picture in homozygous β thalassaemia (Wright's stain×550).

In particular, large hypochromic cells are found, together with small piscine forms which are little more than fragments of stroma. In addition, the number of nucleated red cells is increased and variable numbers of siderocytes are seen in the peripheral blood. Fessas (1963) was the first to point out that after splenectomy ragged inclusion bodies can be seen in the cytoplasm of both nucleated red cells and reticulocytes if the blood is first incubated with methyl violet (Fig. 7.14). These bodies are easily seen on phase-contrast microscopy and also in wet preparations. Although they are most numerous in the peripheral blood of splenectomized subjects they can be found in occasional cells in patients with intact spleens. Recent studies have shown that they consist almost entirely of precipitated α chains (see also Chapter 5) (Fig. 7.15).

Ultrastructural studies of the red cells have been carried out by several groups (Bessis *et al.* 1958; Marinone *et al.* 1958; Nathan & Gunn 1966; Rifkind 1966; Marks & Bank 1971; Polliack & Rachmilewitz 1973; Zaino & Rossi 1974) (see Chapter 5). The most extensive electron-microscopic study was reported by Polliack and Rachmilewitz (1973), who found the most marked changes in splenectomized patients. There is an accumulation of iron, either as free particles or as aggregates of ferritin and haemosiderin, within membrane-bound particles or mitochondria. The cells show gross distortion with infolding of plasma membranes and vacuole formation. Many of them contain inclusion bodies resembling Heinz bodies. However, unlike the latter, the inclusions of thalassaemic cells are not attached to the red-cell membrane. Another prominent feature is the presence of bizarre membrane forms and myelin figures. Polliack and Rachmilewitz (1973) suggest that the latter may represent attempts at autodigestion of intracellular inclusions. The presence of large amounts of ferritin iron has been confirmed using Mössbauer spectroscopy (Bauminger *et al.* 1980).

The absolute reticulocyte count, though elevated, is rarely very high, although it tends to increase after splenectomy.

In well transfused patients the blood picture may look surprisingly normal, with only an occasional abnormal cell, findings which reflect an almost total suppression of endogenous erythropoiesis.

White cells and platelets

The total white-cell count and differential is either normal or possibly slightly elevated. A reduction in white-cell count, particularly if there is a 'shift to the right' with hyperlobulation of the polymorphonuclear leucocytes, is indicative of folate deficiency. Severe neutropenia may occur as part of the picture of severe hypersplenism.

The platelet count is usually normal or slightly elevated; thrombocytopenia usually reflects hypersplenism or folate deficiency. High platelet counts occur after splenectomy, but only tend to persist in those with low haemoglobin levels.

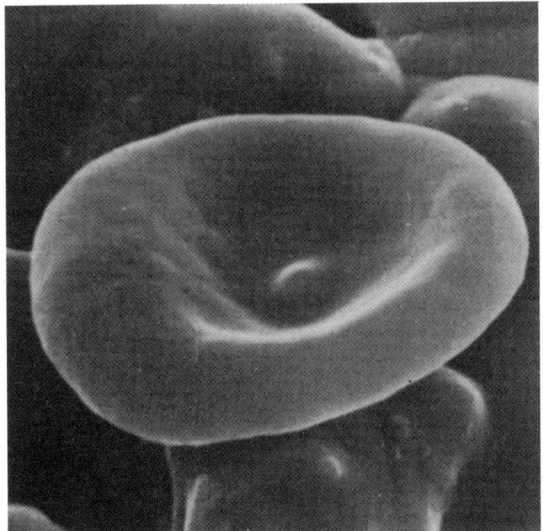

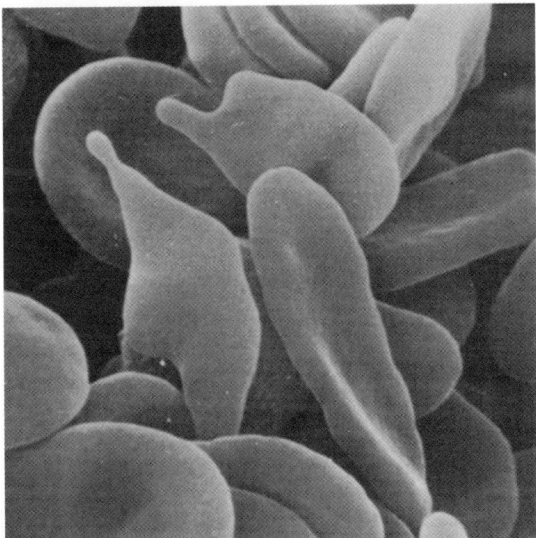

Fig. 7.13 The morphological changes in thalassaemic red cells demonstrated by scanning electron microscopy. Top, target cell; bottom, poikilocytes. Kindly prepared by Drs A. Polliack and E. Rachmilewitz.

Bone marrow

In untransfused patients or those maintained at a low haemoglobin level the bone marrow is extremely cellular due mainly to marked erythroid hyperplasia (Fig. 7.16). There is loss of fat spaces and extension of the erythroid marrow throughout the long bones and skull and, as mentioned earlier, there may be protru-

sion of the marrow through the ribs or inner tables of the skull (see previous section and Chapter 13).

The erythroid hyperplasia is reflected in an alteration in the myeloid/erythroid (M/E) ratio from the normal 3 or 4 to 0.1, or even less. Though there is hyperplasia of all erythroid precursors there is a relative increase in the proportion of basophilic and polychromatophilic normoblasts. All the red-cell precursor series show defective haemoglobinization with reduction in the cytoplasmic diameter, but the size of the nuclei is normal. Staining for iron reveals an abundance in the reticulo-endothelial cells and also in the red-cell precursors but, although some of the iron is distributed in the perinuclear region, abnormal ring sideroblasts are not a feature of thalassaemia.

If the marrow is incubated with methyl violet it is always possible to demonstrate inclusions in the erythroblasts (Fig. 7.17). These are similar to those in the peripheral blood red-cell precursors and mature red cells of patients who have undergone splenectomy. The identification of these bodies as precipitated α chains, the kinetics of their precipitation, their distribution in red cells at different stages of maturation, and the pathophysiological consequences of α-chain precipitation were considered in detail in Chapter 5. The ultrastructure of β-thalassaemia erythroblasts is illustrated in Fig. 5.6, and is also discussed in detail in Chapter 5.

The cytoplasm of thalassaemic erythroblasts shows abnormalities in addition to precipitated α chains. Astaldi *et al.* (1954) noted the presence of periodic acid Schiff (PAS)-positive material in erythroblasts and red cells. It was later shown that this material is glycogen (Matioli & del Pianco 1961; Stegagno & Pollitzer 1963; Fessas & Papayannopoulou 1965). In a further study Yataganas and colleagues (Yataganas *et al.* 1973) found that the glycogen content was most marked in the G_1 phase of early polychromatic erythroblasts. They postulated that the accumulation of glycogen reflects the storage of unutilized energy in erythroblasts that are blocked in the G_1 phase of the cell cycle.

The bone marrow also shows intense phagocytic activity. The presence of large foamy cells resembling Gaucher cells has been demonstrated in the bone marrow and spleen. Zaino *et al.* (1971) and Zaino and Rossi (1974) have shown that they contain intracytoplasmic tubules and phagocytosed mature and immature red cells. Further details of the fine structure of

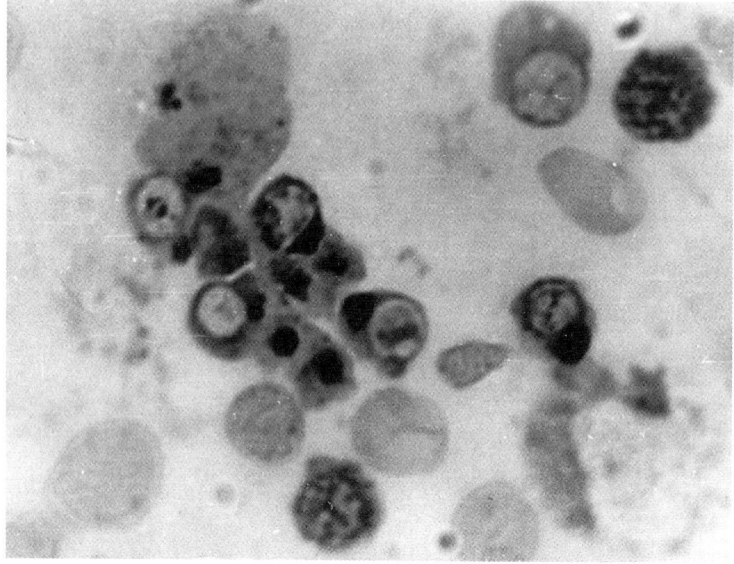

Fig. 7.14 Inclusions in the red-cell precursors in β thalassaemia (methyl violet stain ×500).

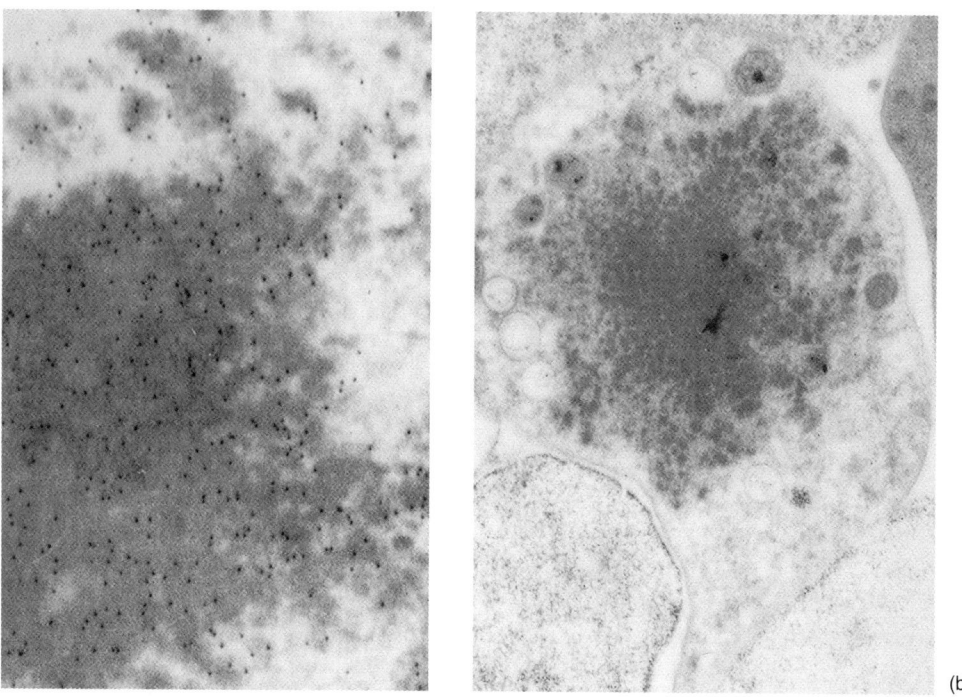

(a)   (b)

Fig. 7.15 Studies of red-cell precursors in β thalassaemia major with specific globin antibodies. (a) Appearances after treatment with anti-α-globin antibody, demonstrating the heavy staining of the inclusions. (b) A similar red-cell precursor treated with anti-β-globin antibody; there is virtually no staining.

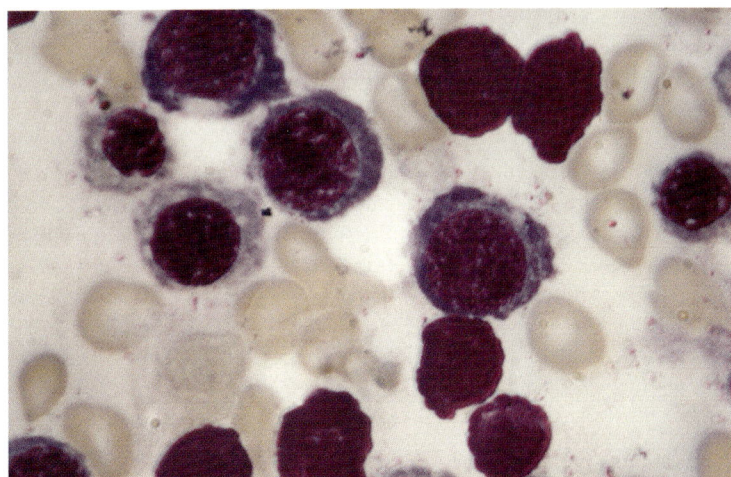

Fig. 7.16 The bone marrow in severe β thalassaemia. There is intense erythroid hyperplasia with many immature erythroid precursors (Leishman stain × 450).

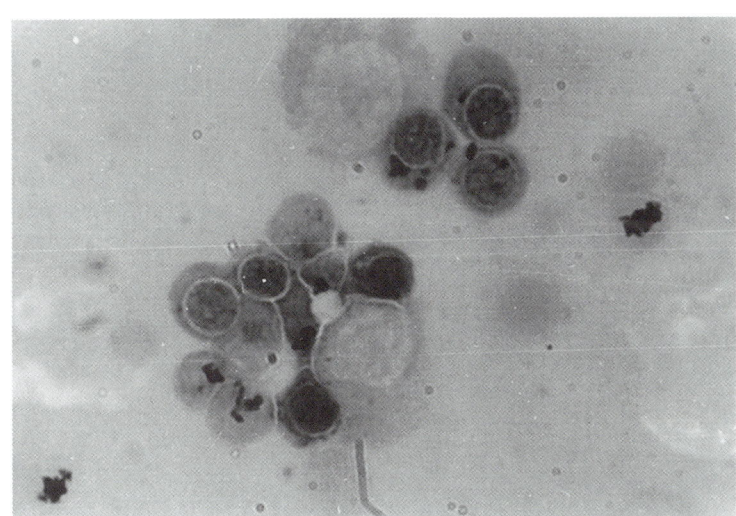

Fig. 7.17 The bone marrow in β thalassaemia major showing inclusions in the red-cell precursors (methyl violet stain × 350).

the macrophages in thalassaemic marrow is given by Wickramasinghe and Hughes (1978).

Hence the bone marrow in thalassaemia is characterized by intense erythroid hyperplasia, intracellular inclusion formation, abnormal accumulation of glycogen in the red-cell precursors and intense phagocytosis. These findings reflect a marked abnormality of proliferation and maturation of red-cell precursors, the basis for which was considered in detail in Chapter 5.

Red-cell survival

Reports of red-cell survival studies using either the Ashby or ^{51}Cr-labelling methods have indicated a reduced survival time ranging from 7 to 22 days (Kaplan & Zuelzer 1950; Sturgeon & Finch 1957; Erlandson *et al.* 1958; Vullo & Tunioli 1958; Blendis *et al.* 1974). Several workers have described survival curves which suggest that there are two populations of red cells, one which is very rapidly destroyed and another with a longer survival (Kaplan & Zuelzer 1950; Bailey & Prankerd 1958; Hillcoat & Waters 1962). The red-cell survival is not directly related to the level of HbF or degree of anaemia (Erlandson *et al.* 1958) but there is evidence, considered in detail in Chapter 5, that the short-lived population contains mainly HbA or α-chain precipitates (Gabuzda *et al.* 1963). Although external scanning suggested that some degree of red-cell destruction occurs in the spleen, the main effect of increasing splenomegaly is trapping of a large number of red cells with consequent hypervolaemia and haemodilution anaemia (Prankerd 1963; Blendis *et al.* 1974).

Red-cell metabolism

There are several distinctive metabolic abnormalities of the red cells in homozygous β thalassaemia. The osmotic fragility is markedly decreased; haemolysis is often incomplete in 0.1% saline. On sterile incubation of thalassaemic red cells, autohaemolysis occurs at the upper limit of normal or at slightly increased rates, and there is a further decrease in osmotic fragility after 24-h incubation (Selwyn 1953). The mechanism is discussed in Chapter 5.

The biochemical characteristics of thalassaemic red cells are discussed in detail in Chapter 5. Morphological and metabolic studies of those from patients who have undergone splenectomy, when separated into young and old populations by centrifugation, have revealed a variety of metabolic abnormalities. Cells from the younger, upper layers contain more inclusion bodies than those lower down the centrifuge tube. The younger cell populations have a lower haemoglobin content and show more crateral distortion than the older cell populations. The younger cells show the more rapid rate of flux of potassium across the membrane and a higher rate of glycolysis and lactate formation with low, unstable levels of ATP (Loukopoulos & Fessas 1965; Nathan & Gunn 1966; Nathan *et al.* 1969). The basis for these changes and their significance in relationship to the degree of haemolysis were considered in Chapter 5.

Since thalassaemic red cells are turning over rapidly they might be expected to show non-specific enzyme changes related to the cell age. This is found in the case of certain enzymes, such as glucose-6-phosphate dehydrogenase, which tend to have higher mean levels in the peripheral blood than normal. The age and degree of membrane and cellular dysfunc-

tion of thalassaemic red cells is also reflected in non-specific abnormalities of glucose utilization and enzyme function (Notario *et al.* 1964a,b, 1976), total lipid composition, and the electrophoretic and sialic acid composition of their membranes (Notario & Meduri 1965; Meduri *et al.* 1973; Notario *et al.* 1974, 1976; Rachmilewitz 1976; Kahane *et al.* 1978). The relationship of these changes to the haemolytic component in the anaemia of β thalassaemia is considered in Chapter 5.

Changes in the red-cell porphyrins have been observed (Sturgeon *et al.* 1958). They include increased concentrations of coproporphyrin and uroporphyrin, with protoporphyrin levels at the upper limit of normal. Elevated levels of free protoporphyrins were also reported by Lyberatos *et al.* (1972).

Anderson and colleagues have studied pyridoxine metabolism in β thalassaemia major (Anderson *et al.* 1975, 1979). Pyridoxine (vitamin B_6) is taken up by red cells and metabolized to pyridoxal via pyridoxine and pyridoxal phosphates. In 25 β-thalassaemia homozygotes the rate of conversion of pyridoxine to pyridoxal varied widely, being normal or elevated (as in other anaemias) in non-transfused cases and low in transfused patients. Anderson *et al.* suggest that the low rate of conversion is inherited independently from the thalassaemia gene and that the two conditions occur together frequently, possibly because they are subject to the same selective forces. This interesting idea requires further study.

Iron metabolism

Iron loading is a constant feature of transfusion-dependent homozygous β thalassaemia. Although the majority of the iron load is derived from blood transfusion there may in certain circumstances be increased gastrointestinal iron absorption. As will be seen in Chapter 13 this is certainly the case in the intermediate forms of β thalassaemia. The clinical consequences of iron overload are discussed earlier in this chapter and the pathophysiology and mechanisms of tissue damage were described in Chapter 5.

Iron absorption

Iron absorption studies have given variable results. Larizza *et al.* (1958) found values at the lower limit of normal, while Smith *et al.* (1957) and Erlandson *et al.* (1962) found increased absorption in anaemic children which became normal after transfusion. Bannerman (1964) found increased absorption in about one-quarter of their cases. Necheles *et al.* (1969) reported high values in about half their cases and Shahid and Abu Haydar (1967) found increased absorption in four anaemic homozygotes. These discrepancies may well have been due to the transfusional status of the patient at the time of study. Indeed, Heinrich *et al.* (1973) found that inorganic iron absorption was markedly increased 64–300 days after transfusion, whereas it fell into the normal range if carried out 3–17 days after transfusion. Presumably the level of iron absorption is related to the degree of ineffective erythropoiesis and erythroid hyperplasia; if this is reduced by transfusion, gastrointestinal iron absorption is reduced. In Heinrich's study food iron absorption followed the same pattern as inorganic iron.

Serum iron

It has long been recognized that the serum iron is elevated in children with homozygous β thalassaemia and that in older children the iron-binding capacity is fully saturated (Smith *et al.* 1950). As described in detail in Chapter 5, the serum of such patients contains 2–7 µmol/l of non-specifically bound iron which is dialysable and can be bound by transferrin from normal sera (Hershko *et al.* 1978).

Serum ferritin

The measurement of plasma or serum ferritin is still the most commonly used estimate of body iron stores in thalassaemia. Earlier in this chapter we discussed the evidence which indicates that there is an imprecise relationship between the serum ferritin and hepatic iron concentrations. It seems likely that the wide fluctuations which occur at high ferritin levels may reflect a variety of mechanisms that alter the concentration independently of the body iron load. These include ascorbate deficiency, acute infection, chronic inflammation, acute and chronic liver damage, haemolysis and ineffective erythropoiesis (Prieto *et al.* 1974; De Virgiliis *et al.* 1980; Roeser *et al.* 1980; Baynes *et al.* 1986).

Thus although it is clear that the majority of severely affected β thalassaemics who are not adequately chelated have elevated serum or plasma ferritin levels, because of these confounding factors, in any individual patient a serum ferritin estimation does not give an accurate indication of the body iron burden (Olivieri *et al.* 1995b). We shall return to this problem when we consider the management of iron overload in Chapter 15.

Other non-invasive estimates of iron loading

A variety of studies have been directed at imaging tissue iron as an indirect approach to assessing the iron load in thalassaemia. These include computed tomography (Houang *et al.* 1979; Long *et al.* 1980; Olivieri *et al.* 1989), nuclear resonance scattering (Wielopolski & Zaino 1992) and magnetic resonance imaging (Stark *et al.* 1985; Gomori *et al.* 1991; Olivieri *et al.* 1992d; Villari *et al.* 1992; Lui *et al.* 1996). In summarizing the results of these and similar studies, Olivieri and Brittenham (1997) conclude that none of them provide measurements of tissue iron that are quantitatively equivalent to those determined directly by biopsy. These authors reach the same conclusions about the relationship between cardiac or pituitary function and body iron burden assessed by these approaches.

Hepatic iron concentration

Currently the measurement of hepatic iron concentration is the most reliable method for determining body iron burden in patients with thalassaemia, particularly with respect to the development of tissue damage (Overmoyer *et al.* 1987; Brittenham 1988; Olivieri *et al.* 1992d). The simplest and most widely available approach is by liver biopsy and direct measurement of the iron concentration. Susceptometry superconducting quantum interference device (SQUID) magnetometry provides an alternative and equally effective approach (Brittenham *et al.* 1982; Brittenham 1988). As already discussed earlier in this chapter, by relating hepatic iron concentration to the risks of tissue damage in patients with primary haemochromatosis it has been possible to derive some guidelines for the prognostic and therapeutic implications of different liver iron levels in β thalassaemia (reviewed in detail by Olivieri and Brittenham (1997) and in Chapter 15). The conclusions from these studies are summarized in Fig. 7.8, p. 296.

In short, because of the vagaries of the serum iron, iron-binding capacity and serum or plasma ferritin values, they can only be used as an approximation of the degree of iron loading in severe forms of β thalassaemia. For a more accurate assessment of the body iron burden, and particularly when trying to relate it to the likelihood of the complications of iron overload, the liver iron concentration is the most accurate indicator of the extent and likely complications of iron loading. Recently it has been demonstrated that there is a linear relationship between total body iron and hepatic iron concentration in patients with thalassaemia major (Angelucci *et al.* 2000).

Ferrokinetics and erythrokinetics

The kinetics of iron metabolism and red-cell precursor turnover were discussed in detail in Chapter 5 and are also considered in Chapter 13; the most direct evidence regarding the degree of effective erythropoiesis in severe β thalassaemia has been obtained from studies of patients with thalassaemia intermedia which are not confounded by the effects of blood transfusion.

Ferrokinetic and erythrokinetic studies (Crosby & Akeroyd 1952; Sturgeon & Finch 1957; Erlandson *et al.* 1958; Larizza *et al.* 1958; Malamos *et al.* 1961; Finch *et al.* 1970) and studies of bilirubin metabolism (Grinstein *et al.* 1960) have provided clear evidence for the existence of a considerable degree of ineffective erythropoiesis in patients with severe β thalassaemia. The remarkable degree of ineffective erythropoiesis which occurs in homozygous β thalassaemia was summarized in the review by Finch *et al.* (1970). Finch's group studied 10 homozygous β thalassaemics and derived the plasma iron turnover (PIT) and erythrocyte iron turnover (EIT) in each case. In thalassaemia the PIT was higher than in any other disease and reached a level of 10 times greater than normal while the EIT was only slightly elevated; this discrepancy represents a massive breakdown of developing red cells in the bone marrow. Similar results have been obtained by others, and a marked suppression of erythropoiesis after blood transfusion has been demonstrated (Cavill *et al.* 1978).

The ferrokinetic and erythrokinetic picture in thalassaemia is therefore one of gross ineffective erythropoiesis. On the one hand there is evidence of increased red-cell and haemoglobin production as judged by bone-marrow hyperplasia, plasma iron turnover and faecal urobilinogen production, while *effective* red-cell production as estimated by the haemoglobin level, absolute reticulocyte count and iron incorporation is not increased, indicating an extreme degree of intramedullary destruction of red cells. Thus, as described in more detail in Chapter 5, the anaemia of thalassaemia is primarily dyserythropoietic, with an added haemolytic component and an element of hypersplenism in some cases.

Other biochemical changes

The haemolytic component of β thalassaemia major is reflected by a mild elevation of unconjugated bilirubin, low or absent haptoglobin and haemopexin (Yamak & Ozsoylu 1969; Cutillo & Meloni 1974), a raised plasma haemoglobin (Crosby & Dameshek 1951) and the occasional presence of methaemalbumin (Fessas & Loukopoulos 1974). There is an increase of urobilinogen in the faeces (Sturgeon & Finch 1957).

There is an increased level of urates in the urine and the serum uric acid levels are higher than in control subjects and, as we saw earlier, gout may occur. Increased nucleoprotein catabolism results in the excretion of large amounts of β-amino isobutyric acid (BAIBA) in the urine. This is a product of thymine catabolism which is not present in heterozygotes and is also absent, or present in only low amounts, postsplenectomy. It has been suggested that this is because the spleen plays a role in trapping and catabolizing normoblasts (Fessas *et al.* 1969).

Another distinctive feature of severe β thalassaemia is the excretion of catabolic products which are not present in appreciable amounts in other haemolytic anaemias. Frequently, thalassaemic patients pass dark-brown urine and this has been attributed to the presence of mesobilifuscins and other dipyrroles (Kreimer-Birnbaum *et al.* 1966, 1969). The mechanism for the production of these unusual pigments, which are also found in the urine of some patients with unstable haemoglobin disorders, is not clear; presumably they reflect the destruction or unusual metabolism of haem or its precursors.

A decrease in serum albumin levels in older children with thalassaemia major was noted by Allamanis (1955).

Details of published data on erythropoietin levels are given in Chapter 5. Because of the problems of relating these values to the transfusion status in severe β thalassaemia, much of this work has been carried out in patients with thalassaemia intermedia; it is discussed further in Chapter 13. In short, the estimation of serum erythropoietin values in transfusion-dependent β thalassaemia is of no practical value.

The changes in vitamin and trace element levels in the serum of thalassaemia patients were reviewed earlier in the chapter. Non-specific changes in the serum lipids were reported by Schwartz-Tiene *et al.* (1953), Rao *et al.* (1972) and Ameri *et al.* (1975).

Serological changes

Giblett and Crookston (1964) noted that the red cells of 17 patients with thalassaemia major who had not been recently transfused reacted as strongly with anti-i as the cells of newborn infants. The amount of i-antigen was not related to the ABO group, the degree of anaemia or the level of HbF. The cells reacted to anti-I as strongly as normal adult cells. The increased reactivity to anti-i is not specific to thalassaemia and has been found in other haemolytic and dyserythro-poietic states and in normal individuals following phlebotomy. Hillman and Giblett (1965) suggest that it is related to the marrow transit time.

Other serological changes in thalassaemic children, related to repeated blood transfusion, are considered in Chapter 15.

Haemoglobin constitution

The red cells in all the severe forms of β thalassaemia contain increased amounts of HbF; this remains the main diagnostic feature (Fig. 7.18). Homozygous β^0 thalassaemics have only HbF and HbA_2; HbA is absent. The level of HbF in β^+-thalassaemia homozygotes is variable but it is always elevated above normal after the first few months of life. Haemoglobin A_2 levels in the homozygous or compound heterozygous states are of no diagnostic value. The only other abnormal finding is the occasional presence of free α chains, which can sometimes be demonstrated using appropriate electrophoretic techniques.

The reader should be aware of the limitations of examination of the haemoglobin pattern in the peripheral blood in severe β thalassaemia. Some widely used methods for measuring HbF tend to give erroneous values, particularly in the high-level range. Once a patient is transfused, endogenous haemoglobin production is depressed and it becomes impossible to determine accurately the amount of Hbs A, F or A_2, even if the estimations are carried out several months after transfusion. Furthermore, the red cells show a remarkable degree of heterogeneity of haemoglobinization, and considerable individual variability in levels of HbF, and probably HbA_2.

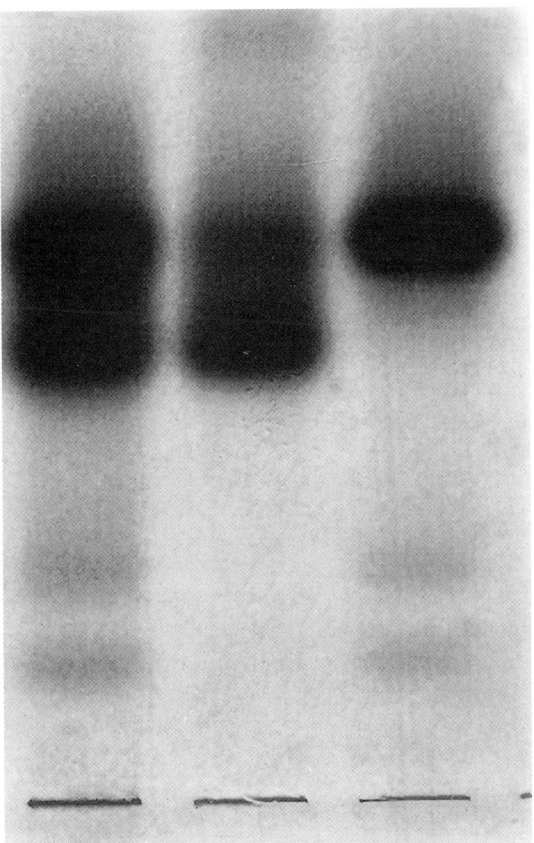

Fig. 7.18 Starch gel electrophoresis of the haemoglobin of a patient homozygous for β^+ thalassaemia (Tris-EDTA-borate system, pH 8.5, amido black stain). The following are shown left to right: 1, β^+-thalassaemia homozygote; 2, cord blood; 3, normal adult.

There are different rates of turnover of Hbs A, F and A_2 in the marrow and peripheral blood. All these factors mean that measurement of Hbs F and A_2 in the blood give limited information about their rates of production in the marrow. For these reasons most studies describing Hbs F and A_2 levels in severe β thalassaemia must be interpreted with caution.

The mechanisms of HbF production in β thalassaemia are discussed in Chapter 5.

Haemoglobin F

After the first description of elevated levels of HbF in thalassaemia by Vecchio (1946) there were many confirmatory reports (Singer *et al.* 1951; Rich 1952; Roche *et al.* 1953; Marinone & Bernasconi 1957; Silvestroni *et al.* 1957, 1968a). Later reports, from studies of either haemoglobin analysis or synthesis, showed unequivocally that some forms of β thalassaemia are associated with a haemoglobin pattern consisting entirely of Hbs F and A_2 (Fessas & Karaklis 1962; Bargellesi *et al.* 1967; Silvestroni *et al.* 1968a; Weatherall *et al.* 1969b; Conconi *et al.* 1970).

Given the many variables which set the final level of HbF in the peripheral blood, discussed in Chapters 5, 10 and 13, it is extremely difficult to make many valid statements about the amount of HbF in the different forms of β thalassaemia. The closest approximation that can be made is to try to measure the percentage HbF by the most accurate method available, to determine the peripheral blood haemoglobin concentration at the same time, and then to describe the level of HbF in g/dl. In fact, in the transfusion-dependent forms of $β^0$ and $β^+$ thalassaemia, once infants have started on regular transfusion, it is almost impossible to determine how much HbF is being produced. Although it is unlikely that the bone marrow is ever fully 'switched off' by blood transfusion we have found that in patients transfused to a haemoglobin level of 9–10g/dl there is very little endogenous haemoglobin production; in patients with HbE β thalassaemia, who in the untransfused state have high levels of HbF, there is a marked reduction in the relative amounts of HbF compared with HbE synthesized at increasing levels of transfusion (Rees *et al.* 1998b). And in well transfused patients, even if they are studied just before their next transfusion, there is always a considerable amount of transfused blood remaining in the circulation. Thus it is not possible to determine the amount of HbF that is produced with any accuracy.

For these reasons we have only the flimsiest idea about the absolute level of HbF production in the severe, transfusion-dependent forms of $β^0$ and $β^+$ thalassaemia. Children homozygous for $β^0$ thalassaemia, examined before their first transfusion, have haemoglobin levels of 6–8g/dl, all of which is HbF (Cao 1988). However, some patients with this disorder produce considerably higher levels of HbF and have thalassaemia intermedia; we shall discuss the possible reasons in Chapter 13. We know even less about the levels of HbF associated with the severe forms of $β^+$ thalassaemia. Again, what is known comes from studies of infants before their first transfusion. In a

series of infants with $β^+$ thalassaemia analysed by Kattamis *et al.* (1975) nearly all had HbF values in excess of 50% of the total haemoglobin. These few observations suggest that some of the very low levels of HbF in severe forms of β thalassaemia reported in earlier studies must be viewed with extreme caution.

The only forms of homozygous or compound heterozygous β thalassaemia for which accurate, steady-state HbF levels in older patients are available are those with the phenotype of β thalassaemia intermedia. The HbF data in these disorders are presented in detail in Chapter 13. In short, some of the milder mutations, in their homozygous or compound heterozygous states, are associated with HbF values in the 15–40% range, notably the homozygous state for the common Mediterranean IVS1-6 T→C mutation. Patients who are homozygous for the mild β-globin-gene promoter mutations, which are found commonly in African populations, have significantly higher HbF values, usually in excess of 50%. But even within these relatively homogeneous groups of patients there is wide variation in HbF levels, perhaps not surprising considering the many different genetic factors which can modify the level of HbF in β thalassaemia; these interactions are discussed in detail in Chapters 10 and 13.

It seems likely therefore that HbF makes up either nearly all or a high proportion of the circulating haemoglobin in the severe transfusion-dependent forms of β thalassaemia. It also constitutes a significant part of the total haemoglobin in the blood of patients with β thalassaemia intermedia. The level is so variable in all these conditions that it is of little diagnostic help, reflecting as it does cell selection, the underlying β-thalassaemia mutation and a variety of other genetic factors which may modify its rate of synthesis.

The alkali-resistant haemoglobin found in β thalassaemia is identical to normal fetal haemoglobin. It has the same electrophoretic, chromatographic, spectroscopic and crystallization properties, and fingerprints and amino acid compositions of its tryptic peptides are identical to those of HbF (Huisman *et al.* 1956; Sturgeon *et al.* 1963; Schroeder *et al.* 1974). As described in Chapter 2, fetal haemoglobin shows structural heterogeneity and consists of two molecular forms, with the formulae $α_2γ_2^{136Gly}$ ($^Gγ$) and $α_2γ_2^{136Ala}$ ($^Aγ$). Thus it can be described by the ratio of $^Gγ/^Aγ$ chains (Schroeder & Huisman 1970). Huisman

The β thalassaemias   329

et al. (1974) examined the $^G\gamma/^A\gamma$ ratios of the HbF of 84 homozygotes and 130 heterozygotes for β thalassaemia. The samples were derived from many different ethnic groups. Heterozygotes tended to fall into two groups, in which the ratio was either 2 to 3, similar to that found in many adults, or about 7 to 3, nearer that which is found in newborn infants. The homozygotes had a broad scatter, with a mean of about 3 to 2 regardless of the findings in the parents. One ethnic group, Kurdish Jews, studied by Rachmilewitz *et al.* (1973) seemed to differ slightly, with a ratio closer to that seen in adults.

More recent studies, discussed in detail in Chapter 10, have provided evidence that the structure of the fetal haemoglobin that is produced both in normal individuals and in those with disorders of β globin is under the influence of a variety of complex genetic factors. Some of these involve polymorphisms of the β-globin-gene cluster while, in the case of β thalassaemia, the situation becomes infinitely more complex because particular mutations may be involved in setting the relative output of the $^G\gamma$ and $^A\gamma$ loci. For this reason it has been easier to try to analyse these interactions in β-thalassaemia heterozygotes (Kutlar *et al.* 1990). When viewed against a background of such complexity it is not surprising that the $^G\gamma/^A\gamma$ ratios in the more severe forms of β thalassaemia show such a broad scatter.

The intercellular distribution of fetal haemoglobin has been assessed using a variety of modifications of the acid elution technique of Kleihauer *et al.* (1957). Several studies (Frazer & Raper 1961; Mitchiner *et al.* 1961; Shepherd *et al.* 1962; Silvestroni *et al.* 1968a; Kattamis *et al.* 1975) have reported that it is heterogeneously distributed among the red cells. It should be remembered that this technique has limitations and, when there are very high levels of HbF and there is marked heterogeneity of haemoglobinization of different red-cell populations, the results may be difficult to interpret. However, there seems little doubt that there is a remarkable variability in the amount of HbF per cell; this indicates that there is a marked variation in the amount of HbF being synthesized in individual red-cell precursors. There is no evidence that fetal haemoglobin synthesis is localized to a single clone of red cells.

Gabuzda *et al.* (1963, 1967), using *in vitro* [^{14}C] glycine labelling of haemoglobin, showed that the turnover of HbF is slower than that of Hbs A and A_2 in thalassaemia major. This is due to the longer sur-vival of cells that contain relatively more fetal haemoglobin. This concept is confirmed by *in vitro* studies of haemoglobin synthesis in the peripheral blood of β thalassaemics. The mechanisms of differential survival and turnover of Hbs A and F in β thalassaemia are discussed in detail in Chapter 5.

It is clear therefore that increased levels of HbF in the red cells is a major feature of both homozygous β^0 and β^+ thalassaemia. In both conditions there is remarkable heterogeneity in the amount of HbF per red cell in the peripheral blood, and clear-cut evidence that those cells which contain the most HbF survive their passage through the bone marrow and in the peripheral blood more effectively.

Haemoglobin A_2

An elevated level of HbA_2, expressed either as a percentage or in picograms (pg) per cell, is an invariable finding in heterozygous β^+ or β^0 thalassaemia. The reported levels in homozygotes or compound heterozygotes have ranged from subnormal, through normal, to elevated (Table 7.7). The difficulties in interpreting these data are similar to those in assessing the level of HbF. Many series have reported levels in patients who have received regular transfusion and even if estimated just before transfusion must have been modified to a varying degree by the presence of transfused blood. In the series of pretransfusion patients described by Kattamis *et al.* (1975), with the mean level of HbA_2 expressed as a percentage of the total haemoglobin in 54 β-thalassaemia homozygotes, of whom 11 were of the β^+ variety, was 3.0% with a range from 0.8 to 5.5%. The absolute value, i.e. converting to pg/cell by calculating the MCH and percentage HbA_2, was not given. However, the mean MCH for the 54 patients was 24.3 pg and hence the mean HbA_2 value was 0.73 pg, very close to the normal value of about 0.75 pg/cell. Even these data, derived from patients who had not received blood transfusion, are difficult to assess. Because of the remarkable cellular heterogeneity in the peripheral blood of homozygous β thalassaemics and the high levels of HbF, it is not clear whether the percentage HbA_2 should be related to the percentage HbA, when it will invariably be raised, or to the total haemoglobin, when it may vary widely, or indeed whether it is valid to express it in pg/cell in a situation where there is such marked heterogeneity of haemoglobinization of cells.

Table 7.7 Some haemoglobin A_2 values in series of patients with homozygous β thalassaemia.

No.	Population	Mean (% HbA_2)	Range (% HbA_2)	Range (% HbF)	Reference
12	Italian and Greek	2.5	1.4–4.1	–	Kunkel *et al.* (1957)
12	Italian	–	<1.5–7.3	–	Carcassi *et al.* (1957a)
8*	Italian	4.2	3.1–5.9	13–57	Marinone & Bernasconi (1957)
8*	Italian	Not detectable	–	70–95	Marinone & Bernasconi (1957)
8*	Italian	1.5	0.5–2.2	57–92	Marinone & Bernasconi (1957)
9*	Italian	2.2	1.5–5.0	27–89	Silvestroni *et al.* (1957)
2	–	1.5 and 5.0	–	27 and 89	Josephson *et al.* (1958)
21*	Greek	–	1.1–13.0	10–70	Fessas (1959)
4*	Black	3.1	2.9–3.5	62–70	Went & MacIver (1961)
12*	–	2.3	1.2–3.5	13–76	Sitarz *et al.* (1963)
54†	Greek	3.0	0.8–5.5	38–92	Kattamis *et al.* (1975)

* Pre-transfusion.
† Before transfusion regimen started.

Table 7.8 Relative amounts of haemoglobins A, F and A_2 in different fractions observed after centrifugation of blood from a patient with β thalassaemia intermedia (untransfused).

Fraction	MCV (fl)	MCH (pg)	MCHC (%)	HbA_2 (%)	HbF (%)	HbA_2 (pg)	HbF (pg)	HbA (pg)
Top	98	27.3	27.7	7.60	62.0	2.07	16.9	8.3
Whole blood	85	26.6	30.4	4.26	75.5	1.10	20.1	5.4
Bottom	83	26.3	31.7	3.17	79.1	0.83	20.8	4.7

MCH, mean cell haemoglobin; MCHC, mean cell haemoglobin concentration; MCV, mean cell volume.

The central question therefore is whether the amount of HbA_2/cell is the same across the heterogeneous population of red cells in the peripheral blood of β thalassaemics and, in particular, whether in those cells which contain predominantly HbF the amount of HbA_2 is the same as in those which contain predominantly HbA. Loukopoulos and Fessas (1965) attempted to measure the absolute amount of HbA_2 in pg/cell in different populations obtained by centrifugation of the peripheral blood of homozygous β thalassaemics. Most of their cases had received transfusions. They concluded that the absolute level of HbA_2 did not vary very much between populations and that there was a slight absolute increase in HbA_2 in each population. Similar studies in the authors' laboratory, using blood from patients with thalassaemia intermedia to overcome the problems of transfused cells, have shown that there is a significant difference in the percentage HbA_2 between HbF-rich and HbA-rich populations, and that there appears to be an absolute decrease in the amount of HbA_2 in the HbF-rich population. A typical experi-

ment is shown in Table 7.8 and in Fig. 5.12, Chapter 5, where this problem is considered in more detail.

It is clear therefore that the HbA_2 level, measured as a percentage of the total haemoglobin, is of no diagnostic help in patients with homozygous β thalassaemia. A reasonable working hypothesis to explain the wide variation in its levels in untransfused patients has evolved, however. There is a significant difference in the absolute amounts of HbA_2 in HbF-rich as compared with HbF-poor cell populations. If those cells that produce relatively large amounts of HbF produce less HbA_2 and vice versa, and if those populations that produce relatively less HbF are preferentially destroyed in the bone marrow or in the peripheral blood, the amount of HbA_2 in the highly selected population that survives in the peripheral circulation may give a totally erroneous indication of the total amount of HbA_2 being synthesized in the bone marrow. If this notion is correct the amount of HbA_2 in the peripheral blood will vary widely according to the degree of destruction of the HbA_2-rich red-cell precursors in the marrow, the amount of

HbA$_2$ being produced in the HbF-rich populations which survive in the peripheral blood, and the activity of the bone marrow, which will in turn depend on the transfusion status at the time of estimation. An experiment which provides some of the evidence in favour of these ideas is shown in Fig. 5.12, Chapter 5. A mechanism of this kind would mean that there should be an inverse relationship between the level of HbF and A$_2$ in β thalassaemia. Such data as there are suggest that this is the case.

The structure of HbA$_2$ from one Afro-American β-thalassaemia homozygote was analysed by isolating the δ chains, peptide mapping and determining the composition of the tryptic peptides (Schroeder *et al.* 1974). They were identical to those of HbA$_2$ from normal individuals.

Occasionally a β-thalassaemia homozygote or compound heterozygote with unusually high levels of HbA$_2$, in excess of 10% of the total haemoglobin, is encountered. This usually occurs in association with forms of β thalassaemia due to deletions which remove the 5′ end of the gene and its associated promoter regions, or in homozygotes or compound heterozygotes for β thalassaemia who also have inherited the genotype associated with HbH disease. These conditions are discussed later in this chapter and in Chapter 13.

Haemoglobin A

In the period before the molecular analysis of the globin genes was possible there was much discussion about whether the 'HbA' observed in β thalassaemia was normal adult haemoglobin or whether it was a variant with a similar charge to normal. However, detailed structural studies showed no differences from normal adult haemoglobin (Guidotti 1962; Schroeder *et al.* 1974).

It is now apparent that there is a broad spectrum of levels of HbA synthesis associated with different mutations of the β-globin genes, ranging from 5–10% of normal in the case of severe alleles, to a modest reduction in the case of the extremely mild or silent alleles (see Chapter 4). Because of the extreme difficulties in measuring the absolute amount of globin synthesis, and because of the difficulty in determining rates of globin synthesis in the blood or marrow in transfused patients, it is probably unwise to make any dogmatic statements about the absolute level of HbA in transfusion-dependent forms of β thalassaemia.

Such evidence as there is, derived from haemoglobin synthesis studies and estimations of the absolute amount of HbA from the steady-state haemoglobin level, indicates that the rate of output of β^A chains in severe forms of β$^+$ thalassaemia may be extremely low, in the range of 3–10% of normal. In the milder, intermediate forms the levels vary between 40 and 80% of the total haemoglobin; these conditions are described in detail in Chapter 13. There we shall see that the levels of HbF also vary widely, even in these milder conditions, and seem to be related to other polymorphisms of the β-globin gene cluster and to the underlying β-thalassaemia mutations. There seems to be a reciprocal relationship between HbA and F production and the final level of HbA must be under the control of a wide range of factors, including the underlying β-thalassaemia mutation and the complex interactions which set the final level of HbF production.

Free α chains

Fresh haemolysates made from the blood of patients with severe forms of β thalassaemia sometimes contain trace amounts of a haemoglobin which migrates more slowly than HbA$_2$ at an alkaline pH. This fraction is best seen if the haemoglobin solutions are prepared without the use of organic solvents. It disappears on the addition of HbH (β$_4$) to the haemolysate (Fessas & Loukopoulos 1964), an observation which suggests that it consists of free α chains which can combine with the β chains of HbH to form HbA. A similar fraction has been found in lysates of red cells containing haemoglobins with an unstable β chain such as Hb Köln. Presumably the α and β chains of these variants dissociate and the unstable β chains precipitate, leaving free α chains in solution.

In vitro haemoglobin synthesis

In vitro globin synthesis studies, described in detail in Chapter 5, have provided a clear picture of haemoglobin production in severe forms of β thalassaemia (Heywood *et al.* 1965; Weatherall *et al.* 1965; Bank & Marks 1966; Bargellesi *et al.* 1967; Modell *et al.* 1969; Weatherall *et al.* 1969b).

In non-thalassaemic reticulocytes α- and β-chain synthesis is synchronous and the cells have only a very small pool of free α chains. If reticulocytes or bone-marrow cells from patients with severe β thalassaemia are incubated with radioactive amino acids for periods ranging from a few minutes to several hours there is always more radioactivity incorporated into the α-chain fraction than into the combined β- and γ-chain fractions (Fig. 7.19), and the ratio of α/β+γ radioactivity varies considerably, with a published range of 1.5–30 (Table 7.9). Imbalanced globin synthesis leads to a substantial amount of free α chains in the red cells and their precursors, which can be demonstrated by both gel filtration (Modell *et al.* 1969) and DEAE-cellulose chromatography (Weatherall *et al.* 1969b) (see Fig. 5.4, Chapter 5). The α chains in this pool exist as both monomers and dimers and can combine with newly made β and γ chains to produce Hbs A and F, respectively (Modell *et al.* 1969). The pattern of haemoglobin synthesis in the bone marrow in the severe forms of β thalassaemia, the reasons for the apparent discrepancies between α/β+γ production ratios between the peripheral blood and marrow, and the fate of excess α

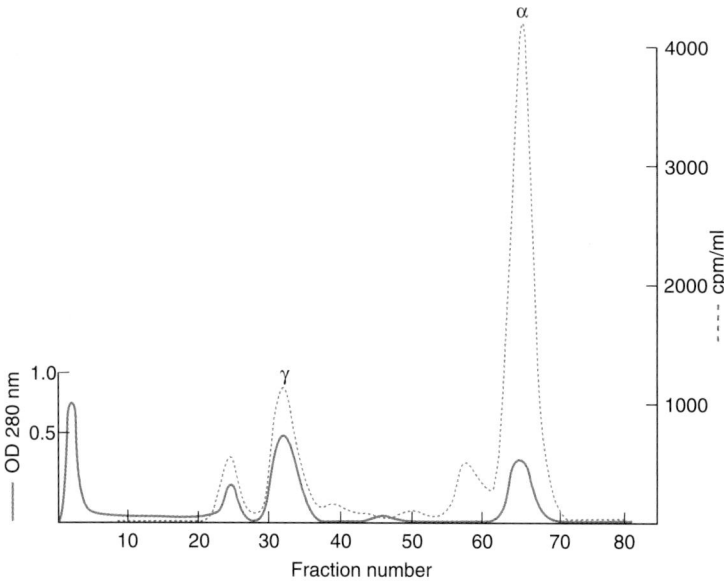

Fig. 7.19 Globin synthesis in the blood of a patient homozygous for β⁰ thalassaemia. The conditions are described in detail in Chapter 5. As shown by the broken line there is considerable globin imbalance, with a major excess of α chains. There is no β-globin-chain synthesis.

Table 7.9 Some typical globin synthesis studies in β thalassaemia.

β Thalassaemia type	Blood			Marrow			Reference
	α/β	α/γ	α/β+γ	α/β	α/γ	α/β+γ	
β⁺	15.0	—	—	9.3	—	—	Braverman & Bank (1969)
β⁺	7.4	—	—	5.1	—	—	
β⁺	8.7	Mean 4.1	—	5.8	Mean 2.2	—	
β⁺	5.0	—	—	4.8	—	—	
β⁺	15.0	—	—	9.9	—	—	
β⁰	—	3.3	—	—	7.7		
β⁰	4.2	—	4.2	3.5	—	3.5	Shchory & Ramot (1972)
	4.5	—	4.4	3.9	—	3.9	
β⁺	4.1	3.7	2.0	2.9	3.2	1.5	Friedman *et al.* (1972)
	4.2	3.0	1.8	2.3	5.2	1.6	
β⁺	3.7	4.7	2.1	3.3	14.0	2.7	
β⁺	3.6	7.1	2.5	6.1	12.5	4.1	Nathan & Benz (1976)
β⁰	—	1/0	1.0	—	5.0	5.0	
β⁰	—	1.5	1.5	—	5.8	5.8	

chains and their role in generating the anaemia of β thalassaemia are discussed in detail in Chapter 5, where the reader will find the range of published globin synthetic ratios derived from bone-marrow studies.

Because of the rapid destruction and turnover of excess α chains in the bone marrow and the heterogeneity of cell populations with respect to γ-chain synthesis, the measurement of globin synthesis ratios in the marrow and blood, if performed in the standard way at a single time-point, does not give information about the *absolute* rates of synthesis of individual chains. Nevertheless, it gives a reasonable indication of the overall severity of the defect in β-globin synthesis. Similarly, provided that the various pitfalls associated with measurements of total counts or specific activities, as outlined in Chapter 5, are taken into consideration, it can be used to monitor the effects of different forms of therapy designed to augment γ-globin synthesis, or other modalities, with a reasonable degree of accuracy.

Heterozygous β thalassaemia

Throughout the early thalassaemia literature, the clinical and haematological heterogeneity of what were later recognized as milder forms of β thalassaemia was stressed. At one end of the scale were individuals with chronic anaemia and splenomegaly associated with skeletal changes characteristic of intermediate or even major forms of the disease. Several less severe forms were recognized. These were characterized by moderate anaemia and splenomegaly, sometimes complicated by leg ulcers or gallstones: a condition which probably corresponds to the Malattia Rietti–Greppi–Micheli of early Italian writers. At the other end of the spectrum were the symptomless carrier states, thalassaemia minima, or microcytaemia, as described in the extensive studies of Silvestroni and colleagues in Italy, and by Neel, Valentine and colleagues in the USA. The story of how the true genetic relationship of these mild conditions to the severe forms of thalassaemia was elucidated is outlined in Chapter 1.

In later years it became apparent that these descriptions included a diversity of disorders, many of which resulted from the interaction of more than one thalassaemia gene. It is now clear that the *true* heterozygous states for the common forms of β thalassaemia are usually symptom free and associated with only a mild degree of anaemia. However, because there are so many different molecular variants of β thalassaemia, their heterozygous phenotypes, though usually mild, show subtle, and occasionally quite marked, differences.

Classification

The heterozygous states for different forms of β thalassaemia are summarized in Table 7.1. The majority are asymptomatic, hence the term β thalassaemia minor, or trait. The most common varieties are associated with an elevated level of HbA$_2$ and a normal or slightly elevated level of HbF. There are rarer variants with unusually high levels of Hbs A$_2$ or F. Another group is characterized by normal levels of HbA$_2$, conditions which are also heterogeneous, particularly with respect to the haematological findings which are either typical of β-thalassaemia trait or normal, or almost so. Finally, there is a much rarer group which is characterized by more severe haematological abnormalities; they result from the co-inheritance of a single β-thalassaemia allele with chromosomes containing extra α-globin genes, or may reflect the action of a genuinely dominant β-thalassaemia allele.

The common forms of heterozygous β thalassaemia

The heterozygous states for most forms of β thalassaemia are characterized by mild anaemia, red-cell abnormalities, an elevated level of HbA$_2$ and a normal or only slightly elevated level of HbF.

Clinical findings

Patients heterozygous for β thalassaemia are symptom free; the condition is usually diagnosed either as part of a family study, as an incidental finding during an intercurrent illness, or as part of a population survey. Occasionally, the mild degree of anaemia brings a carrier to the notice of the physician during a routine health check.

The literature on the 'symptomatology' of heterozygous β thalassaemia is difficult to evaluate. In a series of 123 β-thalassaemia carriers, Gardikas (1968) found that 12 complained of fatigue and lassitude, 22 had symptoms relating to gallstones, and five had mild pyrexia for which no other cause could be found.

In a series of 254 Italian subjects, Mazza *et al.* (1976) noted that 40% of their patients complained of weakness; symptoms were much more frequently observed in females and showed no relationship to the degree of anaemia. These studies were not controlled and hence raise the question of how often such non-specific complaints might be encountered in a non-thalassaemic population. The high frequency of gallstones in the series of Gardikas *et al.* suggests that some of their patients may have had more severe forms of thalassaemia.

Symptoms of this kind were not reported by Pootrakul *et al.* (1973) and Knox-Macaulay *et al.* (1973) in large series of Thai and British subjects. If anything, these reports would have been biased towards symptomatic cases since they were based on hospital practices. The haematological findings were very similar in all these studies and hence the difference in the associated symptomatology is difficult to explain. Whatever the reason, it is now evident that the great majority of patients with heterozygous β thalassaemia are symptomless.

The only common clinical presentation is a refractory anaemia of pregnancy. We shall consider this problem later in this chapter. In the series of Knox-Macaulay *et al.* (1973) several patients had been treated with iron for many years due to the erroneous diagnosis of iron-deficiency anaemia. This is particularly common in populations in which the disease is relatively infrequent. Bannerman and Callender (1961b) reported that, occasionally, heterozygous β thalassaemics may suffer from recurrent attacks of left upper quadrantic abdominal pain, which may result from perisplenitis. This has not been a feature of the larger series quoted earlier and we have never observed this symptom.

The reported physical findings in heterozygous β thalassaemia vary between ethnic groups. In the majority of individuals there are no abnormal physical signs. In the large series reported from Thailand and the UK, splenomegaly was not a feature. The incidence of palpable spleen has varied widely in reports from the Mediterranean region. For example, Fessas (1959) reported that the spleen was palpable in about 50% of cases in Greece, yet Gardikas (1968) observed splenomegaly in only 14 of 123 individuals of the same population group. In the large Italian series of Mazza *et al.* (1976) liver or spleen enlargement was observed in 10% and 19% of cases, respectively. There was no correlation between sex and age

and splenomegaly, nor was there any relationship between the size of the spleen and the degree of anaemia. Certainly, in several hundred β-thalassaemia heterozygotes from many different ethnic groups observed in our clinics, palpable splenomegaly has not been a feature, and it is our practice always to look for another cause if splenomegaly is found in what otherwise appears to be genuine heterozygosity for β thalassaemia.

Haematological findings

Anaemia

The haematological findings are remarkably similar among different ethnic groups. Several reported studies in which data were obtained by electronic cell counting are summarized in Table 7.10. Where a series has been adequately analysed by sex and age it is clear that, although there is a considerable scatter in haemoglobin levels, most heterozygous β thalassaemics have a significant degree of anaemia as compared with 'normal control' individuals from the same population. As pointed out by Castaldi *et al.* (1974, 1975) these large series may not give an entirely representative view of the overall incidence of anaemia in heterozygous β thalassaemia because many of them were derived from hospital-based studies and the ages of the patients were not always given. These workers found that there was a significant degree of anaemia in 86 out of 87 heterozygous β-thalassaemic males and in 61 out of 70 females. Furthermore, Castaldi and Zavagli (1972) noted that there was a significant degree of anaemia in heterozygous β-thalassaemic children aged between 2 and 12 years seen in a hospital population in Rovigo. Weatherall (1964a) observed that the degree of anaemia in β-thalassaemia carriers of African origin is less than that seen in patients from the Mediterranean region, a finding which was confirmed in later series (Charache *et al.* 1974; Millard *et al.* 1977). As we shall see in a later section, this probably reflects the particular mildness of the β-thalassaemia alleles in African populations.

Red-cell indices

The red-cell indices are a valuable diagnostic feature. There is a relatively high red-cell count, which in some cases is of such a magnitude as to suggest the

Table 7.10 Haematological data in heterozygous β thalassaemia.

Population	Sex or age	No.	Hb (g/dl)	RBC (×10^12/l)	MCH (pg)	MVC (fl)	Reference
Greek	Male	85	10.4–16.6 (13.9±1.20)	5.1–7.8 (6.3±0.4)	18–29 (22.0±0.4)	—	Malamos *et al.* (1962)
Thai and Chinese	Male	168	9.25 (12.0±1.38)	4.20–7.87 (5.95±0.78)	16–34 (20.0±3.0)	49–106 (67±9)	Pootrakul *et al.* (1973)
	Female	194	8.25–16.0 (10.78±0.95)	3.29–7.32 (5.21±0.64)			
British	Male	32	8.7–14.7 (11.8±1.50)	4.60–6.60 (5.60±0.60)	18.6–25.6 (21.5±1.3)	63.1–77.1 (70.5±4.2)	Knox-Macaulay *et al.* (1973)
	Female	51	8.4–12.5 (10.8±0.90)	4.30–6.70 (5.10±0.50)	18.8–25.1 (21.8±1.4)	63.0–82.1 (70.3±4.8)	
Italian	Male	82	8.0–15.5 (12.73±1.34)	3.70–6.70 (5.40±0.69)	15–31 (23.5±1.02)	50–98 (76.29±1.03)	Mazza *et al.* (1976)
	Female	69	8.8–14.6 (10.93±1.34)	3.0–7.10 (4.80±0.65)			
	Children	103	9.0–13.0 (11.34±1.04)	3.80–5.70 (4.70±0.58)			
Turkish	Male	64	7.8–15.7 (11.6±1.5)	3.9–6.7 (5.2±0.7)	18–25 (22±2)	66–82 (74±5)	Dinçol *et al.* (1979)
	Children	19	8.0–13.4 (10.5±1.2)	3.6–3.4 (4.9±0.6)	20–23 (21±2)	66–79 (72±4)	
Sardinian	Male	43	11.4–15.3 (13.3±0.8)	5.0–7.0 (6.1±0.5)	14–25 (22±2)	59–85 (66±4)	Galanello *et al.* (1979)
	Female	107	9.1–14.0 (11.8±0.9)	4.0–6.7 (5.4±0.4)	18–26 (22±2)	55–78 (66±4)	

diagnosis of polycythaemia if this is judged by the red-cell count alone! However, the red cells are small and poorly haemoglobinized and, as is demonstrated clearly in Table 7.10, the MCV and MCH are markedly reduced. On the other hand the MCHC is usually in the normal range or only moderately reduced. There seems little doubt that the vast majority of heterozygous β thalassaemics have reduced MCH and MCV values. This is certainly the case if these indices have been obtained from electronic cell counting. For example, in the large Italian series of Mazza *et al.* (1976) the MCV was less than 83 fl in 75% of subjects and the MCH less than 26.5 pg in 86% of cases, i.e. below two standard deviations from the mean for the normal control population. Similar figures were obtained in British subjects (Knox-Macaulay *et al.* 1973), in Greek-Americans (Pearson *et al.* 1974) and in Cypriots (Modell & Berdoukas 1984). Many series showing a wider scatter of values for red-cell indices have not made use of electronic cell counting and hence the figures for the red-cell count must be interpreted with caution. This was pointed out by Pootrakul *et al.* (1973), who found a wide scatter of both MCV and MCH values, which they thought was almost certainly due to the fact that the first half of their series was based on red-cell counts done with a counting chamber. Data on red-cell size distribution, based on electroimpedance, are reported by Tatsumi *et al.* (1992).

The finding of reduced MCV or MCH values in the vast majority of heterozygous β thalassaemics has been used as a basis for population screening for these disorders (Pearson *et al.* 1973, 1974; Klee 1980; Letsky & Weatherall 1998). Provided the electronic cell counter is well calibrated it seems likely that it will pick up somewhere in excess of 95% or more of β-thalassaemia heterozygotes. The MCH and MCV seem to be equally reliable in this respect. In a recent study, directed at analysing the sensitivity of this approach to the diagnosis in pregnancy, it was found that, though it may involve a relatively large number of confirmatory HbA$_2$ estimations, cut-off values for the MCV and MCH of 80 fl and 27 pg, respectively, would detect virtually all affected women (Letsky & Weatherall 1998). As we shall see later, even these values would still miss some carriers of unusually mild β-thalassaemia alleles (see Chapter 14 for a discussion of screening).

Over recent years it has become clear that a number of factors may modify the red-cell indices in heterozygous β thalassaemia. These include the nature of the underlying thalassaemia allele, the co-inheritance of α thalassaemia, and the presence of triplicated or quadruplicated α-globin genes. These factors were not analysed in the large series of β-thalassaemia heterozygotes cited in the previous paragraphs, which may account for some of high red-cell indices that they include. We shall return to this question and discuss its practical implications later in this chapter and in Chapter 14.

Of course, similar red-cell changes are sometimes found in iron-deficiency anaemia. Overall, however, the red-cell indices are different in this condition. The characteristic finding in β-thalassaemia heterozygotes is a very high red-cell count with poorly haemoglobinized cells and only slight anaemia. In iron-deficiency anaemia the red-cell count is lower and there is usually a more severe degree of anaemia if the MCH and MCV are in the β-thalassaemic range. Based on this principle several formulae have been established which relate the MCV, red-cell count and haemoglobin as an approach to discriminating between iron deficiency and thalassaemia. They are discussed in Chapters 14 and 16.

Reticulocyte count

Reticulocyte counts, expressed either as a percentage or in absolute terms, have been reported in several large series (Pootrakul *et al.* 1973; Mazza *et al.* 1976). Both these studies showed that there is a broad range, but that, on average and expressed in either way, there is a slight reticulocytosis of about twice the normal value. In the series of Mazza *et al.* (1976) there was a significant correlation between the absolute reticulocyte value and the haemoglobin level.

Red-cell morphology

There are morphological changes of the red cells in all but the mildest forms of heterozygous β thalassaemia. Characteristically there is microcytosis and hypochromia with some variation in the size and shape of the red cells (Fig. 7.20). The presence of target cells, which was stressed by earlier workers, is very variable and although some may be found their absence is of little diagnostic value. Basophilic stippling is a frequent finding, particularly in Mediterranean patients, although by no means so common in African populations (Weatherall 1964a) or Orientals (Pootrakul *et al.* 1973). After splenectomy small numbers of α-chain inclusions can be found in the

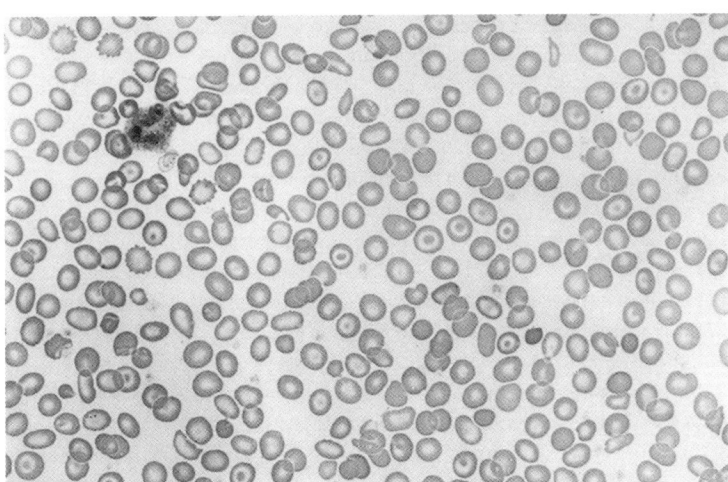

Fig. 7.20 The peripheral blood film in heterozygous β thalassaemia (Wright's stain×232).

peripheral blood although these are not seen in patients with intact spleens (Yataganas & Fessas 1969).

Completely normal red-cell morphology was thought to be extremely uncommon in heterozygous β thalassaemia. In a careful analysis of a large Thai series, Pootrakul and colleagues found only 15 patients in whom they could find no morphological abnormalities of the red cells. They noted that this finding did not run true in their families and reasoned that it resulted from differing expressivity of the thalassaemia genes rather than that normal morphology was the characteristic of a specific form of thalassaemia, as suggested by earlier workers (Ceppellini 1959a; Beaven *et al.* 1964). As we shall see later in this chapter, since the co-inheritance of α and β thalassaemia or the presence of mild β-thalassaemia alleles can modify the degree of haemoglobinization and morphology of the red cells, it seems quite possible that both these explanations for the occurrence of almost normal red-cell morphology may have been correct!

The complex interplay between the high red-cell count and slightly reduced packed cell volume and its effect on whole-blood viscosity is discussed by Crowley *et al.* (1992).

Bone marrow

Excellent descriptions of the bone-marrow appearances in heterozygous β thalassaemia are to be found in the early Italian literature (for example Astaldi *et al.* 1951). There is a variable degree of erythroid hyperplasia, in which polychromatic, pyknotic normoblasts predominate. The cytoplasm is often ragged and shows variable basophilic stippling. Iron is usually plentiful and is distributed normally between the reticulo-endothelial elements and the red-cell precursors. Yataganas and Fessas (1969) found that, on incubation of the marrow with methyl violet, a proportion of the cells show small inclusions similar in type to those seen in abundance in the red-cell precursors of homozygous individuals. This observation was confirmed by electron microscopy (Wickramasinghe *et al.* 1980).

Red-cell survival

The red-cell survival in heterozygous β thalassaemia is normal by the Ashby technique (Kaplan & Zuelzer 1950) and ^{51}Cr half-life times have given mean values just below the normal range in four reported series (Pearson *et al.* 1960; Malamos *et al.* 1961; Gallo *et al.* 1975; Pippard & Wainscoat 1987). Gallo *et al.* were not able to relate the degree of anaemia to the red-cell survival in their small series. Evidence for a small red-cell population with a significantly shortened survival was reported by Honetz *et al.* (1968).

Iron, ferrokinetics and erythropoietin response

Iron status

Serum iron and ferritin estimations have shown that, though there is considerable variability, the mean values are little different from normal (Kattamis *et al.*

1972; Knox-Macaulay *et al.* 1973; Pootrakul *et al.* 1973; Hussein *et al.* 1976; Economidou *et al.* 1980; Pippard & Wainscoat 1987; Galanello *et al.* 1990c). Similarly there are usually no abnormalities of the total iron-binding capacity or per cent saturation of the iron-binding capacity. Information about different molecular forms of serum ferritin is reported by Lasne *et al.* (1991). As will be discussed later, it is not uncommon to find nutritional iron-deficiency anaemia in association with heterozygous β thalassaemia (Kattamis *et al.* 1972; Saraya *et al.* 1984). Galanello *et al.* (1990c) suggest that iron deficiency is less common in children who are β-thalassaemia carriers than in normal children in their population.

Iron loading

Iron loading, as evidenced by an increased serum iron or ferritin levels or iron deposition in the tissues, is unusual. In the series of patients described by Knox-Macaulay *et al.* (1973) five females and four males had iron binding saturations of 50% or more and one 68-year-old woman, who had received iron intermittently for 15 years due to the mistaken diagnosis of iron-deficiency anaemia, had a totally saturated iron binding capacity and clinical evidence of iron overload. Williams and Siemsen (1968) described iron loading in a 30-year-old male who had not received iron therapy. It is not clear why this patient was iron loaded; possibly he had one of the severer forms of β thalassaemia mentioned later in this chapter. Similar patients have been reported by Bowdler and Huehns (1963), Tolot *et al.* (1970) and Parfrey and Squier (1978); the latter workers' patient also had a hepatoma.

In addition to these case reports Fargion *et al.* (1985) described a group of Italian males who had very high serum ferritin levels. Of 101 β-thalassaemia carriers Van der Weyden *et al.* (1989) found 23 individuals with raised plasma ferritin values, 10 of whom also had elevated levels of red-cell ferritin; liver biopsies performed in four showed significant iron overload. The authors emphasize the high incidence of inappropriate iron administration in this group of patients.

It is difficult to evaluate these cases of heterozygosity for β thalassaemia with iron loading. It is possible that some of them result from the administration of oral iron over very long periods because of errors in diagnosis. It is likely that at least some reflect cases of

more severe forms of β thalassaemia, as discussed later in this chapter and in Chapter 13. It is also possible that, since both β thalassaemia and hereditary haemochromatosis are common, the two determinants could be found together in the same individual.

β-Thalassaemia trait and hereditary haemochromatosis

Among populations of north European origin two mutations have been identified at the locus for hereditary haemochromatosis (HFE), the substitution of cysteine for tyrosine at position 282 (C282Y, nucleotide 845) and of histidine for aspartate at amino acid 63 (H63D, nucleotide 187) (Feder *et al.* 1996). Over 90% of patients in north Europe are homozygous for C282Y (Jouanolle *et al.* 1997). In a preliminary examination of 5956 chromosomes (2978 individuals) for the presence of these mutations, Merryweather-Clarke *et al.* (1997) found that the C282Y gene reaches its highest frequency in north European populations and is extremely rare in many Mediterranean countries and in other parts of the world where thalassaemia is common. However, Carella *et al.* (1997) have found that 64% of patients with hereditary haemochromatosis in Italy are homozygous for this allele, 10% are heterozygous and 21% carry the normal allele. The H63D allele is less frequent but has a similar frequency among affected and normal chromosomes. This disease is heterogeneous at the molecular level and different mutations in the HFE gene or other genes may be involved. Furthermore, it is now clear that the H63D mutation does have some functional significance in iron homeostasis (Feder *et al.* 1998), and because this is more widely dispersed in parts of the world where thalassaemia occurs (Merryweather-Clarke *et al.* 1997) the possibility remains that at least some of the variability in iron loading in β-thalassaemia trait may be related to the co-inheritance of one or other allele for hereditary haemochromatosis.

Iron absorption

Iron absorption studies have given variable results. Bannerman and Callender (1961a) reported normal values utilizing food iron and ^{59}Fe-labelled inorganic iron. Crosby and Conrad (1964) found slightly increased iron absorption using a whole-body counter.

Ferrokinetics and erythrokinetics

Iron is rapidly removed from the plasma, the rate of plasma turnover is increased, but iron appears in the red cells relatively slowly, only 50–60% of the initial dose being incorporated in 12–14 days. This figure is intermediate between the very low iron incorporation values obtained in homozygous individuals and the 80–90% incorporation values found in normal persons (Larizza *et al.* 1958; Pearson *et al.* 1960). In a more extensive series of ferrokinetic studies (Pippard & Wainscoat 1987) it was confirmed that the overall efficiency of erythropoiesis is significantly reduced, with a mean of 76±17 standard deviations of normal. In this study values for the total plasma iron turnover were normal or only slightly increased. This suggests a lack of any additional stimulus to erythropoiesis which might normally be expected to compensate easily for the mild degree of anaemia. Interestingly, serum erythropoietin levels are slightly elevated, more so in females than males; there is no correlation with the haemoglobin level (Vedovato *et al.* 1993).

Gallo *et al.* (1975) demonstrated an increased excretion of faecal urobilinogen in heterozygous β thalassaemics. They found a good correlation between the degree of anaemia and the output of faecal urobilinogen in a series of 10 patients. In the same patients the red-cell survival was slightly shortened and did not vary greatly from case to case. This observation led Gallo's group to the conclusion that the observed differences in faecal urobilinogen excretion must reflect differences in the degree of intramedullary destruction of erythroblasts, i.e. ineffective erythropoiesis is largely responsible for the varying severity of the anaemia in this disorder. Pearson *et al.* (1960) and Pippard and Wainscoat (1987) also concluded, using ferrokinetic and red-cell survival studies, that the severity of the anaemia is unrelated to peripheral haemolysis and depends on the relative degree of ineffective erythropoiesis. Similar conclusions were reached earlier by Bruzzese *et al.* (1970, 1973), Rotoli (1976) and Cazzola *et al.* (1979).

The serum bilirubin level shows considerable variation but in the large series of Mazza *et al.* (1976) it was slightly increased and the level correlated significantly with the degree of anaemia. Recent studies have related at least some of this variability to the co-inheritance of the gene for Gilbert's syndrome (see later section).

Complications

The vast majority of patients heterozygous for β thalassaemia go through life without any manifestations that can be ascribed to the disease. The only complication of any importance is a worsening of the anaemia during pregnancy.

Pregnancy

The haemoglobin level may fall to a lower level during pregnancy than in normal women (Meital *et al.* 1961; Pritchard 1962; Ibbotson & Crompton 1963; Beaven *et al.* 1964; Hocking & Ibbotson 1966; Knox-Macaulay *et al.* 1973; Schuman *et al.* 1973; Sicuranza *et al.* 1978; Cooley & Kitay 1984; White *et al.* 1985; Landman 1988). Fleming (1973) noted that the anaemia of pregnancy in β-thalassaemia heterozygotes may sometimes be reflected by placental hypertrophy and fetal distress. However, it is clear that the anaemia is usually mild, and that most of the reports of more severe forms of anaemia in pregnancy reflect the additional complications of either iron or folic acid deficiency (Knox-Macaulay *et al.* 1973; White *et al.* 1985; Landman 1988).

In normal pregnant women there is an increase in both the plasma volume and red-cell mass which commences at about the end of the first trimester. Schuman *et al.* (1973) found that pregnant thalassaemic women are unable to increase their red-cell mass to the same degree as normal women; there is no difference in the degree of expansion of the plasma volume in pregnancy between normal and thalassaemic women. Interestingly, a pregnant β-thalassaemic carrier does show a significant increase in the red-cell mass, though insufficient to match that of her plasma volume. Iron supplements do not improve the erythropoietic response unless, as occurs quite frequently, heterozygous β thalassaemia is complicated by iron deficiency during pregnancy. A single case report, describing the administration of erythropoietin, did not show a convincing response; although there was a small rise in the haemoglobin level this occurred in the third trimester, when this is known to occur in normal pregnancies (Juncà *et al.* 1995).

The haemoglobin levels in two well documented series of pregnant β-thalassaemia heterozygotes are shown in Table 7.11. On average, the decrease in the haemoglobin level between the first and second trimester is comparable with that of normal controls,

Trimester	Normal controls Hb (g/dl)	No.	β-Thalassaemia trait Hb (g/dl)	No.	Reference
1	12.7		10.8		White *et al.* (1985)
2	11.7	6844	9.6	208	
3	12.4		10.1		
1	12.5		10.6		Landman (1988)
2	11.2	160	9.8	48	
3	11.2		9.9		

Table 7.11 Mean haemoglobin levels in two series of pregnant women with β thalassaemia. The series of White *et al.* is drawn from women of 16 ethnic backgrounds in the United Arab Emirates. Those described by Landman are of black and Asian origin.

Table 7.12 Folic acid and vitamin B_{12} status of pregnant women with β-thalassaemia trait drawn from 16 ethnic backgrounds in the United Arab Emirates. No supplementation was given (White *et al.* 1985). Normal ranges: folate <2.0 µg/l; B_{12} <150 ng/l.

	Gestational age (weeks)	Normal (n=784) Mean	Range	% deficient	β thalassaemia (n=97) Mean	Range	% deficient
Folate (µg/l)	20	3.6	0.7–16.5	9.2	3.1	0.4–12.1	8.3
	36	2.9	0.5–12.1	11.2	3.2	–	10.7
B_{12}	20	276	52–744	7.8	296	43–1100	6.7
	36	231	30–512	37.6	228	32–761	33.4

in the range of 7 and 10%, respectively. In the large series of White *et al.* (1985) there were minimal changes in the red-cell indices and Landman (1988) observed only a slight increase in the MCV (mean value 2.8 fl) and the MCH (mean value 0.6 pg). It is clear therefore that any pregnant β-thalassaemia carrier with a haemoglobin value of less than 8–9 g/dl should be investigated for other causes for the anaemia. The likelihood of there being co-existent iron or folic acid deficiency will depend to a large extent on whether the woman has been receiving supplementation and on her social and dietary background. There have been a number of reports of heterozygous β thalassaemia in pregnancy being complicated by iron (Knox-Macaulay *et al.* 1973; Hegde *et al.* 1975) or folate deficiency (Goldberg & Schwartz 1954). In the large series reported by White *et al.* (1985), summarized in Table 7.12, the frequency of folate deficiency was approximately the same in pregnant β-thalassaemia heterozygotes and controls. The role of iron and folate deficiency in aggravating anaemia in pregnancy, particularly in the third trimester, was well documented by Landman (1988). Because of the unreliability of serum iron and iron binding capacity estimations in pregnancy it is impor-

tant to assess the patient's iron status by the estimation of the serum ferritin level.

The finding of a high frequency of apparent vitamin B_{12} deficiency, at least as assessed by the serum vitamin B_{12} level, summarized in Table 7.12 from the large series of White *et al.* (1985), is surprising and difficult to assess. The authors of this report point out that at least some of their patients may have had a dietetic basis for this finding although it should be pointed out that serum vitamin B_{12} levels in pregnancy do tend to fall and there is no evidence that this is associated with functional vitamin B_{12} deficiency.

In two large series in which the maternal outcome was assessed it was concluded that, anaemia apart, β-thalassaemia trait had no deleterious effects on pregnancy, labour or the fetus (Hocking & Ibbotson 1966; Landman 1988).

Folic acid deficiency

Folic acid deficiency has been reported in heterozygous β thalassaemia in non-pregnant persons (Chanarin *et al.* 1959), but this must be extremely rare (Silva & Varella-Garcia 1989). Indeed, it is unlikely that the slightly increased marrow turnover would cause folate deficiency unless the diet is severely depleted in folate (Saraya *et al.* 1984) or there are other complicating factors such as malabsorption or pregnancy. For this reason it seems unnecessary to provide heterozygous β thalassaemics with long-term folate supplements.

Failure of diagnosis

Another notable complication is the suffering experienced by patients in whom the disorder remains undiagnosed for many years. This is more likely to occur in populations in which β thalassaemia is not common and physicians are unaware of the possibility of the diagnosis. In their review of 16 British families Knox-Macaulay *et al.* (1973) found that 14 of the probands and 32 of the 67 affected family members had received a remarkable variety of diagnostic labels before their condition had been recognized for what it was. These included iron-deficiency anaemia, megaloblastic anaemia, sideroblastic anaemia, leukaemia, malabsorption, recurrent blood loss, rheumatic fever, lead poisoning and polycythaemia! Treatment had included iron by various routes for up to 15 years, folic acid, a variety of vitamin injections, liver extracts, corticosteroids and, for good measure, an appendicectomy and hysterectomy! Perhaps not surprisingly, this group of patients had suffered from considerable anxiety and many totally unnecessary investigations. Another common variation on this iatrogenic theme is the unfortunate fact that when a patient is labelled as having heterozygous β thalassaemia any subsequent symptoms may be ascribed to this condition.

Infection

There is no evidence that individuals with β-thalassaemia trait are more prone to infection. Interestingly, there is a report of anaemia in two siblings following human parvovirus infection (Lefrère *et al.* 1986). This is a curious observation in view of the normal or only slightly reduced red-cell survival in β-thalassaemia heterozygotes; severe anaemia due to transient erythroid hypoplasia associated with parvovirus infection is usually only observed in individuals with considerably shortened red-cell survival such as those with sickle-cell anaemia or hereditary red-cell enzyme defects.

Life expectancy

In an extensive study aimed at defining the lifespan of individuals heterozygous for β thalassaemia no significant differences were found between thalassaemics and normals (Gallerani *et al.* 1990). Surprisingly, the same group, in a prospective study of 4401 subjects admitted to St Camillo Hospital, Ferrara, over a 7-year period concluded that male β-thalassaemia heterozygotes showed a significant degree of protection against myocardial infarction (Gallerani *et al.* 1991). Furthermore, the mean age at which myocardial infarction occurred in male heterozygotes was significantly higher than that in normal males; no such differences were found among female subjects. At first sight these findings seem contradictory although it is possible that the relatively small effect on the frequency of myocardial infarction was masked in the life-expectancy survey. These observations require further investigation in other populations.

Haemoglobin constitution

The haemoglobin pattern in heterozygous β thalassaemia is usually characterized by an elevated level of HbA_2 and a slight but significant elevation in the level of HbF in about 50% of cases. Although in the early literature, before methods for determination of Hbs F and A_2 were better standardized, there was considerable scatter in the reported values, this has become less noticeable in recent years.

Haemoglobin A_2

Since the initial observation of Kunkel *et al.* (1957) that the HbA_2 was elevated in β thalassaemia minor, this finding has become the main diagnostic feature. Kunkel and his coworkers found a mean level of HbA_2 of 5.1 (±1.35)% in 34 thalassaemia carriers compared with a value of 2.54 (±0.35)% in 300 normal individuals. These findings were subsequently confirmed by many groups (Carcassi *et al.* 1957a; Silvestroni *et al.* 1957; Gerald & Diamond 1958; Josephson *et al.* 1958; Fessas 1959; Vella 1959; Weatherall 1964a). Haemoglobin A_2 values in β-thalassaemia carriers from different ethnic groups are summarized in Table 7.13. The reader will be struck by the remarkable uniformity of these data. Despite the fact that they are derived from different elec-

Population	No.	HbF (%)	HbA$_2$ (%)	Reference
Greek	85	0.9–8.3 (3.1)	3.6–6.6 (5.2±1.1)	Malamos *et al.* (1962)
British	83	0.5–9.4 (1.8±0.70)	3.8–6.2 (4.9±0.5)	Knox-Macaulay *et al.* (1973)
Thai	310	0–7.8 (1.5±1.5)	3.6–7.1 (5.1±0.6)	Pootrakul *et al.* (1973)
Italian	254	0–14 (1.9±1.5)	3.5–8.0 (5.3±1.1)	Mazza *et al.* (1976)
Afro-American β$^+$	33	0.2–8.0 (1.76±2.1)	3.5–6.4 (4.9±0.7)	Millard *et al.* (1977)
Afro-American β^0	29	0.1–9.2 (1.2±1.9)	3.8–6.9 (5.2±1.2)	Millard *et al.* (1977)
Turkish	164	0.56 (1.2±1.3)	3.8–6.5 (4.7±0.6)	Dinçol *et al.* (1979)
Sardinian	150	0.1–2.5 (1.0±0.50)	4.1–6.6 (4.9±0.5)	Galanello *et al.* (1979)

Table 7.13 Haemoglobin F and A$_2$ values (%) in heterozygous β thalassaemia.

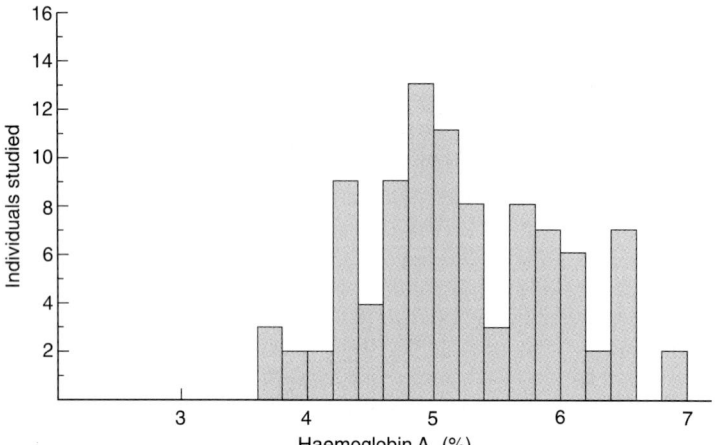

Fig. 7.21 The distribution of HbA$_2$ values in heterozygous β thalassaemia. Data from the authors' laboratory.

trophoretic and chromatographic techniques it appears that the upper limit of normal for HbA$_2$ values is somewhere in the region of 3.3% and that in heterozygous β thalassaemia the range is from 3.5 to 7% with a mean of approximately 5% (Fig. 7.21).

The increased percentage of HbA$_2$ results in an alteration of the HbA/A$_2$ ratio from the normal value of 40 to about 20. Does this reflect a relative or absolute increase in the amount of HbA$_2$? In order to produce a relative increase of HbA$_2$ to twice its normal percentage there would have to be a decrease in the output of HbA of a greater magnitude than that which usually occurs in heterozygous β thalassaemia. Furthermore, several series have shown that there is no relationship between the percentage of

HbA$_2$ and the haemoglobin level. Assuming that the HbA$_2$ is homogeneously distributed among the red cells, the average amount per cell, as derived from the MCH and percentage HbA$_2$, can be computed as approximately 0.7 pg. In an individual with heterozygous β thalassaemia, with an MCH of 20 pg and a HbA$_2$ level of 5.0%, this value increases to a level of approximately 1.0 pg. As pointed out by Weatherall (1964a) there is a reasonable correlation between the percentage HbA$_2$ and the MCH. Thus for any given HbA$_2$ value the absolute amount is increased by about 33%, to about 1 pg.

Another often-asked question is whether the increase in HbA$_2$ results from augmented activity at both δ-chain loci or only at the *cis* locus (i.e. on the same chromosome) to the β-thalassaemia gene. In fact there is excellent evidence that both the *cis* and *trans* (i.e. the gene on the opposite chromosome to the thalassaemia gene) δ-chain loci increase their output. Thus individuals heterozygous for both β thalassaemia and a δ-chain variant, HbA$_2$′ (HbB$_2$), have increased levels of both normal ($\alpha_2\delta_2$) and abnormal ($\alpha_2\delta_2'$) minor haemoglobin components (Ceppellini 1959a; Huisman *et al.* 1961; Weatherall *et al.* 1976; Codrington *et al.* 1990) (see Chapter 3). This finding suggests that although there is defective synthesis at only one β-chain locus the activity of both δ-chain loci is increased. In other words the increased output of δ chains is not just the product of the δ-chain locus adjacent to the β-chain locus carrying the thalassaemia mutation but is due to increased output from both δ-chain loci. As discussed in more detail below, while this is generally true, there are some subtle differences in the relative output from the two δ loci depending on the nature of the β-thalassaemia mutation.

Several workers have noted a tendency for intrafamilial segregation of HbA$_2$ values in heterozygous β thalassaemia (Carcassi *et al.* 1957b; Gerald & Diamond 1958; Weatherall 1964a). This observation suggests that at least some of the factors concerned with the final level of HbA$_2$ in β thalassaemia are genetic in origin. We shall return to this question when we consider the findings in β-thalassaemia heterozygotes with different β-globin-gene mutations.

The level of HbA$_2$ may be reduced in heterozygous β thalassaemics who also have severe iron-deficiency anaemia. It has been reported that the level may fall into the normal range and is restored to its elevated level after iron therapy (Wasi *et al.* 1968a; Kattamis *et al.* 1972), but this must be unusual. What usually seems to happen is that, although the level may fall, it remains elevated in the range found in β-thalassaemia trait (Steinberg 1993).

Why is the level of HbA$_2$ elevated in heterozygous β thalassaemia? Early studies indicated that there is no correlation between the HbA$_2$ level and the haemoglobin level, packed cell volume, red-cell morphology, HbF level or any other associated haematological findings, except the MCH (Fessas 1959; Weatherall 1964a; Pootrakul *et al.* 1973). Thus analyses of this type gave no clue as to the possible mechanism.

Current explanations for the relative reduction in output of δ compared with β chains, which implicate

the defective δ-globin-gene promoter, are discussed in detail in Chapters 2 and 8. Although the precise mechanism for the elevation of HbA$_2$ in β-thalassaemia heterozygotes is not known it seems likely that several factors are involved. One appears to be imbalanced globin synthesis; studies of HbA$_2$ levels in different forms of β thalassaemia, described later in this chapter, indicate that, overall, they seem to be higher in association with more severe β-thalassaemia mutations. This may at least in part reflect a post-translational mechanism. If, as seems likely, α chains combine more readily with β than with δ chains, in the presence of a β-chain deficit there will be a greater likelihood of α chains combining with δ chains and hence an increased level of HbA$_2$ (reviewed by Huisman 1997).

One exception to the observation that HbA$_2$ values tend to be higher in association with severe β-thalassaemia mutations is the finding that relatively high levels also occur in association with mild promoter mutations of the β-globin gene (see later section). This suggests another possible mechanism for the elevation of HbA$_2$. If transcription factors for the globin genes are present in rate-limiting quantities, and if there is inefficient binding to the altered β-globin promoters, this may free more factors for the inefficient δ-globin promoter and hence there may be a relatively high level of HbA$_2$ in the presence of a mild deficit of β-globin production. Evidence that this is the case has been obtained by Codrington *et al.* (1990), who found that, in individuals who are heterozygous for both β thalassaemia and a δ-chain variant, the output from the δ locus *cis* to β-globin-gene promoter mutations is increased relative to that on the other chromosome, even though the output of both δ-globin genes is elevated.

These observations underline the complexity of the regulation of δ-globin-chain production in β thalassaemia and why there may be considerable variability in the levels of HbA$_2$ in heterozygotes.

Haemoglobin F

If an increased level of HbF is demonstrable at all in heterozygous β thalassaemia it is only slightly elevated, and not in every case. In the early study of Beaven *et al.* (1961) of 130 affected individuals, over half had no demonstrable HbF while the remainder had levels in the 1.5% range, with a mean value of 2.1%. Only seven cases had levels of over 5%. Similar data were obtained by Fessas (1959) and Weatherall (1964a). These studies have been confirmed in recent years. In the large series summarized in Table 7.13 there is a remarkable similarity between the mean values for HbF. In the series of Pootrakul *et al.* (1973) and Knox-Macaulay *et al.* (1973) approximately half of the cases had normal values while the remainder were slightly elevated, in the 2–3% range. Similar figures were obtained by Mazza *et al.* (1976). The distribution of HbF levels in over 300 heterozygous β thalassaemics studied in the authors' laboratory is shown in Fig. 7.22.

In all the larger series of HbF levels a few individuals fall outside the distribution of normal to 2–3%, and have values ranging between 4 and 15%. Knox-Macaulay *et al.* (1973) suggested that some β-thalassaemia heterozygotes with unusually high levels of HbF might also be heterozygous for heterocellular HPFH. In fact they were able to show independent segregation of the β thalassaemia and HPFH genes in one of their families. In a retrospective study of all the β-thalassaemia heterozygotes with values of HbF of 4% or over shown in Fig. 7.22 we found that other heterozygotes in the same families had elevated levels of HbF, and in several families it was observed that there is independent segregation of β thalassaemia and elevated HbF levels (Weatherall *et al.* 1980). Mazza *et al.* (1976) found 10 patients with levels of HbF ranging from 4 to 14% in their β-

thalassaemia heterozygotes; four were δβ-thalassaemia heterozygotes while the remaining six were all members of the same family and had values ranging from 5 to 12%. Their clinical and haematological findings were the same as those of other β-thalassaemia heterozygotes in the study. Similarly, in two studies of the interaction of heterocellular HPFH with β thalassaemia it was found that the haematological findings in the doubly affected individuals were the same as those in β-thalassaemia heterozygotes (Wood *et al.* 1976b, 1977b). The interaction of heterocellular HPFH and β thalassaemia is discussed in more detail in Chapter 10.

It is clear therefore that the majority of β-thalassaemia heterozygotes who have levels of HbF in excess of 4–5% also carry one or more genes for heterocellular HPFH. Rarely, as we shall see in a later section, unusually high levels of HbF reflect the direct effect of a β-thalassaemia mutation.

The distribution of fetal haemoglobin within the red cells, as judged by either acid elution or fluorescent antibody techniques, is quite heterogeneous and there is no evidence that it is confined to single red-cell populations (Shepherd *et al.* 1962; Wood *et al.* 1975).

There is no relationship between the level of fetal haemoglobin and the severity of anaemia, red-cell indices or HbA$_2$ values. Weatherall (1964a) found that there was a significant tendency for intrafamilial

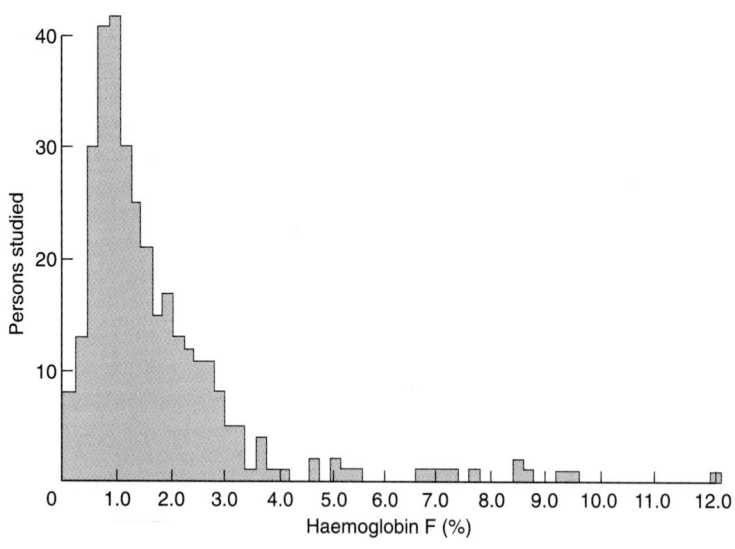

Fig. 7.22 The distribution of HbF values in 331 β-thalassaemia heterozygotes studied in the authors' laboratory.

segregation of HbF values, indicating that several factors are involved in setting the final level, some of which are genetic. There is very little evidence that acquired factors alter the level of HbF to any significant degree in this condition; the only one that has been adequately documented is pregnancy, during which the normal rise of fetal haemoglobin which occurs at mid-term is mirrored in heterozygous β-thalassaemia carriers by an increase at about the same time. It returns to its basal level some time towards the end of pregnancy (Popat *et al.* 1977). The level of HbF is not modified by co-existing iron deficiency (Kattamis *et al.* 1972).

The mechanism for the elevated level of HbF in heterozygous β thalassaemia is considered in Chapter 5. The $^{G}\gamma/^{A}\gamma$-chain composition of the HbF is described earlier in this chapter.

Red-cell metabolism

A variety of metabolic abnormalities of the red cell have been demonstrated. The best known is the decrease in osmotic fragility, which, in contrast to normal red cells, becomes even more marked after sterile incubation for 24 h (Selwyn & Dacie 1954). The addition of glucose during incubation prevents β-thalassaemic cells becoming more resistant to osmotic lysis (Fig. 7.23). The value of the osmotic-fragility test in screening for β thalassaemia is discussed in Chapter 14. The other changes in red-cell metabolism and membrane function are discussed in detail in Chapter 5.

Other biochemical changes

The red-cell free protoporphyrin is elevated (Ziegler & Marti 1966; Lyberatos *et al.* 1972; Hinchliffe *et al.* 1995). As mentioned earlier, plasma ferritin levels are normal or slightly elevated and this may be a useful guide to distinguishing heterozygous β thalassaemia from iron deficiency (Hussain *et al.* 1976; Loria *et al.* 1978). Serum lipid levels, including cholesterol and α and β lipoproteins, are normal (Pantelakis & Doxiadis 1967).

Globin synthesis

The results of studies on the relative rates of α- and β-chain synthesis in the peripheral blood and bone

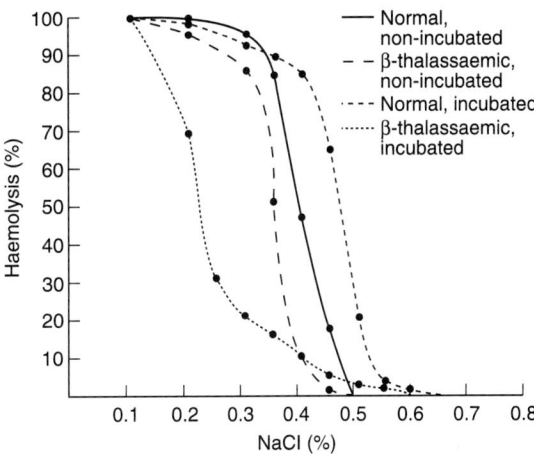

Fig. 7.23 Osmotic-fragility curves of the red cells of a heterozygous β thalassaemic compared with those of a normal individual.

marrow in heterozygous β thalassaemia were discussed in detail in Chapter 5. In summary, there is imbalanced synthesis, with α-/β-chain production ratios ranging from 1.5 to 2.5, both in the bone marrow and in the peripheral blood. Reports of more balanced globin synthesis in the bone marrow were later found to be based on artefacts produced by the presence of radioactively labelled non-globin proteins which cochromatograph with β globin. Hence the measurement of globin synthesis ratios, particularly if peripheral blood reticulocytes are used, provides a valuable confirmatory test for the presence of heterozygosity for β thalassaemia in cases in which the diagnosis is uncertain.

Phenotypic characteristics in relation to different molecular forms of β thalassaemia

Over recent years data have been published which relate the haematological findings and HbA$_2$ and F levels to particular β-thalassaemia mutations. Although this information is limited, it is possible to make some broad generalizations about phenotype/genotype relationships.

Some selected haematological data from β-thalassaemia heterozygotes with different β-thalassaemia alleles, derived from reports from Gonzalez-Redondo *et al.* (1988a,b), Rund *et al.* (1990), Rosatelli *et al.* (1992a) and Stefanis *et al.* (1994), are shown in Tables 7.14–7.16. Although there is some overlap, it is clear that the common, mild β-thalassaemia mutations, notably IVS1-6 T→C, −29 A→G, −87 C→G, and −88 C→T, for example, have slightly higher haemoglobin levels and, more importantly, higher MCH and MCV values than the more severe β⁰- and β⁺-thalassaemia alleles. Similarly, the other mild alleles for which sufficient data are available, including the forms of β thalassaemia associated with Hbs E, Malay and Knossos, are associated with MCH and MCV values that are either normal or only slightly reduced (see also Chapter 13). Indeed, the

pattern that is emerging is of a continuous spectrum of haematological findings, ranging from those associated with severe β⁰- or β⁺-thalassaemia alleles, through milder changes associated with less severe alleles, to complete normality in the silent alleles (see later section). However, because of the wide scatter of values, as indicated in Tables 7.14–7.16, and because of the lack of sufficient published data relating to specific alleles broken down by age, sex and other confounding factors, it is difficult to be dogmatic about the 'typical' red-cell indices associated with a particular allele.

Table 7.14 Average haematological values for β-thalassaemia trait related to genotype. From Gonzalez-Redondo *et al.* (1988a).

Mutation	Subject nos.	Age (yrs)	Hb (g/dl)	PCV (l/l)	RBC ($\times 10^{12}$/l)	MCV (fl)	MCH (pg)	MCHC (g/dl)	HbA$_2$ (%)	HbF (%)	$^G\gamma$ (%)
−29 A→ G (β⁺)	15	2–59	11.7	0.380	5.22	72.8	22.4	30.8	4.75	3.3	68.7
−29 A→ G (β⁺)	4	24–57	10.9	0.360	5.06	71.1	21.5	30.3	5.05	1.3	19.9
−29 A→ G (β⁺)	1	50	12.5	0.380	5.44	70.0	23.0	32.9	4.90	0.6	21.8
−88 C→ T (β⁺)	5	20–75	12.7	0.380	5.22	72.8	24.3	33.4	5.05	3.9	60.9
−88 C→ T (β⁺)	4	24–52	11.8	0.345	4.70	73.4	25.1	34.2	5.40	2.4	14.9
CD24 T→ A (β⁺)	5	4–68	11.5	0.370	4.86	76.0	23.7	31.1	4.15	1.3	70.9
CD24 T→ A (β⁺)	1	30	12.4	0.395	4.95	80.0	25.1	31.4	4.10	0.8	30.6
1.35 kb del (β⁰)*	2	22–30	9.9	0.300	4.80	63.0	20.6	33.0	7.10	3.3	26.0
CD 6 (−A) (β⁰)	2	24–41	12.3	0.410	5.84	69.0	21.0	30.2	5.50	1.1	70.7
CD61 (A→ T) (β⁰)	1	24	11.1	0.380	5.82	65.0	19.1	29.2	4.10	0.8	30.6

MCH, mean cell haemoglobin; MCHC, mean cell haemoglobin concentration; MCV, mean cell volume; PCV, packed cell volume; RBC, red-cell count. * Removes the 5′ end of the β gene.

Table 7.15 A summary of haematological and biosynthesis data for heterozygotes for the three common Greek β-thalassaemia mutations (Stefanis *et al.* 1994).

Parameter range	Subject sex	β⁺⁺ IVS1-6 T→C			β⁺ IVS1-110 G→A			β⁰ CD39 C→T		
		No.	Mean ± SD	Range	No.	Mean ± SD	Range	No.	Mean ± SD	Range
Hb g/dl	M	10	14.58 ± 0.78	13.9–15.8	9	14.33 ± 1.27	11.6–15.6	10	12.73 ± 0.80	11.2–13.8
	F	7	12.25 ± 0.77	10.8–13.1	12	11.91 ± 1.05	10.7–13.9	7	11.94 ± 0.62	11.2–12.8
Haematocrit (%)	M	10	44.36 ± 2.61	41.0–48.0	9	43.22 ± 3.07	37.0–47.0	10	38.80 ± 2.61	35.0–44.0
	F	7	38.50 ± 2.14	35.0–42.0	12	36.75 ± 2.38	33.0–41.0	7	36.75 ± 2.12	34.0–40.0
MVC (fl)	M	10	65.96 ± 6.59	58.3–78.2	9	56.57 ± 2.96	53.5–62.8	9	59.07 ± 4.62	52.4–69.0
	F	7	66.89 ± 8.93	59.3–81.6	10	57.18 ± 2.20	51.5–61.0	7	64.23 ± 2.40	60.7–67.9
	M +F	17	66.32 ± 7.35	58.3–81.6	19	56.89 ± 2.87	51.5–62.8	16	No data	52.4–69.0
MCH (pg)	M	10	21.67 ± 2.00	19.2–25.3	9	18.71 ± 0.76	17.3–20.0	9	19.87 ± 1.81	17.8–23.8
	F	7	21.44 ± 2.12	19.5–25.5	10	18.57 ± 1.24	16.5–20.2	7	20.71 ± 0.78	20.0–22.3
	M +F	17	21.58 ± 1.98	19.2–25.5	19	18.64 ± 1.02	16.5–20.2	16	20.27 ± 1.45	17.8–23.8
α-/non-α biosynthesis ratio		13	2.17 ± 0.34	1.78–2.90	10	2.35 ± 0.28	1.86–2.81	11	2.33 ± 0.35	1.70–2.71

Table 7.16 Haematological features (mean ± 1 SD) in β-thalassaemia heterozygotes in relation to the type of β-thalassaemia mutation. From Rosatelli *et al.* (1992a).

	No. subjects	RBC ($\times 10^{12}$/l)	Hb (g/dl)	PCV (%)	MCV (fl)	MCH (pg)	MCHC (%)	HbA$_2$ (%)
IVS1-110 G→A	34	6.28 ± 0.43	13.2 ± 1.0	40.2 ± 2.9	63.8 ± 1.1	21.1 ± 1.1	32.4 ± 9.0	4.5 ± 0.4
IVS1-1 G→A	10	6.18 ± 0.39	12.8 ± 0.8	39.5 ± 2.9	63.3 ± 3.1	20.3 ± 1.0	30.1 ± 3.1	4.8 ± 0.4
IVS1-6 T→C	11	5.96 ± 0.31	13.8 ± 2.2	42.6 ± 2.2	70.4 ± 1.9	23.3 ± 0.7	32.2 ± 0.7	3.9 ± 0.4
IVS2-745 C→G	11	6.38 ± 0.34	13.1 ± 1.7	39.4 ± 1.7	62.5 ± 3.0	20.3 ± 1.0	31.8 ± 1.4	5.0 ± 0.5
CD6 (−A)	15	6.29 ± 0.66	13.1 ± 1.2	40.0 ± 3.9	63.3 ± 2.8	20.8 ± 1.3	31.1 ± 1.3	5.2 ± 0.3
CD39 C→T	34	6.38 ± 0.34	13.3 ± 0.9	40.8 ± 2.7	62.9 ± 3.0	21.1 ± 1.2	33.0 ± 1.3	5.1 ± 0.4
−87 C→G	11	5.70 ± 0.62	14.1 ± 1.4		74.0 ± 5.2	24.7 ± 1./9		5.3 ± 0.7
Total	126							

PCV, packed cell volume; MCH, mean cell haemoglobin; MCHC, mean cell haemoglobin concentration; MCV, mean cell volume, RBC, red-cell count.

Table 7.17 Haemoglobin A$_2$ levels in β-thalassaemia heterozygotes related to mutations. From Huisman *et al.* (1997).

Mutation	n	HbA$_2$%	Mutation	n	HbA$_2$%
−101 C→T	5	3.50 ± 0.5	IVS1-6 T→C	39	3.60 ± 0.2
−88 C→T	32	5.65 ± 0.3	IVS1-110 G→A	86	4.55 ± 0.2
−29 A→G	64	4.95 ± 0.3	CD36/37 −T	7	5.35 ± 0.3
+22 G→A	5	3.85 ± 0.3	CD38/39 −C	8	5.60 ± 0.3
Initiation CD A→G	4	6.10 ± 0.2	CD39 C→T	81	4.85 ± 0.3
CD8 −AA	28	5.15 ± 0.3	CD41/42 −TTCT	6	5.55 ± 0.4
CD8/9 +G	8	5.25 ± 0.4	CD44 −C	5	5.00 ± 0.3
CD15 TGG-TGA	11	5.10 ± 0.3	CD82/83 −G	8	4.75 ± 0.3
CD16	5	5.50 ± 0.4	IVS2-1 G→A	46	5.10 ± 0.4
CD19 A→G	8	3.65 ± 0.2	IVS2-654 C→T	6	4.55 ± 0.5
CD24 T→A	7	3.90 ± 0.3	IVS2-745 C→G	17	4.95 ± 0.5
CD27 G→T	2	4.4; 4.2	IVS2-849 A→C	2	5.1; 5.7
CD30 G→C	2	5.3; 5.7	IVS2-850 G→A	6	5.5 ± 0.41
IVS1-1 G→A	55	5.00 ± 0.4	CD112 T→A	2	4.7; 4.6
IVS1-1 G→T	10	5.35 ± 0.5	CD121 G→T	11	4.65 ± 0.3
IVS1-5 G→C	15	4.59 ± 0.4	Position +6, 3′ CD147 C→G	4	2.40 ± 0.1

The HbA$_2$ levels found with particular mutations have been reviewed in detail by Huisman (1997). Overall, and though there is considerable overlap, several groups can be defined (Table 7.17). Carriers of β^0- or severe β$^+$-thalassaemia alleles have HbA$_2$ values between 4.5 and 5.5%, whereas those with β$^+$-thalassaemia alleles are between 3.6 and 4.2%. There are exceptions to these findings, however. Carriers of β-globin-gene promoter mutations tend to have relatively high values of HbA$_2$ even though these are mild β-thalassaemia alleles. The highest HbA$_2$ values in heterozygotes appear to be associated with the rare deletional forms of β thalassaemia (reviewed by Thein 1993 and in Table 7.18). In these cases the values have ranged from 5 to nearly 9%, providing further proof that mutations which either involve or remove the β-globin-chain promoters tend to be associated with particularly high values of HbA$_2$.

The levels of HbF in β-thalassaemia heterozygotes associated with different mutations have been reviewed by Gonzalez-Redondo *et al.* (1988a,b) and Kutlar *et al.* (1990) and for the deletional forms of β thalassaemia by Thein (1993). One of the difficulties in assessing results from different laboratories is that the methods used to assess the level of HbF differ considerably in their sensitivity, particularly at low levels. Kutlar and colleagues suggest that high-performance liquid chromatography (HPLC) using a weak cation exchanger is probably the most accurate, and have used this approach to assess the levels of HbF in large numbers of β-thalassaemia heterozygotes. Furthermore, these analyses are complicated by the presence or absence of polymorphisms, particularly C→T at –158 $^G\gamma$, which are thought to modify both the $^G\gamma/^A\gamma$ ratio and level of HbF, under conditions of erythropoietic stress. However it appears that this is not always the case and HbF with a high $^G\gamma$ value is not always associated with unusually high levels of HbF in β-thalassaemia heterozygotes. Nevertheless, within the limit of all these constraints it is possible to make a few generalizations.

It appears that β-thalassaemia heterozygotes with

Table 7.18 Haemoglobin F and A$_2$ values in heterozygotes for deletion forms of β thalassaemia (from Thein 1993). The deletions are defined in Chapter 4.

Deletion	HbA$_2$ (%)	HbF (%)
Asian Indian	4.7–6.2	0.4–1.9
Turkish, Jordanian, Iranian	4.6–8.1	2.7–9.4
Black	8.6	0.2
Black, British	7.2–8.4	1.8–6.9
Croatian	7.6, 8.6	5.8, 8.8
Thai	6.7	4.5
Czech	8.1–9.0	3.3–5.7
Turkish	6.6, 8.5	1.9, 2.0
Asian Indian	7.1–7.8	3.2–4.7
Australian (Anglo-Saxon)	6.4–8.1	2.5–7.2
Dutch	5.3–7.6	5.1–14.4
Vietnamese	2.7–5.1	18.0–27.0
Filipino	7.7, 7.5	1.0, 4.0
Italian		9.0

certain mutations, notably –88 C→T, –29 A→G and IVS1-1 C→A, appear to have relatively elevated levels of HbF independent of the C→T change at –158 $^G\gamma$. On the other hand, carriers of mutations such as IVS1-6 T→C, IVS1-110 G→A, CD24 T→A, CD39 C→T, CD41/42 (–TCTT) and IVS2-745 C→G tend to fall into two groups, that is, with high $^G\gamma$ and low $^G\gamma$ types of HbF; neither are associated with high HbF values. The HbF levels in association with the rare deletional forms of β thalassaemia are summarized in Table 7.18. It is clear that all those which involve the β-globin-gene promoter are associated with unusually high levels of HbF, ranging from 3 to 14%.

It is difficult to summarize these complex issues, particularly in view of the paucity of available data. However, it appears that, overall, point mutations involving the β-globin-gene promoters are associated with slightly higher levels of HbF than other forms of β thalassaemia, that other mutations are usually associated with low levels, and that the only conditions that are regularly found to have unusually high levels are those that are caused by deletions of the β-globin-gene promoters.

Developmental changes in the haematological findings and haemoglobin constitution

Because of the changes which occur both in the red-cell indices and in the haemoglobin pattern of normal infants during the first year of life, studies which set out to describe these changes in β-thalassaemia heterozygotes must be carefully controlled with a population of normal infants at the same stage of development. Haematological and haemoglobin analytical data of this kind have been reported by Galanello *et al.* (1981) and Wood *et al.* (1982b). Galanello *et al.* (1991) have produced percentile curves for red-cell indices in β-thalassaemia heterozygotes in infancy and childhood. Further data on HbF and A$_2$ values during the first year of life are reported by Metaxatou-Mavromati *et al.* (1982). The results of these studies are remarkably consistent and provide a valuable yardstick for the identification of heterozygous β thalassaemia during the first year of life.

The haemoglobin values, red-cell indices and HbA$_2$ and F values obtained in the authors' laboratory (Wood *et al.* 1982b) are summarized in Fig. 7.24. As judged by haemoglobin levels and red-cell indices,

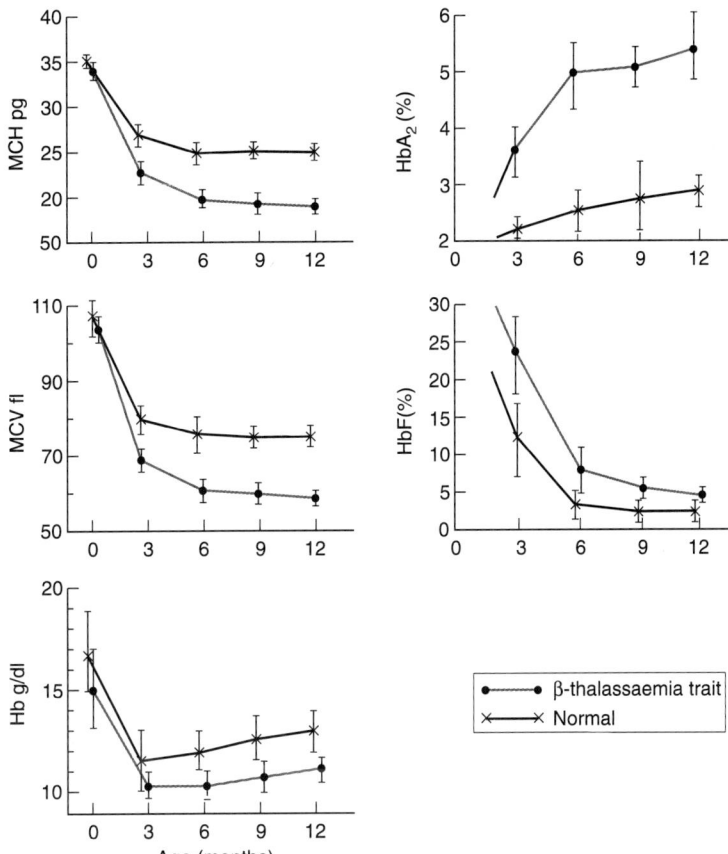

Fig. 7.24 Developmental changes in the red-cell indices and Hbs F and A$_2$ in heterozygous β thalassaemia. Data from Wood *et al.* (1982b).

heterozygous β-thalassaemic newborns do not differ significantly from normal. However, by the age of 3 months clear differences emerge, which become significant by 6 months and remain so during the rest of development. It appears therefore that carrier screening by MCV or MCH determination is feasible from about 3 months onward. Similarly, there is a clear distinction in HbA$_2$ values by 3 months. As shown in Fig. 7.24, and as was observed in all these studies, the rate of decline of HbF is retarded in β-thalassaemia heterozygotes and does not seem to reach its adult level until well into childhood.

Percentile grids for the red-cell indices and HbA$_2$ values during later childhood are reported by Galanello *et al.* (1991). The curves based on their data are particularly interesting in that they show that there is a tendency for the MCV and MCH to rise slightly in β-thalassaemia heterozygotes over the first

10 years of life, mirroring the same changes in normal children but set at a significantly lower level. It is important to remember that during the first year of life and in early infancy the red-cell indices of normal children are significantly lower than during later development. If this fact is overlooked, as it often is, it may lead to a mistaken diagnosis of thalassaemia trait. Thus in assessing the red-cell changes during the first year of life it is important to compare data of the type shown in Fig. 7.24 and the percentile curves published by Galanello *et al.* (1991).

One of the most interesting features of these data is the genuine retardation in the decline in HbF levels in β-thalassaemia heterozygotes. Although this finding remains unexplained, it suggests that the timing of the switch from fetal to adult haemoglobin production can be modified in the presence of abnormal erythropoiesis.

Pathophysiology

The principles of the pathophysiology of β thalassaemia are discussed in detail in Chapter 5. Here we shall simply review those that seem special to the case of β-thalassaemia carriers.

The mild anaemia of heterozygous β thalassaemia is the result of ineffective erythropoiesis secondary to imbalanced α- and β-chain synthesis, with precipitation of the small excess of α chains. Presumably the proteolytic enzymes of the red-cell precursors can almost, but not quite, cope with this α-chain excess. The evidence for there being ineffective erythropoiesis in this condition was summarized in previous sections and seems unequivocal. Interestingly, Gallo *et al*. (1975) found a reasonable correlation between the haemoglobin level and the faecal urobilinogen excretion and also between the haemoglobin level and the α-/β-chain production ratio. Hence the variability in the degree of anaemia presumably reflects differences in the degree of β-chain deficiency. The mild changes in red-cell membrane function probably reflect under-haemoglobinization of the red cells as much as globin precipitation. Certainly the red-cell survival is only slightly shortened and, as discussed earlier, the major cause of the anaemia seems to be ineffective erythropoiesis.

The slightly elevated levels of HbF are probably due to preferential survival of F cells. If blood from heterozygous β thalassaemics is centrifuged the number of F cells and the percentage HbF is always greater in the heavier, older cell population, suggesting that these cells have a preferential survival in exactly the same way as they do in homozygous β thalassaemia (see Chapter 5).

One interesting question, still unanswered, is why individuals with heterozygous β thalassaemia are anaemic. They can elevate their red-cell mass during pregnancy; why don't they do this normally? How well do they compensate for the degree of anaemia? Pearson *et al*. (1977) and Schettini *et al*. (1974) found that 2,3-DPG levels were elevated appropriate to the degree of anaemia but the expected increase in p50 (reduction in oxygen affinity) was not observed. In Pearson's study there was no correlation between 2,3-DPG levels, p50, haemoglobin values or symptoms. Erythropoietin levels are only marginally elevated, and only significantly so in females (Vedovato *et al*. 1993). These curious discrepancies remain unexplained.

Association with other genetic disorders

Because the heterozygous state for β thalassaemia is common it is not surprising that it has been found in association with a variety of other genetic disorders.

In many populations *glucose-6-phosphate dehydrogenase (G6PD) deficiency* and β thalassaemia are found at high frequencies and it is not surprising that they sometimes occur together in the same individual. This interaction was analysed in Sardinia by Piomelli and Siniscalco (1969). The mean haemoglobin levels in hemizygous G6PD-deficient males was 14.1 g/dl, thalassaemic males 13.6 g/dl and males with both disorders 12.5 g/dl. The red-cell indices in thalassaemic males were not altered by co-existent G6PD deficiency. It appeared that the mild degree of anaemia caused by these traits is additive in doubly affected heterozygotes. However, Sanna *et al*. (1980) found no interaction between the two disorders except for slight differences in the MCV between thalassaemics with or without G6PD deficiency. Details of the redox state of red cells associated with this interaction are reported by Magnani *et al*. (1986).

Another common occurrence is the co-inheritance of the genetic determinant for *Gilbert's syndrome* (Galanello *et al*. 1997; Sampietro *et al*. 1997). This interesting observation may explain the variability in bilirubin levels and why it has been difficult to relate it to the degree of ineffective erythropoiesis. There is a polymorphic variation in the promoter of the bilirubin UDP-glucuronosyltransferase gene (UGT-1); the particular motif is A(TA)$_n$TATAA. Several patients with Gilbert's disease have an additional TA in this motif, i.e. the arrangement A(TA)$_7$TATAA rather than the more usual A(TA)$_6$TATAA. It has been found that the expanded variety of the promoter polymorphism occurs commonly in heterozygous β thalassaemics with unusually high bilirubin levels. Interestingly, homozygosity for the (TA)$_7$ motif is not always associated with an elevated bilirubin level in otherwise normal individuals and hence it is likely that the increasing production of bilirubin as a result of the ineffective erythropoiesis in β-thalassaemia heterozygotes is sufficient to cause unusually high blood levels in those with this genetic predisposition.

Several families have been reported in which the genes for *hereditary elliptocytosis* and β thalassaemia were segregating (Aksoy & Erdem 1968a; Swarup-Mitra *et al*. 1969; Frick 1970; Nagaratnam *et al*. 1971; Ros *et al*. 1976; Pavri *et al*. 1977). Because of the considerable clinical and genetic heterogeneity of hereditary elliptocytosis it is difficult to be sure whether the reported cases of 'interaction' of these two genes, with the production of more severe haemolysis, are interpreted correctly or whether they are examples of the severe form of hereditary elliptocytosis in an individual who also happens to have β thalassaemia (Bannerman & Renwick 1962). In one family, reported by Perillie and Chernoff (1965), it appeared as though the presence of both caused summation of the clinical effects of the individual traits but in the other cases cited above this effect was not observed.

A few families have been observed in which the genes for β thalassaemia and *hereditary spherocytosis* have occurred together (Cohen *et al.* 1959; Cunningham & Vella 1967; Aksoy & Erdem 1968b; Swarup-Mitra *et al.* 1969). Their interaction may be associated with relatively severe haemolysis but it is difficult to determine whether this is a true summation effect; hereditary spherocytosis is very variable in its expression even within members of the same family.

Possible examples of the interaction between the genes for β thalassaemia and *pyruvate kinase deficiency* were reported by Baughan *et al.* (1968) and Zoratto *et al.* (1969). The degree of haemolysis is also variable in pyruvate kinase deficiency and it is difficult to determine whether it is worsened by the thalassaemia gene. One family has been reported in which the genes for β thalassaemia and the *Pelger–Huet* abnormality of the white cells were segregating (Tannoia *et al.* 1968). Another entirely coincidental observation with no evidence for interaction was the report of a child with *hereditary methaemoglobinaemia* due to NADH diaphorase deficiency who also happened to be a β-thalassaemia carrier (Kumar *et al.* 1989).

Variant forms of heterozygous β thalassaemia

The variant forms of heterozygous β thalassaemia are summarized in Table 7.1. Although some of them are described in more detail elsewhere in this book, for the sake of completeness we shall briefly summarize their main features in the sections that follow.

Normal haemoglobin A$_2$ β thalassaemia

In previous editions of this book we reviewed the large body of literature which suggested that there must be forms of β thalassaemia in which the HbA$_2$ level in heterozygotes is not elevated. This condition was observed mainly in a setting in which an individual with mild thalassaemia intermedia was found to have one parent with typical β-thalassaemia trait with an elevated HbA$_2$ level, while the other showed either minimal or no haematological abnormalities and a normal HbA$_2$ level. Early reports of this type of patient appeared in the Italian literature, in which they were said to have a form of 'constitutional microcytic anaemia' (Silvestroni & Bianco 1951; Silvestroni *et al.* 1957). Similar families were reported later by workers from other countries (Aksoy 1959; Aksoy *et al.* 1961; Bernini *et al.* 1962). In 1969 Schwartz and colleagues described a family in which two children had a mild form of Cooley's anaemia; the father had a normal haematological picture and normal levels of HbA$_2$ and F, whereas the mother had typical β-thalassaemia trait. On incubation of the father's red cells with radioactive leucine it was found that he had a reduced rate of β-chain synthesis, with α-/β-chain production ratios similar to, although slightly less than, those found in heterozygous β thalassaemia. Schwartz called this mild form of β thalassaemia 'silent' β thalassaemia.

In 1979 Kattamis and colleagues, in a collaborative study with ourselves, analysed nine Greek patients who had β thalassaemia of varying severity, each of whom had one parent with a normal HbA$_2$. On the basis of clinical, haematological and globin synthesis studies these families fell into two groups. Heterozygotes in the six families that comprised group 1 showed minimal red-cell abnormalities though they had imbalanced globin synthesis and hence seemed to correspond to previous descriptions of 'silent' β thalassaemia; compound heterozygotes with typical β-thalassaemia carriers had the clinical picture of mild β thalassaemia intermedia. This condition therefore became known as type 1 normal HbA$_2$ β thalassaemia. The second group was comprised of three families in which the β-thalassaemia heterozygotes with normal HbA$_2$ levels showed more marked red-cell abnormalities and α-/β-globin synthesis ratios typical of β-thalassaemia trait. Compound heterozygotes for this and high HbA$_2$ β thalassaemia were transfusion dependent; heterozygotes of this type were described as having normal HbA$_2$ β thalassaemia, type 2.

Over recent years the heterogeneity and molecular basis for both these have been defined.

Normal haemoglobin A₂ β thalassaemia, type 1: 'silent' β thalassaemia

As its name implies this condition is haematologically silent in carriers and can only be identified clinically when it is found in compound heterozygotes with more severe β-thalassaemia alleles, or in the homozygous state. Globin synthesis usually shows mild imbalance, with α/β production ratios in the 1.2–1.3 range. Since these interactions produce intermediate forms of β thalassaemia of varying severity it is considered in more detail in Chapter 13; the molecular pathology is described in Chapter 4.

In a clinical setting the presence of a silent β-thalassaemia gene should be suspected in a family in which a patient with a mild form of thalassaemia intermedia is found to have one parent who is haematologically normal, or who has children who show no evidence of a high HbA₂ β-thalassaemia trait. The carrier state can only be identified with certainty by globin synthesis studies or by the demonstration of a particular mutation that is known to be associated with silent β thalassaemia. These interactions, and such data as are available about the homozygous state for the silent β thalassaemias, are reviewed in detail in Chapter 13.

Normal haemoglobin A₂ β thalassaemia, type 2

It is now apparent that this is a very heterogeneous condition. One of the commonest underlying genotypes is the compound heterozygous state for both δ and β thalassaemia, a finding which was clarified in extensive family studies by Silvestroni *et al.* (1978). It was clear from this work that the δ-thalassaemia determinant could be *cis* or *trans* to the β-thalassaemia gene.

The molecular basis for the δ thalassaemias is summarized in Chapter 4 and some of the varieties that have been found together with β thalassaemia in individuals with normal HbA₂ β thalassaemia type 2 are shown in Table 7.19. These studies, discussed in more detail in Chapter 8, have confirmed that the δ⁰- or δ⁺-thalassaemia mutations may be *cis* or *trans* to the β-thalassaemia mutation and that in some cases β haplotypes containing β- and δ-thalassaemia genes in *cis* have been disseminated throughout populations. For example, in the mild form of β thalassaemia, Hb Knossos, carriers have minimal haematological changes and low levels of HbA₂ (see Chapter 13). This phenotype results from a mild β⁺-thalassaemia mutation (CD27 G→T) together with a deletion of an A in codon 59 of the δ gene in *cis*, which com-

Table 7.19 Normal haemoglobin A₂ β thalassaemia, type 2 due to compound heterozygosity for β and δ thalassaemia.

No.	β-Thalassaemia mutation	δ-Thalassaemia mutation	HbA₂ level (%) in compound heterozygote
9	IVS2-745 C→G	δ⁺69 G→A (*cis*)	2.53–3.74 (mean 2.97)
1	IVS2-745 C→G	δ⁺27 G→T (probably *cis*)	2.2
1	IVS2-745 C→G	δ⁺27 G→T (*trans*)	2.5
1	CD39 C→T	δ⁺27 G→T (*trans*)	3.4
1	IVS2-745 C→G	δ⁺27 G→T	3.2
1	CD39 C→T	δ⁰59 (–A) (*cis*)	3.5
1	IVS1-110 G→A	δ⁰59 (–A) (*cis*)	3.2
1	IVS1-6 T→C	δ⁺27 G→T (*trans*)	2.7
Many	CD27 G→T (Knossos)	δ⁰59 (–A) (*cis*)	2–3

pletely inactivates it (Olds *et al.* 1991). Haplotype analyses suggest that the $\delta^0 59$ (–A) $\beta^{Knossos}$ allele occurs widely throughout the Mediterranean region.

The same $\delta^0 59$ (–A) mutation which occurs *cis* to β Knossos has been found in *cis* to the $\beta^0 39$ and β^+ IVS1-110 mutations (Tzetis *et al.* 1994) and $\delta^+ CD27$ G→T has been reported in both *cis* and *trans* to the β^+ IVS2-745 mutation (Loudianos *et al.* 1990; Trifillis *et al.* 1991). Other interactions of this type and the associated HbA_2 values are summarized in Table 7.19. Interestingly, while on average the HbA_2 levels fall into the normal range there is considerable scatter and in some cases values in the 3–3.7% range are observed.

Although the diagnosis of co-existent β and δ thalassaemia is best made by direct analysis of the respective globin genes, some clues can be obtained from family studies. Where the two mutations exist in *cis*, that is, on the same chromosome, the condition will be transmitted both vertically and laterally. On the other hand, if the two thalassaemia mutations are in *trans*, that is on opposite pairs of homologous chromosomes, they will separate and individuals with both high HbA_2 and normal HbA_2 thalassaemia may be found in different generations.

Phenocopies of normal haemoglobin A_2 β thalassaemia

Some forms of εγδβ thalassaemia, which involve long deletions of the β-globin-gene complex but which spare the β genes, notably the Dutch, English and Spanish varieties, are characterized by a picture which is indistinguishable from normal HbA_2 β thalassaemia, type 2, in heterozygotes. Similarly, the Corfu form of δβ thalassaemia, in which a 7.2-kb deletion removes part of the δ gene but leaves the β gene intact, is also associated with this phenotype in heterozygotes. This is because the β gene in *cis* to this deletion carries a β-thalassaemia mutation. Interestingly, these two lesions in the β-gene cluster have been described as separate mutations in two different populations; the 7.2-kb deletion starting 3' of the ψβ gene and removing part of the δ gene has been observed in an Italian (Galanello *et al.* 1990a); the normal β gene in *cis* to the 7.2-kb deletion is expressed at normal levels and hence is not associated with a β-thalassaemic phenotype. These conditions are described in detail in Chapter 8.

The homozygous state for α^+ thalassaemia or the heterozygous states for α^0 thalassaemia can also produce a phenotype which is indistinguishable from normal HbA_2 β thalassaemia (see Chapter 11).

Because the forms of this condition that are due to the inheritance of both β and δ thalassaemia can interact with other β-thalassaemia alleles to produce severe, transfusion-dependent diseases the diagnosis may be extremely important for counselling and prenatal diagnosis. Although, as mentioned above, some clues may be obtained from a careful family study the diagnosis can only be established with certainty by globin synthesis studies or by direct DNA analysis of the β- and δ-globin genes.

The problem of a borderline haemoglobin A_2 level

Considering that some forms of normal HbA_2 β thalassaemia are associated with HbA_2 levels which are in the 'no-man's land' between normal and elevated, and that some milder forms of β thalassaemia are associated with slightly elevated levels of HbA_2, as considered earlier in this chapter (Table 7.17) and in more detail in Chapter 13, what action should be taken if, during a screening procedure, an HbA_2 level of this type is encountered? The first thing to do is to repeat the estimation; if a similar value is obtained the finding cannot be ignored.

As a practical approach to this problem Galanello *et al.* (1994) analysed 125 individuals with borderline HbA_2 values as part of their β-thalassaemia screening programme. In 37 cases they were able to detect an underlying molecular defect in the β-, δ- or α-globin genes. In short, seven of the subjects were carriers for the –101 C→T mutation which is associated with 'silent' β thalassaemia (see Chapter 13), 10 carried the mild IVS1-6 T→C allele, 16 were compound heterozygotes for δ and β thalassaemia, two had triplicated α-globin genes, and two had single α-globin-gene deletions. The finding of a relatively high percentage of abnormalities in these individuals, and the fact that many of them can interact with β thalassaemia to produce severe phenotypes, suggests that in any screening programme, particularly when an individual who has a borderline HbA_2 level is planning to have a child with a partner with typical β-thalassaemia trait, it is vital to investigate the case further. Since the only reliable approach to the characterization of the suspect case is by globin-gene analysis, such persons should be referred to a centre which has this capability.

Heterozygous β thalassaemia with unusually high levels of haemoglobin A₂

As discussed earlier, although there is some variation in the elevation of HbA_2 levels in heterozygous β thalassaemia, the values tend to cluster fairly tightly between 3.5 and 6%, with a mean value of about 5%. There is, however, a rare group of β thalassaemias in which levels in excess of these values are found. They all seem to result from deletions of the β-globin gene which remove its 5′ promoter region, including sequences from position –125 to +78 relative to the CAP site; in each case the CACC, CAAT and TATA boxes of the promoter are lost. These deletions, together with original references and descriptions of their boundaries, are described in detail in Chapter 4; the associated HbA_2 levels, which may be as high as 8–9%, are summarized in Table 7.18. It is believed that the unusually high levels of HbA_2 reflect the loss of the β-globin-gene promoter and the release of rate-limiting transcription factors which can interact with the locus control region (LCR) to increase the rates of transcription of the δ- and, as we shall see later, γ-globin genes. As mentioned in an earlier section, the forms of β thalassaemia associated with point mutations in the promoter regions also tend to have slightly higher HbA_2 levels in heterozygotes than other forms of β thalassaemia but it is only in the deletional forms that levels in excess of 6% are encountered.

Heterozygous β thalassaemia with unusually high levels of haemoglobin F

As mentioned earlier and as described in detail in Chapter 10, many β-thalassaemia heterozygotes with HbF in excess of the more usual normal or slightly elevated values appear to also carry genes for one or other form of heterocellular hereditary persistence of fetal haemoglobin (HPFH). Until the molecular basis for heterocellular HPFH is determined this interaction can only be identified by finding raised levels of HbF in relatives who are not β-thalassaemia carriers. The range of HbF values in individuals of this type is summarized in Chapter 10.

It is now apparent that there are rare β-thalassaemia alleles which are associated with unusually high HbF levels. The best documented examples are those which result from deletions that remove the β-globin-gene promoter regions, of the same variety which are also characterized by unusually high HbA_2 values. The HbF levels associated with these deletional forms of β thalassaemia in heterozygotes are summarized in Table 7.18. The first variety to be described, which later became known as the *Dutch form* of β thalassaemia (Went & Schokker 1965; Schokker *et al.* 1966; Van der Ploeg *et al.* 1980), was found in a large kindred with 13 heterozygotes; their HbF values ranged from 5.1 to 14.4% with a mean value of 8.3%. As shown in Table 7.18 similar values have been found in heterozygotes for several other deletional forms of β thalassaemia. As mentioned earlier when discussing the reasons for unusually high HbA_2 levels, it is thought that the high levels of HbF result from the loss of the 5′ promoter region of the β-globin gene, which removes competition for rate-limiting transcription factors which interact with the LCR, resulting in its increased interaction with the γ and δ genes in *cis*, thus enhancing their output.

Another family in which there appeared to be a form of β thalassaemia with high HbF levels in heterozygotes was reported by Weatherall (1964a). A 32-year-old Afro-American woman was found to have a blood picture compatible with heterozygous β thalassaemia although she had 17% HbF and 4% HbA_2. One of her children had sickle-cell thalassaemia with 26% HbF; her other child had the sickle-cell trait with normal levels of HbF. Since at least two deletional forms of β thalassaemia have been found in this ethnic group it is possible that this patient had a lesion of this type; a family study showed no evidence of heterocellular HPFH.

'Isolated' elevated haemoglobin A₂ levels

Since an elevated level of HbA_2 is the hallmark of heterozygous β thalassaemia it is important to consider whether there are any conditions in which this occurs in the absence of defective β-globin synthesis. Increased levels have been described in some acquired conditions such as hyperthyroidism and megaloblastic anaemia (reviewed by Steinberg & Adams 1991). Elevated levels have also been reported in otherwise normal individuals, however. Since the co-inheritance of α thalassaemia with β thalassaemia may result in normalization of the red-cell indices and balanced globin synthesis in heterozygous β thalassaemia, leaving a raised HbA_2 as the sole abnormality, it seems likely that many of the reported cases of isolated high HbA_2 values reflect these interactions (Kanavakis *et al.* 1982; Melis *et al.* 1983). They are described in Chapter 13.

However, there may be another condition associated with a high HbA_2 level in the absence of any demonstrable abnormalities in the α- or β-globin genes. Gasperini *et al.* (1993) described two Sardinian families in which there were individuals with HbA_2 values of 3.9 and 4.7%, respectively, who had normal or almost normal red-cell indices. Detailed structural analyses of their β-globin genes revealed no evidence of a β-thalassaemia mutation and their α-globin genes were normal. Although it is theoretically possible that they might have had a so far undefined form of β thalassaemia together with a non-deletional form of α thalassaemia, globin synthesis studies in their children did not suggest that there were α-thalassaemia alleles in these families. In both cases this abnormality was passed on to a child in the second generation. Although this careful study included a detailed analysis of the δ-globin genes no explanation for the raised HbA_2 values was found.

Heterozygous β thalassaemia with an unusually severe clinical course

As indicated in Table 7.1 there are two main mechanisms whereby heterozygous β thalassaemia may run a more severe course. First, there is a family of dominantly inherited β thalassaemias of varying severity which result from mutations that give rise to products which are able to form inclusion bodies in the red-cell precursors. Second, there is the co-inheritance of a chromosome containing additional α-globin genes, either ααα or αααα. Since the dominant β thalassaemias or interactions with increased numbers of α genes produce the clinical phenotype of β thalassaemia intermedia they are described in Chapter 13.

β Thalassaemia unlinked to the β-globin-gene complex

Several reports have suggested that a form of β thalassaemia segregates independently of the β-globin-gene complex. A mutation of this type was proposed for the findings in a family described by Semenza *et al.* (1984), though further studies suggested that these observations may have resulted from a recombina-

tion event (Schwartz *et al.* 1988). Another family in which the possible β-thalassaemia phenotype caused by a mutation not linked to the β-globin-gene cluster was described by Murru *et al.* (1992). This is an extremely complex three-generation pedigree in which two children with thalassaemia intermedia of varying severity, one of whom had a child with thalassaemia major, were born of parents, one of whom was heterozygous for the β-gene codon 39 nonsense mutation while the other appeared to have a form of β-thalassaemia trait with a normal HbA_2. Because of the remarkable heterogeneity of the clinical findings in the second and third generations the authors speculate that the parent who had the clinical picture of normal HbA_2 β thalassaemia may have passed on a gene for a β-thalassaemia phenotype which is unlinked to the β-globin-gene cluster. There are, however, some very unusual phenotypes in this family, not the least the relative severity of the mother's condition; although she was said to be heterozygous for the β codon 39 nonsense mutation she had a steady-state haemoglobin of 8.1 g/dl and splenomegaly, findings that are unusual for the carrier state for this β-thalassaemia allele. The father and the two patients in the second generation have a rearrangement at position −530 to the CAP site of the β-globin gene but this was not found in the child with thalassaemia major in the third generation of the family. The authors suggest that the existence of another mutation, not linked to the β-globin-gene locus, best explains these findings.

More direct evidence for the existence of a β-thalassaemia-like allele which is not linked to the β-globin-gene cluster was reported in a study by Thein *et al.* (1993). In this four-generation family there were seven individuals who had red cells typical of heterozygous β thalassaemia, with HbA_2 levels ranging from 3.1 to 5.1, and globin synthesis ratios typical of the β-thalassaemia trait. Detailed restriction-fragment-length polymorphism haplotype analysis showed quite clearly that the genetic determinant for this phenotype was not linked to the β-globin-gene cluster. Full sequence analysis of the β-globin genes of these individuals showed no abnormality.

It seems likely that the findings in this family reflect the action of a variant *trans*-acting factor which is involved with β-globin-gene regulation; as described in Chapters 4 and 12 a similar factor has been identified as the basis for the reduced rate of α-globin synthesis in the X-linked α-thalassaemia mental retardation syndrome. It is not clear how common these unlinked forms of β thalassaemia are, though at least two further families have been reported in abstract form (Murru *et al.* 1992; Pacheco *et al.* 1995; Gasperini *et al.* 1998).

Other β thalassaemias of unknown cause

Most laboratories which have sequenced large numbers of β-globin genes during their studies of β thalassaemia have amassed a varying number of cases in which no abnormality has been found. For example, Kazazian (1990) reported that this was the case in nine of the 100 alleles that they had studied in detail with extensive sequence analysis. This kind of figure, or certainly values in excess of 5%, would probably be reported by most laboratories who carry out this kind of work. Since in many cases it is has not been possible to carry out the kind of genetic studies required, it is quite possible that at least some of these undefined disorders reflect the type of unlinked forms of β thalassaemia described above.

Chapter 8
The δβ and related thalassaemias

Introduction

In this chapter we shall consider the thalassaemias that involve the other genes of the β-like globin-gene cluster, either together with the β genes—δβ and εγδβ thalassaemia—or alone as γ or δ thalassaemia.

As we saw in Chapter 1 the story of the δβ thalassaemias dates back to 1958, when Gerald and Diamond discovered Hb Lepore and showed that it is associated with a thalassaemia-like disorder. In 1962 Baglioni found that the non-α chain of Hb Lepore is a δβ fusion chain, which, he suggested, is the product of a δβ fusion gene formed by unequal crossing over between the δ- and β-chain genes. It was shown subsequently that the δβ fusion chain of Hb Lepore is synthesized inefficiently, resulting in a form of thalassaemia in which both β- and δ-chain production is abolished, i.e. a δβ thalassaemia.

At about the same time as Baglioni's studies other workers in the USA described a form of what they thought was β thalassaemia, characterized by a normal level of HbA$_2$ and an unusually high level of HbF in heterozygotes (Zuelzer *et al.* 1961). The condition was subsequently observed in Greeks (Fessas 1961; Gabuzda *et al.* 1963), Afro-Americans (Weatherall 1964a), Italians (Silvestroni *et al.* 1964; Brancati & Baglioni 1966), Thais (Flatz *et al.* 1965b; Wasi *et al.* 1969) and Arabs (Ramot *et al.* 1970). Since this disorder was initially thought to be a form of β thalassaemia it was variously called F thalassaemia, normal HbA$_2$ β thalassaemia or β thalassaemia type 2. However, in 1965 Brancati found that, in the homozygous state, there is no δ- or β-chain synthesis. This observation, together with the finding that compound heterozygotes for this form of thalassaemia and a β structural haemoglobin variant make no HbA, provided unequivocal evidence that it results from defective δ- and β-chain synthesis; that is, it is also a form of δβ thalassaemia.

Hence by the early 1970s it was clear that there were at least two varieties of δβ thalassaemia, one associated with the δβ fusion variant Hb Lepore and another characterized by a complete absence of δ- and β-chain synthesis. The next chapter in this story came from the studies of Schroeder *et al.* (1968), who demonstrated the chemical heterogeneity of HbF. Over the next few years, analyses of the HbF of heterozygotes and homozygotes for δβ thalassaemia for its $^Gγ/^Aγ$-chain composition revealed further heterogeneity of the δβ thalassaemias. At least two clear subgroups were defined: those in which the HbF contains both $^Gγ$ and $^Aγ$ chains, and those in which it contains only $^Gγ$ chains.

Unfortunately, there is no consistency with regard to the nomenclature of the δβ thalassaemias. Once the differences in the composition of the fetal haemoglobin had been recognized, it was customary to call them $^Gγ^Aγ$ or $^Aγ$ δβ thalassaemia. Later this was modified to describe the absence of δ- and β-chain synthesis and the conditions were called $^Gγ^Aγ(δβ)^0$ and $^Aγ(^Gγδβ)^0$ thalassaemia. However, since all the other forms of thalassaemia are designated by the globin that is ineffectively synthesized, it seems more logical, and certainly economical, to call these diseases $(δβ)^0$ and $(^Aγδβ)^0$ thalassaemia, respectively (see also Chapter 3). Similarly, the Hb Lepore thalassaemias are $(δβ)^+$ thalassaemias.

Because of the clinical mildness of some types of δβ thalassaemia, particularly in their heterozygous states, for a while there was considerable confusion in the literature about whether these disorders should be designated δβ thalassaemia or hereditary persistence of fetal haemoglobin (HPFH). In this chapter the different forms of δβ thalassaemia are described. In Chapter 10 we shall summarize the differences between the two conditions and develop the concept that δβ thalassaemia and some, though not all, varieties of HPFH represent the ends of a broad spectrum of disorders of δ- and β-chain synthesis which differ only in the degree to which the defect in δ- and β-chain production is compensated by γ-chain synthesis. Indeed, the major feature of both groups is that the primary genetic defect, as well as resulting in defective δ- and β-chain synthesis, allows variable and functionally significant amounts of γ-chain production to continue into adult life.

There are, in addition, other forms of thalassaemia which involve either all the genes of the εγδβ-globin-gene cluster, or just the γ or δ genes. For convenience sake we shall also describe these rare conditions in this chapter.

The δβ thalassaemias

Classification

It is useful to broadly divide the δβ thalassaemias into the (δβ)⁺ and (δβ)⁰ thalassaemias to indicate whether there is any output of δ and β chains from the affected chromosome (Table 8.1).

Table 8.1 The δβ thalassaemias.

(δβ)⁺ Thalassaemia
  Hb Lepore thalassaemia
    Hb Lepore Washington-Boston
    Hb Lepore Hollandia
    Hb Lepore Baltimore
  Phenocopies of (δβ)⁺ thalassaemia
    Sardinian δβ thalassaemia
    Corfu δβ thalassaemia
    Chinese δβ thalassaemia
    β thalassaemia with δ thalassaemia
(δβ)⁰ Thalassaemia
  Sicilian
  Indian
  Japanese
  Spanish
  Black
  Eastern European
  Macedonian
  Turkish
  Laotian
  Thai
(ᴬγδβ)⁰ Thalassaemia
  Indian
  German
  Cantonese
  Turkish
  Malay 1
  Malay 2
  Belgian
  Black
  Chinese
  Yunnanese
  Thai
  Italian

The (δβ)⁺ thalassaemias fall into two main classes. The first category is comprised of those that result from abnormal crossing over and the production of δβ fusion genes and haemoglobin variants, of which Hb Lepore is the prototype. The second is made up of complex disorders which, in effect, are phenocopies of δβ thalassaemia due to the action of two different mutations in the εγδβ-globin-gene cluster.

The (δβ)⁰ thalassaemias usually result from long deletions involving the εγδβ-globin-gene cluster, which remove the β and δ genes but which leave either one or both of the γ-globin genes intact. As already mentioned they can be divided into the (δβ)⁰ and (ᴬγδβ)⁰ thalassaemias, depending on the length of the deletion, that is, whether the ᴬγ genes are involved or not.

(δβ)⁺ Thalassaemia: the haemoglobin Lepore thalassaemias

In the course of a study of the parents of patients with thalassaemia major, Gerald and Diamond (1958) discovered a new haemoglobin variant associated with a thalassaemia-like disorder. One parent and four other relatives of a child with thalassaemia major had 10% of an abnormal haemoglobin which migrated in a similar position to HbS. This haemoglobin was named Lepore, after the name of the family in which it was first found.

After Gerald and Diamond's initial description, similar variants were found in individuals from many different populations, including Italians (Pearson *et al.* 1959; Silvestroni & Bianco 1963; Wolff & Ignatov 1963; Barkham *et al.* 1964; Silvestroni *et al.* 1965b; Labie *et al.* 1966), Greeks (Fessas *et al.* 1962), Papuans (Neeb *et al.* 1961), Turkish Cypriots (Beaven *et al.* 1964), Afro-Americans (Ranney & Jacobs 1964; Ostertag & Smith 1969), Yugoslavians (Duma *et al.* 1968), Romanians (Rowley *et al.* 1969) and Indians (Chouhan *et al.* 1970). Subsequently it has become clear that Hb Lepore has a world-wide distribution in many different ethnic groups (see later section).

The first definitive chemical studies of Hb Lepore by Baglioni (1962) were carried out on a sample from a patient who came from Washington (Barkham *et al.* 1964). Subsequently, samples were obtained from Boston and it was with these that Baglioni completed the characterization of the variant (Baglioni 1965).

Because of this confusion it has become customary to describe this haemoglobin as either Lepore Washington or Lepore Washington/Boston!

Structure of haemoglobin Lepore

The chemical identity of Hb Lepore Washington/Boston was established by Baglioni (1962, 1965). Initially he found that the α chains were normal while the abnormal β-like globin chains of Hb Lepore comprised an N-terminal δ-like and a C-terminal β-like sequence. Subsequently, he was able to pinpoint the fusion to a region between peptides δ10/11 and β12 (i.e. between residues δ87 and β116) by peptide analysis of carboxymethylated haemoglobin. He also tentatively concluded that the Lepore δβ chain contains the same number of amino acids as β and δ chains. Labie *et al.* (1966) confirmed these findings with a sample of Hb Lepore Washington/Boston from Augusta.

Further studies of Hb Lepore from different ethnic groups showed that there is chemical heterogeneity of variants with similar electrophoretic properties to the original form of Hb Lepore. Three varieties have been defined. As well as Hb Lepore Washington/Boston there is Hb Lepore Hollandia (δ22; β50), first found in a Papuan family (Neeb *et al.* 1961; Barnabus & Muller 1962), and Hb Lepore Baltimore (δ50; β86), first described in a Baltimore black family (Ostertag & Smith 1969). Formerly it was customary to name a newly found Hb Lepore after the area in which the affected individual came from; Hb Pylos found in Greek populations (Fessas *et al.* 1962), Hb Lepore The Bronx (Ranney & Jacobs 1964), and so on. These, and several other variants named in this way, were subsequently found to be identical to Hb Lepore Washington/Boston (Baglioni 1965; Labie *et al.* 1966).

General properties of the Lepore haemoglobins

The three known structural variants of Hb Lepore, Washington/Boston, Baltimore and Hollandia, have similar electrophoretic and chromatographic properties (reviewed by Efremov 1978). Their electrophoretic mobility at an alkaline pH is between that of Hbs A and A_2 and is very slightly faster (i.e. anodal) than HbS. On electrophoresis at pH 6–6.5 they do not separate from HbA. They can be rapidly separated by cation-exchange high performance liquid chromatography (Ou & Rognerud

1993) and the δβ chains can be isolated by chromatography (Clegg *et al.* 1966) or reversed-phase HPLC (Leone *et al.* 1985). The Lepore haemoglobins are stable and do not precipitate on heating or on treatment with isopropanol. Isolated Hb Lepore has normal functional properties (McDonald *et al.* 1975). It shows cooperative ligand binding and a normal Bohr effect but has a slightly higher oxygen affinity than HbA. Hence the rate of dissociation from the Lepore haemoglobins is slower than that from HbA and, conversely, the rate of combination with carbon monoxide is more rapid. The stability of Hb Lepore Boston to mechanical shaking is similar to that of HbA_2 but less than that of HbA.

Technical details of the methods for demonstrating the Lepore haemoglobins are given in Chapter 16.

Immunological studies have shown that all three Lepore haemoglobins induce the formation of a specific antibody in rabbits which does not cross-react with Hbs A or A_2 (Efremov 1978), suggesting the existence of unique antigenic determinants on these hybrid haemoglobins. Interestingly, however, the three Hb Lepore antigens show cross-reactivity with each other; it has not been possible to produce a Hb Lepore type-specific antibody, suggesting that the δβ chains have an altered conformation which is recognized immunologically. A murine monoclonal antibody, specific for the δ chain of HbA_2, reacts with βδ- but not with δβ-hybrid chains, indicating that there is an epitope consisting of positions 116 (Arg) and 117 (Asn) or 125 (Gln) and 126 (Met) of the δ chain (Shyamala *et al.* 1991).

The relationship between the molecular pathology and pathophysiology of the haemoglobin Lepore thalassaemias

All the Hb Lepore variants are inherited in a simple Mendelian manner. In the homozygous state HbA and A_2 are absent and the haemoglobin is made up of Hbs F and Lepore only, findings which indicate that there is a complete absence of β- and δ-chain synthesis directed by the chromosome carrying the Hb Lepore gene.

Structural studies of the Lepore haemoglobins indicate that they have arisen by the fusion of genes controlling the synthesis of the δ and β chains, that part of the gene coding for the 5′ end of δ mRNA (or N-terminal end of the δ chain) being combined with that coding for the 3′ end (C-terminal end of the β-chain mRNA) (see Fig. 4.17, Chapter 4). The resulting δβ-gene product is 146 amino acid residues long, the same as normal δ or β chains.

The genetic mechanism which might result in the production of a δβ fusion gene was first discussed by Baglioni (1962), who took as his model the proposed molecular events leading to the production of the α chain of human haptoglobin (Smithies *et al.* 1962). Because of the close proximity of the δ and β loci, and the similarity of much of their nucleotide sequences, it is likely that during meiosis the δ locus on one chromosome may occasionally misalign itself with the β locus on the partner chromosome. If during this type of displaced synapsis crossing over took place between the coding sequences, a fusion gene would be formed which would direct the synthesis of a chain with the N-terminal δ sequence and the C-terminal β sequence, i.e. a Hb Lepore δβ chain. As the site of crossing over can vary, a series of abnormal genes could be generated in this way. If this is the mechanism whereby the Hb Lepores have been produced, it follows that their counterparts, that is, anti-Lepore haemoglobins which consist of fusion products made up of the 5′ sequences of the β chain and 3′ sequences of the δ chain, should be encountered. Furthermore, the order of genes on a chromosome containing such products would be δ–βδ–β. As we shall see later, a number of anti-Lepore haemoglobin variants have been identified, thus confirming this prediction. These principles are illustrated in Fig. 4.17, Chapter 4.

As discussed in Chapter 4, the crossover region generating Hb Lepore Washington/Boston has been localized to between δ^{87} and β^{IVS2-8} (Baird *et al.* 1981b; Mavilio *et al.* 1983; Fioretti *et al.* 1992; Ribeiro *et al.* 1997). Similarly, the breakpoints for Hbs Lepore Baltimore and Hollandia have been defined as being between codons δ68 and β84, and δ22 and nucleotide 16 of IVS1-β, respectively (Miranda *et al.* 1994; Waye *et al.* 1994d; Huisman 1997; Ribeiro *et al.* 1997).

As we shall see later the δβ chain of Hb Lepore is inefficiently synthesized and this is the basis for the β-thalassaemic phenotype associated with this variant. Why should this be? Since the 5′ sequences of Hb Lepore reflect those of the δ-globin gene, and since HbA_2 is synthesized at a much lower rate than HbA, it has been thought for a long time that the reduced rate of production of Hb Lepore must reflect the properties of its 5′ δ gene sequences. To develop this argument we must digress briefly therefore and

consider what is known about the reasons for the reduced rate of synthesis of HbA_2.

Early experiments on the synthesis of HbA_2 showed that it stops before the reticulocyte stage of red-cell maturation, in contrast to that of HbA, which continues to be made throughout erythroid cell development (Rieder & Weatherall 1965; Winslow & Ingram 1966; Wood *et al.* 1978). It also appears that this decline in δ-chain synthesis is due to instability of δ-chain mRNA so that levels of active δ mRNA are never high in erythroblasts, even when mRNA is being actively synthesized, and fall precipitously when RNA synthesis stops at the intermediate normoblast stage of red-cell development (Roberts *et al.* 1973; Wood *et al.* 1978). Thus when bone-marrow cells from a β-thalassaemia heterozygote were fractionated by age on an albumin density gradient, it was shown that δ-chain synthesis declined very rapidly after the polychromatic stage and was markedly reduced in late normoblasts (Wood *et al.* 1978).

The synthesis of the δβ chains of Hb Lepore and, incidentally, the βδ chains of the anti-Lepore haemoglobins, follow a pattern which is reminiscent of, if not identical to, that of the δ chains of HbA_2. In fact, the synthesis of any globin which is derived from all or part of the δ-chain gene exhibits the same general biosynthetic pattern, again hinting that all their respective mRNAs may be unstable. We suggested that such instability may be related to the 5′ and 3′ non-coding regions of δ mRNA (Clegg & Weatherall 1974).

More recently, attention has turned to the possibility that the δ and, by inference, δβ genes may not be transcribed as effectively as the normal globin genes. The 5′-flanking region regulatory elements of the δ gene have not been fully defined. However, sequence comparisons of the first 100 base pairs of the promoter regions of the human δ- and β-globin genes show a potentially important change in the CAAT box which, in the case of the δ-globin-gene promoter region, has the sequence CCAAC. It has been assumed that this base substitution may be the cause of the low level of expression of the δ-globin gene (Spritz *et al.* 1980). More recently it has been found that the erythroid Krüppel-like factor (EKLF) binding site present in the β gene is missing in the δ-chain gene (Tang *et al.* 1997). Furthermore, by artificially restoring the CCAAC box of the δ-gene promoter to CCAAT, or by similarly creating an EKLF binding site at −85 bp, the expression of the δ-globin gene *in vitro* was increased significantly. These findings suggest that there are several features of the δ-promoter and adjacent regions which could explain the marked reduction in δ-globin-gene transcription and therefore that the reduced rate of production of the Lepore haemoglobins might result from the same structural changes.

There are still many questions that remain unanswered, however. Although other groups have confirmed that the restoration of the EKLF binding site increased expression of the δ-globin gene (Donze *et al.* 1996), it is still not absolutely clear which δ-globin-gene sequences are responsible for its reduced transcription, or which of the ones that have been identified already are the most important. Indeed, there is evidence that additional sequences in IVS2 may be involved; baseline expression of human chimeric β-globin genes containing δ IVS2 in place of β IVS2 show a marked decrease in transcription rates *in vitro* (LaFlamme *et al.* 1987). This suggests that β IVS2 contains an enhancer, presumably missing in δ IVS2. This would explain the higher levels of Lepore compared with HbA_2. On the other hand the apparent decline of messenger RNA during erythroid maturation that best explains the synthesis patterns of both δ and δβ chains is still unexplained. Overall, however, it seems likely that the structural differences between the promoters and the non-coding regions of the δ- and β-globin genes must be a major factor in the reduced output of the δβ chains of the Lepore haemoglobins.

The homozygous state

Some 22 individuals have been reported as being homozygous for Hb Lepore Washington/Boston and two for Hb Lepore Hollandia. The Hb Lepore Washington/Boston homozygotes were from the following populations: one Greek (Fessas & Stamatoyannopoulos 1962), 15 Italian (Quattrin *et al.* 1966b, 1973; Quattrin & Ventruto 1974; Forget *et al.* 1978; Quattrin *et al.* 1980; Pepe *et al.* 1982; Camaschella *et al.* 1989b; Olivieri *et al.* 1997), seven Yugoslavian (Duma *et al.* 1968; Efremov 1978; Efremov *et al.* 1978; Efremov 1990) and one Iranian (Rahbar *et al.* 1975). The two Hb Lepore Hollandia homozygotes were siblings from Papua New Guinea (Neeb *et al.* 1961). Because some of these patients were transfusion dependent, haematological and haemoglobin analytical data are often incomplete.

However, there is sufficient information to allow us to build a reasonable picture of the clinical and haematological manifestations.

Clinical findings

Since Hb Lepore homozygotes synthesize no normal β or δ chains it might be expected that they would have the same degree of clinical disability as homozygous $β^0$ thalassaemics. However, while this has been observed in some patients it is by no means always the case and the small number of homozygotes who have been adequately documented show considerable variability in the severity of their clinical manifestations (Table 8.2).

Detailed clinical descriptions of three Yugoslavian Hb Lepore Boston homozygotes were reported by Duma *et al.* (1968) and some follow-up data on these patients were given by Efremov (1978). Further data on three other Yugoslavian homozygotes were reported by Efremov *et al.* (1978) and Efremov (1978) and on Italians by Quattrin *et al.* (1980) and Olivieri *et al.* (1997). Many of these patients presented within the first 5 years of life, severely anaemic with haemoglobin values ranging from 4 to 7 g/dl. In every case there was significant splenomegaly and hepatomegaly, and skeletal abnormalities indistinguishable from those of homozygous β thalassaemia. Similarly, the bone X-rays showed extensive thalassaemic changes. All these infants and young children required regular blood transfusion and several died within the first 10 years of life. The cause of death is not given in every case, although in one patient in Duma's study it appeared to be infection. The two Italian siblings with Hb Lepore Washington/Boston described by Olivieri *et al.* (1997) were also severely affected and required regular transfusion from early in life. One of them had to stop being transfused after the age of 9 years due to red-cell sensitization; she became profoundly anaemic with massive expansion of the bone marrow with encroachment into both the auditory canals and the orbit (Fig. 8.1).

The clinical picture of some Hb Lepore homozygotes has not been so severe, however. The Greek patient described by Fessas and Stamatoyannopoulos (1962) ran a mild course. He had been anaemic throughout childhood but only required occasional blood transfusions and was well until the age of 20 when he died suddenly: the cause of death was not determined. In reviewing their experience of Hb

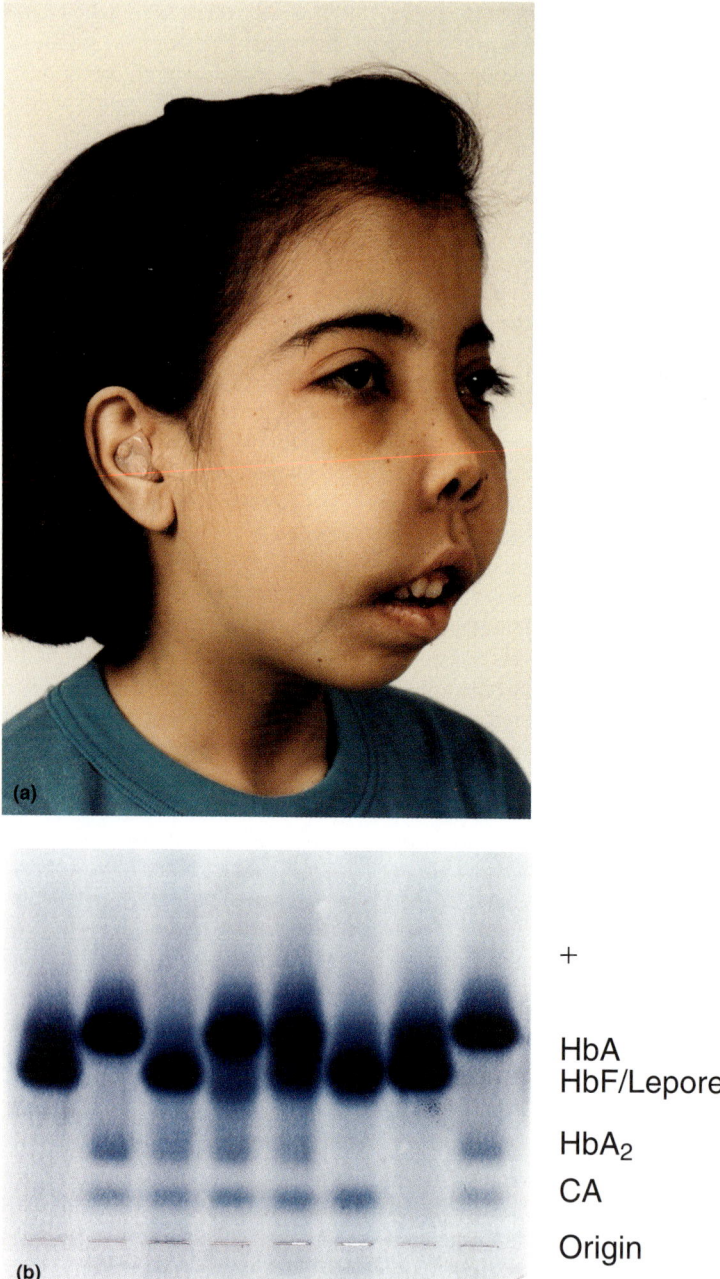

Fig. 8.1 A patient homozygous for Hb Lepore Washington/Boston. (a) This patient had the phenotype of β thalassaemia major. Because of sensitization to blood groups, transfusion became difficult and she developed striking thalassaemic bone changes of the face together with visual deterioration due to compression of the optic nerve. Her deafness was due to encroachment on the auditory canal and middle ear due to bone-marrow expansion. (b) Starch gel electrophoresis (pH 8.5, amido black stain) of haemoglobin from the following (left to right): (1) normal cord blood; (2) normal adult; (3) β^0-thalassaemia homozygote; (4) Hb Lepore trait; (5) Hb Lepore homozygote (transfused); (6) Hb Lepore homozygote shown in (a) (note absence of HbA_2; Hbs F and Lepore separate incompletely under these conditions); (7) normal cord blood; (8) normal adult.

Table 8.2 Findings in haemoglobin Lepore homozygotes.

Population	Age at presentation (years)	Age at death (years)	Clinical features	Transfusion requirements	% Hb Lepore	Reference
Lepore Washington/Boston						
Greek	20	20	Hepatosplenomegaly Bone changes	Occasional	12	Fessas *et al.* (1962)
Italian	4	9	Bone changes	Regular	30	Quattrin & Ventruto (1974)
	3	—	Bone changes	Regular	10	Luppis & Ventruto (1979
	11	—	Bone changes	Nil	20	
	8	—	Hypersplenism	Nil after splenectomy	—	Forget *et al.* (1978)
Iranian	8	—	Hypersplenism	Nil after splenectomy	—	Rahbar *et al.* (1975)
Yugoslavian	2.5	10	Hepatosplenomegaly	Regular	8	Duma *et al.* (1968)
	3.5	9	Hepatosplenomegaly	Regular	9	
	0.5	2	Hepatosplenomegaly	Regular	—	
	1.5	2	Hepatosplenomegaly	Regular	10–15	Efremov *et al.* (1978)
	1	—	Hepatosplenomegaly	Regular		
	5	—	Hepatosplenomegaly	Regular		
Italian	2	—	Bone changes, splenomegaly	Regular	15	Olivieri *et al.* (1997)
	2	—	Splenomegaly	Regular	—	
Lepore Hollandia						
Papuan	5	—	Hepatosplenomegaly	—	24–28	Neeb *et al.* (1961)
	3	—	Bone changes			

Lepore homozygotes in Campania, Quattrin and Ventruto (1974) and Quattrin *et al.* (1980) comment on the relative mildness of some of their cases. One of their patients died as the direct result of splenectomy at the age of 9, but until increasing splenomegaly led to splenectomy he had run the course of a child with thalassaemia intermedia and had required only a few blood transfusions. Two brothers aged 3 and 11 also showed the clinical picture of thalassaemia intermedia, with splenomegaly and a relatively mild anaemia. The Iranian patient reported by Rahbar *et al.* (1975) required a splenectomy at the age of 8. When seen 8 years later he was growth retarded with thalassaemic facies but maintained a haemoglobin level of 10 g/dl. He did not require blood transfusion. Similarly, the 7-year-old Italian female described by Forget *et al.* (1978) was not transfusion dependent until the age of 4. At this time she was found to have a haemoglobin value of 5.2 g/dl and was started on blood trans-

fusion. However, following splenectomy she maintained her haemoglobin at a satisfactory level, in the range 8.1–10 g/dl, and did not require further transfusion.

Very little is known about the two Hb Lepore Hollandia homozygotes except that they presented at the ages of 3 and 5, were profoundly anaemic, and showed marked hepatosplenomegaly and blood changes typical of homozygous β thalassaemia. Their subsequent course is not recorded.

It is clear, therefore, that the homozygous state for Hb Lepore is associated with a severe thalassaemic picture ranging from transfusion-dependent disease, through the more severe spectrum of thalassaemia intermedia, to a milder disorder that appears to be compatible with longevity. However, in the majority of the reports of the milder phenotypes the possibility of ameliorating factors such as α thalassaemia or the segregation of genes for a high level of fetal haemoglobin production have not been excluded. Where they have, in the study of Olivieri *et al.* (1997) for example, the disease appears to be little different from β thalassaemia major.

Haematological findings

The haematological findings have been clouded in some reports by the presence of the transfused blood. There is variable anaemia (see above) and the peripheral blood film is indistinguishable from the severe forms of β thalassaemia. After splenectomy there are large numbers of nucleated red cells in the peripheral blood which contain typical α-chain inclusions. The bone marrow shows marked erythroid hyperplasia with features very similar to those of severe β thalassaemia. Red-cell survival studies have been carried out in three patients, which showed a ^{51}Cr $T_{1/2}$ value of 14–20 days (Efremov *et al.* 1978). Measurements of the levels of erythropoietin and soluble transferrin receptors indicate that there is a high level of erythropoietin production in response to the anaemia, with a major expansion of the erythroid bone marrow (Olivieri *et al.* 1997).

Haemoglobin analysis

The first reported haemoglobin analyses were in Greek and Papuan homozygotes (Neeb *et al.* 1961; Fessas & Stamatoyannopoulos 1962), who had about 12% Hb Lepore, the remainder being HbF. The first report of the homozygote for Hb Lepore Hollandia described a trace of HbA_2 but subsequent analysis showed this to be incorrect; none could be demonstrated (Jonxis 1965) (Fig. 8.1). Later studies of homozygotes from Italy and Yugoslavia confirmed these early findings; the level of Hb Lepore ranges from 8 to 30% with a mean value of approximately 15%. However, as we shall see when we consider the cellular distribution of Hbs F and Lepore, the level of Hb Lepore in the peripheral blood may be determined by the relative survival of red cells containing predominantly one or other haemoglobin, as well as by the amount of Hb Lepore synthesized in the marrow.

Haemoglobin synthesis

In the few homozygotes for Hb Lepore in which *in vitro* haemoglobin synthesis was carried out

(Efremov *et al.* 1978; Forget *et al.* 1978; Wood *et al.* 1978; Luppis & Ventruto 1979; Schiliro *et al.* 1980; Olivieri *et al.* 1997) only Hbs F and Lepore were synthesized (Fig. 8.2).

In the 7-year-old Italian child reported by Forget *et al.* (1978) there was marked imbalance of globin synthesis, reflected by α-/γ- and α-/δβ-chain production ratios of 7 and 13, respectively. The authors noted that there was a small amount of δβ-chain synthesis in the peripheral blood although the child had been splenectomized and they could not rule out the possibility that this was occurring in nucleated red cells. The synthesis of small amounts of Hb Lepore in the peripheral blood of homozygotes is of interest because, as we shall see later, this does not occur in the blood of heterozygotes. In the homozygote studied by Wood *et al.* (1978) the α/non-α and α/δβ ratios were 3.1 and 13.2, respectively. There was 19.2% Hb Lepore in the blood of this patient. These results were similar to those described by Forget *et al*, and again suggested that there was some synthesis of Hb Lepore in the peripheral blood. However, this patient also had been splenectomized so it is possible that at least some of this reflects δβ-chain production in nucleated red cells.

The results of these studies have to be interpreted with caution, not only because of the contribution made by nucleated red-cell precursors but also because, as in homozygous β thalassaemia, the peripheral blood reticulocytes almost certainly represent a highly selected cell population which synthesizes relatively more γ chains. Furthermore, cells which contain relatively more Hb Lepore may be turning over more rapidly than those which contain HbF (see next section). However, it is clear that there is a complete absence of β- and δ-chain production and a marked degree of globin imbalance with excess α chains produced, a picture very similar to homozygous β thalassaemia.

Distribution and structure of haemoglobin F

The bulk of the haemoglobin in the peripheral blood in Hb Lepore homozygotes is HbF. As in β thalassaemia it is heterogeneously distributed among the red cells. This has been demonstrated by examining the relative amounts of HbF and Lepore after centrifugation of the red cells from a Hb Lepore homozygote (Efremov 1978; Efremov *et al.* 1978). In reviewing this experiment Efremov (1978) points out

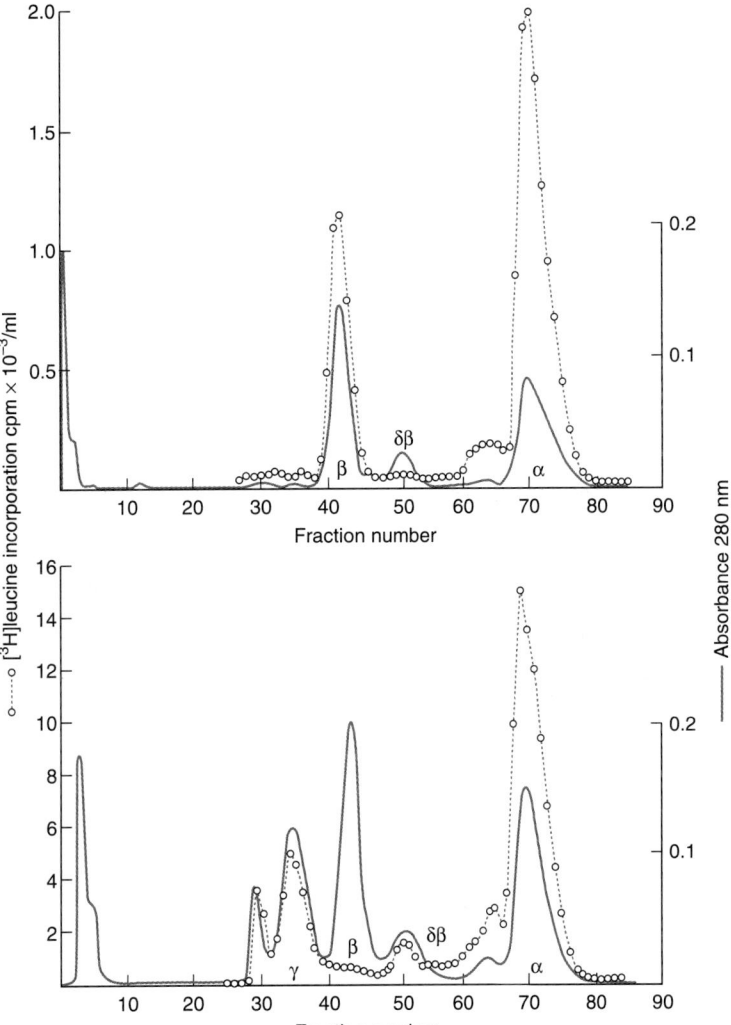

Fig. 8.2 Haemoglobin synthesis in the heterozygous and homozygous states for Hb Lepore. The methods used are as described in Chapter 5. The continuous lines represent protein and the broken, lighter lines show the radioactivity profile. The top graph shows the radioactivity profiles from the cells of a heterozygote showing an absence of δβ-chain synthesis in the peripheral blood. The bottom graph shows the radioactivity profile from the cells of a homozygote, showing a small amount of δβ-chain synthesis in the peripheral blood and the absence of β-chain synthesis (normal adult globin was added to indicate position of elution of β chains). Note the overall imbalance of α- and non-α-chain synthesis in both heterozygote and homozygote.

that the red cells in the younger, lighter population contained higher levels of Hb Lepore, while those from the older cells at the bottom of the centrifuge tube contained predominantly HbF. Unfortunately, absolute values for Hbs Lepore and F were not calculated from the mean cell haemoglobin (MCH), so it is not clear whether the amount of Hb Lepore is constant throughout the cell population or whether there is a reciprocal relationship between the levels of HbF and Lepore. Clearly, however, there is heterogeneity of haemoglobinization; those cells with more HbF survive longer in the peripheral circulation, a situation exactly analogous to that which occurs in β thalassaemia.

The structure of the HbF has been reported by Efremov *et al.* (1974) and Olivieri *et al.* (1997). Both ${}^G\gamma$ and ${}^A\gamma$ chains were present. The ${}^G\gamma/{}^A\gamma$ ratios were either in the range intermediate between that of normal newborns and adults or in the adult range. We shall return to the significance of the production of HbF in the Hb Lepore syndromes later in this chapter.

The heterozygous state

There are numerous single case reports and larger series describing the heterozygous state for Hb Lepore, many of which are based on extensive investigations of the Italian populations of Campania (Quattrin & Ventruto 1974; Marinucci *et al.* 1979b; Quattrin *et al.* 1980; Pepe *et al.* 1982), Yugoslavians (Duma *et al.* 1968; Efremov 1978; Efremov *et al.* 1978; Efremov 1990), Sicilians (Schiliro *et al.* 1980; Mirabile *et al.* 1995) and Spanish and Portuguese populations (Gilsanz *et al.* 1992; Ribeiro *et al.* 1997). These studies show that the condition has a fairly uniform clinical and haematological picture.

Clinical findings

The heterozygous state for Hb Lepore is asymptomatic. In the large Italian series no abnormal physical signs have been reported, but a few of the heterozygotes of Greek and Yugoslavian origin were reported to show slight splenomegaly.

Haematological findings

The haematological findings are very similar to those in heterozygous β thalassaemia. Data from the large series from Italy suggest that heterozygotes are significantly anaemic as compared with control populations in the same countries. This is shown unequivocally in the study by Marinucci *et al.* (1979b), which, although not broken down according to sex, shows a mean haemoglobin value of 12.2 g/dl for 59 Hb Lepore carriers as compared with 15.1 g/dl for the normal control population; the mean haemoglobin level was identical to that of β-thalassaemia carriers

in the same population (Table 8.3). When the red-cell indices are compared with those of β thalassaemics studied in the same laboratory at the same time it is evident that the red-cell size and degree of haemoglobinization are not significantly different in carriers of Hb Lepore and β thalassaemia. The morphological appearance of the blood film is the same in both conditions. Similar conclusions were reported in the large Yugoslavian series of Efremov *et al.* (1978).

Although these findings were consistent, a more recent study of a group of individuals with Hb Lepore trait from the region between Extremadura and Toledo in Spain, in whom haematological findings were compared with heterozygotes for β thalassaemia, reported significantly higher values for haemoglobin, mean cell volume (MCV) and MCH at all ages and in both sexes (Gilsanz *et al.* 1992). It is difficult to reconcile these observations with previously reported data from other populations. Although the differences between Hb Lepore and β-thalassaemia heterozygotes were small, they were significant. Thus whether there are subtle differences in the haemoglobin levels and red-cell indices between these groups remains *sub judice*. However, the overall conclusion that the Hb Lepore trait is similar to that for β thalassaemia appears to hold true.

Such data as are available suggest that there are no major differences in the haematological findings between carriers of the different molecular varieties of Hb Lepore. For example, in an analysis of 12 Hb Lepore Washington/Boston carriers and 11 Hb

Table 8.3 Haematological data and haemoglobin analyses in two large series of haemoglobin Lepore heterozygotes. In the series of Efremov *et al.* normal HbF values are given as < 1%, and 74% of Lepore heterozygotes had elevated levels. In the series of Marinucci *et al.* the mean normal HbF is 0.97%. The mean HbF level for a group of β-thalassaemia heterozygotes studied at the same time was 2.7%. In the series of Marti *et al.* the HbF values were elevated in every Hb Lepore carrier but only in 40% of β-thalassaemia carriers. The figures presented represent the means for each series.

No. cases	Sex	Hb (g/dl)	MCH (pg)	MCV (fl)	HbF (%)	HbA$_2$ (%)	Hb Lepore (%)	Reference
51	Male	13.0 (8.7–15.8)	26 (23–30)	—	2.2	2.5	10.5	Efremov (1978)
52	Female	12.2 (9.0–14.9)	26 (21–30)	—	2.4	2.5	10.7	Efremov (1978)
59	—	12.2	22.3	71.5	3.1	2.2	11.8 (5–18)	Marinucci *et al.* (1979b)
15	—	12.6	25	—	1.1	2.0	9.4	Marti *et al.* (1975)

MCH, mean cell haemoglobin; MCV, mean cell volume.

Lepore Baltimore carriers the haemoglobin levels and red-cell indices were indistinguishable (Ribeiro *et al.*1997).

Red-cell survival and ferrokinetic data have been reported for a few heterozygotes (Pearson & McFarland 1962; Efremov 1978). The red-cell survival is slightly shortened and ^{59}Fe utilization is increased. The findings are similar to heterozygotes for β thalassaemia. Efremov (1978) has described worsening of the anaemia during viral hepatitis.

Haemoglobin analysis

The peripheral blood contains Hbs A, Lepore, A_2 and a variable amount of HbF (Figs 8.1 & 8.3). The values for the relative amounts of the various haemoglobin fractions derived from several large series are summarized in Table 8.3.

Although there is a range of reported levels of Hb Lepore, between 5 and 15%, the majority are closely clustered at approximately 10% of the total haemoglobin (Table 8.3). In a recent study Ribeiro *et al.* (1997) found the levels of Hb Lepore Washington/Boston and Hb Lepore Baltimore were almost identical, with means of 13.9 and 14.9%, respectively. The mean level of HbA_2 is approximately 2%, significantly reduced below normal. However, this represents an increased output from the single δ-chain locus in *trans*. The reported values for HbF range broadly between 1 and 14% (Table 8.3). Overall

there is a significant elevation of HbF; the important question is whether it is greater than in β-thalassaemia heterozygotes.

There are two ways in which this problem can be approached. The first is to analyse the incidence of elevated HbF levels in Hb Lepore heterozygotes. There are extensive data (summarized in Chapter 7) showing that only about 50% of β-thalassaemia heterozygotes have an elevation in their HbF values. On the other hand, of 56 Hb Lepore carriers reported by Duma *et al.* (1968) 54 had significantly raised HbF values. Similar results were reported by Marti *et al.* (1975). In a more detailed analysis of HbF in heterozygotes by Efremov *et al.* (1974) a raised level was observed in all cases with one possible exception. A similar incidence of elevated HbF levels was observed in 59 heterozygotes reported by Marinucci *et al.* (1979b) and by Efremov *et al.* (1978). Thus it appears that a significantly higher proportion of Hb Lepore heterozygotes than β-thalassaemia heterozygotes have raised HbF levels.

In assessing the difference in levels of HbF between the two groups it is essential that the estimations are carried out in the same laboratory using the same technique. There are limited published data that meet this criterion, but the studies of Duma *et al.* (1968), Marti *et al.* (1975), Marinucci *et al.* (1979b), Efremov *et al.* (1978) and Gilsanz *et al.* (1992) (Table 8.3) and our own unpublished observations suggest that there is a higher average level of HbF in Hb

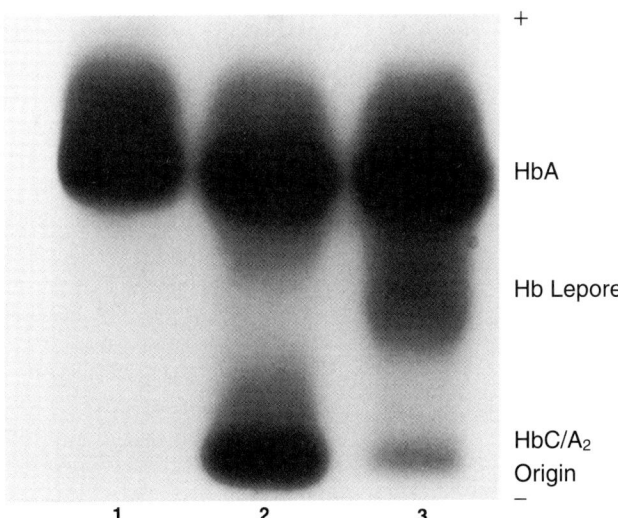

Fig. 8.3 The haemoglobin pattern in the heterozygous state for Hb Lepore. Starch gel electrophoresis (pH 8.5, amido black stain) of the following (left to right): (1), normal adult; (2), HbC trait; (3), Hb Lepore trait.

Lepore heterozygotes than in β-thalassaemia carriers. These observations have been confirmed recently by an analysis of the numbers of F cells, as assessed by fluorescent labelling; the levels are consistent with the raised level of HbF (Olivieri *et al.* 1997).

It appears therefore that in Hb Lepore heterozygotes a raised HbF is the rule rather than the exception, which is quite different from the case in heterozygous β thalassaemia. On the other hand, it is unusual for HbF values to exceed 2 or 4%. Where this has been reported, detailed family analyses have not been available to rule out the presence of a gene for heterocellular HPFH (see Chapter 10). Interestingly, however, in families reported by Duma *et al.* (1968) and Efremov (1978), in which there are heterozygotes with 5 and 13% HbF, several other family members were heterozygous for Hb Lepore with levels in the 1–2% range. Further analyses of this type are required.

In a study which compared the levels of HbF in Hb Lepore Washington/Boston carriers with those for Hb Lepore Baltimore it was found that the former had a mean value of 2.75% while the value in the latter was 4.3% (Lanclos *et al.* 1987). The authors relate the higher level of HbF in the Hb Lepore Baltimore heterozygotes to the presence of the C→T polymorphism at position –158 bp 5′ to the CAP site of the $^G\gamma$-globin gene, the polymorphism identified for *Xmn* I which has been associated with a higher production of HbF in both β thalassaemia and sickle-cell anaemia (see Chapter 10). The increased HbF in the Hb Lepore Baltimore heterozygotes was also associated with significantly higher levels of $^G\gamma$ globin and messenger RNA, which supports this suggestion. There was also a trend to a higher level of HbF in the Hb Lepore Washington/Boston heterozygotes with the haplotypes with the C→T polymorphism at $^G\gamma$ –158.

There is no difference between the Hb Lepore levels of heterozygotes for the different variants. In four heterozygotes for Hb Lepore Baltimore the levels of Hb Lepore were 15% in the original Afro-American patient (Ostertag & Smith 1969), and 8.3–9.8% in the three Yugoslavians reported by Efremov *et al.* (1976). In the Papuans with Hb Lepore Hollandia the range was 7.8–13.8% (Neeb *et al.* 1961).

These observations suggest that the amount of δβ chain produced in heterozygotes, as in the case of homozygotes, varies very little between individuals from different ethic groups or between those with different varieties of Hb Lepore.

Structure of haemoglobin F

The $^G\gamma/^A\gamma$ composition of the HbF of Hb Lepore heterozygotes has been reported by Efremov *et al.* (1974) and Olivieri *et al.* (1997). The ratio of $^G\gamma$ to $^A\gamma$ chains was approximately 1 to 2, which agrees fairly closely with that observed in normal adults (Huisman *et al.* 1977). The higher levels of $^G\gamma$ chains in Hb Lepore Baltimore heterozygotes has already been discussed.

Haemoglobin synthesis

Data have been reported by several groups (Weissman *et al.* 1967; Gill *et al.* 1972; Roberts *et al.* 1972; White *et al.* 1972a,b; Ali & McBride 1973; Weatherall *et al.* 1974a; Efremov 1978; Wood *et al.* 1978; Marinucci *et al.* 1979a; Gilsanz *et al.* 1992). Although the early studies of Weissman and colleagues suggested that there was no significant globin imbalance in the peripheral blood of Hb Lepore heterozygotes this has not been confirmed by subsequent studies and there is now unequivocal evidence that there is an excess of α- over non-α-chain synthesis. Published α-/β + δβ-chain production ratios have ranged from 1.2 to 2.5 with a mean of approximately 1.5. Because of the small numbers of studies from different laboratories it is impossible to determine whether there is a significant difference in the degree of globin imbalance between heterozygous β thalassaemia and Hb Lepore.

The other observation which seems common to all these studies, with the exception of those of Marinucci *et al.* (1979a), is that there is no synthesis of the δβ chains of Hb Lepore in the blood of heterozygotes (Fig. 8.2), a pattern similar to that of the δ chain of HbA_2 (Rieder & Weatherall 1965).

Suggestions that there is balanced globin synthesis in the bone marrow of Hb Lepore heterozygotes (Gill *et al.* 1972; Marinucci *et al.* 1979a) are open to the same criticisms as those discussed earlier for haemoglobin synthesis in the marrow of heterozygous β thalassaemics (Chapters 5 and 7); the arguments stated there seem equally pertinent to the problem of Hb Lepore.

Haemoglobin Lepore in association with β thalassaemia

There are numerous reports of compound heterozygotes for Hb Lepore and β thalassaemia. This condition has been found in Italians and Sicilians (Gerald & Diamond 1958; Pearson *et al.* 1959; Wolff & Ignatov 1963; Silvestroni *et al.* 1965a; Quattrin *et al.* 1967; Quattrin & Ventruto 1974; Marinucci *et al.* 1979a, b; Quattrin *et al.* 1980; Ricci *et al.* 1982; Schiliro *et al.* 1983; Fei *et al.* 1988b), Greeks (Fessas *et al.* 1962), Greek Cypriots (Zachariadis *et al.* 1975), Turkish Cypriots (Beaven *et al.* 1964), Yugoslavians (Duma *et al.* 1968; Efremov *et al.* 1974; Efremov 1978; Efremov *et al.* 1978, 1988; Efremov 1990, 1992), Cubans (Martinez & Colombo 1976), Spaniards (Romero *et al.* 1983) and Algerians (Morlé *et al.* 1984). In every case in which the structure of the Hb Lepore has been analysed it has been of the Washington/Boston variety.

Clinical findings

The clinical picture, though variable, is similar to that of β thalassaemia major. There is usually a history of anaemia from early life, with retardation of growth, thalassaemic bone changes and hepatosplenomegaly. Similarly, the radiological appearances of the bones are indistinguishable from severe β thalassaemia.

The early descriptions of patients with this disorder stressed its clinical variability. At the severe end of the spectrum there are several reports of death in early childhood (Pearson *et al.* 1959; Fessas *et al.* 1962; Wolff & Ignatov 1963). The Greek authors noted that, of 14 children born of one parent with Hb Lepore and the other with β thalassaemia, six died in early life. Of these, two had been splenectomized for severe anaemia and three were known to have severe anaemia, two dying of infection and one following an incompatible blood transfusion. The findings in the nine children reported by Duma *et al.* (1968) and Efremov *et al.* (1978) were indistinguishable from β thalassaemia major, although one of the children showed moderate improvement after splenectomy. Quattrin and Ventruto (1974) were also impressed by the severity of the disease; of their nine cases from the Campania region of southern Italy all showed the clinical picture of β thalassaemia major. On the other hand, Efremov (1978) described a 30-year-old patient with this condition who was not transfusion dependent. In a Greek Cypriot family reported by Zachariadis *et al.* (1975) one sibling had thalassaemia intermedia while the other showed the picture of β thalassaemia major.

The clinical and haematological heterogeneity of the Hb Lepore–β-thalassaemia interactions has been confirmed by more recent observations that have related the phenotype to the particular form of β-thalassaemia mutation that is inherited together with Hb Lepore (Efremov *et al.* 1988). In a group of 10 Yugoslavian patients the disease varied from a transfusion-dependent disorder to a moderate, compensated anaemia without major complications or the need for regular transfusion. All these patients had Hb Lepore Washington/Boston and none had associated α thalassaemia. It was found that, of the six with severe disease, all had inherited a severe β-thalassaemia allele, including IVS1-110 G→A, CD39 C→T, and IVS1-1 G→A. On the other hand, three patients with a milder form of the disease had inherited the allele IVS1-6 T→C, which is known to cause only a modest reduction in β-globin-chain production. Similarly, a patient who had inherited Hb Lepore together with Hb Knossos, which has the phenotype of a particularly mild form of β thalassaemia, had a mild form of thalassaemia intermedia, requiring splenectomy at the age of 53 years.

It is clear therefore that the variable phenotype of the interaction between Hb Lepore and β thalassaemia is related to the severity of the particular β-thalassaemia allele; severe alleles result in a picture of thalassaemia major while milder ones are associated with thalassaemia intermedia of varying severity. The effects of other factors that modify the course of β thalassaemia, co-existent α thalassaemia for example, do not seem to have been defined.

Haematological findings

The published haematological data for this condition are often incomplete and confused by transfused blood. Analysis of reported cases suggests that it is indistinguishable from β thalassaemia major or intermedia. There is variable and sometimes severe anaemia with thalassaemic changes of the red cells and a mild reticulocytosis with nucleated red cells in the peripheral blood, the numbers of which increase after splenectomy.

Haemoglobin analysis

The haemoglobin pattern varies depending on whether the associated β-thalassaemia allele is the $β^0$, severe $β^+$ or mild $β^+$ variety. In cases of the interaction of $β^0$ thalassaemia the haemoglobin consists of F, Lepore and A_2, whereas in interactions with the $β^+$ thalassaemias variable amounts of HbA are present. Overall, the level of Hb Lepore varies between 5 and 15%, while in the $β^+$-thalassaemia interactions HbA has been found in the range 10–40%. The HbA_2 level is usually in the range of 1.2–3%, although in the case of the interaction with Hb Knossos, which is usually found on a chromosome together with $δ^0$ thalassaemia, HbA_2 was absent.

Fetal haemoglobin

The fetal haemoglobin of subjects heterozygous for Hb Lepore and β thalassaemia has been analysed for its $^Gγ/^Aγ$ constitution by Efremov *et al.* (1974). The glycine values fell within the range of 0.5–0.6 residues, intermediate between those of newborn infants and some adults, and similar to those observed in Hb Lepore homozygotes. As expected the distribution of HbF is heterogeneous. Differential centrifugation studies have shown a similar alteration in the distribution of HbF between young and old red cells to that observed in β thalassaemia major (Efremov *et al.* 1974). The older, longer-lived population at the bottom of the centrifuge tube contains significantly more HbF than the lighter, young cell population, which is richer in Hbs Lepore and A_2. These findings indicate that the cells which contain predominantly HbF are protected from the effects of excess α chains, just as they are in homozygous β thalassaemia. The fact that Hb Lepore constitutes about 1% of the haemoglobin at the bottom of the 'spin' and 15% at the top suggests that it may be unevenly distributed, i.e. the HbF-rich population contains less Hb Lepore.

Haemoglobin synthesis

Globin synthesis has been measured in several subjects heterozygous for Hb Lepore and β thalassaemia (Forget *et al.* 1974a; Efremov 1978; Efremov *et al.* 1978; Marinucci *et al.* 1979a). As might be expected there was marked imbalance, with α-/non-α-chain ratios ranging between 1.7 and 5. In one case the β

thalassaemia was of the $β^0$ variety (Forget *et al.* 1974a).

The heterozygous state for haemoglobin Lepore and $(δβ)^0$ thalassaemia

Several well documented examples of this condition have been reported, including Italian patients, heterozygous for both Hb Lepore Washington/Boston and $(δβ)^0$ thalassaemia (Ventruto *et al.* 1967; Quattrin *et al.* 1980), and a Yugoslavian, heterozygous for Hb Lepore Baltimore and $(δβ)^0$ thalassaemia (Efremov *et al.* 1976).

The first reported Italian patient (Ventruto *et al.* 1967), a 32-year-old well developed male from Naples, was found to have an enlarged spleen and liver. The clinical and haematological findings were those of thalassaemia intermedia. His haemoglobin consisted of F (92%) and Lepore (8%); Hbs A and A_2 were absent. His father, two brothers and one daughter were heterozygous for Hb Lepore, while the mother, one brother and another daughter were carriers of δβ thalassaemia. Later reports of other patients from Italy were essentially similar. The 24-year-old Yugoslavian male reported by Efremov *et al.* (1976), heterozygous for Hb Lepore Baltimore and δβ thalassaemia, showed the same clinical picture. His haemoglobin consisted of F and Lepore Baltimore only; the latter comprised about 7% of the total.

Thus the phenotypic expression of these interactions is similar to that of the homozygous state for δβ thalassaemia or the compound heterozygous state for β and δβ thalassaemia (see later section).

The pathophysiology of the haemoglobin Lepore thalassaemias

The basic defect in all the Hb Lepore disorders is the inefficient synthesis of the δβ fusion chain of Hb Lepore, which leads to a variable degree of globin imbalance, excess α-chain production and the clinical phenotype of δβ thalassaemia. The ineffective erythropoiesis and shortened red-cell survival results from the deleterious effects of excess α chains, and the selection of cells which are synthesizing relatively more γ chains follows the same mechanism as occurs in β thalassaemia. This is borne out by the results of the centrifugation experiments cited earlier, which indicate that the cells which contain predominantly

HbF in homozygotes for Hb Lepore, or in compound heterozygotes for Hb Lepore and β thalassaemia, survive longer than those which contain predominantly Hbs A and/or Lepore.

Why is there such remarkable variability in the clinical expression of the homozygous state for Hb Lepore Washington/Boston and in the compound heterozygous state for the Hb Lepores and β thalassaemia? Homozygotes, who make no β or δ chains, would be expected to show the clinical picture of severe homozygous $β^0$ thalassaemia. Similarly, compound heterozygotes should show a similar picture to those for $β^0$ and $β^+$ thalassaemia; as mentioned earlier, much of the heterogeneity reflects the severity of the $β^+$-thalassaemia allele. Genetic analyses are not always available for some of the reported homozygotes and hence it is not possible to rule out co-existent α thalassaemia or heterocellular HPFH. However, it is unlikely that these conditions offer an explanation for the relative mildness of the disorder in all cases. It is possible that the deletion which has resulted in the δβ fusion chain is somehow responsible for increasing the absolute output of γ chains (Olivieri *et al.* 1997), a suggestion that is compatible with the observation that Hb Lepore heterozygotes produce significantly more HbF than β-thalassaemia heterozygotes.

In summary, the Hb Lepore syndromes bear a strong resemblance to the β thalassaemias. As a group, however, they are slightly milder. This raises the possibility that there may be, at least in some cases, a greater overall output of γ chains, related to the deletions which have given rise to δβ chains of the Lepore haemoglobins.

Haemoglobin Lepore in association with structural haemoglobin variants

These interactions are considered in Chapter 9.

The distribution of the haemoglobin Lepore thalassaemias

Haemoglobin Lepore has been found in individuals from a wide variety of ethnic backgrounds, including Italian (Gerald & Diamond 1958; Pearson *et al.* 1959; Silvestroni & Bianco 1963; Wolff & Ignatov 1963; Silvestroni *et al.* 1965a; Quattrin *et al.* 1967; Quattrin & Ventruto 1974; Sasso *et al.* 1975; Marinucci *et al.* 1979b), Greek (Fessas *et al.* 1962), Greek Cypriot (Zachariadis *et al.* 1975), Turkish Cypriot (Beaven *et al.* 1964), Afro-American (Ranney & Jacobs 1964), Yugoslavian (Duma *et al.* 1968; Efremov *et al.* 1978), Romanian (Rowley *et al.* 1969), Jamaican (Ahern *et al.* 1972), Bulgarian, Algerian and French (Tayebi & Labie 1974), French (Labie *et al.* 1971; Beuzard *et al.* 1972), Indian (Saha & Banerjee 1973), Turkish (Çavdar & Arcasoy 1976), Spaniards and Portuguese (Gimferrer *et al.* 1976; Gilsanz *et al.* 1992; Ribeiro *et al.* 1997), Iranian (Rahbar *et al.* 1974, 1975), Cuban (Martinez & Colombo 1973), Indonesian German (Went *et al.* 1975), Scots (Cook & Lehmann 1973), Australian of British stock (Wilkinson *et al.* 1975), English (present authors, unpublished observations), Hungarian (Ringlehann *et al.* 1979) and Brazilian (Miranda *et al.* 1994).

Although in some of these reports the structure of the Hb Lepore was not determined, in the majority of cases in which it was characterized it was Hb Lepore Washington/Boston.

Haemoglobin Lepore Baltimore, which is much less common, has been found in families of Afro-American, Yugoslavian, Sardinian, Portuguese and Spanish origin (Ostertag & Smith 1969; Efremov *et al.* 1976; Marinucci *et al.* 1979a; Miranda *et al.* 1994; Ribeiro *et al.* 1997) while Hb Lepore Hollandia has been found only in families from Papua New Guinea and Bangladesh (Barnabus & Muller 1962; Curtain 1964; Waye *et al.* 1994d).

Precise gene frequencies for Hb Lepore Washington/Boston are not known, but it appears from published series that the disease is relatively common in middle and eastern Europe, central Portugal and Spanish Alta Extremadura. As judged by the extensive studies of Quattrin and colleagues in Naples (Quattrin & Ventruto 1974; Marinucci *et al.* 1979b), it appears to be particularly common among some southern populations of Italy, chiefly Campanians from the Naples and Caserta regions, and also in a few localized parts of Calabria. In an analysis of haemoglobinopathies in the Naples Centre, 2993 cases of abnormal haemoglobin disorders were found in a sample of 42000 persons. The Hb Lepore disorders were found in 117 (3.5%); 91% of cases consisted of various forms of β thalassaemia (Quattrin & Ventruto 1974). The gene also seems to have a relatively high frequency in parts of Yugoslavia and Greece. The distribution in Italy and Yugoslavia is curious because Hb Lepore is not common in other regions with very high frequencies of β thalassaemia

(Duma *et al.* 1968). Malamos *et al.* (1962) found 109 thalassaemia carriers among 1600 Greek Air Force recruits. Two of them were carriers of Hb Pylos (Hb Lepore Washington/Boston), giving an incidence of about 1.2 per 1000. However, this figure, because of the sample size and uneven distribution of the thalassaemia gene in Greece, must be only a very rough approximation of the true gene frequency.

The distribution of the Lepore haemoglobins in central Portugal and in the Spanish Alta Extremadura is of considerable interest (Ribeiro *et al.* 1997). Haemoglobin Lepore is one of the commonest abnormal haemoglobins in this region, with a frequency of 0.28% in a survey of school children. Of a group of 19 Portuguese and 14 Spanish carriers in whom the Lepore variant was characterized at the molecular level it was found that all the Portuguese cases and one Spanish case were heterozygous for Hb Lepore Baltimore, whereas all the other Spanish subjects were Hb Lepore Washington/Boston carriers. To date this is the only region in which a relatively high frequency of Hb Lepore Baltimore has been observed. These two geographical regions have a common border but are isolated by natural barriers, thus limiting the admixture of two populations.

In the last edition of this book we concluded that, although there may have been a founder effect in central and eastern Europe, Hb Lepore Washington/Boston must have arisen in other parts of the world by independent mutation. Analysis of 43 Hb Lepore Washington/Boston $\delta\beta$-globin genes from individuals from Campania and Abruzzo showed heterogeneity of chromosomal background as judged by the associated restriction-fragment-length polymorphism (RFLP) haplotypes (see Chapter 2). Twenty-three of the 31 genes from Campania were associated with the $+ +3'\beta$-globin subhaplotype and framework 1, whereas 12/12 genes from Abruzzo and 3/31 from Campania were associated with the $+ -3'\beta$-globin haplotype and framework 2. In discussing the basis for these observations, Fioretti *et al.* (1992) suggest that second crossover or gene conversion events are a likely cause of these major haplotype differences and that they reflect at least two separate crossover events to generate Hb Lepore Washington Boston in these populations. Lanclos *et al.* (1987) described a third haplotype which seems quite different again. The gene, associated with the $+ -3'/\beta$-globin subhaplotype and framework 2, is virtually restricted to Abruzzo and Yugoslavia. Hence it may have spread from the Balkan countries to Italy, whereas the $++3'/\beta$-globin subhaplotype in framework 1 may have arisen by a second mutation in the Italian population.

The haplotype associated with Hb Lepore Baltimore carriers in the regions of Spain and Portugal, where this condition seems to be relatively common, are homogeneous, but quite different from that described in a Brazilian family of Italian origin (Lanclos *et al.* 1987; Miranda *et al.* 1994; Ribeiro *et al.* 1997). Again, this makes it very likely that this Hb Lepore variant has arisen on more than one occasion.

In short, data from the Balkan countries and parts of Italy are compatible with the notion that Hb Lepore Washington/Boston has arisen on a number of occasions and presumably has reached its relatively high frequency in this curiously patchy distribution by the actions of founder effects, drift and, possibly, local selection by malaria. Indeed, despite the lack of extensive haplotype data the extraordinarily wide distribution of sporadic cases of this variant throughout the world suggests that it may have arisen *de novo* on many different occasions.

The anti-Lepore haemoglobins

Although the anti-Lepore haemoglobins, that is those with non-α chains which have β chain-like residues at the N-terminal ends and δ chain-like residues at their C-terminal ends (see Fig. 4.17, Chapter 4), are not associated with the clinical picture of thalassaemia, we must briefly discuss them here in order to provide a complete picture of the Hb Lepore field.

The different anti-Lepore haemoglobins

The first anti-Lepore, Hb Miyada, was found in a Japanese family (Yanase *et al.* 1968; Ohta *et al.* 1971b). It constituted about 17% of the total haemoglobin and migrated in the same position as Hbs C or E on starch gel electrophoresis at an alkaline pH. None of the carriers of Hb Miyada had any haematological abnormalities, except one who had a slight elevation of HbF. It is difficult to interpret this observation, however, since several normal family members also had a raised HbF level and it was suggested that the gene for heterocellular HPFH (see Chapter 10) was also segregating in this family. Analysis of trypsin digests of the abnormal β-like chain showed that it had an N-terminal β sequence up to residue 12 and a δ-chain sequence beyond residue 22, so the fusion point must be between these residues. These findings are, of course, the opposite of those seen in the Hb Lepores and indicate that the non-α chain of Hb Miyada is a βδ fusion chain, precisely as predicted for an anti-Lepore globin chain.

The second variety was reported by Lehmann and Charlesworth (1970) following their structural analysis of a sample of HbP from the former Belgian Congo, now Zaire (Dherte *et al.* 1959). The abnormal variant was found subsequently in several individuals together with Hbs A and S (Dherte *et al.* 1959; Lambotte-Legrand *et al.* 1960) and was initially thought to be an α-chain mutant. A limited structural analysis of the β-like chain of this variant by Lehmann and Charlesworth (1970) suggested that it might be a βδ fusion variant with a crossover point between residues 30 and 116. Lack of material precluded further analysis.

More detailed studies on another variety of HbP, in this case found in a Nubian living in Cairo, were reported by Badr *et al.* (1973). This variant, which accounted for 21% of the total haemoglobin, was named HbP Nilotic. Analysis of the tryptic peptides of the abnormal βδ chain indicated that the crossover had occurred between residues β22 and δ50. Unfortunately no haematological data were reported. However, Moo-Penn *et al.* (1978a) studied a Mexican-American family in which several members carried HbP Nilotic. While they had completely normal blood pictures there was an unequivocal elevation of HbF as compared with their unaffected relatives. In the studies of Badr *et al.* (1973) and Moo-Penn *et al.* (1978a) it appears that HbP Nilotic had a slightly higher oxygen affinity than HbA and did not interact to the same extent as HbA with 2,3-diphosphoglycerate (2,3-DPG). Haemoglobin P Nilotic shows no significant difference in the degree of cooperativity or Bohr effect as compared with HbA. Other examples of this variant have been observed in Turkish, Sudanese and Kenyan families (Abu-Sin *et al.* 1979; Altay *et al.* 1987; Huisman 1997).

Another anti-Lepore haemoglobin of similar structure to HbP Nilotic was described by Honig *et al.* (1978). This variant, Lincoln Park, in addition to having a non-α chain containing both β and δ sequences, with the fusion point between residues β22 and δ50, differs from HbP Nilotic in that a valine residue is deleted at position 137. The authors speculate that this deletion may have arisen by repeated crossing over between the δ and β genes during meiosis. In fact, to achieve the genotype postulated, three simultaneous crossovers would be required! A more likely explanation is that a gene for HbP Nilotic has, at some time, been involved in a crossover with a δ or β gene carrying the 137 Val deletion, in a manner similar to that proposed to account for β-chain variants with two substitutions. The variant was found in three members of a family originating from southern Mexico. There were no morphological abnormalities of the red cells and the red-cell indices were normal but the reticulocyte counts and their HbF values were elevated significantly as compared with their normal siblings. One of the latter had a slightly raised level of HbF but it appears from the pedigree that he was younger than the propositus, who was himself only 8 years old at the time of study.

The existence of another variety of anti-Lepore haemoglobin, Hb Coventry, was proposed by Casey *et al.* (1978). The situation in this family was extremely complicated because the propositus, a 7-year-old English girl, was found to be heterozygous for two unstable haemoglobins, Sydney and Coventry. Haemoglobin Sydney has a single amino acid substitution, Val→Ala, at position β67. It was found that Hb Coventry has a non-α chain which resembles a $β^A$ chain except that it has a leucine residue deleted at position β141. Furthermore, they suggested that this is, in fact, a βδ fusion chain with the same charge as a $β^A$ chain. This conclusion was based on a structural analysis which appeared to show that the propositus was carrying three different non-α chains, i.e. $β^{Sydney}$, $β^A$ and β (or $βδ)^{Coventry}$. The child's mother carried Hb Sydney and it was assumed that the child's father had Hb Coventry. More recent work suggests that the β chain of Hb Coventry may be a postsynthetic artefact resulting from the oxidation of $β^{141}$ leucine to hydroxyleucine (Brennan *et al.* 1992; George *et al.* 1992b). The same phenomenon is observed in Hb Atlanta. It is suggested that the β75 Leu→Pro substitution in this variant perturbs the haem environment, which, in some way, results in oxidation of the C-terminal leucine. Interestingly, Hb Sydney also has a substitution in the E helix, which might have the same effect, thus explaining the findings in the family with Hb Coventry.

A variant comprising 23% of the total haemoglobin was found in an Indian family; no haematological

Table 8.4 The anti-Lepore haemoglobins.

Haemoglobin	Crossover region	Additional features
Miyada	β12δ22	Migrates as Hb C/E
P Congo	β22δ116	Migrates as HbS
P Nilotic	β22δ50	Migrates as HbS
Lincoln Park	β22δ50	Valine 137 deleted or modified Migrates as HbS
P India*	β87δ116	No data reported
Parchman†	δ12β22 β22δ87	Migrates as HbS

* Reported as abstract only (Préhu *et al*. 1994).
† Double crossover or gene conversion.

studies were reported. DNA analysis suggested that its non-α chain was a βδ hybrid, with a recombination point between β codon 87 and the 8th nucleotide of the δ gene. It was designated HbP India (Préhu *et al*. 1994).

In summary, the anti-Lepore haemoglobins consist of Hbs Miyada, P Congo, P Nilotic, Lincoln Park, which is probably identical to HbP Nilotic except for the deletion of Val 137, and P India (Table 8.4). Haemoglobin Coventry, based on current evidence, is not likely to be a βδ variant, although the β-globin genes of the original propositus have not, to our knowledge, been sequenced.

Molecular analysis

Gene mapping has confirmed that the βδ hybrid gene of HbP Nilotic is the counterpart of the δβ hybrid gene and that it is located between a normal δ and β gene. The crossover point has been pinpointed to a 54-bp region between nucleotides 275 (amino acid residue 31) and 330 (amino acid residue 50), indicating that exon 1 and IVS1 are of β-globin origin, and that exon 2, IVS2 and exon 3 are from the δ-globin gene (Liu *et al*. 1987; Huisman 1997).

The anti-Lepore haemoglobins are usually present in heterozygotes at approximately 15–20% of the total haemoglobin. This suggests that they are synthesized less effectively than HbA. At first sight this is surprising because, unlike the Lepore haemoglobins, the βδ hybrids have normal β-globin-gene promoter sequences. On the other hand, the anti-Lepore haemoglobins have a δ IVS2 sequence and, as mentioned earlier, there is some evidence that this plays a role in the relative inefficiency of δ-chain synthesis.

Thus the presence of this sequence in the genes for the βδ fusion variants may play a role in reducing their level of synthesis as compared with HbA. Because the βδ chains have a similar affinity for α chains to that of β chains it seems unlikely that their relative levels in red cells reflect post-translational modification by differential affinity for α chains.

Haematological findings

Carriers for the anti-Lepore haemoglobins have normal haemoglobin levels and red-cell indices.

Haemoglobin constitution

The anti-Lepore haemoglobins usually constitute between 15 and 20% of the total haemoglobin in carriers. Haemoglobin A_2 levels are in the normal range. In seven HbP Nilotic carriers reviewed by Huisman (1997) the variant haemoglobin constituted approximately 17.8% of the total and the mean HbA$_2$ level was 2.5%.

Haemoglobin synthesis

In the study of the synthesis of Hb Miyada reported by Roberts *et al*. (1973) (Fig. 8.4) there was linear incorporation of isotope into the α and β chains over 2 hours, but virtually no synthesis of the βδ chains. Although when Hbs A and Miyada were separated as intact haemoglobins there appeared to be some synthesis of Hb Miyada, this was found to be due to the exchange of newly labelled α chains between HbA and Miyada. These results are similar to those obtained for the *in vitro* synthesis of Hbs A$_2$ and Lepore. Roberts *et al*. (1973) interpreted these findings as suggesting that the βδ-chain mRNA is relatively less stable than α- or β-chain mRNA. The possible reasons for this will be discussed in a later section. Honig *et al*. (1978) confirmed these observations and showed that, in the reticulocytes of individuals heterozygous for Hb Lincoln Park, α-/non-α-chain synthesis ratios are similar to those in heterozygous β thalassaemia.

The relative rates of α- and non-α-globin synthesis in the cells of individuals heterozygous for HbP Nilotic were studied by Abu-Sin *et al*. (1979). It was found that during short-term incubations, approximately 30 min, there was a mild degree of globin imbalance with an α-/non-α-globin synthesis ratio of

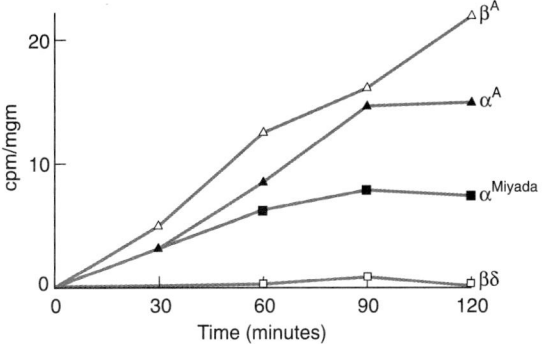

Fig. 8.4 The synthesis of Hb Miyada. Red cells from an Hb Miyada heterozygote were incubated for varying periods of time with ^{14}C leucine and then lysed, Hbs A and Miyada separated, and the α and β or α and βδ chains separated on CM-cellulose chromatography (see Chapter 5). The findings indicate that there is virtually no βδ-chain synthesis in reticulocytes and that any radioactivity incorporated into Hb Miyada is due to the exchange of labelled α chains between Hbs A and Miyada. From Roberts *et al.* (1973).

1.33. At longer periods of incubation there appeared to be a greater degree of chain imbalance, and at 120 min the ratio was 2.02. These authors also confirmed the decline in the relative rates of synthesis of the βδ chains during erythroid maturation. Based on these findings, and on studies of the interaction with HbP Nilotic with β thalassaemia, the authors suggested that the β-chain locus *cis* to the βδ-chain locus is incapable of increasing its output in the presence of a β-thalassaemia gene in *trans*. We shall consider this interesting concept further in the next section.

In summary, there is good evidence that βδ-chain synthesis declines during erythroid maturation at a greater rate than that of α- or β-chain synthesis. In addition, there is some preliminary evidence that the presence of a βδ gene between the δ and β loci on an anti-Lepore chromosome may have some effect on the activity of the linked β-chain locus. Thus it is possible that anti-Lepore heterozygotes may behave phenotypically like extremely mild β-thalassaemia heterozygotes; that is, this could be yet another form of 'silent' β, or δβ, thalassaemia.

Anti-Lepore haemoglobins in association with β thalassaemia

As far as we know there has only been one report of the interaction between an anti-Lepore haemoglobin

and β thalassaemia. Since this combination is of great interest, in that it provides an opportunity for examining the potential for increasing the output of the various non-α-globin genes on the anti-Lepore chromosome, this family warrants careful examination.

The interactions between HbP Nilotic and β^0 thalassaemia was observed in three members of a Sudanese family (Abu-Sin *et al.* 1979). Although the designation of the β-thalassaemia gene as β^0 was not proved conclusively it seems likely that this is the case. The HbP Nilotic heterozygotes had completely normal haematological findings. Interestingly however, the HbP Nilotic β^0-thalassaemia compound heterozygotes had a more severe clinical phenotype than the β-thalassaemia heterozygotes in the same family. The three compound heterozygotes had haemoglobin values ranging from 7.5 to 9.6 g/dl and their red cells were markedly hypochromic with reduced MCH and MCV values (MCH, 18–20.5 pg; MCV, 58–63 fl). The red-cell indices of the two β-thalassaemia heterozygotes in the same family were in a similar range, although they had haemoglobin values of 11.1 and 9.6 g/dl, respectively. The haemoglobin patterns were of particular interest. The carriers of HbP Nilotic had between 25 and 28% HbP, but the compound heterozygotes for HbP Nilotic and β^0 thalassaemia had between 55 and 57% HbP, with elevated levels of HbA_2; on a cellular basis the MCH $\beta\delta^{P \text{ Nilotic}}$ ranged from 4.6 to 5.1 pg and the MCH β^A ranged from 3.1 to 3.2 pg. Furthermore, there was significantly greater overall globin imbalance in the compound heterozygotes than in the heterozygotes for HbP Nilotic or β thalassaemia alone. When the relative rates of synthesis of HbA and HbP Nilotic were compared in the blood and bone marrow of one of the compound heterozygotes it was found that there was a significant decline in the synthesis of HbP Nilotic during erythroid maturation.

Abu-Sin *et al.* (1979) make the point that, in a β^0-thalassaemia heterozygote with a normal δ and β locus in *trans,* there is only mild anaemia and globin imbalance, but when the δ–βδ^P–β complex is in *trans* to a chromosome with β^0 thalassaemia there is more severe anaemia and imbalanced globin synthesis. The inescapable conclusion is that, somehow, the presence of the βδ gene in this complex prevents an increased output of β chains to the extent which is usually achieved by the *trans* chromosome in β^0-thalassaemia heterozygotes. The authors explain these findings by a complicated series of crossing-over events in which there has been loss of a regulatory determinant *cis* to the β gene on the chromosome containing the βδ gene. It is certainly curious that the output of the βδ fusion chain of HbP Nilotic was increased in the compound heterozygotes above that observed in the simple heterozygotes for the variant, whereas that of HbA was, if anything, slightly below that observed in the simple heterozygote. Although the authors' explanation for these findings remains highly speculative this fascinating family raises some fundamental questions about the compensatory mechanisms which occur on the *trans* chromosome in β-thalassaemia heterozygotes. It may be, of course, that these observations simply reflect a positional effect resulting from the insertion of the βδ gene between the β gene and the locus control region (LCR) (see Chapter 2).

A mosaic δβδ haemoglobin variant: haemoglobin Parchman

A variant which comprised 1.6% of the total haemoglobin in a haematologically normal carrier was reported by Adams *et al.* (1982). Gene mapping studies suggested that the non-α chain was the product of a δβδ gene composed of a δβ hybrid (δ12β22) and a βδ hybrid (β22–50 δ87). Although Adams *et al.* proposed that the δβδ gene had most likely arisen by a double crossover, a gene conversion of δ by β seems an equally plausible explanation.

Anti-Lepore haemoglobins in association with other structural haemoglobin variants

These interactions are considered in Chapter 9.

Other possible Lepore- and anti-Lepore-like haemoglobins

In addition to the Hb Lepores and anti-Lepores described above, the existence of other δβ fusion haemoglobins has been predicted (Smithies 1964; Comings & Motulsky 1966; Stamatoyannopoulos *et al.* 1969b).

One set of these putative variants might have the electrophoretic mobility of HbA, while another would behave like HbA_2 and produce a variety of β thalassaemias with unusually high HbA_2 levels. The genetic mechanisms required to produce these haemoglobins are indicated in Table 8.5. Because of the structural similarity between the β and δ chains some of these variants would go undetected. In fact, a δβ fusion occurring before residue 9 will be identical to a normal β chain but its synthesis, by analogy with Hb Lepore, is likely to be drastically reduced. In other words, it would have the phenotype of 'β⁺ thalassaemia' but the affected chromosome would lack a normal δ-chain locus. Conversely, a fusion occurring after residue 126 would produce a 'δβ' chain with a sequence identical to a normal δ chain. The affected chromosome in this case would lack a normal β gene and produce the phenotype of β⁰ thalassaemia with an associated high level of 'HbA_2'.

Although occasional cases have appeared in the literature that have been interpreted as representing the action of δβ fusion genes with products indistinguishable from HbA_2 (Grifoni *et al.* 1975), and there has been considerable discussion about whether

Table 8.5 The Lepore and anti-Lepore haemoglobins and other potential crossover variants. Adapted from Efremov (1978).

Type		
Theoretical or observed	Relative frequency[†]	Charge
δ<9-β	9	β
δ9-β	3	= β
δ12-β	10	= β
δ22-β Hollandia	28	+1
δ50-β Baltimore	36	+1
δ87-β Washington/ Boston	29	+1
δ116-β	1	= δ
δ117-β	7 or 8	= β
δ125-β	1	= δ
δ>126-β 'Lepore'-like	20	δ
β<9-δ 'Miyada'-like	9	δ
β9-δ	3	= δ
β12-δ Miyada	10	= δ
β22-δ P Nilotic Lincoln Park*	28	−1
β50-δ	36	−1
β87-δ	29	−1
β117-δ	7 or 8	= β
β>126-δ Coventry*	20	β

* An additional abnormality is deletion of valine 137 in Hb Lincoln Park and deletion or modification of leucine 141 in Hb Coventry. More recent studies suggest that Hb Coventry may have resulted from a postsynthetic artefact (see text).
[†] Assuming random recombination.

some individuals with β thalassaemia with normal HbA_2 levels might have a Lepore-like variant with the same charge as HbA (Kattamis *et al.* 1978), as far as we know no case of this type has been characterized at the molecular level.

The corresponding anti-Lepore globin chains resulting from the two types of crossovers described above would have sequences indistinguishable from δ and β chains, respectively. In these cases, however, since the anti-Lepore chromosomes also carry normal δ- and β-chain genes, β-thalassaemia phenotypes would not be expected, although at the DNA level affected individuals would appear to have δ- or β-chain gene duplication. On sequencing, the anomalies would be revealed, since the duplicated 'δ' genes would have the associated β non-coding sequences and the duplicate 'β' genes δ non-coding sequences.

One possible example of a duplicate δ gene (i.e. HbA_2-like anti-Lepore haemoglobin) was postulated for a patient with β thalassaemia with an unusually high HbA_2 level of 15% (Schroeder *et al.* 1973a), although the evidence was not conclusive.

Phenocopies: $β^0δ^+$ or $β^+δ^0$ thalassaemia with high levels of haemoglobin F production

There is a heterogeneous group of disorders that resemble the δβ thalassaemias in that they result from the acquisition of two different mutations in the β-globin-gene cluster which may involve the γ-gene promoters, the β genes or the δ genes. The mutations that produce these conditions are described in Chapter 4. Here we shall briefly review the clinical features of this group of phenocopies of the δβ thalassaemias.

Sardinian δβ thalassaemia

In reviewing the different varieties of thalassaemia in Sardinia, Cao and colleagues observed that just over 1% of all the β-thalassaemia-like disorders consisted of a condition with the phenotype of δβ thalassaemia (Cao *et al.* 1982a,b). Heterozygotes have typical thalassaemic blood changes with normal HbA_2 levels and HbF values in the 10–20% range. Analysis of the γCB3 peptide from this HbF gave $^Gγ$ values ranging from 0.02 to 0.14 residues. They also showed that, in the relatively mild form of β thalassaemia that results

from the interaction of this form of δβ thalassaemia with $β^0$ thalassaemia, there is a complete absence of HbA. Thus the chromosome carrying the Sardinian form of $δβ^0$ thalassaemia must not direct the synthesis of any β chains. Furthermore, as judged by the structure of the HbF in heterozygotes, there is a predominance of $^Aγ$-chain production directed by this chromosome.

Structural studies of the β-globin-gene cluster carrying the Sardinian form of δβ thalassaemia revealed two different mutations. The β-globin gene carries the common Mediterranean C→T nonsense mutation at codon 39, while the $^Aγ$-globin gene has a C→T change at position –196 (Guida *et al.* 1984; Pirastu *et al.* 1984a; Ottolenghi *et al.* 1987).

The C→T substitution at position –196 of the $^Aγ$-globin gene has also been detected in Italian populations in association with a form of $^Aγδβ^+$ HPFH (see Chapter 10). It seems likely therefore that the δβ-thalassaemia phenotype in this case results from the over-expression of the $^Aγ$-globin genes associated with the absence of β-globin production due to the presence of a nonsense mutation. The origins of this chromosome have been detailed by Ottolenghi *et al.* (1987). They argue for a single origin of the Italian form of $^Aγ/β^+$ HPFH and suggest that the Sardinian δβ-thalassaemia chromosome has arisen by a crossover, linking together the over-expressed $^Aγ$-globin gene with the β-thalassaemia gene. It is clear from the phenotype of compound heterozygotes for $β^0$ thalassaemia and the Sardinian form of δβ thalassaemia that the high output of γ chains in the latter condition is responsible for the mild clinical course in the compound heterozygotes (Cao *et al.* 1982a,b).

Corfu δβ thalassaemia

This phenocopy of δβ thalassaemia is relatively common in Greek populations. Homozygotes have a mild form of thalassaemia intermedia with typical thalassaemic blood changes and their haemoglobin consists of almost 100% HbF with trace amounts of HbA and no HbA_2 (Traeger-Synodinos *et al.* 1991). Interestingly, heterozygotes show the picture of β-thalassaemia trait with a normal slightly reduced HbA_2 level.

Again, two different types of mutation have been observed on the chromosome that encodes the determinant for Corfu δβ thalassaemia. First, a 7.2-kb deletion removes part of the δ gene, leaving the β gene intact (Wainscoat *et al.* 1984a). In addition, however, the β gene in *cis* has the IVS1-5 G→A β-thalassaemia mutation (Kulozik *et al.* 1988b). As in the case of the Sardinian δβ thalassaemia both these lesions in the β-gene cluster have been described as single, separate mutations in different populations. A 7.2-kb deletion starting 3′ of the ψβ gene and removing part of the δ gene has been found in an Italian individual (Galanello *et al.* 1990a), and the β⁺ IVS1-5 G→A mutation has been found in the Algerian population (Lapoumeroulie *et al.* 1986). Interestingly, when there is a normal β gene *cis* to the 7.2-kb deletion it is expressed at the usual level. Furthermore, homozygotes for the β⁺ IVS1-5 G→A mutation have a severe disease. These observations tell us that the 7.2-kb deletion does not downregulate the β gene in *cis* but, rather, it appears to enhance the expression of the γ genes, thus accounting for the mild phenotype in homozygotes for Corfu δβ thalassaemia.

Chinese δβ thalassaemia

There is a single case report of a Chinese patient with the phenotype of heterozygous δβ thalassaemia, with 22% HbF and a normal HbA$_2$ level, in whom no deletion of the β-globin-gene cluster could be detected (Atweh *et al.* 1986). Both $^G\gamma$ and $^A\gamma$ chains were present in the HbF and partial analysis of the promoters of both γ genes failed to reveal any substitutions. In a later paper it was shown that the β-globin gene carries the –29 A→G β⁺-thalassaemia mutation, but the reason for the normal HbA$_2$ levels and high levels of HbF cannot be explained on these findings. In a further attempt to solve this puzzle (Balta *et al.* 1994) sequenced extensive regions upstream from the $^G\gamma$- and $^A\gamma$-globin genes and the 3′ $^A\gamma$-gene enhancer region. They found a C→T substitution 2401 nucleotides downstream from the $^A\gamma$ gene CAP site. Further studies show that this is not a common polymorphism. Using a number of DNA binding and functional assays Balta and colleagues came to the conclusion that this mutation of the $^A\gamma$-gene enhancer on a chromosome that carries a partially activated β-globin gene may be sufficient to explain the δβ-thalassaemia-like phenotype. It will be important to try to find further examples of this novel combination of mutations to ensure that the downstream enhancer change is the genuine cause of the increased level of HbF in heterozygotes.

β thalassaemia with δ thalassaemia

Strictly speaking, chromosomes that carry both β- and δ-thalassaemia mutations are, in effect, δβ thalassaemias. Depending on the nature of the mutations they may reflect δ⁺β⁰, δ⁰β⁺, δ⁺β⁺ or δ⁰β⁰ arrangements. In practice they give rise to the clinical picture of either normal HbA$_2$ or silent β thalassaemia. In some cases, Hb Knossos for example, the β- and δ-thalassaemia mutations occur on a haplotype which is widespread. However, because of their particular phenotype they are not likely to be confused with the other forms of δβ thalassaemia described in this chapter. The molecular basis for the normal HbA$_2$ β thalassaemias is described in Chapter 4, and the clinical features in Chapter 13. The clinical features of the δ thalassaemias are touched on briefly later in this chapter.

(δβ)⁰ and (ᴬγδβ)⁰ thalassaemia

The δβ thalassaemias are characterized by elevated levels of HbF in heterozygotes and the absence of Hbs A and A$_2$ in homozygotes. As discussed earlier, they are still sometimes classified, by virtue of the structure of the associated HbF, into $^G\gamma^A\gamma$ and $^G\gamma$ varieties. However, to maintain consistency with other forms of thalassaemia it seems more logical to describe them by the loci which are deleted or otherwise inactivated, that is (δβ)⁰ and (ᴬγδβ)⁰ thalassaemia. This nomenclature has been further complicated because the molecular analyses have revealed a remarkable degree of heterogeneity; currently 10 different varieties of (δβ)⁰ thalassaemia and 12 forms of (ᴬγδβ)⁰ thalassaemia have been identified. Hence it is now customary to designate each variety by the ethnic origin of the first patient in whom the condition was characterized at the molecular level (Table 8.1). The molecular pathology of these conditions is considered in detail in Chapter 4. Here we shall describe what is known about their clinical manifestations and their interactions with other forms of thalassaemia.

(δβ)⁰ Thalassaemia

This condition is fairly common in the populations of the Mediterranean region including Sicily, Italy, the Balkans, Hungary, Greece, Turkey, Israel and Egypt. This appears to reflect the fairly widespread distribution of what is now called the Sicilian variety (Fritsch *et al.* 1979; Ottolenghi *et al.* 1979; Henthorn *et al.* 1990; Craig *et al.* 1993). In addition, however, nine other types have been detected in other populations: Indian (Mishima *et al.* 1989; Gilman *et al.* 1992); Japanese (Matsunaga *et al.* 1985; Shiokawa *et al.* 1988); Spanish (Ottolenghi *et al.* 1982a; Baiget *et al.* 1983; Camaschella *et al.* 1987b); Black (Anagnou *et al.* 1985); east European (Palena *et al.* 1992); Laotian (Zhang *et al.* 1988a); Thai (Trent *et al.* 1988); Macedonian (Efremov *et al.* 1986b; Kulozik *et al.* 1992; Craig *et al.* 1995); and Turkish (Öner *et al.* 1996).

The homozygous state

The first description of the homozygous state for δβ thalassaemia was reported by Brancati (1965) in a 31-year-old woman from Calabria and a further description of this patient together with a detailed analysis of her haemoglobin was given by Brancati and Baglioni (1966). It was subsequently observed in Italians (Silvestroni *et al.* 1968b; Russo *et al.* 1973a), Greeks (Fessas 1968; Stamatoyannopoulos *et al.* 1969a; Tsistrakis *et al.* 1974; Amin *et al.* 1979), Arabs (Ramot *et al.* 1970; Amin *et al.* 1979), Turks (Orkin *et al.* 1979a), Indians (Sukumaran *et al.* 1972; Amin *et al.* 1979), Mexicans (Reyes *et al.* 1978), Spaniards (Gimferrer *et al.* 1976; Ottolenghi *et al.* 1982b) and Japanese (Shiokawa *et al.* 1988).

Some of these patients turned out to have $(^A\gamma\delta\beta)^+$ thalassaemia (see later section). It seems likely that many of the earlier descriptions in the Mediterranean populations dealt with what is now known as the Sicilian form of $(\delta\beta)^0$ thalassaemia. The homozygous state has also been fully characterized for the Spanish, Macedonian and Japanese varieties.

Clinical findings

Regardless of the molecular type, there is a mild form of thalassaemia intermedia, similar to that observed in Brancati's first description. All cases have been asymptomatic and nearly all have had only slight hepatosplenomegaly. In a few cases mild radiological changes of the bones have been reported.

Although there have been some reports suggesting that the condition may be more severe, a careful scrutiny does not suggest that this is the case. For example, of three Mexican siblings described by Reyes *et al.* (1978) two were completely healthy, while a third died with the diagnosis of 'thalassaemia major' with a recorded haemoglobin value of 5.3 g/dl; no further clinical details are given. At first sight the clinical history of the Greek patient reported by Tsistrakis *et al.* (1974) also appears to be different. This 22-year-old male was seen during the course of an upper respiratory tract infection and found to have a haemoglobin value of 4.2 g/dl. However it seems likely that this severe anaemia was due to infection because, when he was seen 2 months later, the haemoglobin level was 9 g/dl and he was well. Orkin *et al.* (1978) mention a Turkish family in which there was a child with a 'thalassaemia major-like' disorder with a complete absence of Hbs A and A_2. This child died at the age of 3 years during an intercurrent infection. However, in subsequent papers it appears that she had $(^A\gamma\delta\beta)^0$ thalassaemia (Fritsch *et al.* 1979; Orkin *et al.* 1979a).

Thus, when well defined patients with this condition have been studied in the steady state it appears that it is a uniformly mild form of thalassaemia intermedia and, apart from a drop in haemoglobin during intercurrent infection, is symptomless.

Haematological findings

The haematological data are remarkably homogeneous. There is mild anaemia with steady-state haemoglobin values in the 10–13 g/dl range. The morphological changes are typical of thalassaemia intermedia and the red-cell indices show microcytosis and hypochromia. The reticulocyte count is normal or slightly elevated and, in the few reported cases in which red-cell survival studies have been carried out, it has been found to be slightly shortened or normal.

Haemoglobin analysis

The haemoglobin consists of 100% HbF with a complete absence of Hbs A and A_2. However, there appears to be some heterogeneity in the distribution of HbF among the red cells as judged by their staining properties using the acid elution test.

Structure of haemoglobin F

Extensive studies of the $^G\gamma/^A\gamma$ composition of the HbF have been reported for patients who almost certainly have the Sicilian form of the condition

(Brancati & Baglioni 1966; Silvestroni *et al.* 1968b; Stamatoyannopoulos *et al.* 1971; Ottolenghi *et al.* 1976; Amin *et al.* 1979). The output of $^G\gamma$ and $^A\gamma$ chains is approximately equal and remarkably similar in all these homozygous patients. This is also the case in homozygotes for the Japanese, Spanish and Macedonian forms.

Haemoglobin synthesis

Most studies of globin synthesis in the peripheral blood or bone marrow have demonstrated mild imbalance of a magnitude similar to that observed in heterozygous β thalassaemia (Fig. 8.5). Russo *et al.* (1973a) demonstrated an absence of β- and δ-chain synthesis in the Sicilian $(\delta\beta)^0$-thalassaemia homozygote; the α-/γ-chain synthesis ratio ranged from 1.4 to 1.8. Similar ratios were reported by Shchory and Ramot (1972) in the Arab homozygotes, and we have observed similar ratios in Greek and Arab homozygotes. In the case of the Spanish and Japanese forms the ratios are in the same range (Gimferrer *et al.* 1979; Shiokawa *et al.* 1988).

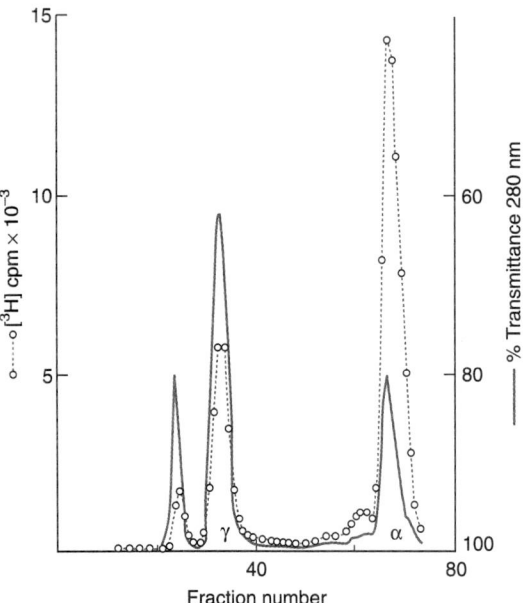

Fig. 8.5 Haemoglobin synthesis in the reticulocytes of a δβ-thalassaemia homozygote. The method is described in Chapter 5. There is an absence of β-chain synthesis and imbalanced globin synthesis with an excess of α over γ chains produced.

It is clear therefore that this form of δβ thalassaemia is associated with very mild globin imbalance; γ-chain synthesis nearly, but not entirely, compensates for the lack of β-chain production.

Heterozygous $(\delta\beta)^0$ thalassaemia

Heterozygous $(\delta\beta)^0$ thalassaemia has been observed in many ethnic groups. Before the different molecular forms were identified, adequate clinical and haematological descriptions were reported in Italians (Zuelzer *et al.* 1961; Wolff & Ignatov 1963; Silvestroni *et al.* 1964, 1968b), Sardinians (Cao *et al.* 1981), Greeks (Fessas 1961; Gabuzda *et al.* 1963; Wolff & Ignatov 1963; Stamatoyannopoulos *et al.* 1969a; Amin *et al.* 1979), Afro-Americans (Weatherall 1964a; Pearson 1969; Zelkowitz *et al.* 1972; Kinney *et al.* 1978), Thais (Flatz *et al.* 1965b; Wasi *et al.* 1969), Arabs (Ramot *et al.* 1970; Amin *et al.* 1979), Indians (Sukumaran *et al.* 1972; Amin *et al.* 1979), Turks (Aksoy *et al.* 1974), Yugoslavians (Efremov *et al.* 1975), Jamaicans (Wood *et al.* 1977a) and Spaniards (Gimferrer *et al.* 1979; Pagnier *et al.* 1979).

The main haematological findings and haemoglobin analyses in heterozygotes for the different molecular forms of $(\delta\beta)^0$ thalassaemia are summarized in Table 8.6.

Clinical and haematological findings

There are no specific clinical features and heterozygotes do not have symptomatic anaemia or splenomegaly. The blood picture is characterized by a normal or slightly reduced haemoglobin level with abnormal morphology of the red cells. The red-cell changes, indistinguishable from those of mild β thalassaemia minor (see Chapter 7), are characterized by mild hypochromia, anisopoikilocytosis and basophilic stippling. The red-cell indices are also similar to those of β-thalassaemia trait although, overall, the MCH and MCV are slightly higher. As shown in Table 8.6, there are no significant differences in the haematological findings in the different molecular forms of the condition.

Haemoglobin analysis

The haemoglobin consists of Hbs A, F and A_2. The HbA_2 value is usually normal or slightly reduced

Table 8.6 Summary of haematological data on (δβ)⁰-thalassaemia heterozygotes defined by molecular analysis.

Type	No of families/ individuals	Hb (g/dl)*	MCV (fl)	MCH (pg)	HbA$_2$ (%)*	HbF (%)	$^G\gamma$ (%)*	α/non-α* synthesis	Distribution/ % F cells
Sicilian	20/24	12.3±1.5	68.2±4.0	22.7±1.8	2.7±0.2	9.6±3.5	43.4±8.2	1.5±0.2	Heterocellular
Laotian	3/3	13.0±1.1	73.7±2.5	23.9±1.8	2.7±0.3	13.8±5.4	60		Heterocellular/52%
E. European	1/5	13.7±0.9	75.7±1.9	24.8±0.8	2.1±0.3	17.7±4.8	71.5±3.5		Heterocellular/67%
Black	1/1	11.6	70.9		1.9	14.7	50		Heterocellular/50%
Macedonian/ Turkish	6/20	12.0±1.0	65.5±6.8	24.5±3.6	2.6±0.4	9.7±2.7	45.6±6.9		Heterocellular
Indian	1/1	11.5	78	26	2.3	16.6	79	1.46	Heterocellular
Spanish	?/?	13.1±1.0	69.0±4.6	23.1±3.0	2.3±0.5	10.1±3.9	35.2±7.1		Heterocellular
Japanese	1/1	12.8	67	21.2	2.9	7.5	49.3	1.37	Heterocellular
Turkish 2	1/2	11.0	64.3±1.8	20.9±0.3	2.5±0.6	10.5±6.3	60		Heterocellular

* Data not necessarily complete for all individuals; extreme outliers omitted.
α Thalassaemia not excluded in all cases; some results obtained after sample had been in transit.
Macedonian and Turkish are identical deletions (Craig *et al.* 1995).
MCH, mean cell haemoglobin; MCV, mean cell volume.

(Table 8.6). In a series of 68 cases reported by Stamatoyannopoulos *et al.* (1969a) the mean HbA$_2$ level was 2.4%, exactly the same as that in the more recent series which relate the different heterozygous phenotypes to the underlying genotype (Table 8.6). However, 2.4% HbA$_2$, with an MCH of 22 pg, constitutes about 0.53 pg HbA$_2$ per cell. Since this represents the output of a single δ-chain locus it appears that δ-chain synthesis from the *trans* chromosome is increased, just as occurs in β thalassaemia. Haemoglobin F values range from 5.4 to 20%. As shown in Table 8.6, there is some variation between the mean level of HbF among heterozygotes for different molecular forms of (δβ)⁰ thalassaemia. It is difficult to be certain of the significance of these observations, however. In some cases the numbers are small, and methodological differences between laboratories may also play a part.

As judged by both the acid elution and fluorescent anti-HbF antibody techniques, the HbF is heterogeneously distributed among the red cells (Fig. 8.6), distinguishing the disorder from heterozygous pancellular HPFH (see Chapter 10). The results of centrifugation studies indicate that the red cells with relatively more HbF survive longer in the circulation (Wood *et al.* 1977a).

Structure of haemoglobin F

The structure of HbF from 32 δβ-thalassaemia heterozygotes from Greece and one from Italy was reported by Stamatoyannopoulos *et al.* (1971). The values for glycine residues in peptide γCB3 ranged from 0.25 to 0.56, indicating that both $^G\gamma$ and $^A\gamma$ chains were present in ratios ranging from 1/3 to 1/1, with an average of about 2/3. Similar findings were obtained in the Yugoslavian series reported by Efremov *et al.* (1975) and in the Spanish families described by Pagnier *et al.* (1979).

More recent information, relating the level of $^G\gamma$ and $^A\gamma$ chains in heterozygotes to individual molecular forms of (δβ)⁰ thalassaemia, is summarized in Table 8.6. Although there is some variation, the numbers are too small in many of the series to be certain about whether this is significant. Huisman *et al.* (1997) suggest that some of this variability may reflect the presence or absence of the *Xmn* I polymorphism at $^G\gamma^{-158}$.

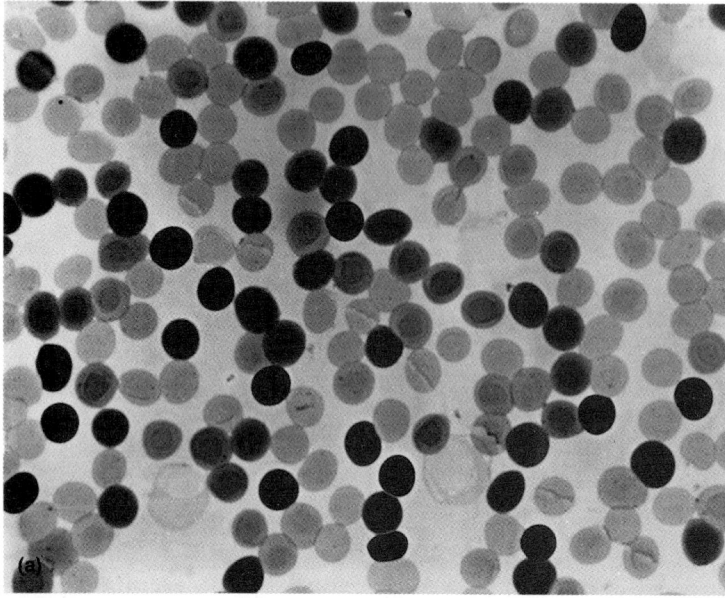

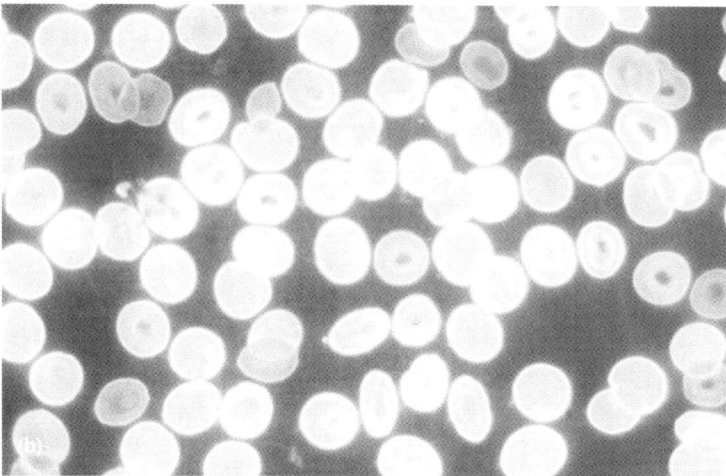

Fig. 8.6 The distribution of haemoglobin F in heterozygous δβ thalassaemia. (a) Acid elution preparation; (b) fluorescent anti-HbF antibody preparation. These preparations were made from carriers with approximately similar levels of HbF. The heterogeneity of distribution is better shown by the acid elution technique, probably because of its lower sensitivity.

Haemoglobin synthesis

Russo *et al.* (1973a) examined *in vitro* globin synthesis in the parents of the children described originally by Silvestroni *et al.* (1968b), who were later shown to have $(\delta\beta)^0$ thalassaemia (Stamatoyannopoulos *et al.* 1971; Ottolenghi *et al.* 1976). Alpha-/beta-chain synthesis ratios ranged from 1.7 to 2.1. In the latter study the α-/β+γ-chain ratios in five cases ranged from 1.59 to 2.04 in the blood and 1.14 to 1.64 in the marrow. These findings have been confirmed in more recent studies in which the specific molecular form of $(\delta\beta)^0$

thalassaemia was defined (see Table 8.6). Overall, they indicate that δβ-thalassaemia heterozygotes have a very mild degree of globin imbalance in their marrow and peripheral blood.

$({}^{A}\gamma\delta\beta)^0$ *Thalassaemia*

In the last edition of this book we reviewed the literature on thalassaemia-like disorders in which the fetal haemoglobin consisted entirely of ${}^{G}\gamma$ chains, and came to the conclusion that these conditions should be classified as forms of δβ thalassaemia rather than

HPFH, largely because of the severity of their homozygous phenotypes. Since then at least 12 different molecular forms of what is now called $(^A\gamma\delta\beta)^0$ thalassaemia have been defined (Table 8.1). These have been designated as follows: Indian (Amin *et al.* 1979; Jones *et al.* 1981a; Trent *et al.* 1984b); German (Anagnou *et al.* 1988); Cantonese (Zeng *et al.* 1985a); Malay 1 (Trent *et al.* 1984b); Turkish (Orkin *et al.* 1978, 1979a; Dinçol *et al.* 1981; Tuan *et al.* 1983); Malay 2 (George *et al.* 1986); Belgian (Losekoot *et al.* 1991a); Black (Henthorn *et al.* 1985); Chinese (Jones *et al.* 1981a; Mager *et al.* 1985); Yunnanese (Zhang *et al.* 1993); Thai (Fucharoen *et al.* 1987); and Italian (De Angioletti *et al.* 1997).

Although only three of these disorders have been encountered in their homozygous states, such information as does exist suggests that the homozygous condition for this form of δβ thalassaemia is more severe than that of $(\delta\beta)^0$ thalassaemia, while, phenotypically at least, the heterozygous states for the two varieties are similar.

Homozygous state

Clinical features

Sukumaran *et al.* (1972) described a 7-year-old Indian child with pallor, mild jaundice and hepatosplenomegaly, with radiological appearances typical of thalassaemia. He required intermittent blood transfusions during periods of severe anaemia due to intermittent bouts of infection. His haemoglobin level was 7.5 g/dl and his blood film showed changes typical of thalassaemia intermedia, with an MCV of 69 fl and an MCH of 21 pg. Haemoglobin analysis showed 100% HbF. The child's parents were both mildly anaemic and they had thalassaemic blood films and MCH values of 25 and 23 pg, respectively. Their HbF values were 8 and 13%, with normal HbA_2 values. Haemoglobin synthesis studies on the relatives of this child were reported in subsequent papers by Altay *et al.* (1977b) and Ringelhann *et al.* (1977). The α-/non-α-chain synthesis ratios ranged from about 1.2 to normal and for this reason the authors felt that this condition should be classified as '$^G\gamma$ hereditary persistence of fetal haemoglobin rather than $^G\gamma\delta\beta$ thalassaemia'. However, because of the clinical phenotype in this child, with the picture of moderately severe thalassaemia intermedia, in the previous edition of this book we felt

that it was more logical to classify it as $(^A\gamma\delta\beta)^0$ thalassaemia.

We subsequently had the opportunity to study two Indian families with three individuals apparently homozygous for $(^A\gamma\delta\beta)^0$ thalassaemia (Amin *et al.* 1979). The propositus in the first family, a 4-year-old boy from the Mohammedan community of Bohra, presented with mild jaundice, anaemia and splenomegaly; he was otherwise well. His haemoglobin level was 8.3 g/dl and there were 15% reticulocytes. The blood film showed changes typical of severe thalassaemia. The diagnosis was confirmed by family study. The propositus from the second family was a 27-year-old male from the same community. He presented with fatigue and gave a previous medical history of two attacks of jaundice and one of pericarditis. His spleen was palpable about 6 cm below the costal margin. The haemoglobin level was 11.2 g/dl with 15% reticulocytes and a typical thalassaemic blood film. The diagnosis was confirmed by family study. We also observed this condition in a 7-year-old child from Kuwait who was anaemic from birth and had required blood transfusion during episodes of infection. The spleen was enlarged 5 cm below the costal margin.

Later reports, which described the homozygous state for forms of $(^A\gamma\delta\beta)^0$ thalassaemia defined at the molecular level, confirmed and extended these observations. In a child homozygous for the Indian deletion (Jones *et al.* 1981a) the clinical picture was of a mild form of thalassaemia intermedia, with hepatosplenomegaly and a steady-state haemoglobin of 9.3 g/dl (Trent *et al.* 1984b). In the homozygote for the Malay 2 variety, an 11-year-old child, there was also hepatosplenomegaly and a steady-state haemoglobin value of 11.8 g/dl (George *et al.* 1986). In the Turkish variety, a homozygote has moderate anaemia, with haemoglobin levels of 8–10.7 g/dl, together with hepatosplenomegaly (Dinçol *et al.* 1981).

Clearly, the homozygous phenotype of this form of thalassaemia shows some variability of clinical phenotype but, overall, it is characterized by a mild to moderate form of thalassaemia intermedia.

Haematological findings

The rather limited clinical data indicate that the haemoglobin levels range from 8 to 11 g/dl, and that the red cells show typical thalassaemic changes and indices.

Haemoglobin analysis and synthesis

As expected, these homozygotes have 100% HbF. The reported α-/γ-globin synthesis ratios for the Indian varieties range from 2.5 to 5.1, with a mean value of 3.9. The homozygote for the Turkish form has an α/γ ratio of 5.

Heterozygous ($^{A}\gamma\delta\beta$)^{0} thalassaemia

The heterozygous state for δβ thalassaemia in which the HbF was of the $^{G}\gamma$ variety has been observed in Chinese (Mann *et al.* 1972), Indians (Sukumaran *et al.* 1972; Amin *et al.* 1979), Afro-Americans (Huisman *et al.* 1975a; Altay *et al.* 1977b; Wood *et al.* 1977a), Arabs (Amin *et al.* 1979) and Turks (Reyes *et al.* 1978; Orkin *et al.* 1979a). More recently, this disease has been dissected into its 12 different molecular forms, and it has been possible to relate the heterozygous phenotypes to the underlying genotypes. These data are summarized in Table 8.7, together with the sources.

Clinical features

No symptoms can be ascribed to this condition and splenomegaly has not been observed.

Haematological findings

As summarized in Table 8.7, the condition is characterized by extremely mild anaemia with typical thalassaemic red-cell indices.

Haemoglobin analysis

Despite the underlying molecular heterogeneity the reported HbF values in heterozygotes have clustered in the 5–15% range. Slightly higher values were found in association with the Cantonese and Malay-1 varieties. The HbF is unevenly distributed among the red cells; the report of the Yunnanese heterozygotes is atypical in that the HbF was said to have a pancellular distribution.

Globin synthesis

The reported globin synthesis ratios are summarized

Table 8.7 Summary of haematological data (mean ± SD) of ($^{A}\gamma\delta\beta$)^{0}-thalassaemia heterozygotes defined by molecular analysis.

Type	No of families/ individuals	Hb (g/dl)	MCV (fl)	MCH (pg)	HbA$_2$ (%)	HbF (%)	$^{G}\gamma$ (%)	α/non-α synthesis*	Distribution/% F cells
Black	20/24	12.6±1.6	74.3±7.4	24.1±2.8	2.4±0.5	11.2±3.4	93.2±4.1	1.43±0.34	Heterocellular
Chinese	5/12	13.9±0.7	72.8±3.8	22.7±1.1	2.5±0.5	11.8±2.1	97.0±2.8	1.38±0.04	Heterocellular/75–90%
Indian	5/16	13.1±1.4	77.1±5.4	24.6±1.3	2.3±0.4	12.9±2.1	99.5±0.5	1.82±0.45	Pancellular
Italian	1/2					14.5±3.5			
Belgian	1/3	13.8±2.5	68.0±6.2	26.3±0.6	2.6±0.2	14.5±0.2		1.68±0.63	Heterocellular/61–94%
Yunnanese	1/6	13.1±1.0	73.5±2.1	22.9±1.0	1.6±0.1	14.5±3.5	82.8±8.8		Pancellular
German	1/3		71.3±4.2		2.5±0.1	11.1±1.8	84		Heterocellular/54–77%
Turkish	2/2	12.5±2.1	72.0±2.8	24.0	2.5±0	11.8±2.5	100	1.96±0.06	Heterocellular/40%
South-east Asian	4/9	12.8±1.5	80.0±2.9	26.4±0.9	2.2±0.5	18.8±2.3	96.4±3.6		Pancellular

*Data not necessarily complete for all individuals; extreme outliers omitted.
α Thalassaemia not excluded in all cases; some results obtained after sample had been in transit.
MCH, mean cell haemoglobin; MCV, mean cell volume.

in Table 8.7. The α-/non-α-chain ratios range from 1.4 to 1.9, reflecting a mild degree of imbalance, probably significantly less than that of heterozygous β thalassaemia.

$(\delta\beta)^0$ or $(^A\gamma\delta\beta)^0$ thalassaemia in association with β thalassaemia

The compound heterozygous state for both β and δβ thalassaemia was first characterized in an Italian family by Zuelzer *et al.* (1961). Further cases were reported in Greeks (Fessas 1961; Gabuzda *et al.* 1963; Wolff & Ignatov 1963; Stamatoyannopoulos *et al.* 1969a; Kattamis *et al.* 1973), Italians (Wolff & Ignatov 1963; Necheles *et al.* 1969; Brancati 1973; Mezzadra *et al.* 1974; Ottolenghi *et al.* 1975), Afro-Americans (Zelkowitz *et al.* 1972; Altay *et al.* 1977b; Kinney *et al.* 1978), Yugoslavians (Efremov *et al.* 1975), Turks (Aksoy *et al.* 1974), Chinese (Mann *et al.* 1972), Indians (Sukumaran & Master 1974) and Spaniards (Romero *et al.* 1976).

The structure of the fetal haemoglobin was only analysed in a few of these early reports. Some of them, Greek and Yugoslavian cases for example, describe the interaction of $(\delta\beta)^0$ thalassaemia with β thalassaemia (Stamatoyannopoulos *et al.* 1971; Efremov *et al.* 1975; Ottolenghi *et al.* 1975). In the Chinese and Afro-Asian families reported by Mann *et al.* (1972) and Altay *et al.* (1977b) the compound heterozygous states for $(^A\gamma\delta\beta)^0$ thalassaemia and β^0 or β^+ thalassaemia, respectively, were described. It is likely that the cases reported from the Mediterranean region and Yugoslavia represent the Sicilian form of the disease.

Since the molecular defects in the different forms of δβ and β thalassaemia have been described, there have been reports of the interaction of the Thai variety of $(^A\gamma\delta\beta)^0$ thalassaemia with the βIVS2-654 C→T mutation (Fucharoen & Winichagoon 1987; Winichagoon *et al.* 1990b) and the Chinese form of the same condition with β^0 thalassaemia (Jones *et al.* 1981b). However, since there are at least 16 different types of δβ thalassaemia, and about 200 varieties of β thalassaemia, the potential for phenotypic variation from these interactions is boundless. In the absence of any large series which have been defined at both the clinical and molecular levels it is only possible to make some generalizations about the clinical features of these disorders.

Clinical and haematological features

Overall, although the clinical manifestations of this condition are extremely variable, the disorder is milder than homozygous or compound heterozygous β thalassaemia and most patients show the clinical picture of thalassaemia intermedia.

In the 21 Greek patients reported by Stamatoyannopoulos *et al.* (1969a), which are likely to reflect interactions of the Sicilian form of $(\delta\beta)^0$ thalassaemia with different varieties of β thalassaemia, the age at presentation ranged from 7 months to 29 years; 12 were more than 10 years old when they were first seen. Nine patients sought medical attention directly as the result of their disorder, five were diagnosed during hospital admissions for other illnesses, and seven were detected during family or population surveys. In those who presented early in childhood the clinical manifestations were similar to severe β thalassaemia intermedia (see Chapter 13). Typical thalassaemic bone changes were only apparent in three children and in most cases there were only minimal deformities. Twelve patients in this series had never received blood transfusion. In the remainder, occasional transfusions were required and only two children needed regular transfusion. In the 11 Greek children reported by Kattamis *et al.* (1973) the clinical picture was similar.

Most of the other clinical descriptions of this disorder in Mediterranean populations involve only one or two cases. Again, there is remarkable heterogeneity of the clinical manifestations. In the early reports of Wolff and Ignatov (1963) one of the patients, a female of Italian extraction aged 2 years, presented with severe anaemia during a 'haemolytic crisis' which resulted in her death after 13 days. On the other hand, the same authors describe a similarly affected Greek who had been followed in their clinic from the age of 6 to 20 years. This patient was dependent on regular transfusions early in life although the transfusion intervals increased from 2 to 4 months as he grew older. In contrast, the Greek patient described by Gabuzda *et al.* (1964) was in reasonable health until the age of 22 years, at which time he underwent splenectomy because of increasing haemolysis. One sibling was similarly affected. The clinical manifestations in the Yugoslavian, Turkish and Italian patients described by Efremov *et al.* (1975), Aksoy *et al.* (1974) and Ottolenghi *et al.* (1975)

were similar to those observed in the Greek population.

It might be expected that the compound heterozygous state for β thalassaemia with $(^A\gamma\delta\beta)^0$ thalassaemia would be more severe. In the Chinese patient reported by Mann *et al.* (1972), in whom the interaction was with β^0 thalassaemia, the child had the phenotype of severe thalassaemia intermedia and became transfusion dependent, even after splenectomy. In the more recent reports of the interaction of the Thai varieties of $(^A\gamma\delta\beta)^0$ thalassaemia with β^0 thalassaemia there was a similar clinical picture (Winichagoon *et al.* 1990b). Earlier reports, backed up by more recent studies, suggested that this interaction is much milder in Afro-American populations. In the patients studied by Zelkowitz *et al.* (1972) there was virtually no anaemia and in one of the two cases the spleen was not palpable. In the patient reported by Altay *et al.* (1977b), a 34-year-old Afro-American female, anaemia was noted for the first time during pregnancy. She had persistent leg ulceration and splenomegaly, and required transfusion at the time of splenectomy for hypersplenism. The 9-year-old boy described by Waye *et al.* (1994a), in whom compound heterozygosity for the mild –29 A→G β-thalassaemia mutation and the Black form of $(^A\gamma\delta\beta)^0$ thalassaemia was defined, had a mild anaemia with thalassaemic red-cell changes; the steady-state haemoglobin level was 9.8 g/dl, with 66% HbF. This child was described as having palpable splenomegaly but no hepatomegaly. Curiously, however, abdominal ultrasound revealed 'no organomegaly'. Since the latter is more sensitive than abdominal palpation for detecting moderate degrees of splenomegaly, these observations are difficult to reconcile.

In short, the reported information on these interactions suggests that they are characterized by the clinical picture of thalassaemia intermedia of varying severity; at the more severe end of the spectrum there are patients with progressive anaemia and splenomegaly who may need transfusion, while at the other end patients may remain symptomless and the condition is only discovered by chance on haematological examination for other reasons. The latter phenotype may reflect interactions with mild β-thalassaemia alleles.

Complications

As already mentioned, some patients with this disorder develop progessive splenomegaly and hyper-

splenism. Chronic leg ulceration has been reported (Mezzadra *et al.* 1974; Altay *et al.* 1977b). As in many patients with thalassaemia intermedia, progressive iron loading may occur (Gabuzda *et al.* 1964). We followed the patient reported by Ottolenghi *et al.* (1975) for many years. At the age of 20 years he had high serum iron and plasma ferritin levels and a liver biopsy showed extensive iron deposition and fibrosis. He responded well to repeated venesection over a 4-year period, during which it is estimated that approximately 25 g of iron was removed. Clearly, more information is needed about the degree of iron loading in this group of patients; we shall return to this question in Chapter 13.

Haemoglobin constitution

The haemoglobin constitution depends on the nature of the associated β-thalassaemia gene, well illustrated in the large series of Stamatoyannopoulos *et al.* (1969a). In 19 patients the mean HbF value was 84.7% with a range from 66 to 98%; in seven, HbA was not detected, while the remainder represented the $(\delta\beta)^0/\beta^+$-thalassaemia genotype. The HbA_2 values in this series ranged from 1.3 to 2.8%, with a mean of 1.9%. A relatively low value seems to be the rule. In the 11 compound heterozygotes reported by Kattamis *et al.* (1973) the mean level of HbF was 70.3% and HbA was absent in five. The findings in both these series reflect the presence of both β^+ and β^0 thalassaemia in the Greek population. It seems probable that the very high levels of HbF in the earlier cases of Wolff and Ignatov (1963) and Gabuzda *et al.* (1964) resulted from $(\delta\beta)^0/\beta^0$- or $(^A\gamma\delta\beta)^0/\beta^0$-thalassaemia genotype and this was also the case in the Italian reported by Ottolenghi *et al.* (1975). In African patients the level of HbF is lower, in the 60% range in the patients described by Zelkowitz *et al.* (1972), Altay *et al.* (1977b) and Waye *et al.* (1994a). These were almost certainly the result of interactions between $(^A\gamma\delta\beta)^0$ thalassaemia and mild forms of β^+-thalassaemia mutations, and proved to be so in the case of Waye *et al.*

The distribution and structure of haemoglobin F

Fetal haemoglobin is heterogeneously distributed among the red cells, as evidenced by differential centrifugation experiments which have shown that the heavier, older cell population at the bottom of a layer of centrifuged blood contains relatively more HbF than that of the lighter, young population (Gabuzda *et al.* 1964). In fact, the classical experiments of Gabuzda and colleagues on the differential turnovers of Hbs A, F and A_2 in β thalassaemia (see Chapter 5) were carried out on a Greek patient who was a compound heterozygote for $(δβ)^0$ and β thalassaemia. They found that the mean lifespan of HbF was 95 days, whereas that of Hbs A and A_2 was 60 days. The HbF-containing populations are longer lived than those which contain predominantly HbA, a situation exactly analogous to that observed in homozygous β thalassaemia.

Curiously, in the compound heterozygote for $(^Aγδβ)^0$ and $β^+$ thalassaemia described by Waye *et al.* (1994a) the HbF was reported to be homogeneously distributed; the level in the peripheral blood was 66%. The child's heterozygous mother had 14.7% HbF, heterogeneously distributed, and confined to about half her red cells.

The structure of HbF was first reported by Stamatoyannopoulos *et al.* (1971). In three Greek patients the glycine residues in peptide γCB3 ranged from 0.5 to 0.61. Interestingly, in each of these cases the glycine value was significantly higher than that found in the heterozygous $(δβ)^0$-thalassaemic relatives. Although at first glance it might be thought that this difference reflects the activity of the γ-chain genes from the chromosome carrying the β-thalassaemia gene this may not be the case; a similar difference in the $^Gγ$ composition of HbF was noted between $(δβ)^0$-thalassaemia heterozygotes and homozygotes for the condition. Similar observations in Yugoslavian patients were reported by Efremov *et al.* (1975).

Analysis of the structure of HbF has been reported for two individuals who were compound heterozygotes for $(^Aγδβ)^0$ thalassaemia and β thalassaemia. In the patient described by Mann *et al.* (1972) the glycine composition of peptide γ15 was 0.94 and the alanine was 2.03, and in the report by Altay *et al.* (1977b) the values were 0.86 and 2.14, respectively. In both studies the heterozygous carriers of $(^Aγδβ)^0$ thalassaemia, as expected, had glycine values of almost 1. These results suggest that there is an important contribution by the γ-chain loci on the chromosome carrying the β-thalassaemia gene in these compound heterozygotes, an observation confirmed by Waye *et al.* (1994a).

Haemoglobin synthesis

There have been only limited studies of globin synthesis in the peripheral blood. Furthermore, they are not comparable because they have been carried out on individuals with different combinations of δβ- or β-thalassaemia genes. In the $(^Aγδβ)^0/β^0$-thalassaemia compound heterozygote studied by Mann *et al.* (1972) the α-/γ-chain production ratio was 2.6 (Fig. 8.7), in the Italian and Sardinian patients with $(δβ)^0/β^0$ thalassaemia reported by Ottolenghi *et al.* (1975) and Cao *et al.* (1981) they were 1.4–4, while in the patient with an undesignated form of δβ thalassaemia interacting with $β^0$ thalassaemia reported by Kinney *et al.* (1978) it was 2.7. A similar value was obtained by Altay *et al.* (1977b) in an Afro-American woman heterozygous for both $(^Aγδβ)^0$ thalassaemia and $β^+$ thalassaemia. These limited data suggest that there is more globin imbalance in this condition than in homozygous $(δβ)^0$ or $(^Aγδβ)^0$ thalassaemia, but less than that found in homozygous β thalassaemia. However, they do not allow any conclusions to be made about the possible differences in the relative degree of globin imbalance in interactions between different genetic variants of δβ and β thalassaemia.

δβ Thalassaemia in association with structural haemoglobin variants

These conditions are considered in Chapter 9.

The pathophysiology of the δβ thalassaemias

The cardinal differences between the β and δβ thalassaemias are the levels of HbF and A_2 in heterozygotes, and the clinical picture of their homozygous states, mirrored by the degree of globin imbalance; in δβ thalassaemia the defect in β-chain production is compensated to a greater degree by an increase in the output of γ chains from the chromosome carrying the thalassaemia determinant.

The homozygous state for $(δβ)^0$ thalassaemia is an extremely mild condition and the degree of anaemia is little more than that observed in some heterozygous β thalassaemics. It appears therefore that the output of γ chains is sufficient to compensate to a considerable degree for the deficiency of β chains. Wood *et al.* (1977a) described *in vitro* incubation and differential centrifugation experiments on the blood of heterozygotes. These studies revealed considerable variability in the distribution of HbF and indicated that those cells which contain more HbF have a longer survival than the predominantly HbA-containing population. The situation is therefore analogous to that observed in β thalassaemia and

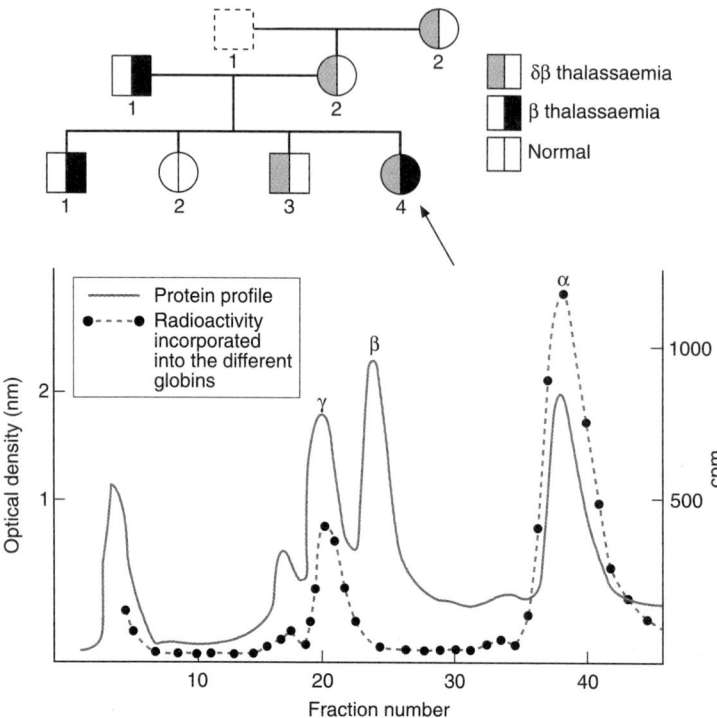

Fig. 8.7 The interaction of $\delta\beta$ thalassaemia and β^0 thalassaemia. Top, inheritance, bottom, globin synthesis in the reticulocytes of the propositus shown in the pedigree (III.4). The experimental conditions are those described in Chapter 5. The continuous line represents the protein profile and the dotted line the radioactivity incorporated into the different globins. There is no β-chain synthesis in the propositus. From Mann *et al.* (1972).

indicates that there is selection for HbF-rich cells in $\delta\beta$-thalassaemia heterozygotes; presumably this also applies to homozygotes. The reason for the uneven distribution of fetal haemoglobin among the red cells in heterozygous and homozygous $\delta\beta$ thalassaemia is still not understood. We shall return to this problem, which is still one of the most perplexing in the entire thalassaemia field, in Chapter 10 when we consider the differences between $\delta\beta$ thalassaemia and HPFH.

Since compensatory γ-chain synthesis is the key factor in producing the mild phenotype of $\delta\beta$ thalassaemia it might be expected that the $(\delta\beta)^0$ thalassaemias would be less severe than the $(^A\gamma\delta\beta)^0$ thalassaemias. As we saw earlier, homozygotes for the latter do seem to be relatively more anaemic than those for $(\delta\beta)^0$ thalassaemia. Curiously, however, these differences do not seem to be clearly reflected in the heterozygous states. Although, if only the larger series are considered, the levels of HbF in $(\delta\beta)^0$-thalassaemia heterozygotes appear slightly higher than those in $(^A\gamma\delta\beta)^0$-thalassaemia heterozygotes (see Tables 8.6 and 8.7), these differences are small and many exceptions have been reported. The reason for this discrepancy is not clear.

The remarkable clinical variability observed in compound heterozygotes for $\delta\beta$ and β thalassaemia is partly explicable by the different severity of the associated β-thalassaemia alleles. In general, patients who have severe β^+- or β^0-thalassaemia alleles interacting with $\delta\beta$ thalassaemia are more seriously affected, although there is considerable heterogeneity among this group. Unfortunately, the published data are not much help in deciding why this might be. In many cases secondary factors such as hypersplenism may have played a role but it is not at all clear from some of the case reports why some patients have shown such severe manifestations. In general, when $(^A\gamma\delta\beta)^0$ thalassaemia interacts with the less severe β^+-thalassaemia mutations found in Afro-Americans, the result is a mild form of thalassaemia intermedia. It might be anticipated that the worst combination of these genes would be $(^A\gamma\delta\beta)^0$ thalassaemia and β^0 thalassaemia. An interaction of this type, reported by Mann *et al.* (1972), resulted in a transfusion-dependent disease from early life; splenectomy had little effect on transfusion requirements. Perhaps we should not draw too many conclusions from one case since there are reports of patients with $(\delta\beta)^0$ thalassaemia and β^+ or β^0 thalassaemia who appeared to be almost as severely affected.

It is quite clear therefore from studies of haemoglobin synthesis and analysis of the distribution and turnover of HbF in these combinations that their pathophysiology resembles β thalassaemia, except that the increased level of γ-chain production, which is presumably the direct result of the $\delta\beta$-thalassaemia mutation, results in an overall amelioration of the $\delta\beta$-thalassaemia syndromes.

The geographical distribution of δβ thalassaemia

In the earlier thalassaemia literature well documented cases of $\delta\beta$ thalassaemia were reported in many different ethnic groups. These include Italians (Zuelzer *et al.* 1961; Wolff & Ignatov 1963; Brancati & Puccetti 1964; Silvestroni *et al.* 1964; Silvestroni & Bianco 1968), Greeks (Fessas 1961; Wolff & Ignatov 1963; Gabuzda *et al.* 1964; Stamatoyannopoulos *et al.* 1969a), Afro-Americans (Weatherall 1964a; Zelkowitz *et al.* 1972; Altay *et al.* 1977b; Kinney *et al.* 1978), Thais (Flatz *et al.* 1965b; Wasi *et al.* 1969), Arabs (Ramot *et al.* 1970; present authors, unpublished observations), Chinese (Mann *et al.* 1972), Indians (Sukumaran *et al.* 1972; Sukumaran & Master 1974; Amin *et al.* 1979), Turks (Aksoy *et al.* 1974), Yugoslavians (Efremov *et al.* 1975), Jamaicans (Ahern *et al.* 1972; Wood *et al.* 1977a), Britons (present authors, unpublished observations), Mexicans (Reyes *et al.* 1978), Spaniards (Pellicer 1967; Gimferrer *et al.* 1979; Pagnier *et al.* 1979) and Sardinians (Cao *et al.* 1981). Other references are cited earlier in the chapter.

More recently, and as a result of the molecular analysis of $\delta\beta$ thalassaemia, it has been possible to obtain further information about the geographical distribution of this condition and to define no less than 22 different varieties based on their identification in different ethnic groups (see Tables 8.1, 8.6 and 8.7).

One of the difficulties in assessing the frequency of this disorder is that the technology employed in many population surveys for thalassaemia may not detect it. This would certainly be the case if osmotic-fragility screening techniques were used, and only those surveys which include a quantitative estimation of HbF, or haemoglobin electrophoresis using a system which separates HbA from F, would provide data about $\delta\beta$-thalassaemia gene frequencies. From the scanty information which is available it looks as

though $\delta\beta$ thalassaemia has its highest incidence in the Mediterranean and eastern European countries; this probably reflects the widespread distribution of the Sicilian variety. It also occurs sporadically in most populations.

By far the most extensive data have come from Greece. In their survey of 1600 healthy young males in the Greek Air Force, Malamos *et al.* (1962) found 109 individuals with a thalassaemia-like blood picture; of these, 11 cases had findings compatible with the heterozygous state for $\delta\beta$ thalassaemia. This must be compared with the finding of 85 β-thalassaemia heterozygotes out of the 109 thalassaemic individuals found in this study. From these data the incidence of β thalassaemia was approximately 5.3%, while that of $\delta\beta$ thalassaemia was 0.6%. However, this was a small population sample and these gene frequencies are only an approximation of the overall figures for the incidence of the different forms of β and $\delta\beta$ thalassaemia in Greece (see Chapter 6).

The condition, again reflecting the Sicilian variety, has been observed repeatedly in Italian populations, although the gene frequency is unknown. In an early population survey in Calabria, Brancati and Puccetti (1964) studied 825 subjects, 58 of whom showed haematological evidence of heterozygous thalassaemia. Of these, 54 were carriers of β thalassaemia and there was one heterozygous for $\delta\beta$ thalassaemia. In their extensive investigations of the population of Campania, Quattrin *et al.* (1973) found 3197 cases of thalassaemia and abnormal haemoglobins out of a total survey of 43 000 persons. Of these, the vast majority were heterozygous β thalassaemics but 56 cases, i.e. 2.5% of the total thalassaemic population, were $\delta\beta$-thalassaemia heterozygotes. This gives an overall incidence of $\delta\beta$ thalassaemia of approximately 0.13%, as compared with 5% for heterozygous β thalassaemia. Cao *et al.* (1982a,b) have estimated a gene frequency of 0.00088 in Sardinia.

Very little is known about the gene frequency for $\delta\beta$ thalassaemia in other populations although the number of reported cases is small compared with β thalassaemia. In the survey of 2790 Thai subjects reported by Flatz *et al.* (1965b) one family with $\delta\beta$ thalassaemia was found. The small number of cases in this and other surveys and the sporadic case reports in the literature suggest that the condition is uncommon outside eastern Europe.

It seems very likely that many of the different forms of $\delta\beta$ thalassaemia have arisen sporadically, possibly by unequal crossing over with the resulting deletion of varying lengths of the $^G\gamma^A\gamma\delta\beta$-gene cluster (see Chapter 4). The most likely crossover events which involve this region are those which produce Hb Lepores, since the δ and β genes have similar nucleotide sequences and lie close together in the β-globin-gene cluster.

$(\varepsilon\gamma\delta\beta)^0$ Thalassaemia

In 1972 Kan and colleagues described a family in which they thought there might be a form of thalassaemia characterized by a deficiency of γ chains *in utero*, and β and possibly δ chains in adult life (Kan *et al.* 1972b). The proband was a full-term female infant of English and German parentage. The child had moderately severe neonatal haemolysis but was also found to have a hypochromic blood picture. There was no evidence of α thalassaemia and studies of globin synthesis revealed a deficiency of γ- and β-chain production relative to that of α chains. As the infant matured, her peripheral blood picture improved but she remained mildly thalassaemic and similar haematological changes were found in her father and in seven of his relatives. The findings in these family members resembled the β-thalassaemia trait except that the HbA_2 level was normal.

Subsequent gene mapping analyses on members of this family revealed that the condition is caused by a deletion of nearly 96 kb which starts approximately 50 kb upstream from the ε gene and finishes in the second exon of the β-globin gene (Orkin *et al.* 1981b). The condition is therefore defined as a form of $(\varepsilon\gamma\delta\beta)^0$ thalassaemia. Based on the ethnic origin of the family it became known as the Anglo-Saxon type of $(\varepsilon\gamma\delta\beta)^0$ thalassaemia.

Several other varieties of $(\varepsilon\gamma\delta\beta)^0$ thalassaemia have been discovered. Although at the molecular level they fall into two distinct categories (see Chapter 4), the associated phenotypes of the two groups seem to be more or less the same. The first group is comprised of conditions rather like the Anglo-Saxon form, in which long deletions have removed all or the greater part of the β-globin-gene cluster. Five further varieties of $(\varepsilon\gamma\delta\beta)^0$ thalassaemia of this kind have been reported: Scottish–Irish (Pirastu *et al.* 1983b; Trent *et al.* 1990); Mexican (Fearon *et al.* 1983); Croatian (Diaz-Chico *et al.* 1988a); Irish (Fortina *et al.* 1991a); and Canadian (Diaz-Chico *et al.* 1988a; Abels *et al.* 1996). The

second group, in which $(\varepsilon\gamma\delta\beta)^0$ thalassaemia has been found in association with intact β-globin genes, is comprised of three forms: Dutch (Van der Ploeg *et al.* 1980); English (Curtin *et al.* 1985); and Hispanic (Driscoll *et al.* 1989). Although the deletions that are involved in the second group leave the β-globin gene intact they still appear to inactivate the entire complex, presumably because of their involvement of the LCR. The molecular basis for these conditions is described in detail in Chapter 4.

Pathophysiology

Presumably because it would not be compatible with fetal survival, the homozygous state for this disorder has not been encountered. Since it inactivates the entire β-globin-gene cluster it might be expected that, in the heterozygous state, it would be phenotypically little different from β^0 thalassaemia. The HbA_2 level would not be elevated because of the loss of one δ-chain locus but otherwise there is no reason why the two conditions should not have a similar phenotype. This is indeed the case in older children and adults. The curious feature, however, is that in the neonatal period it is far more severe than heterozygous β^0 thalassaemia. In the first description by Kan *et al.* (1972b) the baby was quite severely anaemic at birth, with jaundice and a picture similar to haemolytic disease of the newborn. However, the disorder was clearly thalassaemic and globin synthesis studies revealed α-/non-α-chain ratios similar to β-thalassaemia trait.

It is difficult to understand why this condition is more severe in fetal life, particularly since affected infants have two out of the four γ-globin genes intact. It differs, of course, from β thalassaemia, in which there is no globin imbalance *in utero* due to the high level of fetal haemoglobin production. This raises the intriguing possibility that the fetal red cell is much more sensitive than its adult counterpart to the effects of a moderate degree of globin imbalance. Whether this reflects a less effective ability to withstand oxidant stress is not clear but, whatever the mechanism, in many cases this condition is associated with quite severe anaemia at birth.

Clinical features

In newborn babies there may be a moderate degree of anaemia with haemoglobin values in the 7–10 g/dl range. As these patients get older the anaemia becomes less severe. In adult life the disorder is asymptomatic.

One of the remarkable features of this condition is its clinical variability, even within the same family. Trent *et al.* (1990) provide details of six heterozygotes for the Scottish–Irish variety, all from the same family. One of these patients was pale and jaundiced at birth. He had palpable splenomegaly and a cord blood haemoglobin of 13.2 g/dl. The blood picture was typical of thalassaemia. There was no evidence of immune haemolysis and the Coombs test was negative. He required repeated blood transfusions and was discharged from hospital 18 days after delivery with a haemoglobin level of 10.7 g/dl. Twenty-eight days postnatally, his haemoglobin level had fallen to 8.5 g/dl. In contrast, however, two other affected neonates in the same family had completely uneventful postnatal periods and did not require transfusion or hospitalization. As mentioned earlier, the first patient to be described with this disorder had a similar degree of anaemia in the newborn period. A heterozygote for the Canadian form was also found to be moderately anaemic at birth (Diaz-Chico *et al.* 1988a). The proband in the family with the Hispanic form, reported by Driscoll *et al.* (1989), had severe neonatal haemolytic anaemia; at the age of 2 months the haemoglobin level was 7.9 g/dl. Again, it rose and at the age of 11 years the steady-state haemoglobin was 11.6 g/dl.

Haematological findings

Although these patients may be quite anaemic at birth, with typical thalassaemic morphological changes of their red cells, in later life they have a blood picture typical of β-thalassaemia trait but with a normal HbA$_2$ level. Although their haematological findings have not been compared with those of β-thalassaemia heterozygotes in the same laboratory they appear, as a group, to be rather more anaemic and to have more severe microcytosis and hypochromia than many β-thalassaemia heterozygotes.

Haemoglobin analysis

In adult life this condition is associated with HbA$_2$ levels which are normal or at the upper limit of the normal range, and either normal or very slightly elevated levels of HbF. Globin synthesis ratios are in the β-thalassaemia trait range.

Interactions with haemoglobin variants or β thalassaemia

No interactions of this form of thalassaemia with other haemoglobin variants or β thalassaemia in *trans* have been reported. In the family with the Hispanic form the β^S gene was found in *cis* to the deletion but, like the rest of the β-globin-gene complex, it was not expressed (Driscoll *et al.* 1989).

δ Thalassaemia

In 1962 Fessas and Stamatoyannopoulos described a 60-year-old Greek male who had the haematological picture of thalassaemia trait with complete absence of HbA$_2$. Through a normal wife this man had several children, some of whom were normal, others having thalassaemia trait with normal levels of HbA$_2$. These workers concluded that this patient was heterozygous for both a form of thalassaemia associated with defective δ- and β-chain synthesis, δβ thalassaemia, and an inherited defect in δ-chain synthesis, δ thalassaemia. In fact the level of HbF in this patient, 2.5%, was too low for δ thalassaemia and it seems likely that he was homozygous for δ thalassaemia and heterozygous for β thalassaemia.

Thompson *et al.* (1965) reported the combination of δ thalassaemia and HPFH in the same person. Three individuals, born of one parent with HPFH and the other with a low level of HbA$_2$, showed the clinical picture of heterozygosity for HPFH and the absence of HbA$_2$ on starch gel electrophoresis. Since many of the Afro-American forms of HPFH are associated with an absence of β- and δ-chain synthesis, this study indicated that δ thalassaemia, at least in this case, was also associated with a total deficiency of δ-chain synthesis, i.e. this was the first description of δ^0 thalassaemia. A further homozygote for δ thalassaemia was reported by Ohta *et al.* (1971a). Again, no HbA$_2$ could be demonstrated in the proband or in her mother, while the father had reduced quantities and was considered to be heterozygous for δ thalassaemia. Another example of δ thalassaemia, in this case in association with sickle-cell anaemia, was reported by Thompson *et al.* (1966). Further evidence for the existence of this condition was obtained from population surveys in Greece, in which unusually low levels of HbA$_2$ were found in several members of the same family (Fraser *et al.* 1964), and in a later study in Japan, in which five further homozygotes were identified (Yasukawa *et al.* 1980).

Once it became possible to analyse the δ-globin genes directly, more cases of δ thalassaemia were identified, and by 1997 a total of 17 different δ-thalassaemia alleles had been reported. While the bulk of the cases appeared to be δ^0 thalassaemia there were a few reports of δ$^+$-thalassaemia variants (Huisman 1997) (see Chapter 4). Most of these cases were ascertained by analysing the δ-globin genes of individuals who appeared to have the β-thalassaemia trait but with a normal level of HbA$_2$. Others have been identified by the finding of an absence of HbA$_2$ on haemoglobin electrophoresis.

The different varieties of δ thalassaemia are listed in Chapter 4.

Molecular pathology and pathophysiology

The molecular pathology of the δ thalassaemias is described in Chapter 4. Other than reducing the overall output of HbA$_2$ these mutations seem to have no other phenotypic effect.

Haematological findings and haemoglobin analysis

The heterozygous and homozygous states for δ thalassaemia are not associated with any haematological changes. In homozygotes there is no HbA$_2$ while in heterozygotes the level is subnormal, in the range of 0.7–1.6%. There are many examples of δ thalassaemia occurring with β-thalassaemia mutations in the same person. Some typical HbA$_2$ levels are summarized in Chapter 7, Table 7.19. It is clear that the level of HbA$_2$ is reduced from the usual value of 4 to 6% in β-thalassaemia trait to about half this value, i.e. it falls into the normal range or may be slightly elevated. While in some families the δ-thalassaemia mutation is clearly in *trans* to the β-thalassaemia gene, in others the two mutations are in *cis*. For example the δ^{0}CD59 –A mutation is found in *cis* to β^{Knossos} (Olds *et al.* 1991), thus accounting for the silent carrier state of the form of thalassaemia associated with Hb Knossos. The δ^{0}CD59 –A/β^{Knossos} allele is probably quite prevalent throughout the Mediterranean. This form of δ thalassaemia has also been reported in *cis* to the β^{0}CD39 C→T and βIVS1-110 G→A mutations (Tzetis *et al.* 1994). Another δ-

thalassaemia mutation, δ$^+$CD27 C→T, has also been reported in *cis* to a β-thalassaemia gene (βIVS2-745 C→G) in a Greek person with normal HbA$_2$ β thalassaemia. Analysis of the β-globin RFLP haplotypes suggested that this allele has arisen through a crossover between two chromosomes, one carrying δ$^+$CD27 C→T, and the other the IVS2-745 C→G mutation (Loudianos *et al.* 1990). The same mechanism may underlie the other δ thalassaemias that exist in *cis* to β-thalassaemia mutations.

Thus there is little doubt that the co-inheritance of δ thalassaemia accounts for many cases of normal HbA$_2$ β thalassaemia type 2; that is, a condition with the haematological features of β-thalassaemia trait and a normal HbA$_2$ level (for further discussion see Chapter 7).

γ Thalassaemia

As far as is known, there have been no clinical disorders associated with defects that involve the γ genes alone. Indeed, only one form of γ thalassaemia has been defined (Sukumaran *et al.* 1983; Zeng *et al.* 1985b). This results from a deletion of approximately 5 kb which is probably the result of unequal crossover between the ^{G}γ- and ^{A}γ-globin genes, forming a hybrid ^{GA}γ gene. The deletion involves the 3′ end of the ^{G}γ gene and the 5′ end of the ^{A}γ gene, and the region between them.

This anomaly is usually detected by analysis of DNA from newborn babies. At this stage of development the ^{G}γ-chain level is usually in the 65–70% range, but lower values are found in heterozygotes for this variety of γ thalassaemia, usually in the 40% range. This occurs because the hybrid ^{GA}γ gene is expressed as ^{A}γ. Two individuals homozygous for this anomaly have been reported (Zeng *et al.* 1985b).

This condition has to be distinguished from the ^{A}γ^{A}γ-globin-gene arrangement which resembles γ thalassaemia because heterozygous newborns also have HbF with low ^{G}γ values in the 35–40% range (Huisman 1997).

One of the structural variants of HbF, HbF Yamaguchi (α$_2$γ$_2$Ile→Thr; 80 Asp→Asn; 136 Ala) is linked to this type of γ thalassaemia. This unusual condition results in the production of about 30–35% of the γ Yamaguchi chain, which is considerably higher than that expected from a normal γ-gene arrangement (Nakatsuji *et al.* 1984; Wada *et al.* 1986).

Chapter 9
The β and δβ thalassaemias in association with structural haemoglobin variants

Studies of the haemoglobin of individuals heterozygous for both thalassaemia and one of the abnormal haemoglobins have been of great value in elucidating the genetic basis for the thalassaemias. Such an association was first reported in 1946 by Silvestroni and Bianco (1946b), who described the clinical and haematological findings in patients heterozygous for both thalassaemia and the sickle-cell gene; the disorder which resulted from this interaction was called microdrepanocytic disease or sickle-cell thalassaemia. This condition has been studied intensively since then and, as described in Chapter 1, analyses of the haemoglobin of such doubly affected persons, together with the segregation of the sickle-cell and thalassaemia genes in their offspring, provided the basis for much of our subsequent thinking about the heterogeneity and genetics of the thalassaemia syndromes.

The interactions of the thalassaemias with structural haemoglobin variants are also of considerable clinical importance. Although the majority of them are rare, several, notably sickle-cell β thalassaemia and HbE β thalassaemia, cause a considerable public health problem in some parts of the world. Indeed, because of the particularly high frequency of β thalassaemia and HbE in Asia, HbE β thalassaemia will be one of the most important varieties of thalassaemia in the new millennium.

In this chapter we shall review the clinical, haematological and genetic aspects of the various interactions between the different forms of β and δβ thalassaemia and structural haemoglobin variants. For readers who are coming to this subject for the first time it is important to familiarize themselves with the main principles of the structure and function of haemoglobin, and the genetic principles of these interactions, which are outlined in Chapters 2 and 3, before attempting to understand the clinical implications of these complex disorders. References to articles and reviews which deal with the structural haemoglobin variants in greater detail than is possible here are cited in the appropriate sections.

Interactions between the sickle-cell gene and the β and δβ thalassaemias

Sickle-cell β thalassaemia

Introduction

The clinical and haematological findings in patients heterozygous for both thalassaemia and the sickle-cell gene were studied extensively between 1946 and 1955 by Silvestroni and Bianco and summarized in a monograph on the subject in 1955 (Silvestroni & Bianco 1944–45, 1946b, 1952, 1955a,b, 1969). The condition was first recognized in the USA by Powell and colleagues in 1950, and the critically important observation that individuals who receive a sickle-cell gene from one parent and a thalassaemia gene from the other have about 70% HbS and about 30% HbA, i.e. the reverse of that found in sickle-cell trait, was made shortly afterwards by Sturgeon et al. (1952) and Singer et al. (1955). The recognition of this 'interacting' variety of sickle-cell thalassaemia, later identified as sickle-cell β thalassaemia, was soon followed by the description of forms in which such an interaction did not occur; i.e., the doubly affected individuals did not show this reversal of the amounts of Hbs A and S (or C) (Zuelzer & Kaplan 1954; Zuelzer et al. 1956). These, it later transpired, were examples of the inheritance of the HbS or C trait and α thalassaemia. As described in Chapter 1, these observations paved the way for the development of Ingram and Stretton's model of α and β thalassaemia in 1959.

Over subsequent years it has been recognized that sickle-cell β thalassaemia occurs widely in Africa, throughout the Mediterranean, in the Middle East and, sporadically, in India. We shall describe its geographical distribution in more detail later in this chapter.

The clinical and haematological features of sickle-cell thalassaemia have been described most thoroughly in Italians (Silvestroni & Bianco 1944–45,

1946b, 1955a,b, 1959), Afro-Americans (Smith & Conley 1954; Monti *et al.* 1964; Weatherall 1964a; Pearson 1969; Steinberg & Dreiling 1976), Jamaicans (Went & MacIver 1958b; Serjeant *et al.* 1973, 1979), Greeks (Choremis & Zannos 1957), Turks (Aksoy 1959), Indians (Chatterjea 1959; Kulozik *et al.* 1991a), Romanians (Predescu *et al.* 1968) and Saudi Arabians (Pembrey *et al.* 1980). From reading these accounts and the numerous other small series and case reports in the literature, and from our own personal studies, it is clear that sickle-cell thalassaemia is a remarkably heterogeneous disorder. Weatherall (1964a) suggested that the condition can be classified into two broad groups. The first is characterized by a severe course, similar to that found in sickle-cell anaemia; such patients have either no HbA or levels of less than 15% of the total haemoglobin. The second group is associated with a milder course; the haemoglobin consists of 20–30% HbA, the remainder being mainly HbS. Further experience has supported this concept, although there is some overlap between the groups.

The reasons for this clinical heterogeneity became apparent when the molecular basis for the different forms of β thalassaemia had been determined. The form of sickle-cell thalassaemia with a particularly mild phenotype and relatively high levels of HbA, which is most commonly found among those of African origin, results from the interactions of mild β-thalassaemia mutations, particularly those involving the β-globin-gene promoters, which cause only a small reduction in β-globin synthesis. Since this family of mutations are particularly common in Africans, it is now clear why the mild form of sickle-cell β thalassaemia occurs so frequently in these populations. On the other hand, in Mediterranean and other populations, $β^0$ thalassaemia, or more severe forms of $β^+$ thalassaemia, occur more commonly and hence the more severe forms of the disease are seen much more frequently. However, since every population has a mixture of thalassaemia mutations it is not surprising that both mild and severe forms of the disease occur wherever the sickle-cell and β-thalassaemia genes are found together in the same region.

The clinical course of sickle-cell thalassaemia may range from one extreme in which the condition is indistinguishable from severe sickle-cell anaemia to a disorder which is completely symptomless and which

may be found incidentally during a family study or population screening, or presenting as a mild, refractory anaemia in pregnancy. Because the milder forms of the disease are most common in African populations, and have been particularly well documented in Jamaica, it is possible to provide a fairly complete description. However, in other populations the relatively small number of cases and the many different β-thalassaemia mutations involved make it difficult to provide much more than an anecdotal account of the disease.

Molecular pathology and pathophysiology

The molecular and cellular pathology of sickling and the properties of sickle-cell haemoglobin were discussed in Chapter 2. This topic has been reviewed extensively in the last few years (Noguchi *et al.* 1993; Bunn 1997; Hebbel 1997; Hebbel & Vercellotti 1997; Dover & Platt 1998). The factors which combine to account for the different phenotypes of sickle-cell β thalassaemia include the properties of HbS, the relative amounts of Hbs A and S, and those that modify any sickling disorder, in particular the amounts of Hbs S and F that are produced in individual red cells.

Haemoglobin A is much less able to interact in sickling while, as described in Chapter 2, HbF is entirely excluded from polymerization, which, in fact, it inhibits. As discussed in Chapter 2 the double nucleation mechanism, which produces a measurable delay time between the initiation of polymerization and the exponential rise in polymer formation, is a useful reflection of the severity of the sickling process. A variety of kinetic data have shown that both HbS and HbF have a profound, dose-related effect, which is evidenced by an increase in the delay time and decrease in the polymer content of the red cells. For example, compared with pure HbS solutions, mixtures with 15–30% HbA have delay times that are 10 times longer; mixtures with 20–30% HbF have delay times that are 10000 times longer (Sunshine *et al.* 1979). Furthermore, as we shall see later, the red cells in sickle-cell β thalassaemia are not so well haemoglobinized as those in sickle-cell anaemia. It has been found that a fall in the mean cell haemoglobin concentration (MCHC) from 32 to 30 g/dl increases the delay time about threefold (Eaton & Hofrichter 1987). Thus the action of the β-thalassaemia mutation has a twofold effect in modifying the severity of the sickle-cell β-thalassaemia genotype compared with that of sickle-cell anaemia; in the case of the β⁺-thalassaemia alleles it allows the production of HbA, while, overall, it reduces the absolute level of HbS per cell.

The level of HbA in patients with sickle-cell thalassaemia depends on the particular β-thalassaemia mutation. The relative levels of Hbs A and S associated with different mutations are summarized in Table 9.1. The majority of African patients have the –29 A→G or –88 C→T substitutions. These promoter mutations cause a mild reduction in β-chain production and are associated with average levels of HbA in the 20% range. The resulting disease is usually extremely mild. On the other hand, Mediterranean patients with the IVS1-110 G→A mutation have, on average, much lower levels of HbA, in the 10% range. The interaction of IVS2-745 C→G, which is an extremely severe β⁺-thalassaemia mutation, is associated with levels of HbA of about 5% (Gonzalez-Redondo *et al.* 1988b). Finally, at the other end of the spectrum, that is, in patients who inherit β⁰-thalassaemia mutations, there is, of course, no HbA and the haemoglobin constitution is very similar to that of sickle-cell anaemia.

The factors that are responsible for the level of HbF in sickle-cell β thalassaemia are still not well understood. As described in Chapter 2, at least part of the raised level of HbF in this condition can be explained by the selective survival of red cells which produce relatively higher levels of HbF because of the inhibiting effect of the latter on intracellular sickling. Against this background of cell selection, however, a number of other genetic factors are involved, which are probably very similar to those which modify the relative levels of HbF production in β thalassaemia. They are discussed in detail in Chapters 2, 5 and 10. The most striking evidence for the importance of high levels of HbF production in this disease is seen in the populations of Saudi Arabia and Orissa, India, where, despite the inheritance of severe β-thalassaemia alleles, the disease is relatively mild because of the production of unusually high levels of fetal haemoglobin (Pembrey *et al.* 1978; Kulozik *et al.* 1987a). Similarly, the same mechanism underlies the extremely mild interactions between the sickle-cell gene and δβ thalassaemia, described later in this chapter, and those between the sickle-cell gene and hereditary persistence of fetal haemoglobin, described in Chapter 10.

Clinical features

The clinical features of sickle-cell β⁰ and β⁺ thalassaemia are compared in Table 9.2.

Table 9.1 Some interactions between haemoglobin S and different β-thalassaemia alleles. Main sources: Gonzalez-Redondo *et al.* (1988b), Christakis *et al.* (1991), Voskaridou *et al.* (1990) and Huisman *et al.* (1997).

Phenotype	% HbA	Mutation	Population
HbS/β⁺	45	–92 C→T	Italian
HbS/β⁺	20–25	IVS1-6 T→C	Mediterranean, Middle East
HbS/β⁺	18–20	–88 C→T	Afro-American
HbS/β⁺	17–20	–29 A→G	Afro-American
HbS/β⁺	8–14	IVS1-110 G→A	Mediterranean, Middle East
HbS/β⁺	3–5	IVS1-5 G→C	Indian
HbS/β⁺	3–5	IVS2-745 C→G	Mediterranean
HbS/β⁰	0	CD2–4 (–9 bp; +31 bp)	Algerian
HbS/β⁰	0	CD15 G→A	Mediterranean
HbS/β⁰	0	CD25,26 (+T)	Mediterranean
HbS/β⁰	0	IVS1-1 G→A	Indian, Mediterranean, Middle East
HbS/β⁰	0	IVS1-2 T→C	Afro-American
HbS/β⁰	0	CD39 C→T	Mediterranean
HbS/β⁰	0	IVS2-1 G→A	Mediterranean, Afro-American
HbS/β⁰	0	IVS2-849 A→C	Afro-American
HbS/β⁰	0	532-bp deletion	Afro-American
HbS/β⁰	0	1393-bp deletion	Afro-American

Table 9.2 Comparison of some clinical features in haemoglobin S β^0 and in S β^+ thalassaemia. From Serjeant and Serjeant (1982).

	S β^0 thalassaemia ($n=59$)*	S β^+ thalassaemia ($n=71$)*	Significance
Painful crisis			
Patients affected	47 (80%)	54 (75%)	NS
Patients admitted	24 (44%)	14 (19%)	$P<0.01$
Adm/pt admitted	77/24 (3.0)	16/14 (1.3)	—
Leg ulcers (patients > 10 years)	9/40 (23%)	5/59 (8%)	NS
Acute pulmonary episode	14 (24%)	10 (14%)	NS
Priapism	4/28	0/27	NS
Aplastic crisis	2	0	NS
Proliferative retinopathy	2/21 (10%)	8/44 (18%)	NS
Age at menarche (years)	15.35±1.39	14.18±1.33	$P<0.05$
No. of pregnancies	18/14 (1.3)	75/31 (2.4)	—
Fetal loss	1/18 (6%)	10/75 (13%)	—
Hepatomegaly > 3 cm	6	1	$P<0.05$
Splenomegaly	17/5 (33%)	22/70 (31%)	NS
Splenectomy	8 (14%)	1 (1%)	$P<0.05$
Median age	14 years	22 years	—

*Number in parentheses at head of column = n except where denominator appears in table. Denominators for priapism represent total males; for proliferative retinopathy represent all patients with detailed peripheral retinal examination; for pregnancy represent total postpubertal females; and for splenomegaly represent total patients not subjected to splenectomy.

Presentation

As in sickle-cell anaemia, more severely affected individuals tend to present early in life. Of 56 Jamaicans analysed by Serjeant et al. (1973), 21 were discovered incidentally. The latter form of ascertainment was commoner in sickle-cell β^+ thalassaemia than in sickle-cell β^0 thalassaemia. Joint pains in early childhood are the most common presenting symptom in both varieties. In the Jamaican series the hand–foot syndrome (see Chapter 2), osteomyelitis, leg ulcers, splenic infarction, jaundice and pneumonia accounted for the presentation in the majority of patients in early childhood. The hand–foot syndrome, a painful attack of dactylitis leading to swelling of the hands and feet, has been well documented in both Jamaica (Serjeant et al. 1973) and Greece (Karpathios et al. 1977).

Course in childhood

A large cohort study in Jamaica (Stevens et al. 1985; Serjeant 1992) and data from the USA from the Cooperative Study of Sickle-cell Disease (Brown et al. 1994; Gill et al. 1995) are providing valuable information about the evolution of the clinical and haematological findings in sickle-cell β thalassaemia. Overall, the clinical course is less severe in children with the milder form of HbS β^+ thalassaemia than in those with HbS β^0 thalassaemia, which is very similar to sickle-cell anaemia (Table 9.3).

In every variety of the disease there is chronic haemolytic anaemia with a haemoglobin level in the 5–10 g/dl range. As in sickle-cell anaemia this is well tolerated; anaemia *per se* does not often incapacitate patients unless they develop haemolytic or aplastic episodes associated with infection (see later section). Anaemia is more marked in Mediterranean patients than in those of African background (Silvestroni & Bianco 1955b, 1969; Serjeant et al. 1973), reflecting the greater severity of the β-thalassaemia alleles. The major disability in childhood is recurrent attacks of pains in the bones and joints; this occurred in 40 of the 56 Jamaican patients reviewed by Serjeant et al. (1973). They were usually of short duration and relatively mild but were severe enough to lead to hospital admission in 17 of 24 cases. As has been noted with the painful crisis of sickle-cell anaemia, the attacks of bone and joint pain are more common in cold weather and seem to affect sibships quite frequently, suggesting an infective trigger.

Table 9.3 Comparison of some clinical features of sickle-cell (SS) disease and sickle-cell β^0 thalassaemia. From Serjeant *et al.* (1979).

Clinical features	SS disease ($n=123$)	S β^0 thalassaemia ($n=41$)	Significance χ_2	P
Painful crisis				
Patients affected	102 (83%)	33 (80%)	0.13	NS
Patients admitted	48 (39%)	16 (39%)	0.00	NS
Adm/pt admitted	1.71	2.19	—	—
Leg ulcers	42 (34%)	9 (22%)	2.13	NS
Pneumonia	30 (24%)	7 (17%)	0.94	NS
Priapism	5/60 (8%)	2/19 (11%)	0.09	NS
Aplastic crisis	15 (12%)	2 (5%)	1.77	NS
Age at menarche	15.8 years	15.5 years	—	—
No. of pregnancies*	60/49 (1.2)	15/13 (1.2)	—	—
Fetal loss	17/60 (28%)	1/15 (7%)	3.09	NS
Splenomegaly†	7/117 (6%)	10/33 (30%)	15.15	$P<0.01$
Splenectomy	6 (5%)	8 (20%)	8.43	$P<0.001$

* Expressed as proportion of postpubertal women.
† Expressed as proportion of those without splenectomy.

Physical findings

The body habitus is variable and in some reported series growth retardation has been a feature (Silvestroni & Bianco 1955b; Aksoy 1959; Weatherall 1964a; Pearson 1969; Silvestroni & Bianco 1969). In Jamaica, Serjeant *et al.* (1972) found that sickle-cell thalassaemics were significantly lighter and shorter than controls. These findings have been substantiated by studies of patients with both sickle-cell β^0 and β^+ thalassaemia in Italy. Patients were shorter, there was delay in skeletal maturation and the mean age of the menarche was increased. Somatomedin C levels are normal (Caruso-Nicoletti *et al.* 1992). In more severely affected patients there may be some bossing of the skull but the gross skeletal deformities characteristic of homozygous β thalassaemia are rarely seen (Silvestroni & Bianco 1955b, 1969).

Enlargement of the spleen and liver is usual, and the tendency for splenic fibrosis and atrophy, so common in sickle-cell anaemia, seems to be less marked (Serjeant *et al.* 1973). In the Jamaican series half of the patients had hepatomegaly, which did not change much with age; about half the group had palpable spleens. The degree of splenic enlargement is usually moderate but there are well documented cases of massive enlargement with hypersplenism (Silvestroni & Bianco 1955b; Rowley & Jacobs 1972), sometimes necessitating splenectomy (Serjeant *et al.* 1973). In the more severely affected Italian cases of

Silvestroni and Bianco (1955a,b) the spleen became smaller with increasing age, as occurs in sickle-cell anaemia. Generalized lymph-node enlargement was also common in this population.

The notion that splenic function is not lost as early as in sickle-cell anaemia was suggested by the studies of Pearson *et al.* (1985). In a further study in which splenic function was assessed by pitted red-cell counts, Fatunde and Scott (1986) found values of 11.8 ±7.0% in those with sickle-cell anaemia compared with 0.4±0.3% in those with haemoglobin S β^+ thalassaemia; in a later study, the pitted cell counts were 13.8% compared with 2.2% (Barrios *et al.* 1991). These data, which suggest that asplenic function is retained in this condition, relate only to the mild form of sickle-cell β^+ thalassaemia in Africans.

As in sickle-cell anaemia, there is usually a mild degree of cardiac enlargement, which is mirrored by an increased cardiothoracic ratio on chest X-ray. Similarly, soft systolic murmurs are commonly heard. These changes seem to be the result of chronic anaemia; investigation in the Jamaican series (Serjeant *et al.* 1973) showed no evidence of a specific cardiac lesion and the signs were compatible with the degree of anaemia.

Complications

Almost any of the complications which have been reported in sickle-cell anaemia (see Chapter 2) can occur in sickle-cell thalassaemia (Tables 9.2 and 9.3).

Crises

Painful crises associated with widespread bone pain have already been mentioned. More severe vaso-occlusive episodes, including the 'brain syndrome' with convulsions and focal neurological changes, have also been reported (Monti *et al.* 1964; Silvestroni & Bianco 1969). Abdominal pain, occasionally associated with melaena, may follow infarction of areas of bowel (Silvestroni & Bianco 1969). Episodes of pulmonary infarction have also been reported (Steinberg & Dreiling 1976). During infection, particularly associated with parvovirus, there may be aplastic crises in which erythropoiesis is 'shut down', resulting in profound anaemia (Serjeant *et al.* 1973; Brownell *et al.* 1986; Saarinen *et al.* 1986). Sequestration crises, in which there is rapid splenic enlargement and anaemia associated with entrapment of sickled red cells in the spleen, have been reported by Pearson (1969), Serjeant *et al.* (1973) and Solanki *et al.* (1986).

There is increasing evidence that the most serious and life-threatening complications of the sickling disorders, apart from splenic sequestration in early life, are the lung and brain syndromes. The lung syndrome, characterized by pulmonary infiltrates associated with progressive dyspnoea, hypoxia, and sometimes anaemia and thrombocytopenia, is the commonest cause of death in sickle-cell anaemia in Western societies and in Jamaican patients aged over 10 years (Davies *et al.* 1984; Serjeant 1992). Less is known about the frequency of this complication in sickle-cell β thalassaemia, but in an analysis from the USA Cooperative Study of Sickle-cell Disease of a follow-up of 3751 patients with sickling disorders it is quite clear that its frequency is higher in sickle-cell β^0 thalassaemia and that, in this condition at least, it poses a major problem (Castro *et al.* 1994). Similarly, less is known about the frequency of stroke and other neurological disorders, which are now believed to result from narrowing or occlusions of vessels arising from the circle of Willis. Hemiplegia is the most common manifestation, and in patients with sickle-cell anaemia between half and two-thirds of cases recur within 3 years of the initial lesion (reviewed by Serjeant 1992). Although there have been reports of this complication in sickle-cell β thalassaemia, and it

is likely that those with sickle-cell β^0 thalassaemia are at almost as high a risk as those with sickle-cell anaemia, information about this complication is still scanty.

Infection

There are limited data on the frequency of infection in the different forms of sickle-cell β thalassaemia but the pattern seems to be similar to that of patients with sickle-cell anaemia (Serjeant 1992) (see Chapter 2). As is the case for sickle-cell anaemia and β thalassaemia (see Chapter 7), the frequency of positive serology for hepatitis C and resulting liver damage seems to be related directly to the number of blood transfusions received (Hasan *et al.* 1996).

Priapism

As in sickle-cell anaemia, priapism also occurs in sickle-cell β thalassaemia. The pattern and sequelae seem to be identical to other sickling disorders (Fowler *et al.* 1991).

Bones and joints

The sequelae of avascular necrosis of the femoral or humoral heads, observed more commonly in sickle-cell β^0 thalassaemia, may lead to a variety of complications similar to those which occur in sickle-cell anaemia (Goldberg *et al.* 1959; Rand *et al.* 1987; Milner *et al.* 1993) (Table 9.4). In 47 Jamaican patients radiological surveys showed infarction involving the long bones in about a third of the cases and there was metacarpal shortening, presumably a sequela of epiphyseal infarction as part of the hand–foot syndrome, in four patients (Fig. 9.1). Infarction involving the femoral head was observed in three cases and of the humoral head in four (Serjeant & Ashcroft 1973; Serjeant *et al.* 1973) (Fig. 9.2). Severe bone changes of this type have been observed in Mediterranean patients with this disorder (Miotti & Caramello 1968). Osteomyelitis due to salmonella infection or infection with other organisms seems to be similar to that observed in sickle-cell anaemia (Weiss & Katz 1970). The problems of the differentiation between bone infarction and osteomyelitis are discussed by Potente (1988). Symptomatic effusions into the large joints have also been reported (Crout *et al.* 1976; Van Slyck 1976).

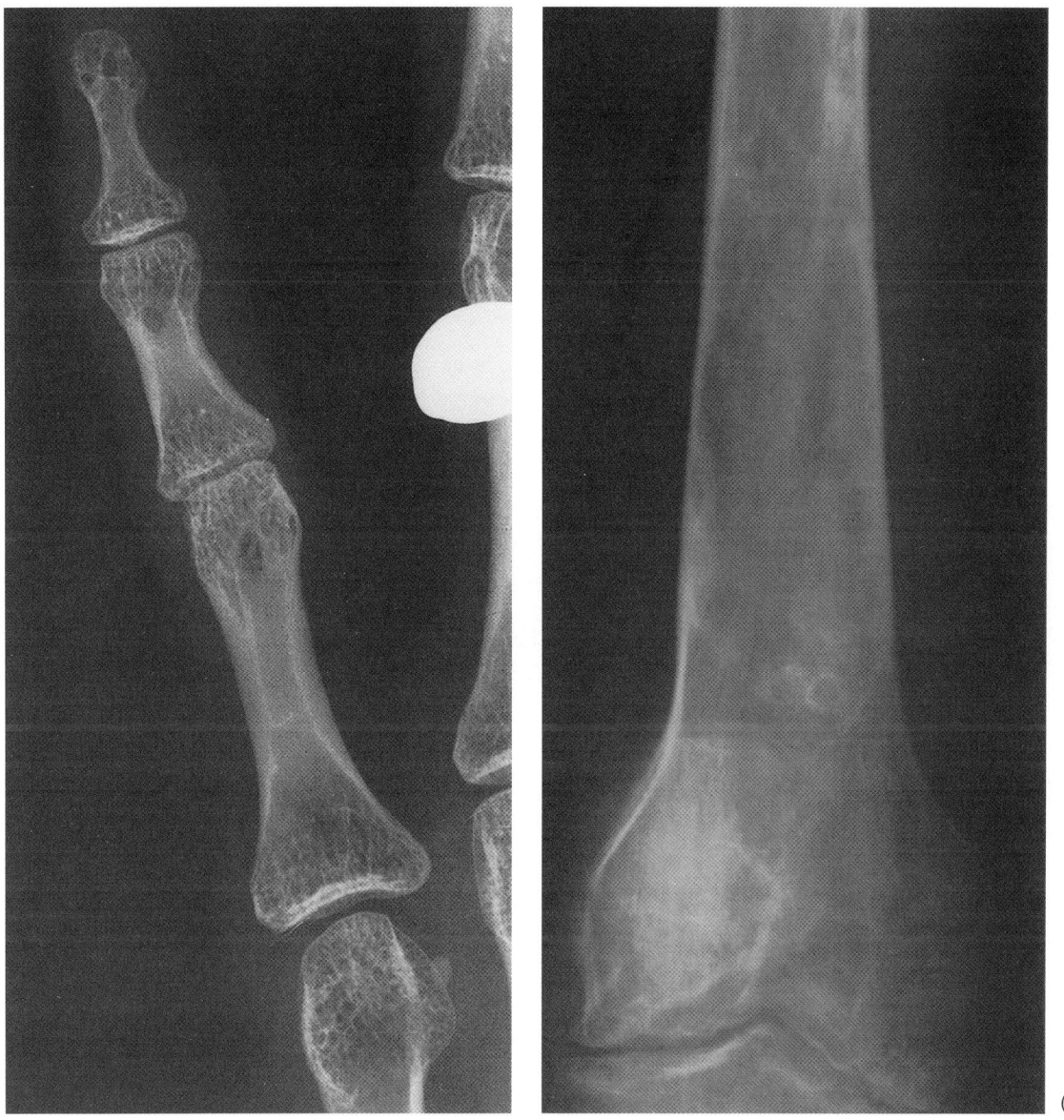

(a)

(b)

Fig. 9.1 Bone changes in sickle-cell β thalassaemia. (a) Phalanges, demonstrating coarse trabecular pattern and wide nutrient foramina. (b) Distal end of the femur showing medullary expansion, cortical thickening and abnormal medullary calcification secondary to a bone infarct. By courtesy of Professor G. Serjeant.

Features	HbS β⁰ thalassaemia (n=14)		HbS β⁺ thalassaemia (n=33)		Significance	
	n	(%)	n	(%)	χ_2	P
Medullary expansion	6	(43%)	7	(21%)	1.35	NS
Coarse trabeculae	8	(57%)	14	(42%)	0.37	NS
Large nutrient foramina	7	(50%)	9	(27%)	1.36	NS
Medullary infarction	5	(36%)	7	(21%)	0.46	NS
Cortical infarction	1	(7%)	1	(3%)	—	—
Thick cortex	4	(29%)	17	(51%)	1.27	NS
Infarction of articular surface	3	(21%)	10	(30%)	0.07	NS
Biconcavity of vertebrae	4	(29%)	13	(39%)	0.14	NS
'Step sign' of vertebrae	5	(36%)	7	(21%)	0.46	NS
Retarded bone age	7	(50%)	3	(9%)	7.53	<0.01

Table 9.4 Comparison of some radiological features in haemoglobin S β⁰ and S β⁺ thalassaemia. From Serjeant *et al.* (1973).

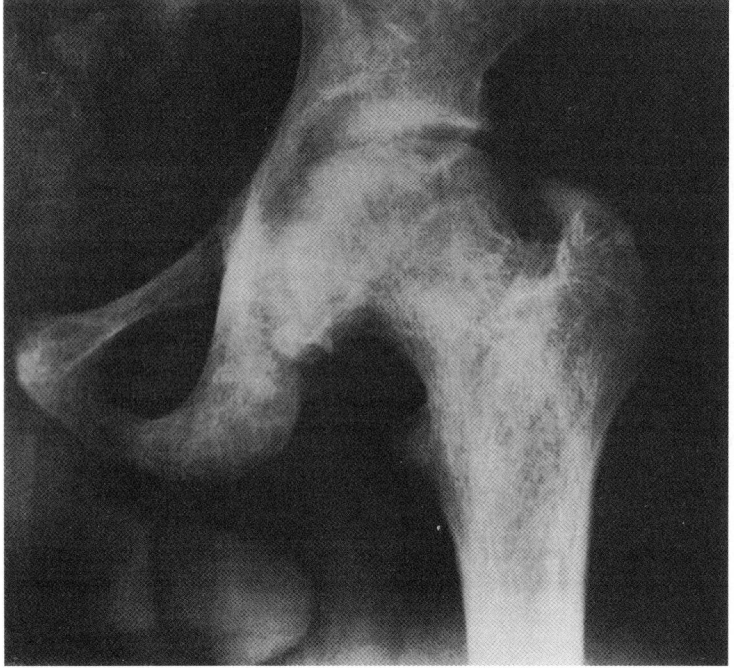

Fig. 9.2 Bone changes in the femoral head in sickle-cell β thalassaemia. The left femoral head in a 42-year-old male patient showing anterosuperior segmental infarction. By courtesy of Professor G. Serjeant.

Bone-marrow or fat embolism

Although this must be a very unusual complication of sickle-cell β thalassaemia, a well documented case report indicates that this condition may be missed and mistaken for pneumonia or a pulmonary sequestration crisis (Zaidi *et al.* 1996). A fatal fat embolism syndrome has also been reported in a child with sickle-cell β⁺ thalassaemia as a complication of an acute parvovirus B19 infection (Kolquist *et al.* 1996). The clinical condition resembled a pulmonary sequestration crisis with anaemia, mental changes and respiratory failure. However, at autopsy widespread fat emboli and bone-marrow necrosis were found. Parvovirus B19 was identified by the polymerase chain reaction from samples obtained from a variety of tissues. A similar complication was reported in a 25-year-old Afro-American with sickle-cell β⁺ thalassaemia by Johnson *et al*. (1994). The patient presented with what was thought clinically to be an asthmatic attack, but later developed widespread bone pain and died suddenly; autopsy showed extensive marrow necrosis and massive fat embolism. Although these events are rare they underline the importance of keeping an open mind about the diagnosis in a patient with sickle-cell β thalassaemia with symptoms suggestive of a pulmonary sequestration crisis; it is clear that both bone-marrow and fat embolism occur occasionally.

Leg ulcers

Leg ulcers are common (Serjeant *et al*. 1973; Eckman 1996). In the large Jamaican series Serjeant *et al*. (1973) described leg ulceration in 27% of patients, which commenced most commonly between the ages of 10 and 15 years. In eight cases the ulcers were small, usually traumatic in origin, and healed within 6 months without recurrence. In the remaining seven patients the ulcer ran a relapsing course over a period of months or years. Leg ulcers seem to be less common in Italian patients (Silvestroni & Bianco 1955a,b). It is likely that patients' lifestyles, and exposure to trauma, play an important role in this complication.

Metabolic changes

During infective episodes sickle-cell thalassaemics may become dehydrated and acidotic. Simon (1972) has described in detail the problem of hyperosmolar diabetic coma in a patient with the disorder.

Ocular changes

Ocular changes have been reported by Smith and Conley (1954), Condon *et al*. (1974), Serjeant *et al*. (1972, 1973) and Friberg *et al*. (1986). These have included tortuosity of the retinal vessels similar to that found in patients with sickle-cell anaemia or haemoglobin SC disease (Fig. 9.3). Of Jamaican patients approximately 14% had some degree of retinitis and this led to transient visual loss associated with vitreous haemorrhage in a few cases. In one case there was a visual field defect associated with an unusual form of chorioretinal degeneration which was thought to result from occlusion of the posterior

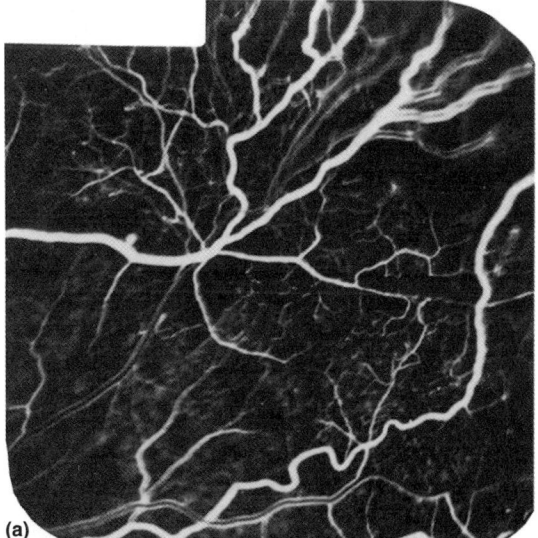

(a)

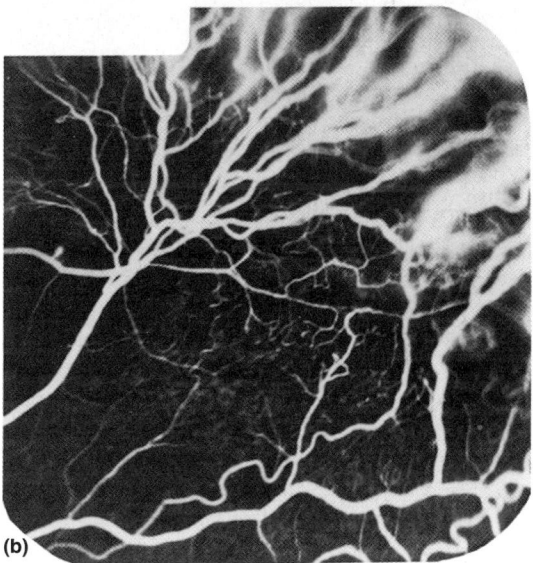

(b)

Fig. 9.3 Retinal changes in sickle-cell β thalassaemia. A fluorescein angiogram in early arterial (a) and venous (b) phases, demonstrating proliferative retinopathy of the superonasal periphery of the right eye in a 19-year-old male patient. By courtesy of Professor G. Serjeant.

choroidal vessels (Condon *et al*. 1973). Angioid streaks, well recognized in sickle-cell anaemia (see Serjeant 1992), were observed in six of 58 patients studied by Aessopos *et al*. (1994).

Gallstones

As in all haemolytic anaemias there is an increased frequency of pigment stones (Steinberg & Dreiling 1976; Bond *et al.* 1987).

Hypersplenism

Gross splenomegaly leading to hypersplenism and regular blood transfusion requirement has been documented by Serjeant *et al.* (1973) and has been observed in several cases by the present authors. This complication seems to occur mainly in childhood. Thrombocytopenia due to hypersplenism has also been reported (Rowley & Jacobs 1972).

Renal complications

As in the other sickling disorders there appears to be a genuine increase in episodes of haematuria in sickle-cell thalassaemia (Smith & Conley 1954; Wilson 1966; Serjeant *et al.* 1973; Steinberg & Dreiling 1976). Early studies suggested that the loss of the ability to concentrate urine, characteristic of sickle-cell anaemia, is not so marked in sickle-cell thalassaemia (Pearson 1969). However, more recent work in Greece, in which the disease tends to be more severe because of the low level of HbA that is produced, suggests that progressive renal damage may be common and follow a similar pattern to that of sickle-cell anaemia. In a study comparing renal function in 41 patients with sickle-cell β thalassaemia, 14 normal controls and eight patients with sickle-cell anaemia, Kontessis *et al.* (1992) found that polyuria, hyposthenuria and mild proteinuria were equally common in the two groups. A renal concentrating defect was observed in all these patients. There was a significant negative correlation between creatinine clearance and age in patients over 30 years. Several other abnormalities were noted; in particular there was a significant positive correlation between tubular reabsorptive capacity for phosphate and the number of painful crises per year. The authors conclude that renal involvement in sickle-cell β thalassaemia, at least in the severe form seen in Greece, is much the same as in sickle-cell anaemia.

Neurological complications

The problem of stroke and other neurological complications was discussed earlier. There are occasional reports of episodes characterized by fits and focal neurological sequelae (Monti *et al.* 1964). Serjeant *et al.* (1973) mention two patients with neurological complications, one with a subarachnoid haemorrhage following delivery and another with a left VIth nerve lesion. Whether these were causally related to the sickling disorder is not clear. The possibility that cerebrovascular accidents in this disease may be associated with the co-inheritance of factor V Leiden has been excluded, at least in African populations (Kahn *et al.* 1997).

Sleep-related upper airway obstruction

This complication, well recognized in patients with sickle-cell disease, appears to be due to hypertrophy of the adenoids and tonsils. It is characterized by episodes of noctural hypoxaemia, potentially deleterious in any sickling disorder. Among the series of patients reported by Samuels *et al.* (1992) there were four with sickle-cell β^0 thalassaemia.

Folic acid deficiency

Folic acid deficiency leading to megaloblastic erythropoiesis and worsening of the anaemia is well documented (Smith & Conley 1954; Walters & Young 1954; Weatherall 1964a; Serjeant *et al.* 1973). This has usually, although not always, been associated with pregnancy.

Fertility and pregnancy

There is little information about fertility and pregnancy in Mediterranean patients with this disorder; presumably pregnancy was less common in the past in these severely affected patients (see Silvestroni & Bianco 1969). This is not the case in individuals of African origin, however. The most extensive information comes from Jamaica (Serjeant *et al.* 1973). Among 21 females aged 20 years or over the mean age of the menarche was 15 years 2 months, similar to that in sickle-cell anaemia but slightly later than in normal Jamaican women. There were a total of 73 pregnancies with 66 live births, eight abortions and one stillbirth. There were two live twin births. There was a significantly higher incidence of abortion and stillbirth among those with sickle-cell β^0 thalassaemia. Remarkably, two of the patients with sickle-cell β^+ thalassaemia each had 10 pregnancies, with 11 and eight live births, respectively! Although pregnancy was well tolerated, complications occurred in the last two trimesters. These included painful crises before or just after delivery, severe postpartum haemorrhage, severe eclampsia and convulsions secondary to a subarachnoid haemorrhage in the postpartum period. Similar experiences have been recorded in smaller series (Brown & Ober 1958; Henderson *et al.* 1962; Monti *et al.* 1964; Dunn & Haynes 1967; Laros & Kalstone 1971; de Hendrickse *et al.* 1972; Jewett 1976).

As in sickle-cell anaemia there appears to be an increased likelihood of crises and worsening of anaemia during pregnancy, and folic acid deficiency is common. There seems to be an increased incidence of fetal morbidity and mortality although precise figures are difficult to obtain.

Bleeding tendency

In the large Jamaican series (Serjeant *et al.* 1973) unexplained epistaxis was observed in two patients; in both cases it was associated with hypersplenism.

Prognosis

Unfortunately, we still do not have adequate information about the prognosis in sickle-cell thalassaemia. This seems to vary between different parts of the world and probably depends on a wide range of factors including the socio-economic background, climate and the particular genetic variety of the disorder. Some of these issues, as they affect different ethnic groups, will be discussed later.

Early reports indicated, as would be expected from what we now know about the β-thalassaemia mutations involved, that the disease is more severe in the Mediterranean population. Thus Silvestroni and Bianco (1955a,b, 1969) reported a high mortality in childhood and found only two adults in a large series of Italian patients. In addition, they reported that successful pregnancies are probably rare in their population. Similarly, Aksoy and Lehmann (1957) mentioned that their Turkish patients had been severely incapacitated due to anaemia. On the other hand, the milder forms of sickle-cell thalassaemia, which are common in the African populations, may be associated with an extremely good prognosis. For example, Singer and his coworkers (Singer *et al.* 1955) described the 'disorder' in a 61-year-old Afro-American with no history of ill health or anaemia. Out of the 16 cases reported by Weatherall (1964a),

eight were over the age of 25 and 12 had never had symptoms of sickling or anaemia. In the 56 cases reported by Serjeant *et al.* (1973), the ages ranged from 3 to 60 years, with 26 patients aged 30 years or above. Serjeant and colleagues did not describe any deaths in their sickle-cell thalassaemia population.

It is clear from these studies and from other smaller series cited in this chapter that there is an extraordinary variability in the severity and prognosis of sickle-cell thalassaemia in different parts of the world. Although detailed longevity studies have not been carried out it seems very likely that these differences reflect both genetic and socio-economic factors. In this sense the problem is very similar to that of sickle-cell anaemia, which is still associated with a high incidence of death in the first few years of life in Africa, while currently in North America the median age of death of patients with sickle-cell anaemia is 42 years for males and 48 years for females (Platt *et al.* 1994). As the prenatal diagnosis of sickle-cell thalassaemia is feasible it is important that we start to re-examine the whole question of the factors which affect the prognosis.

Post-mortem studies

There is very little published information. Some autopsy data are mentioned in the papers of Silvestroni and Bianco cited earlier in this chapter. An excellent account of the post-mortem findings in a single patient is given by Ascenzi and Silvestroni (1957).

Haematological findings

The haematological changes are also very variable (Table 9.5). In the more severely affected there is anaemia, with haemoglobin values of 5–10 g/dl and an associated reticulocytosis in the 10–20% range. The red cells show hypochromia and microcytosis with variation in size and shape and variable numbers of target forms. Sickle cells are sometimes seen on the stained film, which may also show Howell–Jolly and Pappenheimer bodies (Fig. 9.4). There are variable numbers of irreversibly sickled cells in the peripheral blood. There is a reduction in the MCV and MCH, the latter values ranging from 20 to 25 pg, depending on the particular type of β-thalassaemia gene. There may be a slight elevation of the serum bilirubin level.

In the milder forms there may be minimal anaemia with morphological changes of the red cells and a

Table 9.5 Comparison of some haematological findings in sickle-cell β^0 thalassaemia (S β^0) and sickle-cell β^+ thalassaemia (S β^+) over the age of 5 years. From Serjeant and Serjeant (1982).

	S β^0 thalassaemia ($n=59$)		S β^+ thalassaemia ($n=76$)		Significance	
	Mean	$\pm$SD	Mean	$\pm$SD	t	P
HbA$_2$ (%)	5.02	0.56	4.66	0.57	3.59	<0.001
HbF ($\log_e$ (HbF+4))	2.40 (7.0)*	0.42	2.21 (5.1)*	0.42	2.62	<0.01
Hb (g/dl)	8.85	1.13	11.55	1.27	12.54	<0.001
MCHC (g/dl)	0.318	0.018	0.336	0.013	6.55	<0.001
RBC ($\times 10^{12}$/l)	4.03	0.51	4.85	0.49	9.40	<0.001
MCV (fl)	69.3	5.10	73.30	5.20	4.37	<0.001
Reticulocytes ($\log_e$ (% retics+1))	2.10 (7.2)*	0.50	1.27 (2.6)*	0.37	11.00	<0.001

* Bracketed figures represent transformed variables re-expressed as percentages.
MCHC, mean cell haemoglobin concentration; MCV, mean cell volume; RBC, red-cell count.

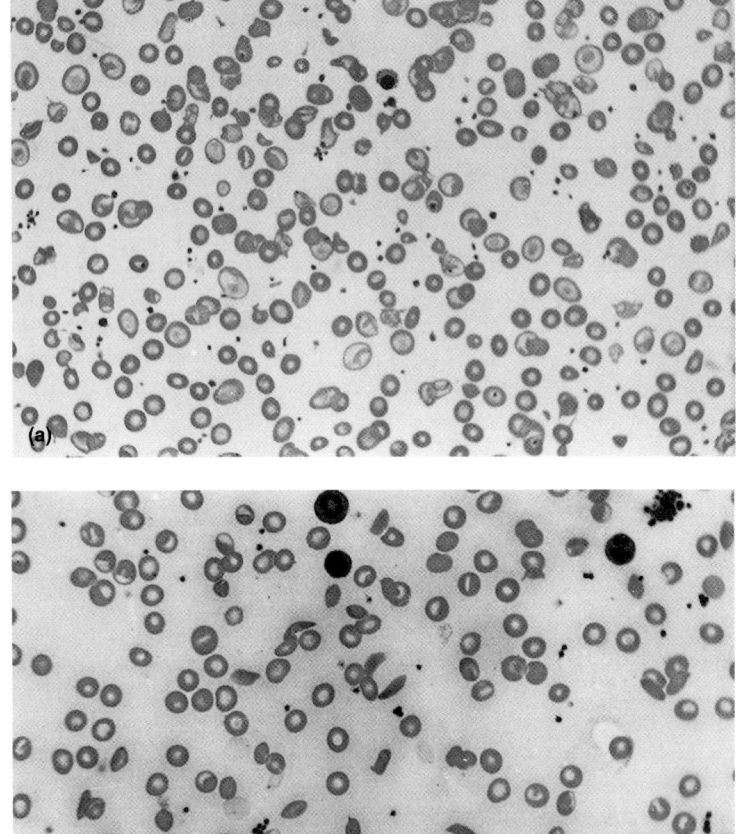

Fig. 9.4 Peripheral blood films of patients with sickle-cell β thalassaemia. (a) The mild form of the disease from an Afro-American patient (Wright's stain); (b) a more severely affected Greek patient with sickle-cell β^0 thalassaemia (Wright's stain). The irreversibly sickled cells in (b) are clearly shown.

reduced mean cell volume (MCV) and mean cell haemoglobin (MCH) as the only abnormal findings. A comparison of the haematological data obtained from patients with sickle-cell β^0 and sickle-cell β^+ thalassaemia in Jamaica is shown in Table 9.5. These data are useful because they give some indication of the two extremes of the condition, i.e. sickle-cell β^0 thalassaemia and the particularly mild forms of the disease in African populations. In Table 9.6 the haematological findings in patients with sickle-cell anaemia are compared with those with sickle-cell β^0 thalassaemia; the main distinguishing feature is the red-cell indices, notably the MCV and MCH (Serjeant *et al.* 1979).

Thus in severely affected patients the haematological picture is similar to sickle-cell anaemia, the main differences being the fewer target forms and the better haemoglobinized red cells in the latter (Serjeant & Serjeant 1972; Steinberg & Dreiling 1976; Serjeant *et al.* 1979; Serjeant & Serjeant 1982). In mild forms the haematological picture may resemble that of heterozygous β thalassaemia. Red-cell fragility is usually reduced (Silvestroni & Bianco 1955a,b).

The bone marrow shows erythroid hyperplasia with poor haemoglobinization of the red-cell precursors. There are no other diagnostic features. Yataganas and Fessas (1969) found typical α-chain inclusion bodies in the nucleated red cells.

Red-cell survival data have been reported by Malamos *et al.* (1963), Monti *et al.* (1964) and Joishy *et al.* (1976). The survival time of ^{51}Cr-labelled red cells was extremely variable, with a $T_{1/2}$ ranging from 7 to 24 days, but on average the survival was about half that of normal red cells. Malamos *et al.* also studied ^{59}Fe incorporation and found that it was rapidly cleared from the plasma, but only about 70% of the initial dose was incorporated into the red cells. Surface counting suggested that there is a group of rapidly destroyed cells or that siderotic granules are removed from the newly labelled and released cells. Red-cell destruction occurred in both the spleen and liver in these series.

Haemoglobin constitution

The action of the β-thalassaemia gene in individuals heterozygous for both β-thalassaemia and sickle-cell genes is to reduce the output of β^A chains as compared with β^S chains. Thus the level of HbS exceeds that found in the sickle-cell trait (Fig. 9.5), comprising more than 50% of the total haemoglobin. In addition there is a variable increase in HbF and HbA$_2$.

Haemoglobin A

In the early analyses of the haemoglobin of patients with sickle-cell thalassaemia it was noted that

Table 9.6 Comparison of haematological indices in sickle-cell (SS) disease and haemoglobin S β^0 thalassaemia. From Serjeant *et al.* (1979).

Variable	SS disease			S β^0 thalassaemia			Significance	
	n	Mean	SD	*n*	Mean	SD	*t*	*P*
Age (years)	123	19.2	12.2	41	19.1	13.0	—	—
HbA$_2$ (%)	123	2.87	0.64	41	5.04	0.42	−20.3	<0.001
Log$_e$ (HbF+4)	122	2.147 (4.56)*	0.368	41	2.288 (5.86)	0.366	−2.1	<0.05
Hb (g/dl)	123	7.83	0.96	41	8.55	0.95	−4.2	<0.001
Hct (ratio)	123	0.242	0.032	41	0.282	0.029	−7.1	<0.001
MCHC (g/dl)	123	32.61	1.88	41	30.32	1.52	7.1	<0.001
RBC ($\times 10^{12}$/l)	121	2.82	0.53	41	4.03	0.50	−12.8	<0.001
MCV (fl)	121	85.9	8.1	41	68.9	6.0	12.3	<0.001
MCH (pg)	121	28.5	3.3	41	21.3	1.9	13.2	<0.001
Log$_e$ (% retics+1)	115	2.414 (10.18)	0.364	31	2.098 (7.15)	0.391	4.2	<0.001
Log$_e$ (absolute retics)	113	5.636 (280)	0.335	31	5.663 (288)	0.443	−0.4	NS
Log$_e$ (ISC+10)	116	2.870 (7.64)	2.89	39	2.516 (2.37)	0.136	7.4	<0.001

*Figures in parentheses are means of transformed values re-expressed in original units.

Hct, haematocrit; ISC, irreversibly sickled cells; MCH, mean cell haemoglobin; MCHC, mean cell haemoglobin concentration; MCV, mean cell volume; RBC, red blood cells; retics, reticulocytes.

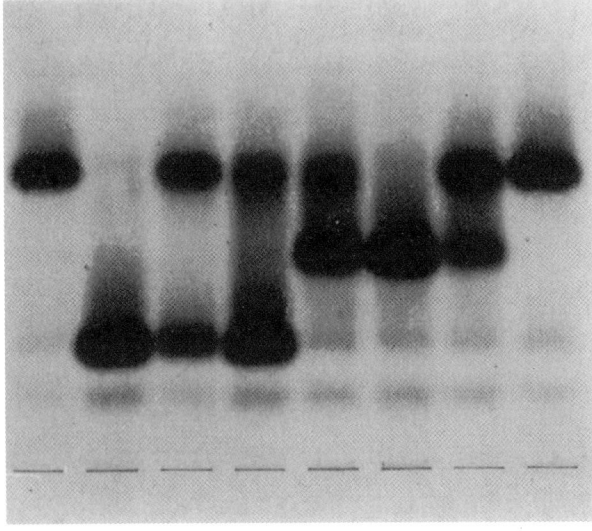

+

HbA

HbS

HbC/A₂

Origin

–

Fig. 9.5 Haemoglobin electrophoresis in sickle-cell β thalassaemia and HbC β thalassaemia. Starch gel electrophoresis (pH 8.5, amido black stain), left to right: 1, normal adult; 2, HbC disease; 3, HbC trait; 4, HbC β⁺ thalassaemia; 5, sickle-cell β⁺ thalassaemia; 6, sickle-cell disease; 7, sickle-cell trait; 8, normal adult.

two main haemoglobin patterns occur: SAF and SF (Sturgeon *et al.* 1952; Singer *et al.* 1955). In 1964 Weatherall pointed out that these run true within sibships. In the first edition of this book (Weatherall 1965) all the available sibships were analysed and the results suggested that the HbA- and non-HbA-producing varieties of sickle-cell thalassaemia were distinct genetic entities. Subsequent series confirmed this observation (Serjeant *et al.* 1973). It also became clear that there is wide variation in the relative amounts of HbA in sickle-cell β⁺ thalassaemia. Weatherall (1964a) noted that in Afro-Americans the level of HbA was usually in the 20–30% range but reported one patient with approximately 5% HbA; similar observations were made by Pearson (1969). In their extensive study of the disorder in Jamaica Serjeant *et al.* (1973) found that the haemoglobin pattern fell into three groups, characterized by the presence of no HbA, or 5–15% and 20–30% HbA. The mean levels of HbA in the latter groups were 12 and 24%, respectively; the β⁺-thalassaemia gene in the individuals with the lower level of HbA came from non-African sources.

The reasons for these early observations on the levels of HbA in sickle-cell β⁺ thalassaemia became apparent once it was possible to define the nature of the β-thalassaemia allele at the molecular level (Gonzalez-Redondo *et al.* 1988b; Christakis *et al.* 1991; Kulozik *et al.* 1991a). The relative levels of HbA found in association with different β-thalassaemia mutations in sickle-cell β⁺ thalassaemia are summarized in Table 9.1. For example, inheritance of the IVS2-745 C→G mutation in Greek and Turkish populations is associated with levels of between 3 and 5%, and the IVS1-110 G→A mutation in the Mediterranean population with levels of 8–14%. On the other hand, in individuals of African origin with the mutations –88 C→T or –29 A→G, levels of 18 to 25% haemoglobin A are observed. The highest level that has been reported is approximately 45% in a compound heterozygote for the β –92 C→T mutation, which results from an extremely mild reduction in β-globin chain synthesis (Divoky *et al.* 1993a; Rosatelli *et al.* 1995).

In short, there is a continuous spectrum of HbA levels, ranging from close to 50% to 1–2%, depending on the activity of the β⁺-thalassaemia allele.

Haemoglobin F

The level of HbF in sickle-cell thalassaemia is also very variable. For example, in the 56 patients reported by Serjeant *et al.* (1973) it ranged from 0.5 to 21.2%, with a mean of approximately 5% in sickle-cell β⁺ thalassaemia, and means of 4.3 and 7.3% for males and females, respectively, in sickle-cell β⁰ thalassaemia. The sex difference was only significant for the latter group.

Unusually high levels of haemoglobin F

Although it is unusual to find HbF levels in excess of

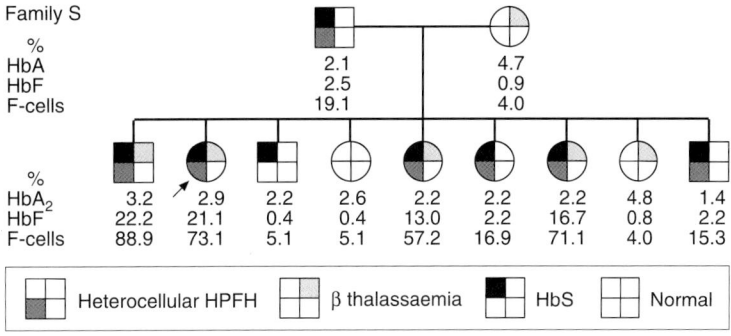

Family S

%			
HbA	2.1	4.7
HbF	2.5	0.9
F-cells	19.1	4.0

%									
HbA$_2$	3.2	2.9	2.2	2.6	2.2	2.2	2.2	4.8	1.4
HbF	22.2	21.1	0.4	0.4	13.0	2.2	16.7	0.8	2.2
F-cells	88.9	73.1	5.1	5.1	57.2	16.9	71.1	4.0	15.3

Heterocellular HPFH   β thalassaemia   HbS   Normal

Fig. 9.6 A family pedigree showing the inheritance of heterocellular hereditary persistence of fetal haemoglobin together with the sickle-cell and β-thalassaemia genes to produce sickle-cell β thalassaemia with unusually high levels of HbF. Data from Family S reported by Wood *et al.* (1976b).

10% in patients with sickle-cell thalassaemia there are many reported exceptions. In the series of Jamaican and Greek cases reported by Serjeant *et al.* (1973) and Choremis and Zannos (1957) there were several patients with levels in the 19–25% range. However, they were found in infants or young children. It has been established that there is a decline in HbF levels in the sickling disorders over the first 15 years of life (Pembrey *et al.* 1978; Hayes *et al.* 1985) and this appears to be the case in sickle-cell thalassaemics in Greece (Choremis & Zannos 1957).

There are, however, several reported instances of unusually high levels of HbF in adults with sickle-cell thalassaemia. Weatherall (1964a) described an 18-year-old boy with sickle-cell thalassaemia who had 26% HbF. The boy's mother was a β-thalassaemia heterozygote with 17.8% HbF. It was suggested that the mother was also homozygous for heterocellular hereditary persistence of fetal haemoglobin (HPFH) and that the boy was heterozygous for HPFH as well as having sickle-cell thalassaemia.

The interaction between sickle-cell β⁺ thalassaemia and heterocellular HPFH was reported by Wood *et al.* (1976b, 1977b) (see also Chapter 10). Three Indian siblings with sickle-cell β⁺ thalassaemia had HbF values of 22–31%, and were symptom free. The family pedigree is shown in Fig. 9.6. It is clear that a heterocellular HPFH gene is segregating within this family and that it has been inherited by the three children with sickle-cell β thalassaemia. It is probable that the patient described by Martinez and Colombo (1974) is another example of this interaction. It appears therefore that heterocellular HPFH, if inherited together with sickle-cell β thalassaemia, can produce HbF levels in the 15–30% range.

Another group of patients with unusually high HbF levels was found in the oasis populations of eastern Saudi Arabia (Pembrey *et al.* 1980). Eighteen patients with sickle-cell β⁰ thalassaemia were studied. They had remarkably mild clinical courses. Their HbF values ranged from 4.8 to 27.2% with a mean of 17.3%. This unusual ability to increase HbF production in the presence of the sickle-cell gene has been well documented in patients with sickle-cell anaemia in this population (Perrine *et al.* 1972; Pembrey *et al.* 1978). The genetic basis is not yet clear but it seems to be a characteristic of both sickle-cell anaemia and sickle-cell thalassaemia among the population of eastern Saudi Arabia. The same finding has been reported in Iran (Haghshenass *et al.* 1977) and in Indian populations in Orissa (Kulozik *et al.* 1987a). The possible relationship of the high levels of HbF to the β-globin restriction-fragment-length polymorphism (RFLP) haplotype in these populations, and the $^G\gamma$–158 polymorphism that it carries, is discussed in Chapter 10.

The reader should not be misled into believing that this account of the distribution of HbF levels in sickle-cell thalassaemia is the whole story. While, in general, low levels of HbF, i.e. less than 10%, are found in African and Mediterranean sickle-cell thalassaemics after the first few years of life, unusually high levels in these populations are sometimes associated with a heterocellular HPFH gene, and high levels are the rule in eastern Saudi Arab and some Indian populations, there are many exceptions to these generalities. It is not uncommon to find African or Mediterranean patients with HbF levels in the 15–25% range for which there is no obvious explanation (Serjeant *et al.* 1973; Shaeffer & Moake 1975; Steinberg & Dreiling 1976; present authors, unpublished data). In general, such patients run a relatively mild course, like those of eastern Saudi Arabia, but again there are exceptions.

Cellular distribution of haemoglobin F

The intercellular distribution of HbF, as judged by the acid elution technique, is heterocellular (Shepherd *et al.* 1962). Evidence in support of this observation has been obtained from differential centrifugation experiments in which the distribution of HbF in the young and older cell populations was analysed (Wood *et al.* 1977b). There was a major increase in the amount of HbF in the older cell populations, suggesting that the cells which contain relatively more HbF survive longer in the peripheral blood. These findings suggest that these cells are relatively protected from the effects of HbS and therefore that at least part of the elevation of HbF can be ascribed to selective survival of F cells.

Haemoglobin A_2

Increased levels of HbA_2 in sickle-cell thalassaemics have been well documented (Aksoy 1963; Huisman 1963; Weatherall 1964a). In the 56 cases reported by Serjeant *et al.* (1973) the HbA_2 values ranged from 4.7 to 5.4%; the distribution was very similar to that seen in heterozygous β thalassaemia.

An elevated level of HbA_2 is not always found in sickle-cell β thalassaemia, however. The exception to the rule is seen in individuals with unusually high levels of HbF, in particular those who have also inherited a heterocellular HPFH gene. In the three siblings reported by Wood *et al.* (1977b) the HbA_2 values were within the normal range. One possible explanation is that the cells which contain predominantly HbF have a relatively low amount of HbA_2, similar to the findings in homozygous β thalassaemia (see Chapters 5 and 7). Indeed, the differential centrifugation studies reported by Wood *et al.* (1977b) showed that there is an absolute increase in HbA_2 in the younger (HbF-poor) cell population as compared with the older (HbF-rich) population. In 16 Saudi Arabian patients reported by Pembrey *et al.* (1980) the HbA_2 levels ranged from 1.46 to 5.87% and eight of the subjects had levels in the normal range. There was a significant negative correlation between the levels of HbF and A_2 in these patients, regardless of whether the HbA_2 was expressed as a percentage of the total haemoglobin or of the HbS alone. This finding provides further evidence that the cells which contain relatively high levels of HbF have lower levels of HbA_2, and that the average level of HbA_2 in

the peripheral blood cells may vary widely, depending on the contribution made by the HbF-rich as compared with the HbF-poor population.

In short, in genetically proven cases of sickle-cell β thalassaemia the percentage HbA_2 may sometimes be normal; this usually occurs in cases with unusually high levels of HbF.

In vitro haemoglobin synthesis

Haemoglobin synthesis has been studied in the peripheral blood of individuals of African, Italian, Greek, Arab and Sicilian origin (Weatherall *et al.* 1969b; Conconi *et al.* 1970; Clegg & Weatherall 1972; Bank *et al.* 1973; Gill & Schwartz 1973; Joishy *et al.* 1976; Steinberg & Dreiling 1976). In these experiments the relative rates of α- as compared with non-α-, i.e. $β^A$-, $β^S$- and γ-, chain synthesis were measured. In all cases reticulocytes showed an overall imbalance of globin synthesis. The α-/non-α-chain production ratios in a series of sickle-cell $β^+$ thalassaemics ranged from 1.2 to 2.2, with mean values in the series of Gill and Schwartz, Bank *et al.* and Steinberg and Dreiling of 1.5, 1.4 and 1.7, respectively. The ratios were not significantly different in sickle-cell $β^0$ thalassaemia. In identical twins studied by Joishy *et al.* (1976) the α-/non-α-chain ratios were identical, at 1.7. These findings are remarkably consistent and indicate that the overall degree of globin imbalance in sickle-cell $β^0$ or sickle-cell $β^+$ thalassaemia is approximately that observed in the heterozygous states for these forms of β thalassaemia. The presence of a relatively large pool of free α chains in the cells of sickle-cell β thalassaemics was demonstrated by Weatherall *et al.* (1969b).

In the studies of Gill and Schwartz (1973) and Bank *et al.* (1973) it was found that there was balanced globin synthesis in the bone marrow of sickle-cell thalassaemics while there was clear-cut imbalance of globin production in reticulocytes. The problem of apparent balance of globin synthesis in the bone marrow in thalassaemia was discussed in Chapter 5. The same problems may be relevant to the experiments described in these two studies.

In a study of haemoglobin synthesis in the bone marrow and peripheral blood of a young Arab boy with sickle-cell thalassaemia (Clegg & Weatherall 1972) it was found that the relative specific activities of HbA and S remained similar throughout erythroid maturation. These findings indicated that Hbs A and

S are produced in reticulocytes at the same rate as they are synthesized in the bone marrow and, at the time, did not support the notion that the deficiency of β^A-chain production in sickle-cell β^+ thalassaemia is due to the relative instability of β^A mRNA as compared with normal mRNA (i.e. in this case β^S mRNA). More recent knowledge of the molecular pathology of β^+ thalassaemia is, of course, in keeping with this interpretation.

Interactions between sickle-cell β thalassaemia and α thalassaemia

In an attempt to understand the clinical heterogeneity of sickle-cell anaemia several studies have been carried out to determine whether the phenotype can be modified by the co-inheritance of α thalassaemia (Embury *et al.* 1982; Higgs *et al.* 1982; Embury *et al.* 1984). The effect of the co-inheritance of the homozygous state for α^+ thalassaemia ($-\alpha/-\alpha$) is not particularly marked; the frequency of the acute chest syndrome and leg ulceration is less and persistent splenomegaly is more common (see Chapter 11).

There has been less opportunity to study the interaction of sickle-cell β thalassaemia with α thalassaemia. Persistent splenomegaly and splenic sequestration is more common in subjects with four α-globin genes and the co-inheritance of α thalassaemia results in a slightly increased haemoglobin level and decreased reticulocyte response. Interestingly, the MCH and MCV were also higher, as has been found in other interactions with α and β thalassaemia (see Chapter 13). Overall, however, the effect of the co-inheritance of α thalassaemia seems to be small (Steinberg *et al.* 1984; Vyas *et al.* 1988). In the study of Gonzalez-Redondo *et al.* (1988b), which described 25 patients with sickle-cell β thalassaemia associated with the -29 A→G β-thalassaemia allele, 11 had single α-gene deletions ($-\alpha/\alpha\alpha$). No clinical details are given but the haematological findings, though not significantly different, show the same trend as in the other two series; a single missing α gene was associated with a slightly higher haemoglobin level, MCV and MCH.

Population distribution and clinical variability

Sickle-cell thalassaemia is widely distributed, especially among individuals of African and Mediterranean origin. The disease has been well documented in persons of many ethnic backgrounds: Italians (Silvestroni & Bianco 1944–45, 1955a,b, 1969); Sicilians (Silvestroni & Bianco 1955a,b; Signorelli 1966; Silvestroni & Bianco 1969; Conconi *et al.* 1970; Caruso-Nicoletti *et al.* 1992; Mirabile *et al.* 1997), Sardinians (Sansone *et al.* 1967); Greeks (Choremis & Zannos 1957); Afro-Americans (Smith & Conley 1954; Singer *et al.* 1955; Monti *et al.* 1964; Weatherall 1964a; Pearson 1969; Steinberg & Dreiling 1976; Gonzalez-Redondo *et al.* 1988a); West Africans (Watson-Williams 1965; Gatti *et al.* 1967; Konotey-Ahulu & Ringelhann 1969; Bienzle *et al.* 1983a); Jamaicans (Went & MacIver 1958a; Serjeant & Serjeant 1972; Serjeant *et al.* 1973, 1979; Serjeant 1992); Guadeloupeans (Romana *et al.* 1996); Indians (Chatterjea 1959; Devi *et al.* 1969; Saha & Banerjee 1973; Kulozik *et al.* 1991a); Libyans (Jain 1985); Turks (Aksoy & Lehmann 1957; Aksoy 1959; Aksoy *et al.* 1963); Romanians (Bratu & Predescu 1969); Tunisians (Roche *et al.* 1956; Fattoum *et al.* 1991); Jordanians (Barkawi *et al.* 1991; Bashir *et al.* 1992a); Algerians (Belhani *et al.* 1977; Trabuchet *et al.* 1977b); Israelis (Divlansky *et al.* 1976); Chileans (Rona *et al.* 1973); Brazilians (Zago *et al.* 1983); Saudi Arabians (Pembrey *et al.* 1980; El-Hazmi & Al-Swailem 1987); Sudanese (Weatherall *et al.* 1971) and Indonesians (Wahidijat *et al.* 1974). The authors have also observed sickle-cell thalassaemia in patients from Cyprus, the Lebanon and Sri Lanka.

Sickle-cell thalassaemia does not reach a high frequency in any population. It has been estimated that sickle-cell β^0 thalassaemia occurs approximately once in every 23 000 Afro-Americans (Steinberg & Dreiling 1976), and has a frequency in Jamaica of one in 6750 (Serjeant *et al.* 1979). The disorder is seen quite frequently in Sicily, Greece and north Africa, particularly in Algeria, and probably in Sudan. It also occurs relatively frequently in the oasis regions of eastern Saudi Arabia and in the Orissa populations of India. Gene frequencies have not been determined for any of these populations.

In all the populations in which sickle-cell β thalassaemia is found both sickle-cell β^+ and β^0 thalassaemia have been observed. As mentioned earlier, the different clinical expressions probably explain at least some of the differences in severity between different races. Hence the disease is generally milder in American, Jamaican and African populations, in which the mild β^+-thalassaemia promoter mutations are common. More severely affected Africans have sickle-cell β^0 thalassaemia or the sickle-cell gene interacting with the more severe forms of β^+ thalassaemia. The latter interactions are the rule in the Mediterranean region. This also accounts for the very severe clinical course which was recorded in the early descriptions of the disease by Silvestroni and Bianco in southern Italy and Sicily, and by Choremis and Zannos and later workers in Greece.

As mentioned earlier, in the studies in Jamaica of Serjeant *et al.* (1979) there were only minimal differences in the clinical phenotypes between sickle-cell anaemia and sickle-cell β^0 thalassaemia (see Tables 9.3 and 9.6). Broadly, the same conclusions have been drawn from this kind of comparison in Algeria (Belhani *et al.* 1984) and Saudi Arabia (El-Hazmi 1987). Similarly, it is clear that in patients with sickle-cell β^+ thalassaemia in whom the β-thalassaemia allele is severe the phenotype differs very little from sickle-cell anaemia. For example, in a comparison of Orissan Indian patients with sickle-cell β^+ thalassaemia, in which the β-thalassaemia allele in each case was the severe IVS1-5 G$\rightarrow$C variety associated with only 3–5% HbA production, there were no significant clinical differences (Kulozik *et al.* 1991a). On the other hand, studies of the interaction of the common Mediterranean β-thalassaemia allele, IVS1-110 G$\rightarrow$A, in which the output of HbA in sickle-cell β^+ thalassaemia is in the 8–14% range, suggested that this interaction is significantly milder than sickle-cell anaemia in the Greek population. This was evidenced by a higher steady-state haemoglobin level and lower reticulocyte count, together with a milder clinical course (Christakis *et al.* 1991). Similar conclusions were drawn from a study in the population of southeast Sicily by Schiliro *et al.* (1995).

A word of caution is necessary in assessing these ethnic variations in the severity of sickle-cell thalassaemia. In certain populations, notably those of the eastern province of Saudi Arabia (Perrine *et al.* 1972), Iran (Haghshenass *et al.* 1977), Kuwait (Pearson & Al-Rasheid 1987) and Orissa State, India (Kar *et al.* 1986; Kulozik *et al.* 1991a), there is a milder form of sickle-cell anaemia associated with unusually high levels of fetal haemoglobin and a high frequency of α thalassaemia. Thus, though comparisons of the phenotypes of sickle-cell anaemia and sickle-cell β^0 thalassaemia may not show significant differences in these populations, overall the latter tends, like sickle-cell anaemia, to run a milder course.

In short, the ethnic and individual variability in the phenotype of this disease seems to be based largely on the frequency and severity of particular β-thalassaemia alleles in the population together with other factors that modify the expression of the sickle-cell gene.

Inheritance

In earlier editions of this book we analysed all the published family pedigrees of individuals with sickle-cell thalassaemia. Before the DNA era a study of the offspring of patients with this condition born of normal individuals was the only approach to trying to determine the chromosomal location of the β-thalassaemia gene. The fact that all these children are either HbS or β-thalassaemia carriers indicated that the two conditions are either alleles or closely linked. We now know, of course, that they are alleles; there have been no families reported with independent segregation of the sickle-cell and β-thalassaemia genes although, as mentioned in Chapter 4, there appear to be rare forms of β thalassaemia that are not encoded in the β-globin-gene complex.

The β^S gene which also carries a β-thalassaemia mutation

In our last edition we speculated about the phenotype which might result if a β-thalassaemia gene was in *cis* to the β^S mutation, i.e. a β-globin gene containing mutations for both β thalassaemia and sickle haemoglobin (see Chapter 3). The predicted phenotype was the sickle-cell trait with an extremely low level of HbA and the haematological picture of β-thalassaemia trait. Gratifyingly, this combination has now been found in the real world! The proband has the phenotype of β-thalassaemia trait with an HbA$_2$ level of 6.2% and an HbS level of 11.4%. The β-thalassaemia mutation was found to be the β –88 C$\rightarrow$T. This combination should be suspected in any individual with the sickle-cell trait with an unusually low level of HbS together with thalassaemic red-cell indices (Baklouti *et al.* 1987, 1989).

Problems for genetic counselling

As we have seen, as a general rule the mild forms of sickle-cell β^+ thalassaemia in African populations are, as a group, remarkably innocuous conditions compared with the more severe forms of sickle-cell β^+ and

β^0 thalassaemia observed in other ethnic groups. The problem for counselling families with potential children with these conditions is that there are always exceptions in any of these different groups. For example, some patients with the interactions of the milder β-thalassaemia alleles, although they may run a fairly trouble-free course, are not free from some of the more serious complications of the disease. Indeed, in some cases the condition may be as severe as sickle-cell anaemia. Atweh and Forget (1987), describing a patient like this, suggest that sometimes the antisickling effect of the high level of HbA may be counterbalanced by a higher haemoglobin level with increased blood viscosity and a greater propensity for sickling. Interestingly, the milder sickling disorders found in the eastern provinces of Saudi Arabia are also characterized by higher haemoglobin levels and, although there may be fewer painful crises or other complications, there is a relatively high frequency of severe bone disease. Thus, for reasons that we still don't understand, even forms of sickle-cell β thalassaemia which should, based on current evidence, be mild may occasionally be quite severe. Similarly, what are usually more severe forms of the condition may occasionally run an extremely mild course.

For these reasons genetic counselling in sickle-cell thalassaemia is, like that in sickle-cell anaemia, rather imprecise. Probably the only safe statement is that the great majority of patients of African origin with the interaction of the mild promoter mutations are, as a group, unlikely to suffer much disability from their disease. In all other forms of sickle-cell β thalassaemia the chances are that the condition will behave like sickle-cell anaemia.

The interactions of the sickle-cell gene and the δβ thalassaemias

As described in Chapter 8, the δβ thalassaemias consist of the $(\delta\beta)^+$ thalassaemias, or Hb Lepore disorders, and a series of conditions characterized by the complete absence of δ- and β-chain synthesis associated with the production of variable amounts of HbF with either $^G\gamma$ and $^A\gamma$ or only $^G\gamma$ chains, the $(\delta\beta)^0$ and $(^A\gamma\delta\beta)^0$ thalassaemias, respectively. Because these conditions are relatively uncommon, there have been few opportunities for studying their interactions with the sickle-cell gene. From what little is known it appears that they are variable in their clinical expression, particularly in the case of the sickle-cell Hb Lepore disorders.

Haemoglobin S in association with haemoglobin Lepore

The interaction of the sickle-cell and Hb Lepore genes was first described in a Greek family by Stamatoyannopoulos and Fessas in 1963, and subsequently in Italians by Silvestroni *et al.* (1965a) and in Jamaicans by Ahern *et al.* (1972). The identity of the particular form of Hb Lepore (see Chapter 8) was not reported in these early studies, though the variety described in the family of Stamatoyannopoulos and Fessas, which they originally called Hb Pylos, was subsequently identified as Hb Lepore Washington/Boston (Stamatoyannopoulos *et al.* 1971). In all the other examples of this combination that have been reported subsequently the Hb Lepore has been identified as Washington/Boston. This interaction has been studied in detail in Jamaican families (Stevens *et al.* 1982), Afro-Americans (Headings *et al.* 1983; Fatunde & Scott 1986), Greeks (Voskaridou *et al.* 1995), Sicilians (Mirabile *et al.* 1995) and an individual of mixed Italian/Moroccan descent (Huisman 1997). The haematological findings in these cases are summarized in Table 9.7.

Clinical features

Even though there are relatively few reports of this condition, and in some the clinical data are scanty, it appears that the clinical picture is extremely variable. This is well exemplified in the first reported family of Stamatoyannopoulos and Fessas (1963). One of the siblings had typical thalassaemic bone changes with pallor, icterus and marked hepatosplenomegaly. She also had bone pains and other sickling symptoms and a steady-state haemoglobin of 8.6 g/dl with typical thalassaemic red-cell indices. On the other hand, her brother, a 12-year-old boy, had been well all his life except for one episode of bone pain. He had slight splenomegaly, and a steady-state haemoglobin of 12.3 g/dl, again with thalassaemic red-cell changes. The 6-year-old propositus in the Italian family described by Silvestroni *et al.* (1965a) was also severely anaemic from early in life, necessitating regular transfusions. She was pale and had typical thalassaemic bone changes and marked hepato-

Table 9.7 Findings in haemoglobin S/haemoglobin Lepore compound heterozygotes.

Race	Age	Sex	Hb (g/dl)	MCV (fl)	Reticulocytes (%)	Hb Lepore (%)	HbF (%)	HbA$_2$ (%)	Reference
Greek	12	M	12.5	78	7	10.5	25.0	1.8	Stamatoyannopoulos & Fessas (1963)
Greek	13	F	8.6	81	33	10.2	9.6	0.9	
Italian	Adult	F	9.0	80	8	10.0	9.3	1.8	Silvestroni et al. (1965a)
		F	8.0	83	8	10.0	9.7	0.9	
Jamaican	76	F	10.6	78	4	10.1	10.4	2.6	Ahern et al. (1972)
Jamaican	8	M	7.3	7.1	11	8.7	6.1	2.2	Stevens et al. (1982)
	7	F	9.1	68	4	10.6	9.6	2.7	
Afro-American	8/12	M	87	83	5.9	—	40.2	2.9	Headings et al. (1983)
Afro-American	9	F	11.3	68	5.6	12.0	14.0	3.0	Wessels et al. (1986)
Afro-American	10	M	9.7	7.1	5.9	11.1	8.7	2.3	Seward et al. (1993)
Afro-American	11	M	10.6	74	5.0	10.0	15.6	2.2	
Italian/Moroccan	19	M	12.5	79	—	15.4	14.6	2.3	Huisman (1993)
Greek	19	M	13.4	68	6	8.5	3.6	1.9	Voskaridou et al. (1995)
Greek	21	M	13.8	65	15	10.5	3.5	1.6	
	53	M	13.8	76	3	8.5	16.3	2.2	
Sicilian	7	M	7.4	70	—	11.5	8.7	2.3	Mirabile et al. (1995)
	3	M	10.9	73	—	13.5	15.5	3.0	
	14	M	13.5	85	—	16.3	5.9	3.0	
	13	M	12.6	80	—	15.9	6.8	3.1	
	3	M	11.7	68	—	15.2	33.0	3.0	
Afro-American	23	M	9.9	78	—	12.0	8.0	2.0	Fairbanks et al. (1997)
	26	M	10.4	75	—	11.0	7.0	4.0	
	16	M	11.9	66	—	20.0	5.0	3.0	

splenomegaly. After splenectomy she no longer required blood transfusions and her haemoglobin levelled at 9 g/dl.

At the other end of the clinical spectrum the Jamaican patient described by Ahern *et al.* (1972) was a 76-year-old woman who had lived for 60 years in a hilly rural community 2000 ft above sea level and had led a very active life. She had had five successful pregnancies and no abortions. She had never had any symptoms suggestive of a sickling disorder although, at the age of 70, she developed an ulcer over the left lateral malleolus. Her steady-state haemoglobin level was 10.6 g/dl with thalassaemic red-cell indices.

The children reported by Voskaridou *et al.* (1995) are described as having a clinical picture ranging from 'mild to severe', although no details are given except that one of them had been totally free of symptoms all his life. In the Sicilian patients reported by Mirabile *et al.* (1995) there is, again, clinical heterogeneity. One 7-year-old male had a clinical picture similar to that of moderately severe sickle-cell anaemia, with painful crises, haemolytic anaemia and hepatomegaly, but no splenomegaly. Similarly, 22- and 23-year-old males had a severe clinical picture and suffered from frequent painful crises; their younger brother, aged 12, with the same genotype, was almost completely asymptomatic.

It appears therefore that even in this very small series of patients there is quite remarkable heterogeneity. At its worst, this condition is characterized by a picture very similar to severe sickle-cell anaemia, with added thalassaemic features, while, at the other end of the spectrum, it appears to be a symptomless disorder associated with mild anaemia. As in sickle-cell anaemia, regression of the spleen appears to occur in severe cases, though in the majority splenomegaly persists.

Haematological changes

The haematological changes in some of the reported families are summarized in Table 9.7. The steady-state haemoglobin levels range from 7 to 14 g/dl although in most cases there is mild anaemia, with haemoglobin values in the 9–10 g/dl range. The red cells tend to be moderately hypochromic and microcytic. Although there is some variation in reticulocyte counts, when reported, they are always elevated though they tend to be lower than in patients with sickle-cell anaemia. In the few cases for whom serum

iron or ferritin data are given it has been normal or marginally elevated. Red-cell density distribution data are given by Voskaridou *et al.* (1995).

Haemoglobin pattern

The haemoglobin consists of S, Lepore, F and A_2. The level of Hb Lepore is fairly consistent, in the 9–15% range. There is remarkable variability in HbF values. As a group they are similar to those of patients with sickle-cell anaemia. But, as shown in Table 9.7, a few patients have unusually high levels in the 20–30% range, although the one patient with a level in excess of 30% was only 3 years old, and another with a relatively high level was 12 years old. The HbA_2 levels tend to be normal or slightly reduced.

Course and prognosis

There are too few reported patients or families with this condition to provide any data about prognosis.

Problems in diagnosis

Haemoglobins S and Lepore migrate in approximately the same position under some electrophoretic conditions; they are best separated by isoelectric focusing (Voskaridou *et al.* 1995; Huisman 1997). The condition should be suspected in a patient with apparent sickle-cell anaemia with thalassaemic red-cell indices and a normal or low–normal HbA_2 level. It can be confirmed, of course, by a family study, which will reveal Hb Lepore in one or other parent or in siblings.

Pathophysiology and phenotype/genotype relationships

It is very difficult to account for the extraordinary heterogeneity of this disease. As discussed in Chapter 8, Hb Lepore is synthesized at a reduced rate and behaves like a relatively severe δβ thalassaemia. Thus the clinical picture of this interaction might be expected to resemble sickle-cell $β^+$ thalassaemia due to a moderately severe $β^+$-thalassaemia allele. From a careful analysis of the reported cases there does not appear to be any particular relationship between the steady-state level of HbF and the clinical phenotype. The state of the α-globin genes has not been reported so it is not possible to rule out the co-existence of α thalassaemia in some of these cases. From what is known about the level of HbF production in the Hb Lepore disorders (see Chapter 8) it is, perhaps, surprising that the levels are not higher in these patients. While they are in a few cases, as a group HbF production seems to be little different from that in sickle-cell anaemia. However, this analysis is again bedevilled by the small numbers of patients involved.

In short, from the published data it is not possible to draw any conclusions about the mechanisms for the quite remarkable heterogeneity of this disorder.

Sickle-cell $(\delta\beta)^0$ or $(^A\gamma\delta\beta)^0$ thalassaemia

As described in Chapters 4 and 8 there is a family of $\delta\beta$ thalassaemias, all of which result from long deletions of the β-globin-gene cluster. Depending on whether they remove the $^A\gamma$ gene or not, they are divided into the $(\delta\beta)^0$ and $(^A\gamma\delta\beta)^0$ thalassaemias.

In the period before it was possible to define the different molecular forms of $\delta\beta$ thalassaemia, its combination with HbS was observed and well characterized in Sicilian, Italian, Greek, Arab and Afro-American individuals (Russo *et al.* 1963; Silvestroni & Bianco 1964; Stamatoyannopoulos *et al.* 1967; Zelkowitz *et al.* 1972; Altay *et al.* 1977b; Belhani *et al.* 1977; Kinney *et al.* 1978). When it became possible to subdivide these disorders according to the structure of the fetal haemoglobin it was found that the Greek cases had HbF with both $^G\gamma$ and $^A\gamma$ chains and hence this condition could be classified as $(\delta\beta)^0$ thalassaemia. On the other hand, in the Afro-American family reported by Altay *et al.* (1977b) the HbF was of the $^G\gamma$ variety. Although there was some discussion as to whether this latter condition should be classified as $\delta\beta$ thalassaemia or HPFH, later studies at the molecular level, together with further clinical analyses of a large number of cases, indicated that this condition is a form of $(^A\gamma\delta\beta)^0$ thalassaemia (Henthorn *et al.* 1985).

Sickle-cell $(\delta\beta)^0$ thalassaemia

It seems likely that the early reports of the Greek, Sicilian and Italian patients with this disorder represented the interaction of the Sicilian (Mediterranean or southern Italian) form of $(\delta\beta)^0$ thalassaemia which results from a 13 377-bp deletion spanning δ-IVS2 to 26 kb 3' to the termination codon of the β gene (see

Chapter 4). This condition is widely distributed in Mediterranean populations. There have been more recent reports of patients with this form of $\delta\beta$ thalassaemia interacting with HbS in which this deletion has been demonstrated by DNA analysis (Trent *et al.* 1986b; Mirabile *et al.* 1995).

From the limited clinical and haematological data that are available it appears that this is a relatively mild sickling disorder. Although in one case there was a history of painful crises, several others have not given a history of any features suggestive of a sickling disorder. Splenomegaly seems to be present in some but not all patients. Haemoglobin values range between 10 and 12 g/dl, with a significant reduction in the MHC and MCV. In each case the haemoglobin has consisted of S, F and A_2, with HbF values ranging from 9 to 25%.

Sickle-cell $(^A\gamma\delta\beta)^0$ thalassaemia

This genetic combination was first reported by Altay *et al.* (1977b) in the Afro-American siblings. Further families were reported by Henthorn *et al.* (1985) and haematological data on this condition are given by Huisman *et al.* (1997). No clinical data are presented in the more recent papers but in the study of Altay *et al.* the three children were originally thought to have sickle-cell anaemia. They had pain in the limbs or in the abdomen at approximately monthly intervals. These symptoms were severe enough to require hospital admission on several occasions. No abnormal physical signs were described; presumably this means that they did not have palpable splenomegaly.

The haematological findings have been fairly consistent between different reports. The haemoglobin values range from 9 to 12 g/dl and there are slightly reduced MCH and MCV values. The blood films show slight hypochromia and microcytosis. The haemoglobin consists of S, F and A_2. Haemoglobin F values range from 17 to about 25%. Haemoglobin A_2 values have been in the normal range. Globin synthesis studies have shown mild imbalance, with α-/non-α-chain production ratios in the range 1.7–1.9.

In the report of Henthorn *et al.* (1985) and Huisman (1997) one of the patients was also heterozygous for α^+ thalassaemia, as evidenced by a globin synthesis ratio of 0.9.

Phenotype/genotype relationships for the haemoglobin S δβ thalassaemias

Because of the paucity of published clinical data, and the small number of cases that have been described, it is not possible to draw any firm conclusions about the severity of these combinations or about whether the two different forms differ significantly. It might be expected that the interactions with $(^A\gamma\delta\beta)^0$ thalassaemia might be more severe and would be associated with a lower output of HbF. Overall, however, the relatively high output of fetal haemoglobin in these conditions would be expected to place them at the milder end of the spectrum of the different sickling disorders.

Haemoglobin C thalassaemia

The association of the genes for thalassaemia and HbC in one individual was first described in an Afro-American patient by Zuelzer and Kaplan in 1954 (Zuelzer & Kaplan 1954) and by Karl Singer and his coworkers in the same year (Singer *et al.* 1954). In the following years the condition was well characterized in Afro-Americans (Singer *et al.* 1954, 1957; Smith & Krevans 1959; Weatherall 1964a). During this period the condition was also found in Italians (Erlandson *et al.* 1956; Perosa *et al.* 1961), north Africans (Portier *et al.* 1960) and Turks (Göksel & Tartaroglu 1961). More recently it has been further defined in Italians (Polosa *et al.* 1966; Blatrix *et al.* 1970; Polosa *et al.* 1970), north Africans (Baumes 1972; Belhani *et al.* 1977), West Africans (Konotey-Ahulu & Ringelhann 1969; Willcox 1983), Sicilians (Coquelet *et al.* 1970), Spaniards (De Pablos *et al.* 1987), Afro-Americans (Maberry *et al.* 1990) and Tunisians (Fattoum *et al.* 1993). The case of Kaplan and Zuelzer differed from the others in that the level of HbA exceeded that of HbC and was almost certainly an example of HbC α thalassaemia. The other reported cases have all been examples of the interaction of HbC and different forms of β thalassaemia.

Pathophysiology

The pathophysiology of HbC is outlined in Chapter 2.

One of the interesting features of this disorder is the remarkable clinical heterogeneity and the striking differences in the clinical and haematological manifestations between different ethnic groups. It is now apparent that, as in the case of sickle-cell β thalassaemia, much of this variability reflects the particular variety of β-thalassaemia gene which is interacting with HbC. The forms of β^+ thalassaemia common to African populations produce an extremely mild clinical disorder, while HbC β^0 thalassaemia or HbC associated with the forms of β^+ thalassaemia with very low levels of HbA production causes a more severe condition.

Although studies at the molecular level are limited, there are sufficient data to indicate that the levels of HbA in HbC β thalassaemia reflect the action of different β-thalassaemia alleles (Table 9.8). Gonzalez-Redondo *et al.* (1988b) have found that the milder forms of the disease with 20–30% HbA found in African populations are associated with the β –29 A→G and β –88 C→T mutations, whereas the levels of HbA in the intermediate range, 10–11%, are associated with the β IVS1-110 G→A mutation. Haemoglobin C β^0 thalassaemia has been found in association with the β codon 39 C→T mutation in Mediterranean populations (Huisman 1997), and together with a 532-bp deletion of the 5′ end of the β-globin gene by Waye *et al.* (1991).

Clinical and haematological findings

The HbC thalassaemias fall into several different clinical groups depending on the particular genetic interactions outlined above.

Table 9.8 Some interactions between haemoglobin C and β thalassaemia. Sources Gonzalez-Redondo *et al.* (1988b) and Huisman *et al.* (1997).

Phenotype	% HbA	Mutation	Population
HbC/β^+	16–18	–88 C→T	Afro-American
HbC/β^+	16–20	–29 A→G	Afro-American
HbC/β^+	11	IVS1-110 G→A	Mediterranean
HbC/β^0	0	CD39 C→T	Mediterranean
HbC/β^0	0	532-bp deletion	Afro-American

The mild form of haemoglobin C β⁺thalassaemia in African populations

The clinical and haematological manifestations of this disorder have been well documented in Africans and Afro-Americans by Singer *et al.* (1954, 1957), Smith and Krevans (1959), Weatherall (1964a) and Willcox (1983), and in Tunisians by Fattoum *et al.* (1993). There is a mild degree of anaemia similar to that observed in β-thalassaemia heterozygotes. The condition is symptomless except for the occurrence of a mild iron-refractory anaemia during pregnancy (Singer *et al.* 1954; Weatherall 1964a; Maberry *et al.* 1990). There are no abnormal physical findings and the spleen is not usually enlarged. The red cells show some variation in shape and size with many target cells, ranging from 20 to 50% of the total red-cell population (Fig. 9.7). The MCH and MCV are reduced to the range usually seen in heterozygous β thalassaemia. Indeed, the blood film looks very like that of the latter disorder except for the unusually large number of target cells. There are no complications except for a mild anaemia of pregnancy, although the authors have observed worsening of the anaemia with iron deficiency and nutritional folate deficiency.

Haemoglobin C β⁰ thalassaemia in African populations

With the exception of three children of a patient with Hb Leslie β⁰ thalassaemia (see below) described by Lutcher *et al.* (1976) and a report from Israel by Ozsoylu *et al.* (1989) we have not been able to find any good clinical descriptions of this condition in African populations and therefore we shall briefly describe a patient who was referred to us with this disorder. She was a 34-year-old woman who presented with refractory anaemia in pregnancy. On clinical examination she was pale and mildly icteric and her spleen was palpable 6 cm below the costal margin. There were no bone changes on either clinical or radiological examination. She was anaemic, with a haemoglobin level of 9.3 g/dl and 14% reticulocytes, and her red-cell indices indicated that she had small red cells with a markedly reduced MCH. She developed severe anaemia during her first pregnancy, which had necessitated blood transfusion in the postpartum period. After the delivery of her second infant her haemoglobin level rose to 11.3 g/dl but a reticulocytosis of 9–10% persisted. A study of her haemoglobin synthesis is shown in Fig. 9.8.

Afro-American siblings with HbC β⁰ thalassaemia were described briefly by Lutcher *et al.* (1976). One of them was admitted to hospital with pneumonia at the age of 3 years but otherwise they were in good health. Apparently they did not have palpable spleens. Their haemoglobin values ranged from 10.0 to 10.3 g/dl and they had markedly reduced MCH and MCV values. Curiously, in the two cases in whom reticulocyte counts were recorded, they were hardly elevated, both being 1.1%. It is clear from these brief clinical descriptions that the degree of haemolysis in these children was not as severe as in the patient described above. Thus there seems to be heterogene-

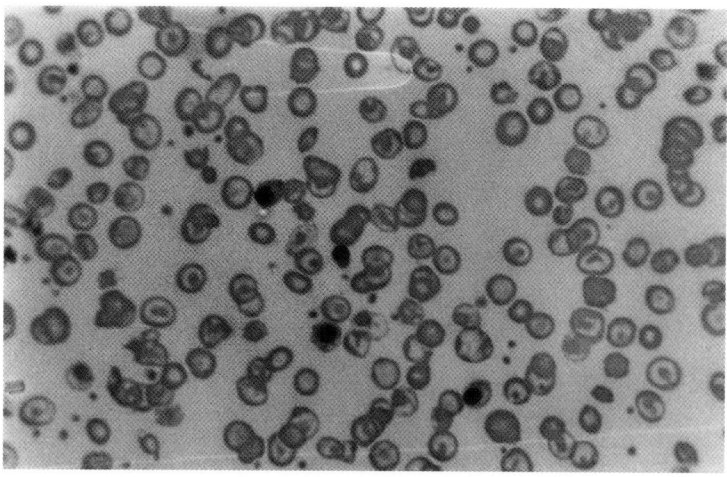

Fig. 9.7 Peripheral blood film of a patient with HbC β⁺ thalassaemia (×420).

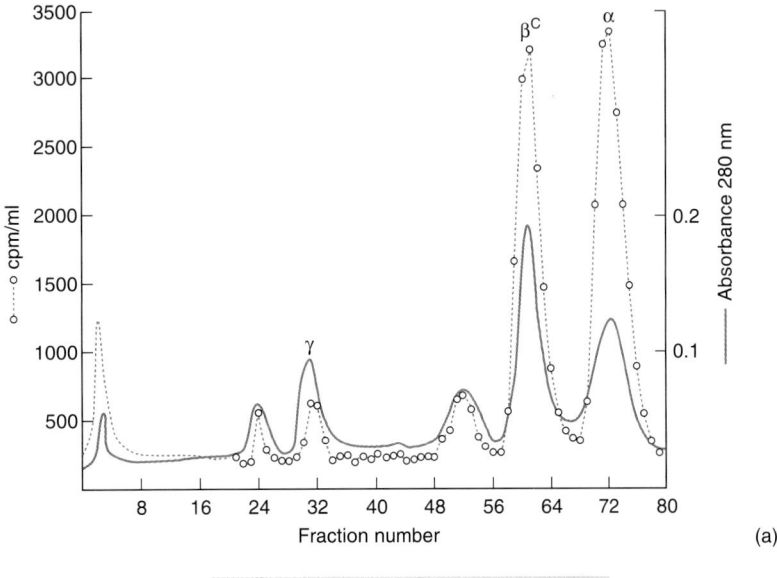

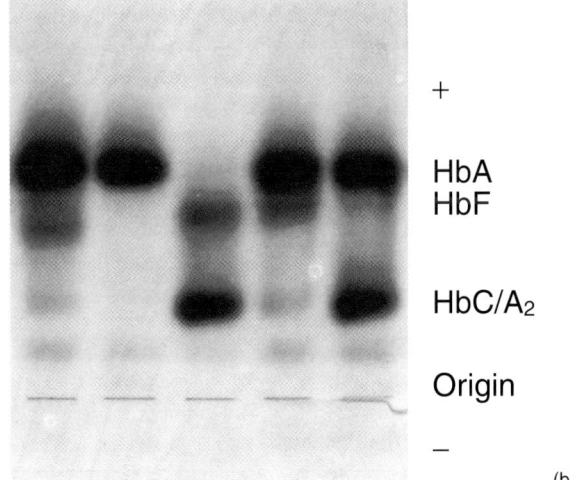

Fig. 9.8 The haemoglobins in the HbC β or δβ thalassaemias. (a) Haemoglobin synthesis in HbC β^0 thalassaemia. The radioactive profile, shown by the broken line, indicates that there is no HbA production but that there is minimal overall globin imbalance. (b) Haemoglobin electrophoresis (starch gel, pH 8.5, amido black stain) of the following, left to right: 1, δβ-thalassaemia trait; 2, normal; 3, HbC δβ thalassaemia; 4, δβ-thalassaemia trait; 5, HbC trait.

ity of HbC β^0 thalassaemia, even within those of African origin.

Severe haemoglobin C β^+ or β^0 thalassaemia in other population groups

Again, though good data are extremely sparse, it appears that this condition is more severe in Mediterranean populations because it usually results from the interaction of severe β^+- or β^0-thalassaemia alleles. The low levels or absence of HbA in these

compound heterozygotes reported in some of the later descriptions of the disease are in keeping with this suggestion, though molecular data on these interactions are not available.

Excellent clinical descriptions of more severe HbC β thalassaemia have been reported in Italians and Sicilians (Erlandson *et al.* 1956; Polosa *et al.* 1966, 1970; Pich *et al.* 1973), Turks (Göksel & Tartaroglu 1961), Algerians (Portier *et al.* 1960; Belhani *et al.* 1977) and Spaniards (Casado *et al.* 1978). In the early reports it was not absolutely clear whether these were cases of HbC β^0 thalassaemia, or β^+ thalassaemia of the severe variety. However, in later studies from Sicily, Algeria and Tunisia (Polosa *et al.* 1970; Belhani *et al.* 1977; Boreux *et al.* 1978; Fattoum *et al.* 1993) it became clear that both of these varieties of HbC β thalassaemia occur in Mediterranean populations. The clinical findings in these patients are characterized by moderate to severe anaemia, icterus, bone changes similar to those of thalassaemia intermedia and, almost invariably, moderate to marked splenomegaly. Although it is difficult to determine the prognosis, and the picture is clouded by the poor social conditions in which some of them have been found, it seems likely that there is an increased infant mortality (Belhani *et al.* 1977).

The blood picture shows a variable degree of anaemia with haemoglobin values in the 7–10 g/dl range and morphological changes of the red cells and red-cell indices typical of those of β thalassaemia. However, there are large numbers of target cells and moderate numbers of microspherocytes, many of the cells showing a characteristic folded appearance. The reticulocyte count is usually elevated, in the 5–20% range.

From these limited data there does not appear to be a major phenotypic difference between HbC β^0 thalassaemia and the interactions of the more severe forms of β^+ thalassaemia. The clinical findings are very similar to those described above for this interaction in African populations. However, as is always the case in the thalassaemia field, there are exceptions, and Belhani *et al.* (1977) have documented cases with almost normal PCV and haemoglobin levels. The reasons for this remarkable heterogeneity are not clear; there are no published data on family studies which have looked for other possible ameliorating factors such as the co-existence of α thalassaemia and the relative level of HbF.

The bone marrows of patients with more severe forms of HbC β thalassaemia show marked erythroid hyperplasia. Ultrastructural studies have been reported by Wickramasinghe (1990). As well as erythroid hyperplasia the red-cell precursors show intracytoplasmic α chains in polychromatic erythroblasts and reticulocytes. These abnormal erythroblasts show a marked depression or complete failure of incorporation of ^{3}H-leucine into protein. In addition, there is marked phagocytic activity in the marrow, similar to that observed in other forms of β thalassaemia.

Patients with more severe forms of HbC β thalassaemia are subject to a variety of complications. They may undergo aplastic crises during episodes of infection and the marked splenomegaly may result in secondary hypersplenism necessitating splenectomy. We have already mentioned the moderately severe degree of anaemia which can occur in pregnancy. However, these patients are able to have children; in the family originally reported by Portier *et al.* (1960) and on which further data were presented by Belhani *et al.* (1977), a woman with HbC β^+ thalassaemia (in which the β^+-thalassaemia gene was of the severe variety) was able to produce no fewer than 14 children! Maberry *et al.* (1990) provide further information about HbC thalassaemia in pregnancy in Black populations.

Haemoglobin analysis

The electrophoretic findings depend on whether the associated thalassaemia gene is of the β^+ or β^0 variety (see Table 9.8). In African cases of HbC β^+ thalassaemia there is usually between 65 and 80% HbC, the remainder being HbA with a very low level of HbF, in the 2–5% range (Fig. 9.5). The HbF is distributed heterogeneously throughout the red cells (Shepherd *et al.* 1962).

Because of the similar electrophoretic mobilities of Hbs C and A_2 the earlier accounts of this condition did not report the level of HbA_2. More recently, by separating Hbs A, F, C and A_2 by cation-exchange high-performance liquid chromatography, it has been found that the HbA_2 level is elevated to about twice normal (Gonzalez-Redondo *et al.* 1988b).

In HbC β^+ thalassaemia in which the β-thalassaemia gene is of the more severe variety (see earlier section and Table 9.8) the HbA level varies between 5 and 12% (Erlandson *et al.* 1956; Belhani *et al.* 1977). It seems likely that this was the type of HbC thalassaemia described in the Turkish sibship of Göksel and Tartaroglu (1961). In HbC β^0 thalassaemia only Hbs C and F are demonstrable on haemoglobin electrophoresis. The HbF values range from 3 to 10% and appear to be significantly higher than those found in the HbC β thalassaemia of African populations.

Haemoglobin synthesis

Haemoglobin synthesis does not seem to have been examined very often in this condition. The findings in an African woman with HbC β⁰ thalassaemia studied in the authors' laboratory are summarized in Fig. 9.8. There was absent β^A-chain synthesis and only β^C, γ and α chains were produced. Interestingly, there was very little overall globin imbalance. The total amount of γ chain synthesized in the peripheral blood as compared with β^C chain was approximately 8%. However, there was 16% HbF in the blood, suggesting that there is selection of HbF-containing cells. The data presented in Fig. 9.8 are also of interest in relation to the synthesis of HbC. While there were more total counts incorporated into the α chains than into the β^C chains (α-/β^C-production ratio, 1.1) the specific activities of the β^C chains were significantly greater than those of the α chains (α-/β^C-chain ratio, 0.86). These results indicate that the β^C chains may not have been present in the peripheral blood in the quantities in which they were being synthesized and suggest that HbC may be slightly unstable. Further work on the synthesis of HbC is required.

Pathophysiology

As outlined in Chapter 2, the basis for the shortened red-cell survival in HbC disease is understood, at least in part. The clinical manifestations of the HbC disorders are dependent on the physical properties of HbC and, particularly, on its overall concentration in the red cells. An individual with HbC disease will have approximately 27 pg HbC per cell. In HbC β⁰ thalassaemia this figure drops to about 18 pg but as the cells are smaller the concentration of HbC may be similar to that in homozygotes. On the other hand in HbCβ⁺ thalassaemia of the mild variety there is only approximately 13 pg of HbC per cell, which is not much greater than the 10–12 pg found in HbC carriers. Furthermore the red cells are larger in this form of thalassaemia. Thus it seems likely that the degree of haemolysis in HbC β⁰ thalassaemia is similar to that observed in HbC disease because of the relatively high intracellular concentration of the variant. The haemolysis may be accentuated by the mild degree of globin imbalance in the thalassaemic cells, which may also result in a moderate degree of ineffective erythropoiesis (Wickramasinghe 1990).

The level of HbF is higher in HbC β⁰ thalassaemia than in HbC disease. This probably reflects globin imbalance with selective survival of F cells.

Inheritance

One parent has HbC and the other is heterozygous for β thalassaemia. The children of HbC thalassaemics through a normal partner show either the HbC or β-thalassaemia trait.

Geographical distribution

We have already outlined the distribution of HbC thalassaemia. In summary, it occurs predominantly in individuals of West African origin, where the HbC gene has its highest incidence. It has been well documented in various Italian populations (Erlandson *et al.* 1956; Polosa *et al.* 1966, 1970), is seen occasionally in Sicily, Sardinia (Cataldo *et al.* 1977) and north Africa (Portier *et al.* 1960; Belhani *et al.* 1977), and probably occurs sporadically as far east as Turkey (Göksel & Tartaroglu 1961).

Haemoglobin C with haemoglobin Lepore or δβ thalassaemia

Presumably because of the relative rarity of Hb Lepore and δβ thalassaemia in West African populations there have been few opportunities for studying their interaction with HbCs.

Haemoglobin C in association with haemoglobin Lepore

The simultaneous occurrence of Hbs C and Lepore was described in a 17-year-old Afro-American boy by Ranney and Jacobs (1964). He had no symptoms and was found to be mildly anaemic with no other abnormal physical signs. The haemoglobin level was 10.7 g/dl with a slightly elevated reticulocyte count. The peripheral blood film appearances were similar to HbC disease, with numerous target cells and many cells with the typical folded appearance of that disorder. On starch gel electrophoresis Hbs C and Lepore were demonstrated together with small quantities of HbF. Quantification showed Hbs C 80%, Lepore 14% and F 6%. No HbA was demonstrable and the level of HbA₂ could not be determined. Chemical studies showed that this form of Hb Lepore, initially called Hb Lepore The Bronx, was identical to Hb Lepore Washington/Boston. Family studies showed that the patient's mother was heterozygous for Hb

Lepore while the father was not available for study. The patient's daughter was heterozygous for HbC.

Two similarly affected Jamaican siblings were described by Ahern *et al.* (1972). A 57-year-old male had been completely symptom free all his life except for chronic leg ulceration, starting at the age of 50 years, while his 60-year-old brother had had no symptoms. Clinical examination was normal in both cases and there was no splenomegaly. Their blood counts showed slightly reduced haemoglobin values in the 12–13 g/dl range, with a reduced MCH and MCV. In both cases the haemoglobin consisted of C (77 and 80%), Lepore (10.6 and 10.3%) and F (9.2 and 12.1%). Both these patients had blood films typical of an HbC disorder, with many target cells, occasional spherocytes and very occasional nucleated red cells. The ^{51}Cr red-cell survival in one case was 22 days. The findings in an Afro-American male (Schoentag *et al.* 1985) and in an Algerian family (Francina *et al.* 1985) were similar.

In short, the combination of HbC with Hb Lepore Washington Boston produces an extremely mild disorder which is similar to the variety of HbC β^+ thalassaemia found in African populations.

Haemoglobin C δβ thalassaemia

This is an extremely rare disorder, which has not yet been studied in patients in whom the particular form of δβ thalassaemia has been characterized at the molecular level. In two early reports, which include full clinical and haematological descriptions, both of the patients were Afro-Americans. In the patient described by Wood *et al.* (1977a) the γ chains consisted entirely of the $^G\gamma$ variety and it seems likely that this represented the interaction between black $(^A\gamma\delta\beta)^0$ thalassaemia and HbC. Certainly in both cases the genetic evidence for the inheritance of δβ thalassaemia, rather than HPFH, was quite clear.

The patient described by Zelkowitz *et al.* (1972) was a 68-year-old black male. No clinical details are given. He had a haemoglobin value of 14.7 g/dl with an MCV of 80.5 fl. The peripheral blood film showed marked morphological changes characterized by target cells, microspherocytes and hypochromia. The patient described by Wood *et al.* (1977a) was a 20-month-old boy of West Indian origin who presented with tonsillitis and an infected foot. Clinical examination was otherwise normal and his spleen was not palpable. There were no radiological abnormalities of

his bones. His blood picture showed a haemoglobin of 8.4 g/dl, MCV 67 fl, MCH 19.4 pg and morphological changes of the red cells. It appears therefore that neither of these patients was incapacitated by his disease and splenomegaly and bone changes were not observed.

In both cases the haemoglobin consisted of C and F; the levels of HbA$_2$ were not determined (Fig. 9.8). The level of HbF in the 68-year-old male was 26.1% and in the 20-month-old child was 23.9%. In both studies the HbF was unevenly distributed among the red cells. As mentioned earlier, structural analysis of the HbF in the patient described by Wood *et al.* (1977a) showed that the γ chains consisted entirely of the $^G\gamma$ variety.

Globin synthesis was carried out on the peripheral blood of the 20-month-old child. Only α, β^C and γ chains were synthesized; there was a complete absence of β^A-chain production. The α/non-α ratio was approximately 2.3. The proportion of γ chain synthesized relative to β^C chain was less than the relative proportions of Hbs F and C in the peripheral blood. This finding was supported by specific-activity data which showed that that of the γ chain was only about half that of the β^C chain. This indicates that the relative turnover rate of HbF is slower than that of HbC in the peripheral blood of this patient, suggesting preferential survival of the HbF-rich cell population.

Complete genetic studies were not carried out on either of these families. In the family reported by Wood *et al.* (1977a) the mother of the propositus had δβ-thalassaemia trait with an HbF value of 11.3%; the father was not available. In the family described (Zelkowitz *et al.* 1972) the 68-year-old male had one child with HbS δβ thalassaemia. No lateral relatives were studied.

From these limited data it appears that HbC δβ thalassaemia is a milder disorder than HbC disease and HbC β^0 thalassaemia. The two reported patients have a disorder of similar severity to HbC β^+ thalassaemia of the African variety. It seems likely that the relatively high level of HbF reduces the severity of the haemolytic process consequent on the presence of HbC. The biosynthetic studies show quite clearly that there is preferential survival of the red cells which contain relatively more HbF, presumably as a result of the globin imbalance caused by the δβ-thalassaemia gene. The combination of the δβ-thalassaemia mutation, which allows relatively high levels of HbF production, together with the differential survival of HbF-rich populations, results in a higher level of HbF in this disorder than that observed in the different forms of HbC β thalassaemia.

Haemoglobin E β thalassaemia

In the previous edition of this book we wrote 'although a great deal is known about the clinical manifestations and complications of this disorder it is a remarkable fact that although we have known of its existence for over 20 years it is still far from clear why the interaction of HbE and β thalassaemia produces such a severe clinical disorder. This is an area of the thalassaemia field that has been seriously neglected.' Unfortunately, as we review this field nearly another 20 years on, the situation has not changed all that much. This is particularly regrettable, since it is now clear that HbE β thalassaemia will pose a major public health problem in the Far East and in parts of India, Pakistan and Bangladesh in this new millennium. Indeed, globally, it is one of the most important varieties of thalassaemia (Weatherall & Clegg 1996).

Early descriptions and the development of knowledge about haemoglobin E β thalassaemia

The first description of HbE β thalassaemia appeared in a paper by Virginia Minnich and colleagues in 1954 under (at that time) the rather surprising title 'Mediterranean anaemia; a study of 32 cases in Thailand'! The first electrophoretic identification of HbE was reported independently by Chernoff and Sturgeon and their colleagues in the same year (Chernoff *et al.* 1954; Sturgeon *et al.* 1955). Interestingly, both these reports characterized HbE in combination with thalassaemia. In 1956 Chernoff and colleagues re-examined some of the cases of thalassaemia first described in Thailand by Minnich and colleagues and discovered that they were a mixed bag of disorders made up of classical β thalassaemia major, HbH disease and HbE β thalassaemia. Amoz Chernoff's paper should be read by anyone interested in the thalassaemia field because it contains some of the best clinical descriptions of the disease which have ever been published. Haemoglobin E β thalassaemia was further characterized in large-scale clinical studies in Thailand (Na-Nakorn 1959; Wasi *et al.* 1969) and in many other parts of south-east Asia and the Indian subcontinent (Sturgeon *et al.* 1955; Punt & Van Gool 1957; Vella 1958a; Chatterjea 1959; De Silva *et al.* 1959; Lie-Injo 1959b; Chatterjea 1966).

More recently there have been further descriptions of the disease in Thailand (Fucharoen & Winichagoon 1987; Winichagoon *et al.* 1993), India (Swarup-Mitra 1988; Agarwal *et al.* 1997), Vietnam (Khanh *et al.* 1990), Malaysia (George & Wong 1993), Vietnamese immigrant populations in the USA (Marsh *et al.* 1983; Sandhaus *et al.* 1983) and Bangladeshi immigrants in the UK (Rees *et al.* 1998c). The authors have had the opportunity to study over 150 patients with the condition in Sri Lanka.

Molecular pathology and pathophysiology

Haemoglobin E

Haemoglobin E comigrates with Hbs A_2 and C on routine electrophoresis, although these haemoglobins can be separated by isoelectric focusing (Basset *et al.* 1978) or high-performance liquid chromatography (Huisman 1993). The variant haemoglobin makes up approximately 25–30% of the total haemoglobin in heterozygotes.

At least *in vitro*, HbE appears to be mildly unstable and precipitates in solution at 50–60°C or at a reduced pH (Yuthavong *et al.* 1975). It shows slightly increased sensitivity to oxidants (Frischer & Bowman 1975; Yuthavong *et al.* 1975; MacDonald & Charache 1983) and, like other unstable haemoglobins, precipitates in 70% isopropanol (Ali *et al.* 1980). In the presence of oxidative products of fava beans the red cells of HbE carriers may be more resistant to *Plasmodium falciparum* malaria (Kitayaporn *et al.* 1992). It also appears to dissociate into monomers more readily than HbA (Ruenwongsa & Yuthavong 1975). Whole-blood oxygen dissociation curves of homozygotes for HbE appear to be shifted slightly to the right (Kolatat 1964; Bellingham & Huehns 1968; Fairbanks *et al.* 1980). On the other hand, purified HbE has a normal oxygen affinity, Bohr effect and reactivity with 2,3-diphosphoglycerate (Bunn *et al.* 1972; Gacon *et al.* 1974).

While these observations suggest that HbE is mildly unstable *in vitro*, there is no evidence that this is the case *in vivo*, at least in the heterozygous and homozygous states; the red-cell survival in homozygotes is normal (Fairbanks *et al.* 1980). On the other hand, the early studies of Chernoff *et al.* (1956) and Lehmann and Singh (1956) suggested that patients with HbE disease have a mild anaemia and microcytic red cells with a significantly reduced MCH and MCV. These findings were confirmed by Fairbanks and his colleagues and others, who, in an extensive series of studies of Asian immigrants to the USA, found that heterozygotes have a mild microcytosis while homozygotes have morphological changes of their red cells and red-cell indices very similar to those of heterozygous β thalassaemia (Fairbanks *et al.* 1979, 1980; Wong & Ali 1982). In the papers from Fairbanks' group there are summaries of all the haematological data in the HbE disorders published up to that time and it is quite clear that this condition is associated with hypochromic, microcytic red cells which seem to survive normally. They did not find elevated HbF levels in homozygotes, though in a study by Dorléac *et al.* (1984) it was slightly raised, at about 3%.

In short, therefore, the inheritance of HbE produces the phenotype of an extremely mild form of β thalassaemia. In homozygotes this is very similar to β-thalassaemia trait, with a mild anaemia and little or no elevation of HbF; the red-cell precursors show scanty inclusions resembling α-chain precipitates (Wickramasinghe *et al.* 1984). Subsequently, studies at the molecular level have provided the mechanisms for these thalassaemic changes.

Molecular pathology of haemoglobin E

Studies of haemoglobin synthesis in HbE homozygotes demonstrated imbalanced globin synthesis, with α-/β-chain production ratios very similar to those of heterozygous β thalassaemia (Pagnier *et al.* 1974; Fairbanks *et al.* 1980; Traeger *et al.* 1980; Wong & Ali 1982). Furthermore, reticulocytes from heterozygotes synthesize significantly less HbE than HbA (Feldman & Rieder 1973). Further studies showed that there are decreasing levels of β^E messenger RNA in the cells of heterozygotes and homozygotes during erythroid maturation (Traeger *et al.* 1980; Benz *et al.* 1981; Traeger *et al.* 1982). It was subsequently found that the base substitution at codon 26, GAG→AAG, that gives rise to HbE, β26 Glu→Lys, also activates a cryptic splice site that causes abnormal messenger RNA processing; since the usual donor site has to

compete with this new site, the level of normally spliced, that is, β^E, mRNA is reduced (Orkin *et al.* 1982b). The abnormally spliced mRNA is non-functional since part of exon 1 is missing and a new stop codon is generated (see also Chapter 4). Thus the β^E chain is produced in reduced amounts and results in a β-thalassaemic phenotype.

In short, HbE is ineffectively synthesized and shows some evidence of instability *in vitro* but not *in vivo*. In addition, it is likely that its final level in the red cell may also reflect a relatively ineffective combination of α and β^E as compared with α and β^A chains, a phenomenon which, as we shall discuss in Chapter 11, is accentuated by α-chain deficiency due to the co-inheritance of α thalassaemia.

β-Thalassaemia alleles in haemoglobin E β thalassaemia

There have been extensive studies of the different thalassaemia alleles that interact with HbE in Thailand (Fucharoen *et al.* 1989b; Petmitr *et al.* 1989; Thein *et al.* 1990b; Winichagoon *et al.* 1990a, 1992b), Malaysia (Yang *et al.* 1989; George *et al.* 1992a), India (De *et al.* 1997), Indonesia (van Solinge *et al.* 1996), Bangladesh (Rees *et al.* 1998c) and Sri Lanka (De Silva *et al.* 2000; Fisher *et al.* 1999). The consequences of some of these interactions are summarized in Table 9.9. The majority of the β-thalassaemia alleles that are commonly found with HbE are of the β^0 or the severe β^+ variety; mild β-thalassaemia alleles are relatively uncommon in populations in which HbE occurs.

Cellular pathophysiology

The central problem in trying to understand the pathophysiology of this disease is why the interaction of HbE—which in the homozygous state is associated with an extremely mild form of thalassaemia with insufficient globin imbalance to cause any selective increase in the level of HbF—with β-thalassaemia alleles produces the profound degree of anaemia that is observed in many compound heterozygotes. As we shall see later, there is marked ineffective erythropoiesis and a shortened red-cell survival, comparable with that observed in homozygous β thalassaemia. Similarly, there is evidence of oxidant damage to the red-cell membranes and widespread tissue damage due to iron accumulation, also of a similar pattern to

Table 9.9 Some interactions between haemoglobin E and β thalassaemia. Main sources are Lynch *et al.* (1988), Fucharoen *et al.* (1989b), Fucharoen & Winichagoon (1992), Yang *et al.* (1989), Thein *et al.* (1991), Winichagoon *et al.* (1990a, 1992b), Ghanem *et al.* (1992), Huisman *et al.* (1997), Rees *et al.* (1998c), unpublished data from our laboratory.

Phenotype	% HbA (Hb Malay*)	% HbF	Hb (g/dl)	Mutation	Population
HbE/β⁺	25–30	8–13	8–10	–28 A→G	Thailand
HbE/Hb Malay	37–43*	3–4	9–10	CD19 A→G	Malaysia, Thailand
HbE/β⁺	41	8	9–10	Poly(A), A→G	Malaysia
HbE/β⁺	4–6	30–65	6–8	IVS1-5 G→C	Thailand, Malaysia, Bangladesh, India, Sri Lanka
HbE/β⁺	4–6	30–55	6–7	IVS2-654 C→T	Thailand, Malaysia, China
HbE/β⁰	0	30–70	4–7	CD41/42 –TCTT	Thailand, Malaysia, China, Indonesia
HbE/β⁰	0	40–70	5–7	CD17 A→T	Thailand, Malaysia
HbE/β⁰	0	—	—	CD26 G→T	Thailand
HbE/β⁰	—	30–70	5–8	IVS1-1 G→T	Malaysia, Thailand
HbE/β⁰	0	—	—	CD22 G →T	Reunion Island
HbE/β⁰	0	30–70	4–8	IVS1-1 G→A	India, Sri Lanka
HbE/β⁰	0	59	7	CD95 +A	Thailand
HbE/β⁰	0	—	4–8	CD71/72 +A	Thailand, China
HbE/β⁰	0	60	3–8	CD123/124/125 –ACCCCACC	Thailand
HbE/β⁰	0	—	—	CD35 C+A	Thailand, Malaysia
HbE/β⁰	0	—	—	CD14/15 +G	Thailand
HbE/β⁰	0	20–50	5–7	CD8/9 +G	Sri Lanka
HbE/β⁰	0	20–60	4–7	CD15 –T	Sri Lanka
HbE/β⁰	0	—	—	CD41 –C	Thailand

* Hb Malay is, like HbE, produced at a slightly reduced rate due to activation of a cryptic splice site.

that seen in other forms of β thalassaemia. Malasit *et al.* (1997) have also found IgG, IgM, IgA, C3 and potentially cytolytic C5b-9 on the surface of the red cells; the significance in relationship to the haemolytic component is not clear. But is the reduced rate of production of β^E globin sufficient in itself to produce these severe interactions with different β-thalassaemia alleles, or does some additional property of HbE also contribute to the severity of the disease?

Could the instability of HbE play any role in contributing to the severity of HbE β thalassaemia? As mentioned earlier, there is very little evidence for the instability of HbE *in vivo*. There has been one report of dapsone-induced haemolysis in an HbE carrier (Lachant & Tanaka 1987), and Rees *et al.* (1996) demonstrated marked instability of HbE in a patient who had also inherited 5′ nucleotidase deficiency. Since the precise mechanism of haemolysis associated with this enzyme deficiency is uncertain it is not clear whether this observation is relevant to HbE β thalassaemia, except that it has been suggested that enzyme-deficient cells of this type may be under

increased oxidant stress. In studies of the stability of HbE in HbE β thalassaemia, encompassing both *in vitro* haemoglobin synthesis and differential centrifugation experiments to assess the relative stability of Hbs A and E in the blood, no evidence for instability of HbE in the steady state was obtained (Rees *et al.* 1998a). These findings are compatible with electron-microscopic and immunocytochemical studies reported by Wickramasinghe and Lee (1997), who demonstrated that the erythroblast inclusions in the bone marrow of patients with HbE β thalassaemia consist entirely of precipitated α chains; there is no evidence of coprecipitation of β^E chains.

On the other hand, if biosynthetic experiments are carried out at temperatures ranging from 38 to 41°C there is marked instability of HbE, a finding which is also seen in red cells from HbE homozygotes (Rees *et al.* 1998a). Although the clinical significance of this observation remains to be determined, these temperatures are frequently encountered even during mild infections in patients in tropical countries where HbE β thalassaemia is particularly common.

Taken together, these findings suggest that, while in

a steady state, instability of HbE does not play a major role in the anaemia of HbE β thalassaemia, under certain conditions it may be of considerable importance.

Phenotypic heterogeneity

Several studies have been carried out to try to explain the marked phenotypic variability of this disease, asking similar questions to those which have been addressed to try to understand the clinical heterogeneity of the homozygous or compound heterozygous states for β thalassaemia (see Chapters 5 and 13) (Fucharoen *et al.* 1984, 1985; Wasi *et al.* 1985; Fucharoen *et al.* 1988b; Winichagoon *et al.* 1993; Kalpravidh *et al.* 1995; Rees *et al.* 1998c). A sib-pair analysis by Fucharoen *et al.* (1984) suggested that multiple genetic factors must be involved in determining the clinical variability. It appears that co-inheritance of different α-thalassaemia alleles or increased level of HbF production, at least as evidenced by the presence or absence of the *Xmn* I polymorphism –158 to the $^{G}\gamma$ globin gene (see Chapters 10 and 13), may play a minor role in modifying the phenotype. Occasionally, mild disease may reflect the interaction of a mild β-thalassaemia allele (see Table 9.9), though these are quite rare in India and south-east Asia, where the disease is particularly common. There is no evidence that variability in the relative rates of removal of excess α chains is involved (Kalpravidh *et al.* 1995).

Other mechanisms must play a role in the clinical heterogeneity of this disease. In the studies of Rees *et al.* (1998c) in patients from Bangladesh, in whom there was a very low frequency of α thalassaemia and who were all heterozygous for the *Xmn* I –158 polymorphism, there was still marked phenotypic variability, with haemoglobin levels ranging from 5 to 10 g/dl. The only factor which seemed to account for the clinical diversity was the steady-state level of HbF. The possible mechanisms involved are similar to those discussed for the variability of HbF production in the other β haemoglobinopathies, as discussed in Chapters 10 and 13.

With the possible exception of the interaction of the rarer mild forms of β^+ thalassaemia (Table 9.9) there seems to be very little relationship between the remarkable phenotypic variation of this disease and the particular β-thalassaemia allele that has been inherited. For example, in a study from Uttar Pradesh, Agarwal *et al.* (1997) were able to divide

their patients into severe transfusion-dependent and milder cases with no or rare transfusion requirements. In each group the severe β-thalassaemia allele, IVS1-5 G→C, was found in almost equal numbers; we have observed similar clinical heterogeneity in patients from Bangladesh and Sri Lanka with the same β-thalassaemia allele.

Clinical features

As already stressed, HbE β thalassaemia shows remarkable clinical variability. At its worst it is very similar to the severest forms of β thalassaemia. We cannot do better than to quote the description of children with this disorder from the paper of Chernoff *et al.* (1956):

> . . . the small stature, wasted extremities, and poor body development stood out in marked contrast to the huge protuberant abdomen, which completely dominated their physical appearance. So great was the abdominal enlargement that many children of five and six years of age found it necessary to arch their backs to maintain their balance in the erect position. In many ways this stance resembled that of a pregnant woman. The abdominal enlargement, coupled with the generalized wasting, dry, wrinkled skin, sunken eyes and wizened expression frequently suggested a diagnosis of progeria.

Clearly this description (see also Fig. 1.10, Chapter 1) is remarkably similar to that of the poorly transfused homozygous β-thalassaemic children which we discussed in Chapter 7.

As many of these children grow older they develop the features of severe thalassaemia (Fig. 9.9). There are marked skeletal deformities with typical thalassaemic facies (Fig. 9.10). In a review of 408 patients (Wasi *et al.* 1969) thalassaemic changes of the bones of the face were described in 81% of cases and radiological bone changes in 92%. There is nearly always marked pallor of the skin and mucous membranes and the conjunctivae show a variable degree of icterus. Cardiomegaly is usually present, together with systolic flow murmurs. These findings are roughly proportional to the severity of the anaemia (Chernoff *et al.* 1956). The latter workers also noted that a generalized lymphadenopathy was common in these patients; this has not been a feature of the disease in Sri Lanka. The liver was enlarged in all of

Fig. 9.9 A child with severe HbE β thalassaemia. (a) This Sri Lankan child has a typical thalassaemic facial appearance with massive enlargement of the spleen and liver and the characteristic stance associated with this degree of hepatosplenomegaly. (b) A demonstration of the lower edge of the spleen.

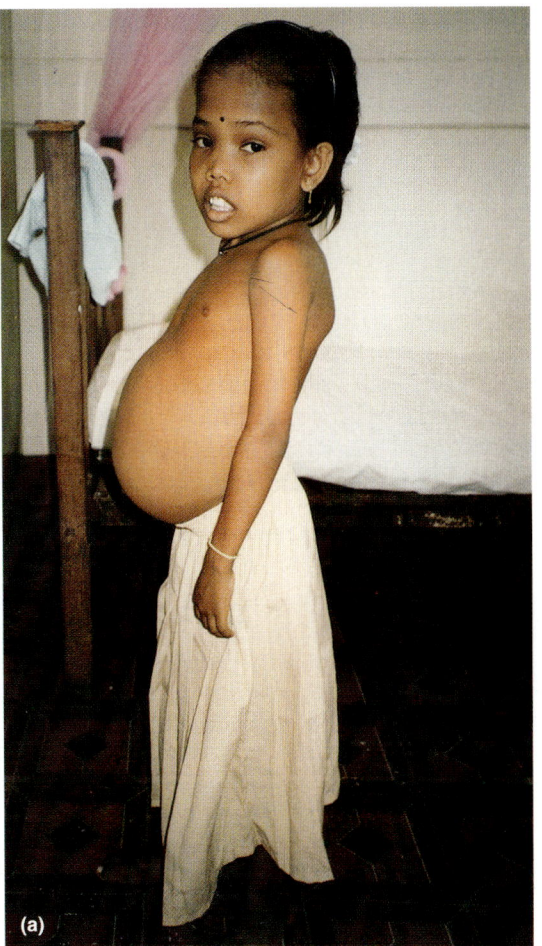

(a)

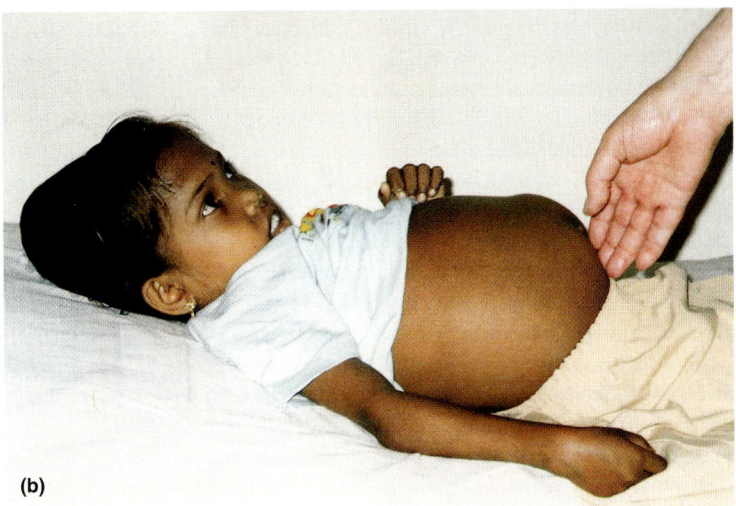

(b)

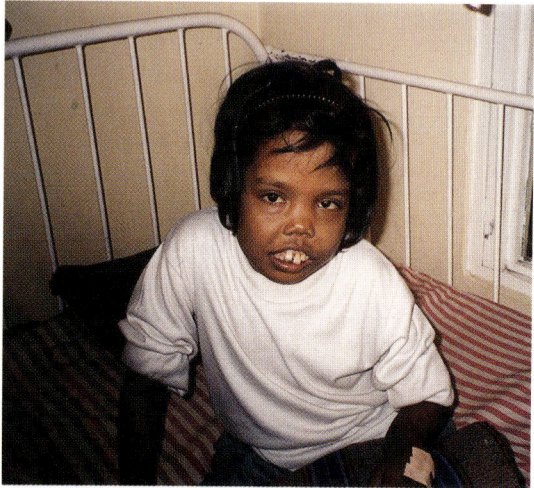

Fig. 9.10 Facial appearance in severe HbE β thalassaemia.

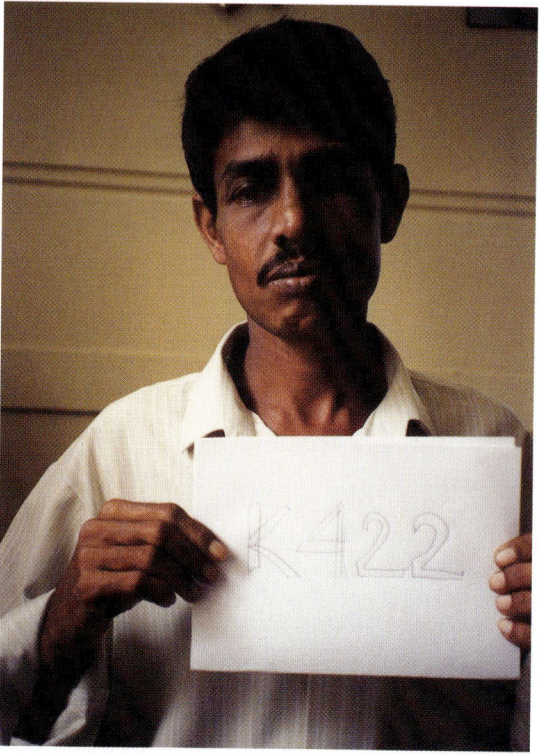

Fig. 9.11 A patient with mild HbE β thalassaemia. This Sri Lankan patient was aged 45 years at the time that he was studied. He had grown and developed normally with no symptoms and had mild hepatosplenomegaly. He has the same haemoglobin genotype as the child shown in Fig. 9.9.

the patients described by Chernoff's group and in 92% of the larger series of Wasi and his coworkers. Similarly, splenomegaly was present in the vast majority of cases. It is rare to find a spleen which is enlarged much less than 5 cm below the costal margin and not at all uncommon for it to descend below the umbilicus or even into the pelvis.

The severity of the disorder as just described was confirmed in clinical descriptions from other population groups (Chatterjea 1959; De Silva *et al.* 1959; Lie-Injo 1959b). Later descriptions of the disease in Thailand (Wasi *et al.* 1969), Vietnam (Khanh *et al.* 1990) and India (Agarwal *et al.* 1997) all underline how severe this disease may be. The clinical pictures at the severe end of the spectrum are indistinguishable from those of the homozygous or compound heterozygous states for severe β thalassaemia.

However, it is clear from all these accounts, and from more recent studies of immigrants in the West (Rees *et al.* 1998c) and a large population of patients in Sri Lanka (authors' unpublished observations) that the disease is extremely variable in its phenotype. In every population some patients remain independent of transfusion with relatively normal growth and development (Fig. 9.11). This was the case in approximately half of the cases reported from Uttar Pradesh by Agarwal *et al.* (1997) and has been observed in our recent studies in Sri Lanka. The spectrum of severity in these patients is very similar to that described for β thalassaemia intermedia (see

Chapter 13), ranging from a disorder that presents late and requires occasional transfusion to a completely symptomless condition which may be found by a chance blood examination or during a family study (Fig. 9.11).

We have recently had the opportunity to study a number of these older and less severely affected patients in the Bangladeshi population in the UK (Rees *et al.* 1998c), in the Indian immigrant population in the UK (unpublished observations) and in a cross-sectional study of patients in different age groups in Sri Lanka (unpublished observations). These patients, whose ages range between 25 and over 50 years, appear to have grown and developed normally, although their final height may be short, an observation which is difficult to interpret because of lack of developmental data in their particular ethnic groups. Most of them were sexually mature and many of them had had children. They had encountered some of the complications outlined in the sections which follow, notably progressive splenomegaly which, in many cases, had led to splenectomy. In some cases they had never attended a hospital at all and were ascertained by family studies or by chance. Although some of them had mild bone changes, severe thalassaemic facial abnormalities were not a feature. In short, while these individuals have steady-state haemoglobin levels little higher than the most severely affected children with this condition, they seem to have grown and developed normally and to have had very few symptoms ascribable to thalassaemia.

Course and complications

Many children with HbE thalassaemia go through childhood in chronic ill health due to severe anaemia and suffer a variety of complications, many of which are similar to those which occur in β thalassaemia major (see Chapter 7). It is important to realize, however, that the bulk of the literature on this disease reflects hospital-based cases. As discussed above, it is now becoming clear that this condition has an extremely variable course and that some patients, particularly in the emerging countries, never present to hospital and many of those that do have a much milder illness.

Age at diagnosis

Although there are few published data, it is clear that the age of presentation of this disease is, overall, later than that of the more severe forms of β thalassaemia. For example, in 120 patients studied in Sri Lanka, the age of presentation ranged from 1 to 54 years, and even the more severely affected children tended to present later than homozygotes or compound heterozygotes for β thalassaemia (unpublished observations).

Growth retardation

Retardation of growth and development was noted in the early descriptions of the disease by Chernoff *et al.* (1956) and has been well documented in later series. For example, Wasi *et al.* (1969) noticed defective development in 57% of their 408 patients. The relationship of growth retardation in terms of both

height and weight to the haemoglobin level was examined by Israngkura *et al.* (1978a,b). These workers divided their patients into three groups, maintained at haemoglobin levels of 8–10, 6–8 and 4–6 g/dl, respectively; they found reduction of height and weight in approximately 35, 60 and 80% of cases in the high, moderate or low haemoglobin level groups, respectively. There was a similar correlation between the size of the liver and spleen, with significantly greater hepatosplenomegaly in the most anaemic group. There was a less impressive correlation between haemoglobin level and bone age. It should be noted that this study was carried out in children aged between 1 and 14 years; it is not clear whether they proceeded to a normal adolescent growth spurt or whether even some of those with a relatively high haemoglobin level did not attain a normal adult height, as appears to be the case in some well transfused homozygous β thalassaemics (see Chapter 7).

More recently, preliminary studies on the patterns of development on groups of patients in Sri Lanka suggest that much more needs to be learnt about the relationship between the steady-state haemoglobin level and growth and sexual maturation in this disease (Olivieri *et al.* 1998b). Two groups of patients were compared with respect to their rates of growth, sexual maturation and bone age. In one, the patients had been maintained on low-level transfusion and many of them had undergone splenectomy, while a second group had presented much later and had had virtually no medical intervention. This study suggested that, even in the absence of specific therapy, including transfusion and splenectomy, and though maintained at a haemoglobin level of 5–6 g/dl throughout development, skeletal maturation and growth, though it may be delayed, appears to be relatively normal by the age of 20 years or more. By the third decade most patients had achieved a normal adult bone age. Clearly it is very important that larger studies of this type are carried out in order to try to develop some better guidelines for the management of this disease (see Chapter 15).

Infection

Children with HbE β thalassaemia are prone to infection and this is probably the commonest cause of death at all ages (see later section) (Fig. 9.12). The increased incidence of infection was first described

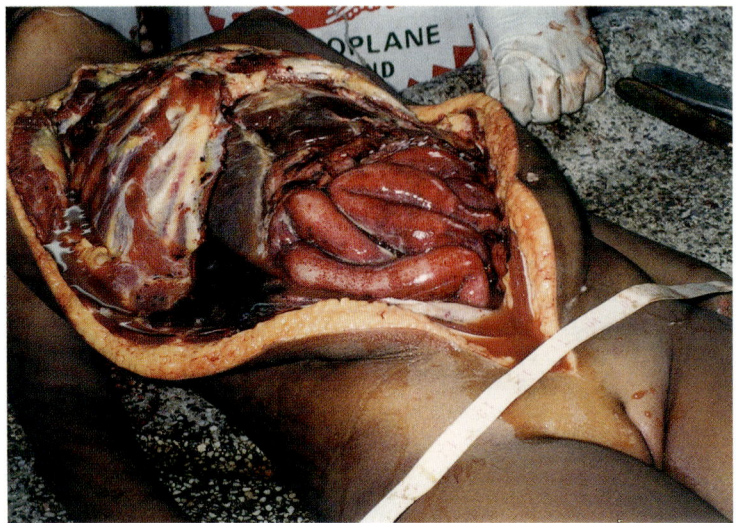

Fig. 9.12 Severe haemorrhagic peritonitis found at autopsy in a child with HbE β thalassaemia. This child, who had previously undergone a splenectomy, died within 12 h of a fulminating septicaemia with assumed disseminated intravascular coagulation.

by Chernoff *et al.* (1956) and highlighted in subsequent reports (Wasi *et al.* 1969; Tanphaichitr *et al.* 1978). These early studies were followed up by an extensive series of investigations into the frequency and varieties of infection in Thailand (Aswapokee *et al.* 1988a,b; Issaragrisil *et al.* 1988; Wasi *et al.* 1988). Overall, they have demonstrated an increased susceptibility to a wide variety of infections in patients compared with controls and, interestingly, this included both bacterial and viral illnesses. In the latter case patients appeared to be more prone to Coxsackie B virus but not to rubella, herpes simplex, cytomegalovirus, adenovirus or *Mycoplasma pneumoniae*. Although there is a clear relationship between splenectomy and increased propensity to infection this was not shown for viral illnesses. In an analysis of 51 deaths from infection it was possible to identify a causative organism in 22 cases; these included *Klebsiella pneumoniae*, *Escherichia coli*, *Pseudomonas aeruginosa* and *Streptococcus pneumoniae*. As in other transfusion-dependent populations, infection with hepatitis B and C or evidence of previous infection is relatively common in this disorder (Thakerngpol *et al.* 1992; George & Wong 1993; Laosombat *et al.* 1997). These patients also seem predisposed to infections with *Campylobacter jejuni* (Jackson *et al.* 1997).

Apart from the effect of splenectomy, and neutropenia associated with hypersplenism, attempts to demonstrate a cellular or humoral basis for increased propensity to infection have, as in other forms of tha-

lassaemia, not provided any clear-cut answers. Humoral immunity seems to be intact and though a variety of non-specific changes in lymphocyte populations have been observed, including reduced levels of T cells (Swarup-Mitra 1988), a reduction in the relative numbers of OKT3+ and subsets of OKT4+ and OKT8+ and a significant decrease in the OKT4+/OKT8 ratio (Boonpucknavig *et al.* 1988), these findings were not observed in patients studied by Wanachiwanawin *et al.* (1996). The latter workers found, however, that without mitogen, lymphocytes from their patients incorporated more tritiated thymidine than those from normal controls, suggesting that lymphocytes from thalassaemic patients are activated *in vivo*. Whether or not these cells are less efficient in their response to new or previously exposed antigens remains to be determined. Swarup-Mitra (1988) observed some non-specific defects in phagocytic function of polymorphonuclear leucocytes. All in all, however, these studies do not explain such a high rate of infection in this particular form of thalassaemia.

There have also been isolated reports of seronegative rheumatoid arthritis and of atypical forms of glomerulonephritis (De Silva *et al.* 1988; Ongajyooth *et al.* 1995).

Hypersplenism

Massive enlargement of the spleen with hypersplenism is well documented (Chernoff *et al.* 1956;

Chatterjea 1959; Wasi *et al.* 1969). Apart from discomfort due to a large spleen, progressive splenomegaly may cause worsening of anaemia, thrombocytopenia and neutropenia. In most reported series of splenectomies there has been some overall improvement in the haemoglobin level; this occurred in 16 of the 18 cases reported by Chatterjea (1959) and in a significant proportion of the 143 patients reviewed by Wasi *et al.* (1969). However, the steady-state haemoglobin levels before surgery and the length of follow-up afterwards are not mentioned in either of these series.

Hepatomegaly

In the early descriptions of this disease by Chernoff *et al.* (1956) it was noted that some of the children developed considerable hepatomegaly, particularly after splenectomy. Although this complication has been mentioned in the literature occasionally, it has not been well documented. We have observed it not infrequently in children in Sri Lanka, particularly in those who have undergone splenectomy. The liver may become quite massively enlarged, a finding that has also been noted in patients with other severe forms of β thalassaemia (see Chapter 7). Whether this reflects a major increase in hepatic extramedullary erythropoiesis or the trappage of abnormal red cells in the liver is not known. Recently, we have had the opportunity to study liver biopsies from patients of this type in Sri Lanka. There is marked extramedullary erythropoiesis, largely involving red-cell precursors, which often involves the liver sinusoids. There is a varying degree of haemosiderosis and in some cases there are inflammatory changes associated with early fibrosis and cirrhosis; viral hepatitis is not common in this population. It appears therefore that extramedullary erythropoiesis plays an important part in the hepatomegaly observed in this disease, but that inflammatory change and the early stages leading to hepatic fibrosis may also be a factor.

Aplastic crises

Temporary aplasia of the bone marrow with worsening of the anaemia has been well documented (Chatterjea 1959). In his excellent description Chatterjea described the reticulocytopenia and relative hypocellularity of the bone marrow in association with infection. Although this complication can probably occur with a variety of different infective organisms, in Chatterjea's paper a particularly interesting feature was the association with an acute episode of malaria.

Megaloblastic anaemia

Megaloblastic anaemia was reported from India by Chatterjea in 1959. It was not clear whether this was due to folic acid or vitamin B_{12} deficiency. Low serum vitamin B_{12} and serum folate levels were found in a high proportion of Chatterjea's cases but it should be remembered that nutritional deficiency of both these vitamins is relatively common in parts of India. However, it seems likely that folic acid requirements are markedly increased. In a study of 53 patients in Thailand, serum folate levels were lower than 3 ng/ml in 33%, and red-cell folate values of less than 180 mg/ml were found in 28% (Vatanavicharn *et al.* 1978). Thus it appears that in Thailand, as in India, folate deficiency is quite frequent.

Extramedullary bone-marrow 'tumours'

As in all forms of severe thalassaemia intermedia, large tumour masses may be caused by extension of bone marrow due to massive erythroid hyperplasia (Fig. 9.13). This may result in a mediastinal mass on chest X-ray (De Costa *et al.* 1974). Large bone-marrow masses may result in a cerebral tumour or cause a severe paraplegia (Fucharoen *et al.* 1981a). The latter complication has also been documented by Mihindukulasuriya *et al.* (1977). Another example of an intracranial mass, presenting with epilepsy, was reported by Fucharoen *et al.* (1985), and an obstructive uropathy due to a pelvic mass of extramedullary tissue was described by Intragumtornchai *et al.* (1993). A variety of tumour masses of this kind are illustrated in the atlas of thalassaemia pathology prepared by Sonakul (1989).

Myelofibrosis

Myelofibrosis has been reported in a patient with HbE β thalassaemia (Aksoy *et al.* 1978b), though it seems likely that this was a chance association.

Iron loading

There is good evidence that severe iron loading may occur in HbE β thalassaemia. An increased rate of

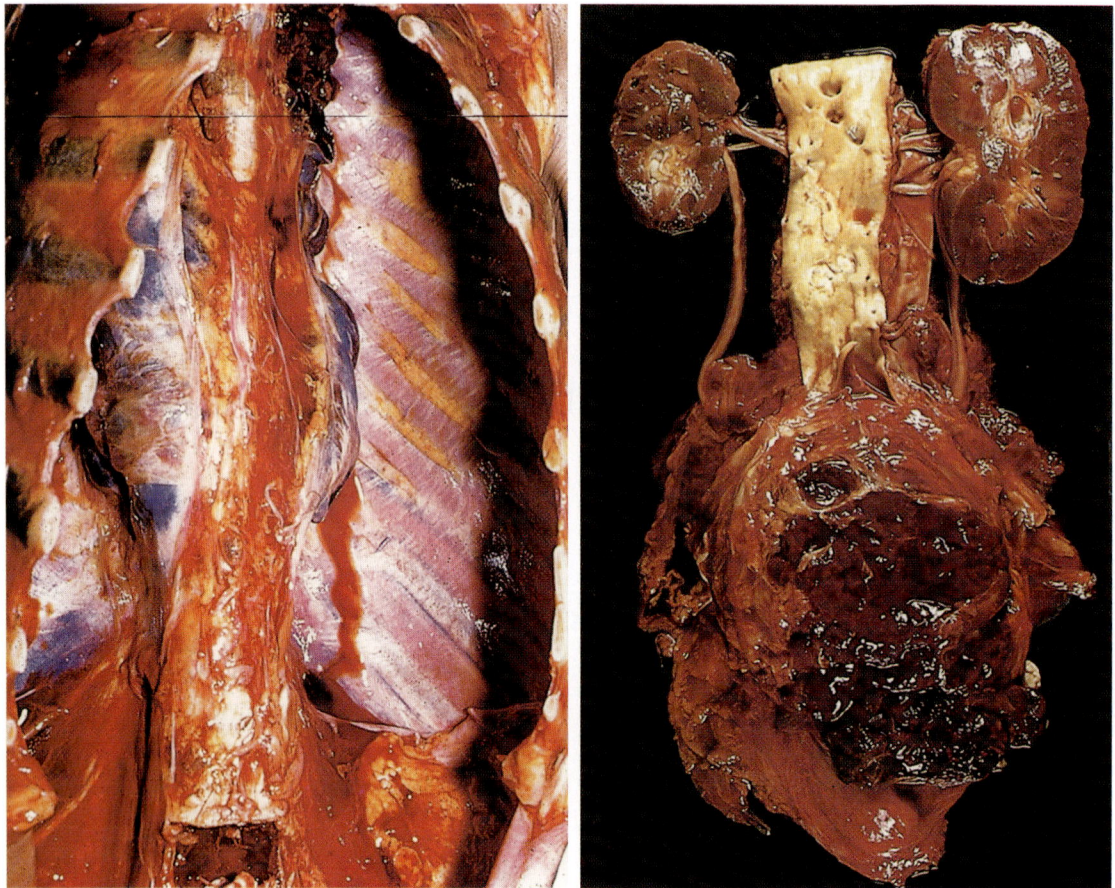

Fig. 9.13 Extramedullary haemopoiesis in HbE β thalassaemia. (a) Paravertebral mass; (b) mass in presacral region. From Sonakul (1989), with permission.

iron absorption, apparently greater in splenectomized patients than in those with intact spleens, was reported by Vatanavicharn *et al.* (1983). In an extensive erythrokinetics study, Pootrakul *et al.* (1988) showed that there was a consistent relationship between the degree of expansion of erythropoiesis and the rate of radioiron absorption. Even in non-transfused patients there is an increase in serum ferritin levels related to age (Fouladi *et al.* 1998) and the levels of non-transferrin plasma iron concentrations show a significant increase in older patients, which appears to be more marked in those who have undergone splenectomy (Anuwatanakulchia *et al.* 1984). We have observed extremely high hepatic iron concentrations in some older patients in Sri Lanka who have received very few transfusions during their

life. The purification and characterization of tissue ferritins obtained from the heart and pancreas is described by Tran *et al.* (1990a,b).

The histological changes in liver biopsies from patients with severe HbE β thalassaemia, examined by both light and electron microscopy, are reported by Thakerngpol *et al.* (1992). They are compatible with cirrhosis of varying degrees. Cirrhosis of the liver has also been reported from patients in India (Mitra *et al.* 1996). In a series of over 60 liver biopsies obtained from patients of different ages in Sri Lanka we have observed a variety of changes ranging from increased iron deposition, through early inflammatory appearances and fibrosis, to frank cirrhosis.

Pathological data have been reported by Chatterjea (1959), Bhamapravati *et al.* (1967) and Sonakul

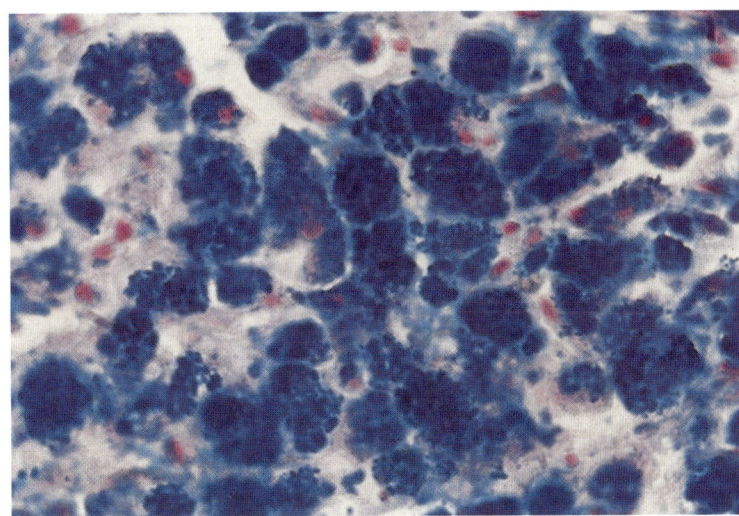

Fig. 9.14 Heavy iron loading of the liver in HbE β thalassaemia (Prussian blue stain ×450). From Sonakul (1989), with permission.

et al. (1978, 1984), and are illustrated in a monograph by Sonakul (1989). In each series there was extensive iron loading of the tissues, the liver being most heavily involved (Fig. 9.14). Sonakul and colleagues noted that the degree of hepatic fibrosis did not always correlate with the amount of iron, and suggested that some of the changes may have been due to viral hepatitis. Interestingly, cirrhosis seemed to be more common in splenectomized patients. Other organs with gross haemosiderosis included the spleen, lymph nodes, pancreas, adrenals, kidneys, alimentary tract and heart, in that order of severity. The degree of myocardial iron loading was not very impressive. The earlier studies of Chatterjea (1959) on the Indian population showed similar abnormalities. Many of the Thai patients in these studies had been infrequently transfused and it seems certain therefore that the bulk of the excess iron was derived from increased absorption from the alimentary tract.

Despite evidence of considerable liver damage it is unusual to observe patients with liver failure or portal hypertension in the Thai population (Fucharoen & Winichagoon 1997).

Cardiopulmonary dysfunction

While the cardiological complications resulting from iron loading of the myocardium in heavily transfused patients with HbE β thalassaemia may be similar to those described in Chapter 7 for transfusion-dependent β thalassaemia major, as is the frequent occurrence of pericarditis (Fucharoen & Winichagoon 1997), there appear to be several cardiopulmonary manifestations which are different from the other forms of β thalassaemia. As mentioned earlier, severe iron loading of the myocardium as a result of increased iron absorption in patients who have not been regularly transfused does not seem to be a major problem.

In the late 1970s and early 1980s a series of papers from Thailand described pulmonary arterial obstruction, pulmonary hypertension, chronic hypoxaemia and right-heart failure in patients with HbE β thalassaemia, particularly after splenectomy. Furthermore, these changes could be partially reversed by the administration of aspirin (Sonakul *et al.* 1980; Fucharoen *et al.* 1981b; Winichagoon *et al.* 1981; Wasi *et al.* 1982). It was suggested that these findings reflected chronic right ventricular strain and hypoxia, possibly as the result of high platelet counts after splenectomy, leading to platelet aggregation in the pulmonary arterial vessels. Later, autopsy studies revealed obliterative changes in the pulmonary arterioles (Fig. 9.15) and, in some cases, evidence of large pulmonary embolic lesions (Sonakul *et al.* 1984). These early studies were followed by a series of papers dealing with various aspects of cardiopulmonary function in this disease. The presence of obliterative changes in the pulmonary arterioles and larger pulmonary obstructive lesions caused, presumably, by recurrent thromboembolism were confirmed

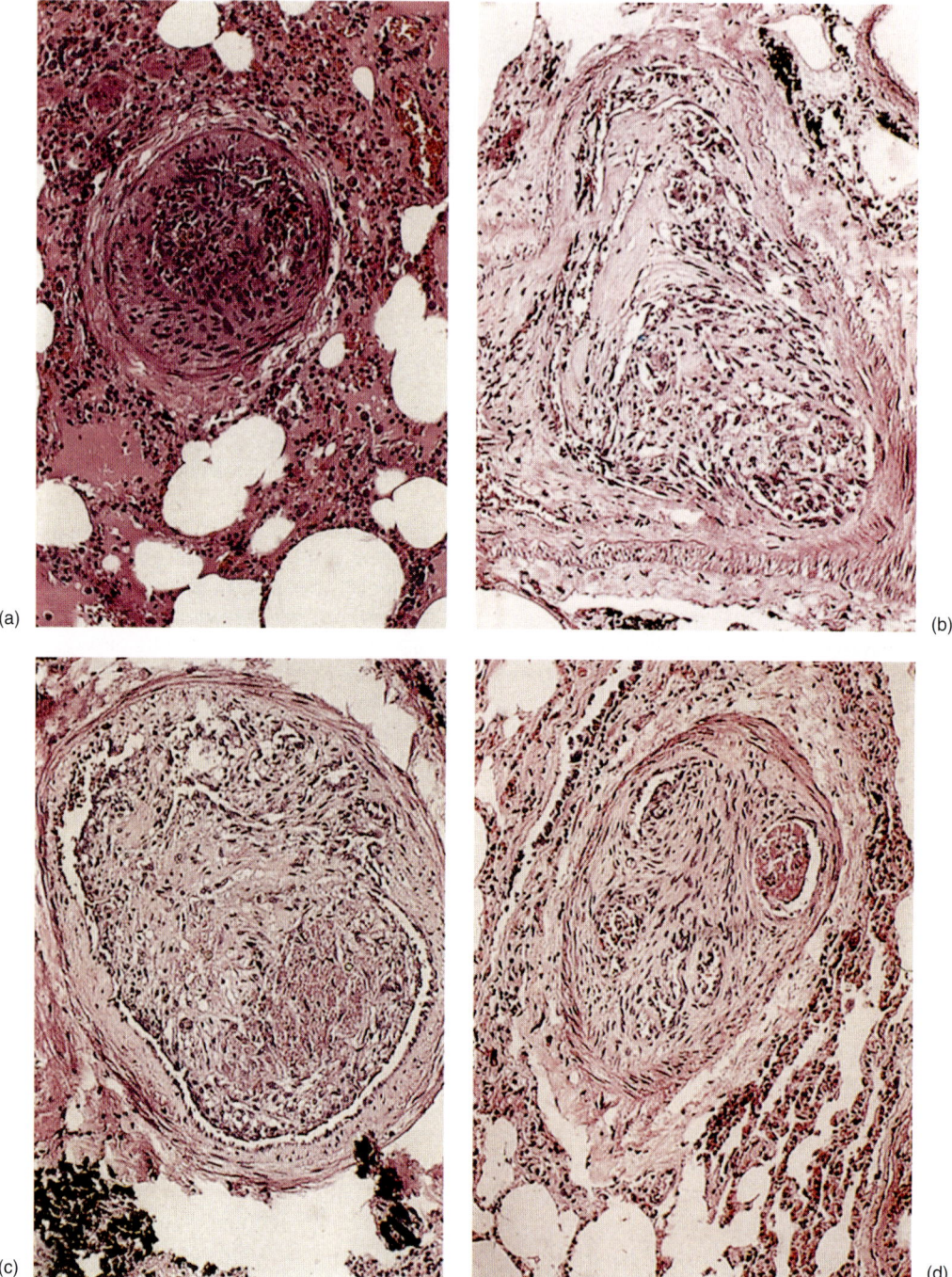

(a)

(b)

(c)

(d)

Fig. 9.15 The pulmonary arteries in an autopsy of a patient with HbE β thalassaemia. Thrombus or embolus in small pulmonary arteries: (a) with early recanalization; (b) canalized thromboembolus with the formation of septa; (c,d) recent thromboemboli superimposed on old recanalized thromboemboli. From Sonakul (1989), with permission.

by Sonakul *et al.* (1988a,b). Pulmonary function tests showed an extremely complex pattern of abnormalities consistent with both restrictive and obstructive defects, or both (Youngchaiyud *et al.* 1988). In a study of splenectomized thalassaemic children it was found that about half had arterial hypoxaemia, together with a wide variety of pulmonary function defects and abnormalities of platelet function (Israngkura *et al.* 1988).

In a study of eight Thai adults, all but one of whom had undergone splenectomy, admitted with congestive cardiac failure, it was found that the systemic blood pressure was low normal, the electrocardiograms showed sinus rhythm with right axis deviation and right atrial enlargement, and echocardiograms revealed right-sided abnormalities with pericardial effusion. Cardiac catheterization demonstrated moderate to marked hypoxaemia. It was concluded that all these patients, with one exception, had clear-cut evidence of pulmonary hypertension, and that right-heart failure secondary to pulmonary artery obliteration disease is a major complication of HbE β thalassaemia in this population (Jootar & Fucharoen 1990). A further analysis of the cardiac status of 25 patients, using two-dimensional echocardiography followed by a stepwise multiple regression analysis, suggested that the steady-state haemoglobin level was the major determinant of cardiac enlargement, while the ejection fraction and percentage fractional shortening were significantly associated with the transferrin-bound iron saturation (Intragumtornchai *et al.* 1994). In many of these studies the additional complication of pericardial effusion or fibrinous pericarditis was present in a varying number of cases.

It is still difficult to obtain a clear picture of the mechanisms of cardiopulmonary disease in HbE β thalassaemia. There is undoubtedly an element of cardiac disease due to iron loading in transfusion-dependent patients and, in addition, there is evidence of right-heart disease due to recurrent thromboembolism and/or the results of platelet aggregation in the pulmonary circulation. There may also be the additional complication of iron-mediated lung disease, as described in Chapter 7. The clinical relevance of these complications is still not absolutely clear, although it appears that there are well documented cases of right-heart failure. Why, therefore, have these changes not been observed in other populations or in individuals with other forms of thalas-

saemia intermedia after splenectomy? The recent observation of this type of problem in other forms of thalassaemia, discussed in Chapters 7 and 13, suggests that they may have been overlooked. Have they not been looked for or is there something quite unusual about patients with HbE β thalassaemia which results in a hypercoagulable state? These are extremely important questions which still require clarification.

Coagulation abnormalities

From the preceding discussion it appears that, from the Thai experience, there may be a state of hypercoagulability and/or platelet dysfunction in patients with HbE β thalassaemia, particularly after splenectomy. Related complications have also been reported in patients of other ethnic origins (Wijburg *et al.* 1988); two Chinese patients developed cerebral infarction due to occlusion of their extracranial carotid vessels.

As in other forms of thalassaemia, many abnormalities of platelet numbers and function, or of clotting factors and their antagonists, have been reported in HbE β thalassaemia, although no clear-cut pattern has emerged. These include an increase in spontaneous platelet aggregation (Laosombat *et al.* 1992; Opartkiattikul *et al.* 1992a), a variety of abnormalities of platelet aggregation and function (Visuphiphan *et al.* 1994), reduced levels of proteins C and S (Shirahata *et al.* 1992), changes in platelet factor III availability (Opartkiattikul *et al.* 1992b) and an acquired abnormality of von Willebrand factor (Benson *et al.* 1990). As was described in Chapter 5, it has also been suggested that abnormalities of the erythrocyte membranes may play a role in activating the coagulation system.

Clearly, as discussed in Chapter 5, we do not understand the hypercoagulable state associated with the thalassaemias; the case of HbE β thalassaemia is no exception. But enough evidence is amassing to suggest that it exists and may have important implications for the management of this disease, particularly in splenectomized patients.

Endocrine dysfunction

Several Thai groups have studied endocrine dysfunction consequent on iron loading (Tuchinda *et al.* 1978; Vannassaeng *et al.* 1978). There was some diminution in growth hormone release after insulin stimulation. Most patients studied were hypogonadal and had low 17-ketosteroid levels. All were euthyroid. Serum cortisol levels were low or in the low-normal range while 17-oxycorticoids were in the normal range. ACTH stimulation tests were normal and the metyrapone test showed either an adequate or slightly slow response. In 12 out of 16 cases the insulin response to an oral glucose load was diminished and in one case there was clinical diabetes mellitus. The significance of the growth hormone studies remains to be determined. The development of diabetes may have serious consequences. In an analysis of 166 patients in Thailand, Piankijagum *et al.* (1978) described three splenectomized patients with severe diabetes and repeated diabetic acidosis; ultimately all of them died from septicaemia.

These studies, although rather limited, indicate that the iron loading may produce some degree of endocrine insufficiency although its full clinical spectrum remains to be determined (see Chapter 7).

Chronic leg ulcers

Chronic ulceration of the lower legs and ankles is common in some populations (Wasi *et al.* 1969), though is seen less frequently in immigrant populations in the West. For example, we have observed it frequently in patients in Sri Lanka, yet in the Bangladesh population of the UK, who have identical genotypes, it is rare.

Bone disease

The marked skeletal deformities described in the early reports of HbE β thalassaemia were mentioned earlier in this chapter. Although there have been few systematic studies it appears that there is increasing reduction in bone density as patients grow older, which may be associated with an increasing tendency to spontaneous fractures (Pootrakul *et al.* 1981a; Fucharoen & Winichagoon 1997).

Gallstones

This is a particularly common complication. In one series ultrasonography showed gallstones in about 50% of cases (Chandcharoensin-Wilde *et al.* 1988).

Hyperpyrexial reaction after blood transfusion

Of eight patients described by Wasi *et al.* (1978) with the strange syndrome of post-transfusion hypertension, convulsions and cerebral haemorrhage in thalassaemic patients after multiple blood transfusions, six had HbE β⁰ thalassaemia. Autopsy findings in six fatal cases were reported by Sonakul and Fucharoen (1992). The brains were oedematous and congested, with visible cerebral haemorrhages in three cases. Microscopically, they showed small focal or perivascular haemorrhages but no lesions characteristic of hypertensive cerebral damage. No underlying vascular disease was found.

Further cases of this syndrome were reported by Chuansumrit *et al.* (1986) and Thirawarapan *et al.* (1989) although, again, no underlying mechanisms were suggested. This type of clinical picture does not seem to have been encountered in other centres with transfusion-dependent patients. We have observed one patient in Sri Lanka who died after an episode which was very similar, and which followed within 12 h of a blood transfusion. But in this case, although there were haemorrhagic lesions similar to those reported from Thailand, it was clear that the death was due to an overwhelming infection, possibly contracted at the time of blood transfusion.

Prognosis

There have been no longitudinal studies of survival patterns in HbE β thalassaemia, but from the limited data that are available it is clear that the condition has a very variable prognosis. There is no doubt that, in some populations, it is associated with a considerable mortality in childhood. However, it is not clear how many patients survive to adult life or the extent to which much of the mortality in early life is due, at least in part, to the poor socio-economic conditions in which many affected children live in south-east Asia and India.

In their descriptions of the disease in early childhood in Thailand Chernoff and colleagues reported that there was a high mortality and, as far as they could tell, the majority of deaths were due to infection. In their analysis of 20 autopsies, Bhamapravati *et al.* (1967) noted that the age at death ranged from 2 to 38 years and that all but six died under the age of 14 years, many in the first 8 years of life. Nearly all the deaths in early childhood in this series were due to infection and, of the total, over half had an infective basis. Death due to hypertension, convulsions and cerebral haemorrhage after blood transfusion has already been mentioned. Another curious syndrome which has been observed by the Thai physicians is characterized by progressive wasting. Patients with this complication are usually between the ages of 15 and 35 years and suffer from severe weakness, weight loss and general malaise for which no obvious cause can be found (Fucharoen & Winichagoon 1997). We have observed something similar in Sri Lanka. It is possible that it reflects multiorgan failure due to extensive iron loading, though this needs to be explored by adequate autopsy studies. Curiously, apart from patients dying from congestive cardiac failure associated with severe anaemia, cardiac deaths of the type observed in well transfused and poorly chelated homozygous β thalassaemics (see Chapter 7) are rare (Yipintsoi *et al.* 1968).

The severity of this disorder is also reflected in a report from Bangkok by Piankijagum *et al.* (1978). These authors analysed 166 cases who were admitted to the adult medical service at Siriraj Hospital between 1964 and 1966. Although the age distribution is not given it is presumed that most of them were aged 14 years or over. During the 2-year period there were 17 deaths. The mortality rate was very much higher in those who had been splenectomized (13 out of 53 cases) as compared with those with intact spleens (4 out of 113 cases). Infection was the major cause of death in the splenectomized group.

It seems likely, however, that all these reports are biased towards the severe end of the spectrum of this disease. As mentioned earlier, it is becoming clear that some patients go through childhood and adolescence relatively symptom free and that some survive relatively fit and well into adult life. In the authors' recent studies in Sri Lanka a number of patients with HbE β thalassaemia were ascertained by carrying out family studies of patients who were attending the clinic in Kurunegala. These individuals had never been incapacitated by their disease. Similarly, in the Asian immigrant populations in the United Kingdom, Canada and America increasing numbers of adults with the disease are being encountered who have run a similar course (Fouladi *et al.* 1998; Rees *et al.* 1998c). Thus, although the disease may kill in infancy or adolescence, there is no doubt that it is compatible with survival into adult life.

Clearly our current picture of the overall severity and natural history is limited and clouded by the socio-economic backgrounds of many of the patients. More information is needed about this important problem.

Haematological findings

There is a variable and sometimes severe degree of anaemia from early life. In the series reported by Chernoff *et al.* (1956) the haemoglobin level ranged from 2.3 to 7 g/dl. In 408 patients reviewed by Wasi *et al.* (1969) the mean haemoglobin level was 6.4 g/dl, in the 166 cases described by Piankijagum *et al.* (1978) it ranged from 1.8 to 11.7 g/dl (mean 6.3±1.9 g/dl), and in the 802 cases reviewed by Fucharoen *et al.* (1988b) it ranged from 2.5 to 13.5 g/dl. It is not clear from these reports whether the haemoglobin levels were taken in a steady state, or what the relationship to transfusion was. As shown in Table 9.10, even in those who are untransfused there is a wide scatter of haemoglobin values; as a group they are mainly in the 5–7 g/dl range.

The red-cell indices are similar to those in homozygous β thalassaemia. This is also true of the red-cell morphology, which shows marked aniso- and poikilocytosis, moderate hypochromia and microcytosis, some target cells and polychromasia (Fig. 9.16). Basophilic stippling is very variable, being marked in some patients and almost absent in others. Chernoff *et al.* (1956) noted moderate numbers of spherocytes on the blood film in some cases. The reticulocyte count is moderately elevated, in the 4–6% range, though sometimes higher. Nucleated red cells are almost invariably present in the peripheral blood and may reach extremely high levels after splenectomy. Target-cell counts are variable and in the series of Chernoff *et al.* (1956) ranged from 5 to 25% of the red cells on the stained blood film; the largest numbers were seen in patients with co-existent liver disease or who had undergone splenectomy. The white-cell count is usually normal or elevated. Chernoff and colleagues noticed that about half their patients had somewhat reduced platelet counts. Following splenectomy many of the nucleated red cells show inclusion bodies similar to those observed in homozygous β thalassaemia. This phenomenon was observed by Chernoff and Na-Nakorn in their early studies in Thailand but its significance was not appreciated until the report of Fessas (1963) which suggested that these inclusions are precipitated α chains.

Table 9.10 Haemoglobin levels in untransfused patients with haemoglobin E β thalassaemia in a steady state.

Population	No.	Age range	Haemoglobin (g/dl)	β-Thalassaemia mutation	Reference
Malaysian	6	2–3	5.6–7.1	IVS1-5 G→C	George & Wong (1993)
Malaysian	6	19–32	7.3–9.4	IVS1-5 G→C	George & Wong (1993)
Uttar Pradesh	15	4–38	7.3–10.8	IVS1-5 G→C CD30 G→C CD15 G→A CD 41/42 (–TCTT)	Agarwal *et al.* (1997)
Bangladeshi	25	1–60	4.6–10.5	IVS1-5 G→C	Rees *et al.* (1998c)
Sri Lankan	102	1–56	3.2–8.5	IVS1-5 G→C IVS1-1 G→A Others	Unpublished data

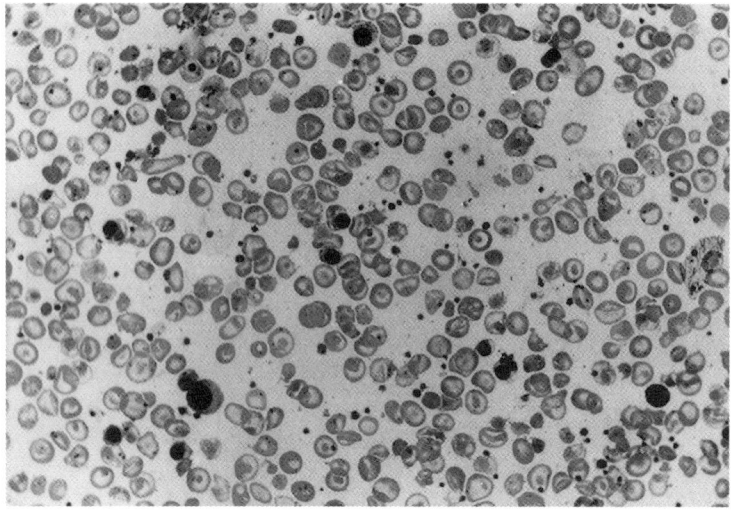

Fig. 9.16 The peripheral blood film in HbE β thalassaemia (Leishman stain × 400). There are many nucleated red cells and target cells.

The bone marrow shows intense erythroid hyperplasia and many intracellular inclusions in the normoblasts. The inclusions consist solely of precipitated α chains (Wickramasinghe & Lee 1997).

The red-cell survival time is considerably shortened (Swarup *et al.* 1961; Feldman & Rieder 1973). Red-cell osmotic fragility curves show a skewed pattern representing mixed cell populations, some of which show increased osmotic fragility, some of which fall within the normal range, and some of which have decreased osmotic fragility (Chernoff *et al.* 1956). A similar pattern was noted by De Silva *et al.* (1959). The rate of autohaemolysis is increased (Swarup *et al.* 1960b).

Chatterjea (1959) gives extensive data on serum bilirubin and plasma haemoglobin levels. As might be expected there is considerable variability but the serum bilirubin is almost invariably elevated and there is usually a slight elevation of the plasma haemoglobin level, indicating some degree of intravascular haemolysis. Evidence for splenic sequestration of red cells has been reported by Ruymann *et al.* (1978).

Metabolic abnormalities of the red cells

Metabolic abnormalities of the red cells were first described by Chatterjea's group in Calcutta (Swarup *et al.* 1960a,b; 1966a,b). They used the glutathione stability test, developed by Beutler and colleagues for the demonstration of sensitivity to oxidant stress in red cells which are glucose-6-phosphate dehydrogenase (G6PD) deficient, to examine the cells of patients with HbE β thalassaemia. They found that despite normal or increased G6PD levels the cells of these patients showed significantly reduced glutathione stability. In their later papers this group described a reduced level of red-cell NADP, and

reduced levels and stability of ATP (Swarup *et al.* 1966a,b).

Haemoglobin analysis

Most cases of HbE β thalassaemia in south-east Asia and India are due to the interaction of β^0 or severe types of β^+ thalassaemia with HbE. Hence the haemoglobin consists of E, F and A_2, and HbA is absent or present in low amounts (Fig. 9.17). The level of HbF in

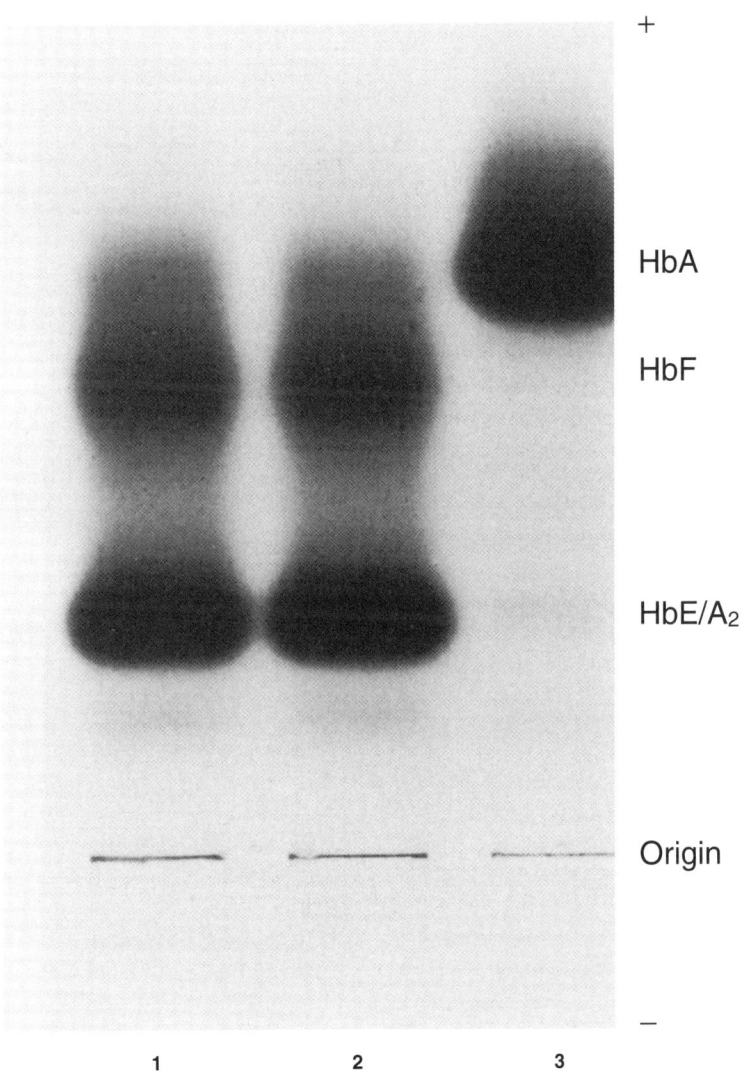

Fig. 9.17 The haemoglobin pattern in HbE β thalassaemia. Starch gel electrophoresis, pH 8.5, amido black stain, of red-cell lysates from the following (left to right): 1 and 2, HbE β^0 thalassaemia; 3, normal adult.

the peripheral blood shows wide variation; from 5 to 85% in the series of Chernoff *et al.* (1956), 10–87% (Vella 1958b), 7–58% (Chatterjea 1959) and 2–49% (Lie-Injo 1959b). In 132 patients studied by Wasi *et al.* (1969) the mean level of HbF was 48% with a standard deviation of 10.5%. It is heterogeneously distributed among the red cells (Rakshit *et al.* 1973).

Although it is usual to find high levels of fetal haemoglobin in this condition, it is becoming clear that there are well documented instances when the HbF level is less than 5% of the total (Krishnamurti *et al.* 1998). We have also seen examples of this type of patient in Sri Lanka. We shall discuss the diagnostic importance of this unusual variety of the disorder in a later section.

Some of the reported haemoglobin patterns associated with interactions of the different molecular forms of β^+ thalassaemia with HbE are shown in Table 9.9.

Haemoglobin synthesis

Studies of haemoglobin synthesis in the peripheral blood of patients with HbE β thalassaemia have been carried out in individuals of Thai, Burmese, Laotian and Bangladeshi backgrounds (Weatherall *et al.* 1969b; Feldman & Rieder 1973; Testa *et al.* 1980; Rees *et al.* 1998c) (Fig. 9.18). In most cases examined, no β^A-chain production could be demonstrated. In the

authors' cases there was a large excess of α chains produced as compared with the combined amounts of γ and β^E chains. The degree of globin imbalance was comparable with that found in homozygous β thalassaemia. Free α chains can be demonstrated, both by DEAE-cellulose chromatography and by Sephadex gel filtration (Weatherall *et al.* 1969b). Curiously, there was much less globin imbalance in the patient studied by Feldman and Rieder (1973); we can offer no explanation for this discrepancy. Haemoglobin synthesis studies in a patient who has HbE β^+ thalassaemia are shown in Fig. 9.18. In the study of Testa *et al.* (1980), in which synthesis was examined at different stages of erythroid maturation, the findings suggested that most of the HbF in the blood reflects selective survival of HbF-containing precursors.

Genetic findings and diagnosis in the newborn period

The usual finding in the families of individuals with HbE β thalassaemia is the HbE trait in one parent and β-thalassaemia trait in the other. Occasionally, one parent may have HbE β thalassaemia and the other HbE trait. The latter form of inheritance can cause counselling or diagnostic difficulty, particularly if the parent with HbE β thalassaemia has an extremely low level of HbF, in which case the condi-

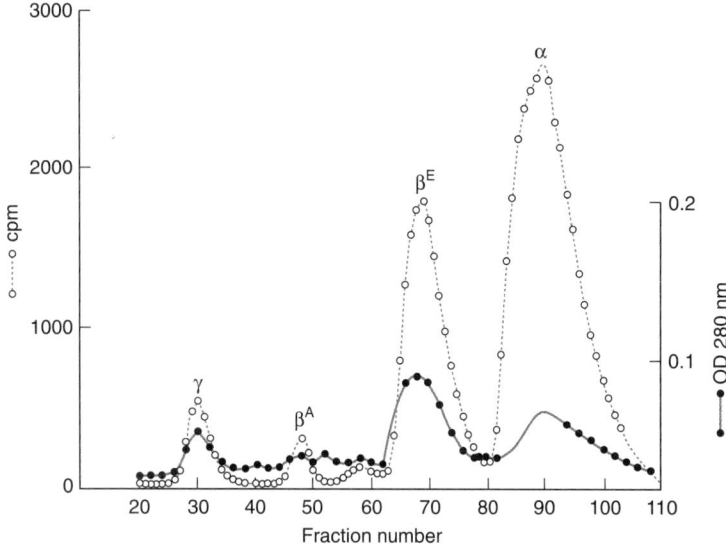

Fig. 9.18 Haemoglobin synthesis in HbE β thalassaemia. The method is described in Chapter 5. The open dotted line represents the radioactivity tracing, which indicates that there is marked globin imbalance. In this particular patient there was a small amount of β^A-chain synthesis.

tion may be misdiagnosed as the homozygous state for HbE (Krishnamurti *et al.* 1998). The diagnostic problems and best approaches to managing newborn children of individuals of these unusual matings are reviewed in detail by Weatherall (1998b).

Geographical distribution and prevalence

Haemoglobin E β thalassaemia is spread widely throughout south-east Asia and the Indian subcontinent. There are few figures available for its prevalence. From approximate frequencies for the genes for HbE and β thalassaemia Wasi *et al.* (1969) estimated that there were somewhere in the region of 49 000 patients, or potential patients, with HbE β thalassaemia in Thailand. It has been estimated recently that approximately 3000 new cases are being added to the population of Thailand each year (Dr Suthat Fucharoen, personal communication). These figures give some estimate of the public health problem which this disease will cause in south-east Asia, particularly as socio-economic conditions improve and these children survive the infections which almost certainly killed many of them in early life in the past.

The disease is widespread in other parts of south-east Asia including Vietnam (Khanh *et al.* 1990), Malaysia (Vella 1958b; Bolton & Eng 1969; George & Wong 1993), Indonesia (Punt & Van Gool 1957; Lie-Injo 1959b; Oman & Wiradisuria 1969) and Burma (Lehmann *et al.* 1956; Aung-Than-Batu & Hla-Pe 1971). It is also extremely common in parts of the Indian subcontinent. Thus in 1966 Chatterjea was able to describe 526 cases investigated in Calcutta among Indian Hindus, with the following distribution: Bengalese 508, Oriahs 10, Biharis 4, Assamese 2, Punjabi 1, south Indian 1. In addition there were 48 cases among Bengalese Muslims. Later accounts of the distribution of HbE β thalassaemia in the Indian subcontinent were given in reviews by Saha and Banerjee (1973), and Agarwal *et al.* (1997). It is common in Sri Lanka (Ellepola *et al.* 1980), where it constitutes between 10 and 40% of the severe forms of β thalassaemia (De Silva *et al.* 2000).

A case of HbE β thalassaemia has been reported in Eti-Turks (Okcuoglu *et al.* 1965) and further cases were reported in a Turkish immigrant family in Greece (Aksoy *et al.* 1963) and in a Greek family (Gouttas *et al.* 1960).

Unresolved problems

As we recently pointed out (Weatherall & Clegg 1996) HbE β thalassaemia will constitute an extremely important public health problem in the new millennium. As recently exemplified from studies in Sri Lanka, in populations where there is a relatively high frequency of β thalassaemia the presence of the HbE gene, even at a low frequency, may greatly magnify the number of patients in the population with serious forms of thalassaemia (De Silva *et al.* 2000).

The major gaps in our knowledge of the natural history and pathophysiology of this disease, as outlined in this section, are making it very difficult to evolve effective approaches to management, a subject to which we shall return in Chapter 15. One of the most important unresolved problems is our lack of understanding of the reasons for its remarkable clinical heterogeneity. As discussed earlier, there is some evidence that its course may be affected by the co-inheritance of α thalassaemia, increased numbers of α-globin genes, an increased propensity for synthesizing HbF, and a variety of other factors, some of which may be environmental. However, none of these factors fully explain the variable clinical course. And there are still major gaps in our understanding of why this disease may be so severe in the first place, information which is badly needed if we are to be able to manage the increasing numbers of patients with this disorder, particularly in south-east Asia.

Haemoglobin E and δβ thalassaemia

There have been very few opportunities to study the interactions of HbE with different forms of δβ thalassaemia of either the deletional or non-deletional types.

Haemoglobin E with haemoglobin Lepore

One family was observed in Thailand in which there was a woman who was a compound heterozygote for HbE and Lepore (Boontrakoonpoontawee *et al.* 1988). This 36-year-old female presented with symptoms of anaemia and was found to have mild hepatosplenomegaly. Her blood picture showed a haemoglobin value of 11.4 g/dl with typical thalassaemic red-cell changes; the haemoglobin consisted of Hbs F, Lepore and E. The different haemoglobins were fractionated by DEAE-cellulose chromatography and the following values were obtained: HbE 53%, Hb Lepore 12.7% and HbF 34%. Partial structural studies indicated that this was a form of Hb Lepore although it was not characterized further. The mildness of this interaction, which is surprising, may have depended, at least in part, on a relatively high level of HbF.

Haemoglobin E and deletional forms of δβ thalassaemia

Haemoglobin E δβ thalassaemia was described by Wasi *et al.* (1969). In this Thai family there were four affected individuals. Two siblings showed a mild thalassaemia-like disorder, with haemoglobin values of 12.7 and 9.7 g/dl, respectively. They had only Hbs E and F on electrophoresis. Both had children, one through an individual with HbE trait and the other through a normal individual. In the former mating there were two children with HbE δβ thalassaemia, two HbE homozygotes and one with HbE trait. In the latter mating one child had HbE trait and two had typical δβ-thalassaemia trait, with 8 and 13% HbF, respectively. The variety of δβ thalassaemia that was segregating in this family is not known.

The interaction of $(^A\gamma\delta\beta)^0$ thalassaemia of the Malay 1 variety (see Chapter 8) and HbE was reported by Trent *et al.* (1984b). The proband in this family, the compound heterozygote, had a haemoglobin value of 11.4 g/dl and thalassaemic red-cell changes. Haemoglobin analysis showed only Hbs F and E, with an HbF value of 46%. Similar findings were reported in a Chinese compound heterozygote for $(^A\gamma\delta\beta)^0$ thalassaemia and HbE (Fucharoen & Winichagoon 1987). In this case the deletion appears to have been the Chinese variety (see Chapter 8).

Clearly, the clinical phenotype of the interactions of $(^A\gamma\delta\beta)^0$ thalassaemia with HbE is characterized by a much milder disease than HbE β thalassaemia. The haemoglobin composition in the two conditions may be very similar, however. It seems likely that the phenotypic difference reflects the greater absolute amount of γ-chain production associated with δβ thalassaemia; in HbE β thalassaemia there is much more chain imbalance and the high levels of HbF probably reflect cell selection rather than a high basal rate of production.

Haemoglobin D Los Angeles β thalassaemia

Haemoglobin D Los Angeles (D Punjab) ($\beta^{121\ Glu\to Gln}$) has an incidence of 2–3% in the Sikhs of the Punjab and has been found throughout the world, usually but not always in individuals with Indian backgrounds. Its distribution was reviewed in detail by Vella and Lehmann (1974). It has been found together with β thalassaemia on many occasions.

After the early reports of Hynes and Lehmann (1956) and Sukumaran *et al.* (1960) the interaction was well documented in other populations (Preto *et al.* 1961; Cortesi *et al.* 1966; Quattrin *et al.* 1966a; Thompson *et al.* 1966; Marengo-Rowe *et al.* 1968; Schneider *et al.* 1968; Jain *et al.* 1970; Oldrini *et al.* 1972; Rohne *et al.* 1973; Tsistrakis *et al.* 1975; Rieder *et al.* 1976; Ballas *et al.* 1977; Castro *et al.* 1979). In some of these cases the 'HbD' was analysed chemically and found to be identical to HbD Los Angeles (Marengo-Rowe *et al.* 1968; Schneider *et al.* 1968; Rohne *et al.* 1973; Rieder *et al.* 1976; Ballas *et al.* 1977). In well documented cases the findings have been fairly consistent (Table 9.11). There is mild anaemia, occasional splenomegaly, haemoglobin values ranging between 8 and 12 g/dl, and typical thalassaemic indices and morphological changes of the red cells. Haemoglobin F values are only slightly elevated, in the 1–7% range. In most cases the interaction was with β^0 thalassaemia. In the patient described by Schneider *et al.* (1968) there was 7% HbA, suggesting that the interaction involved a severe form of β^+ thalassaemia. In two cases in which globin synthesis was carried out there was a moderate degree of imbalance, with α-/non-α-globin-chain ratios similar to that of β-thalassaemia heterozygotes (Rieder *et al.* 1976; Ballas *et al.* 1977).

From these reports it is clear that the degree of disability caused by HbD Los Angeles β^0 or β^+ thalassaemia is little greater than in HbD homozygotes or in heterozygous β thalassaemics.

β Thalassaemia in association with rare structural β-chain variants

The chance interaction in one person of one or other form of β thalassaemia with a rare structural β-chain haemoglobin variant might, at first sight, be considered to be an interesting collector's item of no clinical

Table 9.11 Findings in some reported cases of haemoglobin D Los Angeles ($^{121\ Glu\rightarrow Gln}$) β thalassaemia. In the cases of Rieder *et al.* (1976) and Ballas *et al.* (1977) α-/non-α-globin chain synthesis ratios were about 2.

Population	Hb (g/dl)	MCH (pg)	MCV (fl)	Retics (%)	HbF (%)	HbA₂ (%)	HbA (%)	HbD (%)	Clinical findings	Reference
Indian	9.1	20	60	4.1	5	5.3	7.0	82.7	Splenomegaly, anaemia	Schneider *et al.* (1968)
Indian	12	23	70	2	1.2	3.0	0	95.0	Nil	Marengo-Rowe *et al.* (1968)
Greek/Italian	—	24.3	78	4.2	'Normal'	6.4	0	93.6	Splenomegaly	Rieder *et al.* (1976)
Indian	8.3	16.9	52	4.9	7	5.0	0	82.0	Splenomegaly	Ballas *et al.* (1977)

MCH, mean cell haemoglobin; MCV, mean cell volume; Retics, reticulocytes.

or biological significance. There are many reports of this kind but, unfortunately, quite often insufficient clinical or haematological data are given to provide a clear picture of the interaction (or lack of) between the genes. However, there are a few such interactions that will repay a brief examination, in part because of their severity, but also because of the information that they yield about the pathophysiology of β thalassaemia in general. Some of them are summarized in Table 9.12.

Mild interactions

It is evident that the compound heterozygous states for some β-chain variants with β thalassaemia are associated with no more disability than the heterozygous carrier states for β thalassaemia alone (Table 9.12).

Haemoglobin O Arab β thalassaemia

The distribution of this variant, $β^{121\ Glu\rightarrow Lys}$, is discussed by Efremov *et al.* (1977) and Huisman *et al.* (1998). It has been found in Afro-Americans, Romanies, Arabs, Egyptians and Pomaks, a population group in the Balkans. It seems to occur at a high frequency in the Burgas district of Bulgaria; Kantchev *et al.* (1975) described the findings in 12 families from this region in whom there were 44 HbO Arab heterozygotes and 16 compound heterozygotes for HbO Arab and $β^0$ thalassaemia. The latter appeared to have a moderately severe disorder with a phenotype not dissimilar to the milder forms of HbE thalassaemia. Their haemoglobin values ranged from 6 to 8 g/dl, with reticulocyte values ranging from 3.5 to 8.2%. The blood films showed marked thalassaemic

changes and in every case normoblasts were present. All the patients had splenomegaly, ranging from 2 to 5 cm below the costal margin. However, there were no bone changes typical of β thalassaemia on radiological examination. These patients seemed to be largely asymptomatic except that they had exacerbations of haemolysis associated with pains in the joints and over the liver and spleen, which were usually provoked by infection. The haemoglobin consisted of HbO with no HbA; HbF and A₂ values were not given. In the report by Huisman *et al.* (1997) in which the interaction was with a mild form of $β^+$ thalassaemia due to a promoter mutation, the haematology was close to normal; no clinical details are given.

The homozygous state for HbO Arab is characterized by a mild to moderate microcytic anaemia. The patient described by Kantchev *et al.* (1975), a 15-year-old girl, had splenomegaly, mild jaundice and a haemoglobin level of 7.0 g/dl. A second homozygote was reported by Efremov *et al.* (1977). In this case the proband was an 18-year-old girl of Romany origin from Yugoslavia. She had mild anaemia and splenomegaly although the picture seemed to be clouded by the presence of liver disease. The peripheral blood picture showed a haemoglobin value of 11.2 g/dl and a film with anisocytosis, poikilocytosis, polychromasia and many target cells.

It is still not absolutely clear why interaction between $β^0$ thalassaemia and HbO Arab can be so severe. Homozygotes for this variant are clearly more severely affected than those for HbE, although heterozygotes seem to show the mild haematological changes similar to HbE heterozygotes. Haemoglobin O Arab is not unstable and its underlying mutation is not likely to cause reduced β-globin synthesis. Thus this question remains open.

Table 9.12 Interactions between β thalassaemia and some rare haemoglobin variants.

Variant	Functional properties	Hb (g/dl)	MCV (fl)	MCH (pg)	Retics (%)	β-thalassaemia allele	HbF (%)	HbA$_2$ (%)	Variant (%)	Clinical features	Reference
Abruzzo β143 His→Arg	OA↑	17–18	80–82	—	—	β⁰	1.5	5–6	93–97	Splenomegaly	Chiarioni et al. (1974)
Arta β45 Phe→Lys	OA↓ U	8.7	68	22	3.3	β39 (C→T)	3.2	4	90+	Well Mild splenomegaly	Vassilopoulos et al. (1995)
Beograd β121 Glu→Val	N	9.6 7.3 10.8	— 66 —	— 18 —	9.0 8.4	β⁰ β⁰	6.5 14.7 3.0	7.4 6.5 5.2	87.1 79 86.0	Anaemia Splenomegaly Thal. intermedia Thal. intermedia	Rudivic et al. (1975) Aksoy et al. (1984)
City of Hope β69 Gly→Ser	N	7.0	62	21	—	β⁰	4.0	7.0	90+	No other details	Kutlar et al. (1989a)
Crete β129 Ala→Pro	OA↑ MU	14.5	69	—	3.0	β⁰	10.3	5.1	84.6	No clinical details	Maniatis et al. (1979)
D Iran β22 Glu→Gln	N	10.5	60	—	—	β⁰	1.3	4.2	94.5	Normal	Rohne et al. (1973) De Marco et al. (1994)
Dhonburi β126 Val→Gly	U	9.2	55	17	—	IVS1-5 (G→C) + Hb Baden	—	6.0	98	Not given	Divoky et al. (1994)
Duarte β62 Ala→Pro	OA↑ MU	15.1	68	26	10.4	?	2.6	5.8	?	Splenomegaly	Beutler et al. (1974)
E Saskatoon β22 Glu→Lys	N	13.5	61	—	0.6	IVS1-6 (T→C)	1.6	5.8	71	No clinical details	Gurgey et al. (1990)
G Ferrara β57 Asn→Lys	MU	—	—	—	—	β⁰	2	6	92	Morphological changes in red cells	Tentori et al. (1975)
G San Jose β7 Glu→Gly	U	11.0	66	19	—	β⁰	0.1	6.1	92.3	No clinical findings	Brancati et al. (1978) Musumeci et al. (1979b)
G Siriraj β7 Glu→Lys	?	11.9	66	24	3.0	β⁰	4.0	4.0	92	Splenomegaly	Tuchinda et al. (1964)
G Szuhu β80 Asn→Lys	N	11.7	61	17	2.1	β⁰	4.1	6.9	92	β thal. trait	Romero et al. (1985)
Hofu β126 Val→Glu	MU	94	65	19.7	—	CD 8/9 (+G)	1.8	6.2	92	Transfusion in pregnancy. Spleen not mentioned	Pande et al. (1995); Arends et al. (1985)
J Baltimore β16 Gly→Asp	N	10.1–10.8 10.6–13.1	66–73 61–3	19–21 19	— 0.1	β⁰ β⁰	— 1.0	9–11 4–4.5	89 81–87	No clinical findings Normal	Wilkinson et al. (1967) Arribalzaga et al. (1996)
J Calabria β64 Gly→Asp	OA↑ MU	—	—	—	—	β⁺	—	Increased	86	Haemolytic anaemia	Tentori et al. (1975)

Variant									Clinical findings	Reference
La Desirade β129 Ala→Val	OA↑ MU	12.7	64	20	0.9	β0	2.2	91.9	No clinical findings	Merault et al. (1986)
Leiden β6 or 7 Glu→O	U	9.2	74	21	11.2	β0	7.1	86.5	Splenomegaly	Lie-Injo et al. (1977)
Lulu Isalnd β107 Gly→Asp	U	8.5	78	20	—	CD15 (G→A)	2.7	~90	Splenomegaly Splenectomy	Gray et al. (1995)
Mississippi β44 Ser→Lys	MU	7	68	—	2–6	β+	18		Splenomegaly Thal. intermedia	Steinberg et al. (1987)
Monroe β30 Arg→Thr	U	8.6	80	25.6	—	-29 (A→G)	16.5	—	Thal. major Regular transfusion	Gonzalez-Redondo et al. (1989c)
N Baltimore β95 Lys→Glu	N	12	90	27	—	-29 (A→G)	4.7	~65	No clinical findings	Huisman et al. (1997)
New York β113 Val→Glu	OA↑ MU	—	—	—	—	β0	2–3	92	No clinical findings	Zeng & Huang (1982)
O Arab β121 Glu→Lys	N	6–13	—	—	3–8	-29 (G→C)	—	80–90	Splenomegaly Variable anaemia	Kantchev et al. (1975); Haji et al. (1985)
P Galveston β117 His→Arg	N	12 / 10.4 / 9.2	71 / 72 / 66	27 / 23 / 20	— / 1.3 / 1.1	— / β0 / β0 / β0	6.6 / 4.7 / 5.7	~60 / 94 / 93	No clinical findings	Huisman et al. (1997); di Iorio et al. (1975)
Pôrto Alegre β9 Ser→Lys	N	10–13	63–68	18–19	—	β0	5–6	90+	No clinical findings	Malcorra-Azpiazu et al. (1993)
Riyadh β120 Lys→Asn	N	11.0	68	22	—	β0	<1.0	95.4	Thal. trait	Pinkerton et al. (1979)
Roseau-Pointe à Pitre β90 Glu→Gly	OA↑ MU	10.8	69	23	3.3	β+	17	62	Age 6 months Normal	Merault et al. (1985)
Saki β14 Leu→Pro	U	11.1	69	22	9.2	—	0.4	—	Splenomegaly	Milner et al. (1976)
Siirt β27 Ala→Gly	U	8.2	60	—	—	CD5 (−CT)	5.5	~90	Splenomegaly Thal. intermedia	Bianco et al. (1997b)
Tak β+11 residues	OA↑ MU	6.3	79	26	2.3	β0	—	6.3	Anaemia Splenomegaly	Lehmann & Lang (1975)
Shelby β131 Gln→Lys	MU	7.7 / 10–11	72 / 80	20 / 18–19	— / 5–12	β0 / CD15 (G→A)	9.5 / 4–7	77.2 / 85–88	No clinical details Splenomegaly	Carcassi et al. (1980); Çürük et al. (1992a) Originally described as Hb Leslie by Lutcher et al. (1976)
Valetta β87Thr→Pro	N	—	68	—	—	IVS1-6 (T→C)	—	29–34	Not described	Scerri et al. (1993)
Vancouver β73 Asp→Tyr	OA↓	9–12	—	61	19	β0	5.4	89.5	Splenomegaly	Gray & Marion (1978)

N = normal; U = unstable; MU = mildly unstable; OA = oxygen affinity.

Interactions of β thalassaemia with unstable haemoglobin variants

There have been many opportunities to study the interaction of unstable haemoglobin variants with different forms of β thalassaemia (Table 9.12). Overall, the resulting clinical disorders show, not unexpectedly, a wide range of phenotypes. One of the first to be described, that of Hb Duarte ($\beta^{6 \text{ Ala} \rightarrow \text{Pro}}$) (Beutler *et al.* 1974), was of particular interest in that the phenotype is so mild, despite the fact that this variant shows typical changes of instability. It is interesting that it also has a high oxygen affinity and whether this is partly responsible for the higher haemoglobin level is not clear. The affected individual also had a splenomegaly and episodic jaundice with the passage of dark urine. The interaction of β^+ thalassaemia with Hb Saki ($\beta^{14 \text{ Leu} \rightarrow \text{Pro}}$), described by Milner *et al.* (1976), is also instructive. Although this patient's haemoglobin was relatively high he had persistent splenomegaly with a reticulocyte count of 9% and suffered from bouts of severe anaemia associated with intercurrent infection. This seems to be a particularly common complication in interactions of this type.

At the severe end of the spectrum these conditions can mimic symptomatic forms of β thalassaemia although it is clear that the haemolytic component is more marked. This is well documented in the case of Hb Leiden (β^6 or $\beta^{7 \text{ Glu} \rightarrow \text{O}}$) (Lie-Injo *et al.* 1977). The compound heterozygote had severe anaemia and hepatosplenomegaly and was observed at the age of 8 years to have a haemoglobin value of 3.7 g/dl with a reticulocyte count of 51%. Following splenectomy he improved considerably, transfusion requirements diminished, and when seen at the age of 15 years the haemoglobin level was 9.2 g/dl, with 11.2% reticulocytes. The interaction of β thalassaemia with Hb Mississippi ($\beta^{44 \text{ Ser} \rightarrow \text{Lys}}$) also seems to produce a severe phenotype, despite the fact that this variant is only mildly unstable on *in vitro* testing (Steinberg *et al.* 1987). On the other hand the different interactions of Hb Shelby ($\beta^{131 \text{ Gln} \rightarrow \text{Lys}}$) seem to show quite a wide variation, even when the β-thalassaemia alleles are severe (Adachi *et al.* 1993). The interaction of Hb Lulu Island ($\beta^{107 \text{ Gly} \rightarrow \text{Asp}}$) also seems to have been severe enough to require splenectomy (Gray *et al.* 1995).

In short, these interactions are remarkably variable and it is not apparent why some are more severe than others. It may reflect the fact that some unstable variants are more prone to oxidant damage in the environment of severe globin imbalance, and the relative oxygen affinity of the variant may also play a role in setting the final haemoglobin level. But because most of these abnormal haemoglobins are extremely rare there is insufficient experience to be able to predict the likely clinical consequences of interactions of this type.

Interactions of β thalassaemia with haemoglobin variants with an abnormal oxygen affinity

A few interactions between β thalassaemia and haemoglobin variants with abnormal oxygen-carrying properties have been reported (Table 9.12). The combination of β^0 thalassaemia and Hb Crete ($\beta^{129 \text{ Ala} \rightarrow \text{Pro}}$) was reported by Maniatis *et al.* (1979). Although the compound heterozygote had 85% Hb Crete, and the latter has a high oxygen affinity, his haemoglobin level was 14.5 g/dl which is only just outside the upper end of the range for a heterozygous β^0-thalassaemic male. A relative with $\delta\beta^0$ thalassaemia/Hb Crete was polycythaemic. The combination of β thalassaemia with the low-oxygen-affinity variant, Hb Hope ($\beta^{136 \text{ Gly} \rightarrow \text{Asp}}$), is associated with a normal haemoglobin level (Charache *et al.* 1979).

β Thalassaemia in association with β-chain variants in *cis*

Earlier in this chapter we described the findings in individuals who had a sickle-cell gene which also carried a β-thalassaemia mutation. Adams *et al.* (1981) in describing Hb Vicksburg ($\beta^{79 \text{ Leu} \rightarrow \text{O}}$) suggested that one of the reasons for the extremely low level of this variant in heterozygotes, approximately 7.6%, might be that a β^+-thalassaemia mutation is present in *cis* to the structural variant. As far as we know this has not been confirmed. In a particularly interesting family study reported by Divoky *et al.* (1992) a carrier of the common IVS1-5 G→C β-thalassaemia mutation was also found to have a GTG→ATG mutation at codon 18 of the β-globin gene, resulting in the replacement of a valine residue by a methionine residue. This variant, which was called Hb Baden, was present at only 2–3% in this individual and in a child who was heterozygous for both the doubly affected chromosome and Hb Dhonburi ($\beta^{126 \text{ Val} \rightarrow \text{Gly}}$). Presumably the very low level of Hb Baden reflects the extreme severity of the IVS1-5 mutation, which is associated with a very low output of HbA.

β Thalassaemia in association with α-chain haemoglobin variants

It was originally thought that there would be no 'interaction' between the β thalassaemias and α-chain haemoglobin variants, i.e. in the presence of a β-thalassaemia gene the relative levels of HbA and an α-chain variant would remain the same as in the heterozygous state for the α-chain variant alone. Indeed, early studies suggested that this was the case (Fessas *et al.* 1965; Lee & Huisman 1965; Atwater *et al.* 1970). However, it became apparent later that this is not always so and that when a carrier for an α-chain variant also has a β-thalassaemia gene the level of the α-chain variant is usually lower in the doubly affected individual than in the simple heterozygote. This phenomenon will repay a brief examination because it provides useful information about the post-transcriptional regulation of haemoglobin synthesis.

α-Chain variants in association with homozygous β thalassaemia

Probably the first description of a combination of an α-chain haemoglobin variant with the homozygous state for β thalassaemia came from Silvestroni, Bianco and their colleagues in 1960 with the description of HbL Ferrara in combination with homozygous β thalassaemia. The patient is described in their original paper (Silvestroni *et al.* 1960) and further information about this interaction is summarized in a monograph by the same workers, *Le Emoglobine Umane*, published in 1963 (Silvestroni & Bianco 1963). These studies suggest that individuals with HbL Ferrara who also have β thalassaemia have a reduced amount of HbL Ferrara as compared with heterozygous carriers for this haemoglobin variant.

Alberti *et al.* (1975) later described the interaction between an α-chain variant Hb Hasharon ($\alpha^{74\,Asp\rightarrow His}$) (which turned out to be the same as HbL Ferrara) and β thalassaemia. They also pointed out that in homozygous β thalassaemics who are carriers of Hb Hasharon the amount of the α-chain variant is markedly reduced. Similarly, in Hb Hasharon carriers who are also heterozygous for β thalassaemia there is a significant reduction in the amount of the variant.

This phenomenon was studied in detail by Conconi *et al.* (1978) and del Senno *et al.* (1979). They found that, as expected, there is marked imbalance of globin synthesis in homozygous β thalassaemics who are also heterozygous for Hb Hasharon. Furthermore, although the synthesis of the normal and abnormal α chains occurs at much the same rate, there is a much more rapid removal of the excess of mutant α chains from the red cells than is the case for the excess of normal α chains. They argued that the differential affinity of normal and variant α chains for non-α chains and the preferential removal of the variant α chains explains the reduced level of Hb Hasharon found in subjects who also carry the gene for β thalassaemia. The difference in the relative amounts of Hb Hasharon in the cells of simple heterozygotes, heterozygotes for both the α-chain variant and β thalassaemia, and in homozygous β thalassaemics who also carry Hb Hasharon is illustrated in Fig. 9.19.

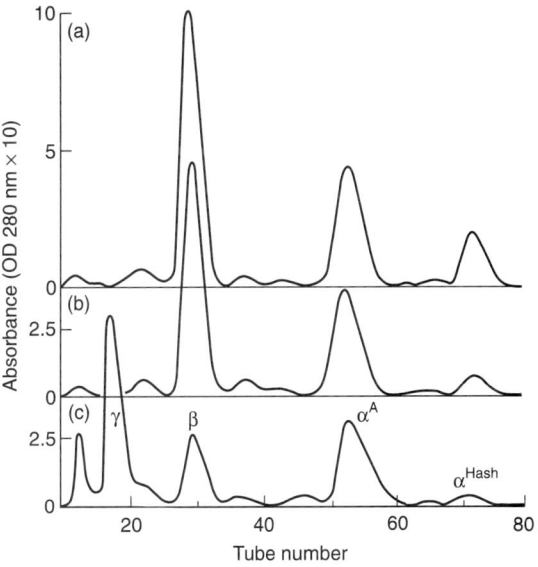

Fig. 9.19 The effects of β thalassaemia on the relative production of haemoglobins A and Hasharon. The figure shows the elution profiles obtained by separating the globins by CM-cellulose chromatography (see Chapter 5) from globin prepared from the following: (a) Hb Hasheron heterozygote; (b) an individual heterozygous for Hb Hasheron and β thalassaemia; (c) an individual homozygous for β thalassaemia and heterozygous for Hb Hasheron. Note that there is a marked reduction in the α Hasheron chain in the presence of β thalassaemia. Adapted from Conconi *et al.* (1978).

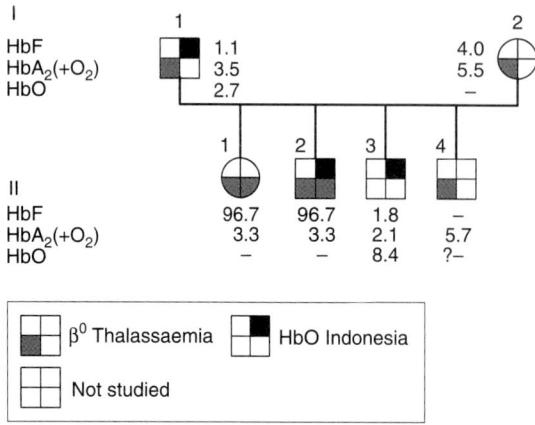

Fig. 9.20 Family pedigree showing the inheritance of HbO Indonesia and β thalassaemia. The propositus (II.2) and his sister are both homozygous for β thalassaemia; electrophoretic analysis failed to demonstrate HbO Indonesia in either of them. A brother (II.3) is an HbO Indonesia carrier with 8.4% of the variant. The father is heterozygous for β thalassaemia and HbO and has 2.7% of the latter in his peripheral blood. The data shown in Fig. 9.21 provide clear evidence that II.2 is synthesizing the α chains of HbO Indonesia but they are not forming a viable haemoglobin in the presence of severe β thalassaemia.

Several years ago we had the opportunity of studying a family in which the genes for β thalassaemia and HbO Indonesia ($\alpha_2^{116\ Glu \rightarrow Lys}\beta_2$) were segregating (unpublished observations). There were two siblings homozygous for β^0 thalassaemia whose haemoglobin electrophoretic patterns showed Hbs F and A_2 with no other abnormal components. The father, a heterozygote for both β thalassaemia and HbO Indonesia, had approximately 2.7% HbO Indonesia while a brother, who was an HbO Indonesia carrier, had approximately 8.4% HbO Indonesia. However, when globin synthesis studies were carried out on the β-thalassaemia homozygotes it was clear that one of them was synthesizing $\alpha^{o\ Indonesia}$ chains although no HbO Indonesia was present in his red cells. These findings are illustrated in Figs 9.20 and 9.21. It is clear therefore that in the presence of homozygous β^0 thalassaemia, the $\alpha^{O\ Indonesia}$ chains were rapidly destroyed and the expected variant, $\alpha_2^O\gamma_2$, was not produced. The message from this study is clear. It may be impossible to determine whether a homozygous β thalassaemic is carrying an α-chain variant by simple haemoglobin analysis, and it is necessary to carry out complete family studies or to examine globin synthe-

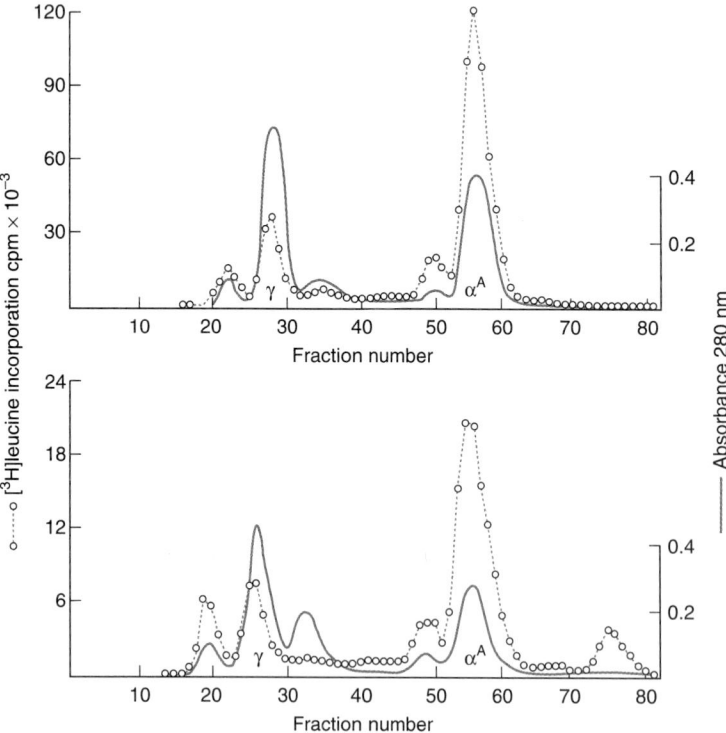

Fig. 9.21 Haemoglobin synthesis in individuals with β thalassaemia and HbO Indonesia. The conditions are as described in Chapter 5. The upper graph shows the radioactive elution profile from the cells of individual II.1 from the pedigree shown in Fig. 9.20. The pattern is typical of homozygous β^0 thalassaemia. The lower graph shows the elution pattern from individual II.2. He is also homozygous for β thalassaemia (the small optical density peak in the β-chain region is from transfused blood) but in addition there is a second radioactive α-chain peak which represents the α chains of HbO Indonesia. Thus this child is homozygous for β^0 thalassaemia and heterozygous for HbO Indonesia but the latter does not form a viable haemoglobin in the presence of a marked deficiency of β chains.

sis using radioactive amino acids. A similar phenomenon was described in a β-thalassaemia homozygote who was also heterozygous for HbG Waimanalo
($\alpha_2^{64\,Asp\rightarrow Asn}\beta_2$) (Baine *et al*. 1979).

The reason for the preferential loss of the variant α
chains is not clear. It seems quite likely that, with a
limited number of non-α chains, normal α chains will
be bound preferentially by β (and γ) chains; if there
is a severe degree of globin imbalance virtually no
variant α chains combine with the limited number of
β or γ chains. Presumably, the excess variant α chains
are precipitated or subjected to proteolytic degradation in the red-cell precursors. The HbO Indonesia
interaction, described above, was associated with a
form of thalassaemia intermedia and this raises the
fascinating possibility that these abnormal α chains
may be subjected to more rapid proteolytic degradation, resulting in relatively less inclusion-body formation and hence in a milder degree of ineffective
erythropoiesis. However, this is highly speculative
and the clinical manifestations of interactions of this
type require further study.

α-Chain variants in association with heterozygous β thalassaemia

Although the earlier studies of Fessas *et al*. (1965),
Lee and Huisman (1965) and Atwater *et al*. (1970) did
not suggest that there was any alteration in the
haemoglobin constitution of carriers for α-chain variants if they also had β thalassaemia, this is not usually
the case. The data summarized in Table 9.13 show that

there is often a reduction in the amount of the α-chain
variant in doubly affected persons. This has been
shown quite convincingly for the interaction of β
thalassaemia with HbQ India ($\alpha_2^{64\ His\rightarrow Asp}\beta_2$)
(Sukumaran *et al*. 1972), Hb Inkster ($\alpha_2^{85\ Asp\rightarrow Val}\beta_2$)
(Reed *et al*. 1974), Hb Hasharon ($\alpha_2^{47\ Asp\rightarrow His}\beta_2$)
(Alberti *et al*. 1975), HbJ Paris ($\alpha_2^{12\ Ala\rightarrow Asp}$ or
$^{54\ Gln\rightarrow Glu}\beta_2$) (Marinucci *et al*. 1977), HbJ Rovigo
($\alpha_2^{53\ Ala\rightarrow Asp}\beta_2$) (Moo-Penn *et al*. 1978b), HbG
Waimanalo ($\alpha_2^{64Asp\rightarrow Asn}\beta_2$) (Tan *et al*. 1978), Hb
Rampa ($\alpha_2^{95\ Pro\rightarrow Ser}\beta_2$) (Huisman *et al*. 1978), HbO
Indonesia ($\alpha_2^{116\ Glu\rightarrow Lys}\beta_2$) (present authors, unpub-
lished observations; Casoni *et al*. 1977; Marinucci
et al. 1978a,b) and HbQ Thailand ($\alpha_2^{74\ Asp\rightarrow His}\beta_2$)
(Lehmann & Lang 1975). Curiously this was not the
case in individuals heterozygous for HbJ Sardegna
($\alpha_2^{50\ His\rightarrow Asp}\beta_2$) or G Philadelphia ($\alpha_2^{68Asn\rightarrow Lys}\beta_2$) and
β thalassaemia (Gallo *et al*. 1972; Huisman *et al*. 1978).

It seems likely that the reduction in the level of the
α-chain variant follows the same mechanism as outlined in the previous section. Huisman *et al*. (1978)
observed that in individuals heterozygous for HbG
Philadelphia and β thalassaemia the level of HbG
Philadelphia was the same as that in simple heterozygotes for the α-chain variant. On the other hand they
found a marked reduction in the amount of the α-
chain variant Hb Rampa in the double heterozygote
as compared with the simple heterozygote. In a series
of *in vitro* mixing and reassociation experiments
Huisman and colleagues showed that β chains have
a similar affinity for α^A and $\alpha^{G\ Philadelphia}$ chains,
whereas they have a much greater affinity for α^A than

Table 9.13 The quantities of 10 different α-chain variants in heterozygotes with and without an additional β thalassaemia allele. From Molchanova and Huisman (1998).

Variant	Mutation	Amino-acid replacement	Helix; contact	Without β thalassaemia		With β thalassaemia	
				n	%	*n*	%
J Paris I	α_2; GCG→GAC	12 Ala→Asp	A10; external	5	25.6	1	28.5
J Oxford	α_1; GGT→GAT	15 Gly→Asp	A13; external	29	23–31	3	24.8
J Sardegna	n.d.	50 His→Asp	CE8; salt bridge	3	16–30	3	21–24
J Meerut	α_2; GCG→GAG	120 Ala→Glu	H3; external	3	19.2	2	20.2
Hasharon	α_2; GAC→CAG	47 Asp→His	CE8; external	7	18.9	1	10.5
Q India	α_1; GAC→CAC	64 Asp→His	E13; external	17	17.0	5	9.2
Q Thailand	α_1; GAC→CAC	74 Asp→His	EF3; external	6	27.4	2	14.7; 16.5
G Philadelphia	$\alpha_2\alpha_1$; AAC→AAG	68 Asn→Lys	E17; external	Many	29–35	2	33.5; 44.5
Inkster	α_2; GAC→GTC	85 Asp→Val	F6; external	12	21–23	2	19.0; 21.0
Rampa	n.d.	95 Pro→Ser	G2; α1β2	1	20.0	3	5–7.

n.d., no data.

α^{Rampa} chains. Thus in the presence of a relative deficiency of β chains it might be expected that the relative amounts of Hbs A and G Philadelphia would remain unaltered while the relative level of Hb Rampa might be markedly decreased. Recently, Huisman has revisited this problem and has confirmed that differential affinity of different α chains for β chains occurs, provided further molecular data on the reasons for these differences, and hypothesized that these changes may also reflect the underlying mechanism for the relative quantities of β-chain variants in heterozygotes (Molchanova & Huisman 1997). Some of these data are summarized in Table 9.13.

There has been at least one opportunity to look at the interaction of an α-chain variant with homozygous $β^0$ thalassaemia in an infant. The variant was HbJ Oxford and, as expected, the patient, in addition to having HbF, had an abnormal fetal haemoglobin component with the molecular structure $\alpha_2^J\gamma_2$ (Schiliro et al. 1976).

δβ Thalassaemia or haemoglobin Lepore in association with rare haemoglobin variants

There have been very few reported instances of the interaction of δβ thalassaemia with rare haemoglobin variants. The combination of δβ thalassaemia with HbD Ibadan ($\alpha_2\beta_2^{Thr\rightarrow Lys}$) was described in a 58-year-old black male by Castro et al. (1979). The interaction produced no clinical abnormalities and the patient had HbD Ibadan together with 17% HbF and a normal level of HbA_2. The combination of Hb Crete ($\alpha_2\beta_2^{129\ Ala\rightarrow Pro}$) with δβ thalassaemia was reported by Maniatis et al. (1979). This 30-year-old Greek male was found to be polycythaemic on routine examination and haematological studies showed that he had a haemoglobin level of 19.6 g/dl with a PCV of 57%. Haemoglobin analysis showed 66.8% Hb Crete and 13.0% HbF. As mentioned earlier, Hb Crete has a high oxygen affinity and these two haemoglobins in combination resulted in a blood p50 of 11.2 mmHg. Presumably this high-oxygen-affinity state resulted in a marked degree of secondary polycythaemia. Details of another association between δβ thalassaemia, in this case shown to be the Indian form of $(^A\gamma\delta\beta)^0$ thalassaemia, and a high-oxygen-affinity variant, Hb Headington ($\beta^{72\ Ser\rightarrow Arg}$), is reported by Rochette et al. (1994). This interaction produced a marked erythrocytosis with a concomitant increase in the level of the variant haemoglobin.

The interaction between Hbs Lepore and J Oxford ($\alpha_2^{15\ Gly\rightarrow Asp}\beta_2$) was reported by Ventruto et al. (1970) and further reviewed by Quattrin and Ventruto (1974). Since HbJ Oxford is an α-chain variant it would not be predicted that this interaction would produce any more clinical disability than the Hb Lepore trait and this was the case. Interestingly, however, the level of HbJ Oxford was reduced to about 15%, which seems to bear out the general rule that α-chain variants occur at a relatively low level in individuals who have any form of β or δβ thalassaemia.

Haemoglobin Lepore Washington/Boston was found in association with Hb Peterborough by King et al. (1972). Haemoglobin Peterborough ($\beta^{111\ Val\rightarrow Phe}$) is an unstable variant which precipitates on heating, or in vivo after the administration of drugs, e.g. sulphonamides. The doubly affected child was mildly anaemic with a haemoglobin value of 10 g/dl and 20% reticulocytes. The haemoglobin was made up of about 70% Peterborough and 30% Lepore Washington/Boston. Presumably Hb Peterborough is stable enough in the absence of oxidants for the child to maintain an adequate haemoglobin level. It has a low oxygen affinity, which can reduce the rate of red-cell production by decreasing the hypoxic drive to erythropoietin synthesis.

The interaction of Hb Lepore and O Arab ($\alpha_2\beta_2^{121\ Glu\rightarrow Lys}$) was described by Rajevska et al. (1978).

The association of β or δβ thalassaemia with δ-chain haemoglobin variants

The commonest δ-chain variant is HbA_2' (otherwise called HbB_2), which has the structure $\alpha_2\delta_2^{16\ Lys\rightarrow Arg}$. This occurs most commonly in parts of West Africa where it may reach an incidence of 1–2% (Weatherall et al. 1971; Vella 1977). The findings in individuals heterozygous for both β thalassaemia and HbB_2 were first reported by Ceppellini (1959a,b) and later by Huisman et al. (1961) and many others; the families in which both these genes segregated were reviewed by Weatherall et al. (1976) and Stamatoyannopoulos et al. (1977). Although HbB_2 has no clinical significance it is a useful marker of the δ-chain locus. The fact that β-thalassaemia heterozygotes who also carry

Table 9.14 Delta-chain haemoglobin variants associated with β thalassaemia.

Haemoglobin	Mutation	Phenotype	References
A$_2$ Adria	δ51 Pro→Arg	β-thalassaemia trait	Alberti *et al.* (1978)
A$_2'$ (B$_2$)	δ16 Gly→Arg	β-thalassaemia trait	Horton *et al.* (1961); many others
A$_2$ Canada	δ99 Asp→Asn	β-thalassaemia trait	Salkie *et al.* (1982)
A$_2$ Coburg	δ116 Arg→His	β-thalassaemia trait	Sharma *et al.* (1975)
A$_2$ Indonesia	δ69 Gly→Arg	β-thalassaemia trait	Ganeson & Lie-Injo (1978)
A$_2$ NYU	δ12 Asn→Lys	β-thalassaemia trait	Ranney *et al.* (1969); Schiliro *et al.* (1991)
A$_2$ Parkville	δ47 Asp→Val	β-thalassaemia trait	Leung *et al.* (1991)
A$_2$ Puglia	δ26 Glu→Asp	β-thalassaemia trait	Loudianos *et al.* (1993)
A$_2$ Pylos*	δ11 Val→Gly	δ-thalassaemia trait, β thalassaemia, normal HbA$_2$	Drakoulakou *et al.* (1997)
A$_2$ Victoria	δ24 Gly→Asp	β-thalassaemia trait	Brennan *et al.* (1984)

* Low level in heterozygotes. May be unstable.

this variant have an elevated level of both HbA$_2$ and B$_2$ is the best evidence we have that the elevation of HbA$_2$ in β thalassaemia occurs both in *cis and* in *trans,* i.e. the activity of both δ-chain loci are increased (see Chapters 3 and 7).

Some other δ-chain variants that have been found in association with β thalassaemia are summarized in Table 9.14.

The interaction of δβ thalassaemia with HbB$_2$ was reported by Comings and Motulsky in 1966. The doubly affected individual had Hbs A, F and B$_2$ and a complete absence of HbA$_2$. The HbB$_2$ comprised about 3% of the total haemoglobin. The fact that the HbB$_2$, which was the product of only one δ-chain locus, was present at the same level as HbA$_2$ in normal individuals indicated that the *trans* δ-chain gene in heterozygous δβ thalassaemia behaves in a similar way to that in β thalassaemia and directs the production of increased amounts of δ chains. Later, HbA$_2$ Zagreb ($\alpha_2\delta_2^{125\ \text{Gln}\rightarrow\text{Glu}}$) was found in association with δβ thalassaemia (Juricic *et al.* 1983).

Chapter 10
Hereditary persistence of fetal haemoglobin

Hereditary persistence of fetal haemoglobin (HPFH) is the name given to a group of conditions characterized by persistence of fetal haemoglobin synthesis into adult life in the absence of significant haematological manifestations. As we intimated in earlier editions of this book, it has much in common with the β and δβ thalassaemias. More recent experience has confirmed that this is the case and it is becoming increasingly doubtful whether some of the better defined forms of HPFH should be separated from the δβ thalassaemias, which they resemble closely. Indeed, we shall develop the concept that disorders of δ- and β-chain synthesis exist in a continuous clinical spectrum; at one end there is β^0 thalassaemia, in which fetal haemoglobin production is usually inadequate to compensate for the deficiency of adult haemoglobin, while at the other extreme there are forms of HPFH in which fetal haemoglobin is almost, although not entirely, able to make up for the deficit. However, to complicate matters it has become apparent in recent years that there are some types of HPFH which do not fulfil the criterion required of a thalassaemia-like disorder, i.e. imbalanced globin synthesis.

In this chapter we shall review the various types of HPFH and then attempt to summarize current views about their relationship to the thalassaemias. As this is such a complicated subject, and not only for those meeting it for the first time, it may be useful to begin with a brief description of how we reached our present state of understanding about the nature of HPFH. Some of these issues were touched on briefly in Chapter 1.

The development of the concept of hereditary persistence of fetal haemoglobin

In 1955 Edington and Lehmann described two healthy adults in West Africa who, because they had only Hbs S and F in their red cells, appeared to be homozygous for HbS. They wondered if they might in fact be heterozygous for both sickle-cell and thalassaemia genes, and they noted that 'the only resort is still the family study' (Edington & Lehmann 1955). In the event they discovered that each of the patients had at least one child who did not have sickle-cell haemoglobin, showing that they had transmitted a gene other than that for HbS. Furthermore, these children each produced a considerable amount of HbF, which led the authors to conclude that the parents and children carried a thalassaemia-like gene (Edington & Lehmann 1955). In 1958 Jacob and Raper found a similar group of patients in Uganda and showed quite clearly that these individuals (who, incidentally, had a mild sickling disorder) had inherited the sickle-cell gene from one parent and a gene for a high level of HbF from the other. Even more importantly, they described how the carriers for the latter trait have HbF in the 20% range, with no haematological evidence of thalassaemia. In a very thoughtful discussion Jacob and Raper decided that the genetic determinant responsible for the high level of HbF, while thalassaemia-like, did not produce the haematological picture of thalassaemia and therefore introduced the descriptive term 'hereditary persistence of fetal haemoglobin'.

A similar condition was reported by Went and MacIver (1958b) in Jamaica, and in the early 1960s workers at Johns Hopkins Hospital characterized the condition extensively in Baltimore Afro-Americans and showed that its genetic determinant behaves as an allele of the β structural locus (Bradley et al. 1961; Herman & Conley 1960; Bradley et al. 1961). The homozygous state was described in the same population in 1961 by Wheeler and Krevans (1961) and was characterized by the absence of Hbs A and A_2, the affected child having 100% HbF. In 1963 Conley and his coworkers reviewed their large experience of the condition in Baltimore and confirmed that heterozygotes have between 20 and 30% HbF, that the genetic determinant behaves as an allele of the β-chain gene and is associated with a complete absence of δ- and β-chain synthesis in *cis*, and that, while in the heterozygous state there are no haematological abnormalities, homozygotes have a mild thalassaemia-like blood picture (Conley *et al.* 1963).

In 1964 Fessas and Stamatoyannopoulos described a similar disorder in Greek populations and summarized the main differences between the Greek and African forms of HPFH.

Reports of the condition in other population groups also started to appear at about the same time: Portuguese Indians (Barkham & Adinolfi 1962); Italians (Manganelli *et al.* 1962; Quattrin *et al.* 1973; Quattrin & Ventruto 1974); Sicilians (Motta & Polosa 1966); Chinese (Wong 1966; Blackwell *et al.* 1971); South Africans (Jenkins & Stevens 1970); Indians (Sukumaran *et al.* 1961; Bird *et al.* 1964; Sukumaran *et al.* 1972; Schroeder *et al.* 1973b); and Turks (Yamak *et al.* 1973). Most of these papers described conditions similar to those found in the Afro-American populations. The two homozygous children reported by Motta and Polosa (1966) were anaemic with splenomegaly and also had 100% HbF with no HbA or A_2; these clinical findings suggest that these children may have been $\delta\beta$-thalassaemia homozygotes.

Further progress followed the discovery by Schroeder *et al.* (1968) that human fetal haemoglobin consists of two separate forms, differing only at position 136 in the γ chain. Structural analysis of HbF from individuals with HPFH allowed its further classification into those varieties in which the HbF contains both types of HbF molecules, i.e. $^G\gamma^A\gamma$ HPFH, and those in which there is only $^G\gamma$ or $^A\gamma$ HbF, i.e. $^G\gamma$ or $^A\gamma$ HPFH (Huisman *et al.* 1969, 1974). During the 1970s, and in the period up to the time when it was possible to analyse these conditions at the molecular level, further attempts were made to characterize their heterogeneity and to speculate about their underlying cause. It is beyond the scope of this chapter to cover the vast literature of this period in detail. Readers who are interested are referred to the previous edition of this book and to the extensive writings of Huisman, Schroeder and others who did so much to develop this subject (Huisman *et al.* 1969, 1970a; Schroeder & Huisman 1970; Huisman *et al.* 1971; Sukumaran *et al.* 1972; Schroeder *et al.* 1973b; Huisman *et al.* 1974, 1975a; Altay *et al.* 1977b; Ringelhann *et al.* 1977).

A typical feature of HPFH, first defined by the Johns Hopkins group (Shepherd *et al.* 1962), is the relatively homogeneous distribution of HbF throughout the red cells. This characteristic is still used to distinguish HPFH from disorders such as thalassaemia and sickle-cell anaemia in which the HbF is more or less heterogeneously distributed among the red cells. Indeed, this and the absence of haematological changes in heterozygotes have been the hallmarks of HPFH.

In the years during which the African and Greek forms of HPFH were being defined, another condition associated with an increased level of HbF in adult life was described. In 1963 Marti, in the course of studies on Swiss army recruits, noted that a small percentage had slightly elevated levels of HbF and that this appeared to be genetically determined. Unlike the African and Greek forms of HPFH the HbF was distributed unevenly among the red cells. This condition, which became known as the 'Swiss' form of HPFH, attracted little notice for about 10 years. But in the mid-1970s there was a reawakening of interest when it became apparent that if it was found together with the β-thalassaemia or sickle-cell traits it produced higher levels of HbF than are usually found in these conditions.

Because of the increasing heterogeneity of the entities which were encompassed by the general title HPFH, Boyer *et al.* (1977) proposed that they be classified into two main groups, i.e. pancellular, in which the HbF is uniformly distributed among the red cells, and heterocellular, in which it is distributed heterogeneously. Later it became clear that pancellular HPFH is very closely related to $\delta\beta$ thalassaemia, while at least some forms of heterocellular HPFH seem to be different conditions altogether, probably unrelated to the thalassaemias. As we shall see later in this chapter, it is still not clear whether the division of HPFH has any real biological meaning or whether it simply reflects the varying sensitivity of the methods used to study the intracellular distribution of HbF (Wood *et al.* 1979).

Over the last 15 years it has been possible to obtain a clearer picture of the different varieties of HPFH by defining their molecular basis and then relating genotype to phenotype. Although this has allowed us to characterize many different forms, in truth we still have very little insight into the mechanisms of the persistent fetal haemoglobin production.

Classification

The different forms of HPFH are shown in Table 10.1. Broadly, they are now classified into deletional and

Table 10.1 Hereditary persistence of fetal haemoglobin.

Deletion

$(\delta\beta)^0$

  Black (HPFH 1)
  Ghanaian (HPFH 2)
  Indian (HPFH 3)
  Italian (HPFH 4 and 5)
  South-east Asian

$(^A\gamma\beta)^+$ (Hb Kenya)

Non-deletion

  Linked to β-globin-gene cluster (pancellular*)

$^G\gamma\beta^+$

  Black $^G\gamma$–202 C→G
  Tunisian $^G\gamma$–200 +C
  Black/Sardinian $^G\gamma$–175 T→C
  Japanese $^G\gamma$–114 C→T
  Australian $^G\gamma$–114 C→G

$^A\gamma\beta^+$

  Greek/Sardinian/Black $^A\gamma$–117 G→A
  British $^A\gamma$–198 T→C
  Black $^A\gamma$–202 C→T
  Italian/Chinese $^A\gamma$–196 C→T
  Brazilian $^A\gamma$–195 C→G
  Black $^A\gamma$–175 T→C
  Black $^A\gamma$–114 to –102 (del)
  Georgia $^A\gamma$–114 C→T

$^G\gamma^A\gamma\beta^+$

  Linked to β-globin-gene cluster (heterocellular*)
    Atlanta
    Czech
    Seattle
    Others (including some cases of $^G\gamma$–158 T→C)†

  Unlinked to β-globin-gene cluster (heterocellular*)
    Chromosome 6
    Others

*The intercellular distribution of HbF is not always reported and there are some inconsistencies within groups.
† See Table 10.7.

non-deletional types. For want of a better approach, where the underlying deletion or point mutation in the non-deletional forms is known, they are designated by the ethnic origin of the individuals in whom they were first characterized. Originally it was thought that there might be deletional forms of HPFH which either left both the $^G\gamma$- and $^A\gamma$-globin genes intact or which removed the $^A\gamma$- as well as the δ- and β-globin genes, and hence which were called $^G\gamma^A\gamma$ and $^G\gamma$ HPFH, respectively. It is now known that

nearly all the deletions that remove the $^A\gamma$- and δ- and β-globin genes are associated with the phenotype of δβ thalassaemia. Thus the only deletional form of HPFH is in fact $^G\gamma^A\gamma (\delta\beta)^0$ HPFH. This condition can either be designated in this way or, more simply, $(\delta\beta)^0$ HPFH. Indeed, the only deletional form of HPFH with persistent $^G\gamma$-chain synthesis is that associated with the γβ fusion variant, Hb Kenya. The best characterized non-deletional forms of HPFH are all due to point mutations in the promoter regions of either the $^G\gamma$- or $^A\gamma$-chain genes. They are associated with persistent $^G\gamma$- or $^A\gamma$-chain production with β- and δ-chain synthesis in *cis*; they are therefore called $^G\gamma\beta^+$ and $^A\gamma\beta^+$ HPFH, respectively, and further classified by the underlying mutation and ethnic origin of the individual in whom they were first described.

In addition to these well defined types of HPFH there is a heterogeneous group of non-deletional forms which may or may not behave as alleles of the β-globin-gene cluster and for which, in most cases, the underlying molecular mechanisms remain to be determined.

Deletional forms of hereditary persistence of fetal haemoglobin

$(\delta\beta)^0$ *Hereditary persistence of fetal haemoglobin*

By a combination of molecular and haematological studies it has been possible to identify six different forms of $(\delta\beta)^0$ HPFH (Table 10.1). They are most easily defined by findings in heterozygotes; there are no haematological abnormalities, the levels of HbF are increased in the 15–30% range, the HbF is pancellular in distribution, and there are significantly reduced levels of HbA_2. All of these conditions result from partial deletions of the β-globin-gene cluster, described in detail in Chapter 4. The best characterized at the clinical and haematological level are the Black (HPFH 1) (Huisman *et al*. 1971; Tuan *et al*. 1980; Jagadeeswaran *et al*. 1982; Tuan *et al*. 1983; Kutlar *et al*. 1984; Adams *et al*. 1985; Feingold & Forget 1989; Martínez *et al*. 1990; Stolle *et al*. 1990) and Ghanaian (HPFH 2) (Ringelhann *et al*. 1977; Tuan *et al*. 1983; Kutlar *et al*. 1984; Bakioglu *et al*. 1986; Collins *et al*. 1987) types. The other forms of $(\delta\beta)^0$ HPFH, which have only been encountered in a few families, include: Indian (HPFH 3) (Schroeder *et al*. 1973b; Kutlar *et al*. 1984; Wainscoat *et al*. 1984b;

Henthorn *et al.* 1986); Italian (HPFH 4 and 5) (Saglio *et al.* 1986; Camaschella *et al.* 1990c); and south-east Asian (Motum *et al.* 1993a).

The clinical and haematological descriptions that follow are based mainly on studies of the disease in families of African origin, that is the Black and Ghanaian types. There appear to be no major phenotypic differences between these conditions. What little is known about the phenotypic expression of the rarer forms of HPFH is summarized, where appropriate, in the following sections.

Homozygous state

At least nine Afro-Americans have been described in whom there was good evidence for homozygosity for $(\delta\beta)^0$ HPFH. Although because reports of the same individual appear in different papers and at different times it is sometimes difficult to be certain about their identity, it is clear that these descriptions encompass both the Black (HPFH 1) (Wheeler & Krevans 1961; Forget *et al.* 1976; Fritsch *et al.* 1979) and Ghanaian (HPFH 2) varieties (Ringelhann *et al.* 1970; Acquaye *et al.* 1977; Ringelhann *et al.* 1977; Huisman *et al.* 1981; Kutlar *et al.* 1984). Other well documented cases include those of Siegel *et al.* (1970) and Reyes *et al.* (1978). Although some of these reports contain limited clinical and haematological data, it is still possible to compile a fairly comprehensive picture of this condition.

Clinical findings

Homozygosity for $(\delta\beta)^0$ HPFH was first observed in a male Afro-American child in Baltimore, who was 15 months old when first studied (Wheeler & Krevans 1961). He was born of a full-term delivery, and growth and development were completely normal. He was anaemic when first seen but this was ascribed to iron deficiency and he had an excellent response to iron therapy. Follow-up studies on this child were reported by Conley *et al.* (1963), Charache and Conley (1969) and Charache *et al.* (1976). His subsequent growth and development were completely normal and he had no symptoms ascribable to his condition.

The homozygotes who were described subsequent to the Baltimore child presented at various ages and in no case were there any symptoms or signs suggestive of thalassaemia. In particular, growth and development were completely normal and hepatosplenomegaly was not reported.

Haematological findings

The haematological findings at various stages of development in the patient first described by Wheeler and Krevans are summarized in Table 10.2. They are similar to those observed in the seven other homozygotes; a composite summary of the haematological findings of this group of patients is presented in Table 10.3.

There are relatively high haemoglobin levels (range 14.8–18.2 g/dl; mean 16.3 g/dl) and the red cells are small and poorly haemoglobinized (MCH 23–27 pg, mean 24.9 pg; MCV 68–84 fl, mean 75 fl). These changes are reflected in the blood films, which show slight but unequivocal microcytosis and minimal hypochromia with variation in shape and size of the red cells. The reticulocyte counts range between 1 and 2%, with a mean of 1.2%. The white-cell and platelet counts are normal.

Table 10.2 Haematological data from the Baltimore HPFH homozygote (Charache *et al.* 1976).

Age (years)	RBC ($\times 10^{12}$/l)	Hb (g/dl)	PCV (%)	MCV (fl)	MCH (pg)	MCHC (%)
1	6.06	13.3	43.2	71	22	31
4	6.23	15.2	44.4	71	27	34
6	6.12	15.0	45.6	75	24	33
7	6.35	14.3	44.1	70	23	32
11	6.24	14.1	42.8	68	23	33
13	6.73	15.3	46.4	69	23	33
14	6.71	15.9	46.5	69	24	34
15	6.40	15.9	43.2	68	25	37

MCH, mean cell haemoglobin; MCHC, mean cell haemoglobin concentration; MCV, mean cell volume; PCV, packed cell volume; RBC, red-cell count.

Table 10.3 Summary of haematological data and haemoglobin analysis for $(\delta\beta)^0$ HPFH homozygotes (references in text).

Number of cases	8
Hb (g/dl)	14.8–18.2 (16.3)
Mean cell volume (fl)	68–84 (75)
Mean cell haemoglobin (pg)	23–27 (24.9)
Reticulocytes (%)	1–2 (1.2)
$^G\gamma$	0.52–0.65 (0.59)
α-/γ-chain synthesis	1.4–3.3 (2.0)*

*If one unusually high value of 3.3 (Ringelhann *et al.* 1977) is excluded, the mean ratio is 1.7.

There have been few studies to determine whether there is a haemolytic element. Charache *et al.* (1976) found that the bilirubin and haemopexin levels were normal. These findings, together with normal reticulocyte counts, suggest that this is unlikely.

Haemoglobin analysis

Haemoglobin analysis by electrophoresis or chromatography shows 100% HbF (Fig. 10.1); this has been confirmed by analysis of the globin by chromatography in 8M urea mercaptoethanol buffer systems. Details of these studies are given in the papers of Conley *et al.* (1963), Siegel *et al.* (1970), Ringelhann *et al.* (1970, 1977) and Charache *et al.* (1976).

Structure of haemoglobin F

The first structural analysis of the HbF was carried out by Baglioni (1963). He confirmed that the haemoglobin of these patients consists only of HbF and showed that the constitution of the γ-chain peptides is identical to those of umbilical cord blood. The HbF was analysed for its $^G\gamma^A\gamma$-chain composition by Huisman and his colleagues (Huisman *et al.* 1969; Ringelhann *et al.* 1970; Huisman *et al.* 1971; Ringelhann *et al.* 1977). Although several papers gave

discrepant results of the analysis of the HbF from the Ghanaian family of Kamuzora *et al.* (1974, 1975), the situation was later resolved (Ringelhann *et al.* 1977) and it is quite clear that in the seven cases where this analysis has been carried out adequately the HbF contains both $^G\gamma$ and $^A\gamma$ chains; the glycine composition of peptide γCB3 has ranged from 0.52 to 0.65 residues, suggesting that these chains are present in approximately equal proportions.

The HbF associated with the Black deletion has a higher $^G\gamma$ composition than that in the Ghanaian deletion in heterozygotes. This may be because the former is found on a chromosome with the C→T change at position −158 in the $^G\gamma$ gene, known to be associated with relatively high levels of $^G\gamma$-chain production (Bakioglu *et al.* 1986). However, there is no difference in the proportion of $^G\gamma$ chains among homozygotes for the two types, with values of 0.60 and 0.57 for the Black and Ghanaian forms, respectively.

Haemoglobin synthesis

Charache *et al.* (1976) first reported that HPFH homozygotes have imbalanced globin synthesis and that for that reason, and because of the haematological changes, the condition is, in effect, a mild form of δβ thalassaemia (Fig. 10.2). This observation was con-

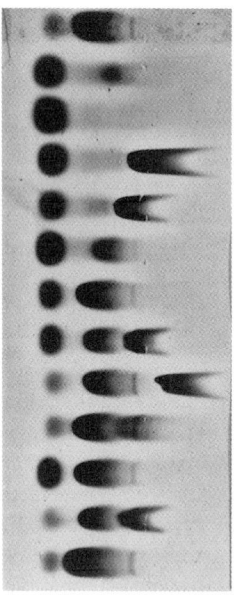

Normal adult	1
Normal umbilical cord blood	2
F. Homozygote	3
C–F. Doubly abnormal heterozygote	4
S–F. Doubly abnormal heterozygote	5
F– Thalassemia. doubly abnormal heterozygote	6
A–F Heterozygote	7
A–S Heterozygote (3 month old infant)	8
A–C Heterozygote	9
A–S Heterozygote	10
A–S Heterozygote	11
A–S Heterozygote	12
Normal adult	13

Fig. 10.1 Agar gel electrophoresis (citrate buffer, pH 5.9) of red-cell lysates from individuals with different combinations of the gene for hereditary persistence of fetal haemoglobin (HPFH). Top to bottom: 1, normal adult; 2, normal cord blood; 3, HPFH homozygote; 4, HPFH/HbC compound heterozygote; 5, HPFH/HbS compound heterozygote; 6, HPFH/β-thalassaemia compound heterozygote; 7, HPFH heterozygote; 8, sickle-cell trait in a 3-month-old infant; 9, HbC heterozygote; 10, HbS heterozygote; 11, HPFH heterozygote; 12, sickle-cell heterozygote; 13, normal adult.

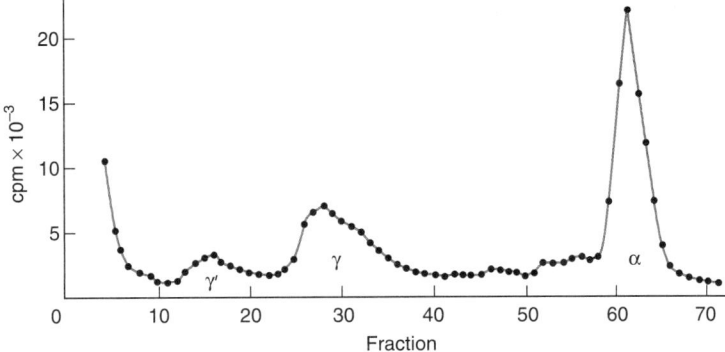

Fig. 10.2 Haemoglobin synthesis in a homozygote for hereditary persistence of fetal haemoglobin. Reticulocytes from the peripheral blood of the first reported Baltimore homozygote were incubated with radioactive leucine for 1 h and the globins separated by CM-cellulose chromatography. The figure shows the profile of the radioactivity from the column; there is no β-chain synthesis. It is also clear that there is a mild degree of imbalanced globin synthesis with an excess of α over γ chains produced. From Charache *et al.* (1976).

firmed in subsequent studies (Forget *et al.* 1976; Ringelhann *et al.* 1977; Orkin *et al.* 1978). The α-/non-α-globin synthesis ratios have usually ranged from 1.4 to 2.0, although Ringelhann *et al.* (1977) described one individual in whom it was 3.3. The mean ratio for all the cases studied to date is 2.0 if the latter case is included, and 1.7 if it is excluded. Hence the degree of globin imbalance is similar to that observed in heterozygous β thalassaemia.

Other properties of the red cells

In an adult with 100% fetal haemoglobin it is of interest to know whether the other red-cell proteins which change during the transition from fetal to adult life are present in normal adult proportions. In the Baltimore homozygote the non-haemoglobin pattern of the red-cell lysates is similar to that of an adult, i.e. carbonic anhydrases 1 and 2, which are present in low amounts in cord blood and reach an adult level at about 2–3 years (Weatherall & McIntyre 1967), are present in normal quantities (Conley *et al.* 1963). Other parameters which change during development such as the i antigen, glutathione peroxidase activity, red-cell esterases and immunoglobulins are of the adult variety or level (Charache & Conley 1969).

The oxygen affinity of the Baltimore homozygote's red cells and haemoglobin was analysed by Charache *et al.* (1976). The p50 of the whole blood was 17.8 mmHg as compared with 26–27 mmHg in normal adults. This was associated with a slightly elevated 2,3-DPG level. However, the p50 of his stripped haemoglobin, i.e. haemoglobin in solution separated from small molecular weight components such as 2,3-DPG, showed no difference from the intact cell. Therefore the high oxygen affinity of this patient's blood reflects the fact that it consists of 100% HbF. The latter interacts poorly with 2,3-DPG. Thirty per cent of this child's haemoglobin is the acetylated form (HbF₁), more than that usually found in cord blood, and since this fraction is totally unreactive with 2,3-DPG, this may also contribute to the marked increase in oxygen affinity.

Pathophysiology

HPFH homozygotes suffer no clinical disability. However, one feature that they all have in common is an erythrocytosis with a high haemoglobin level. Presumably this is related directly to the high oxygen affinity of their blood. In discussing this problem Charache *et al.* (1976) pointed out that the Baltimore homozygote has a haemoglobin concentration of 16 g/dl, whereas a p50 of 17.8 mmHg would predict a higher haemoglobin level, somewhere in the range of 18 g/dl. However, there is a reasonable explanation for this discrepancy. As shown by the same workers, and in the subsequent studies outlined above, HPFH homozygotes have imbalanced globin synthesis. It seems likely that the resulting mild degree of ineffective erythropoiesis does not allow them to achieve the level of haemoglobin which would be compatible with their p50 values. Another possibility is that there is a low-grade haemolysis although, as already mentioned, there is no evidence that this is the case.

Inheritance

In those families in which appropriate relatives were available for study both parents have been carriers for HPFH (Fig. 10.3). In the remarkable family reported by Ringelhann *et al.* (1977) the 54-year-old propositus had a total of 10 children through two wives; eight were HPFH heterozygotes and two were homozygotes. Presumably his second wife was also an HPFH heterozygote!

Relationship to (δβ)⁰ thalassaemia

It is clear from the mild thalassaemic red-cell changes and globin imbalance in the homozygous states for this condition that it is, in effect, a form of δβ thalassaemia in which the output of $^G\gamma$ and $^A\gamma$ chains is sufficient to almost, but not completely, compensate for the absence of β- and δ-chain production.

Heterozygous state

There have been numerous studies of the heterozygous states for (δβ)⁰ HPFH, though the only large series are of Afro-Americans, representing HPFH types 1 and 2. They are asymptomatic and are usually ascertained by a population survey or family study. The findings in the different molecular forms are summarized in Table 10.4.

Haematological findings

In early studies it was thought that there were no haematological changes whatever (Conley *et al.* 1963). However, these reports appeared before the availability of the more sophisticated electronic cell counters. In Table 10.4 the red-cell indices in the larger published series of heterozygotes of known genotype are summarized. It appears that there may be a slightly reduced MCV. These values must be interpreted with caution, however; iron deficiency and α thalassaemia have not always been excluded. By and large the red-cell findings are almost normal.

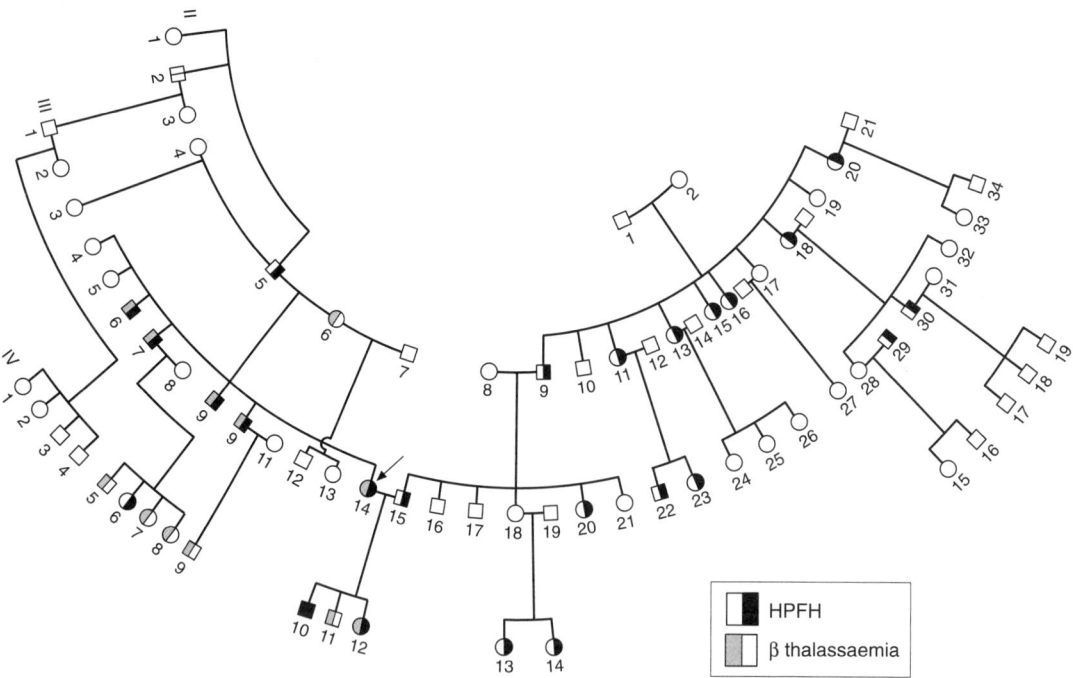

Fig. 10.3 The family pedigree of the first reported homozygote for hereditary persistence of fetal haemoglobin (IV.10). The pedigree is an extension of that reported by Wheeler and Krevans (1961). The further data were kindly supplied by Dr Samuel Charache.

Table 10.4 Summary of haematological data on deletion HPFH heterozygotes defined by molecular analysis.

Condition	No of families/ individuals	Hb* (g/dl)	MCV† (fl)	MCH† (pg)	HbA₂* (%)	HbF (%)	Gγ* (%)	α/non-α* synthesis	Distribution
Black HPFH	40/53	12.4 ± 2.2	83.7 ± 4.8	27.1 ± 3.6	1.7 ± 0.4	24.8 ± 3.1	50.7 ± 4.3	—	Pancellular
Ghanaian HPFH	35/64	13.8 ± 1.3	80.3 ± 5.0	25.7 ± 1.6	2.3 ± 0.3	24.5 ± 2.8	32.3 ± 4.8	1.23 ± 0.25	Pancellular
Indian HPFH	5/8	14.1 ± 1.1	90.7 ± 5.6	28.5 ± 1.6	1.8 ± 0.3	22.5 ± 2.6	70.9 ± 2.9	1.2	Pancellular
Italian HPFH	4/9	13.4 ± 1.6	81.8 ± 5.9	27.2 ± 2.7	1.8 ± 0.1	24.7 ± 5.5	35.0 ± 3.2	1.12 ± 0.05	Pancellular
Sicilian HPFH	1/2	13.8 ± 0.3	79.5 ± 2.9	26.0	3.6 ± 0.3	18.0 ± 2.8	16.0 ± 1.4	1.15	Pancellular
SE Asian HPFH	4/13	13.2 ± 1.8	85.0 ± 7.9	24.6 ± 1.6	3.8 ± 0.6	20.7 ± 3.8	61.6 ± 1.7	1.46	Pancellular

* Data not necessarily complete for all individuals; extreme outliers omitted.

† α Thalassaemia not excluded in all cases; some results obtained after sample had been in transit.

Haemoglobin constitution

Haemoglobin F and A₂ values for heterozygotes of known genotype are summarized in Table 10.4. Haemoglobin F in heterozygotes for HPFH types 1 and 2 ranges from 13 to 30%, with a mean value of about 25%. It is similar in the other varieties. Haemoglobin A₂ is significantly reduced (Fig. 10.4). Haemoglobin F is present in every cell if blood films are examined by an immunofluorescence technique (Wood *et al.* 1975) (Figs 10.5 and 10.6). Similarly, on acid elution all the cells seem to contain some HbF, although there may be variation in staining from cell to cell, suggesting some heterogeneity of distribution (Thompson *et al.* 1961; Shepherd *et al.* 1962). Interestingly, in individuals who are severely iron deficient the level of HbF is decreased (Adams *et al.* 1985).

Differential centrifugation experiments have also indicated that there may be some heterogeneity of distribution of HbF in this condition; cells obtained from the bottom of the centrifuged column of blood contain slightly more HbF than those at the top of the spin. However, this effect is much less marked than in the red cells of patients with β or δβ thalassaemia (Gabuzda *et al.* 1963; Abraham *et al.* 1975).

Haemoglobin synthesis

Haemoglobin synthesis has been studied in the peripheral blood of Afro-American HPFH heterozygotes by Natta *et al.* (1974), Huisman *et al.* (1975a) and Friedman *et al.* (1976b). Natta *et al.* and Huisman

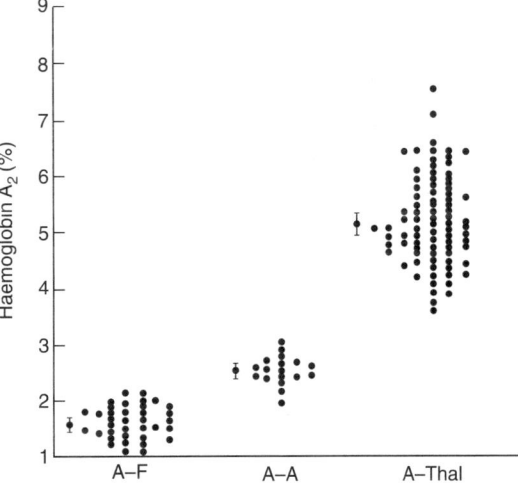

Fig. 10.4 HbA₂ values in hereditary persistence of fetal haemoglobin. The HbA₂ levels in heterozygotes (A–F) are compared with normal persons (A–A) and β-thalassaemia heterozygotes (A–Thal).

et al. found that globin synthesis was more or less balanced. Friedman and colleagues found balanced synthesis in 10 cases but in two there was a slight but significant excess of α chains produced. Unfortunately, however, the synthesis ratios in the latter study were, in many cases, only reported in terms of α/β rather than α/β+γ and so the results are difficult to interpret. It appears that in most cases there is minimal globin imbalance in HPFH heterozygotes. Ringelhann *et al.* (1977) added a note of caution in

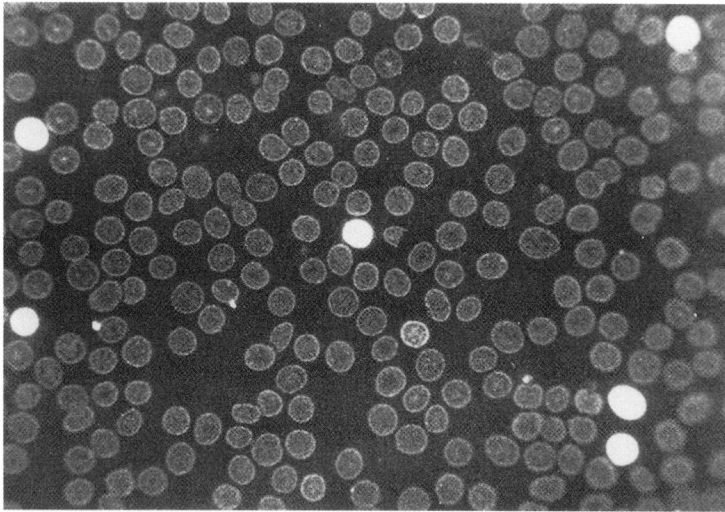

Fig. 10.5 Normal blood film treated with a fluorescently labelled anti-HbF antibody. A few F cells are labelled.

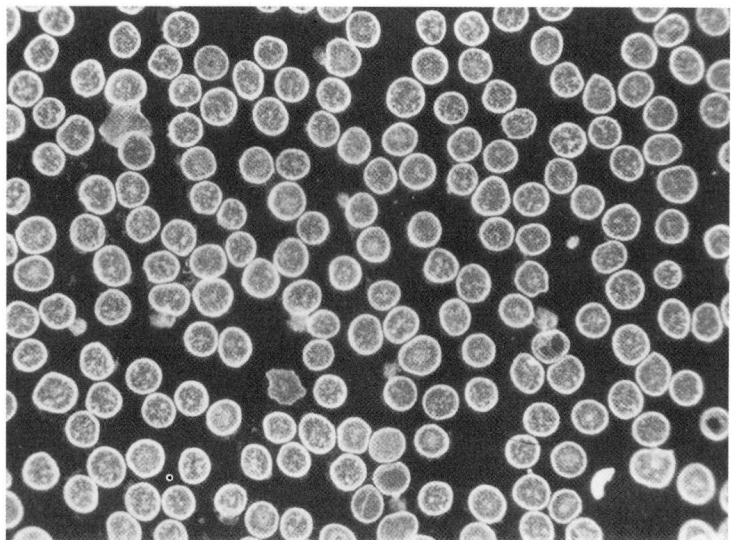

Fig. 10.6 The distribution of HbF in heterozygous $(\delta\beta)^0$ hereditary persistence of fetal haemoglobin. Staining conditions similar to Fig. 10.5.

interpreting this type of data, suggesting that γ-chain synthesis may decline more rapidly than β-chain synthesis during erythroid development, a mechanism which is reflected by the changes in γ- and β-globin-gene expression in early progenitors maintained in cell culture (Huisman *et al*. 1979; Papayannopoulou *et al*. 1979).

Structure of haemoglobin F

The relative amounts of $^{G}\gamma$ and $^{A}\gamma$ chain in the HbF of $(\delta\beta)^0$-thalassaemia heterozygotes varies significantly between the different molecular forms (Table 10.4). In the African varieties heterozygotes for HPFH 1 have, on average, about equal amounts of $^{G}\gamma$ and $^{A}\gamma$ chains while heterozygotes for HPFH 2 have $^{G}\gamma$ values of about 32%. Heterozygotes for HPFH 3, 4 and 5 have $^{G}\gamma$ values of approximately 69%, 30% and 15%, respectively.

Heterozygous state with haemoglobin S

This combination, first described by Edington and Lehmann in 1955, was subsequently the subject of many other reports (Griggs & Harris 1956; Jacob & Raper 1958; Went & MacIver 1958a; Bradley *et al.* 1961; Herman & Conley 1960; Motulsky 1960; MacIver *et al.* 1961; Thompson *et al.* 1961; Thompson & Lehmann 1962; Conley *et al.* 1963; Watson-Williams 1965; Huisman *et al.* 1969; Natta *et al.* 1974; Bethlenfalvay *et al.* 1975; Friedman *et al.* 1976b).

It is very likely that the majority of these reports describe the interaction of either HPFH 1 or HPFH 2 with the sickle-cell gene. The haematological and haemoglobin findings in the few reports in which the underlying molecular lesion has been defined are summarized in Table 10.5 and are mentioned, where appropriate, in the sections which follow.

Clinical and haematological findings

Although these compound heterozygotes have haemoglobin constitutions similar to some patients with sickle-cell anaemia, they are generally quite healthy. There are usually no symptoms that can be attributed to anaemia and few episodes suggesting sickle-cell crises, although occasional mild bone or joint pains have been reported. Interestingly, although splenomegaly has not been a regular feature of this condition in the USA, Konotey-Ahulu (1973) noted it in about 40% of cases in West Africa, and in this series about 25% of cases had occasional mild crises. Aseptic necrosis of the femoral heads, similar to that found in sickle-cell disease, has been described (Jacob & Raper 1958; Conley *et al.* 1963). Uncomplicated pregnancy has been the rule (Jacob & Raper 1958; MacIver *et al.* 1961; Conley *et al.* 1963).

There is usually no anaemia and little evidence of haemolysis. The haemoglobin level in 18 cases reviewed by Conley *et al.* (1963) was usually greater than 14 g/dl and only in four was it below 12 g/dl. These findings were substantiated in later studies (Natta *et al.* 1974; Friedman *et al.* 1976b). The peripheral blood film shows moderate anisopoikilocytosis with variable numbers of target cells. The reticulocyte count is usually normal or slightly elevated and the serum haptoglobin level is normal. The red-cell osmotic fragility is normal or decreased. The plasma clearance times for ^{59}Fe are normal (Bradley *et al.* 1961), as is the survival time of red cells, both when transfused into normal recipients (Conley *et al.* 1963; Watson-Williams 1965) and by ^{51}Cr-labelling (Watson-Williams 1965).

Table 10.5 Summary of haematological data on deletion HPFH heterozygotes' interactions with haemoglobin S, haemoglobin C and β thalassaemia.

Condition	No. of families/ individuals	Hb* (g/dl)	MCV† (fl)	MCH† (pg)	HbA$_2$* (%)	HbF (%)	G$_\gamma$* (%)	α/non-α*	Distribution
Black or Ghanaian HPFH	35/64	13.8 ± 1.3	82.3 ± 4.9	25.7 ± 1.6	2.3 ± 0.3	24.7 ± 3.0	32.3 ± 4.8 or 50.7 ± 4.3	1.23 ± 0.25	Pancellular
HPFH/HbS‡	19/44	13.7 ± 1.6	79.7 ± 5.6	26.6 ± 3.1	2.0 ± 0.5	29.5 ± 5.9	44 ± 5	1.1 ± 0.2	Pancellular
HPFH/HbC‡	7/12	13.0 ± 1.2	73.2 ± 7.9	26.4 ± 1.6	—	33.9 ± 4.1	50 ± 4		Pancellular
HPFH/β$^+$ thal.‡	9/12	12.1 ± 1.8	73.3 ± 7.3	23.9 ± 1.9	2.9 ± 0.8	67.3 ± 4.5	67 ± 7	1.7	Pancellular
Indian HPFH	5/8	14.1 ± 1.1	90.7 ± 5.6	28.5 ± 1.6	1.8 ± 0.3	22.5 ± 2.6	70.9 ± 2.9	1.2	Pancellular
Indian HPFH/β$^+$ thal.	4/4	7.4 ± 1.6	63.0 ± 8.2	20.8 ± 6.4	2.8 ± 0.5	79.9 ± 10.3	72 ± 3	4.2	Pancellular

* Data not necessarily complete for all individuals; extreme outliers omitted.

† α Thalassaemia not excluded in all cases; some results obtained after sample had been in transit.

‡ Molecular basis unknown (except for three HPFH/HbS cases that were of the Ghanaian type (Huisman *et al.* 1981; Anagnou *et al.* 1985)); all cases are of African origin and therefore presumably carry the Black or Ghanaian deletions.

Haemoglobin constitution

The haemoglobin constitution is shown in Fig. 10.1 and, in cases in which the molecular form of the HPFH deletion was characterized, in Table 10.5. Only Hbs S, F and A_2 are present; no HbA is produced. The latter finding was further demonstrated by electrophoresis on both starch gel and agar gel, by column chromatography using Amberlite IRC-50 (Conley *et al.* 1963) and by globin synthesis (Natta *et al.* 1974; Friedman *et al.* 1976b). The level of HbF varies between 15 and 42%. Taking together the series reviewed by Conley *et al.* (1963) with later cases reported by Huisman *et al.* (1969), Wrightstone and Huisman (1974), Natta *et al.* (1974), Friedman *et al.* (1976b) and Huisman *et al.* (1981), the mean level of HbF is about 29%. This is significantly higher than in HPFH heterozygotes. In cases in which the molecular basis of the HPFH has been identified, both Ghanaian (HPFH 2), the HbF levels were 22% (Anagnou *et al.* 1985) and 33% (Huisman *et al.* 1981; Kutlar *et al.* 1984).

The HbF is distributed more or less homogeneously among the red cells (Bradley *et al.* 1961; Thompson *et al.* 1961; Shepherd *et al.* 1962; Abraham *et al.* 1975) (Fig. 10.7). The level of HbA_2 is normal or slightly reduced (Herman & Conley 1960; Thompson *et al.* 1961; Watson-Williams 1965; Huisman *et al.* 1969; Natta *et al.* 1974; Wrightstone & Huisman 1974; Friedman *et al.* 1976b).

Haemoglobin synthesis

Globin synthesis has been analysed in a few cases

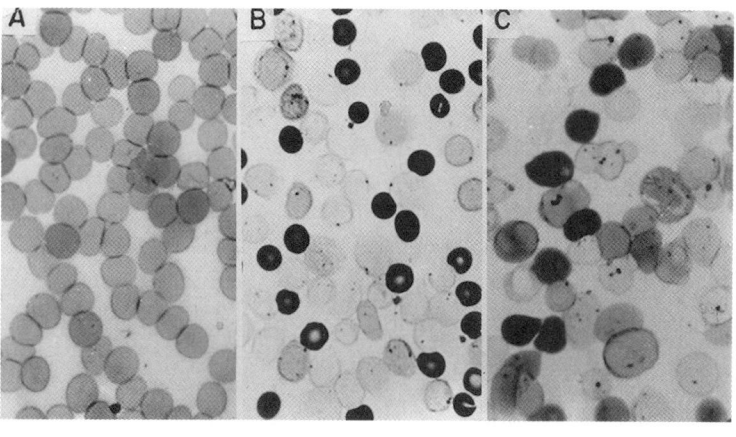

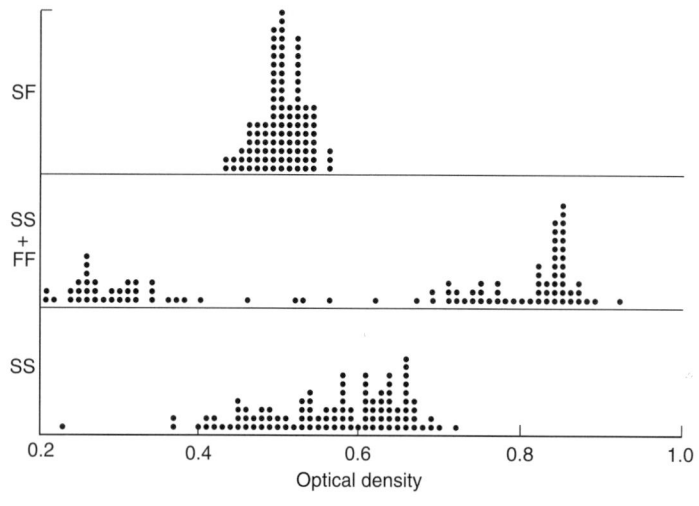

Fig. 10.7 Acid elution patterns of the following: (A) compound heterozygous state for the sickle-cell and HPFH genes; (B) an artificial mixture of cord blood cells and cells from an individual with sickle-cell anaemia; and (C) sickle-cell anaemia. The plots are photodensitometric readings of individual cells from (A), (B) and (C), respectively, showing the homogeneous distribution of HbF in (A) compared with a heterogeneity of distribution in (C). From Shepherd *et al.* (1962).

(Natta *et al.* 1974; Friedman *et al.* 1976b). Natta *et al.* found balanced synthesis in both marrow and blood while Friedman *et al.* found a slight excess of α-chain synthesis in a few cases. Natta *et al.* (1974) noted that α/β ratios were significantly lower than 2/1 and concluded that balanced synthesis was achieved by an increased output of β chains from the normal allele in addition to that from the γ gene *cis* to the HPFH determinant. It appears therefore that globin synthesis is balanced in the majority of cases, and this may be in part due to increased output from the normal β-chain allele in *trans* to the HPFH determinant. The corollary of this is that the γ-chain locus (or loci) *cis* to the HPFH determinant is unable to compensate completely for the loss of output from the adjacent δ and β loci. This notion is supported by the results of globin synthesis analysis in homozygotes, referred to earlier, which show unequivocal imbalance, in the range observed in β-thalassaemia heterozygotes.

Structure of haemoglobin F

The $^{G}\gamma^{A}\gamma$ composition of the haemoglobin F shows a higher proportion of $^{G}\gamma$ chains compared with relatives who are simple HPFH heterozygotes (Huisman *et al.* 1981).

Inheritance

When full family studies have been performed one parent has always had the sickle-cell trait and the other has been heterozygous for HPFH. The children of matings with normal persons are heterozygous for either HPFH or the sickle-cell trait; no normal or doubly affected individuals have been described.

A comparison of the pathophysiology of sickle-cell disease with heterozygosity for both hereditary persistence of fetal haemoglobin and the sickle-cell gene

Both experimental and epidemiological studies have shown that elevated levels of HbF tend to reduce the severity of sickle-cell anaemia. As described in Chapter 2, and shown in Fig. 10.7, the intercellular distribution of HbF is quite heterogeneous in sickle-cell disease; red cells that contain relatively lower levels have a shorter survival (Singer & Fisher 1952; Bradley *et al.* 1961). Irreversibly sickled cells tend to

have low levels of HbF (Bertles & Milner 1968). In populations such as those of eastern Saudi Arabia and Orissa, India, in which patients with sickle-cell anaemia tend to have higher levels of HbF, the disease tends to run a milder course, although painful crises still occur and bone disease may be quite severe (Perrine *et al.* 1972; Padmos *et al.* 1991). These early observations have been substantiated by more recent epidemiological studies (Powers *et al.* 1984; Platt *et al.* 1991; Noguchi *et al.* 1993).

At least some understanding of the way in which fetal haemoglobin modifies the phenotype of the sickling disorders has been obtained over recent years (reviewed by Noguchi *et al.* 1993 and Dover & Platt 1998). An increase in the proportion of non-sickle haemoglobins, particularly HbF, within red cells is beneficial because it reduces the intracellular concentration of HbS. Furthermore, mixed hybrids of Hbs S and F do not enter into the formation of the polymers which underlie sickling. This, in turn, has a beneficial effect on the abnormal rheological properties of the sickle cell.

As already mentioned, patients with sickle-cell anaemia from populations such as eastern Saudi Arabia or Orissa who have unusually high levels of HbF still have many of the complications of sickle-cell anaemia, particularly bone disease, and their course is not as mild as that of compound heterozygotes for HbS and HPFH. It seems likely that the major reason for the difference between these two phenotypes lies in the cellular distribution of HbF (Fig. 10.7). Even in patients with sickle-cell anaemia with unusually high levels of HbF the cellular distribution is quite heterogeneous and not as uniform as in compound heterozygotes for HPFH and HbS. It is the *uniformly* high level of HbF per cell that renders the interaction with HPFH and HbS so mild. This is an important observation because it provides valuable insights into the level of HbF in each red cell that would be required to control sickle-cell anaemia by the pharmacological stimulation of HbF synthesis.

Heterozygous state with haemoglobin C

Like HbS, reports of this interaction are almost certainly restricted to the HPFH 1 and 2 varieties. Data from the few reports in which the underlying molecular defect has been described are summarized in Table 10.5.

Clinical and haematological findings

This combination is found in West Africans and Afro-Americans, usually by chance on haemoglobin electrophoresis (Motulsky 1960; Kraus *et al.* 1961; MacIver *et al.* 1961; Schneider *et al.* 1961; Thompson & Lehmann 1962; Conley *et al.* 1963; Huisman *et al.* 1969; Bethlenfalvay *et al.* 1975). The ages of reported cases have ranged from 9 to 70 years and none have had any symptoms suggesting a haematological disorder. In four, splenomegaly was present. The haemoglobin levels have ranged from 11.3 to 15 g/dl and in three cases there was a slight reticulocytosis. The red cells show moderate variation in shape and size with many target cells, and the morphological changes are more marked than in the HbC trait. The serum haptoglobin levels were reduced in one case, as was the ^{51}Cr red-cell survival (Conley *et al.* 1963). Thus the clinical and haematological findings are compatible with a mild, compensated haemolytic process.

Haemoglobin constitution

The fetal haemoglobin level ranges from 27 to 39% (Fig. 10.1) and it is distributed uniformly throughout the red cells (Shepherd *et al.* 1962). Although there is considerable reported variation, the level of HbF seems to be significantly higher than in heterozygotes for HPFH or in compound heterozygotes for HPFH and HbS. The remainder of the haemoglobin is HbC and, presumably, HbA_2 although, since the latter has a similar electrophoretic mobility to HbC, the level of HbA_2 is not usually determined. It was suggested by McCormick and Humphreys (1960), Kraus *et al.* (1961) and Schneider *et al.* (1961) that variable quantities of HbA may be present in this condition, but detailed electrophoretic analysis on agar gel (Fig. 10.1) and examination by a variety of chromatographic studies did not confirm these findings (Conley *et al.* 1963); the disorder is characterized by a total absence of HbA production. In retrospect, it seems likely that the cases described by McCormick and Humphreys and Schneider *et al.* were examples of $^{G}\gamma\beta^{+}$ HPFH together with HbC (see later section).

Structure of haemoglobin F

The $^{G}\gamma^{A}\gamma$ composition of the HbF in this condition is similar to or higher than that found in HPFH het-

erozygotes in the same family (Huisman *et al.* 1969) (Table 10.5).

Inheritance

In families in which both parents have been available for study, one showed HPFH trait and the other HbC trait. Children born of matings between individuals of the C–F genotype and normal persons show either HbC or are heterozygous for HPFH.

Heterozygous state with haemoglobin E

In the early descriptions of this combination it was not absolutely clear whether interactions that were being described were between HPFH and HbE, or between $\delta\beta$ thalassaemia and HbE (Wasi *et al.* 1968b; Altay *et al.* 1977b; Ringelhann *et al.* 1977). Recently more data have been published from the family reported by Wasi *et al.* (1968b). Two family members, neither of whom was anaemic, had only HbE and F, and thalassaemic morphology of their red cells. Both $^{G}\gamma$ and $^{A}\gamma$ chains were demonstrated, with a pancellular distribution of HbF. One sibling had normal haematological findings, with an HbF of 21.2% and a pancellular distribution of HbF. Later, Southern blot analysis demonstrated a large deletion similar to the Indian form of $(\delta\beta)^{0}$ HPFH (Fucharoen & Winichagoon 1997).

From this limited information it appears that this is a mild interaction which is of little more clinical significance than the HbE trait.

Heterozygous state with β thalassaemia

This combination has been most thoroughly characterized in Afro-American families (Kraus *et al.* 1961; Wheeler & Krevans 1961; Conley *et al.* 1963; Becker & Rossi 1966; Huisman *et al.* 1971; Natta *et al.* 1974; Bethlenfalvay *et al.* 1975; Rothschild *et al.* 1976). All these studies described examples of interactions of the HPFH gene with β^{+} thalassaemia. An example of an Afro-American family in which there was an individual heterozygous for both HPFH and β^{0} thalassaemia was reported by Fogarty *et al.* (1974). In assessing these interactions it should be remembered that more recent information indicates that the commonest forms of β^{+} thalassaemia in patients of African origin are due to mild promoter mutations. Thus, with one exception, these descriptions largely deal with the interactions of $(\delta\beta)^0$ HPFH 1 and 2 with extremely mild forms of β thalassaemia. Several patients have been described who are compound heterozygotes for the Indian form of $(\delta\beta)^0$ HPFH and severe β^+-thalassaemia alleles (Schroeder *et al.* 1973b; Wainscoat *et al.* 1984b).

Clinical and haematological findings

Most of the reported Afro-American patients with $(\delta\beta)^0$HPFH/β^+ thalassaemia have been symptom free, although in the early series reviewed by Conley *et al.* (1963) one complained of attacks of pain attributable to an enlarged spleen. Interestingly, this is the only reported instance in which the spleen was palpable; in all the other cases either no mention was made of the physical findings or there were no clinical abnormalities. These individuals show either no anaemia, or only a slightly diminished haemoglobin level similar to that found in heterozygous β thalassaemia. The red-cell indices are also similar to the latter condition, with a high red-cell count for the haemoglobin level and a reduced MCH. The MCV is also diminished and is in the β-thalassaemia range. In a few reported cases there has been a slight elevation in the reticulocyte count and serum bilirubin level. Thus the clinical and haematological findings are very similar to those of heterozygotes for β or $\delta\beta$ thalassaemia.

The patient reported by Fogarty *et al.* (1974) who was heterozygous for both $(\delta\beta)^0$ HPFH and β^0 thalassaemia, though only limited clinical data are given, also seems to have been very mildly affected. She was a 69-year-old Afro-American who was reported to have been mildly anaemic in the past but at the time of study had a haemoglobin level of 12.4 g/dl with typical thalassaemic red-cell indices. Her only complaint was some chronic abdominal pain, which was thought to be due to a markedly enlarged spleen. Unfortunately, no other clinical data are given and so it is difficult to explain the considerable splenomegaly with a steady-state haemoglobin of 12.4 g/dl. However, it appears that this is a mild interaction.

Schroeder *et al.* (1973b) described three Indian patients with $(\delta\beta)^0$HPFH/β^+ thalassaemia. Again, although there are few clinical data it appears that this was a relatively severe interaction because the haemoglobin values in the three children were 5.5, 6.7 and 9.0 g/dl. Wainscoat *et al.* (1984b) described

another Indian patient with what was initially characterized as $(\delta\beta)^0$ HPFH/β^+ thalassaemia. The patient had the clinical picture of relatively severe β thalassaemia intermedia, and a falling haemoglobin level necessitated splenectomy at the age of 5 years, after which her haemoglobin level stabilized at about 8.0 g/dl. Other complications included recurrent infections and an episode of severe bleeding following tonsillectomy. This child had typical thalassaemic red-cell changes and an HbF value of 64.5%, very similar to that described in the families of Schroeder *et al.* Subsequent molecular characterization of these families demonstrated that they had the same deletion, but one that differs from either of the two Black varieties (Wainscoat *et al.* 1984b; Henthorn *et al.* 1986). Hence it was designated as the Indian form of $(\delta\beta)^0$ HPFH, or HPFH 3. Clearly its interaction with what were almost certainly severe β^+-thalassaemia alleles produces a severe form of thalassaemia intermedia.

Haemoglobin constitution (Table 10.5)

In the review of Conley *et al.* (1963), which covered the cases described up to 1963, the HbF level ranged from 67 to 71%. These findings were confirmed in a later paper by Huisman *et al.* (1971), who reported levels ranging from 60 to 78%, and in subsequent studies (Natta *et al.* 1974; Bethlenfalvay *et al.* 1975). One of the exceptions was a patient described by Rothschild *et al.* (1976) who was reported to have only a trace of HbA and between 85 and 95% of HbF. This is quite different from the other cases and, if the haemoglobin data are correct, suggests that this may represent the interaction between HPFH and a more severe form of β^+ thalassaemia. The other unusual case was a 69-year-old Afro-American female who clearly was heterozygous for HPFH and β^0 thalassaemia (Fogarty *et al.* 1974) (see above). She had 98.1% HbF and 1.9% HbA$_2$; there was no HbA. The HbF is more or less equally distributed among the red cells (Shepherd *et al.* 1962) in these patients.

Haemoglobin A$_2$ levels are variable. In some cases they are elevated while in others they appear to be normal. Rothschild *et al.* (1976) reviewed the literature relating to 28 reported cases (some of which we have not been able to trace) and noted that seven had elevated levels of HbA$_2$ while the rest were normal. As described in Chapter 7, it is more meaningful to calculate the output of HbA$_2$ in terms of pg per cell.

Unfortunately, it is not always possible to do this from published data, but in the series of Huisman *et al.* (1971) the HbA$_2$ values range from 2.7 to 5.1%, or from 0.62 to 1.0 pg. However, the average haemoglobin A$_2$ in this series, and in those reported elsewhere in the literature, is approximately 3%, or about 0.7 pg per cell. Since this represents the output from only one δ-chain locus it means that δ-chain production is increased by at least twofold, and sometimes even threefold.

Haemoglobin synthesis

Natta *et al.* (1974) studied haemoglobin synthesis in the peripheral blood of a patient heterozygous for both HPFH and β thalassaemia. The α-/non-α-globin synthesis ratio was 1.7, in the range usually found in β-thalassaemia heterozygotes.

Structure of haemoglobin F

The structure of HbF was examined in six individuals heterozygous for HPFH and β thalassaemia by Huisman *et al.* (1971). The glycine composition of peptide γCB3 ranged from 0.58 to 0.78 residues. Huisman and colleagues suggest that, from analysis of these figures together with those obtained from the γCB3 peptides of the parents of some of their cases, it is possible to calculate that most of the excess HbF in compound heterozygotes for HPFH and β thalassaemia over that found in the simple HPFH heterozygotes is derived from the chromosome carrying the β-thalassaemia determinant.

In the HPFH β^0-thalassaemia compound heterozygote described by Fogarty *et al.* (1974) γCB3 contained 0.77 residues of glycine. The HPFH heterozygotes had only 0.11–0.17 glycine residues, particularly low for this condition. The authors suggested that the higher glycine values in the compound heterozygote result from the output of mainly ^{G}γ chains from the β^0-thalassaemia chromosome.

In the compound heterozygotes for the Indian form of HPFH and β$^+$ thalassaemia reported by Schroeder *et al.* (1973b) the HbF contained 0.70–0.75 glycine residues, little different from the heterozygotes in the same family.

Inheritance

In families in which good genetic data have been available, one parent has shown β-thalassaemia trait and the other the HPFH trait (Fig. 10.3). Children of these compound heterozygotes have had either β thalassaemia minor or HPFH.

Pathophysiology

In the majority of African patients with this disorder the level of γ-chain production is sufficient to almost completely compensate for defective β-chain production. The interactions between HPFH 3 and β$^+$ thalassaemia are interesting in this respect. This seems to always result in a fairly severe form of β thalassaemia intermedia; the phenotype is much more severe than the interaction of the Black form of (δβ)^0 thalassaemia with β^0 thalassaemia. It was the difficulty in reconciling these observations that led Wainscoat *et al.* (1984b) to characterize the form of HPFH which is observed in Indian populations as a variety of (δβ)^0 thalassaemia. These observations are particularly surprising because the heterozygous state for HPFH 1, 2 and 3 have an almost identical phenotype, with very similar levels of HbF; the HPFH 3 heterozygotes have relatively normal red-cell indices.

Association with rare structural haemoglobin variants

(δβ)^0 HPFH of an undetermined variety was found in association with HbJ Lomé ($α_2β_2^{59\ \text{Lys→Asn}}$) by Amegnizin *et al.* (1979). The compound heterozygote had no clinical or haematological abnormalities and her haemoglobin consisted of 82% Hb Lomé, 15% HbF and 2.8% HbA$_2$. She had six children through two husbands. One was dead, two were HPFH heterozygotes and three were heterozygous for Hb Lomé.

Association with haemoglobin A$_2$ variants

The association of HPFH and HbA$_2$′ (a δ-chain variant, now usually called B$_2$) in the same individual was first reported by Kraus *et al.* (1961). The authors described an HPFH heterozygote with both Hbs A$_2$ and B$_2$. However, when re-examined the haemoglobin pattern showed only Hbs A, F and B$_2$ (Conley *et al.* 1963). This finding provided evidence that the δ-chain gene in *cis* to the HPFH determinant is completely inactive (or absent). Two Afro-American women with similar findings were reported by Bethlenfalvay *et al.* (1975). Between them they produced 11 offspring, of which five had HPFH and six

HbB₂; there were no normal children. Two further individuals heterozygous for both HPFH and HbB₂ were described by Huisman *et al.* (1976) and again HbA₂ was absent. All these reports provided evidence for the complete absence of δ-chain synthesis *cis* to the HPFH determinant; the segregation data given in the families of Bethlenfalvay *et al.* (1975) are compatible with current knowledge about the molecular basis for $(\delta\beta)^0$ HPFH.

Association with δ thalassaemia

Thompson *et al.* (1965) described three children heterozygous for HPFH who had no HbA₂. One parent was heterozygous for HPFH and the other, who was haematologically normal, had a reduced level of HbA₂. The findings in the parents suggest that the three children are heterozygous for both HPFH and a form of δ thalassaemia.

$(^A\gamma\beta)^+$ *Hereditary persistence of fetal haemoglobin (haemoglobin Kenya)*

An abnormal haemoglobin associated with HPFH was reported by Huisman *et al.* (1972). This variant, which was designated Hb Kenya, was further charac-

terized by Kendall *et al.* (1973) and Smith *et al.* (1973). Haemoglobin Kenya turned out to contain normal α chains combined with non-α chains which are γβ fusion chains. Thus, it has much in common with Hb Lepore, which has α chains combined with δβ fusion chains. After its original discovery further examples of HPFH associated with this variant were reported by Nute *et al.* (1976) and Wood *et al.* (1977a).

Clinical and haematological features

Haemoglobin Kenya carriers have normal or near-normal haematological findings. In the compound heterozygous state for Hbs Kenya and S there is very slight anaemia but the red cells are normochromic and normocytic and the blood films show only occasional target cells. The MCH values may be slightly reduced (Waye *et al.* 1992). The reticulocyte counts are not elevated.

Haemoglobin constitution

Haemoglobin Kenya carriers have in addition to HbA, Hbs F, Kenya and A₂ (Fig. 10.8). In 12 carriers reported by Smith *et al.* (1973) the HbF values ranged from 5.0 to 9.0% (mean 6.5%), the Hb Kenya levels from 6.9 to 12.4% (mean 9.6%) and the HbA₂ values

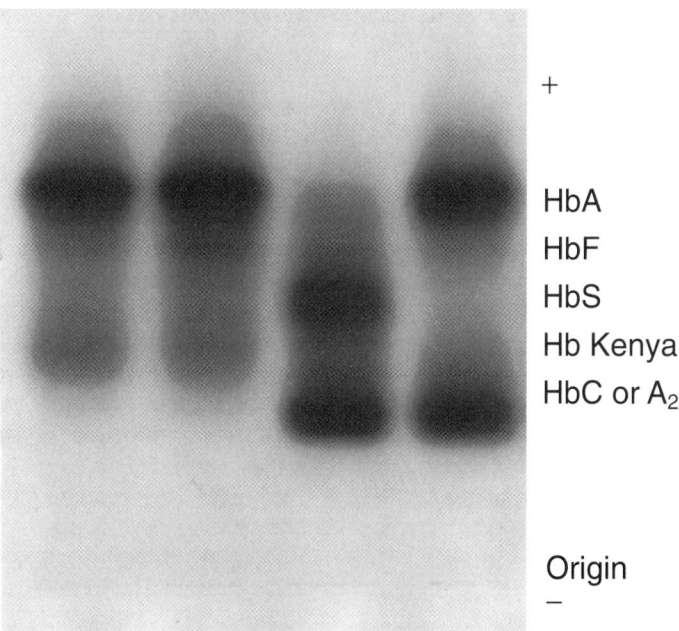

+

HbA
HbF
HbS
Hb Kenya
HbC or A₂

Origin
–

Fig. 10.8 Starch gel electrophoresis (pH 8.5, amido black stain) showing Hb Kenya. Left to right: 1 and 2, Hb Kenya heterozygotes; 3, Hb SC disease; 4, HbC trait.

from 1.39 to 1.84% (mean 1.5%). Similar values were reported by Kendall *et al.* (1973) but in the family of Nute *et al.* (1976) and some of those of Smith *et al.* (1973), while the levels of HbF were similar, the levels of Hb Kenya were higher, ranging from 20 to 23%. In the three individuals with Hbs Kenya and S described by Kendall *et al.* (1973) the HbS values ranged from 62 to 69% and HbF from 6.6 to 11.0%. The Hb Kenya levels ranged from 17.6 to 19.0% and HbA was absent in each case. The haemoglobin constitution of Hb Kenya heterozygotes is summarized in Fig. 10.8.

More recent data on heterozygotes, or compound heterozygotes with HbS, are essentially the same (Huisman *et al.* 1997).

In the cases reported by Kendall *et al.* (1973) and Smith *et al.* (1973) the HbF was shown to be relatively homogeneously distributed among the red cells of Hb Kenya carriers using the acid elution technique. This observation was confirmed by Nute *et al.* (1976) using an immunofluorescent method.

Haemoglobin synthesis

Haemoglobin synthesis was studied in the peripheral blood of an Hb Kenya carrier by Wood *et al.* (1977a) (Fig. 10.9). Globin synthesis was balanced and Hb Kenya was synthesized in reticulocytes at a rate compatible with its level in the peripheral blood.

It appears that there is compensating β-chain

synthesis from the normal β gene in *trans* to the Hb Kenya determinant; in Hb Kenya/HbS compound heterozygotes the combined $^{G}\gamma + \gamma\beta$-chain production is only 60% of the output of normal non-α genes.

Structure of haemoglobins F and Kenya

The HbF in Hb Kenya heterozygotes is all of the $^{G}\gamma$ type (Kendall *et al.* 1973; Smith *et al.* 1973). The non-α chain of Hb Kenya has a γ-chain sequence for residues 1–80 and a β-chain sequence for residues 87–146 (see Fig. 4.17, Chapter 4). Presumably its genetic determinant has arisen by non-homologous crossing over between the $^{A}\gamma$ and β loci, with the result that the δ-chain locus and parts of the $^{A}\gamma$ and β loci are deleted, leaving only the $^{G}\gamma$ and $^{A}\gamma\beta$ fusion genes on the chromosome. This interpretation is supported by Southern blotting analysis (Ojwang *et al.* 1983).

Frequency of deletional forms of hereditary persistence of fetal haemoglobin

The incidence of the different deletional forms of HPFH is not known. Conley *et al.* (1963) estimated that HPFH occurs in approximately 0.1% of the Baltimore Afro-American population. A similar figure was suggested by Thompson *et al.* (1965) from a survey in the southern USA.

Since the HPFH genes came to North America

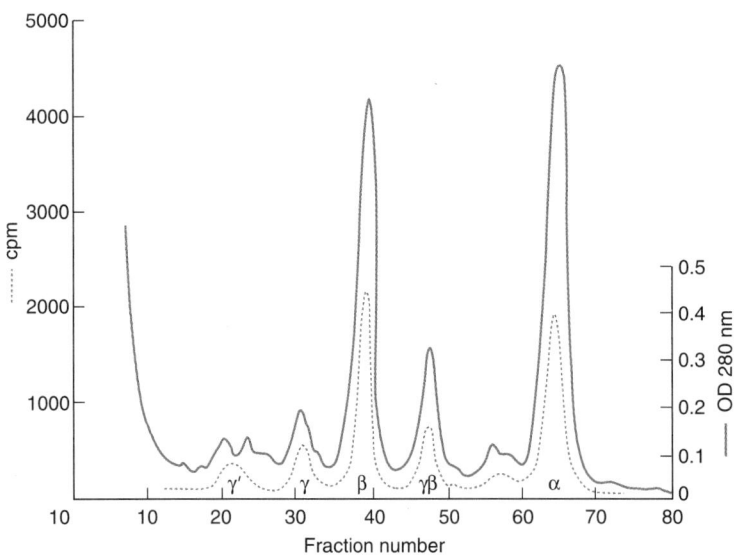

Fig. 10.9 Haemoglobin synthesis in the reticulocytes of an Hb Kenya heterozygote. It is clear that the γβ chains of Hb Kenya are synthesized in the peripheral blood.

from Africa, it would be of interest to obtain approximate gene frequencies in the latter population. Unfortunately, there are only limited data. Jacob and Raper (1958) estimated that there might be about one case per 300 of the population of Uganda. Watson-Williams (1965) found HPFH in four out of 9618 Nigerians whose haemoglobin was subjected to routine electrophoresis because their red cells sickled. Watson-Williams argues that this frequency, i.e. about 1 in 2000 Nigerians from Ibadan and district, is a reasonable approximation of the gene frequency for HPFH in the Nigerian population. In their small-scale surveys of some African populations, Weatherall *et al.* (1971) found one case of HPFH out of 574 samples from Lagos (0.2%), four cases out of 464 samples from south Ghana (0.8%) and one case out of 224 samples from north Ghana (0.4%). Thus the HPFH genes seem to occur widely in West Africa, but probably at a low frequency.

Non-deletional forms of hereditary persistence of fetal haemoglobin

As shown in Table 10.1, the non-deletional forms of HPFH can be divided into those in which there is a mutation in either the $^G\gamma$- or $^A\gamma$-gene promoters associated with persistent $^G\gamma$ or $^A\gamma$ fetal haemoglobin production and β- and δ-chain synthesis in *cis*, that is $^G\gamma\beta^+$ HPFH and $^A\gamma\beta^+$ HPFH, and the heterogeneous group of conditions that are characterized by persistent low levels of fetal haemoglobin synthesis in the apparent absence of any structural change in the β-globin-gene cluster.

$^G\gamma\beta^+$ *Hereditary persistence of fetal haemoglobin*

Of the four families in which this disorder was first characterized (Huisman *et al.* 1975b; Friedman *et al.* 1976b; Tatsis 1978; Higgs *et al.* 1979a), the HPFH gene was found together with HbS in three, and in the fourth with HbC. In two of the families α thalassaemia was also present. In the report of Tatsis (1978) the HbF was not analysed chemically but the phenotype was very similar to the other cases in which its structure was determined. The characteristic finding is the presence of significant amounts of HbA in compound heterozygotes for this form of HPFH and the β-chain haemoglobin variants, S and C.

Later studies, which related this form of HPFH to promoter mutations of the $^G\gamma$ genes, suggested that at least some of the Afro-American or Caribbean families in which the condition was first characterized may have had either the $^G\gamma$ –175 T→C mutation (Surrey *et al.* 1988) or the $^G\gamma$ –202 C→G mutation (Collins *et al.* 1984).

Subsequently, it became clear that this condition is not restricted to African populations and different molecular forms were identified elsewhere: Tunisia, $^G\gamma$ –200 +C (Pissard *et al.* 1996); Japan, $^G\gamma$ –114 C→T (Fucharoen *et al*, 1990f); and Australia, $^G\gamma$ –114 C→G (Motum *et al.* 1994). In addition, the $^G\gamma$ –175 T→C mutation has been observed in Sardinian populations (Ottolenghi *et al.* 1988); it is therefore sometimes designated the Black/Sardinian variety. The findings in heterozygotes for the different molecular forms are summarized in Table 10.6.

Black $^G\gamma\beta^+$ HPFH –202 C→G

This condition has been fully characterized in a few Afro-American families (Huisman *et al.* 1975b; Collins *et al.* 1984; Yang *et al.* 1988). Heterozygotes are haematologically normal (Table 10.6). They have between 16 and 21% fetal haemoglobin, which is nearly all of the $^G\gamma$ variety, together with HbA$_2$ values which range between 1.3 and 2.2%, with a mean of approximately 1.7%. This reflects about 0.5 pg HbA$_2$ per cell, which is slightly reduced, suggesting that the output of both the β and δ chains *cis* to this HPFH determinant have a lower output than normal.

This condition has been observed in the compound heterozygous state with HbS in a few individuals. They are not anaemic, their red-cell indices show only a very slight reduction in the MCH and MCV, and there are no significant morphological changes of the red cells. The HbF values range from 18 to 22% with a mean of approximately 20%; the average HbA$_2$ value is approximately 2.3%. The HbA values range from 24 to 36% with a mean of approximately 30%. It appears that the β^S gene in these individuals produces about 14 pg of HbS per cell, while the β^A gene *cis* to the HPFH determinant produces only about 7–8 pg per cell, or approximately half the amount of a normal β^A gene.

In both heterozygotes and compound heterozygotes the distribution of HbF, as determined by the acid elution technique, is relatively homogeneous although there is some variability in staining from

Table 10.6 Summary of haematological data (mean ± SD) on non-deletional HPFH heterozygotes defined by molecular analysis.

Condition	Mutation	No. of families/individuals*	Hb (g/dl)	MCV† (fl)	MCH† (pg)	HbA$_2$ (%)	HbF (%)	$^G\gamma$ or $^A\gamma$ (%)	α/non-α synthesis	Xmn I at −158 in cis	Distribution
$^G\gamma$*Mutations*											
Black	−202 C→G	1/5	13.3±1.3	82.0±6.5	27.7±2.0	1.7±0.4	15.6±1.2	99.0±0.5	0.87±0.02	−	Pancellular
Tunisian	−200 +C	1/5	13.1±0.9	95.9±1.8	31.9±0.4	1.5±0.3	25.2±4.1	100±0		+	
Black/Sardinian/British	−175 T→C	2/3	12.7±1.1	85.2±3.1	28.4±1.8	1.3±0.2	20.3±2.8	94.0±5.2	0.97±0.17	−	Pancellular
Japanese	−114 C→T	1/2	12.5±2.1	89.0±4.2						+	
Australian	−114 C→G	1/1	14.2	92		2.3	8.6	90		−	
$^A\gamma$*Mutations*											
Black	−202 C→T	1/5	12.9±0.9	84.4±5.9	30.0±2.3	2.7±1.0	2.5±0.9	92.8±2.8		−	
British	−198 T→C	3/22	14.2±1.2	83.1±3.3	29.0±1.0	2.5±0.4	6.9±2.2	92.2±1.8	1.05±0.13	−	Heterocellular
Italian/Chinese	−196 C→T	4/8	Normal	Normal	30.0±0.9	1.8±0.6	13.7±2.0	95.0±0.2	1.06±0.05	−	Heterocellular
Brazilian	−195 C→G	1/3	Normal	Normal	Normal	2.1	5.4±1.4	89.0±2.5			
Black	−175 T→C	3/7	Normal	Normal	Normal	1.5±0.2	37.4±1.0	78.0±5.5		+	Pancellular
Cretan‡	−158 C→T	3/3	13.9±0.7	84.5±6.0	27.3±1.0	2.8±0.2	3.7±1.2	43.3±8.6		+	
Greek/Black/Sardinian	117 G→A	64/144	14.2±1.1	85.9±4.5	28.4±2.4	2.0±0.3	12.1±2.8	93.4±4.7	0.95±0.10	−	Pancellular
Black§	−114 to −102	2/2	11.4±2.9	75.5±2.1	26.8±0.3	2.1±0.0	31.0±1.2	85.7±5.7		−	
Georgia	−114 C→T	1/2	Normal	Normal	Normal	2.5±0.4	3.8±1.3	90.9±0.8		−	

* Data not necessarily complete for all individuals; extreme outliers omitted.
† α Thalassaemia not excluded in all cases; some results obtained after sample had been in transit.
‡ This mutation in the $^A\gamma$ gene is the same as that occurring as a polymorphism in the $^G\gamma$ gene.
§ Described only in combination with HbS.

cell to cell. Using the more sensitive immunofluorescent technique, all the red cells appear to contain some HbF. The differential centrifugation experiments reported by Huisman *et al.* (1975b) show no significant difference in the amount of HbF in the young and old red-cell populations, whether its level was determined as a percentage or in pg per cell. These observations provide further evidence for the relative uniformity of the distribution of HbF among red cells.

In the family of Huisman *et al.* (1975b) heterozygotes had almost balanced globin synthesis and this was also the case in compound heterozygotes, although in a few of the family members there appeared to be an α-thalassaemia gene segregating, which complicated the interpretation of the data.

Tunisian $^G\gamma\beta^+$ HPFH –200 +C

This is the only form of $^G\gamma\beta^+$ HPFH that has been identified in the homozygous state. So far only one family with this condition has been reported (Pissard *et al.* 1996).

Homozygous state

Pissard *et al.* described a family in which both parents and all of the five offspring had elevated levels of HbF in the absence of any clinical or haematological abnormalities. Three of the five children had values ranging from 18 to 27%, while in two it was approximately twice this level, 48% and 49%, respectively. These observations, together with a genetic analysis using restriction-fragment-length polymorphism (RFLP) haplotypes, provided clear evidence that the two children with higher levels of HbF are homozygous for this form of HPFH. Neither of them were anaemic, with haemoglobin levels of 13.6 and 13.7 g/dl, respectively, nor were there any abnormalities of their red cells. Their HbA$_2$ levels were slightly reduced.

Heterozygous state

The five heterozygotes in this family have completely normal haematological findings with levels of HbF ranging from 18 to 27%. No further clinical data are given but it appears that this condition is not associated with any clinical or haematological abnormalities.

Black/Sardinian $^G\gamma\beta^+$ HPFH –175 T→C

This condition has been characterized in both Afro-American (Friedman *et al.* 1976b; Surrey *et al.* 1988) and Sardinian families (Ottolenghi *et al.* 1988). It has been observed in the heterozygous state and in the compound heterozygous state with either HbS or β^0 thalassaemia.

Heterozygous state

Heterozygotes have normal haematological findings and an elevated level of HbF of approximately 30%; the HbA$_2$ values are slightly reduced.

Compound heterozygosity with haemoglobin S

This combination is not associated with any clinical or significant haematological changes. The HbF level is approximately 30%, while Hbs A and S account for about 27 and 41%, respectively. The HbA$_2$ level is slightly reduced at just under 2%.

Compound heterozygosity with β^0 thalassaemia

In a later study of the original Sardinian family (Ottolenghi *et al.* 1988) the interaction of this form of HPFH with β^0 thalassaemia was described. The 27-year-old man was not anaemic, with a steady-state haemoglobin level of 13.1 g/dl, and red-cell indices typical of β-thalassaemia trait. The haemoglobin composition was: HbA$_2$ 2.5%, HbF 64% and the remainder HbA. The α-/non-α-globin synthesis ratio was 1.8, and the composition of the γ chain remained at 100% $^G\gamma$ (Pistidda *et al.* 1997). These studies suggest therefore that the combined output of the γ and β chains from the non-deletion HPFH chromosome must closely approximate the output from a normal β-globin gene.

Japanese $^G\gamma\beta^+$ HPFH –114 C→T

This condition has only been observed in the heterozygous state in one Japanese family (Fucharoen *et al*, 1990f). There were no haematological changes and the heterozygotes had 11.0 and 14.0% HbF, respectively. The HbA$_2$ levels were not reported. The proband was also homozygous for the C→G polymorphism at $^G\gamma$–158.

Australian $^G\gamma\beta^+$ HPFH –114 C→G

This condition has been reported in one Australian male. Apart from the fact that this 54-year-old man had insulin-dependent diabetes no further clinical details are given. He was haematologically normal with normal red-cell indices and his HbF value was 8.6% with an HbA_2 value of 2.3%. He was also heterozygous for the C→T polymorphism at $^G\gamma$ –158 (Motum *et al.* 1994).

Other forms of $^G\gamma\beta^+$ HPFH

The family reported by Indrak *et al.* (1991) is sometimes included in classifications of these conditions. However, the phenotype is completely different from those described above and we shall return to discussion of this condition in a later section which deals with the hereditary persistence of low levels of fetal haemoglobin.

The action of the $^G\gamma\beta^+$ HPFH determinant

It is probable that the different $^G\gamma$-gene promoter mutations are the cause of persistent production of $^G\gamma$ chains, which in turn is responsible for reduced β-chain synthesis in *cis* (see Chapter 4). There is also reduced δ-chain synthesis *cis* to the $^G\gamma\beta^+$ HPFH determinant, a conclusion which is strengthened by the finding of reduced levels of HbA_2 in the Tunisian homozygotes. Curiously, however, there appeared to be no difference between the mean levels of HbA_2 in homozygotes and heterozygotes in this family. From analyses of globin synthesis in compound heterozygotes it seems likely that the chromosome carrying the $^G\gamma\beta^+$ determinant produces more or less equal amounts of β^A and γ chains, the combined output being slightly less than the normal output of the non-α genes on one chromosome. The balance is presumably made up from the normal β gene in *trans* to the HPFH determinant.

$^A\gamma\beta^+$ *Hereditary persistence of fetal haemoglobin*

The discovery by Fessas *et al.* (1961) of a relatively common form of HPFH in the Greek population was an important landmark in our understanding of this condition. It was clearly different from the varieties that were being characterized in Afro-American populations at about the same time, and it always seemed likely that it might be characterized by at least some β-chain synthesis *cis* to its determinant. Many years later it was found to result from a point mutation in the $^A\gamma$-globin-gene promoter, a G→A substitution at position –117 (Collins *et al.* 1985). In 1988 the frequent occurrence of an identical condition was described in the population of northern Sardinia (Ottolenghi *et al.* 1988). A single Afro-American family has also been reported with this form of HPFH; haplotype analysis suggested that it was a new mutation (Huang *et al.* 1987).

Over recent years several other molecular varieties of $^A\gamma\beta^+$ HPFH have been identified (Table 10.6). However, none appear to be common, and the Greek/Sardinian form is the only one to have been found to be distributed widely.

Greek/Sardinian/Black $^A\gamma\beta^+$ HPFH ($^A\gamma$–117 G→A)

Homozygous state

Two Sardinian families have been identified in which there was one individual who was clearly homozygous for $^A\gamma\beta^+$ HPFH (Camaschella *et al.* 1989a). Although few clinical details are given in this paper it is clear that this condition is not associated with any clinical manifestations. In one of the families the homozygote, who had a completely normal haematological picture, produced four heterozygous children through a normal partner. In the other, an individual who also had completely normal haematological findings was born of parents both of whom were heterozygous for $^A\gamma\beta^+$ HPFH.

The red-cell indices in these homozygotes appear to be relatively normal except that in one case there is a slightly reduced MCV and MCH; no details of the iron status of this person are given.

The haemoglobin findings are characterized by elevated levels of HbF of about 24% (double the mean level of 12.1% in heterozygotes) and reduced levels of HbA_2 of about 0.8%. These observations suggest that this form of $^A\gamma\beta^+$ HPFH is characterized by persistent $^A\gamma$-chain synthesis with reduced β- and δ-chain synthesis *cis* to the HPFH determinant.

Heterozygous state (Table 10.6)

In 33 Greek HPFH heterozygotes studied by Fessas and Stamatoyannopoulos (1964) there were no clinical abnormalities and the haematological findings were completely normal. In particular there was no microcytosis and the MCH values were within the normal range. These findings were confirmed in subsequent reports. In the Greek study the HbF values ranged from 10 to 19.4%, with a mean of 14.5%, while the HbA_2 values ranged from 1.6 to 2.8% with a mean of 2.1%, just significantly lower than those of their normal siblings and other unaffected family members. These findings were confirmed by Sofroniadou *et al.* (1975), Clegg *et al.* (1979) and Huang *et al.* (1987). Essentially similar data have been reported more recently in Sardinian populations (Ottolenghi *et al.* 1988; Camaschella *et al.* 1989a). In 72 heterozygotes the mean level of HbF was 11.9% and that of HbA_2 was 1.99%, findings in close agreement with those of earlier studies in Greek populations.

The distribution of HbF as judged by acid elution is relatively homogeneous, although there is some variation in staining from cell to cell. It is also more or less homogeneous when assessed with an immunofluorescent anti-HbF antibody (Clegg *et al.* 1979). The latter workers also showed that there is very little difference in the amount of HbF in young and old red cells, although there appears to be slightly more in the older population.

In vitro haemoglobin synthesis was studied in three Greek heterozygotes by Sofroniadou *et al.* (1975). The mean α/non-α ratio was 0.97, indicating balanced synthesis of α and non-α chains. Similar results were obtained by Camaschella *et al.* (1979). In the two heterozygotes studied by Clegg *et al.* (1979) the α/non-α ratios were 1.23 and 1.61, respectively; in these cases there appeared to be a slight but significant imbalance of globin synthesis with an excess of α-chain production.

Huisman *et al.* (1970b) studied the structure of the HbF in seven Greek heterozygotes and found that the γCB3 peptide gave glycine values ranging from 0.05 to 0.13 residues. This observation, together with the results of Edman degradation analyses, led Huisman and colleagues to conclude that the γ chains were all of the $^Aγ$ variety. However, a different conclusion was reached by Clegg *et al.* (1979). These workers found approximately 10% glycine in peptide γCB3, and a detailed chemical analysis suggested that this was not derived from contamination by extraneous sources but was an integral part of the HbF, i.e. it contained about 10% $^Gγ$ chains. A variety of control experiments provided circumstantial evidence that at

least some of the $^Gγ$ chains were derived from the same chromosome as the $^Aγ$ chains. Thus these findings suggested that this form of HPFH is characterized by the production of predominantly $^Aγ$ chains, though there may be a slight increase in $^Gγ$ chains. As far as we know this observation has not been followed up in more recent studies of the condition, which have all focused on analysis at the DNA level.

The heterozygous state with β thalassaemia

This disorder has been well characterized by Fessas and Stamatoyannopoulos (1964), Sofroniadou *et al.* (1975), Clegg *et al.* (1979), Gelinas *et al.* (1985), Collins *et al.* (1985), Ottolenghi *et al.* (1988) and Pistidda *et al.* (1997). The association does not cause a symptomatic clinical disorder. In each case the body habitus and facies have been normal although there is usually slight pallor, icterus and splenomegaly. X-rays of the bones have revealed mild osteoporosis in a few cases but no changes compatible with the more severe form of β thalassaemia.

There is usually a mild anaemia, with haemoglobin values in the 9–11 g/dl range. The red cells show typical thalassaemic indices, with reduced MCV and MCH values in the 58–70 fl and 19-21 pg range, respectively, and abnormalities of shape and size with marked hypochromia. Fetal haemoglobin levels range from 25 to 45% with a mean value of approximately 30%. The HbA_2 values are nearly always elevated, in the range 3.8–5.2%. Fetal haemoglobin appears to be present in most of the red cells although there is considerable variation in the amount from cell to cell. This observation has been confirmed by differential centrifugation studies (Sofroniadou *et al.* 1975; Clegg *et al.* 1979). For example, in the experiments reported by Clegg *et al.* (1979) the amount of HbF in the younger, lighter cell populations ranged from 24 to 36% (5.1–7.0 pg per cell), while in the older, more dense, cell populations HbF values ranged from 46.5 to 57% (8.7–10.7 pg per cell). These observations indicate that there is heterogeneity of distribution of HbF in this disorder and that the red cells which contain relatively more fetal haemoglobin survive longer, either in the bone marrow or in the peripheral blood (or in both sites).

In the haemoglobin synthesis studies of Sofroniadou *et al.* (1975) and Clegg *et al.* (1979) the α/non-α chain ratios in five Greek HPFH/β-thalassaemia compound heterozygotes ranged from 1.6 to 3.4. These results indicate that there is a significant degree of globin imbalance, with an excess α-chain production slightly greater than that observed in β-thalassaemia heterozygotes. This finding was confirmed by Sofroniadou *et al.* (1975), who found that there was a pool of free α chains of similar magnitude to that found in β-thalassaemia heterozygotes.

The HbF has been examined chemically by Huisman *et al.* (1970b) and Clegg *et al.* (1979) with comparable results. The glycine composition of peptide γCB3 ranged from 0.22 to 0.33 in Huisman and colleagues' study and 0.28-0.32 in Clegg and colleagues' study. These findings indicate that there is a significantly higher proportion of $^G\gamma$ chains in compound heterozygotes as compared with the simple heterozygotes. Similar results were obtained in a single patient studied by Sofroniadou *et al.* (1975).

Sofroniadou and Clegg and their colleagues also examined the structure of HbF after the red cells had been separated into young and old fractions by centrifugation. This was done to see if the older HbF-rich population, which would be expected to contain HbF derived largely from the chromosome carrying the β-thalassaemia gene, might be richer in $^G\gamma$ chains. Surprisingly, this was not the case, and the $^G\gamma/^A\gamma$ ratios were almost identical between young and old cells in both studies.

These findings raise some important questions about the consequences of the interaction of $^A\gamma\beta^+$ HPFH and β thalassaemia. They suggest, in effect, that in these compound heterozygotes the factors that determine the amount of γ-chain production per cell act in *cis* and *trans*, i.e. on both homologous chromosomes, to maintain the same $^G\gamma/^A\gamma$ ratio whether there is 5 or 10 pg HbF per cell. Clearly there are several complex interacting factors responsible for the levels and distribution of HbF in the different $^A\gamma\beta^+$ HPFH genotypes (Clegg *et al.* 1979).

Genetics

Compound heterozygotes for Greek/Sardinian $^A\gamma\beta^+$ HPFH and β thalassaemia result from matings between HPFH heterozygotes and β thalassaemics. Of children studied from matings with normal individuals (Fessas & Stamatoyannopoulos 1964; Huisman *et al.* 1970b; Sofroniadou *et al.* 1975), eight were HPFH heterozygotes and four were β-thalassaemia heterozygotes, the type of segregation

that is expected now that it is established than this HPFH determinant results from a mutation within the γ–δ–β gene complex.

British $^A\gamma\beta^+$ HPFH ($^A\gamma$ –198 T→C)

Both homozygotes and heterozygotes for this condition were reported in a large British family by Weatherall *et al.* (1975) and the underlying mutation in the promoter region of the $^A\gamma$ genes was characterized by Tate *et al.* (1986). Further families with this condition were identified by Donald *et al.* (1988) and Harvey *et al.* (1992). Family P of Huisman *et al.* (1970a) was later shown to have the same mutation (Yang *et al.* 1988).

Homozygous state

Three homozygotes were identified in the original family reported by Weatherall *et al.* (1975). They had approximately twice the level of HbF of their heterozygous relatives and all their four children, born of matings with normal individuals, were HPFH heterozygotes. Their haematological findings were completely normal. Haemoglobin F values were 19.4%, 19.6% and 20.4%, respectively (Fig. 10.10). There was a slight but significant reduction in the percentage HbA_2 values. When these figures are converted to absolute values, that is, pg/cell, it is clear that they have a significant reduction in their output of HbA_2, with a mean of 0.4 pg as compared with the normal of 0.75 pg.

Heterozygous state

Thirty-four heterozygotes have been identified for this condition in three families. There are no haematological abnormalities and the mean HbF level is 6.9%, with a mean HbA_2 value of 2.5%.

Weatherall *et al.* (1975) carried out a carefully controlled series of experiments to analyse the cellular distribution of HbF in this condition (Fig. 10.11). Surprisingly, it is quite uneven, i.e. heterocellular; there was a marked difference between acid elution preparations from both homozygotes and heterozygotes in this family and artificial mixtures of cord blood and adult cells. This was confirmed by immunofluorescence (Boyer *et al.* 1977; Wood *et al.* 1982a), which demonstrated a significant correlation between percentage HbF as F cells ($r=0.94$).

(a)

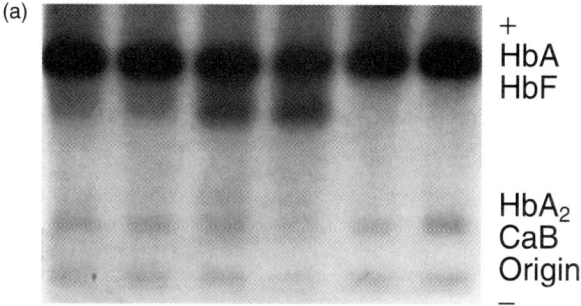

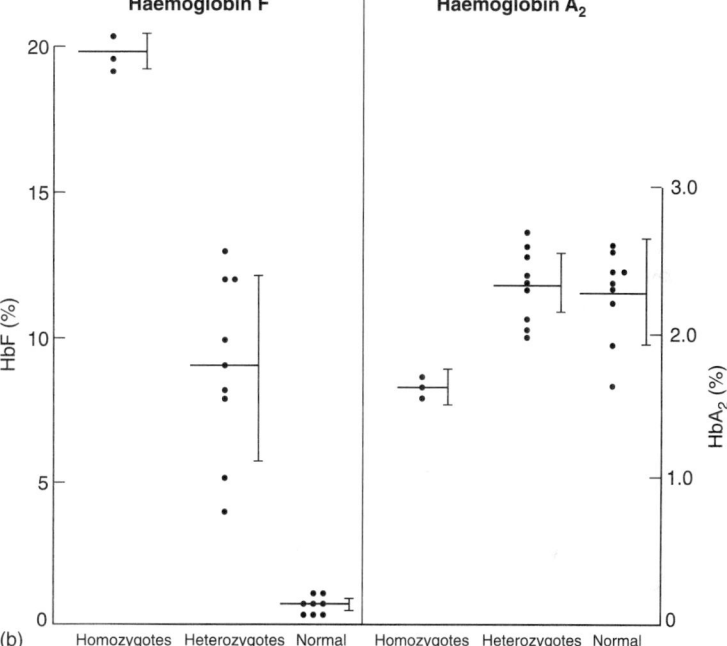

Fig. 10.10 The British form of $^A\gamma\beta^+$ hereditary persistence of fetal haemoglobin. (a) Starch gel electrophoresis (pH 8.5, amido black stain) of the following, left to right: 1 and 2, British HPFH heterozygotes; 3 and 4, British HPFH homozygotes; 5 and 6, normals. (b) HbF and HbA$_2$ levels in homozygotes, heterozygotes and normals.

Compound heterozygous state with β thalassaemia

This interaction produces a clinical phenotype that is very little different from that of the carrier state for β thalassaemia alone. However, the HbF level is elevated at approximately 8%; nearly 100% is of the $^A\gamma$ variety (Donald *et al*. 1988).

Mechanism of action of the hereditary persistence of fetal haemoglobin determinant

It was possible to study the pattern of $^G\gamma$- and $^A\gamma$-globin chain production in two offspring of one of the homozygotes in the original British family (Wood *et al*. 1982a). The HbF levels in cord bloods were within the normal range, as was the $^G\gamma/^A\gamma$ ratio, suggesting that the –198 $^A\gamma$ mutation has little effect when the γ-globin genes are operating maximally in fetal life. On the other hand, the postnatal decline in HbF output was slower than in normal infants and was accompanied by a sharp fall in the $^G\gamma/^A\gamma$ ratio.

Black $^A\gamma\beta^+$ HPFH ($^A\gamma$–202 C→T)

The phenotypic effects of this mutation were characterized in a single Afro-American family by Hattori *et al*. (1986) and Gilman *et al*. (1988a). There were no haematological abnormalities; the condition was

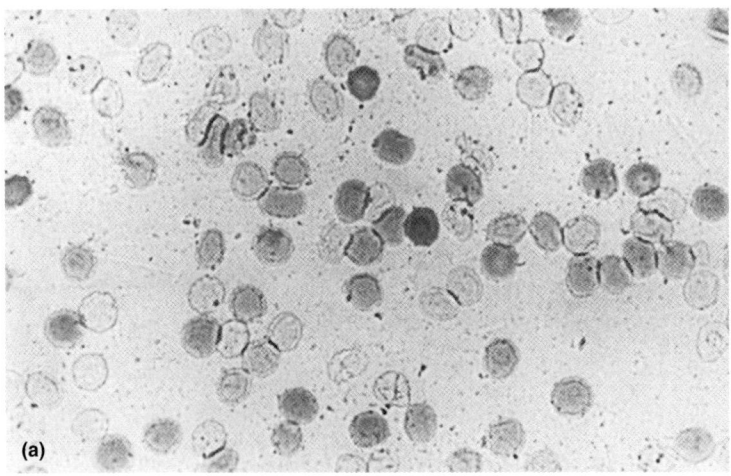

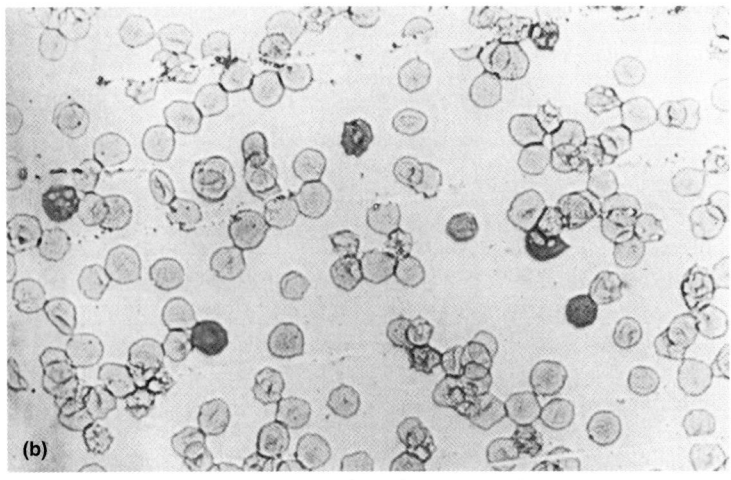

Fig. 10.11 An acid elution preparation showing heterogeneous distribution of HbF in British hereditary persistence of fetal haemoglobin. (a) Homozygote; (b) heterozygote.

found in individuals with the sickle-cell trait. Haemoglobin F values ranged from 1.6 to 3.9%; HbA$_2$ values were normal.

Italian/Chinese $^A\gamma\beta^+$ HPFH (−196 C→T)

This condition has been observed in several Italian families and in one Chinese family (Giglioni *et al.* 1984; Gelinas *et al.* 1986; Yang *et al.* 1988). There are no haematological abnormalities and the HbF values in heterozygotes range from 12 to 16%. In two Italian patients this mutation has been found in *trans* to a β-thalassaemia gene, resulting in HbF levels of 21.7 and 23.4%. The clinical picture was one of mild anaemia with slight enlargement of the spleen (Camaschella *et al.* 1979). Haemoglobin A$_2$ values are normal.

The mutation has also been found on the same chromosome as a severe β^0-thalassaemia allele (CD39 C→T) (see Sardinian δβ thalassaemia, Chapter 8). This association produces a mild form of thalassaemia intermedia with HbF values of approximately 40%, and elevated HbA$_2$ levels of approximately 4%.

Brazilian $^A\gamma\beta^+$ HPFH ($^A\gamma$−195 C→G)

This condition has been observed in a single Brazilian family of European descent (Costa *et al.* 1990). There were no haematological abnormalities and the HbF values in three heterozygotes ranged from 4.5 to 7.0%. The HbA$_2$ values were normal.

Black $^A\gamma\beta^+$ HPFH ($^A\gamma$ –175 T→C)

This mutation has been observed in Afro-American families (Stoming *et al.* 1989; Coleman *et al.* 1993). There appear to be no haematological abnormalities in heterozygotes, in whom HbF levels range from 36% to 38%. When found in combination with Hbs S and C the HbF values were 37.3 and 40.4%, the HbA$_2$ values 1.6 and 1.9%, and HbS and C values 41 and 45.4%, respectively. Interestingly, these individuals, who appeared to be both clinically and haematologically normal, had significant levels of $^G\gamma$ chains, ranging from 18.1 to 38% of the total γ-chain output. Coleman *et al.* (1993) explained this finding by the presence of the additional $^G\gamma$ –158 C→T mutation, which has been associated with elevated $^G\gamma$-chain production in adult life in response to stress. They go further, and propose calling this constellation of linked mutations $^G\gamma^A\gamma\beta^+$ forms of HPFH (see below).

Black $^A\gamma\beta^+$ HPFH ($^A\gamma$ –114 to –102 deletion)

The single report of the discovery of this mutation (Gilman *et al.* 1988b) describes its interaction with HbS in two individuals in an Afro-American family. No clinical or haematological details are given. The HbF values were 31.8 and 30.1%, and the HbA$_2$ values were both 2.1%. Haemoglobin S was estimated to be approximately 44 and 47%, and $^A\gamma$ chains constituted 80–90% of the fetal haemoglobin. Each of these individuals produced HbA, at a level of 21 and 20%, respectively.

Georgia $^A\gamma\beta^+$ HPFH ($^A\gamma$ –114 C→T)

This condition has been reported in one Afro-American family from Georgia (USA) (Öner *et al.* 1991b). There are no haematological abnormalities in the two heterozygotes. The HbF values are elevated at 4.7 and 4.8%, with a major preponderance of $^A\gamma$ chains. The HbA$_2$ levels are in the normal range. The cellular distribution of HbF is not reported.

$^G\gamma^A\gamma\beta^+$ HPFH

As mentioned above, the form of $^A\gamma\beta^+$ HPFH that results from a T→C substitution at $^A\gamma$ –175 is associated with unusually high levels of HbF, in either heterozygotes or compound heterozygotes with Hbs

S and C. One possible explanation for this observation, suggested by Coleman *et al.* (1993), is that this mutation is also found on a chromosome with the –158 C→T polymorphism, which has been associated with elevated $^G\gamma$-chain production in adult life, although usually in response to stress. However, heterozygotes for this condition have, unlike other forms of $^A\gamma\beta^+$ HPFH, between 18 and 38% $^G\gamma$ chains. Thus, strictly speaking, this is a form of $^G\gamma^A\gamma\beta^+$ HPFH, although whether these observations can be ascribed entirely to the presence of the polymorphism at $^G\gamma$ –158 is not clear. The position will only be clarified when this particular $^A\gamma$ promoter mutation is found on a chromosome without the $^G\gamma$ –158 polymorphism. It should be noted, however, that in most forms of $^A\gamma\beta^+$ HPFH, with the exception of the Brazilian and Georgian forms, which have not been evaluated in this way, the –158 C→T change is not present on the linked $^G\gamma$ gene.

Other inherited conditions associated with increased haemoglobin F in adults

In addition to the reasonably well defined forms of HPFH described in the previous sections, in which the pattern of inheritance is clear-cut, there is an extremely heterogeneous group of conditions in which there appears to be a genetically determined increase in HbF production in adult life. In most cases they are characterized by only a modest increase, rarely above 5% of the total haemoglobin, and, in themselves, are of no clinical importance. However, there is evidence that they may play a significant role in modifying the phenotype of β thalassaemia or sickle-cell anaemia, and hence they are of relevance to the thalassaemia field.

Although these conditions are frequently lumped together as 'Swiss HPFH', so named after the original report of Marti (1963), or heterocellular HPFH, since in most cases the distribution of HbF is quite uneven among the red cells (Boyer *et al.* 1975), in truth these terms are not of great value in trying to define or dissect out this mixed group of conditions. However, for the want of anything better, we shall use 'heterocellular HPFH' throughout this section, though simply as a descriptive term. What is known of the molecular pathology of these conditions is summarized in Chapter 4. They are listed in Table 10.7.

Table 10.7 Summary of different forms of heterocellular HPFH or other possible genetic causes of an increased propensity for haemoglobin F production in children and adults.

Structural changes within the β-globin-gene cluster
Seattle HPFH
Czech HPFH
$C \rightarrow T - 158\,^{G}\gamma$
$C \rightarrow T - 158\,^{G}\gamma\,C \rightarrow T - 158\,^{A}\gamma$ (Cretan HPFH)
$A \rightarrow G - 161\,^{G}\gamma$

γ-Globin gene rearrangements
Atlanta HPFH $^{G}\gamma\text{-}^{G}\gamma/C \rightarrow T - 158\,^{G}\gamma$
$^{G}\gamma\text{-}^{G}\gamma\text{-}^{A}\gamma/C \rightarrow T - 158\,^{G}\gamma$
$^{G}\gamma\text{-}^{G}\gamma\text{-}^{G}\gamma\text{-}^{A}\gamma$

Unlinked to the β-globin-gene cluster
FC locus on Xp22.2
Locus at 6q.23
Others

The development of knowledge about the inheritance of haemoglobin F in normal adults, and its relationship to heterocellular hereditary persistence of fetal haemoglobin

Every study of the level of HbF, or HbF-containing cells (F cells), in adult life has shown a skewed distribution, with a varying though small proportion of values above the arbitrary cut-off point for the normal level of HbF, approximately 1% (see Chapter 2). The skew to a higher level is more marked during the first year of life and in most studies there has been a clear tendency for the values in females to be skewed further to the right than those in males. Clearly, from a mechanistic viewpoint it is important to determine whether this difference between the sexes is present throughout development or only appears at puberty. Information on this fundamental question is rather limited. Rutland *et al.* (1983) showed that there was a slightly higher fetal haemoglobin level in females than males throughout life. Similarly, Mason *et al.* (1982) observed higher levels of HbF in females than males aged 1–6 years in normal controls, but not in patients with sickle-cell anaemia.

There seems little doubt that the level of HbF or the number of F cells during later development is under genetic control. In the study of Zago *et al.* (1979), of 750 samples from normal blood donors, six (0.8%) had HbF levels in excess of 1.1%, which put them at the upper end of the continuous distribution curve for adult values. In each case there was a significantly elevated number of F cells. There was a good correlation between the percentage HbF and the number of F cells, indicating that the increased amount of HbF could be ascribed entirely to the higher numbers of F cells which are produced. In other words, this form of 'HPFH' is characterized by an increase in F-cell numbers and the F cells contain about the same amount of HbF, approximately 3 pg, as they do in normal adults. These persons had no haematological abnormalities, and although the $^{G}\gamma/^{A}\gamma$ composition of the HbF was variable, both types of chains were always present. In these studies, and in the earlier studies of Marti and colleagues, there was a tendency for one or other parent of individuals with high values for HbF or F cells to have increased levels, although these observations did not fall into any clear-cut pattern of genetic transmission. Recently, extensive twin studies have shown that the relative numbers of F cells has a strong genetic component (Garner *et al.* 2000).

There have been several attempts to establish the chromosomal location of the genetic control of F cells and, by inference, the form of heterocellular HPFH characterized by values outside the normal range. For example, a study of HbF levels in healthy Japanese adults suggested that the high-normal F-cell or HbF-level phenotype might be an X-linked trait, 11% of males and 21% of females being carriers (Miyoshi *et al.* 1988).

The possibility of there being a regulatory locus for HbF or F-cell production on the X chromosome has been explored further in an extensive series of studies by Dover and colleagues. By analysis of the relative numbers of F cells and F reticulocytes (reticulocytes that contain HbF) in individuals with the sickle-cell trait, they were able to divide males into two phenotypes for F reticulocytes: low, less than 12%; and high, greater than 12%. On the other hand, in females three phenotypes were observed: low, less than 12%; high, 12–24%; and very high, greater than 24%. Using segregation analysis based on these phenotypes a putative locus has been identified at Xp22.2, which may be involved in the regulation of F-cell production and hence has been called the FC locus (Dover *et al.* 1992). This work, and its relationship to the Japanese studies quoted earlier, remains to be confirmed. It will be extremely interesting to determine the nature of this particular locus.

In short, therefore, there is considerable evidence that the levels of HbF and F cells in apparently normal adults are under genetic control and that there is, in every normal population studied, a small group of individuals with significantly higher levels of HbF or F cells (Fig. 10.10). Currently, the site of the genetic locus, or loci, involved in the control of F cells in this form of heterocellular HPFH is uncertain.

Further reports of heterocellular hereditary persistence of fetal haemoglobin

As well as Marti's original survey of Swiss army recruits there have been many reports of families in which a gene for heterocellular HPFH is segregating. Betke (1960) described seven affected adults with HbF values ranging from 1.2 to 6.2%. Pedigrees with slightly elevated levels of HbF in adults were reported by Horton *et al.* (1965) and Pawlack and Kozlowska (1970); the increased levels of HbF appeared to follow an autosomal dominant pattern of inheritance. Similar findings were reported by Ohta *et al.* (1971a), Pembrey *et al.* (1973) and Knox-Macaulay *et al.* (1973). In one of these studies it was shown that globin synthesis was balanced and that both $^G\gamma$ and $^A\gamma$ chains were present in the HbF (Pembrey *et al.* 1973). Boyer *et al.* (1977) reported a small-scale survey of F-cell values in normal adults and noted that the individuals with the highest numbers had family members with similar values. A further series of families in which more than one member have slightly elevated levels of HbF is reported by Huisman (1997).

There is abundant evidence therefore that families with slightly increased levels of HbF are encountered quite commonly; because the levels are not high, and overlap with the normal, it has been extremely difficult to study the genetic transmission and the possible relevance to the genetic control of HbF and F-cell production in normal individuals. One approach to this problem has been to examine the interaction of these forms of heterocellular HPFH with the β-chain disorders. Some of these conditions were touched on earlier, in Chapters 2, 4, 7 and 9.

Heterocellular hereditary persistence of fetal haemoglobin with β-globin disorders

The association of heterocellular HPFH with HbS or β thalassaemia has been reported in many families (Knox-Macaulay *et al.* 1973; Makler *et al.* 1974; Martinez & Colombo 1974; Stamatoyannopoulos *et al.* 1975; Wood *et al.* 1975; Altay *et al.* 1976-77; Wood *et al.* 1977b; Cappellini *et al.* 1981; Gianni *et al.* 1983; Giampaolo *et al.* 1984b; Martinez *et al.* 1989; Thein & Weatherall 1989). Typical family pedigrees are shown in Fig. 10.12.

In all these families there are normal individuals with slightly elevated levels of HbF in the 2–3% range. Offspring of persons who have received a β-thalassaemia gene together with this type of HPFH from one or other parent produce considerably higher levels of HbF than are usually observed in β-thalassaemia heterozygotes. Furthermore, individuals with the sickle-cell trait with slightly elevated levels of HbF, presumably due to the action of this gene, may have children with sickle-cell anaemia or sickle-cell thalassaemia with unusually high levels of HbF, often in the 16–25% range.

Genetic analyses of these family pedigrees leave little doubt that there is interaction between this form of HPFH and β thalassaemia. Such interactions were studied in detail by Wood *et al.* (1976b, 1977b) and Cappellini *et al.* (1981). The HbF per F cell in the HPFH heterozygotes appears to be normal and hence, as mentioned earlier, the condition is characterized by an increased number of F cells rather than an increased production of HbF per F cell. While there is no evidence for selective survival of F cells in normal individuals, heterozygotes for both heterocellular HPFH and β thalassaemia have increased numbers of F cells in their older cell populations. Hence it appears that the unusually high level of HbF in compound heterozygotes is the direct result of globin imbalance caused by the β-thalassaemia gene. This leads to selection of F cells, since those red-cell precursors that synthesize relatively more γ chains will have relatively less globin imbalance. This implies that heterozygous β thalassaemics with this form of HPFH have a larger F-cell pool for selection to act on and hence produce relatively more HbF. A mechanism of this type would tend to favour F cells with relatively large amounts of HbF; in fact the amount of HbF per F cell is increased in these compound heterozygotes.

There is also interaction of heterocellular HPFH with HbS. In these families sickle-cell carriers with 2–3% HbF have children with sickle-cell anaemia with HbF values in the 19–30% range. These individuals also have an increased amount of HbF per F cell.

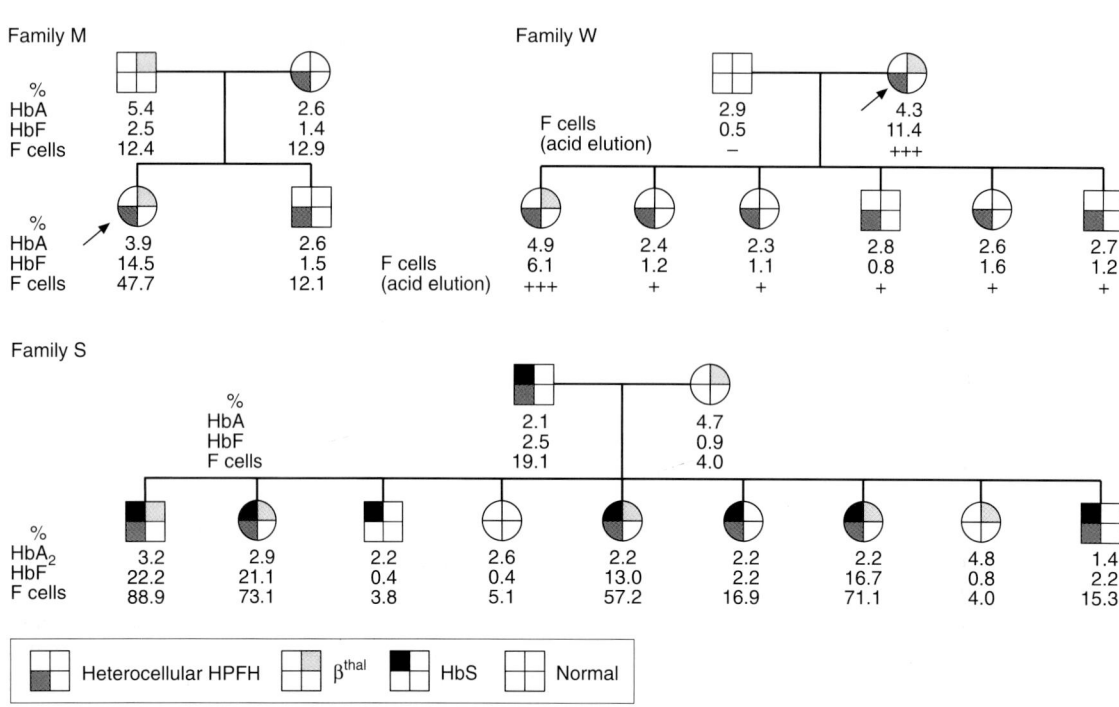

Fig. 10.12 Three pedigrees showing the interactions of heterocellular hereditary persistence of fetal haemoglobin with either β thalassaemia or HbS. From Wood *et al.* (1976b).

Since it is well known that there is selection of F cells in the sickling disorders it seems likely that either F cells with relatively high levels of HbF are preferentially selected or that there is interaction between the sickle-cell (and for that matter β-thalassaemia) genes and heterocellular HPFH which results in an increased number of F cells as well as an increased amount of HbF per F cell. In an attempt to test the notion that patients with sickle-cell anaemia who have unusually high levels of HbF have inherited an HPFH gene, Serjeant *et al.* (1977) examined HbF values in the parents of 16 patients with sickle-cell anaemia with HbF levels greater than 10% which persisted beyond the age of 10 years. They found significantly elevated values in one or other parent of 14 of the 16 patients and in only two cases were HbF values normal in both parents.

The interaction of sickle-cell β thalassaemia and heterocellular HPFH is shown in Fig. 10.12, taken from the studies of Wood *et al.* (1976b, 1977b). Again it is quite clear that individuals who inherited an HPFH gene had considerably higher levels of HbF than is usually found in sickle-cell β thalassaemia in

African populations. Similarly, in the family reported by Makler *et al.* (1974) it was found that, in individuals with HbSC disease in whom there was evidence for a co-existent heterocellular HPFH gene, the level of HbF is greater than that usually seen in HbSC disease.

Genetics and further characterization of heterocellular hereditary persistence of fetal haemoglobin

As pointed out earlier, the levels of HbF in the normal population and in those who appear to have heterocellular HPFH form a continuum. Therefore it is very difficult to be absolutely certain about the designation of any particular family member; when levels of HbF are in the 2–3% range it is relatively easy to trace the gene through a family, but it is never certain whether critical family members might have lower levels and hence how they should be categorized.

The earlier studies of Swiss HPFH suggested an autosomal dominant form of inheritance. By combining published pedigrees Wood *et al.* (1976b) attempted to analyse linkage relationships between β thalassaemia or HbS and heterocellular HPFH. Although a number of putative recombinants were observed the data suggested, albeit tentatively, that at least in some families the determinant may be close to the β-globin-gene complex. However, later studies suggested that there is genetic heterogeneity, and several families were described in which this phenotype clearly segregates independently from the β-globin-gene cluster (Gianni *et al.* 1983; Giampaolo *et al.* 1984b; Martinez *et al.* 1989; Thein & Weatherall 1989).

Studies over recent years leave little doubt about the remarkable heterogeneity that underlies the term 'heterocellular HPFH'. It is clear that there are varieties that are encoded within or near to the β-globin-gene cluster and there is now unequivocal evidence that there are other forms which are determined by genes which are not part of this cluster.

Heterocellular hereditary persistence of fetal haemoglobin due to determinants in the β-globin-gene cluster (Table 10.7)

Several families have been described in which a small increase in the level of HbF is inherited in a pattern that suggests that its determinant is within the β-globin-gene cluster.

In the *Atlanta* variety of heterocellular HPFH, levels of HbF in the 2–4% range, with a high proportion of $^G\gamma$ chains, are found (Altay *et al.* 1976–77). Molecular studies indicate that in these individuals the usual $^G\gamma$–$^A\gamma$ gene arrangement is changed to $^G\gamma$–$^G\gamma$, each of which carries the T→C mutation at position −158 which is thought to increase the propensity for fetal haemoglobin production, at least in conditions of erythroid stress (Gilman *et al.* 1984).

In the *Czech* form of heterocellular HPFH, possibly something of a misnomer because the HbF value in heterozygotes is normal, the fetal haemoglobin is nearly all of the $^G\gamma$ variety, presumably resulting from an underlying A→C change at $^G\gamma$ −110. When this mutation is found in the compound heterozygous state with β⁰ thalassaemia the clinical picture is identical to β-thalassaemia trait with an HbF value of 3.1%, again nearly all of the $^G\gamma$ variety.

In the so-called *Cretan* type of HPFH, three unrelated adults were observed with slightly increased HbF levels of 2.9, 3.1 and 5.1%. All three carried a

C→T substitution at position −158 of the $^A\gamma$ gene in *cis* to the common $^G\gamma$ −158 C→T change, presumably as a result of gene conversion. The $^G\gamma$/$^A\gamma$ ratios ranged from 49 to 66% $^G\gamma$. None of 180 normal individuals had this mutation. It would appear therefore that the effect of these combined substitutions in *cis* causes small overall increases in HbF (Patrinos *et al.* 1998).

In the *Seattle* form of heterocellular HPFH, two individuals with sickle-cell trait were found to have unusually high levels of HbF, 3–8%, with almost equal numbers of $^G\gamma$ and $^A\gamma$ chains. In addition there was a relative with sickle-cell disease and 20% fetal haemoglobin (Stamatoyannopoulos *et al.* 1975). Sequencing of the γ-chain promoters failed to identify any abnormality (Gelinas *et al.* 1988). Evidence for linkage to the β-gene cluster is not very strong in this case. In a similar family, in which individuals with the sickle-cell trait had raised HbF and those with sickle-cell β thalassaemia carried between 13 and 22%, the increased HbF levels may have been due to the β^S gene being carried on an Asian RFLP haplotype bearing the *Xmn*I site at $^G\gamma$ −158 (Old *et al.* 1982a).

The role of the C→T change at $^G\gamma$ −158 in families with slightly elevated levels of fetal haemoglobin in adult life is unclear. It has been implicated as a possible cause in some cases (Efremov *et al.* 1987; Sampietro *et al.* 1992). However, this is not a consistent finding, the substitution is not present in all affected family members and, conversely, it is found in some individuals with normal HbF levels (Economou *et al.* 1991). As a group, otherwise normal individuals with this polymorphism have a significantly higher level of F cells than those who do not, but there is a major overlap between them (Sampietro *et al.* 1992).

In short, it is likely that the $^G\gamma$ −158 C→T change predisposes towards increased HbF production in adult life, particularly in conditions of erythroid stress, but, alone, it does not always produce increased levels of HbF. Interestingly, a G→A substitution at −161 5′ to the $^G\gamma$ gene is also associated with high proportions of $^G\gamma$-chain production and slightly elevated levels of HbF, in the 1–2% range (Gilman 1987). There is also evidence that triplication of the γ-globin genes may, under certain circumstances, be associated with a slight elevation of HbF in adult life. For example, the arrangement $^G\gamma$–$^G\gamma$–$^A\gamma$ appears to result in levels of HbF in the 3–6% range provided that the C→T mutation at γ−158 is present in both $^G\gamma$ genes (Efremov *et al.* 1986a). A few individuals have been identified in which there is quadruplication or quintruplication of the γ-globin genes. Although this has been found in association with a mild elevation of fetal haemoglobin, the affected individuals have had a β-thalassaemia mutation on the same chromosome and hence it is difficult to determine the significance of this observation (Yang *et al.* 1986). The rearrangements or duplications of the γ-globin genes associated with heterocellular HPFH are summarized in Table 10.7.

Heterocellular hereditary persistence of fetal haemoglobin not linked to the β-globin-gene cluster

There is now strong evidence that at least some forms of heterocellular HPFH are determined at loci that are not part of the β-globin-gene cluster. Over recent years there have been intensive studies in the authors' laboratory on an extremely large kindred in which the genes for β thalassaemia and a form of heterocellular HPFH are segregating (Thein & Weatherall 1989; Thein *et al.* 1994; Craig *et al.* 1996). By a variety of statistical treatments it was possible to exclude β thalassaemia or the C→T polymorphism at position γ–158 as the major factors in the elevation of HbF in this family, and a third determinant for HbF production was defined on chromosome 6. By extensive linkage analyses using minisatellite and other markers this locus has been further localized to a region on chromosome 6q23, with a lod score of over 13.

By using the same approach it has been possible to study other extensive pedigrees with heterocellular HPFH. In these families there has been no evidence for linkage of HPFH to chromosome 6 and therefore it is clear that there must be further heterogeneity of this condition; the chromosomal location of the determinants is yet to be determined (Craig *et al.* 1997).

The FC locus on the X chromosome, described earlier, while it may modify the numbers of F cells, has not been directly related to the genesis of heterocellular HPFH.

Variation in haemoglobin F production in sickle-cell anaemia and β thalassaemia

Another approach to searching for putative determinants for heterocellular HPFH is to analyse the variability in the levels of HbF that are produced in

sickle-cell anaemia or β thalassaemia. Although, as mentioned earlier, family studies have shown quite unequivocally that there is interaction between heterocellular HPFH and these β-chain haemoglobinopathies, a great deal of work has been done over recent years to try to further define the genetic factors that are involved in setting the level of HbF in these conditions. Progress in this extremely complex field is discussed in Chapter 2 and is summarized by Wood (1993).

It is well established that there are considerable differences in the mean HbF levels in patients with sickle-cell anaemia from different parts of the world, even though there is a wide range in all populations. In those of African origin the level ranges between 5 and 10% (Serjeant 1985), while in India the mean is about 17% (Kulozik *et al.* 1987a) and in eastern Saudi Arabia it is 20%, or greater (Perrine *et al.* 1972; Pembrey *et al.* 1978) (Fig. 10.12). One approach to determining the basis for this variability has involved the analysis of the β-globin-gene cluster RFLP haplotypes and, more recently, the γ-globin-gene promoter sequences. The β^S mutation has arisen independently at least twice, and possibly more often, on different β-haplotype backgrounds (Wainscoat *et al.* 1983c; Antonarakis *et al.* 1984; Pagnier *et al.* 1984; Chebloune *et al.* 1988; Flint *et al.* 1998) (see Chapter 6). It is commonly found on five different haplotypes, two of which, the Senegal and Arab/Indian, are closely related.

An association between a β-globin-gene cluster and a high proportion of ^Gγ chains was noted by Gilman *et al.* (1984) and then, as mentioned earlier in this chapter, shown to be related to the polymorphism for the enzyme *Xmn* I at position –158 (Gilman & Huisman 1985). Analysis of fetal haemoglobin levels in patients with sickle-cell anaemia of different haplotypes has shown that those containing the Arab/Indian and Senegal haplotypes have significantly higher HbF levels than the others. Both these contain the C→T substitution at position –158, yet those with the Arab/Indian haplotype have considerably higher levels of HbF than those with the Senegal haplotype. Thus while a C→T substitution at –158 may contribute to higher levels of fetal haemoglobin production in sickle-cell anaemia it cannot be the only factor. However, sequence analysis of γ-globin-gene promoters has shown that this is the only difference between any of these haplotypes in at least 300 nucleotides upstream from the messenger

RNA CAP site (Miller *et al.* 1987). Furthermore, in the Senegal and Arab/Indian haplotypes both γ genes are identical in their upstream regions up to –1200 as well as throughout the genes themselves (Lanclos *et al.* 1991).

The sickle-cell gene in Orissa, India, and in eastern Saudi Arabia is found almost exclusively on the same haplotype but it is not clear whether the higher levels of HbF found in patients with sickle-cell anaemia in these populations are due to other substitutions within the cluster or whether there are other factors involved. The fact that in Saudi Arabia the sickle-cell trait is associated with a significantly higher number of F cells than in African populations (Wood *et al.* 1980) (see Fig. 10.13) suggests that a determinant in the β-globin-gene cluster may be involved. Interestingly, it appears that one copy of the Arab/Indian or Senegal haplotype is sufficient to produce the relatively high levels of HbF in sickle-cell anaemia; that is, it is behaving as a dominant genotype.

Studies of HbF levels in β thalassaemia also point to the influence of the β-globin-gene haplotype. In analysing HbF production in β thalassaemia it is important to consider the underlying mutation before looking for other factors. For example, HbF levels tend to be higher in those alleles that are due to a deletion of the β-globin gene or a point mutation in its promoter. Slight differences in HbF levels in heterozygotes have been observed in different β-thalassaemia alleles (Kutlar *et al.* 1990), although this may be due to the influence of the haplotype on which the alleles occur (Gonzalez-Redondo *et al.* 1988a).

A minority of β^0-thalassaemia homozygotes run a mild course and at least some of them are homozygous or heterozygous for a haplotype closely related to the Asian/Senegal haplotypes seen in sickle-cell disease, that is, those which carry the –158 C→T substitution (Labie *et al.* 1985b; Thein *et al.* 1987b). It appears therefore that this mutation, while it has little effect in normal individuals or in β-thalassaemia heterozygotes, under the influence of more severe anaemia may play a role in substantially increasing HbF production to levels which may alleviate clinical severity. This cannot be the whole story, however. High fetal haemoglobin levels and a mild clinical course have also been observed in homozygotes for β-thalassaemia mutations on other haplotypes. While some of these have involved β-globin-gene promoters, which are known to be associated with higher levels of fetal haemoglobin

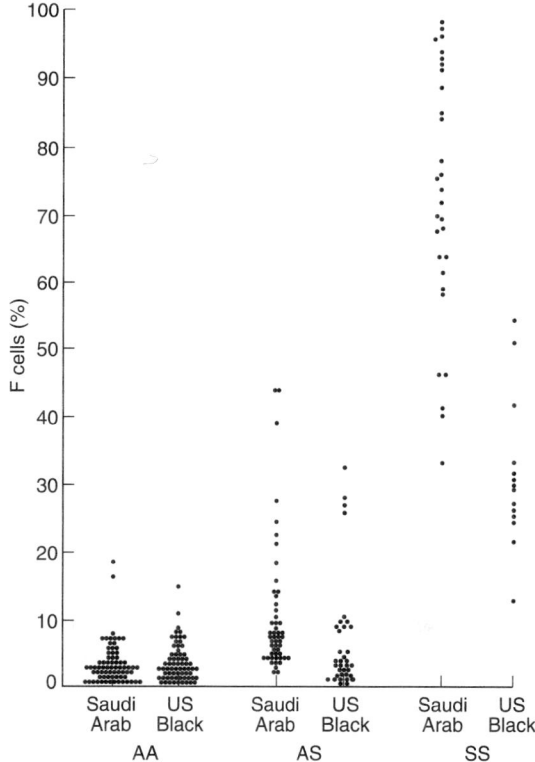

Fig. 10.13 Distribution of F-cell numbers in Saudi Arabian sickle-cell anaemia patients compared with those of Afro-Americans. Clearly there are a few normal individuals in both populations who have F-cell numbers significantly above the norm for the population. This is also well shown in the sickle-cell carriers. It is also clear that the baseline HbF production in the Saudi sickle-cell trait population is higher than that among Afro-Americans, reflecting the increased output of HbF in patients with sickle-cell anaemia in this group. Data from Pembrey *et al.* (1978).

production (Camaschella *et al.* 1990a), otherwise unexplained high levels of fetal haemoglobin production have also been found in patients with thalassaemia intermedia who are homozygous for more severe thalassaemia alleles (Ho *et al.* 1998a).

Because it has been clear for some time that there are still many cases of β thalassaemia and sickle-cell anaemia in which detailed studies failed to reveal the reasons for unusually elevated levels of HbF, further efforts have been made to identify alterations in the β-globin-gene cluster that might be responsible. The results of these studies have been summarized by Steinberg (1996), Labie and Elion (1996) and

Plonczynski *et al.* (1997). They have included extensive sequence analysis of hypersensitive (HS) sites 2 and 3 in the locus control region (LCR) and, in addition, of phylogenetically conserved sequences within the LCR but outside the cores of HS 2 and 3. However, they have not revealed any structural changes which can be unequivocally related to an increased propensity for γ-globin synthesis in the sickling disorders or β thalassaemia.

Comment

It is now apparent that HPFH constitutes an extremely heterogeneous group of conditions. But, as emphasized in Chapter 2, despite our detailed knowledge of the molecular basis of many of the different varieties, this information has shed very little light on the reasons for persistent γ-globin chain synthesis.

It is quite clear that the deletional forms of HPFH are very similar to, and form a continuum with, the δβ thalassaemias (Fig. 10.14). As shown in Fig. 10.15 there is a remarkable consistency in the composition of the HbF in the deletional forms of HPFH, though less in δβ thalassaemia. This may be because in the former the HbF is mainly the product of the affected chromosome, while in the latter, because of greater

chain imbalance, the output is from both chromosomes and there is selection of F cells. On the other hand, $^{G}\gamma\beta^{+}$ and $^{A}\gamma\beta^{+}$ HPFH do not show the features of thalassaemia, in that there is no associated globin imbalance. These conditions do show, however, the characteristic reciprocity between the γ- and β-globin chain loci, and undoubtedly the output of β chains from the loci *cis* to the determinants for these forms of HPFH is reduced. The other curious finding in these varieties of HPFH is that there is a remarkable variation in the intercellular distribution of HbF. Thus, while in some forms it is relatively homogeneous, in others, notably the British type, it is quite heterogeneous, a finding which cannot be explained entirely by the level of HbF. Although this characteristic has not been well defined in some reports, it is clear that within the same class of HPFH it is possible to find completely different cellular distributions of HbF.

The situation regarding the less well defined forms of heterocellular HPFH, and the mechanisms for unusually high production of HbF in β thalassaemia and sickle-cell anaemia, remains extremely complex and unsatisfactory. What the vast amount of work in this field seems to be telling us is that there are several, and perhaps many, genetic and acquired

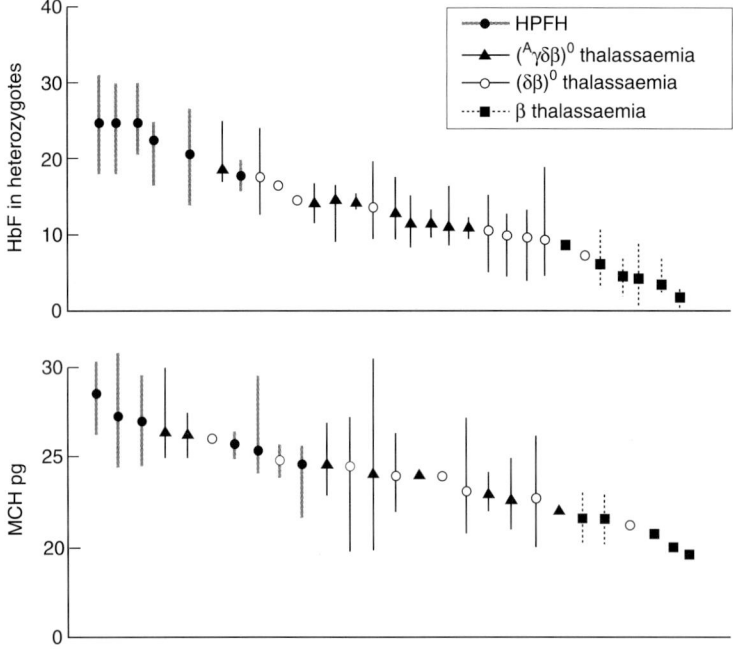

Fig. 10.14 Comparison of HbF and MCH values for different forms of thalassaemia and hereditary persistence of fetal haemoglobin. The data show the mean ±1 SD.

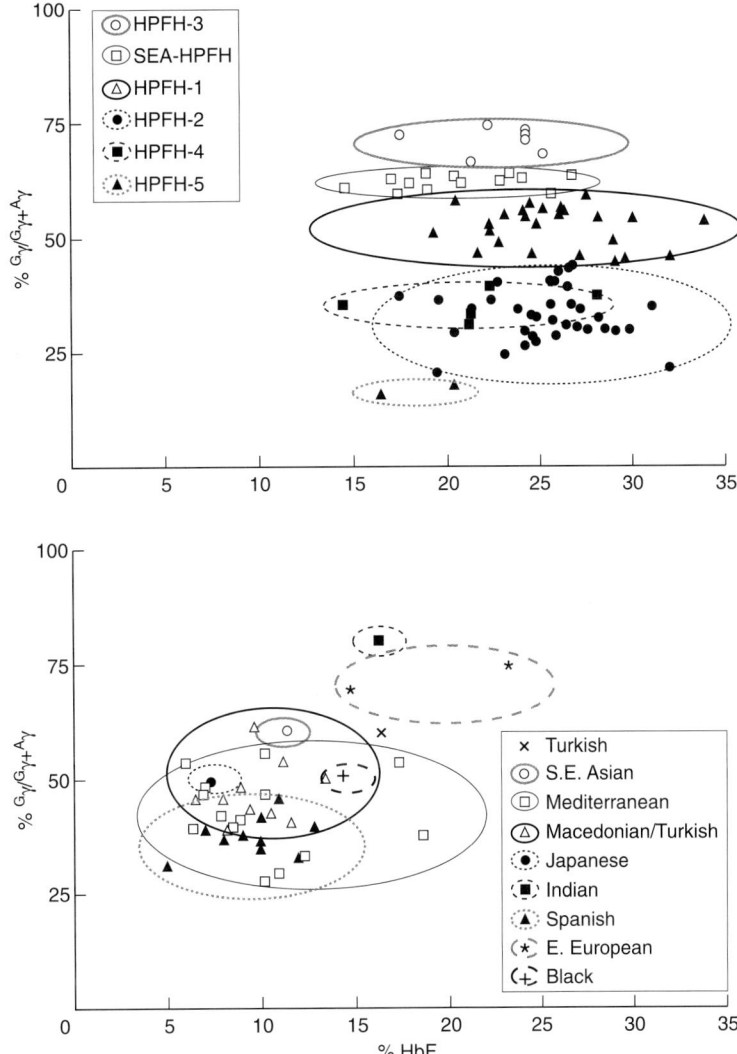

Fig. 10.15 Comparison of the $^{G}\gamma/^{A}\gamma$ composition of HbF in different types of hereditary persistence of fetal haemoglobin and δβ thalassaemia. The upper figure shows the data for HPFH, the lower the data for δβ thalassaemia.

factors that are involved in fine-tuning the level of HbF in adult life. And what is equally clear is that some of these still remain to be identified. It is important that work continues in this difficult area. We need to identify these loci and understand their mode of action, both for prognostic purposes and for the better understanding of the regulation of the switch from fetal to adult haemoglobin.

Chapter 11
The α thalassaemias and their interactions with structural haemoglobin variants

Introduction

The α thalassaemias are probably the commonest monogenic diseases; yet, because of the restricted distribution of their more severe forms, they pose a less serious global health problem than the β thalassaemias. However, even their milder alleles, which reach extremely high frequencies in some populations, are important. Because many of them result in varying degrees of hypochromic anaemia they are very frequently mistaken for iron deficiency, an error which can lead to an incorrect assessment of the nutritional status of a community. Furthermore, they may have quite profound effects on the phenotypes of different varieties of β thalassaemia, an issue to which we shall return in Chapter 13.

In previous editions of this book it was only possible to describe the clinical phenotypes of the α thalassaemias and to try to explain their remarkable diversity by making an educated guess about the nature of their underlying genotypes (see Chapter 1). Now that their molecular pathology has, at least to a large extent, been clarified, much of this uncertainty no longer remains. As described in Chapters 3 and 4, when we talk about α-thalassaemia alleles we are, in effect, describing haplotypes, that is, the state of the linked pair of α-globin genes on chromosome 16. As is the case for all the thalassaemias, the severity of the α thalassaemias is largely related to the degree of imbalanced globin production. There are potentially several hundred different interactions between the large number of α-thalassaemia alleles that have now been described. The spectrum of different clinical disorders that comprise the α thalassaemias correlates well with the number of affected α-globin genes, that is, from the normal complement, αα/αα, to the loss of all four, −−/−−.

As described in earlier chapters, there are two major classes of α thalassaemia, α^0 and α^+ thalassaemia. In α^0 thalassaemia both α-globin genes are inactivated, −−/, whereas in α^+ thalassaemia only one of the pair is defective, due either to a deletion ($-\alpha$),

or to another form of mutation ($\alpha^T\alpha$ or $\alpha\alpha^T$). As we shall see, there are several phenotypic differences reflecting a variation of output of α-globin genes from alleles which contain the $-\alpha$ as compared with the $\alpha^T\alpha$ or $\alpha\alpha^T$ determinants. But, overall, the α thalassaemias can be looked on as a spectrum of conditions that reflect gene dosage effects resulting from the loss of function of variable numbers of α-globin genes.

The important differences between the α and β thalassaemias are, as described in detail in Chapter 5, a reflection of the different properties of the particular globin that is produced in excess in the two conditions. Unlike the β thalassaemias, in which unbound α chains are unstable and precipitate in the red-cell precursors, the excess γ and β chains that are produced in the α thalassaemias form γ_4 or β_4 tetramers, Hbs Bart's and H, respectively. It is the functional properties of these homotetramers, together with their inherent instability, particularly in the case of HbH, that are the major determinants of the pathophysiology of all the α thalassaemias.

The different interactions of the better characterized α-thalassaemia alleles are summarized in Fig. 11.1. In this chapter we shall describe the associated clinical disorders. Readers who are new to the field should familiarize themselves with the main features of the pathophysiology of α thalassaemia, described in Chapter 5.

Haemoglobin Bart's hydrops fetalis syndrome

The combination of generalized oedema, ascites and pleural and pericardial effusions in a developing fetus that is encompassed by the term hydrops fetalis may occur in a wide variety of fetal and maternal disorders (Holzgreve *et al*. 1984; Nicolaides *et al*. 1985; Jauniaux *et al*. 1990; Arcasoy & Gallagher 1995). The predominant causes vary from one population to another. In the West, rhesus immunization used to be very common, but, with the widespread introduction

		αα	α⁺				α⁰	
			ααᵀ	-α	αᵀα	-αᵀ	(αα)	--
α⁰	--	T	H	H	H, Hy			Hy
	(αα)	T	H					
α⁺	-αᵀ	T		H	T	H		
	αᵀα	T		T	H			
	-α	T		T				
	ααᵀ	T						
	αα	N						

Fig. 11.1 Interactions producing the phenotype of α thalassaemia. Abbreviations: (αα), non-deletion α⁰ thalassaemia; --, deletion α⁰ thalassaemia; H, HbH disease; Hy, Hb Bart's hydrops fetalis syndrome; N, normal; T, α-thalassaemia trait.

of immunoprophylaxis and the decline in rhesus isoimmunization (Clarke & Whitfield 1977), 'non-immune' causes, including intrauterine infection, chromosomal abnormalities and congenital cardiac and renal defects, now account for 75% of cases (Machin 1981; Nicolaides *et al.* 1985). In south-east Asia, 60–90% of cases are caused by α thalassaemia, which leads to the Hb Bart's hydrops fetalis syndrome (Lie-Injo 1959a; Thumasathit *et al.* 1968; Liang *et al.* 1985; Tan *et al.* 1989; Ko *et al.* 1991).

Throughout south-east Asia, where the frequency of α⁰-thalassaemia trait (--/αα) is high (see Chapter 6), between 1/200 and 1/2000 infants inherit no functional α genes (--/--) from their parents. Since α-globin chains are normally produced throughout development, contributing to embryonic ($\alpha_2\epsilon_2$), fetal ($\alpha_2\gamma_2$) and adult ($\alpha_2\beta_2$) haemoglobins, they suffer from severe anaemia *in utero* which causes hypoxia, heart failure and, consequently, hydrops fetalis (Fig. 11.2). They produce large amounts of Hb Bart's (γ_4) and small amounts of the embryonic haemoglobin, Hb Portland ($\zeta_2\gamma_2$), which may allow sufficient tissue oxygenation for them to survive until the third trimester of pregnancy, at which time they are usually born prematurely and die.

Clinical and autopsy findings

Presentation

Following a gestation of about 33 weeks (range 23–43 weeks) infants with the Hb Bart's hydrops fetalis syndrome usually die *in utero*, during delivery or within an hour or two of birth (Thumasathit *et al.* 1968; Liang *et al.* 1985; Vaeusorn *et al.* 1985; Nakayama *et al.* 1986; Chui & Waye 1998). Occasionally, and even without

specific treatment, they survive for a few days (Israngkura *et al.* 1987).

Clinical features

Typically, these infants are pale, slightly jaundiced, growth retarded and oedematous (see Fig. 11.2). The skin may be affected by a 'blueberry muffin' rash caused by subcutaneous nodules of extramedullary haemopoiesis (Beutler *et al.* 1995). The abdomen is usually distended due to a combination of ascites and hepatosplenomegaly. An observation reported in some of the early descriptions of the disease (Wong 1966), and still unexplained, is that hepatomegaly is usually more marked than splenomegaly, a finding which is different from that in severe hydrops fetalis resulting from Rh or ABO blood-group incompatibility. In the series reported by Wong (1966) it was pointed out that most of these babies have low birth weights despite the added burden of accumulated oedema fluid. However, gross fluid overload of this kind is not invariable, and some of these infants are not severely hydropic (Chui & Waye 1998). The placenta is greatly enlarged and friable. In one study the placenta/fetal weight ratio ranged from 0.37 to 1.16 (mean 0.68), compared with the normal ratio of 0.15–0.25 (Liang *et al.* 1985).

Developmental abnormalities have been reported in up to 17% of cases (Guy *et al.* 1985; Liang *et al.* 1985; Nakayama *et al.* 1986). They include hydrocephaly (Liang *et al.* 1985), microcephaly (Liang *et al.* 1985), abnormal limb development (Liang *et al.* 1985; Carr *et al.* 1995; Harmon *et al.* 1995; Abuelo *et al.* 1997; Chitayat *et al.* 1997) and urogenital abnormalities, including undescended testes, variable degrees of hypospadias, ambiguous genitalia and even male

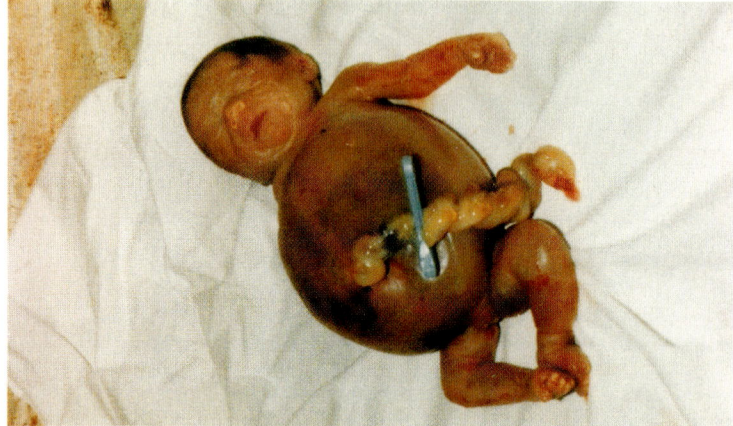

(a)

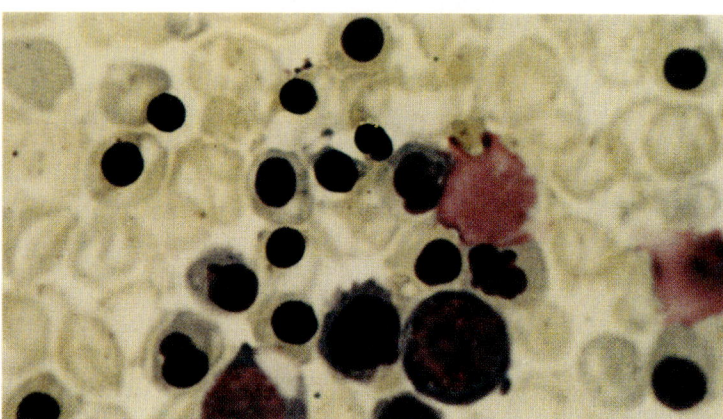

(b)

Fig. 11.2 The Haemoglobin Bart's hydrops syndrome. (a) Stillborn hydropic infant; (b) peripheral blood film with many immature red-cell precursors and hypochromic, microcytic, red cells showing anisocytosis and poikilocytosis.

pseudohermaphroditism (reviewed in Wasi *et al.* 1969, 1974; Ongsangkoon *et al.* 1978; Liang *et al.* 1985; Israngkura *et al.* 1987; Abuelo *et al.* 1997).

Autopsy findings

Ascites is usually pronounced and there are often pleural and pericardial effusions. There are widespread petechial haemorrhages. Organ weights are usually reported with respect to gestational age, body weight and body length (Fig. 11.3). The combination of oedema and disturbed growth can severely distort these relationships. With this caveat, enlargement of the heart, liver and to a lesser degree the spleen is usually observed, whereas there is retarded development of the lungs, thymus, adrenals and kidneys (Wasi *et al.* 1969, 1974; Vaeusorn *et al.* 1985; Nakayama *et al.* 1986). Particularly notable is the progressive decrease in brain weight relative to that

expected for gestational age, from about 8 weeks of gestation (see Fig. 11.3). Again, many abnormalities of the organs have been noted, including cardiac defects (Liang *et al.* 1985; Vaeusorn *et al.* 1985), pulmonary hypoplasia (Vaeusorn *et al.* 1985) and undescended and intra-abdominal testes (Nakayama *et al.* 1986; reviewed in Abuelo *et al.* 1997).

Histologically, interstitial oedema is present in all tissues. There are multiple sites of extramedullary erythropoiesis; up to 60–70% of the liver parenchyma may consist of developing red cells. The placenta is vascular and oedematous and contains many nucleated red cells. It has been suggested that the haematological changes (see below) may cause occlusion of small blood vessels with subsequent disruption of end organs leading, for example, to abnormal limb development (Chitayat *et al.* 1997).

It is interesting that, even though the majority of infants with hydrops fetalis have an identical geno-

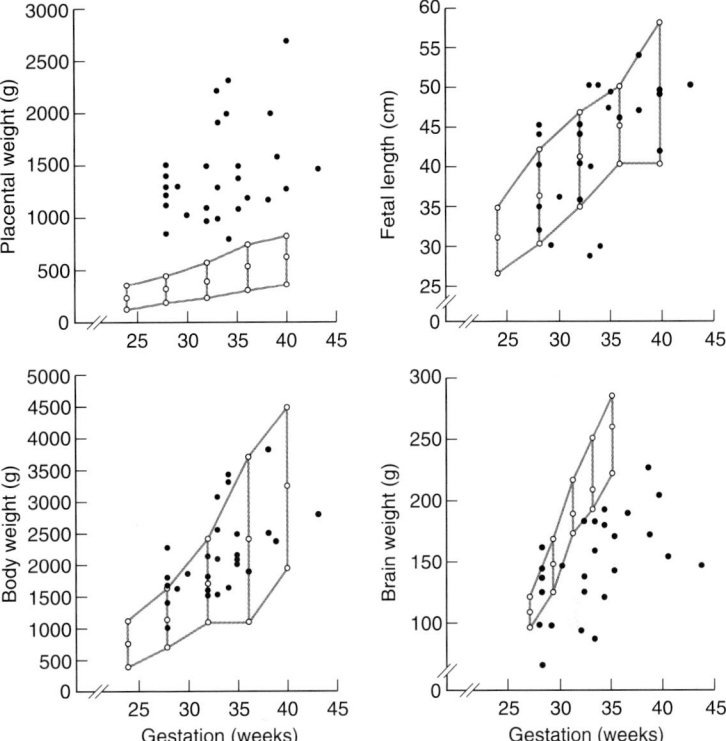

Fig. 11.3 The placental weight, body weight, fetal length and brain weight of infants with the haemoglobin Bart's hydrops fetalis syndrome. The open circles represent the mean values and 95% confidence limits. Redrawn, with permission from S. Fucharoen, from Vaeusorn *et al.* (1985).

type ($-$−^{SEA}/$-$−^{SEA}), there is considerable variation in the pace and extent of abnormal development in each fetus.

Maternal complications

Mothers of infants with this disorder often give a history of previous stillbirths or neonatal deaths; early miscarriages are probably uncommon. All reports point to an increased incidence of serious maternal complications (Table 11.1) (Liang *et al.* 1985; Vaeusorn *et al.* 1985; Nakayama *et al.* 1986).

In the antenatal period symptoms first arise in the third trimester, at which time some mothers note a cessation of fetal movements. Common complications include anaemia, pre-eclampsia characterized by hypertension and fluid retention with or without proteinuria, polyhydramnios (excessive accumulation of amniotic fluid), oligohydramnios (decreased amniotic fluid), antepartum haemorrhage and the premature onset of labour. Less common medical and obstetric complications have also been reported

(Guy *et al.* 1985; Liang *et al.* 1985; Vaeusorn *et al.* 1985; Nakayama *et al.* 1986).

Labour and delivery may be particularly difficult, and assistance in the form of embryotomy, breech delivery, forceps or Caesarean section is required in approximately 50% of cases. Postpartum complications include retained placenta, haemorrhage, eclampsia with fits and coma, sepsis and anaemia.

It has been suggested that, without medical care, up to 50% of women carrying these fetuses would die as a direct result of their pregnancy (Vaeusorn *et al.* 1985). However, to date, there have been no retrospective studies of maternal mortality rates in communities in which medical assistance is unavailable.

Long-term survival

As already noted, there is considerable variability in the clinical course of infants with this condition. Although most die *in utero*, during delivery or within one or two hours of birth others may survive for

Reference	Hydrops (%)			Non-hydrops (%)*
	1	2	3	1 and 4
Antepartum				
Anaemia	65			17
Pre-eclampsia	61	75	35	7
Eclampsia	0	1.5		<1
Polyhydramnios	59	3	17.5	<1
Antepartum haemorrhage	6.5	11†		3
Placenta praevia	4.3			
Abruptio placentae	‡		10	
Premature delivery	93		35	5–10
Delivery and postpartum				
Malpresentation	37			<5
Assisted vaginal delivery	35	34		5
Caesarean section	17	14		2–3
Retained placenta	‡			‡
Postpartum haemorrhage		11†		5
Anaemia	46			‡

Table 11.1 Maternal complications in the haemoglobin Bart's hydrops fetalis syndrome.

* These figures are only a guide since they will vary greatly depending on the population studied and the level of antenatal care provided.
† Includes ante- and postpartum haemorrhage.
‡ Recorded but figures not given.
Data compiled from the following references:
1 Liang *et al.* (1985).
2 Vaeusorn *et al.* (1985).
3 Nakayama *et al.* (1986).
4 Llewellyn-Jones (1969).

several days (Israngkura *et al.* 1987): in some cases the diagnosis may not be immediately obvious in a newborn infant. It is therefore not surprising that during the last 10 years, as neonatal care has continued to improve, several homozygotes for α^0 thalassaemia have survived, either as a result of treatment prior to confirmation of the diagnosis or as a result of preplanned intervention.

Currently we know of nine such cases (Table 11.2) (see also Chapter 15). Most have been delivered prematurely by Caesarean section and transfused soon after birth; two received transfusions *in utero* from ~25 weeks onwards. They had a difficult postnatal period with cardiopulmonary complications and, as mentioned earlier, there is a disturbingly high frequency of congenital abnormalities including patent ductus arteriosus (PDA), limb deformities and urogenital abnormalities in male infants. Subsequent development has been abnormal in at least half of the children, and all have required regular blood transfusion and chelation therapy.

Haematological findings

The peripheral blood film shows large, hypochromic red cells and marked anisopoikilocytosis (Fig. 11.2). Some elongated cells are said to have the appearance of 'sickle cells' (Wasi *et al.* 1974). Typical haematological findings are summarized in Table 11.3. There is severe anaemia, with a mean haemoglobin level of 6.5 g/dl (Vaeusorn *et al.* 1985), and an increased mean cell volume (MCV). The reticulocyte count is raised (Wasi *et al.* 1974) and the blood contains many nucleated red cells (Fig. 11.2). The bone marrow is hyperplastic and there are many sites of extramedullary haemopoiesis, which is predominantly erythropoietic, with widespread deposition of haemosiderin.

Haemoglobin constitution

Haemoglobin pattern at birth

In the original report of Lie-Injo and Jo (1960a,b) a very high proportion of Hb Bart's was found in the

Table 11.2 Summary of clinical and haematological data of infants who have survived the haemoglobin Bart's hydrops fetalis syndrome.

Case	Sex	Delivery (weeks of gestation)	Method	First transfusion	Neonatal problems	Hb at birth (g/dl)	Weight at birth (g)	Hb Portland (%)	Subsequent development	References
1	M	34	CS	Interuterine at 25 weeks	Missing one-third of foot, syndactyly, hand defects, hypospadias, incompletely descended right testicle	Transfused	2100	Transfused	Psychological testing at 21/12 showed developmental delay ≡ 16 months. Motor delay at 21/12. Growth below the 3rd percentile at 21/12	Carr et al. (1995); Abuelo et al. (1997)
2	M	32	CS	At birth	Cardiopulmonary, convulsions, PDA, hypospadias, cholestatic jaundice, subarachnoid haemorrhage	9.7	2300	20	At 14 months ≡ 6–9 months. At 6 years, delay in speech and hearing. Height at the 10th percentile. Weight at the 5th percentile	Beaudry et al. (1986); Jackson et al. (1990a)
3	F	28	CS	At birth	Respiratory distress, jaundice	(Hct 29.1%)	1080	19	At 5 years normal development, height 50%, weight 25%	Bianchi et al. (1986); Fischel-Ghodsian et al. (1987); Jackson et al. (1990a)
4	NR	28	PV (breech)	At birth	NR	NR	NR	7	Gross motor delay at 10 months, height 50%, weight 25%	Jackson et al. (1990a)
5	F	31	CS	At birth	Jaundice, PDA, heart failure	7.9	1600	NR	At 27 months, growth retarded (less than 3rd percentile); spastic quadraplegia and profound developmental delay	Lam et al. (1992)
6	M	33	CS	At birth	Jaundice, metabolic instability, cortical infarcts on CT scan, right inguinal hernia	9.7	1850	17*	Spastic diplegia at 20 months. Mild global development delay	S. Howarth (1996) and C. Cole (1998) (personal communication)
7	F	32	PV	At birth	PDA, cardiopulmonary, 'blueberry muffin' rash	~7.0	1623	10	Severe growth retardation, asymmetry in hand size. Limited neuropsychiatric assessment appears normal at 5 years	D.K. Bowden (1992, unpublished)
8	M	35	PV	At birth	Penoscrotal hypospadias	(Hct 30%)	1900	22	At 6/12, weight at the 10th percentile, length at the 3rd percentile	C.K. Li (personal communication)
9	NR	37	CS	Intrauterine at 26 weeks	Cardiopulmonary, thrombocytopenia, left portal vein obstruction	NR	NR	NR	Neurologically normal at 3 years	Naqvi et al. (1997)

* Not confirmed as Hb Portland.
CS, Caesarian section; HCT, haematocrit; NR, not recorded; PDA, patent ductus arteriosus; PV, per vaginam.

Table 11.3 Haematology in the normal developing fetus and in those with the haemoglobin Bart's hydrops fetalis syndrome.

Age (weeks)	RBC ($\times 10^{12}$/l)	Hb (g/dl)	Hct (%)	MCV (fl)	MCH (pg)	Retic. (%)	Hb Bart's (%)	Hb Portland (%)	Reference
Non-thalassaemic									
30–31	4.79±0.74	19.1±2.2	60±8	127±12.7	38*	5.8±2			Nathan & Oski (1987)
~40	5.14±0.7	19.3±2.2	61±7.4	119±9.4	34*	3.2±1.4	<1		Nathan & Oski (1987)
~40	4.7±0.8	16.5±3.0	51±9	108±10	34±3				Dallman (1977)
Hydrops fetalis									
28–43	2.2±0.8	6.5±2.3	30.4±13.8	136±23	31.9±9		86.9±5.1	13.1±5.8	Vaeusorn *et al.* (1985)
30–40		6.7		100–190		Variable may be >60%	70–80		Wasi *et al.* (1974)
28–38		4.9 (3–8.5)	21.3						Thumasathit *et al.* (1968)

Mean values±SD.
* Calculated MCH.
Hct, haematocrit; MCH, mean cell haemoglobin; MCV, mean cell volume; RBC, red-cell count; Retic., reticulocytes.

cord blood. This observation was subsequently confirmed by many others, and a detailed analysis of the haemoglobin of these infants was reported by Weatherall *et al.* (1970) and Todd *et al.* (1970). The starch gel electrophoretic pattern of lysates obtained from two of these infants is shown in Fig. 11.4a. The haemoglobin consists mainly of Hb Bart's with traces of HbH. Electrophoretic analysis at a variety of pH conditions confirmed the absence of HbA. In addition, there is a variable amount of Hb Portland, ranging from approximately 10 to 20% of the total haemoglobin.

Haemoglobin composition during development

Presumably the embryonic haemoglobins, Hbs Gower 1 ($\zeta_2\varepsilon_2$) and Portland I ($\zeta_2\gamma_2$), are produced normally in the first few weeks of life, although there can be no Hb Gower 2 ($\alpha_2\varepsilon_2$). Severe anaemia probably develops at around 6–7 weeks' gestation when the switch from embryonic (ζ and ε) to fetal (α and γ) gene expression occurs (Peschle *et al.* 1985). In the absence of α-chain synthesis no HbF ($\alpha_2\gamma_2$) is made and excess γ chains form soluble tetramers (γ_4, Hb Bart's), which constitute 80–90% of the total haemoglobin, the remainder being Hb Portland. Towards the end of gestation, as the fetal (γ) to adult (β) switch

occurs, small amounts of HbH (β_4) appear in the fetal blood, together with Hb Portland II ($\zeta_2\beta_2$) (Randhawa *et al.* 1984).

Haemoglobin synthesis

Haemoglobin synthesis was studied in the cells of an infant who was liveborn and from whom blood samples were obtained at exchange transfusion (Weatherall *et al.* 1970). The elution pattern after chromatography of the radioactively labelled globin is shown in Fig. 11.4b. It can be seen that there is no α-globin synthesis and that both γ- and β-globin production are active, with γ-chain synthesis predominating. Under these conditions the ζ chains of Hb Portland are not recovered and so it is not possible to determine the level of ζ-chain synthesis.

Genetic findings and heterogeneity

Since the Hb Bart's hydrops fetalis syndrome nearly always results from the inheritance of two α^0-thalassaemia alleles the parents of these babies have haemoglobin changes typical of the heterozygous state (see later section). The nomenclature for the deletional forms of α^0 thalassaemia is described in Chapters 3 and 4.

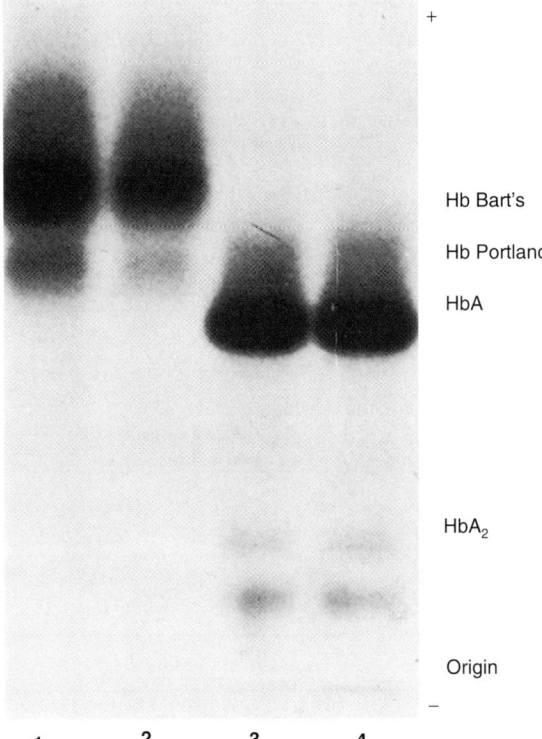

Fig. 11.4 (a) Haemoglobin analysis in the haemoglobin Bart's hydrops fetalis syndrome. Starch gel electrophoresis (pH 8.5, amido black stain) of red-cell lysates from the following (left to right): 1 and 2, Hb Bart's hydrops fetalis syndrome; 3 and 4, normal adults.

In south-east Asia, $--^{SEA}/--^{SEA}$ is the most common genotype but in areas where the $--^{FIL}$ (Fischel-Ghodsian *et al.* 1988), $--^{THAI}$ (Fischel-Ghodsian *et al.* 1988) and $--^{HW}$ (Waye *et al.* 1992) determinants occur some hydropic babies may be compound heterozygotes ($--^{FIL}/--^{SEA}$ and $--^{THAI}/--^{SEA}$). These three, less common alleles ($--^{FIL}$, $--^{THAI}$ and $--^{HW}$) remove both the α and ζ genes. Since homozygotes, $--^{FIL}/--^{FIL}$ for example, do not produce any embryonic haemoglobin they must die very early in gestation (Fischel-Ghodsian *et al.* 1988).

Alpha zero thalassaemia is much less common in other parts of the world. Nevertheless, occasional cases of Hb Bart's hydrops fetalis have been reported in Greeks ($--^{MED}/--^{MED}$) (Diamond *et al.* 1965; Sharma *et al.* 1979; Kattamis *et al.* 1980; Pressley *et al.* 1980c), Cypriots ($--^{MED}/--^{MED}$, $--^{MED}/-(\alpha)^{20.5}$, $-(\alpha)^{20.5}/-(\alpha)^{20.5}$) (Sophocleous *et al.* 1981; Nicholls *et al.* 1985), Sardinians ($--^{MED}/--^{MED}$) (Galanello *et al.* 1990b), Turks ($-(\alpha)^{20.5}/-(\alpha)^{20.5}$) (Gurgey *et al.* 1989) and Asian Indians ($--/--$) (Dr J.M. Old, personal communication). Many of these cases occur in restricted population groups or, in some cases, result from consanguineous marriages. Given the large number of α^{0}-thalassaemia mutations that have been described (see Chapter 4) it is important to be aware of the possibility of this condition in any family with a history of recurrent stillbirths, particularly of hydropic infants.

Very rarely, severe fetal anaemia with or without overt hydrops fetalis may also result from the co-inheritance of α^{0} and non-deletional α^{+} thalassaemia (Fig. 11.1), an interaction that normally causes HbH disease. The best examples were described by Chan *et al.* (1985), who have reported two cases of HbH hydrops fetalis.

Haemoglobin H hydrops fetalis

There have been three reports describing seven neonates with severe anaemia and changes associated with hydrops fetalis due to the co-inheritance of α^{0} and α^{+} thalassaemia (Chan *et al.* 1985; Trent *et al.* 1986c; Ko *et al.* 1991; Chan *et al.* 1997). In three well characterized cases the α^{+} thalassaemia resulted

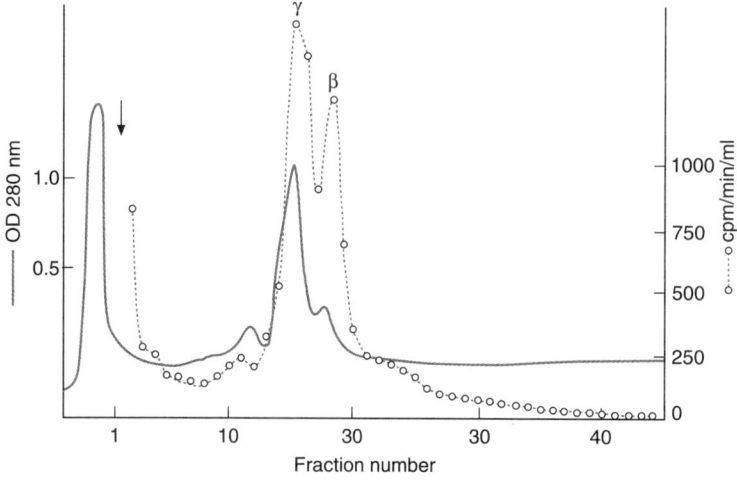

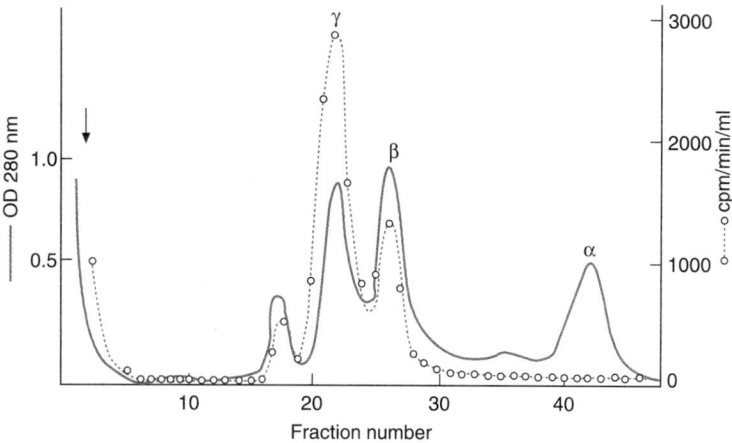

Fig. 11.4 (b) Globin synthesis in the Hb Bart's hydrops fetalis syndrome. Top, blood samples were obtained from a hydropic infant delivered at 36 weeks by Caesarean section. The red cells were incubated with [^{3}H] leucine and the globins were separated by CM-cellulose chromatography. Bottom, before the globin was fractionated adult haemoglobin was added as a carrier to mark the position of the α and β chains. The cord blood sample shows γ- and β-chain synthesis and no radioactivity eluting with the carrier α-chain peak. From Weatherall *et al.* (1970).

from mutations in the α2 gene associated with highly unstable α-globin variants ($--/\alpha^{\Delta30}\alpha$, $--/\alpha^{59\,Gly\rightarrow Asp}\alpha$, $--/\alpha^{125\,Leu\rightarrow Pro}\alpha$, $--/\alpha^{66\,Leu\rightarrow Pro}$) (Ko *et al.* 1991; Chan *et al.* 1997; Fairweather *et al.* 1999) (these variants are described in Chapter 4).

Mothers of some of these children gave a history of previous neonatal deaths due to anaemia. At birth all the infants were anaemic, with haemoglobin values ranging from 3.4 to 9.7 g/dl, with large amounts of Hb Bart's (31–65%); five died at birth and three survived following intrauterine blood transfusion but have remained transfusion dependent.

These cases reflect the transition between severe, transfusion-dependent HbH disease (see later section) and Hb Bart's hydrops fetalis. As accurate molecular diagnosis becomes more common, further cases of this kind are likely to be identified. It is not

clear why some infants with α^0/α^+ thalassaemia interactions should be so severely affected while others with an identical genotype (see Ko *et al.* 1991) may survive normally.

Diagnosis

The combination of a hydropic infant with a very high proportion of Hb Bart's in the peripheral blood is found in no other condition. Except in those rare cases that reflect more severe forms of HbH disease, the diagnosis can be confirmed by the demonstration of the heterozygous state for α^0 thalassaemia in both parents (see later section). Indeed, as mentioned earlier, it is important to screen both partners in any family of the appropriate ethnic background in which there is a history of recurrent stillbirth. The condition can be identified towards the end of the first trimester by chorion villus sampling, and later by amniotic fluid DNA analysis or fetal blood sampling (see Chapter 14). Using ultrasound, Lam and Tang (1997) report that they can identify 62% of cases at 13–14 weeks' gestation and 75% of cases at 17–18 weeks' gestation, as judged by a cardiothoracic ratio of greater than 0.05.

Pathophysiology

The general features of the pathophysiology of the α thalassaemias were considered in Chapter 5. Most of the features of the Hb Bart's hydrops syndrome can be ascribed to profound intrauterine hypoxia. This accounts for the gross pallor, generalized oedema, widespread extramedullary haemopoiesis, and the numerous nucleated red cells in the peripheral circulation. The increased drive to haemopoiesis also accounts for the hepatosplenomegaly, due largely to persistent extramedullary haemopoiesis.

Why are these babies so hypoxic? At first sight this is surprising considering that their haemoglobin values at birth, in the range of 6–8 g/dl, are compatible with survival in other forms of intrauterine anaemia. The answer almost certainly lies in the properties of Hb Bart's, which shows no haem/haem interaction or Bohr effect and binds oxygen very tightly, as in the R state of normal haemoglobin (see Chapter 2). In effect, its oxygen dissociation curve resembles that of myoglobin. Although the precise levels in early development are not known, at birth these babies have approximately 20% Hb Portland, an embryonic haemoglobin with physiological oxygen-transporting properties. However, in absolute terms, at a haemoglobin level of 8 g/dl, Hb Portland would only constitute 1.6 g/dl of the circulating haemoglobin. It is almost inconceivable that a fetus could survive with a functional haemoglobin of this level; either there must be a greater proportion of Hb Portland during the earlier months of pregnancy, or some oxygen must be extracted from Hb Bart's under these extreme conditions.

As discussed earlier, and as confirmed by ultrasound studies (Lam & Tang 1997), it is very likely that a severe degree of anaemia is established by 8–10 weeks' gestation in these babies. Whether early intrauterine hypoxia is responsible for the high frequency of other congenital abnormalities is not clear, and is a question of considerable importance for our broader understanding of the mechanisms of defects in fetal development.

The molecular and cellular basis for persistent ζ-globin expression is also not understood. A very small increase in ζ-globin chains is seen in some carriers of deletions that cause $α^0$ thalassaemia and, superficially, this resembles the persistent γ-globin expression that accompanies some deletions that remove the β-globin genes to cause hereditary persistence of fetal haemoglobin (HPFH) (Chui *et al.* 1986, 1989; Kutlar *et al.* 1989b; Tang *et al.* 1992; Ausavarungnirun *et al.* 1998) (see Chapters 4 and 10). However, the levels of ζ globin observed in carriers of $α^0$ thalassaemia (<1%) are much lower than levels of γ globin in HPFH. It seems likely that mechanisms other than increased ζ-globin-gene transcription, cell selection or alterations in ζ-globin mRNA stability for example, must be operating to allow such high levels of Hb Portland to accumulate. However, it is interesting that Hb Gower 1 ($ζ_2ε_2$) does not persist in this condition, suggesting that, whatever the mechanism, it acts specifically on ζ-globin genes rather than reflecting a more general effect on embryonic (ζ and ε) globin-gene expression.

Haemoglobin H disease

As discussed earlier, interactions between the many determinants of α thalassaemia (Fig. 11.1) lead to a broad spectrum of clinical and haematological phenotypes, ranging from normal to the Hb Bart's hydrops fetalis syndrome. Persons over the age of 6 months with sufficient globin imbalance to produce readily detectable levels of HbH, that is, greater than 1–2% in their peripheral blood, together with inclusion bodies in their red cells, are said to have HbH disease.

Not surprisingly, defined in this way the condition spans a wide range of clinical phenotypes. The majority of those affected are healthy and the epithet HbH 'disease' is inappropriate. Some have thalassaemia intermedia, while the most severe forms may be lethal late in gestation or in the perinatal period, a condition called HbH hydrops fetalis, which was described in the previous section.

Most patients with HbH disease originate from the populations of south-east Asia, the Mediterranean basin and the Middle East (see Chapter 6). This geographical distribution is easily explained now that we understand its molecular basis (Fig. 11.1). It most commonly results from the interaction of α^0 and α^+ thalassaemia. Although α^+ thalassaemia is common throughout all tropical and subtropical regions, α^0 thalassaemia, and hence HbH disease, is found predominantly in the Mediterranean region and southeast Asia. In the latter, the most common genotype is $--^{SEA}/-\alpha$, whereas in the Mediterranean $--^{MED}/-\alpha$ and $-(\alpha)^{20.5}/-\alpha$ predominate (see Chapter 4). Less often HbH disease results from the interaction of α^0 thalassaemia with non-deletional forms of α^+ thalassaemia ($--/\alpha^T\alpha$). It can also occur in homozygotes for some non-deletional forms of α^+ thalassaemia, $\alpha^T\alpha/\alpha^T\alpha$. Again, these molecular forms are most frequently seen in south-east Asia and the Mediterranean, though they also occur at high frequencies in some parts of the Middle East (see Chapter 6).

Despite these useful geographical rules of thumb, the reader should be aware that α^0-thalassaemia trait and HbH disease have been described in almost every ethnic group; patients originating from regions in which α thalassaemia is otherwise rare are often found to have unusual and biologically informative molecular pathology.

Although HbH disease is quite common, there have been relatively few systematic studies of its natural history or the relationship between genotype and phenotype. Much of the discussion about its clinical features which follows is based on the large series of patients reported from Thailand (Wasi *et al.* 1969, 1974; Wasi 1983) and from smaller series from elsewhere (Weatherall & Clegg 1981; Wong 1984; Kattamis *et al.* 1988; George *et al.* 1989; Galanello *et al.* 1992; Styles *et al.* 1997).

Presentation

In the series reported by Wasi *et al.* (1974) the age of presentation ranged from birth to 74 years, with more than half older than 20 years. At birth, infants destined to develop HbH disease have near-normal haemoglobin levels and no hepatosplenomegaly; the diagnosis can only be made by haemoglobin analysis (see later section). The clinical features evolve slowly over the first year of life.

Patients most frequently come to medical attention because they are found to have a hypochromic, microcytic anaemia during routine haematological investigation for other reasons, or because they develop the symptoms of either acute or chronic anaemia; presentations with more acute forms of anaemia are more common in childhood. Less common presentations include anaemia of pregnancy or symptoms associated with gallstones (Piankijagum *et al.* 1978).

Clinical findings

The most common clinical findings are mild pallor, scleral icterus and hepatosplenomegaly. In the series reported by Wasi *et al.* (1974) approximately 70% of patients had hepatomegaly and more than 80% had enlarged spleens. In our more limited experience of patients of other racial groups hepatomegaly is much less common and splenomegaly, while it is almost invariably present, rarely attains the magnitude of that seen in the more severe forms of β thalassaemia.

Approximately one-third of patients with HbH disease in the Thai population are reported to have bone changes typical of thalassaemia (Wasi *et al.* 1969). Usually these are mild but may occasionally cause facial deformities. In the Thai series only 1% of patients had evidence of impaired physical development.

Course and complications

Course

Most patients go through life with a variable degree of anaemia; the haemoglobin level may fluctuate and, occasionally, fall quite dramatically, resulting in episodes of profound weakness and pallor requiring hospital admission and blood transfusion (Wasi *et al.* 1974). The cause of these fluctuations, the severity of which seems to vary between different populations, is not understood (see later section). They may occur after exposure to oxidant drugs such as sulphonamides (Rigas & Koler 1961), infection or transient aplasia, again possibly due to intercurrent viral infection (Dr Donald Bowden, personal communication).

It is unusual for patients with HbH disease to require regular blood transfusion and, even where this is thought to be necessary, it is not always clear what criteria have been used. There is some evidence that transfusion dependence is related to particular genotypes (see later section). There have been no studies of longevity.

Complications

Hypersplenism

Although this may be one of the commonest complications there are no extensive studies of splenic function or plasma volume levels. Wasi *et al.* (1974) thought that hypersplenism, leading to significant aggravation of the anaemia and a reduced platelet and white-cell count, occurs in about 10% of patients. In an earlier study, Wasi *et al.* (1969) reported that they had carried out splenectomy in 50 patients and that the levels of haemoglobin were raised, on average, 2–3 g/dl. Hathirat *et al.* (1978) reported similar findings in a much smaller series.

Gallstones

As in other haemolytic anaemias there is an increased frequency of gallstones. Fucharoen and Winichagoon (1997) report a frequency of about 35%. Of 95 patients followed for 2 years by Piankijagum *et al.* (1978) there were four episodes of cholecystitis associated with gallstones.

Leg ulcers

There have been occasional reports of chronic leg ulcers, as in other forms of thalassaemia (Daneshmend & Peachey 1978).

Infection

Although it has been the impression that patients with HbH disease have an increased frequency of infection there have been no prospective, controlled studies of this relationship. Piankijagum *et al.* (1978) followed 95 patients between 1964 and 1966. About a third suffered from infective episodes; upper and lower respiratory tract infections were by far the most common. They also observed that these episodes were associated with a significant fall in the haemoglobin level. However, in an uncontrolled study of this type it is not certain whether the frequency of infections would have been greater than that in the general population. Only one severe episode of septicaemia was observed, in a patient who had undergone splenectomy. Wasi *et al.* (1974) suggest that patients with HbH disease may be more susceptible than

normal to streptococcal infection. The incidence of tuberculin reactivity and white-cell function as judged by the NBT (nitro-blue tetrazolion) test are normal (Serirodom *et al.* 1972; Tanphaichitr *et al.* 1973). It has also been the impression that infection is commoner in patients with HbH disease in populations other than those of Thailand (Cao *et al.* 1991).

Folate deficiency

There have been no reports of clinical folate deficiency in HbH disease, possibly because in populations in which the disease is particularly common dietary folate deficiency is relatively uncommon. However, Vatanavicharn *et al.* (1978) observed significant reductions in serum folate levels in 8% and in red-cell folate in 30% of their patients.

Iron loading

The different varieties of tissue damage to the liver and endocrine organs which are characteristic of the transfusion-dependent forms of β thalassaemia are not a feature of HbH disease except in those cases in which it has been necessary to resort to regular blood transfusion. However, there is some evidence that older patients may accumulate considerable amounts of iron, presumably by increased absorption from the gastrointestinal tract. Hence the potential for the development of complications due to increased levels of tissue iron should not be overlooked in this age group; we shall return to this question later in this section.

Venous thrombosis

In the last edition of this book we described a patient with HbH disease who, following splenectomy, developed the unusual combination of superficial migrating thrombophlebitis, deep venous disease and major pulmonary emboli, which led to his death. He was one of a series reported by Hirsh and Dacie (1966), which described subjects who had been splenectomized for different forms of haemolytic anaemia and how, after surgery, there was an inverse relationship between the haemoglobin level and platelet counts; those with higher platelet counts seemed to be at risk of pulmonary embolic disease. Subsequently, we have seen several more patients of this type, one of whom we have followed for over 15 years and who has had many attacks of superficial and deep venous thrombosis together with life-threatening pulmonary emboli. A detailed analysis of his coagulation profile has revealed no other abnormalities. A small group of similarly affected patients was reported from Hong Kong by Tso *et al.* (1982). Although, as described in Chapters 5 and 7, thrombotic disease is being recognized with increasing frequency in the β thalassaemias, this particular constellation of superficial and deep venous thrombosis does not appear to have been reported in conditions other than HbH disease. It has not been identified in Thailand, where HbH disease is so common (Prawase Wasi, personal communication). However, venous thrombotic disease in general is unusual in that population. What little is known of the underlying mechanisms for increased thrombosis in different forms of thalassaemia is discussed in Chapter 5.

Extramedullary haemopoietic masses

Because the severe forms of HbH disease are associated with a clinical picture of thalassaemia intermedia, and because the production of extramedullary haemopoietic masses is relatively common in this condition (see Chapter 13), it is surprising that this complication has not been observed more frequently in patients with this disorder. It was not mentioned by Sonakul (1989) in her extensive study of extramedullary haemopoiesis at autopsy, a series which included several patients with HbH disease.

Pregnancy

There have been no consecutive studies of haemoglobin levels during pregnancy although early reports suggested that it may fall into the 4–5 g/dl range (White & Jones 1969; Wasi *et al.* 1974; Ong *et al.* 1977). However, in these cases it is clear that both iron and folate deficiency were common and it is unclear to what extent this complicated the picture. In a more recent study Galanello *et al.* (1992) described the outcome of 58 pregnancies in 24 women; seven (12%) miscarried, 10 (16%) were found to have haemoglobin values of less than 7.5 g/dl, and five (8%), in whom transfusion was thought necessary, had values of less than 6.0 g/dl. In our experience it is unusual to observe haemoglobin values below 7 g/dl. This limited information suggests that, although the haemoglobin level may fall as it does in normal women in pregnancy, profound anaemia is unusual and, when it is observed, it is important to look for complicating factors such as iron or folic acid deficiency.

Haematological findings

The early series from Thailand reported that patients with HbH disease are always anaemic, although there was a very broad scatter in haemoglobin levels; the means of two large series were 7.4 and 7.8, respectively (Piankijagum *et al.* 1978; Wasi *et al.* 1979). More recent data comparing the haematological findings in individuals with one functional α gene ($--/-\alpha$) with normal persons ($\alpha\alpha/\alpha\alpha$) are shown in Table 11.4 and Fig. 11.5. Those who inherit only a single α gene have lower levels of haemoglobin, a reduced mean cell haemoglobin (MCH) and MCV, but higher red-cell counts (RBC). These differences are seen at all stages of development (see Table 11.4), although there are no substantial data on infants with HbH disease in the perinatal period or during the early months of life. The most important finding is that, using data accumulated from a variety of surveys (see Table 11.4), patients with HbH disease are anaemic with, on average, haemoglobin values of approximately 3 g/dl less than age- and sex-matched normals. It has been noted in some surveys that there may be major fluctuations in the level of haemoglobin measured sequentially in the same individual over the course of several years (Wasi *et al.* 1974; Piankijagum *et al.* 1978), although in our experience this is not common. These wide fluctuations may have been partly due to concomitant iron and folate deficiency, or intercurrent infection (see later section).

The peripheral blood film shows hypochromia and polychromasia with variable anisopoikilocytosis, basophilic stippling and target cells (Fig. 11.6). The reticulocyte count is usually raised to around 3–6%, although higher counts may be observed. Nucleated red cells may be present (Wasi *et al.* 1974) but in our experience this is quite rare except after splenectomy.

An important characteristic of the peripheral blood is that it is always possible to generate multiple, ragged inclusions in the red cells after incubation with brilliant cresyl blue for 20 min or more at room temperature or at 37°C (reviewed by Gibbons *et al.* 1991). These bodies are artefacts produced by the redox action of the dye (Fig. 11.6), and even after pro-

Table 11.4 Hematological data for Mendelian α thalassaemia. The number of samples (N), mean (μ) and unbiased estimate of the standard deviation (SD) are shown for the nine possible combinations of the αα, –α, $\alpha^T\alpha$ and –– genotypes (excluding ––/––), in increasing order of severity, for the age groups (years) 1–4, 5–9, 10–15 and ≥16 (adult). The normal data are derived from Dallman (1977), Dallman and Siimes (1979) and Lubin (1987); the principal sources for the α-thalassaemia data are described in the text. In addition to the unpublished data sets acknowledged in Higgs *et al.* (1989), further valuable series were contributed by C.C. Thompson (Hamilton, Ontario) and T. Sophocleous (Nicosia). Because of significant sex differences, the Hb and *red-cell count* (RBC) are tabulated separately for adult males and females; although both mean cell volume (MCV) and mean cell haemoglobin (MCH) tend to be slightly higher in males than females, the relative differences are much smaller (~1 fl and ~0.5 pg, respectively), so these data are pooled, as are the α-/β-globin-chain synthesis ratios for all ages.

α-Globin genotype	Age (years)		Hb (g/dl) M	F	RBC (×10^{12}/l) M	F	MCV (fl)	MCH (pg)	HbH (%)	α/β Ratio
αα/αα	1–4	N	—		—		—	—	—	
		μ	12.6		4.55		79	27.5	0	
		SD	0.8		0.35		4	2.0	—	
	5–9	N	—		—		—	—	—	
		μ	13.2		4.6		81.5	28.5	0	ine up
		SD	0.8		0.3		4	2.0	—	
	10–15	N	—		—		—	—	—	
		μ	13.9		4.7		84	29.5	0	
		SD	1.0		0.3		4.5	2.0	—	
	≥16	N	—	—	—	—	—	—	—	27
		μ	15.5	14.0	5.2	4.6	90	30	0	1.06
		SD	1.0	1.0	0.35	0.3	5	2.0	—	0.11
–α/αα	1–4	N	55		52		55	52	—	
		μ	10.9		4.74		73.0	23.2	0	
		SD	1.2		0.53		6.4	2.5	—	
	5–9	N	49		49		49	49		
		μ	11.8		4.87		76.4	24.5	0	
		SD	0.86		0.50		5.6	2.2	—	
	10–15	N	42		42		42	42	—	
		μ	12.5		5.00		80.2	25.2	0	
		SD	1.2		0.48		6.1	1.8	—	
	≥16	N	81	106	77	102	191	184	—	29
		μ	14.3	12.6	5.42	4.88	81.2	26.2	0	0.87
		SD	1.4	1.2	0.58	0.53	6.9	2.3	—	0.12
$\alpha^T\alpha/\alpha\alpha$	10–15	N	4		4		4	4	—	
		μ	12.8		5.3		71.7	24.2	0	
		SD	0.2		0.26		2.4	1.3	—	
	≥16	N	22	17	21	17	39	38	—	12
		μ	14.5	12.5	5.76	5.21	75.5	24.8	0	0.75
		SD	0.9	0.6	0.49	0.50	6.48	1.7	—	0.12
–α/–α	1–4	N	10		10		10	10	—	
		μ	10.1		5.08		63.0	19.9	0	
		SD	1.7		0.30		6.1	6.1	—	

Continued

Table 11.4 *Continued.*

α-Globin genotype	Age (years)		Hb (g/dl) M	F	RBC (×10¹²/l) M	F	MCV (fl)	MCH (pg)	HbH (%)	α/β Ratio
	5–9	N	7		7		7	7	—	
		μ	10.8		5.0		66.2	21.5	0	
		SD	1.4		0.5		3.0	0.9	—	
	10–15	N	14		14		14	14	—	
		μ	12.0		5.47		72.1	22.1	0	
		SD	0.9		0.49		8.7	2.3	—	
	≥16	N	31	45	30	45	77	75	—	8
		μ	13.9	12.0	5.98	5.30	71.6	22.9	0	0.72
		SD	1.7	1.0	0.81	0.49	4.1	1.3	—	0.12
−−/αα	1–4	N	6		5		6	5	—	
		μ	11.2		5.79		60.7	19.6	0	
		SD	0.6		0.58		4.9	1.2	—	
	5–9	N	8		7		8	7	—	
		μ	11.0		5.47		62.5	20.3	0	
		SD	0.8		0.48		3.4	0.8	—	
	10.15	N	13		14		14	13	—	
		μ	12.2		5.83		67.5	21.4	0	
		SD	1.0		0.70		3.4	1.8	—	
	≥16	N	63	83	54	71	145	130	—	31
		μ	13.7	12.1	6.28	5.65	69.1	21.7	0	0.65
		SD	1.1	1.1	0.63	0.49	4.4	1.7	—	0.12
αᵀα/−α	1–4	N	1		1		1	1	—	
		μ	10.8		5.78		59	18.7	0	
		SD	—		—		—	—	—	
	5–9	N	1		1		1	1	—	
		μ	11.4		5.79		60.2	19.7	0	
		SD	—		—		—	—	—	
	≥16	N	6	6	5	6	12	12	—	4
		μ	12.3	10.6	5.78	5.10	66.1	21.0	0	0.8
		SD	1.05	0.65	0.80	0.37	3.3	1.5	—	0.06
αᵀα/αᵀα	1–4	N	2		2		2	2	2	
		μ	7.9		4.25		63.3	18.9	14.2	
		SD	3.2		2.30		2.9	2.8	5.3	

Continued

longed incubation, it is unusual to find them in every cell; the reason for this heterogeneity is not clear, a problem to which we shall return when we consider the pathophysiology of HbH disease. The picture is different after splenectomy. In this case a proportion of the cells contain single, large Heinz bodies which stain with methyl violet and which are present in the majority but not all of the cells (Fig. 11.7). These single bodies are preformed and quite unlike the ragged, multiple inclusions which occur after incuba-

Table 11.4 *Continued.*

α-Globin genotype	Age (years)		Hb (g/dl) M	F	RBC (×10^{12}/l) M	F	MCV (fl)	MCH (pg)	HbH (%)	α/β Ratio
	5–9	N	1		1		1	1	1	
		μ	6.9		3.5		68	19.7	8.4	
		SD	—		—		—	—	—	
	10–15	N	3		3		3	3	3	
		μ	10.7		5.97		58.3	17.8	7.6	
		SD	2.8		0.82		5.7	2.8	8.0	enlarge
	≥16	N	2	3	2	3	6	6	5	5
		μ	11.2	9.9	5.82	5.21	60.5	18.9	10.5	0.47
		SD	0.5	1.4	0.35	0.56	4.77	1.2	7.6	0.18
–α/––	1–4	N	17		16		17	16	13	
		μ	9.6		5.77		57.7	17.0	5.7	
		SD	0.8		0.66		8.5	2.2	3.4	
	5–9	N	11		11		11	11	10	
		μ	9.6		5.52		58.7	17.7	4.8	
		SD	0.8		0.86		6.4	2.5	4.0	
	10–15	N	19		18		19	18	15	
		μ	9.5		5.47		59.3	17.7	5.1	
		SD	0.8		0.76		5.6	1.3	2.4	
	≥16	N	28	59	24	58	121	120	110	32
		μ	11.1	9.4	6.1	5.14	64.8	19.1	7.0	0.44
		SD	1.1	1.2	0.82	0.78	7.2	2.3	4.8	0.20
α^{T}α/––	1–4	N	4		3		4	3	3	
		μ	7.8		5.16		67.4	16.6	19.6	
		SD	1.4		1.13		16.7	5.3	2.1	
	5–9	N	8		8		8	8	8	
		μ	8.8		4.69		66.6	19.3	13.4	
		SD	1.9		1.23		7.7	2.5	7.2	
	10–15	N	8		8		8	8	8	
		μ	9.2		5.03		66.1	17.8	22.8	
		SD	0.9		0.49		3.4	1.5	3.5	
	≥16	N	6	5	3	5	14	14	13	17
		μ	10.5	8.5	5.1	4.68	68.0	18.7	22.3	0.32
		SD	1.0	0.7	0.31	0.66	5.9	1.5	6.5	0.15

tion with brilliant cresyl blue, and which are due to the precipitation of HbH. Electron-microscopic analysis of the single inclusions show that they are distributed round the periphery of the cell (see Fig. 5.15, Chapter 5).

The bone marrow shows marked erythroid hyperplasia. A few inclusions can be seen on light microscopy after staining with methyl violet (Fessas & Yataganis 1968). Electron microscopy shows them to be highly condensed, branching, intracytoplasmic structures in early and late polychromatic erythroblasts and reticulocytes (Fig. 11.8). In addition, autora-

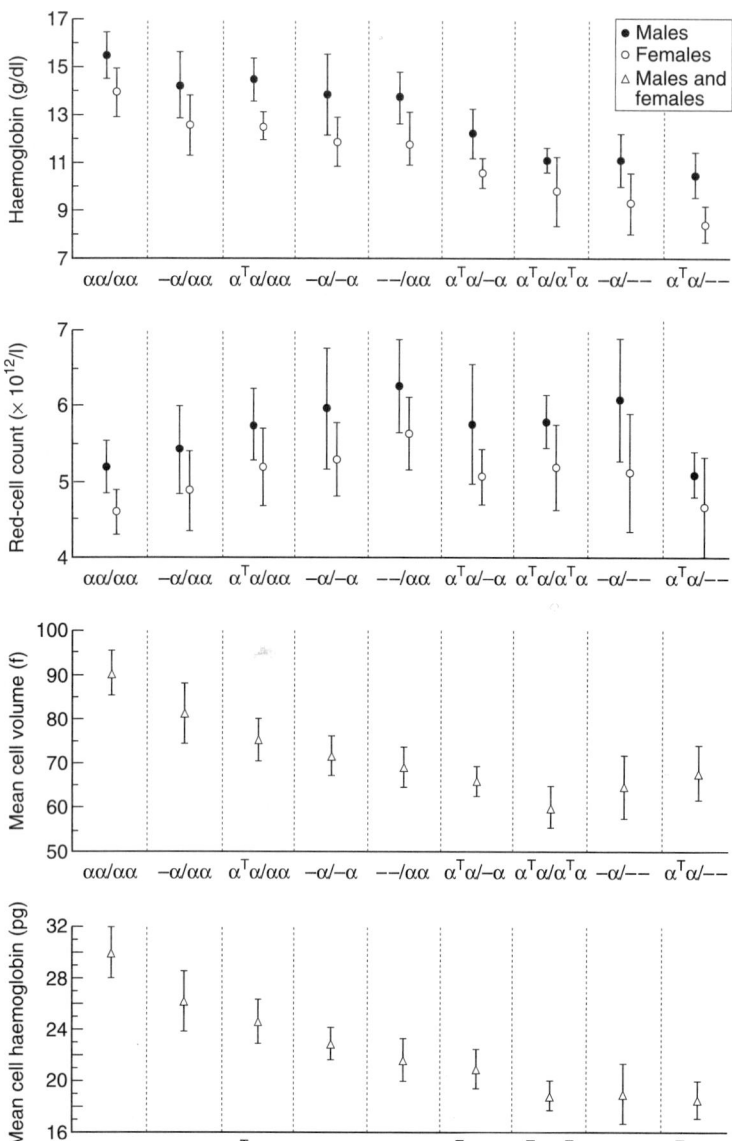

Fig. 11.5 The red-blood-cell indices in patients with various α-thalassaemia genotypes. For each set of data the mean and 1 SD are shown. For the level of haemoglobin and estimates of red-cell count, differences between males and females are shown. Data are from Wilkie (1991).

diographic analysis has demonstrated the addition of newly synthesized protein, possibly β chains, on to these inclusions (Wickramasinghe *et al.* 1980).

Haemoglobin constitution

On electrophoresis at alkaline pH HbH migrates more rapidly than HbA and has a similar mobility to haemoglobin I (Fig. 11.9). On electrophoresis at pH 6.5 it can be clearly distinguished from other haemoglobin variants by its anodal migration. On storage at 4°C or after freezing it is relatively unstable and tends to precipitate. Haemolysates which have been made for some time produce a series of bands in the general position of HbH; it is best stored in the carbonmonoxy form and can be kept in this state for long periods without loss of clarity of the bands on electrophoresis.

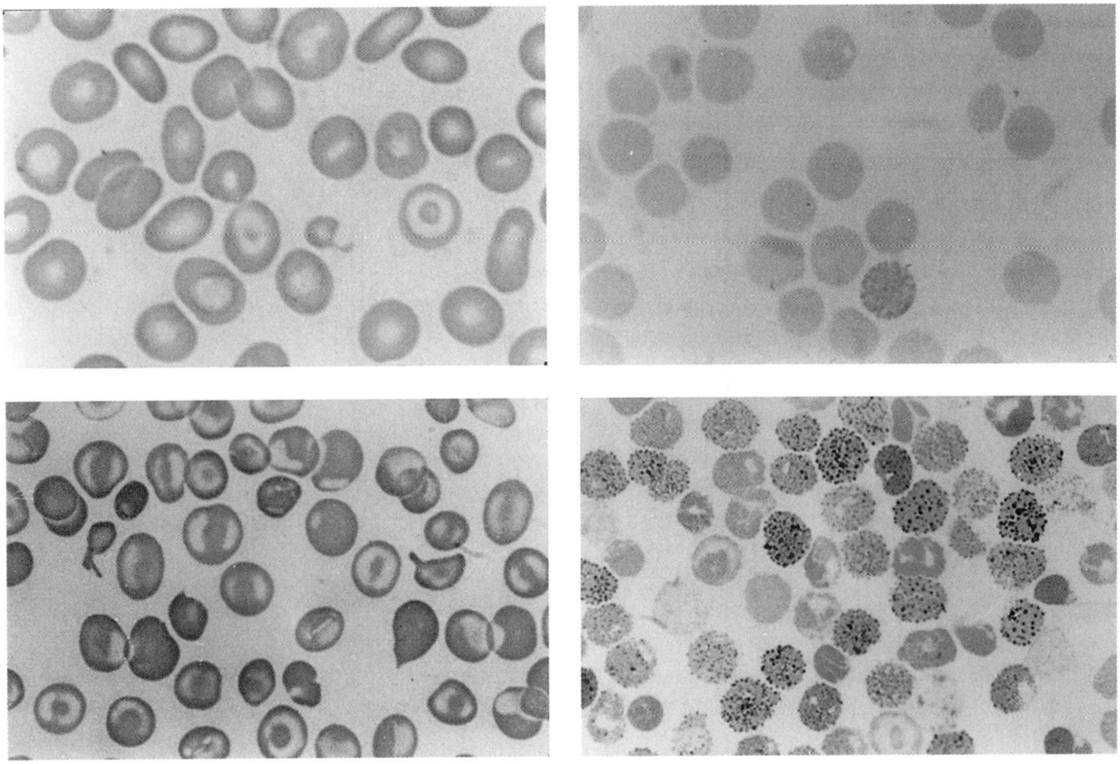

(a)

(b)

(c)

(d)

Fig. 11.6 Red cells in heterozygous α^0-thalassaemia trait and haemoglobin H disease. (a) A peripheral blood film from an individual with α^0-thalassaemia trait showing mild morphological abnormalities. (b) A brilliant cresyl blue preparation of the red cells of an individual with α^0-thalassaemia trait showing very occasional cells which contain inclusion bodies. (c) The blood film from a patient with HbH disease. (d) A brilliant cresyl blue preparation of the red cells of a patient with HbH disease showing numerous inclusions generated by the dye.

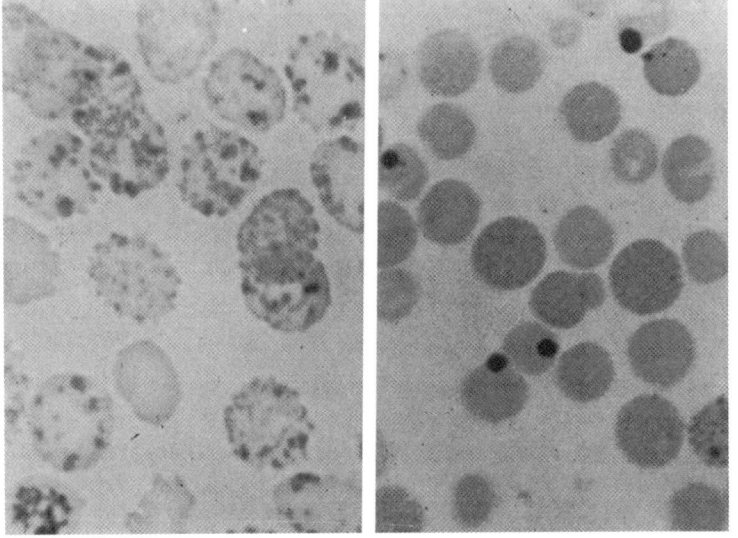

Fig. 11.7 Inclusion bodies in haemoglobin H disease after splenectomy. The figure on the left shows a brilliant cresyl blue preparation similar to that shown in Fig. 11.6. On the right is a blood film from a patient with HbH disease after splenectomy stained with methyl violet. Large, preformed inclusions are present.

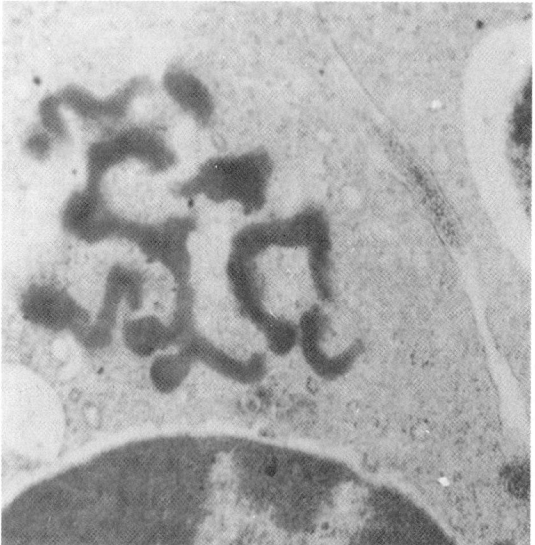

Fig. 11.8 Inclusions in the bone marrow in haemoglobin H disease. Precipitation of HbH in erythroblasts in the bone marrow of a patient with HbH disease (×22815). By courtesy of Professor Sunitha Wickramasinghe. (See also Fig. 5.15, Chapter 5.)

In many patients there is a second rapidly migrating component which moves more slowly than HbH at pH 8.6 and nearer the anode than HbH at pH 6.5 (Fig. 11.9). This fraction was identified as Hb Bart's (Ramot *et al.* 1959; Fessas 1960; Sturgeon *et al.* 1961). Using combined chromatographic and electrophoretic techniques a third haemoglobin was isolated from the blood of a patient with HbH disease (Dance *et al.* 1963). This fraction consists entirely of the δ chains of HbA_2, although it is not certain whether it has the molecular formula δ_4 since its molecular weight was not determined.

The relative amount of HbH varies from less than 1% to 40%. The range in 69 cases reported by Na-Nakorn *et al.* (1965) was 2–24% with a mean of 9.0%, while the mean level in 260 patients examined by Wasi *et al.* (1969) was 8%. The latter workers found Hb Bart's in 67 out of 130 cases studied, with a mean level of 4.8%. The HbA_2 value is always diminished; the mean figure for Wasi's series was 1.55%. The level of HbH may drop in association with iron deficiency and rise again after iron therapy (O'Brien 1973). In a proportion of patients in south-east Asia, and occasionally elsewhere, about 2% Hb Constant Spring is found. This variety of HbH disease, together with the differences in the findings associated with the differ-

ent genotypes that underlie the condition, will be considered later in this chapter.

The relative amounts of haemoglobins Bart's and H during development and in adults

Infants who were later to develop HbH disease were studied from birth by Pootrakul *et al.* (1967b), Wasi *et al.* (1969, 1974) and Pootrakul *et al.* (1970). At birth there was 19–27% Hb Bart's; during development the level gradually fell and it was replaced by variable amounts of HbH. In many cases the level of Hb Bart's at birth exceeded that of HbH in adult life (Table 11.4). This may reflect both the fact that there is normally a very mild degree of globin-chain imbalance at birth, with a slight excess of γ and β chains (see Chapter 5), and the fact that HbH is less stable than Hb Bart's.

In most cases the level of HbH exceeds that of Hb Bart's in adults although occasionally the fetal type of haemoglobin pattern persists and Hb Bart's levels may exceed those of HbH (Ramot *et al.* 1959). The reasons for this variability are not known but it probably reflects the activity of the γ-chain loci in later life. If these remain unusually active and relatively large amounts of γ chains are produced, both β and γ chains will be competing for a depleted pool of α chains. Since α chains associate with β chains in preference to γ chains, the overall result may be a greater excess of γ than β chains, with the production of more Hb Bart's than H.

The instability of haemoglobin H

Haemoglobin H is unstable and thermolabile (Scott *et al.* 1970). As mentioned earlier, it tends to precipitate out of haemoglobin solutions kept at 4°C, and it is more stable in the cyan- and carbonmonoxy-haemoglobin forms. It contains two reactive SH groups per β chain; the β chains in HbA have only one reactive SH group per chain in the oxy form. Gabuzda (1966) suggested that the relative susceptibility of HbH to oxidation might result from the presence of the eight free thiols, which might confer a lower net reduction–oxidation potential on the molecule.

As mentioned in Chapters 2 and 5, the formation of haemichromes may be an important intermediate stage in the denaturation of various types of haemoglobin and its subunits. Electron paramagnetic spin resonance (PER or ESR) were used to charac-

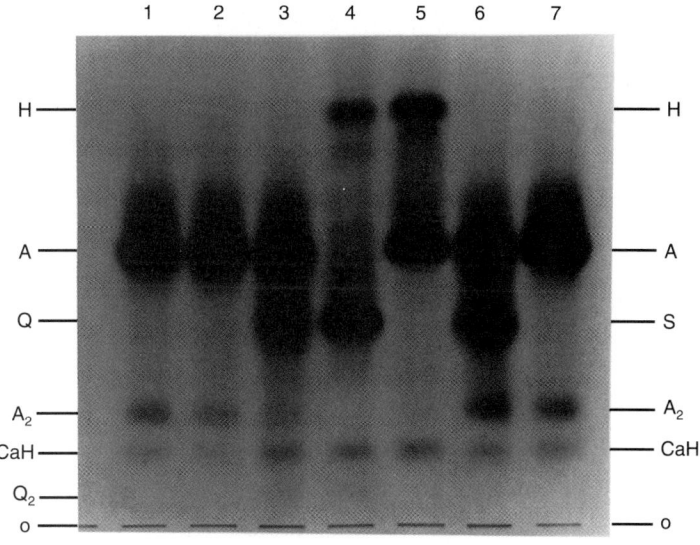

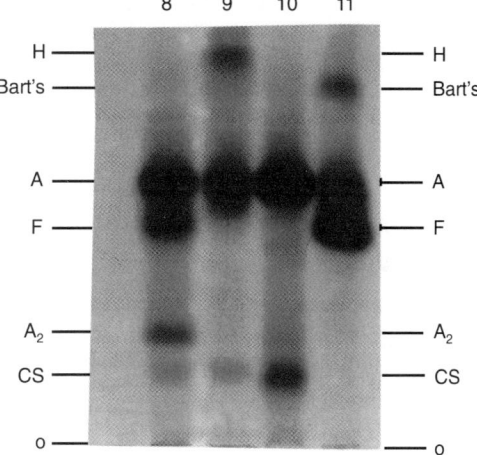

Fig. 11.9 Haemoglobin electrophoresis (Coomassie Blue stain) in different forms of α thalassaemia. The following are shown: normal (1, 2 and 7); a heterozygote for HbQ (3); HbQ-H disease (4); HbH disease (5 and 9); a heterozygote for HbS (6); a homozygote for Hb Constant Spring (CS) (10); and a cord blood with an elevated level of Hb Bart's (11). o denotes the origin and CaH indicates the position of carbonic anhydrase.

terize these intermediates (Rachmilewitz 1969; Rachmilewitz *et al.* 1969). The bonding of the distal histidine imidazole to the oxidized haem results in the transition from high-spin to low-spin states, giving a characteristic ESR signal. This type of haemichrome (haemichrome 1) is reversible and, on reduction of the haem iron to the ferrous state, deoxyhaemoglobin is formed. However, further distortion of subunit conformation allows other groups to form an internal bond with the haem, resulting in the formation of an irreversible haemichrome, which again can be distinguished by its ESR spectrum. The formation of irreversible haemichrome is accompanied by precipitation of the haemoglobin.

It has been found that HbH forms haemichromes much more rapidly than HbA (Rachmilewitz 1969; Rachmilewitz *et al.* 1969). Furthermore, Rachmilewitz and Harari (1972) have shown that the rate of haemichrome formation of Hb Bart's is considerably slower than that of HbH and have suggested that this is the reason for its greater stability.

Functional properties

Haemoglobin H shows no haem–haem interaction or Bohr effect and has an oxygen affinity 10 times that of HbA. Thus the oxygen dissociation curve of purified HbH is a rectangular hyperbola (Benesch *et al.* 1961).

The curve of whole blood of patients with HbH disease may show two components due to the combined presence of Hbs A and H. It follows from these observations that patients carrying large amounts of HbH have a whole-cell oxygen dissociation curve which is shifted to the left; less oxygen is given up at physiological tensions, a factor which causes further problems for patients who are already anaemic.

2,3-Diphosphoglycerate (2,3-DPG) binds equally to the oxy and deoxy forms of HbH (Benesch *et al.* 1968a,b). In other words the interaction of 2,3-DPG with HbH is not oxygen linked. This is because HbH does not change its quaternary conformation on oxygenation.

Clearly therefore HbH is useless as an oxygen carrier, a point which is considered in more detail in Chapter 5.

Red-cell survival and erythrokinetics

Red-cell survival as judged by ^{51}Cr studies is shortened, reported figures ranging from 8.1 to 17 days for the ^{51}Cr half-life (Rigas & Koler 1961; Pearson & McFarland 1962; Woodrow *et al.* 1964; Knox-Macaulay *et al.* 1972). The red-cell survival curve in HbH disease is much more uniform than that found in β thalassaemia, reflecting the more homogeneous nature of the cell population being destroyed (Malamos *et al.* 1962; Nathan & Gunn 1966). External scanning studies have shown that the spleen is the site of much of the red-cell destruction (Rigas & Koler 1961; Woodrow *et al.* 1964).

Utilizing 2-[^{14}C]-glycine as a label the rates of turnover of Hbs H and A were examined *in vivo* by Gabuzda *et al.* (1965). These studies showed that Hbs H and A have different turnover times and that HbH disappears more rapidly from the circulation than HbA.

Iron kinetic and erythrokinetic studies have shown a rapid disappearance of ^{59}Fe from plasma to bone marrow but more than 50% of the injected dose is found in red cells and much of this is present in haemoglobin (Pearson & McFarland 1962). Srichaikul *et al.* (1984) performed full erythrokinetic studies on nine non-splenectomized patients. They demonstrated an increased red-cell mass and plasma volume and a reduced red-cell survival, of 6–19.5 days (normal range 25–32 days), with sequestration of ^{51}Cr-labelled red cells in the liver and spleen. In addition there was a rapid clearance of ^{59}Fe with relatively good ^{59}Fe incorporation into red cell compared with patients with β thalassaemia. They also found that the packed cell volume (PCV) correlated with the red-cell survival. Together, these findings suggest that both haemolysis and ineffective erythropoiesis contribute to anaemia in HbH disease, but that the predominant factor is haemolysis.

Iron status

The clinical manifestations of iron overload frequently encountered in patients with β thalassaemia intermedia and major (see Chapters 5, 7 and 13) are rarely seen as a result of HbH disease (Weatherall & Clegg 1981; Wasi 1983; Tso *et al.* 1984; Chim *et al.* 1998). Except in cases of co-existent iron deficiency bone-marrow iron stores are usually normal and there is less tissue haemosiderosis at autopsy in patients with HbH disease than in those with homozygous β thalassaemia (Sonakul *et al.* 1978). Ferrokinetic studies have suggested that, although iron absorption is increased (Lin *et al.* 1992a), its utilization appears normal, consistent with this being primarily a haemolytic anaemia (Srichaikul *et al.* 1984; Lin *et al.* 1992a).

Most young patients with HbH disease have normal (Galanello *et al.* 1983a) or only slightly raised levels of serum ferritin (Anuwatanakulchia *et al.* 1984; Tso *et al.* 1984). However, significantly raised levels may be found in older patients (Fig. 11.10), those treated with regular blood transfusion and those given inappropriate medication with iron (Galanello *et al.* 1983a). In the study of Galanello *et al.* (1992) no difference in the levels of serum ferritin was and seen between patients with deletional and non-deletional HbH disease.

As is the case for β thalassaemia (see Chapter 7), HbH disease may co-exist with the common form of hereditary haemochromatosis (Feder *et al.* 1996), which could account for unexplained iron overload in occasional patients (Lin *et al.* 1990; Galanello *et al.* 1992).

In vitro haemoglobin synthesis

The rate of α- and β-chain production has been studied in reticulocytes and bone marrow obtained from patients with HbH disease using [^{14}C]- or [^{3}H]-leucine (Weatherall *et al.* 1965; Clegg & Weatherall 1967; Kan *et al.* 1968; Schwartz *et al.* 1969; Knox-

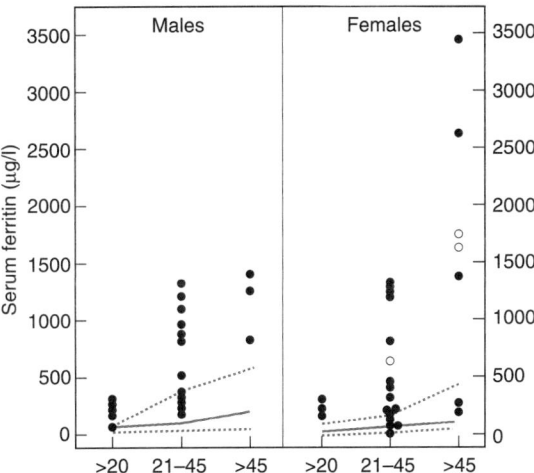

Fig. 11.10 Serum ferritin levels of patients with haemoglobin H disease according to sex and age. The solid lines connect the median control values of the different age groups and the dotted lines the upper and lower values of the corresponding control range. Splenectomized subjects are shown as open circles. Redrawn from Tso (1994).

Macaulay *et al.* 1972; Shchory & Ramot 1972; Ramot *et al.* 1973; Russo *et al.* 1973b; Wood & Stamatoyannopoulos 1976-77; Hunt *et al.* 1980). In all these studies there has been a marked imbalance of globin synthesis, α/β ratios ranging from 0.2 to 0.5 with a mean of approximately 0.4, mirroring the reduction in α-globin mRNA levels (see Fig. 5.14, Chapter 5). In a study in which globin synthesis was examined both in bone-marrow cells of different ages separated by centrifugation and in peripheral reticulocytes, Wood and Stamatoyannopoulos (1976–77) showed that the α-/β-globin production ratio is similar at all stages of erythroid maturation.

These findings, together with further studies of the kinetics of globin synthesis in this disorder described in Chapter 5, provide a fairly clear picture of the formation of Hbs A and H in HbH disease. There is imbalanced globin synthesis and the excess of β chains exist in two forms. The majority of them form the β₄ tetramers of HbH but there is a small intracellular pool which is capable of combining with newly made α chains as these become available. Furthermore, there is clear-cut evidence that HbH is not present in the blood in amounts reflecting the rate at which it is synthesized, indicating that it must be lost from the red cells during their time in the circulation.

Red-cell metabolism

The metabolic properties of red cells in HbH disease have been studied by Gabuzda (1966), Nathan *et al.* (1969), Scott *et al.* (1970) and Knox-Macaulay *et al.* (1972).

The rates of glucose utilization and lactate formation are two to three times normal, a finding which must in part reflect the young cell population. Both young and old cells have increased cation permeability, the most marked change being in the older population, which contains single inclusion bodies in splenectomized individuals. It is possible that the rapid rate of glucose utilization is partly due to the stimulation of the cation pump as a result of these changes in membrane permeability. Red-cell ATP levels are normal or slightly reduced and fall more rapidly than those in normal red cells after sterile incubation. The red cells also have an increased rate of methaemoglobin production.

Reduced glutathione (GSH) levels are lower in the older cell population than in young red cells. Furthermore, hexose monophosphate shunt (HMPS) activity is more marked in the older population. It has been suggested that, since HbH is particularly sensitive to oxidative precipitation, its reactive thiols may participate in cellular reduction reactions and thus substitute for glutathione. Thus HMPS activity would be reduced in a situation in which glutathione is spared, i.e. in the younger cell population, but increased with cell ageing as HbH precipitates and becomes less available. Some glutathione may well precipitate with haemoglobin.

A totally unexplained metabolic abnormality of the red cells was reported by Beutler *et al.* (1977). It was found that the level of glutathione peroxidase is markedly elevated, in the range found in association with glucose-6-phosphate dehydrogenase deficiency.

The functional significance of these changes in relationship to the pathophysiology of α thalassaemia is discussed in Chapter 5.

Genotype/phenotype relationships

Although there are still only a limited number of studies, such information as there is suggests that there are subtle differences between the clinical manifestations of HbH disease, depending on the underlying genotype.

Haematological findings

Several studies have compared the haematological findings in patients with deletional forms of HbH disease ($--/-\alpha$) and those with non-deletional forms, including $--/\alpha^{CS}\alpha$ (HbH/Hb Constant Spring) (Fucharoen et al. 1988a; Styles et al. 1997) and $--/\alpha^{Hph}\alpha$ (Galanello et al. 1983a, 1992). It appears that in the forms of HbH disease due to the interaction of non-deletional alleles there is a significantly lower haemoglobin level and red-cell count and a higher mean cell haemoglobin (MCH).

Haemoglobin constitution

In the relatively small numbers of patients studied it appears that HbH disease due to interactions of the non-deletional forms of α thalassaemia, notably that associated with Hb Constant Spring, is characterized by significantly higher levels of HbH and numbers of red cells containing HbH inclusions (Winichagoon et al. 1980; Styles et al. 1997).

Overall clinical severity

From these limited data it appears that there may be significant variability in the clinical course among these different genetic forms of HbH disease. These differences were particularly marked in the study of Styles et al. (1997); in comparing the deletional forms of HbH disease with HbH/Hb Constant Spring she found that patients with the latter genotype were more likely to have splenomegaly or have undergone splenectomy, and to have received transfusions.

Clearly more data on larger series of patients with different molecular forms of HbH disease are needed before any definitive conclusions can be drawn. But from such evidence as there is it appears that interactions of the non-deletional forms of α thalassaemia are, overall, associated with a more severe phenotype.

Pathophysiology

The pathophysiology of α thalassaemia is described and contrasted with that of β thalassaemia in Chapter 5. We saw how the anaemia of HbH disease is the result of a mild degree of ineffective erythropoiesis associated with a shortened red-cell survival due to the damaging effects of the interaction between pre-cipitated β chains and the red-cell membrane, combined with the physical barriers encountered by older red cells containing inclusions of precipitated HbH during their passage through the microcirculation, particularly in the spleen. We also considered the abnormal functional properties of Hbs H and Bart's, a topic to which we alluded earlier in this chapter.

Throughout the literature from Thailand, which we considered earlier in this section, fluctuations in the haemoglobin level are emphasized, a finding which we have not observed frequently in patients with this disorder in Western countries. Although it is possible that some of this variability reflects superimposed folate or iron deficiency, the Thai writers have been struck by the importance of infection in determining a fall in the steady-state haemoglobin level. One possibility, which has not been fully explored, is that the marked heat lability of HbH might cause its in vivo precipitation at high body temperatures. In Chapter 9 we raised the same question in the case of HbE, pointing out that that variant is also heat labile and suggesting that it has the potential for increased instability at body temperatures only slightly above normal. In a report by Chinprasertsuk et al. (1994) it was found that, in a series of patients with pyrexial illnesses with body temperatures ranging from 38 to 41°C, there was a drop in mean haemoglobin levels from 8.6 to 5.6 g/dl, splenic enlargement and a significant increase in the numbers of preformed inclusion bodies. Further work on the precise relationship between the instability of HbH and different temperatures needs to be carried out together with appropriate in vivo studies of its level in the peripheral blood during periods of raised body temperature at different levels.

Pathophysiological considerations have important implications for the assessment of the function of patients with α thalassaemia, at any stage of development. We have already seen how, because of the properties of Hb Bart's, infants who are homozygous for α^0 thalassaemia are much more hypoxic than their peripheral blood haemoglobin values would suggest. The same discrepancy is sometimes observed in adults with HbH disease. If, for example, their steady-state haemoglobin level is 8 g/dl, and they have 20% HbH in their red cells, they are, in effect, functioning with a haemoglobin value of 6.6 g/dl. While these subtleties may not be important in young people they may be of considerable importance to older patients with a compromised coronary artery circulation. We have, for example, observed an elderly patient with an acquired form of HbH disease (see Chapter 12) who, with a steady-state haemoglobin level of over 9 g/dl and with 40% HbH, suffered all the symptoms of profound anaemia together with severe angina. As mentioned earlier, there is increasing evidence that the slightly lower haemoglobin levels and higher values of HbH associated with interactions of the non-deletional forms of α thalassaemia result in more severe clinical phenotypes, which, in some cases, are transfusion dependent (Styles *et al.* 1997). Thus, in assessing any patient with HbH disease it is not sufficient to simply determine the steady-state haemoglobin but it is also important to measure the level of HbH on a carefully prepared red-cell lysate.

Autopsy findings

There have been very few reports of the autopsy findings in this condition. In her atlas showing autopsy changes in different forms of thalassaemia, including HbH disease, Sonakul (1989) provides some data about the distribution of iron in different tissues.

Prognosis

Although it is known that most patients with HbH disease survive into adult life, as far as we know there have been no long-term studies which analyse longevity compared with normal individuals in the same population.

The milder α-thalassaemia phenotypes

In previous editions we described how, spanning the clinical and haematological gap between patients with HbH disease and normal individuals, there is a wide range of hypochromic anaemias of different severity which almost certainly reflect the action of different α-thalassaemia alleles. Up to the early 1980s it was only possible to characterize these conditions by their associated haematological findings (Pornpatkul *et al.* 1969), the presence of raised levels of Hb Bart's at birth (Hunt & Lehmann 1959; Weatherall 1963), the presence of HbH inclusions in adult blood (McNiel 1968; Pornpatkul *et al.* 1978) or the demonstration of a reduced α-/β-globin synthesis ratio (Kan *et al.* 1968). Unfortunately, these diagnostic criteria failed to identify a significant proportion

of α-thalassaemia carriers and, in addition, could not discriminate between those with different forms of the disease. The application of these 'blunt' diagnostic tools led to a large volume of confusing literature, some of which is outlined in Chapter 1 and which was reviewed in detail in the last edition of this book.

The reasons for these difficulties soon became apparent once it was possible to define the different molecular forms of α thalassaemia. For, as it became feasible to study reasonable numbers of individuals with well defined α-globin genotypes, it became apparent that there is an overlapping continuum of haematological findings and haemoglobin constitutions stretching across these interactions of milder α-thalassaemia alleles. Essentially, this reflects the heterozygous and homozygous states for the deletional forms of $α^+$ thalassaemia ($-α/αα$ and $-α/-α$), the heterozygous state for $α^0$ thalassaemia ($--/αα$), the equivalent states for non-deletional forms of $α^+$ thalassaemia ($α^Tα/αα$ or $α^Tα/α^Tα$) and the various compound heterozygous states for the deletion and non-deletional forms of $α^+$ thalassaemia ($-α/α^Tα$).

We shall discuss this complex problem by first comparing and contrasting the findings in the different mild forms of α thalassaemia and then summarizing their main diagnostic features. It is important to emphasize at the outset that virtually none of them can be identified with certainty except by DNA analysis.

Because of the greater heterogeneity of the non-deletional forms of $α^+$ thalassaemia ($α^Tα/α^Tα$), or compound heterozygotes for the deletion and non-deletional forms of $α^+$ thalassaemia ($-α/α^Tα$), we shall consider first the effect of α-globin-gene deletions, comparing normal persons ($αα/αα$) with those with the heterozygous ($-α/αα$) or homozygous state ($-α/-α$) for $α^+$ thalassaemia, or the heterozygous state for $α^0$ thalassaemia ($--/αα$). As discussed by Ganczakowski *et al.* (1995) and Williams *et al.* (1996b) we make no distinction between the $-α^{3.7}$ and $-α^{4.2}$ forms of $α^+$ thalassaemia. Although the haematological effects of such deletions will be illustrated by reference to specific studies, it is important to remember that these measurements can vary from one normal ($αα/αα$) population to another (Owen & Yanochik-Owen 1977) and, in practice, slight variations may also be obtained even in healthy, non-thalassaemic individuals (Ross *et al.* 1988).

Haematological changes

The heterozygous and homozygous states for deletional forms of α^+ thalassaemia, and heterozygous α^0 thalassaemia

Adult values

In general, those with simple gene deletions ($-\alpha/\alpha\alpha$, $-\alpha/-\alpha$ and $--/\alpha\alpha$) have lower levels of total haemoglobin, MCHC, MCV and mean cell haemoglobin (MCH), but higher RBC than normal (see Table 11.4 and Fig. 11.5).

The degree of abnormality varies from one parameter to another. The greatest differences are seen in MCH; those with α thalassaemia clearly make less haemoglobin per cell than normal. Nevertheless, adequate haemoglobin levels are maintained, within ~1.0–1.5 g/dl of normal, at all stages of development (Table 11.4). It appears that the main compensatory mechanism for the underproduction of haemoglobin is an increase in the production of red cells, in a similar way to that described for β-thalassaemia heterozygotes in Chapter 7.

There is now adequate information to compare the haematological findings in adults with these deletional forms of α^0 and α^+ thalassaemia (Table 11.4 and Fig. 11.5). Although there is a good correlation between the predicted reduction in α-chain synthesis and haemoglobin, MCV, MCH there is considerable overlap. Therefore these parameters are of only limited value in distinguishing one genotype from another. However, it is clear that, with the exception of the $-\alpha/\alpha\alpha$ genotype, most homozygotes for deletional types of α^+ thalassaemia, or heterozygotes for α^0 thalassaemia, can be distinguished from normal on the basis of their MCH, which is usually less than 26 pg and always below 27 pg (Higgs *et al.* 1989; Higgs 1993).

The peripheral blood film is also quite variable from one genotype to another but usually shows hypochromia, with occasional poikilocytes and target cells (Fig. 11.6). The reticulocyte count is usually raised, in the 2–3% range. As discussed in more detail in a later section, it is possible to generate HbH inclusions in a few red cells in α^0 thalassaemia carriers ($--/\alpha\alpha$), but rarely in heterozygotes or homozygotes for α^+ thalassaemia. Red-cell survival and erythrokinetic studies have not been carried out in many of these mild α thalassaemias. The red-cell ^{51}Cr half-life

estimates in two α-thalassaemia carriers reported by Wasi *et al.* (1974) were 25 days and 29.5 days (normal range 25–30 days).

Changes during development

Developmental changes in the haematological findings follow the same patterns as those of normal individuals ($\alpha\alpha/\alpha\alpha$) (Fig. 11.11). The haemoglobin level, PCV, MCH and MCV fall rapidly after birth and begin to rise slowly in the second year. Throughout development it is possible to distinguish the haematological findings in patients with $\alpha\alpha/\alpha\alpha$, $-\alpha/\alpha\alpha$ and $-\alpha/-\alpha$ genotypes. For all parameters there is a greater difference between those with $-\alpha/-\alpha$ and $-\alpha/\alpha\alpha$ genotypes than those with the $-\alpha/\alpha\alpha$ and $\alpha\alpha/\alpha\alpha$ genotypes. The smaller data set for individuals with the $--/\alpha\alpha$ genotype most closely resembles the $-\alpha/-\alpha$ genotype. Few differences are seen between males and females prior to puberty, after which there are significant sex-dependent differences in all genotypic groups (Table 11.4).

Changes during pregnancy

The changes in the haemoglobin levels and red-cell indices in women heterozygous or homozygous for the deletional form of α^+ thalassaemia, taken from a study of Dr. Mary Ganczakowski and present authors (unpublished), are shown in Fig. 11.12. They mirror those observed in heterozygotes for β thalassaemia (see Chapter 7). There is a fall in the haemoglobin level, starting towards the end of the first trimester, which mirrors that in normal women. There are no major changes in the red-cell indices between the pregnant and non-pregnant state. Just as the case for heterozygous β thalassaemia, it is clear that severe anaemia does not occur in these milder forms of α thalassaemia during pregnancy and, when it is found, complicating factors such as folate or iron deficiency should be sought.

Heterozygous non-deletion α^+ thalassaemia and compound heterozygosity for deletional and non-deletional forms of α^+ thalassaemia

As shown in Table 11.4 and Fig. 11.5, as a group, the heterozygous states for the non-deletional forms of α thalassaemia ($\alpha^T\alpha/\alpha\alpha$) show slightly more marked haematological changes than those for the deletional

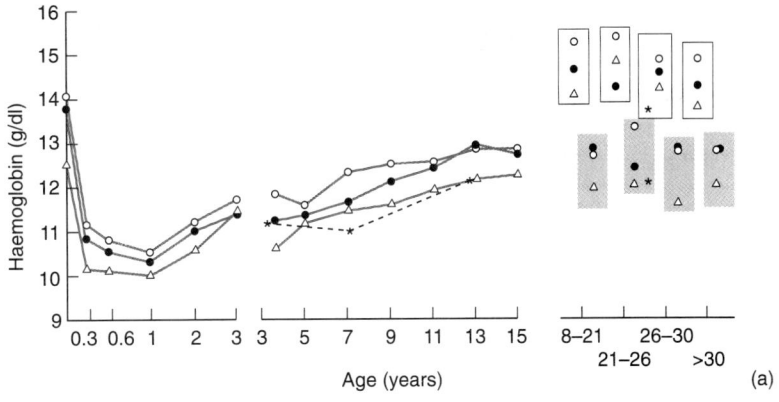

(a)

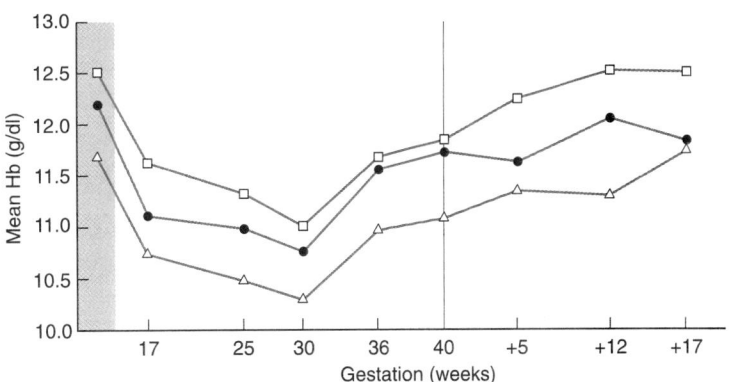

(b)

Fig. 11.11 Developmental changes in the haemoglobin (a) and MCH (b) in individuals with the αα/αα (○), –α/αα (●) and –α/–α (△) genotypes. The data indicated by stars are for the ––/αα genotype. Open boxes, males; stippled boxes, females.

Fig. 11.12 Changes in the level of haemoglobin in pregnant women with the αα/αα (□), –α/αα (●) and –α/–α (△) genotypes. Results in shaded area indicate normal values prior to pregnancy. The vertical line denotes the usual time of birth. From Dr M. Ganczakowski and the authors (unpublished).

forms. However, the numbers are relatively small and there is a considerable overlap between genotypes. Similarly, the haematological findings in compound heterozygous states for the deletion and non-dele-

tional forms ($\alpha^T\alpha/-\alpha$) are very similar to those in the heterozygous states for the deletional forms of α^0 thalassaemia.

The homozygous states for the non-deletional

forms of α^+ thalassaemia ($\alpha^T\alpha/\alpha^T\alpha$) have very variable haematological changes. As shown in Fig. 11.5 and Table 11.4 the degree of haemoglobinization of the red cells and other haematological findings are very similar to those of patients with HbH disease. Indeed, as we saw in an earlier section, there are several varieties of HbH disease associated with this genotype. Those due to the chain termination mutations produce a completely different clinical picture, which is described later in this chapter.

Haemoglobin analysis

The heterozygous and homozygous states for deletional forms of α^+ thalassaemia, and heterozygous α^0 thalassaemia

Adults

The haemoglobin constitution of adults with these conditions is indistinguishable from normal, although as a group they may have slightly lower levels of HbA_2. However, in a small survey (Maude *et al.* 1985) there appeared to be no significant differences in the levels of Hbs A_2 and F between those with $\alpha\alpha/\alpha\alpha$, $-\alpha/\alpha\alpha$ and $-\alpha/-\alpha$ genotypes at different stages of development (Fig. 11.13).

In the previous edition of this book we discussed the value of the demonstration of a few HbH inclusions as a diagnostic aid to some of the carrier states for α thalassaemia. Galanello *et al.* (1984) found that occasional cells containing HbH can be detected in up to 65% of individuals who must have been carriers for different forms of α thalassaemia. In our experience, using standard HbH preparations (Gibbons *et al.* 1991) inclusions are usually found in heterozygotes for different forms of α^0 thalassaemia ($--/\alpha\alpha$) (Fig. 11.6) but rarely in heterozygotes or homozygotes for the deletional forms of α^+ thalassaemia. However, various modifications of the standard HbH preparation may significantly increase the sensitivity of this assay (Maungsapaya *et al.* 1985; Kuptamethi *et al.* 1988). Although it has been found that some adult α-thalassaemia carriers may have trace amounts of Hb Bart's which can be demonstrated in an immunological assay (Wasi *et al.* 1979), and small amounts of embryonic ζ-globin chains can be detected in carriers for α^0 thalassaemia (Chui *et al.* 1986), which, it has been suggested, can be used as a simple assay for detecting some forms of α-

thalassaemia carrier states (Ausavarungnirun *et al.* 1998), neither of these approaches have been widely used. Their value in clinical practice remains to be substantiated.

Changes during development

Before the application of molecular genetic methods for the diagnosis of α thalassaemia there was good evidence that a raised level of Hb Bart's (γ_4) in the neonatal period (Fig. 11.13) reflects the presence of α thalassaemia (Weatherall 1963 and reviewed in Wasi *et al.* 1974). The mechanisms involved, and the reasons why Hb Bart's is not replaced by HbH in later development in the milder forms of α thalassaemia, are discussed in Chapter 5. However, while it was clear that normal infants produce traces of Hb Bart's at birth it was not known whether all individuals with α thalassaemia have a raised level of Hb Bart's at this stage of development. Similarly, the relationship between the amount of Hb Bart's and the underlying α-thalassaemia genotype was uncertain.

These issues have now been clarified by studies correlating the level of Hb Bart's with the α-globin genotype. Most surveys using assays that are sufficiently sensitive to detect a minimum of 0.5–1% Hb Bart's at birth detect a large proportion of neonates with α thalassaemia but do not identify all cases of the $-\alpha/\alpha\alpha$ genotype (Higgs *et al.* 1980b; Bowden *et al.* 1987a; Zhao *et al.* 1988). Therefore, surveys based solely on the presence of Hb Bart's in the cord blood consistently underestimate the frequency of α^+ thalassaemia. Furthermore, although the levels of Hb Bart's are generally related to the degree of α-chain deficit they do not accurately distinguish the various α genotypes (see later section). For example, even though homozygotes for the leftward, 4.2-kb, deletion ($-\alpha^{4.2}$), have significantly higher levels of Hb Bart's at birth than homozygotes for the rightward, 3.7-kb, deletion ($-\alpha^{3.7}$), there is considerable overlap between the groups.

During the first 6 months after birth, the level of Hb Bart's in babies with α thalassaemia declines (Fig. 11.13) and eventually becomes undetectable by conventional assays (Weatherall 1963) although, as mentioned earlier, minute amounts may be detected in adults with α thalassaemia using an immunological assay (Wasi *et al.* 1979). Similarly, small amounts of embryonic ζ chains can be detected in some adults

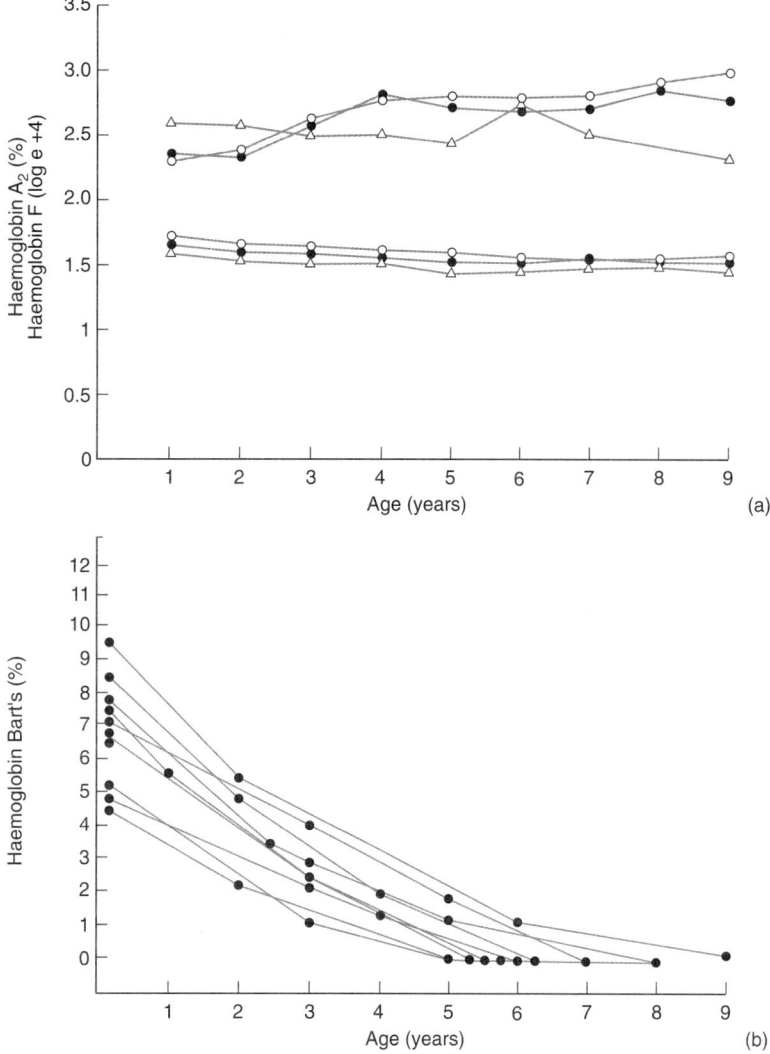

Fig. 11.13 Developmental changes in the haemoglobin constitution in α thalassaemia. (a) HbA$_2$ (above) and HbF (below) in patients with the αα/αα (○), –α/αα (●) and –α/–α (△) genotypes (data from Maude *et al.* 1985). (b) The level of Hb Bart's in infants with α thalassaemia during the first few months of life. Redrawn from Weatherall (1963).

with α thalassaemia (Chui *et al.* 1986). The problems of detecting HbH inclusions in relationship to different genotypes was discussed earlier.

Deletional forms of α$^+$ thalassaemia commonly occur in areas where β-globin variants (e.g. Hbs S, C and E) are also found at a high frequency. The presence of α thalassaemia can alter the proportion of variant haemoglobin found in the peripheral blood and therefore, where α thalassaemia co-exists with β variants, the proportion of Hb variant can be a useful guide to the presence of α thalassaemia (see below).

Heterozygous non-deletion α$^+$ thalassaemia and compound heterozygosity for the deletional and non-deletional forms of α$^+$ thalassaemia

Adults

With the exception of those cases which are due to mutations of the α-globin-chain termination codon, the heterozygous states for the non-deletional forms of α$^+$ thalassaemia (α^{T}α/αα) are not associated with any changes in the haemoglobin constitution in adult life. In carriers for the α-globin chain termination mutants trace amounts of the variant can be demonstrated, although they are usually missed unless a sensitive electrophoretic technique is used (see later section). In our experience, using standard HbH preparations, inclusions are usually found in those with the genotypes $\alpha^T\alpha/\alpha\alpha$ and $-\alpha/\alpha^T\alpha$.

The haemoglobin findings in homozygotes for the non-deletional forms of α thalassaemia ($\alpha^T\alpha/\alpha^T\alpha$) are extremely variable. In some cases there are no abnormalities except, possibly, for a slightly reduced level of HbA_2. However, in others the degree of α-chain deficiency may be such as to result in the haemoglobin findings typical of HbH disease (see earlier section), while in the case of the homozygous state for the α-chain termination mutation which causes Hb Constant Spring, there may be persistent Hb Bart's together with a relatively high level of the variant; we shall return to this condition later in this chapter. In those with no changes in the haemoglobin pattern it is usually possible to demonstrate HbH inclusions.

The haemoglobin findings associated with the non-deletion α^+ thalassaemias that result from the production of highly unstable α-chain variants (see Chapter 4) are also variable. Just as described for the dominant β thalassaemias in Chapters 4, 5 and 13, there seems to be a continuum of disorders reflecting the degree of instability of the α-gene product. In some cases, Hbs Agrinio (Hall *et al.* 1993b) and Lleida (Ayala *et al.* 1996) for example, it is impossible to detect any abnormal haemoglobin and its structure is assumed from the abnormal DNA sequence. In other cases, Hbs Sallanches (Morlé *et al.* 1995) and Suan Dok (Sanguansermsri *et al.* 1979) for example, trace amounts of the haemoglobin variant can be found in the peripheral blood. However, in many cases these variants can only be detected by isoelectric focusing.

α-/β-*Globin mRNA estimation and globin synthesis*

Assays using heterologous cell-free assays consistently showed that mRNA from reticulocytes of patients with α thalassaemia direct the synthesis of less α than β globin (Benz *et al.* 1973; Grossbard *et al.* 1973; Gambino *et al.* 1974; Pritchard *et al.* 1974). Subsequently, it has been found that this results from under-representation of accumulated mRNA in most determinants of α thalassaemia (Housman *et al.* 1973; Kacian *et al.* 1973; Kan *et al.* 1974d; Natta *et al.* 1976).

Hunt *et al.* (1980) were the first to analyse the α-/β-globin mRNA ratios in carriers of α thalassaemia and, although the precise genotypes of the patients studied were not known, they demonstrated clear differences between normal individuals and obligate carriers (Fig. 11.14).

Subsequently, studies using reverse transcription PCR-based quantification of α- and β-globin mRNA in patients with accurately known genotypes have confirmed these observations (Lin *et al.* 1994; Smetanina *et al.* 1996). Although Hunt *et al.* (1980) showed no overlap in the α-/β-globin mRNA ratios of normal individuals and those with α-thalassaemia genotypes, the more recent studies demonstrated wider variation (Lin *et al.* 1994; Smetanina *et al.* 1996). Nevertheless, Smetanina *et al.* (1996) confirmed that the α-/β-globin mRNA ratios of those with two functional α-globin genes ($-\alpha/-\alpha$ and $--/\alpha\alpha$) are quite distinct from normal.

The α-/β-chain biosynthesis ratios in patients with different α-globin genotypes, measured by *in vitro* haemoglobin synthesis (Clegg & Weatherall 1967; Pootrakul *et al.* 1967b; Kan *et al.* 1968; Weatherall *et al.* 1970), broadly reflect the α-/β-globin mRNA ratios.

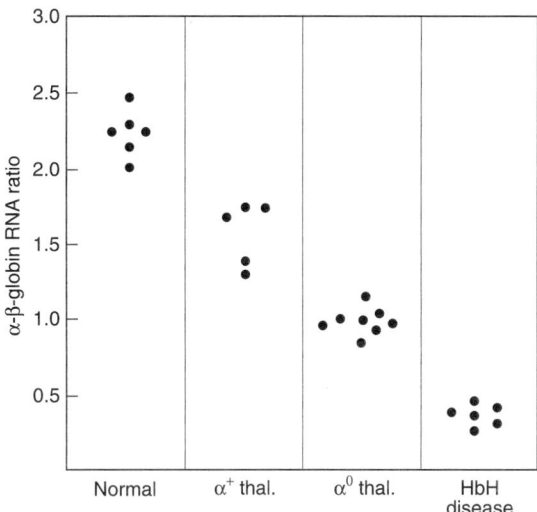

Fig. 11.14 α-/β-globin messenger RNA ratios. The results were obtained by cDNA hybridization with total RNA prepared from the peripheral blood of non-thalassaemics or obligate carriers with mild (α thalassaemia 2) or severe (α thalassaemia 1) α-thalassaemia trait, or HbH disease. Redrawn from Hunt *et al.* (1980).

Data accumulated from the current literature are summarized in Table 11.4 and Fig. 11.15. Again, those with two functional α genes (−α/−α and −−/αα) can be clearly distinguished from normal.

It is interesting that the same trends in α-/β-globin mRNA, globin synthesis and red-cell indices are seen when comparing individuals with four, three or two functional α genes. In each case those with two α-globin genes can be clearly distinguished from those with four genes. The values in those with three genes (−α/αα) overlap the two groups, but are more closely related to those with four genes (αα/αα).

The clinical heterogeneity of the homozygous states for non-deletional α⁺ thalassaemia

As a group, the homozygous states for the non-deletional forms of α⁺ thalassaemia are extremely heterogeneous (Table 11.4). As we have seen, in some cases the overall deficit of α-chain production is sufficient to result in the phenotype of HbH disease. In others the phenotype is closer to that of the homozygous state for α⁺ thalassaemia or the heterozygous state for α⁰ thalassaemia, although the degree of anaemia and hypochromia may be more severe (Paglietti *et al.* 1986). Finally, patients homozygous for the α-chain termination mutations, which result in the production of elongated α-chain variants, the commonest of which is Hb Constant Spring, are associated with a clinical phenotype which is quite different from that of any other form of α thalassaemia.

Haemoglobin Constant Spring and associated α-chain termination variants

The relationship between Hb Constant Spring and HbH disease was first reported by Milner *et al.* (1971) and its structure was described by Clegg *et al.* (1971b).

The homozygous state for Hb Constant Spring was first described by Lie-Injo *et al.* (1974) and further details of this patient were reported by Weatherall and Clegg (1975). The condition was found in a 12-year-old Malay boy who had no symptoms and was ascertained during a population study because his younger brother was found to have Hbs Constant Spring and Bart's at birth. Subsequently, several other homozygotes were described (Lie-Injo *et al.* 1975; Pongsamart *et al.* 1975; Pootrakul *et al.* 1981c).

Clinical features

None of the homozygotes were symptomatic. In all cases there was mild pallor and scleral icterus, and there was splenomegaly with mild hepatomegaly in about half of them. Heterozygotes are asymptomatic.

Haematological findings

The haematological changes in homozygotes are unusual for patients with α thalassaemia. The haemoglobin level ranges from 9 to 11 g/dl. The red-cell count is relatively low, $3.9 \pm 0.9 \times 10^{12}$/l, and the MCV tends to be normal, 88 ± 6 fl, while the MCH is only slightly reduced, 26 ± 3 pg. The peripheral blood

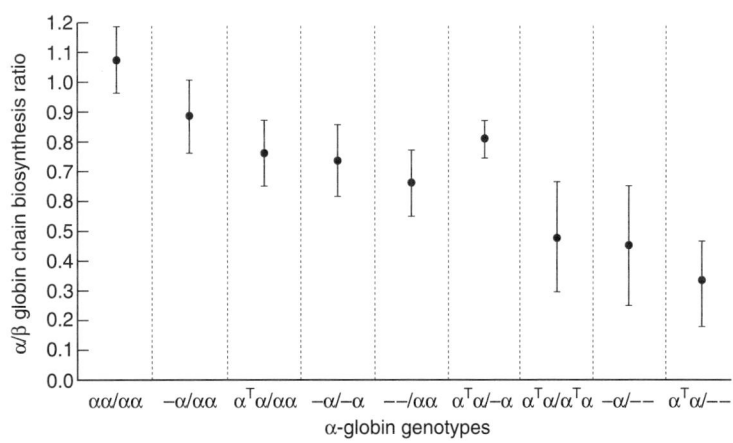

Fig. 11.15 The α-/β-chain biosynthesis ratios in different α-globin genotypes. The data are derived from the references in the legend to Table 11.4.

514   *Chapter 11*

film shows mild anisocytosis and hypochromia, with anisochromia and a few fragmented red cells. Approximately 6% of the cells show marked basophilic stippling. The reticulocyte count is consistently raised in the region of 6.0±3.3%. The serum haptoglobin level is reduced and the ^{51}Cr red-cell survival time is shortened, with values of 17.3 and 20.5 days, in two patients. Taken together, these findings suggest that these patients have a mild haemolytic anaemia.

The haematological findings in heterozygotes are typical of the genotype $\alpha\alpha/\alpha^T\alpha$ (see Table 11.4).

Haemoglobin constitution

In homozygotes the haemoglobin consists of Hbs A, A$_2$, and Constant Spring with small amounts of Hb Bart's. Haemoglobin Constant Spring can be seen as two discrete bands migrating more slowly than HbA$_2$ on electrophoresis at alkaline pH (Fig. 11.16). Overall, the levels of Hb Constant Spring have varied between 2.6 and 11.6%, while those of Hb Bart's ranged from 1.8 to 3.6%. One newborn infant with this condition had 14.2% Hb Bart's at birth, which fell to 4.6% at 8 months (Lie-Injo *et al.* 1975).

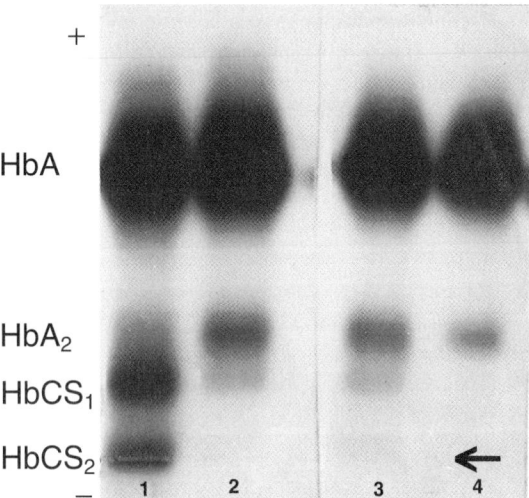

Fig. 11.16 The homozygous state for haemoglobin Constant Spring. Starch gel electrophoresis (pH 8.5, benzidine stain) of red-cell lysates from the following (left to right): 1, Hb Constant Spring homozygote; 2 and 3, the heterozygous parents; 4, normal adult. The arrow shows the position of the application of the haemoglobin to the gel.

In heterozygotes or in compound heterozygotes with α^0 thalassaemia trace amounts of variant are seen on electrophoresis, though they are easily overlooked (Fig. 11.17). At birth there is an elevated level of Hb Bart's, in the range 1–4% (Pootrakul *et al.* 1975b).

Structure

The isolation, purification and characterization of Hb Constant Spring was described in detail by Clegg *et al.* (1971b) and Weatherall and Clegg (1975). It is an α-chain variant which is elongated by 31 residues at its C-terminal end. This unusual 'tail' has several sites which are susceptible to proteolytic attack and hence it tends to break up into smaller components, either *in vivo* or after various manipulations or storage *in vitro* (Fig. 11.18). The components most easily observed on electrophoresis are the version with 31 additional residues, αCS_1, and that missing the terminal tripeptide Val-Phe-Glu, αCS_2. αCS_3, which has a shortened α chain ending at the tryptophan residue at position α154, migrates slightly faster than HbA$_2$, while αCS_4 can be observed as a very faint band migrating more slowly than αCS_2.

Haemoglobin synthesis

A surprising finding is that the α-/β-globin synthesis ratios in homozygotes are 1.5±0.16 rather than the reduced figure that would be expected in α thalassaemia. This probably reflects the fact that globin synthesis only remains linear in the cells of Hb Constant Spring homozygotes for approximately 30 min. This, together with the rapid removal of excess β chains, probably accounts for the relatively high α-/β-chain synthesis ratios observed in longer incubations (Derry *et al.* 1984). Similar mechanisms, together with the instability of Hb Constant Spring mRNA, probably reflect the wide range of α-/β-globin synthesis ratios observed in heterozygotes and compound heterozygotes (Fig. 11.19) (Weatherall *et al.* 1973; Pongsamart *et al.* 1975). The pathophysiological significance of these unexpected observations was discussed in Chapter 5.

Pathophysiology

More recent insights into the pathophysiology of the red-cell changes associated with Hb Constant Spring

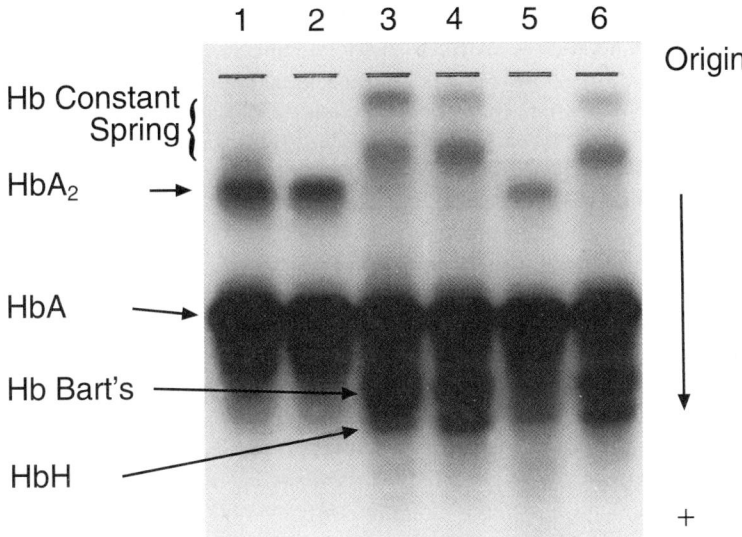

Fig. 11.17 Haemoglobin Constant Spring associated with haemoglobin H disease. Overloaded descending starch gel electrophoresis (pH 8.5, benzidine stain) of the following lysates (left to right): 1, Hb Constant Spring carrier; 2, normal; 3 and 4, Hb Constant Spring/HbH disease; 5, HbH disease without Hb Constant Spring; 6, HbH disease with Hb Constant Spring.

are discussed in Chapter 5 and by Schrier (1997) and Schrier *et al*. (1997). In short, the erythrocytes of patients with the forms of HbH disease associated with Hb Constant Spring are even more overhydrated than those of patients with other forms of HbH disease. This probably accounts for the relatively higher MCV. Furthermore, the membranes of the red cells containing Hb Constant Spring are even more rigid and hyperstable than in other forms of α thalassaemia. These changes have been related to both the accumulation of excess β chains and the attachment of partially oxidized $α^{CS}$ chains to the red-cell membrane and its skeleton. As suggested in Chapter 5, these changes may reflect the slow association of $α^{CS}$ with β chains and the early association of $α^{CS}$ chains with the membranes of the red-cell precursors. However, once $α^{CS}$ and β chains have associated to form Hb Constant Spring the variant appears to be relatively stable.

Other α-chain termination mutations

The clinical phenotypes associated with the other α-chain termination mutations have not been studied in the same detail as those for Hb Constant Spring. The homozygous state for Hb Koya Dora and the interactions of this variant with different α-thalassaemia

alleles and with Hbs S and E have been characterized, at least to some extent (de Jong *et al*. 1975; Gupta *et al*. 1991; Çürük *et al*. 1993a). It appears that the homozygous state is characterized by similar haematological changes and levels of the variant haemoglobin to those for Hb Constant Spring. Heterozygotes have extremely mild haematological changes and approximately 0.5–2% of the variant. Hb Icaria has been observed only in the heterozygous state (Fig. 11.20) or in its interaction with different α-thalassaemia alleles (Clegg *et al*. 1974; Efremov *et al*. 1990; Traeger-Synodinos *et al*. 1993; Kanavakis *et al*. 1996). Heterozygotes have extremely mild haematological changes and approximately 0.5% of the α-chain variant. Similar observations have been made in the case of heterozygotes for Hbs Seal Rock and Paksé.

Diagnostic problems and other practical issues

It is quite clear from this review of the homozygous and heterozygous states for the milder α-thalassaemia alleles that they cannot be identified with certainty at any stage of development other than by direct analysis of the α-globin genes. Unfortunately, many routine diagnostic laboratories may not

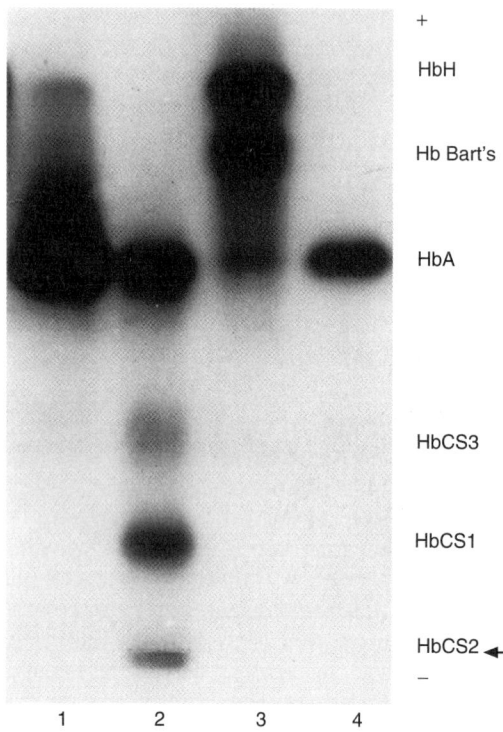

(a)

141
.......Tyr.Arg.GLN. ALA.GLY. ALA.SER. VAL. ALA.
... — α^A ⬏

149   —— CS 3 ⌐
VAL.PRO.PRO.ALA.ARG.TRP.ALA. SER.

157
GLN.ARG. ALA. LEU. LEU.PRO.SER.LEU.

165   —— CS 2 ⌐   172
HIS.ARG.PRO.PHE.LEU.VAL. PHE.GLU.

+

HbH

Hb Bart's

HbA

HbCS3

HbCS1

HbCS2 ◂
–

(b)   1   2   3   4

Fig. 11.18 The structure of haemoglobin Constant Spring.
(a) The structure of the elongated α chain. The normal α
chain ends with the arginine residue at position 141, while
Hb Constant Spring is elongated by 31 residues. The Hb
Constant Spring components 2 and 3 are probably
generated by enzymatic degradation at the sites indicated.
(b) Electrophoretic analysis of the various Hb Constant
Spring components prepared by exchange chromatography.
Lane 2 shows the purified Hb Constant Spring fraction
showing the three main components indicated in A; there is
a small amount of contaminating HbA. Lane 1 shows
mainly HbA, while lane 3 contains mainly Hbs H and
Bart's. Lane 4 is an HbA marker.

have the facilities for this type of analysis and hence
we thought it would be useful to discuss some guidelines for helping to deal with these thorny diagnostic
problems.

The α thalassaemias pose particular difficulties in
certain settings: an unexplained mild hypochromic
anaemia on routine blood testing; a mild hypochromic anaemia with normal HbA$_2$ level in a parent
whose partner has a typical β-thalassaemia trait as
part of prenatal counselling; during studies of the
relatives of patients with HbH disease; and as part of
a screening programme for thalassaemia in newborn
infants. In all these situations there are some clues as
to the presence of α thalassaemia and the likely identity of the particular allele.

The finding of a microcytic, hypochromic anaemia
in an individual who is iron replete, and in whom the
HbA$_2$ level is normal, should always raise the possibility of α thalassaemia. This is particularly the case if
the MCH and MCV are low and the red-cell count
is high; as discussed in Chapter 7 in the case of β-
thalassaemia trait, iron deficiency, when it causes the
MCV and MCH to fall into the thalassaemic range, is
nearly always associated with a more severe degree
of anaemia. The distinction between β thalassaemia
with a normal HbA$_2$ level and one or other form of α
thalassaemia can usually be made by globin synthesis.
If this suggests α thalassaemia the ethnic background
of the patient may be helpful in establishing which
type. A hypochromic microcytic picture of this kind in
individuals of African origin, where α^0-thalassaemia
trait (−−/αα) is extremely uncommon, nearly always
reflects the homozygous state for α$^+$ thalassaemia
of the deletional variety (−α/−α). On the other hand,
in persons of Mediterranean or south-east Asian
descent, where both α$^+$ and α^0 thalassaemia are
common, it is not safe to make this distinction
without globin-gene analysis.

In prenatal counselling there are two important
questions relating to putative α thalassaemia. First,
there is the common problem in which one parent
has typical β-thalassaemia trait and the other has a
similar blood picture but with a normal HbA$_2$. While,
as discussed in Chapter 7, it may be possible to identify the co-existence of β and δ thalassaemia in the
latter case by a family study, this is not always the
case. The most direct approach here, in the absence of
DNA analysis, is to distinguish between normal
HbA$_2$ β thalassaemia and α thalassaemia by globin
synthesis. A related problem is to determine whether

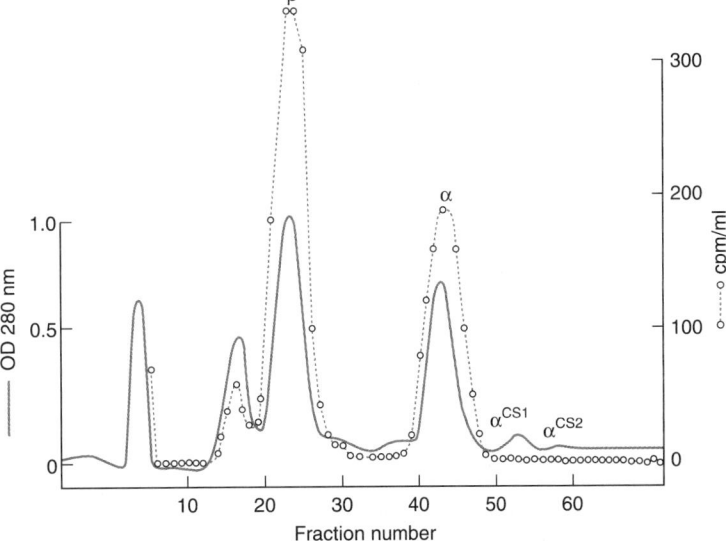

Fig. 11.19 The synthesis of haemoglobin Constant Spring. The experimental conditions are described in Chapter 5. The figure shows haemoglobin synthesis in the reticulocytes of a compound heterozygote for Hb Constant Spring and α^0 thalassaemia (Hb Constant Spring/HbH disease). It is clear that there is no synthesis of Hb Constant Spring in the peripheral blood. As discussed in Chapter 4 this probably reflects the instability of Hb Constant Spring messenger RNA.

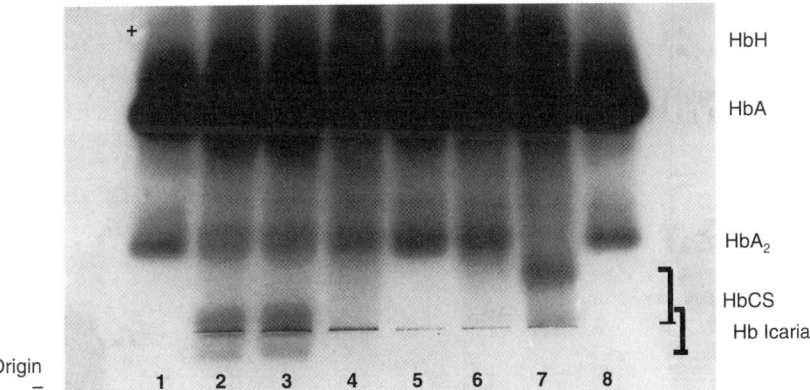

Fig. 11.20 Haemoglobin Icaria. Starch gel electrophoresis (pH 8.5, benzidine stain) of the following (left to right): 1, normal adult; 2 and 3, Hb Icaria heterozygotes; 4, Hb Constant Spring heterozygote; 5, normal adult; 6, Hb Constant Spring heterozygote; 7, Hb Constant Spring homozygote; 8, normal adult.

partners who both have thalassaemic red-cell changes with normal HbA_2 levels are at risk for having an infant with the Hb Bart's hydrops syndrome. Here the difficulty is to decide whether both of them are carriers for α^0 thalassaemia or whether one or other of them is a homozygote for α^+ thalassaemia. Although the ethnic background of the persons may be of some help, if this is not the case the only approach is to refer blood samples to a laboratory which is able to analyse the α-globin genes.

Some laboratories still use the level of Hb Bart's at birth as an indicator of the presence of different α-thalassaemia alleles. While it is now clear that low levels, in the 1–2% range, usually reflect the heterozygous state for α^+ thalassaemia, the absence of detectable Hb Bart's does not rule out this diagnosis. By and large, higher levels, in the 4–10% range, usually indicate the heterozygous state for α^0 thalassaemia or the homozygous state for α^+ thalassaemia. Higher levels, in excess of 12%, suggest that an infant may go on to develop one or other form of HbH disease. But, as is clear from discussions in the previous sections, these figures only reflect a general rule of thumb, and there is a great deal of overlap in the levels of Hb Bart's at birth between different α-thalassaemia genotypes.

Interactions between α thalassaemia and haemoglobin structural variants

Historically, interactions between α thalassaemia and structural variants of the α and β globins were of considerable importance in helping us to understand the genetics of haemoglobin and the thalassaemias (see Chapter 1).

Interactions between α thalassaemia and α-globin structural variants

When a patient with a normal β-globin genotype (β^A/β^A) and a full complement of α genes inherits one structural α-chain variant ($\alpha\alpha/\alpha^V\alpha:\beta^A/\beta^A$ or $\alpha\alpha/\alpha\alpha^V:\beta^A/\beta^A$) the amount of abnormal haemoglobin produced will depend on the rate at which it is synthesized, its stability, its affinity for β^A chains (see below) and on whether the mutation affects the α2 or α1 gene. As discussed in Chapters 2 and 4, although the ratio of α2/α1 mRNA is 3/1, there is still some dis-

agreement about the relative contributions of the two α-globin genes to the overall level of haemoglobin production. In addition, there is considerable methodological variation in the quantification of haemoglobin variants. Not surprisingly, the reported proportions of α-globin variants range from 0% in the case of the highly unstable Hb Quong Sze to ~35% for HbJ Toronto, with an average value of about 25%. Even if the highly unstable α-chain variants are excluded there is still considerable variation but, in general, mutations affecting the α2 gene are found at higher levels than those affecting the α1 gene (Huisman *et al.* 1997). Most α-globin variants are symptomless, although some are associated with a high oxygen affinity, congenital cyanosis or haemolytic anaemia (see Chapter 2). Some heterozygotes for highly unstable variants, Hb Quong Sze for example, may have the phenotype of α thalassaemia and hence they are best considered as determinants of non-deletional forms of α thalassaemia. They were considered in an earlier section.

The effect of co-inheriting α thalassaemia with α-chain variants is to increase the proportion of the variant and to reinforce any associated clinical phenotype (Table 11.5). These principles are exemplified by HbG Philadelphia ($\alpha^{68(E17) \; Asn \to Lys}$) (see also Chapter 3). Carriers of this common α-chain variant may have a full complement of four α genes

Table 11.5 Interactions between α-globin variants and α thalassaemia.

		Predicted* % of variant Hb	Haematological phenotype
$\alpha\alpha/\alpha^V\alpha$	β^A/β^A	25†–37.5‡	Normal
$\alpha\alpha/\alpha\alpha^V$	β^A/β^A	12.5†–25‡	Normal
$\alpha\alpha/\alpha^V\alpha^V$	β^A/β^A	50	Normal
$-\alpha/\alpha^V\alpha$	β^A/β^A	30†–50‡	α-Thalassaemia trait
$-\alpha/\alpha\alpha^V$	β^A/β^A	16.6†–30‡	α-Thalassaemia trait
$-\alpha/\alpha^V\alpha^V$	β^A/β^A	66	α-Thalassaemia trait
$--/\alpha\alpha^V$	β^A/β^A	30†–50‡	α-Thalassaemia trait
$-\alpha^V/\alpha\alpha$	β^A/β^A	50	α-Thalassaemia trait
$-\alpha^V/-\alpha$	β^A/β^A	50	α-Thalassaemia trait
$--/\alpha^V\alpha$	β^A/β^A	50†–70‡	α-Thalassaemia trait
$-\alpha^V/-\alpha^V$	β^A/β^A	100	α-Thalassaemia trait
$--/-\alpha^V$	β^A/β^A	100	HbH disease

* Assuming that the α^V variant is synthesized efficiently, completely stable and associates with β^A chains with the same kinetics as α^A chains.
† Assuming that the relative contribution of α2 and α1 is 1/1.
‡ Assuming that the contribution of α2 and α1 is 3/1.
By reference to Huisman *et al.* (1996), all of these assumptions almost never apply to any known variant and estimated values often differ greatly from these predicted values.

($\alpha^G\alpha/\alpha\alpha$), 20–25% of the variant haemoglobin, and no haematological abnormalities (Bruzdzinski *et al.* 1984; Molchanova *et al.* 1994a). In some, the HbG Philadelphia mutation is on a $-\alpha^{3.7}$ haplotype ($-\alpha^G$), giving rise to $-\alpha^G/\alpha\alpha$, $-\alpha^G/-\alpha$ and $-\alpha^G/-\alpha^G$ genotypes, which are associated with 30–35%, ~45% and 100% HbG Philadelphia, respectively (Milner & Huisman 1976; Sancar *et al.* 1980; Pardoll *et al.* 1982): such patients have the haematological phenotypes of heterozygous or homozygous α^+ thalassaemia. Rarely, the $-\alpha^G$ haplotype may interact with α^0 thalassaemia to produce HbH disease ($--/-\alpha^G$). Such patients produce only Hbs H and G and have the typical clinical and haematological findings of HbH disease, a condition called HbG-H disease (Rieder *et al.* 1976; Sancar *et al.* 1980).

An account of all the mutations linked to an α-thalassaemia determinant is given in Chapter 4; their interactions with other α-globin haplotypes are very similar to those just described above for HbG Philadelphia.

The interaction between HbI ($\alpha^{16Lys\rightarrow Glu}$) and α thalassaemia was initially very puzzling (Atwater *et al.* 1960; Schwartz & Atwater 1972). Most often this variant accounts for 24–28% of the total haemoglobin (Huisman *et al.* 1996). However, in the family first reported by Atwater and colleagues, in which there was also evidence for α thalassaemia, the level was 70%. It is now known that, rarely, the HbI mutation may occur on both the α2 and α1 genes on the same chromosome, presumably as a result of gene conversion (Liebhaber *et al.* 1984). Thus the patient with the $-\alpha/\alpha^I\alpha^I$ genotype had ~70% HbI, as we would now predict.

The interactions between α thalassaemia and highly unstable α-globin variants were described earlier in this chapter and in Chapter 4. In general, the $-\alpha/\alpha^V\alpha$ and $-\alpha/\alpha\alpha^V$ genotypes in these cases

give rise to α-thalassaemia trait, and the $--/\alpha^V\alpha$ genotype is associated with HbH disease. There is a tendency for such interactions to fall at the severe end of the clinical spectrum of patients with HbH disease, including HbH hydrops (see earlier section).

Interactions between α thalassaemia and β-globin structural variants

Pathophysiology

When a person inherits a normal α-globin genotype ($\alpha\alpha/\alpha\alpha$) and two β genes, one of which encodes a structural variant (β^A/β^V), the amount of abnormal haemoglobin produced will depend on its rate of synthesis, stability and the pattern of subunit assembly to form αβ dimers (Bunn & McDonald 1983; Bunn 1987). It is not surprising therefore that, just as is the case for α-globin variants, heterozygotes for β-chain variants show a wide range of different levels of the abnormal haemoglobin (Huisman *et al.* 1996). Some are synthesized less efficiently than β^A and represent less than 50% in heterozygotes, while others are unstable and may be present at 30% or less. Differences in the rates of αβ-subunit assembly also account for the lower levels of variant haemoglobins in heterozygotes.

The formation of αβ dimers is a rate-limiting step in the assembly of haemoglobin. This process is thought to be facilitated by the electrostatic attraction between positively charged α globin and negatively charged β-globin subunits. Many common β-globin variants acquire a positive charge (e.g. $\beta^{S:\ 6Glu\rightarrow Val}$) thereby reducing their ability to compete with β^A chains for α chains. In such cases less variant haemoglobin than HbA accumulates; the opposite

Table 11.6 Proportion of haemoglobin variant and haematological phenotypes in patients with positively charged β-globin variants.

		Predicted level of variant	Hb haematological phenotype
$\alpha\alpha/\alpha\alpha$	β^A/β^V	50%*	Normal
$-\alpha/\alpha\alpha$	β^A/β^V	↓	α-Thalassaemia trait
$-\alpha/-\alpha$	β^A/β^V	↓↓	α-Thalassaemia trait
$--/\alpha\alpha$	β^A/β^V	↓↓↓	α-Thalassaemia trait
$--/-\alpha$	β^A/β^V	↓↓↓↓	HbH disease

* Assuming that the variant is synthesized efficiently, is completely stable and associates with α^A chains with the same kinetics as β^A chains.

situation is seen with negatively charged β-globin variants (Fig. 11.21). These observations are supported by *in vitro* subunit competition assays using mixtures of normal (β^A) and variant (e.g. β^S and β^C) subunits (Bunn & McDonald 1983; Bunn 1987).

In the presence of α thalassaemia, in which limiting amounts of α chains are synthesized in the red cell, these effects are exaggerated. The accumulated levels of positively charged β variants are further decreased in proportion to the deficit in α-globin chains (Bunn & McDonald 1983; Bunn 1987). In contrast the levels of negatively charged variants may increase. This is a good rule of thumb although there are exceptions, HbN Baltimore for example, and the situation becomes complex when more than one β variant is involved or if α-globin variants are also present.

The co-inheritance of α thalassaemia may influence the levels of HbA_2 in the presence of β-globin variants. The δ-globin subunit is considerably more positively charged than the β-globin subunit. In α thalassaemia the amount of HbA_2 should decrease therefore, and, in general, this is what is found (Wasi *et al.* 1969, 1974). However, in the presence of a variant, positively charged β-globin subunit which has less affinity for α subunits, there may be sufficient free α chains to interact with all δ subunits, thereby increasing the level of HbA_2. Such increases have been observed in individuals with sickle-cell trait (Whitten & Rucknagel 1981) and sickle-cell disease (see below).

The presence of α thalassaemia may also influence the levels of HbF ($\alpha_2\gamma_2$) and Hb Bart's (γ_4) in some interactions. Several observations suggest that αγ dimers form less readily than αβ dimers. As discussed earlier there is more Hb Bart's in newborns with α thalassaemia than HbH in adults with the same genotype. There is some evidence that the proportion of HbF in newborns is lower in infants with α thalassaemia than those with four α genes (Stallings *et al.* 1983). Chui *et al.* (1990) described an Italian boy who co-inherited HbH disease (––/–α) and the –117 $^A\gamma$-globin HPFH mutation (see Chapters 4 and 10). They found that approximately 90% of the α chains combined with β-globin chains to form HbA (~78%), and 10% of the α chains associated with γ chains to form HbF (9.5%). Although there were sufficient free γ chains to produce approximately 11% Hb Bart's, there were insufficient free β chains remaining to produce detectable amounts of HbH on electrophoresis, although HbH inclusions were found.

Taken together these findings support the hypothesis that α globin has a higher affinity for β than γ globin. However, the interpretation of these complex interactions is by no means certain, since there are other patients with similar interactions who produce different patterns of haemoglobin expression (see e.g. Rombos *et al.* 1989).

Clinical phenotypes of patients with α thalassaemia and β-globin variants

The clinical phenotype of patients with α thalassaemia and stable β-chain variants is, as shown in Table 11.6, determined by the particular α-thalassaemia allele. In general, heterozygotes for β-chain variants who are also heterozygous for α^+ thalassaemia of the deletion or non-deletional varieties, –α/αα or $\alpha\alpha^T$/αα, show minimal haematological changes and, as a group, a slightly lower level of the β-chain variant than normal. Those that are homozygous for the deletional forms of α^+ thalassaemia, –α/–α, have hypochromic, microcytic red cells and mild anaemia, and significantly lower levels of the β-chain variant, while those who inherit the α-thalassaemia genotype associated with HbH disease, ––/–α, have the clinical picture of this condition associated with extremely low levels of the β-chain variant. The same general principles apply to the co-inheritance of the non-deletional forms of α^+ thalassaemia.

Heterozygous or homozygous α^+ thalassaemia in carriers for β-chain structural variants

Before it was possible to analyse the α-globin genes directly, extensive evidence accumulated which suggested that individuals with the sickle-cell or HbC trait who had hypochromic, microcytic red cells, with or without mild anaemia, and significantly reduced levels of the β-chain variant had co-inherited one or other form of α thalassaemia (Weatherall 1963; Tuchinda *et al.* 1964; Weatherall 1964b; Wasi *et al.* 1969; Charache *et al.* 1974; Steinberg *et al.* 1975; Henson & Huisman 1978). This suggestion was confirmed when it became possible to analyse the α-globin genes (Higgs *et al.* 1979b) (Fig. 11.21). Those who had inherited the sickle-cell trait together with the heterozygous or homozygous states for α^+ thalassaemia, –α/αα or –α/–α, had significantly reduced levels of HbS compared with those with the sickle-cell trait alone; those homozygous for α^+ thalas-

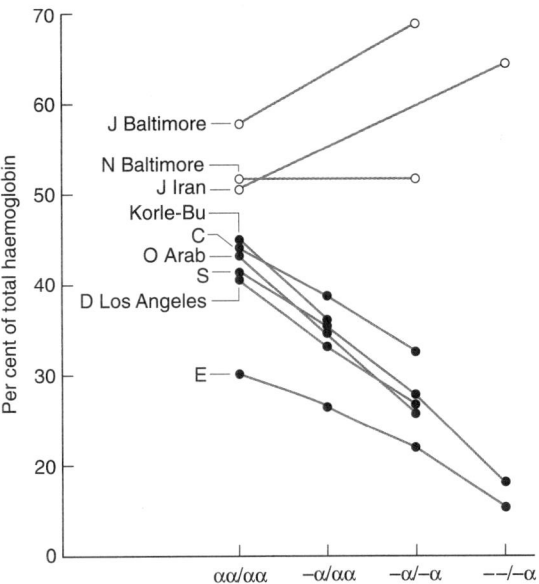

Fig. 11.21 Effect of α thalassaemia on the proportion of negatively charged (○) and positively charged (●) β-globin variants in heterozygotes. In all cases HbA constitutes the bulk of the remaining haemoglobin. In three-gene deletion α thalassaemia, a small amount of HbH (β₄) is present. Redrawn from Bunn (1987).

saemia had a significant reduction in the MCH and MCV and were mildly anaemic.

This type of interaction should be suspected, therefore, in any individual who is heterozygous for a β-chain structural haemoglobin variant and, in the absence of iron deficiency, has a hypochromic microcytic blood film and an unusually low level of the particular variant. Because of the considerable overlap in haematological values and the levels of the variant haemoglobins between different α-thalassaemia genotypes, a precise diagnosis can only be made by direct DNA analysis.

Heterozygosity for β-chain variants and the genotype of haemoglobin H disease

When a patient inherits only one functional α gene (or its equivalent) and a β-globin variant they usually have the clinical and haematological picture of HbH disease. Splenomegaly is particularly prominent in some patients (Giordano *et al.* 1996). Such interactions have been described with HbC (Giordano *et al.* 1996), HbE (Thonglairuam *et al.* 1989), HbS

(Matthay *et al.* 1979; Weatherall & Clegg 1981) and Hb Hope (Dr D.K. Bowden, personal communication). Haemoglobin analysis usually demonstrates HbA with a very reduced amount (10–20%) of the variant haemoglobin. The reported levels of HbH are quite variable in this interaction and sometimes undetectable by routine Hb electrophoresis. Nevertheless, HbH inclusions can usually be demonstrated following incubation with brilliant cresyl blue. Haemoglobin Bart's may be detectable and is characteristically found at levels of 1–6% in carriers for HbE with HbH disease, a condition referred to as A + E + Bart's disease (−−/−α, β^A/β^E or −−/α^{CS}α, β^A/β^E) (Thonglairuam *et al.* 1989) (see below).

Rare interactions between HbH disease and β-globin variants support the electrostatic model for haemoglobin subunit assembly. Su *et al.* (1992) reported HbH disease in a Chinese patient with Hb Hamilton (β$^{145\,Val→Ile}$), which has the same charge as HbA, and it appeared that the level of this variant was not significantly reduced. Rahbar and Bunn (1987) described an Iranian female with HbH disease and HbJ/Iran (β$^{77His→Asp}$), a negatively charged subunit. In this case the interaction with α thalassaemia produced an increased level (65%) of the variant haemoglobin.

Finally, Chan *et al.* (1987b) described a Chinese female with a severe transfusion-dependent haemolytic anaemia (Hb 3.4–6.8 g/dl) resulting from the interaction of HbH disease with Hb New York (β$^{113\,Val→Glu}$), an unstable, negatively charged β-globin variant. In this case the co-inheritance of α thalassaemia increased the formation of Hb New York and thus exacerbated the haemolytic anaemia.

Interactions of α thalassaemia with the common β-chain variants

Because Hbs S and E occur at such high frequency in some populations (see Chapter 6), and because there is also a high frequency of α thalassaemia in at least some of them, it is quite common for individuals to inherit both types of disorders. For this reason we shall describe some of the more clinically important interactions of this type (Table 11.7).

Haemoglobin A + E + Bart's disease

This condition, which reflects the heterozygous state for HbE in association with genotypes which cause

Genotype	Clinical findings	Haemoglobin
$\alpha\alpha/\alpha\alpha, \beta\beta^E$	Normal Red cells slightly hypochromic	A + E (HbE about 27%)
$-\alpha/\alpha\alpha, \beta\beta^E$	Normal Hypochromic red cells	A + E (HbE 20–25%)
$--/\alpha\alpha, \beta\beta^E$	Normal Hypochromic red cells	A + E (HbE about 17–20%)
$--/-\alpha, \beta\beta^E$	Similar to HbH disease	A + E + Bart's (HbE about 14%)
$-\alpha/\alpha\alpha, \beta^E\beta^E$	As for HbE disease	E + trace Bart's
$--/-\alpha, \beta^E\beta^E$	Severe thalassaemia intermedia	E + F + Bart's (HbE 80%, HbF 13%)
$--/\alpha^{CS}\alpha, \beta\beta^E$	Similar to HbH disease	A + E + Bart's + Constant Spring (as for $--/-\alpha, \beta\beta^E$ above with 1–2% Hb CS)
$--/\alpha^{CS}\alpha, \beta^E\beta^E$	Similar to HbH disease	E + Bart's (1–2% Hb CS)
$--/-\alpha, \beta^E\beta^0$	Severe thalassaemia intermedia	E + F + Bart's
$--/\alpha^{CS}\alpha, \beta^E\beta^0$	Severe thalassaemia intermedia	E + F + Bart's (1–2% Hb CS)

Table 11.7 Some interactions of haemoglobin E with α thalassaemia.

HbH disease, $--/-\alpha$ or $--/\alpha^{CS}\alpha$, occurs frequently in Thailand and other parts of south-east Asia (Wasi *et al.* 1967, 1974; Thonglairuam *et al.* 1989). The clinical manifestations are similar to those of HbH disease. There is a variable degree of anaemia and splenomegaly. In a series of 70 patients with this genotype the mean haemoglobin value was 7.3 g/dl and the red-cell morphology was similar to that seen in HbH disease (Wasi *et al.* 1974). However, unlike the latter disorder, there are relatively few red-cell inclusion bodies. The haemoglobin pattern consists of Hbs A, E, Bart's and F, and, occasionally, small amounts of HbH are found. Haemoglobin Bart's is usually found in adults with this disorder, constituting about 8% of the total haemoglobin; the average amount of HbE is in the region of 14%.

It has never been adequately explained why adults with this condition produce Hb Bart's rather than HbH. Elevated levels of HbF are very commonly found, but only in the range of 1–2% of the total haemoglobin. Clearly the γ-chain genes remain active and thus γ, β^A and β^E chains are competing for a limited number of α chains. Since β^A chains compete better than β^E chains for the relatively few available α chains this may result in an excess of γ and β^E chains. While the γ_4 tetramer is stable the β_4^E tetramer is probably not (Tuchinda *et al.* 1967) and so these patients have Hbs Bart's and E.

α Thalassaemia in homozygotes for β^E and compound heterozygotes for β^E and β^0 thalassaemia

Homozygotes for HbE are usually mildly affected but compound heterozygotes for β^E and β^0 thalassaemia display a wide variety of phenotypes and some may be as severely affected as patients with homozygous β thalassaemia (see Chapter 9). A study by Winichagoon *et al.* (1985) investigated whether the co-inheritance of α thalassaemia contributed to the variable phenotype. Among 42 β^E/β^0 thalassaemia compound heterozygotes they found seven with α thalassaemia ($-\alpha/\alpha\alpha$, β^E/β^0). The mean level of haemoglobin was higher in patients with α thalassaemia than in patients with four α genes ($\alpha\alpha/\alpha\alpha$, β^E/β^0) and their condition was thought to be clinically milder since they had not required blood transfusion, had less splenomegaly and attended the clinic less frequently. Although the haematological and clinical characteristics of patients with $-\alpha/\alpha\alpha$, β^E/β^0 thalassaemia were shifted to the mild end of the spectrum, this study could not clearly differentiate these patients from many others with HbE β thalassaemia without α thalassaemia (see Chapter 9).

Less commonly, patients with the genotype of HbH disease co-inherit two β^E alleles or β^E and β^0-thalassaemia alleles (Fucharoen *et al.* 1988c). To date four genotypes have been identified ($--/-\alpha$, β^E/β^E; $--/-\alpha$, β^E/β^0; $--/\alpha^{CS}\alpha$, β^E/β^E; and $--/\alpha^{CS}\alpha$, β^E/β^0), although many other interactions are possible. In a study of 19 patients by Fucharoen *et al.* (1988c), it was not possible to distinguish the clinical findings associated with these genotypes from others with β^E/β^0 thalassaemia ($\alpha\alpha/\alpha\alpha$, β^E/β^0), HbA + E + Bart's disease ($--/-\alpha$, β^A/β^E) or HbH disease ($--/-\alpha$, β^A/β^A). The haemoglobin levels ranged from 6.1 to 10.4 g/dl. The MCV (58–74 fl) and MCH (15–21 pg) values were markedly reduced in all cases. Reticulocyte counts were raised, 0.8–11.4%, and the peripheral blood films showed anisopoikilocytosis, polychromasia and target cells. Haemoglobin analysis characteristically showed HbE (67.7–94.5%), with HbF (1.3–24.9%) and Hb Bart's (1.2–7.3%). Hence this group of inter-actions are also referred to as HbE + F + Bart's disease (Wasi *et al.* 1974; Weatherall & Clegg 1981).

When Hb Constant Spring is one of the α-thalassaemia determinants it may also be present in the range 0.3–4.3%. Like HbA + E + Bart's disease, HbH inclusions are rare in E + F + Bart's disease, further evidence that β^E chains do not form homotetramers.

α *Thalassaemia and sickle-cell anaemia*

The pathophysiology and clinical features of the sickle-cell disorders were summarized in Chapter 2.

Wherever sickle-cell disease occurs α thalassaemia nearly always co-exists, so that it is common to co-inherit the two conditions. There have been many studies over the past 10–15 years to evaluate the influence of α thalassaemia on sickle-cell disease. The haematological effects are now well characterized and reasonably well understood. On the other hand the effects of α thalassaemia on the clinical manifestations of sickle-cell disease are subtle and have been inconsistent between different studies (Table 11.8).

Patients with α^+ thalassaemia and sickle-cell disease ($-\alpha/\alpha\alpha$, β^S/β^S and $-\alpha/-\alpha$, β^S/β^S) have higher levels of haemoglobin and higher red-cell counts

Table 11.8 The influence of α thalassaemia on the clinical features of sickle-cell disease.

Clinical feature	Reported effect of α thalassaemia	References
Painful crisis	No direct effect	Higgs *et al.* (1982); Steinberg *et al.* (1984); Platt *et al.* (1991)
Acute chest syndrome	Less frequent; no effect	Higgs *et al.* (1982); Steinberg *et al.* (1984)
Leg ulceration	Less frequent; no effect	Higgs *et al.* (1982); Steinberg *et al.* (1984)
Peptic ulceration	No significant effect	Higgs *et al.* (1982)
Aplastic crisis	No significant effect	Higgs *et al.* (1982)
Splenectomy	No significant effect	Higgs *et al.* (1982)
Splenic sequestration	More frequent; no effect	Mears *et al.* (1982); Emond *et al.* (1984)
Splenomegaly	More common	Higgs *et al.* (1982)
Hepatomegaly > 3 cm	Reduced	Higgs *et al.* (1982)
Priapism	No effect	Higgs *et al.* (1982)
Peripheral retinal closure	Reduced	Fox *et al.* (1993)
Proliferative sickle retinopathy	No effect	Fox *et al.* (1993)
Obstetric complications	No effect	Higgs *et al.* (1982)
Physical development	No effect	Higgs *et al.* (1982)
Stroke	Possibly reduced risk	Piomelli *et al.* (1986); Miller *et al.* (1988b); Adams *et al.* (1994)
Aseptic necrosis	Increased	Steinberg *et al.* (1984); Ballas *et al.* (1989); Milner *et al.* (1991)
Survival	Prolonged; no effect	Higgs *et al.* (1982); Mears *et al.* (1983)

than patients without α thalassaemia (αα/αα, β^S/β^S). In addition they have lower reticulocyte counts and levels of serum total bilirubin, suggesting that α thalassaemia reduces haemolysis. This has been confirmed by studies of red-cell survival in both –α/–α, β^S/β^S (deCeulaer *et al.* 1983) and –α/αα, β^S/β^S (Serjeant *et al.* 1996) genotypes.

The co-inheritance of α thalassaemia results in relatively lower MCH and MCV values in patients with sickle-cell disease. However, the main mechanism by which α thalassaemia is thought to reduce haemolysis is by decreasing the concentration of HbS in the red cell, thereby reducing polymerization. The red cells of patients with both conditions have a reduced MCHC and, as judged from density gradient studies, are better hydrated (Embury *et al.* 1984, 1985a) with fewer dense forms (Noguchi & Schechter 1981). As a consequence, the red cells are deformable and have a greater membrane redundancy so that they are better protected against sickling-induced membrane stretching and cation loss (reviewed in Steinberg 1991). Consistent with these findings, patients with α thalassaemia and sickle-cell disease have fewer irreversibly sickled cells in their peripheral blood (Higgs *et al.* 1982).

By the same logic that explains how α thalassaemia reduces haemolysis in sickle-cell disease it would be predicted that it might also reduce microvascular disease. Certainly, vaso-occlusive events may be marginally less frequent, as is the case for the acute chest syndrome and ankle ulceration. However, the frequency of painful crises is unaffected and aseptic necrosis of bone may be more frequent (see Table 11.8), possibly because improvements in red-cell deformability are offset by the rheological consequences of an increased packed cell volume. Although it has been suggested that α thalassaemia prolongs survival in patients with sickle-cell disease (Mears *et al.* 1983), this is an extremely difficult question to answer in a highly selected clinical population; this effect is not observed in all studies (Higgs *et al.* 1982).

The co-inheritance of α thalassaemia alters the haemoglobin composition of patients with sickle-cell disease. As already explained, the relatively low affinity of β^S for α-globin subunits may release sufficient α chains to combine with all available δ chains, accounting for the increased levels of HbA$_2$ observed in patients with –α/αα, β^S/β^S and –α/–α, β^S/β^S genotypes. There are less consistent alterations in the levels of

HbF compared with patients with sickle-cell anaemia without α thalassaemia. They may be elevated (Embury *et al.* 1982), unchanged (Steinberg *et al.* 1984) or reduced (Higgs *et al.* 1982). The level of HbF in patients with sickle-cell disease is the end result of several complex interactions (see Chapters 4, 9 and 10). The simplest explanation for the small effect of α thalassaemia is that, by inhibiting haemolysis, it reduces the selective pressure for cells containing HbF, which survive longer because of their ability to resist intracellular sickling.

The haematological differences between sickle-cell homozygotes with or without α thalassaemia evolve over the first few years of life; those in MCV are present from birth and in red-cell count by 1 month. Patients with α thalassaemia have reduced numbers of reticulocytes from 3 months (Stevens *et al.* 1986). The differences in haemoglobin levels develop more slowly; in the study of Stevens *et al.* (1986) no difference was seen by 8 years of age, whereas Felice *et al.* (1987) observed characteristically higher levels in children with the –α/–α, β^S/β^S genotype from the age of 8 years onwards. Elevated levels of HbA$_2$ were observed in patients with α thalassaemia by the age of 1 year, but HbF levels did not differ significantly, even at the age of 15 years, in the study of Felice *et al.* (1987).

Other interactions between α thalassaemia and haemoglobin S

Because of the rarity of α^0-thalassaemia alleles in African or Indian populations in which the sickle-cell gene is common, the association of the genotype for HbH disease with the sickling disorders is unusual. It is most likely to occur either in persons of mixed ethnic background or in populations such as those of Saudi Arabia and other countries in which there is a high frequency of the sickle-cell gene and non-deletional forms of α$^+$ thalassaemia which, in the homozygous state, result in HbH disease.

A description of what was almost certainly an example of the interaction of the homozygous state for α$^+$ thalassaemia and homozygosity for the sickle-cell gene was reported by Weatherall *et al.* (1969a). The patient was a 4-year-old girl from the oasis population of eastern Saudi Arabia. She was mildly anaemic with hypochromic red cells. Haemoglobin analysis revealed Hbs S, F and Bart's, in the proportions 40.7, 43.7 and 14%, respectively. Both the child's parents had the sickle-cell trait and both showed marked hypochromia and variation in the shape and size of their red cells. The unexpectedly high levels of Hbs F and Bart's in this child are not surprising, considering that relatively high levels of HbF are extremely common in the sickle-cell population of eastern Saudi Arabia (see Chapters 4 and 10). Although this child was studied before direct DNA analysis of the α-globin genes was possible, subsequent studies in Saudi Arabia showed that all cases of HbH disease result from the homozygous state for a non-deletional form of α thalassaemia (Pressley *et al.* 1980b).

The association of the sickle-cell trait with HbH disease has been reported in individuals from two populations, one of mixed Chinese and African origin (Matthay *et al.* 1979), the other from eastern Saudi Arabia (Weatherall & Clegg 1981). The findings in both these patients were similar, with one exception. Both had mild to moderate hypochromic anaemias with haemoglobin values in the 7–9 g/dl range. In both cases red-cell inclusions were generated after incubation with brilliant cresyl blue. Their haemoglobin patterns consisted of approximately 60% HbA, 15–17% HbS and 5–10% HbF. In the child reported by Matthay *et al.* no HbH could be demonstrated, although there was 3.4% Hb Bart's. In the Saudi patient there was approximately 10% HbH. It is not clear why in one case of this interaction the patient produced only Hb Bart's while in the other there was a relatively high level of HbH. In the child of Chinese and African origin the genotype was $--/-\alpha$, whereas in the Saudi child the genotype was, presumably, $\alpha^T\alpha/\alpha^T\alpha$. However these differences are not really accounted for by the molecular pathology and, as is the case for HbH disease in general (see earlier section), it is not absolutely clear why some patients make predominantly Hb Bart's while others produce HbH.

In none of these patients with co-existing sickling disorders and α thalassaemia has it been possible to identify haemoglobins with the structure β_4^S. Molecules with this structure were described by Huisman (1960a,b) and called Hb Augusta 1, but they do not appear to have been identified subsequently.

Postscript

Over the past 20 years we have obtained a comprehensive picture of the molecular basis of α thalassaemia and we now know that a substantial proportion of the world's population has one or other of the genetic conditions summarized in this chapter. Because α thalassaemia is so common, the chance finding of a hypochromic, microcytic anaemia is often the cause of inappropriate investigation and concern for unaware or inexperienced physicians. Fortunately, once the diagnosis has been made, only a small proportion, albeit large numbers, of patients need further attention. Most patients with HbH disease are well, whereas a few have thalassaemia intermedia. There is a need to document the natural history of HbH disease and to establish more fully the correlation between genotype and phenotype to improve our ability to predict clinical severity. Ultimately, this would enable more precise prenatal counselling and would allow us to develop the best strategies for managing the relatively few patients who will be severely affected by this disorder.

The most important task for the future is to establish cheap, effective screening programmes to avoid pregnancies leading to the lethal Hb Bart's hydrops fetalis and the rare HbH hydrops fetalis syndromes, which also impose considerable risk on the mother. At-risk couples are still not always identified, even in countries with advanced medical services.

Current observations on the clinical and haematological interactions of α thalassaemia with β thalassaemia (Chapter 13) and β-chain abnormalities such as sickle-cell disease suggest that reducing α-globin synthesis may offer another therapeutic approach to the amelioration of these conditions. Hopefully, such approaches should evolve from our continued attempts to understand more completely the mechanisms by which the α-globin genes are regulated.

Chapter 12
α Thalassaemia with mental retardation or myelodysplasia

Introduction

All the different forms of α thalassaemia described in the previous chapters follow a simple Mendelian pattern of inheritance and, although they can occur in any population, are only found at high frequencies in parts of the world where malaria was, or in some cases still is, a major killer. As we saw in Chapter 6, there is now very substantial evidence that these high gene frequencies are related to resistance on the part of individuals with the milder forms of α thalassaemia to malarial infection.

It has been apparent for some time, however, that there are other forms of α thalassaemia which do not have any particular geographical pattern of occurrence and which are not inherited in the usual Mendelian way. Since the last edition of this book was written it has become clear that there are two conditions in which mild forms of α thalassaemia are associated with mental retardation. Studies of these disorders have provided valuable information about the regulation of the α-globin genes and, in addition, are starting to offer important insights into the pathogenesis of some forms of mental retardation and developmental abnormalities. Another unusual form of α thalassaemia, that associated with myelodysplasia, has been recognized for much longer. Although less progress has been made towards an understanding of its pathogenesis and relationship to haemopoietic neoplasia, it too has important implications for our further understanding of the regulation of the α-globin genes and, perhaps more importantly, for providing some badly needed insights into the aetiology of the myelodysplasias. X

In this chapter we shall review what is known of these unusual forms of α thalassaemia and what their study is telling us about the regulation of the α-globin genes. It should be emphasized that these disorders are completely unlike the other forms of thalassaemia described in this book. The thalassaemic phenotype is not the main feature of these conditions. Rather it is a result of situations in which the α-globin genes, as innocent bystanders, have been caught up in a pathological process that leads to a completely different disorder.

α Thalassaemia and mental retardation

The rare association between α thalassaemia and mental retardation might easily have been dismissed as the chance occurrence of two common conditions. However, when Weatherall *et al.* (1981a) described three mentally retarded children with α thalassaemia and a variety of developmental abnormalities interest was stimulated by the unusual nature of the α thalassaemia.

The children were of North European origin, where α thalassaemia is uncommon (see Chapter 6), and, although it might have been expected that there would be clear signs of this inherited anaemia in their parents, in the event it appeared to have arisen *de novo* in the affected offspring. It was concluded that the combination of α thalassaemia and mental retardation, together with the associated developmental abnormalities, represented a new syndrome and that a common genetic mechanism might be responsible for these diverse clinical manifestations.

It is now clear that these original suspicions were well founded, although it has subsequently emerged that there are two distinct syndromes in which α thalassaemia is associated with mental retardation (ATR) (Wilkie *et al.* 1990a,c). The first, ATR-16, is characterized by large (1–2 Mb) chromosomal rearrangements that delete many genes from the short arm of chromosome 16: it is therefore an example of a contiguous gene syndrome. In the second, ATR-X, a complex phenotype, including α thalassaemia, results from mutations in an X-encoded factor which is a putative regulator of gene expression. Mutations in this gene downregulate α-gene expression and also perturb the expression of other, as yet unidentified, genes.

The ATR-16 syndrome

To date we know of 17 individuals who have the ATR-16 syndrome (Table 12.1). Often, clinicians have been alerted to this condition by observing the unusual association of α thalassaemia and mental retardation in persons originating from outside the areas in which thalassaemia commonly occurs (see Chapter 6). There are two common patterns of inheritance. In 11 cases neither parent has α thalassaemia (αα/αα×αα/αα) and the affected offspring has the phenotype of severe α-thalassaemia trait (genotype −−/αα). In five cases one parent has the phenotype of mild α-thalassaemia trait, while the other is normal (−α/αα×αα/αα); the child has HbH disease (genotype −−/−α). In all such cases initial molecular genetic analyses have shown that the patients fail to inherit the entire ζα-globin cluster from one or other of the parents.

Clinical features

For reasons which are described below, the clinical features, including the degree of mental retardation, are extremely diverse. The main findings in the cases reported to date are summarized in Table 12.2.

Chromosomal abnormalities

In some cases conventional cytogenetic analysis may immediately demonstrate the underlying genetic abnormality. Since the α-globin complex lies very close to the 16p telomere (Fig. 12.1) any chromosomal abnormality affecting this region may give rise to α thalassaemia (Wilkie *et al.* 1990a). In some patients with ATR-16 gross chromosomal abnormalities resulting in deletions (Wilkie *et al.* 1990a), the formation of ring chromosomes (e.g. Neidengard & Sparkes 1981; Quintana *et al.* 1983; Callen *et al.* 1989)

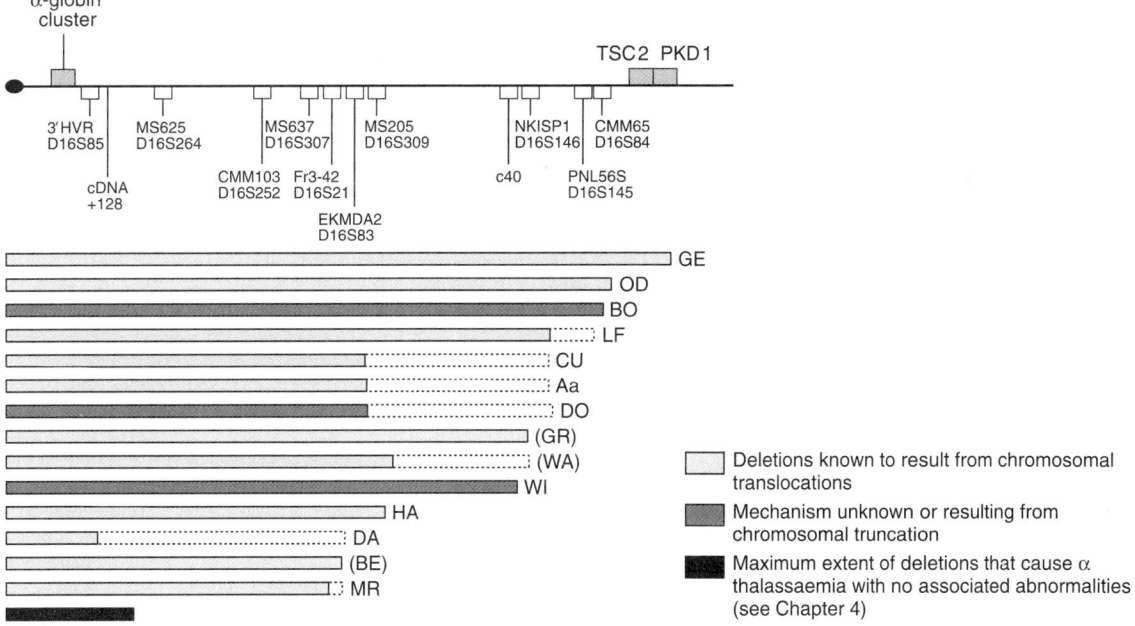

Fig. 12.1 Summary of ATR-16 deletions. Above, the 16p telomere is indicated as a black oval and the positions of the α-globin cluster and the genes encoding tuberous sclerosis (TSC2) and the adult form of polycystic kidney disease (PKD1) are indicated. The positions of other 'anchor' markers are also shown. Below, the extent of each deletion is shown with the patient code alongside (see Table 12.1). Solid bars indicate regions known to be deleted and broken lines indicate the region of uncertainty of the breakpoints (S. Horsley *et al.* 2001; R. Daniels *et al.* 2001).

Table 12.1 Cytogenetic and haematological data and origin of ATR-16 mutations.

Case	Sex	MR	Phenotype	Genotype	Conventional cytogenetics	Chromosomal abnormality	Origin	Parental mechanism	Reference
OD	M	Moderate	HbH	--/-α	Normal	46,XY −16, +der(16)t(1;16)(p36p13.3)	Maternal	Inherit 16:1 unbal trans	Lamb et al. (1989); Wilkie et al. (1990a)
DA	M	Mild	Trait	--/αα	Abnormal	45,XY −15, −16 +der(16)t(15;16)(q13.1p13.3)	Paternal	De novo	Wilkie et al. (1990a)
CU	M	Mild	Trait	--/αα	Abnormal	46,XY −16 +der(16)t(9;16)(21.2;p13.3)	Maternal	De novo	Wilkie et al. (1990a); Rack et al. (1993)
MR	F	Mild	Trait	--/αα	Abnormal	46,XX −16, +der(16)t(9;16)(21.2:13.3)	Paternal	De novo	Rack et al. (1993)
Aa	F	Borderline	Trait	--/αα	Abnormal	46,XX −16, +der(126)t(10:16)(q26.13;p13.3)	Maternal	Inherit 16:10 unbal trans	Buckle et al. (1988); Wilkie et al. (1990a)
BO	M	Mild	HbH	--/-α	Normal	46,XY del(16)(p13.3)	Paternal	De novo truncation	Wilkie et al. (1990a); Lamb et al. (1993)
DO	F	Mild	HbH	--/-α	Normal*	46,XY del(16)(p13.3) +?	Maternal	Unknown	Wilkie et al. (1990a)
HA	M	Borderline	HbH	--/-α	Normal	46,XY del(16)(p13.3) +?	Paternal	Unknown	Wilkie et al. (1990a)
WI	M	Borderline	Trait	--/αα	Normal	46,XY del(16)(p13.3) +?	Paternal	Unknown	Wilkie et al. (1990a)
LF	M	Unknown	NA	NA	Abnormal	46,XY −16 +der(16)t(X;16)(p11.4;p13.3)	Maternal	Inherit unbal trans	K. May (personal communication)
CH(BE)	F	NA	Trait	--/αα	Normal	46,XX +der(16)t(16;16)(q24p13.3)	Unknown	Inversion/deletion	Rönich & Kleihauer (1967) and unpublished
W(BE)	M	NA	Trait	--/αα	Normal	46,XX +der(16)t(16;16)(q24p13.3)	Unknown	Inversion/deletion	Rönich & Kleihauer (1967) and unpublished
C(WA)	F	Borderline	Trait	--/αα	Normal	46,XX −16, +der(16)t(16;20)(p13.3;q13.3)	Maternal	Inherit unbal trans	Unpublished
M(GR)	M	Borderline	Trait	--/αα	Normal	46,XY del(16)(p13.3) +?	Maternal	Inherit 16:21 unbal trans	Unpublished
J(GR)	F	Borderline	Trait	--/αα	Normal	46,XY del(16)(p13.3) +?	Maternal	Inherit 16:21 unbal trans	Unpublished
C(BE)	F	MR+	HbH	--/-α	Normal	46,XX +der(16)t(16;16)(q24p13.3)	Maternal	Inversion/deletion	Rönich & Kleihauer (1967) and unpublished
GE	M	Severe	Trait	--/αα	NA	45,XY −16 −22 +der(16)(16qter-16p13.3::22q11.21-22qter)	Maternal	Inherit unbal trans	European Polycystic Kidney Disease Consortium (1994)

* At low resolution.
MR, mental retardation; trans, translocation; unbal, unbalanced.
MR+, mental retardation not classified.
NA, not assessed.

Table 12.2 Clinical findings in patients with ATR-16 syndrome.

Case†	MR	Normal BW	Neonatal problems	Microcephaly	Short stature	Facial dysmorphism	Genital abnormalities	Skeletal abnormalities	Miscellaneous abnormalities
OD	Moderate	+	+	-	-	+	+	-	CAL
DA	Mild	+	+	-	-	+	+	+	SPC, HT
CU	Mild	+	-	-	-	+	-	+	SPC
MR	Mild	+	-	-	+	+	-	+	SPC
Aa	Borderline	+	+	-	-	+	-	-	UG, HPN
BO	Mild	+	-	+	-	+	+	+	IC, P
DO	Mild	+	+	-	+	+	-	-	IC
HA	Borderline	+	+	-	-	+	-	+	E
WI	Borderline	+	-	-	-	+	+	+	AN, IC
LF	U	NA	NA	NA	NA	+	+	NA	T, CS, CHD, H
CH(BE)	NA	NA	NA	NA	NA	+	NA	NA	NA
W(BE)	NA	NA	NA	NA	NA	+	NA	NA	NA
C(BE)	+*	-	+	-	NA	+	-	NA	S
C(WA)	Borderline	+	+	-	+	+	-	+	S, PVC, LFW, SD, NW
M(GR)	Borderline	+	+	-	-	+	-	+	
J(GR)	Borderline	+	+	+	-	+	-	+	CHD
GE	Severe	NA	-	-	-	-	-	-	TS, RC, E

+* Mental retardation not classified. † See also Table 12.1.

AN, accessory nipple; BW, birth weight; CAL, café au lait patches; CHD, congenital heart disease; CS, choanal stenosis; E, epilepsy; H, hydrocephalus; HPN, high-placed nipples; HT, hypoplastic enamel of teeth; IC, impaired coordination; LFW, left facial weakness; M, myopia; MR, mental retardation; NA, data not available; NW, neck webbing; P, ptosis; PL, pigmented lesions (hypo- and hyper-); PVC, paralysed vocal cord (unilateral); RC, renal cysts; S, strabismus; SD, sacral dimple; SPC, single palmar crease; T, tracheobronchomalacia; TS, tuberous sclerosis; U, unable to assess at time of death; UG, unsteady gait.

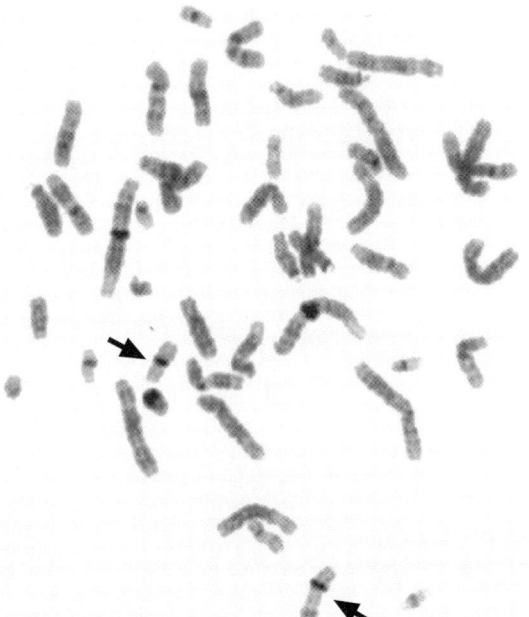

Fig. 12.2 High-resolution cytogenetic analysis in an individual with ATR-16 syndrome demonstrating a translocation between chromosomes 9 and 16. The normal and abnormal copies of chromosome 16 are arrowed.

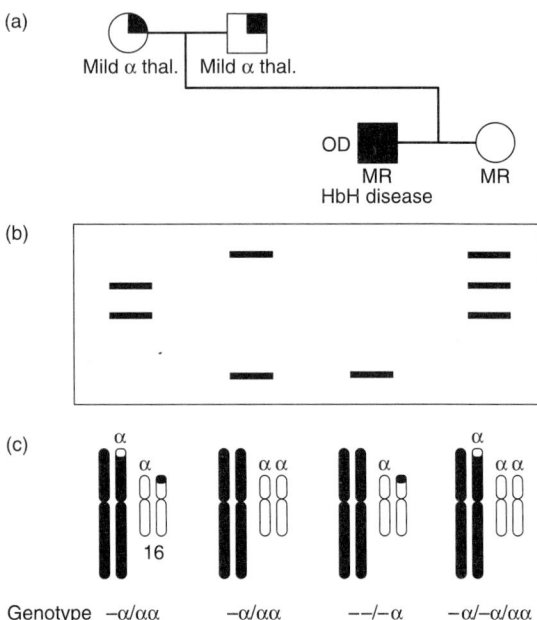

Fig. 12.3 Familial subcytogenetic translocation (from Lamb *et al.* 1989). (a) Pedigree showing parents with mild α thalassaemia only, a son (OD) with mental retardation and severe α thalassaemia (HbH disease), and a daughter with mental retardation. (b) Schematic representation of restriction fragment length polymorphism analysis using a fully informative marker closely linked to the α-globin cluster. Each track corresponds to the individuals shown above. (c) Segregation of 1:16 translocation and α-globin complex (α) in each family member. The resulting genotype is shown. Note that both children have inherited the paternal chromosome carrying the (–α) allele; it has not been determined whether the mother's normal or translated chromosome 16 bears her (–α) allele.

and translocations (e.g. Buckle *et al.* 1988) have been observed. Although such abnormalities may arise as *de novo* genetic events, often one parent carries a pre-existing balanced translocation which the child inherits in an unbalanced fashion (see Figs 12.2 and 12.3 for examples), resulting in monosomy for 16p and loss of the α-globin-gene cluster.

In many cases of ATR-16 initial high-resolution cytogenetic analysis appears entirely normal. However, it is important to remember that even chromosomal rearrangements involving large fragments of DNA (5–10 Mb) may not be detected by routine cytogenetics. In this situation the pattern of inheritance of variable-number tandem repeats (VNTRs) (as defined in Chapter 2) within the α cluster may reveal the underlying molecular defect. In the example given in Fig. 12.3 (originally described in Lamb *et al.* 1989) the parental 16p alleles can be distinguished from each other. The mother in this family carries an unbalanced (16:1) translocation which both of her children inherited in an imbalanced fashion. Her son OD (Table 12.1) is monosomic for

16p, and therefore has α thalassaemia (in this case HbH disease), whereas her daughter is trisomic for 16p. Both children have mental retardation, dysmorphic facies and a variety of associated developmental abnormalities.

VNTRs are not always informative and, more recently, fluorescence *in situ* hybridization (FISH) studies have been used to analyse ATR-16 families. In this type of analysis large segments (~40 kb) of chromosome 16 in cosmid vectors are used as probes to demonstrate the presence or absence of the corresponding sequences in the 16p telomeric region with fluorescence microscopy (Buckle & Kearney 1994). By analysing the chromosomes of both parents and the affected child it is possible to define the extent of 16p monosomy and the mechanism by which it has arisen. In the example shown in Fig. 12.4a FISH analysis demonstrated that the mother of children with the ATR-16 syndrome carries a 5:16 translocation (unpublished observation) which was inherited in an unbalanced fashion, as in Fig. 12.3, by her offspring. In the second example (case HA in Wilkie *et al.* 1990a) both parents were shown to be normal but FISH analysis demonstrated a *de novo* loss of material from the end of chromosome 16 (Fig. 12.4b) in their child HA (Table 12.1). These types of chromosomal abnormality that can only be detected by FISH or molecular analyses are referred to as 'cryptic' chromosomal abnormalities.

Using a combination of conventional cytogenetics, FISH and molecular analysis, at least three types of chromosomal rearrangements — inherited or *de novo* translocations, inversion/deletions and truncations — have now been found in patients with ATR-16 (Fig. 12.1 and Table 12.1). At present none of the breakpoints associated with the 16p translocations has been sequenced. Similarly, the inversion/deletion event (CHBE, WBE, CBE) has only been partially characterized. The telomeric truncation seen in BO (Table 12.1) has been fully analysed (Lamb *et al.* 1993). In this important case it appears that the chromosome was broken, truncated and 'healed' by the direct addition of telomeric repeats $(TTAGGG)_n$ (Fig. 12.5), as described for some less extensive 16p deletions in Chapter 4.

A review of the literature has also identified other less well characterized chromosomal abnormalities that may cause the ATR-16 syndrome. For example, Pawlowitzki *et al.* (1979) described a child with the unbalanced karyotype 46,XX, −16,+der(16),t(16;20)(p13;q11) who at the age of 9 months had severe hypochromia (MCH was 17.6 pg): it is likely that this child had α thalassaemia, but this was not investigated. There are a number of other reports of possible chromosome 16p deletions, including ring (16), associated with mental retardation, but haematological data were either not given (Pergament *et al.* 1970; Bauknecht *et al.* 1976; Golden *et al.* 1981; Nielsen *et al.* 1983; Quintana *et al.* 1983; Anneren & Gustavson 1984; Nazarenko *et al.* 1987; Chodirker *et al.* 1988) or were equivocal (Neidengard & Sparkes 1981; Emanuel *et al.* 1982). Further analysis of DNA from the ring (16) patient of Neidengard and Sparkes (1981) indicates that the

α-globin complex has been deleted from the ring chromosome (Callen *et al.* 1989), the breakpoint lying between EKMDA2 and NIKSP1 (see Fig. 12.1; unpublished results), and the ring (16) patient of Quintana *et al.* (1983) is also missing the α-globin complex from the involved chromosome (Callen *et al.* 1989).

Although such cases of α thalassaemia and mental retardation have doubtless been overlooked, it is nevertheless likely that the syndrome is rare, because each case found to date has been the result of a unique and independent chromosome mutation.

How do chromosomal abnormalities give rise to the ATR-16 syndrome?

In the light of these observations it is clear that individuals with ATR-16 may have quite variable degrees of chromosomal imbalance and consequently it is not surprising that there is considerable variation in the associated clinical phenotypes (Table 12.2). The degree of 16p monosomy varies from ~1 to 2 Mb (Fig. 12.1) but at least 11 patients have additional chromosomal aneuploidy; in some cases imbalance of the non-16 material may dominate the clinical picture. For example in DA (Table 12.1) loss of material from chromosome 15, while forming the abnormal derivative t(15:16) chromosome, produced the striking phenotype associated with the Prader–Willi syndrome.

In only one patient (BO) can all of the clinical features be attributed solely to loss of material from 16p (Lamb *et al.* 1993). However, in two other patients (DO and WI, see Fig. 12.1 and Table 12.1) current data suggest that the predominant abnormality may similarly result from 16p monosomy. Several of these patients have a similar facial appearance, similar degrees of mild mental retardation and some associated developmental abnormalities in common (Fig. 12.6 and Table 12.2).

By studying such a group of patients it should be possible to understand how 16p monosomy gives rise to the associated developmental abnormalities. Initially it seemed possible that hemizygosity for the embryonic ζ-globin gene might give rise to neonatal hypoxia and consequent developmental abnormalities. However, we now know that many patients with relatively small (up to 200-kb) deletions (see Chapters 4 and 11 and Fig. 12.1) including the entire ζ–α cluster may be developmentally normal. Another

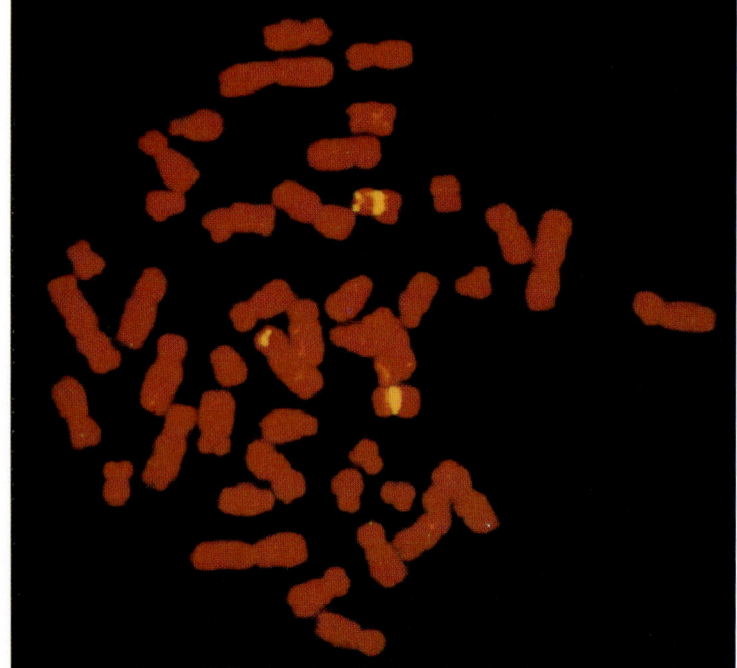

(a)

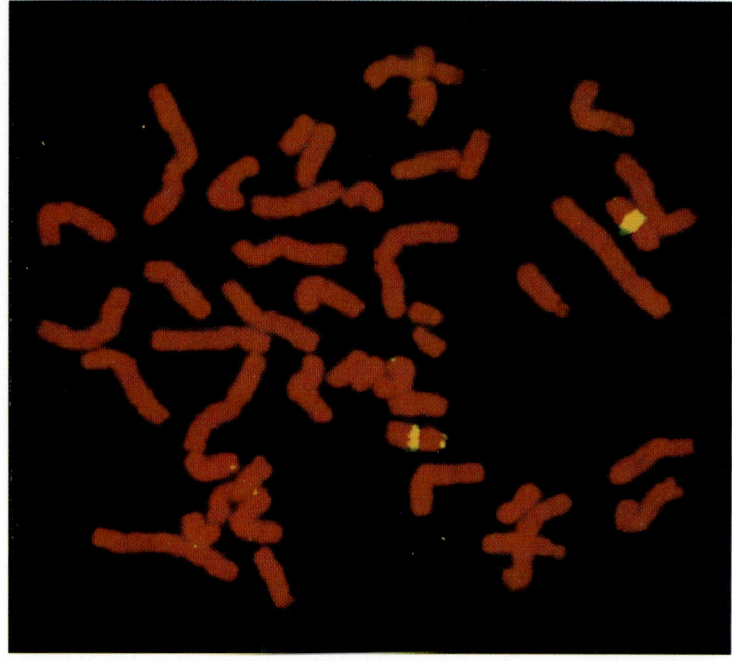

(b)

Fig. 12.4 Cytogenetic findings in ATR-16 syndromes. (a) An example of an unbalanced translocation in a parent of a child with the ATR-16 syndrome. (b) Loss of 16p material in an individual with the ATR-16 syndrome.

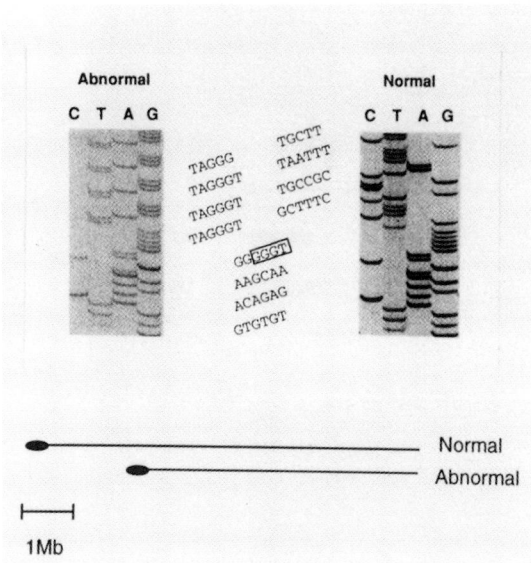

Fig. 12.5 Sequence analysis of the BO breakpoint. The chromosome has broken and been 'healed' directly by the addition of telomeric (TTAGGG) repeats (see Lamb *et al.* 1993). (See also Fig. 12.1.)

possibility is that deletion of a large number of genes from one copy of chromosome 16 could unmask mutations in its homologue; the more genes that are deleted the greater the probability of this occurring. However, this is unlikely to be the explanation for most ATR-16 cases since it is estimated that normal individuals only carry a few harmful mutations of this type in the entire genome (Vogel & Motulsky 1986). A further possibility is that some genes in 16p are imprinted (Hall 1990) so that deletions could remove the only active copy of the gene. At present there is no evidence for imprinting of the 16p region (reviewed by Schneider *et al.* 1996), and in the few ATR-16 cases we have analysed there appear to be no major clinical differences between patients with deletions of the maternally or paternally derived chromosomes (Table 12.1). It therefore seems more likely that there are some genes in the 16p region that encode proteins whose effect is critically determined by the amount produced; so-called dosage-sensitive genes (see Fisher & Scambler 1994). Examples include those encoding proteins that form heterodimers, those required at a critical level for a rate-determining step of a regulatory pathway, and

tumour suppressor genes, TSC2 for example (see below). Removal of such critical, dosage-sensitive genes might account for many of the clinical effects seen in patients with ATR-16.

Some of these points can be addressed from currently available data. It is clear that removal of up to ~250kb of 16p, including an estimated 20 genes (Horsley *et al.* 2001), has little or no effect on phenotype other than producing α thalassaemia (see Chapter 4 and Fig. 12.1 for summary). Furthermore, patients with deletions of up to 1 Mb of 16p may be quite mildly affected (Daniels *et al*, in preparation). However, the single patient with 16p monosomy for the terminal 2 Mb of 16p (BO) is more severely affected (IQ 53). One patient (GE) whose deletion extends just beyond the BO breakpoint was shown to have the phenotype of severe mental retardation, tuberous sclerosis and polycystic kidney disease (European Polycystic Kidney Disease Consortium 1994). Subsequently, patients with even quite small interstitial deletions (3–6kb) around the TSC2 and PKD1 loci have been shown to have the variable but often severe syndrome of tuberous sclerosis (European Chromosome 16 Tuberous Sclerosis Consortium 1993), providing clear examples in which removal of a critical gene from the terminal region of 16p can account for most, if not all, of the clinical features.

These findings suggest that the accumulated loss of many genes from chromosome 16p may have a relatively mild effect. However, this region may contain less abundant, critical genes that exert a severe effect when only one copy is deleted. Characterization of further patients with 16p monosomy and identification of all expressed sequences within 16p13.3 will be of considerable help in localizing such critical genes in this area.

The ATR-16 syndrome has served as an important model for improving our general understanding of the molecular basis for mental retardation. It provided the first examples of mental retardation due to a cryptic chromosomal translocation and truncation. Further work has shown that such telomeric rearrangements may underlie a significant proportion of unexplained mental retardation (Flint *et al.* 1995). The current challenge is to understand in detail the mechanisms by which monosomy causes developmental abnormalities; the ATR-16 syndrome provides an excellent model for addressing this issue.

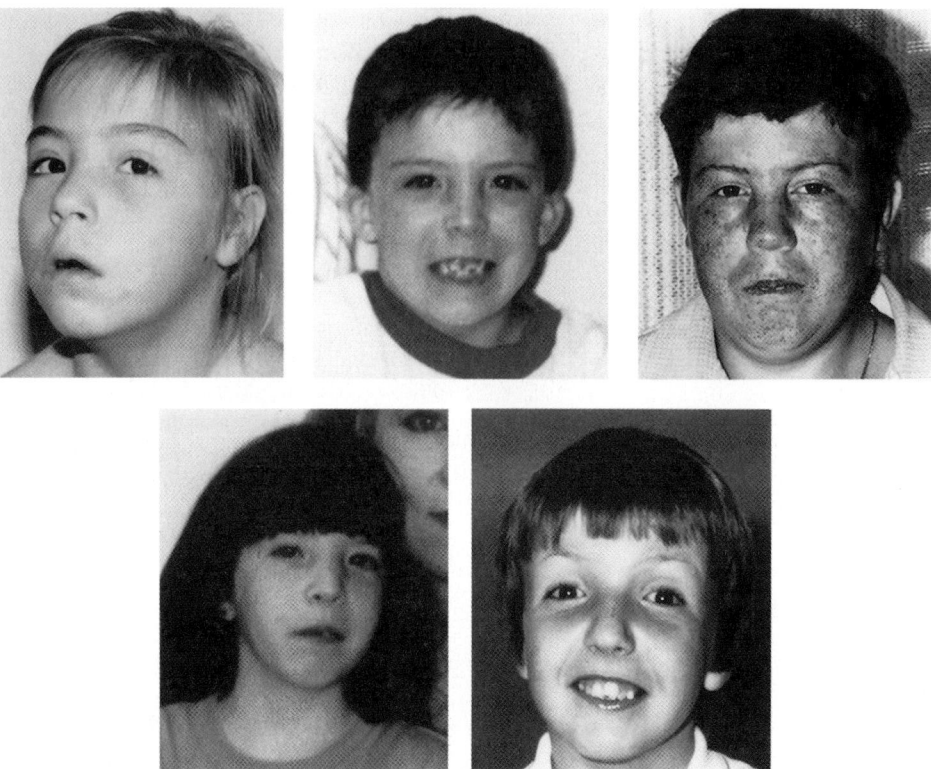

Fig. 12.6 The facial appearance of patients with the ATR-16 syndrome. Common features include relative hypertelorism, a small chin and mouth, a 'beaked' nose, downslanting palpebral fissures and crowded teeth.

The ATR-X syndrome

As further patients with α thalassaemia and mental retardation were identified throughout the 1980s, it became clear that a distinct group exists in whom no structural abnormalities of the α cluster or 16p can be found. In contrast to the ATR-16 syndrome, patients in this 'non-deletional' group are phenotypically uniform: they are male and have severe mental retardation with a remarkably similar facial appearance (Wilkie *et al.* 1990c; Gibbons *et al.* 1991). That this group constitutes a distinct and recognizable dysmorphism was confirmed when additional cases were identified on the basis of their facial features alone (Wilkie *et al.* 1991c). Ultimately, it was shown that this unusual syndrome of α thalassaemia with severe mental retardation results from an X-linked abnormality and the condition is now referred to as the ATR-X syndrome.

Clinical and haematological features

Over 100 cases of the ATR-X syndrome from over 70 families have now been characterized and a definite phenotype is emerging (Table 12.3). The majority of children have profound and global developmental delay. They have marked hypotonia as neonates and in early childhood, and all milestones are delayed. Some are never able to walk and in most cases speech is not developed, and there is only situational understanding with complete dependence for almost all activities. However, in one family with four affected male cousins, one has profound mental retardation, whereas the others have IQs of 41, 56 and 58 (Guerrini *et al.* 2000). The basis for this marked variation is unknown but indicates that mutations in the ATR-X gene may be responsible for a wider spectrum of intellectual disability than previously thought.

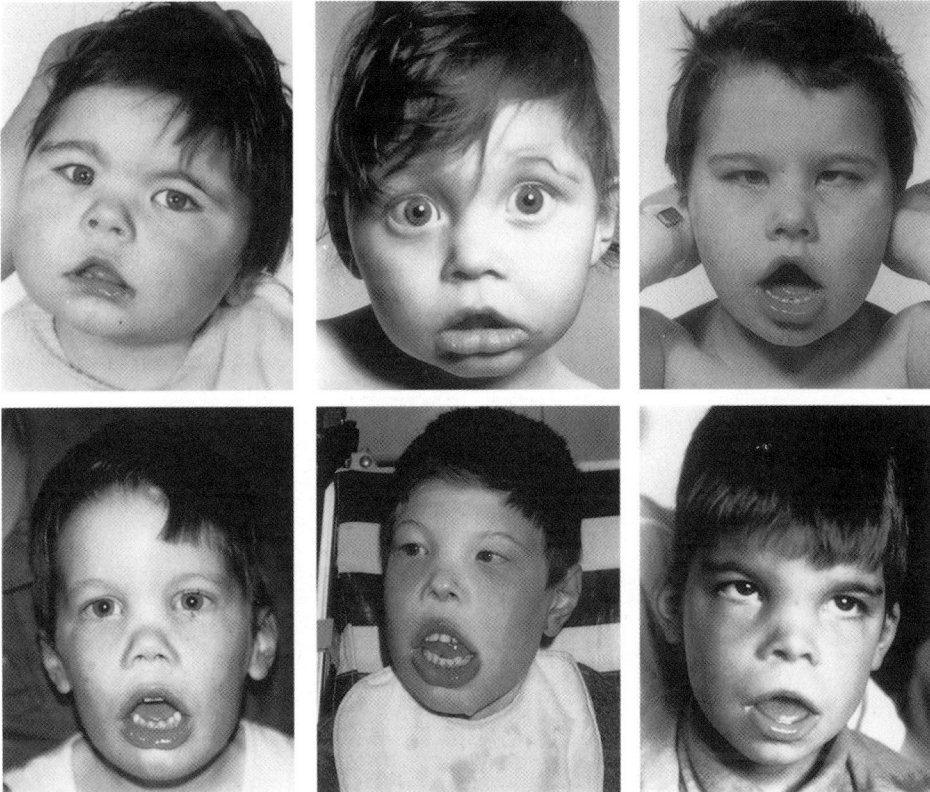

Fig. 12.7 The facial appearance of patients with the ATR-X syndrome. The main features are described in the text.

Table 12.3 Summary of the major clinical manifestations of the ATR-X syndrome.

Clinical feature	Total*	%
Severe mental retardation†	108/110	98
Normal birth weight	65/72	90
Neonatal hypotonia	59/68	87
Seizures	36/104	35
Characteristic face	86/96	90
Microcephaly	67/88	76
Genital abnormalities	83/94	88
Skeletal abnormalities	83/91	91
Cardiac defects	21/98	21
Renal/urinary abnormalities	16/98	16
Gut dysmotility	66/86	77
Short stature	51/74	69

112 patients

*Total represents no. of patients on whom appropriate information is available and includes patients who do not have thalassaemia but in whom ATR-X mutations have been identified.

†Two patients too young (<1 year) to assess degree of mental retardation.

In early childhood the facial features are quite distinctive (Fig. 12.7): the frontal hair is often upswept, there is telecanthus, epicanthic folds, a flat nasal bridge and mid-face hypoplasia, and a small triangular, upturned nose with the alae nasi extending below the columella and septum. The upper lip is tented, and the lower lip full and everted, giving the mouth a 'carp-like' appearance. The frontal incisors are often widely spaced, the tongue protrudes and there is excessive dribbling. There is a wide spectrum of associated abnormalities affecting many systems (Table 12.4), the most striking of which are the genital abnormalities seen in almost all children (Gibbons *et al.* 1995a). These may be very mild, undescended testes for example, but the spectrum of abnormality extends through hypospadias and micropenis to external female genitalia and male pseudohermaphroditism. These abnormalities tend to segregate within families (McPherson *et al.* 1995). Recurrent vomiting or regurgitation, sometimes requiring fundoplication, is a common feature and seems likely to

Table 12.4 Clinical manifestations of the ATR-X syndrome.

Genital abnormalities	Small/soft testes, cryptorchidism, gonadal dysgenesis, inguinal hernia, micropenis, hypospadias, deficient prepuce, shawl scrotum, hypoplastic scrotum, ambiguous genitalia, female external genitalia
Skeletal abnormalities	Delayed bone age, tapering fingers, drumstick distal phalanges, brachydactyly, clinodactyly, bifid thumb, fixed flexion deformities of joints, overriding toes, varus or valgus deformities of feet, scoliosis, kyphosis, hemivertebra, segmentation defects of the vertebrae, spina bifida, coxa valga, chest wall deformity
Renal/urinary abnormalities	Renal agenesis, hydronephrosis, small kidneys, vesico-ureteric reflux, pelvo-ureteric junction obstruction, exstrophy of bladder, urethral diverticulum, urethral stricture
Cardiac defects	Atrial septal defect, ventricular septal defect, patent ductus arteriosus, tetralogy of Fallot, transposition of the great arteries, dextracardia with situs solitus, aortic stenosis, pulmonary stenosis
Gut dysmotility	Discoordinated swallowing, eructation, gastro-oesophageal reflux, vomiting, hiatus hernia, recurrent ileus/small bowel obstruction, volvulus, intermittent diarrhoea, severe constipation
Miscellaneous	Apnoeic episodes, cold/blue extremities, blepharitis, conjunctivitis, entropion, cleft palate, pneumonia, umbilical hernia, encephalitis, optic atrophy, blindness, sensorineural deafness, prolonged periods of screaming/laughing, self injury

be a manifestation of a more generalized dysmotility of the gut (Table 12.4). An apparent reluctance to swallow probably reflects the dyscoordinated swallowing that has been observed. A tendency to aspiration is commonly implicated as a cause of death in early childhood.

CT or MRI brain imaging frequently shows no abnormality, though mild cerebral atrophy may be seen and in two cases partial or complete agenesis of the corpus callosum has been reported.

Despite the fact that these children have α thalassaemia the haematological findings are surprisingly normal. The haemoglobin level and mean cell haemoglobin are not as severely affected as in the common forms of α thalassaemia (Fig. 12.8), reflecting, perhaps, the different pathophysiology of the conditions. Where there is more than one affected member in a family there is often a marked variation in the frequency of cells with HbH inclusions. In one French family (Lefort *et al.* 1993) two third-degree relatives had 30% and 13% of cells with HbH inclusions, respectively, whereas an affected fifth-degree relative had less than 0.001% cells with inclusions. This suggests that the haematological picture is complicated by other variables, possibly genetic.

Evidence that the ATR-X syndrome is X linked

The five original 'non-deletion' cases described by

Wilkie *et al.* (1990c) were sporadic and, apart from them all being male, there were no immediate clues to the mode of transmission. Somatic cell hybrids composed of mouse erythroleukaemia cell lines containing each copy of chromosome 16 from an affected boy produced human α globin in a manner indistinguishable from similar hybrids containing chromosome 16 from normals. It seemed likely therefore that the defect in globin synthesis lay in *trans* to the α-globin cluster. This was confirmed in a family with four affected siblings in which the condition segregated independently of the α-globin cluster (Donnai *et al.* 1991).

Preliminary observations suggested that the syndrome mapped to the X chromosome and hence it was named the ATR-X syndrome. Subsequent linkage analysis of 16 families localized the disease to the region Xq13.1–q21.1, confirming that the associated α thalassaemia results from a *trans*-acting mutation (Gibbons *et al.* 1992).

The ATR-X syndrome behaves as an X-linked recessive disorder; only boys are affected. Female carriers have a normal appearance and intellect, although approximately one in four have subtle signs of α thalassaemia, with very rare cells containing HbH inclusions (Gibbons *et al.* 1992). Almost all carriers have a highly skewed pattern of X inactivation, observed in leucocytes (derived from mesoderm), hair roots (ectoderm) and buccal cells (endoderm).

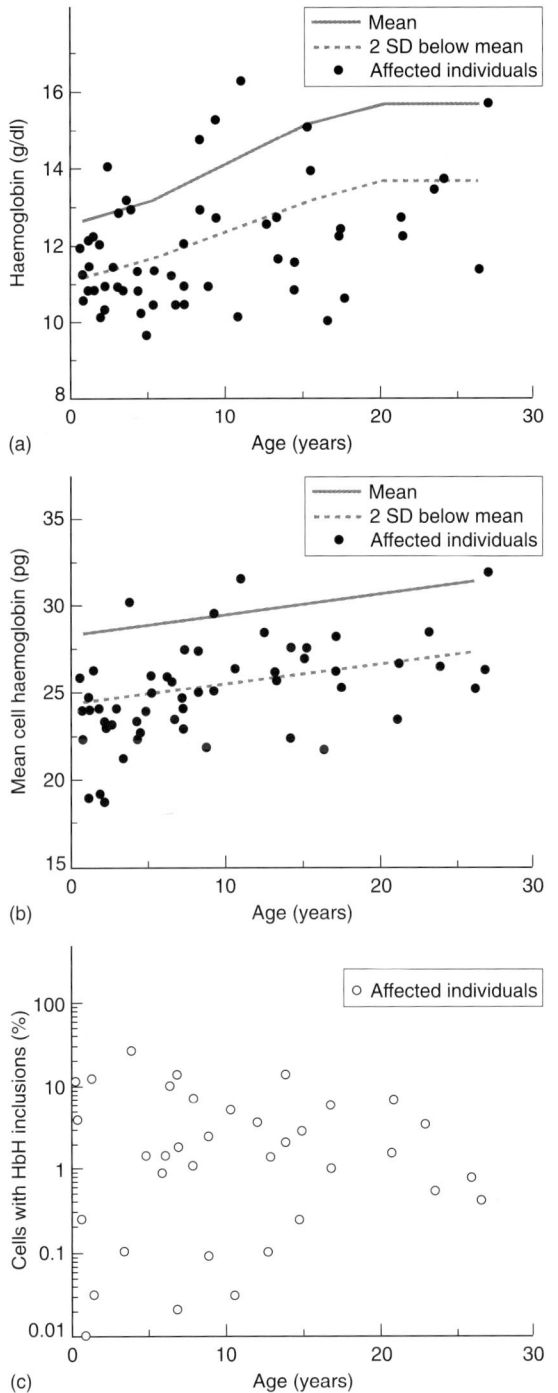

Fig. 12.8 Haematological findings in the ATR-X syndrome. (a) Haemoglobin levels and (b) mean cell haemoglobins in subjects with ATR-X syndrome at various ages. The solid line indicates the mean and dashed line 2 SD below the mean (Dallman 1977). For any subject only one result within each consecutive 5-year period is given. (c) Proportion of red cells with HbH inclusions in subjects with ATR-X syndrome after 1% brilliant cresyl blue incubation at room temperature. Only one result is given for each subject. The percentage of positive cells is plotted on a logarithmic scale.

In each case the disease-bearing X chromosome is preferentially inactivated. In one exception, a developmentally normal 3-year-old female carrier, there was a balanced pattern of X inactivation and almost as many HbH inclusions as her affected brother (Gibbons *et al.* 1992).

Characterization of the ATR-X gene and the potential role of its product in gene expression

The identification of the ATR-X gene is described by Gibbons *et al.* (1995b). It spans about 300 kb of genomic DNA and contains 36 exons (Picketts *et al.* 1996). It encodes at least two alternatively spliced ~10.5-kb mRNA transcripts which differ at their 5′ ends and are predicted to give rise to slightly different proteins of 265 and 280 kDa, respectively (Fig. 12.9).

The ATR-X protein can be broadly divided into three regions (Fig. 12.9): an N-terminal hydrophilic segment (~1640 amino acids), a central region containing alternating hydrophilic and hydrophobic stretches (~855 amino acids) and a C-terminal domain (~135 amino acids). Within the N-terminal region there is a complex cysteine-rich segment (ZFM, Fig. 12.9) part of which shows striking similarity to a PHD finger domain (Gibbons *et al.* 1997). A PHD finger is a putative zinc binding domain (Cys_4-His-Cys_3), 50–80 amino acids in length, which has been identified in a growing number of proteins, many of which are thought to be involved in chromatin-mediated transcriptional regulation (Aasland *et al.* 1995). In particular, the PHD finger of ATR-X is very similar to the PHD domains of Mi-2 (Zhang *et al.* 1998b), a protein involved in nucleosome remodelling, and DNMT3B, which is important for *de novo* methylation (Okano *et al.* 1999). The

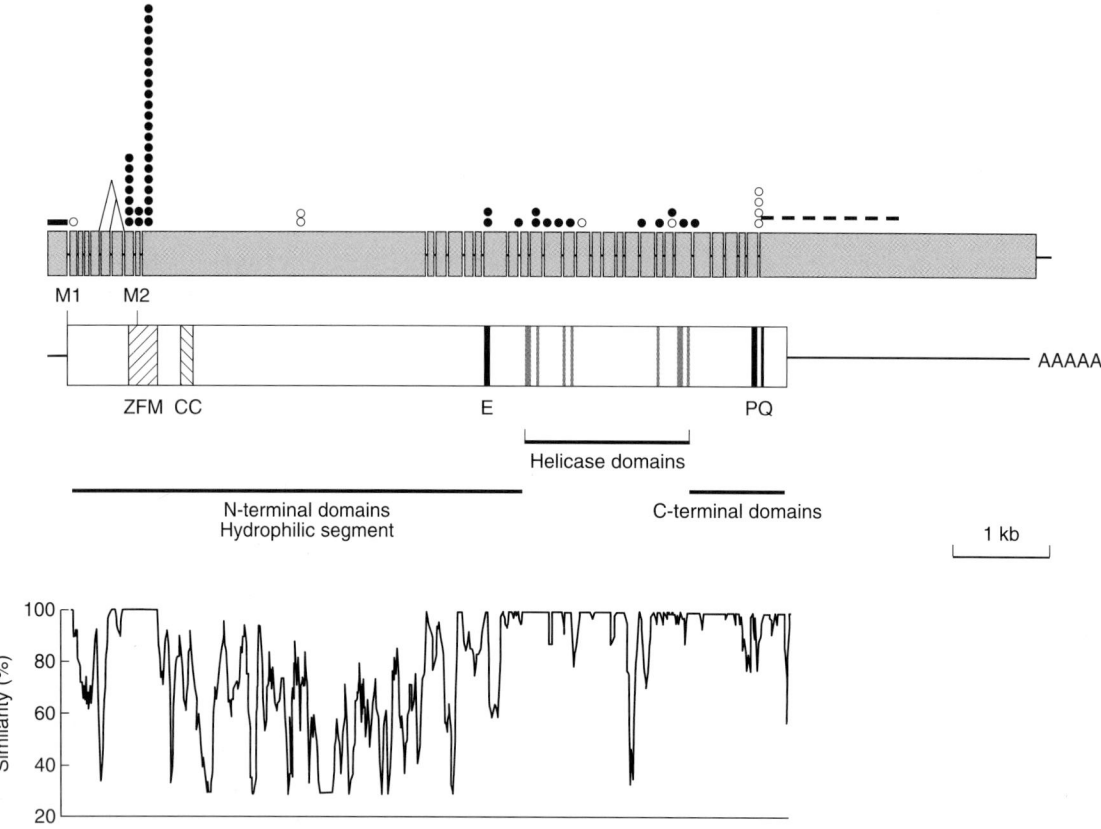

Fig. 12.9 Schematic diagram of complete ATR-X cDNA. The boxes represent the 36 exons and thin horizontal lines represent the introns (not to scale). The largest open reading frame is shown as an open box (lower figure) with the 5′ and 3′ UTR sequences as black lines with the poly(A) tail denoted (AAA . . .). The positions of the mutations are shown by circles; open circles indicate mutations that would cause protein truncation. The alternate splicing that results in transcripts lacking exons 6 and 7, or lacking exon 7 only, is shown by inverted Vs. The alternate initiation codons are labelled M1 and M2. The principal domains, the N-terminal hydrophilic domain, the central domain containing the highly conserved helicase motifs, and the C-terminal domain, are indicated. Additional domains are shown as black boxes and include the zinc finger motif (ZFM), the potential coiled coil (CC), a stretch of 21 glutamic acid residues (E), the P box (P) and a glutamine-rich region (Q). In the lower part of the figure is a graphical representation of the amino acid similarity between human and mouse ATR-X proteins.

functional importance of the segment containing the PHD domain is demonstrated by the high degree of conservation between human and mouse (97 of 98 amino acids) and the fact that it represents a major site of mutations in patients with ATR-X syndrome, containing over 60% of all mutations (Fig. 12.9 and see below).

Also within the N-terminal region is a segment of protein that has a high probability of forming a coiled coil, a structure implicated in protein/protein interactions. Although this resides in an evolution-

arily less conserved region a similar coiled coil is predicted in the mouse protein (Picketts *et al.* 1998). Two reports of proteins that interact with ATR-X involve this region (Le Dourain *et al.* 1996; Ohsawa *et al.* 1996). Using the yeast 2-hybrid approach to identify proteins that interact with the mouse chromatin-associated protein mHP1α, Le Dourain and colleagues identified a partial mouse ATR-X sequence corresponding to this region. Cardoso *et al.* (1998) explored the protein interactions of this region further in a yeast system and showed binding to the SET domain of the polycomb-like protein EZH2.

The central and C-terminal regions show the greatest conservation between mouse and human sequences (94%) (Picketts *et al.* 1998). The central portion of the molecule contains motifs that identify ATR-X as a novel member of the SNF2 subgroup of a superfamily of proteins with similar ATPase and helicase motifs. Other members of this subfamily are involved in a wide variety of cellular functions including the regulation of transcription (SNF2, MOT1 and Brahma), control of the cell cycle (NPS1), DNA repair (RAD16, RAD54 and ERCC6) and mitotic chromosome segregation (Lodestar) (see Lewin 1997). An interaction with chromatin has been shown for SNF2 and Brahma and may be a common theme for all this group (reviewed in Carlson & Laurent 1994). The helicase domains may be interchanged between members of the same group without substantially changing the specific function of the protein, indicating that regions outside this central domain may be responsible for the individual properties of these proteins (Carlson & Laurent 1994). The ATR-X protein, although showing marginally higher sequence homology to RAD54 than other members of this group, does not obviously fall into a particular functional category by virtue of homology in these flanking segments. There is no clinical evidence for ultraviolet sensitivity or the premature development of malignancy in the ATR-X syndrome that might point to this being a defect in DNA repair. Furthermore, cytogenetic analysis has not demonstrated any evidence of abnormal chromosome breakage or segregation. Rather, the consistent association of ATR-X with α thalassaemia suggests that the protein normally exerts its effect at one or more of the many stages involved in gene expression.

The extreme C terminus of ATR-X encodes two additional domains of potential functional importance which are highly conserved in mouse. The P box (Fig. 12.9) is an element conserved among other SNF2-like family members involved in transcriptional regulation, and a stretch of glutamine residues (Q box) represents a potential protein interaction domain.

It is interesting that ATR-X mutations appear to downregulate expression of the α- rather than the closely related β-globin genes. Activation of the α- and β-globin genes involves a common group of lineage-restricted (GATA-1 and NF-E2) and ubiquitous (CACC box) DNA binding factors (see Chapter 2). A key difference, however, is that the α-globin genes lie in a region of constitutively 'open', transcriptionally active chromatin and their expression is regulated by a remote, tissue-specific enhancer, whereas the β-globin genes lie within a segment of chromatin that is 'closed' in non-erythroid cells but which 'opens' in a tissue-specific manner under the influence of a remote locus control region (Vyas *et al.* 1992; Craddock *et al.* 1995). It is conceivable that the ATR-X protein acts to derepress or activate the α-globin genes by interaction with chromatin, whereas these functions are subserved by alternative mechanisms in the β-globin cluster. The analysis of α-globin regulation and its perturbation by ATR-X mutations offers a unique opportunity for understanding exactly how the protein regulates gene expression.

As patients with the ATR-X syndrome have multiple associated congenital abnormalities, it seems likely that ATR-X mutations exert pleiotropic effects. By analogy with SNF2, for example, ATR-X may regulate expression of a restricted class of genes; perturbation in expression of these 'target' genes could affect development of many different systems, including the central nervous system.

ATR-X is a candidate for playing an important part in the development of the central nervous system. It is widely expressed with relatively high levels in brain, heart and skeletal muscle compared with lung and liver. Its murine homologue *Mxnp* is expressed in the early primitive streak (7.0 days postcoitum) which represents the earliest stage of mouse development at which *Mxnp* expression has yet been studied (Stayton *et al.* 1994). Although its expression is widespread, there are considerable changes in the levels in different cell types during development.

Intracellular distribution of ATR-X protein

Recently we have developed a panel of antibodies to the N-terminal region of the ATR-X protein (McDowell *et al.* 1999). In interphase it appears that the protein occurs entirely within the nucleus where it is found in discrete regions associated with pericentromeric heterochromatin. In metaphase, ATR-X is similarly found close to the centromeres of many chromosomes but, in addition, is found at the stalks of acrocentric chromosomes, where the rDNA genes are located. These physical localizations have provided important clues to another potential role of ATR-X protein in the establishment and/or maintenance of methylation in the genome (see below).

Mutations of the ATR-X gene

Now that the ATR-X gene has been fully characterized (Gibbons *et al*. 1995b; Picketts *et al*. 1996) it will be important to establish the full range of disease-causing mutations to facilitate genetic counselling and to identify functionally important aspects of the protein. To date, 33 different mutations have been documented (Table 12.5 and Fig. 12.9): 20 mis-sense; four nonsense; one 3-bp insertion; six splicing defects, of which four cause frameshifts and protein truncation, and two deletions (see Chapter 4 for description of different mutations). The mis-sense mutations, in particular, are clustered in two regions, the zinc finger motif and the helicase domain.

Analysis of the mutations and their resulting phenotypes allows important conclusions to be drawn. A number of mutations predicted to cause protein truncation are scattered throughout the gene (Fig. 12.9). Where this leads to the loss of critical domains loss of function would be expected. Similarly, in the case of a 3′ deletion, ATR-X mRNA is reduced to less than 1% of normal and this may represent a null mutation (Gibbons *et al*. 1995a,b). Nevertheless it is clear that these mutations are not lethal. Furthermore, the resulting phenotype is similar to that seen for the other mutations and this is consistent with the view that the common final pathway of these mutations is a decrease in ATR-X activity. In some of the splicing mutations, including those presented here, the levels of normal ATR-X mRNA range from <1 to 30% (Villard *et al*. 1996c). The fact that key features of the ATR-X syndrome are found in the presence of substantial amounts of normal ATR-X mRNA suggests that the target pathways are sensitive to the dosage of this protein. One reason for such sensitivity could be that, like the related SNF2 protein (Peterson & Herskowitz 1992; Wilson *et al*. 1996), ATR-X may be required in carefully controlled stoichiometric amounts for the formation of multi-protein complexes.

Recently, an important new finding points to a role for the ATR-X protein in establishing or maintaining the pattern of methylation in the human genome. Mutations of ATR-X cause consistent changes in the patterns of methylation of rDNA (where the protein has been shown to bind, see above), Y-specific repeats and subtelomeric repeats. One possibility is that ATR-X alters access of the *de novo* methylase (DNMT3) to its binding sites. Alternatively ATR-X (like Mi-2) might be a member of a protein complex (so-called HDAC/MBD complexes) involved in establishing or maintaining the pattern of methylation in the genome (Gibbons & Higgs 2001).

Phenotype/genotype relationships

Since the discovery of the ATR-X gene most new cases of ATR-X syndrome are defined on the basis of severe mental retardation with the typical facial appearance associated with a mutation in the ATR-X gene. This allows a less biased evaluation of the effect of ATR-X mutations on the commonly associated clinical features.

There are now six different mutations associated with the most severe urogenital abnormalities (Table 12.5). One represents the putative null mutation (see above). In three of the others, the protein is truncated, resulting in the loss of the C-terminal domain including a conserved element (P in Fig. 12.8) and polyglutamine tract (Q in Fig. 12.9). These mutations may therefore have the greatest potential to disrupt ATR-X function. From the available data it appears that in the absence of significant ATR-X function, particularly that of the C-terminal domain, severe urogenital abnormalities are inevitable. Consistent with this prediction, in families with such mutations severe urogenital abnormalities breed true (McPherson *et al*. 1995) and an identical, independently arising nonsense mutation gives rise to a similar phenotype. Interestingly, in one family with a splicing defect that produces variable amounts of normal ATR-X mRNA (Mutation 23 in Table 12.5), urogenital abnormalities were only seen in the patient with the least amount of normal ATR-X mRNA (Lefort *et al*. 1993; Villard *et al*. 1996c).

The relationship between ATR-X mutations and α thalassaemia is less clear. Since the presence of excess β chains (HbH inclusions) was originally used to define the ATR-X syndrome, current observations are inevitably biased. Nevertheless, there is considerable variability in the degree to which α-globin synthesis is affected by these mutations. Some patients do not have HbH inclusions (Villard *et al*. 1996a,b,c) although this does not rule out downregulation of α-globin expression since inclusions may not appear until there is a 30–40% reduction in α-chain synthesis (Higgs *et al.* 1989). There appears to be no consistent relationship between the degree of α thalassaemia and the predicted severity of the ATR-X mutations and therefore no correlation with abnormal sexual differentiation.

It is interesting that patients with identical mutations may have very different, albeit stable, degrees of α thalassaemia, suggesting that the effect of ATR-X protein on α-globin expression may be modified by other genetic factors. This is most clearly illustrated by comparing the haematology of cases with identical mutations (Table 12.5). In the 3′ splicing mutation (Mutation 4, Table 12.5), whereas cases in pedigrees 12, 46 and 49 have α thalassaemia, in the affected individual in pedigree N17 no HbH inclusions could be detected. Furthermore, comparison of the 21 pedigrees with the common C1073T mutation (12, Table 12.5) shows a variation in frequency of HbH inclusions of over four orders of magnitude. This may be analogous to mutations of other members of the SNF2 family whose effects are known to be modified by a variation in many genes encoding proteins that interact with SNF2-like proteins (Hirschhorn *et al.* 1992; Carlson & Laurent 1994).

Recently it has been shown that phenotypic variability extends to the degree of intellectual disability (see above). A nonsense mutation in exon 2 (2, Table 12.5) has been identified in an ATR-X pedigree in which the degree of mental retardation in four affected individuals varies from mild to severe. The basis for this variation is not understood but it suggests that the clinical spectrum for ATR-X mutations may be considerably broader than previously defined. Mutation in the ATR-X gene has been identified in a case of Juberg–Marsidi syndrome (severe mental retardation, variable degree of sensorineural deafness, hypogenitalism and short stature: 28, Table 12.5) and in a number of other cases in which α thalassaemia appears not to be present. However, given that these features are seen within the spectrum of abnormalities associated with a single mutation, the case for phenotype splitting is not persuasive.

Systematic mutation analysis of a broad population of patients with learning difficulties should help determine the extent of the phenotypic spectrum associated with ATR-X mutations and their prevalence.

Postscript

From the initial simple clinical observations made almost 20 years ago in patients with unusual forms of thalassaemia two important genetic mechanisms by which mental retardation may arise have been elucidated.

Further analysis of the ATR-16 syndrome will provide some answers as to how chromosomal imbalance may give rise to developmental abnormalities.

Understanding the ATR-X syndrome has opened up many new questions. It seems likely that mutations in this class of genes, which appear to regulate many other genes, may be a common cause of syndromal mental retardation and, it is hoped, over the next few years, using information gathered from the ATR-X syndrome, we shall identify similar conditions. At the same time it shall be important to identify the 'target' genes that are regulated by ATR-X. Finally, having established that ATR-X is almost certainly involved in the normal regulation of α-gene expression we shall have to try to understand exactly what role it plays in this process.

The acquired form of α thalassaemia associated with myelodysplasia (ATMDS)

Very rarely, patients with myelodysplasia develop an unusual form of HbH disease with a severe hypochromic microcytic anaemia, HbH inclusions and detectable levels of HbH in the peripheral blood. Most are of North European origin and in all cases for which archival data are available there is no evidence of pre-existing α thalassaemia.

The first cases to be reported (Table 12.6) were diagnosed as having a variety of haematological malignancies including leukaemias, myelofibrosis, myeloproliferative diseases and acquired sideroblastic anaemias. Most of these reports preceded the accurate definition of myelodysplasia (MDS) set out by the French/American/British (FAB) group (Bennett *et al.* 1982). A recent review of 14 patients (Craddock 1994) demonstrated that all of them have one or other form of MDS and therefore we now refer to this condition as the α thalassaemia/myelodysplasia syndrome (ATMDS).

Table 12.5 Summary of ATR-X mutations.

Mutation no.	Case	Nucleotide	Amino acid	Mutation*	De novo†	Genital abnormality‡	HbH inclusions cells (%)	Reference
1	Ped N1,DL	1–213		D		++	0	Unpublished
	Ped N1,ML	1–213		D		++	nd	Unpublished
	Ped N1,JP	1–213		D		++	0	Unpublished
2	Ped 59,III-M	324	37	N;C→T;Arg→stop		Normal	0.006	Unpublished
	Ped 59,II-F	324	37	N;C→T;Arg→stop		Normal	0.003	Unpublished
	Ped 59,II-S	324	37	N;C→T;Arg→stop		Normal	0	Unpublished
	Ped 59,III-A	324	37	N;C→T;Arg→stop		Normal	0	Unpublished
3	Ped 29,GH	866	177	I;CAA,Q		+	0.12	Gibbons et al. (1997)
	Ped 29,JH	866	177	I;CAA,Q		+	0.003	Gibbons et al. (1997)
	Ped 29,GC	866	177	I;CAA,Q		+	nd	Gibbons et al. (1997)
4	Ped 12, case 3	869–931	178–198	S:deletion 63 bp; in frame A873G	+	+	0.1	Picketts et al. (1996)
	Ped N17	869–931	178–198	S:deletion 63 bp; in frame A873G	+		0	Picketts et al. (1996)
	Ped 46	869–931	178–198	S:deletion 63 bp; in frame A873G		++	0.4	Gibbons et al. (1997)
	Ped 49	869–931	178–198	S:deletion 63 bp; in frame A873G	+	Normal	1.5	Gibbons et al. (1997)
5	Ped 51	905	190	M;C→G;Pro→Ala		++	4.8	Gibbons et al. (1997)
6	Ped 39	913	192	M;G→C;Leu→Phe		Normal	<0.01	Gibbons et al. (1997)
7	Ped 35	936	200	M;G→C;Cys→Ser	+	++	31.5	Gibbons et al. (1997)
8	Ped 32	995	220	M:T→C;Cys→Arg		++	0.01	Gibbons et al. (1997)
9	Ped 50	1002	222	M;G→C;Trp→Ser		++	0.003	Gibbons et al. (1997)
10	Ped 30,232	1054	239	M;C→A;Phe→Leu		nd	2	Unpublished
11	Ped 19	1056	240	M;G→T;Cys→Phe	+GS	++	6	Gibbons et al. (1997)
12	Ped 9, case 1	1073	246	M;C→T;Arg→Cys		++	1.4	Gibbons et al. (1997)
	Ped 9, case 2	1073	246	M;C→T;Arg→Cys		++	0.8	Gibbons et al. (1997)
	Ped 4	1073	246	M;C→T;Arg→Cys	+	++	5.2	Gibbons et al. (1997)
	Ped 7	1073	246	M;C→T;Arg→Cys		++	14	Gibbons et al. (1997)
	Ped 8, RH	1073	246	M;C→T;Arg→Cys		++	14	Gibbons et al. (1997)
	Ped 8, MC	1073	246	M;C→T;Arg→Cys		+	3.5	Gibbons et al. (1997)
	Ped 16	1073	246	M;C→T;Arg→Cys		++	1	Gibbons et al. (1997)
	Ped 18	1073	246	M;C→T;Arg→Cys		++	1.8	Gibbons et al. (1997)
	Ped 6	1073	246	M;C→T;Arg→Cys		+	6.8	Gibbons et al. (1997)
	Ped 24	1073	246	M;C→T;Arg→Cys	+	+	0.05	Gibbons et al. (1997)
	Ped 24	1073	246	M;C→T;Arg→Cys	+	+	0.1	Gibbons et al. (1997)
	Ped 25,SG	1073	246	M;C→T;Arg→Cys		+	0.01	Gibbons et al. (1997)
	Ped 25,JL	1073	246	M;C→T;Arg→Cys		++	0.25	Gibbons et al. (1997)
	Ped 31	1073	246	M;C→T;Arg→Cys		nd	3	Gibbons et al. (1997)
	Ped 33	1073	246	M;C→T;Arg→Cys		++	0.006	Gibbons et al. (1997)
	Ped 34	1073	246	M;C→T;Arg→Cys	+	nd	nd	Gibbons et al. (1997)
	Ped 43	1073	246	M;C→T;Arg→Cys		++	2.2	Gibbons et al. (1997)
	Ped 48	1073	246	M;C→T;Arg→Cys		+	0.4	Gibbons et al. (1997)
	Ped 55	1073	246	M;C→T;Arg→Cys		nd	4.2	Gibbons et al. (1997)
	Ped 62 IV:11	1073	246	M;C→T;Arg→Cys		++	+	Unpublished
	Ped 62 IV:7	1073	246	M;C→T;Arg→Cys		+	+	Unpublished

	Pedigree/case			Mutation*	†,‡	HbH inclusions	α/β ratio	Reference
13	Ped 36	1076	247	M:A→G; Asn→Asp		++	+	Unpublished
14	Ped 11, case 1	1083	249	M:G→A; Gly→Asp	+GL	++	2.5	Gibbons et al. (1997)
	Ped 11, case 2	1083	249	M:G→A; Gly→Asp	+GL	nd	3.9	Gibbons et al. (1997)
15	Ped 10, case 1	2064	576	N:C→A; Ser→stop		+++	2.8	Unpublished
	Ped 10, case 2	2064	576	N:C→A; Ser→stop		+	2.1	Unpublished
	Ped 10, case 3	2064	576	N:C→A; Ser→stop		++	10	Unpublished
	Ped 10, case 4	2064	576	N:C→A; Ser→stop		++	1.4	Unpublished
	Ped 58, CB	2064	576	N:C→A; Ser→stop		++	2.2	Unpublished
	Ped 58, MR	2064	576	N:C→A; Ser→stop		Normal	nd	Unpublished
16	Ped 20, case 11	4654		S:G→A; insertion 53 bp; frameshift		+++	3.6	Picketts et al. (1996)
	Ped 20, case 12	4654		S:G→A; insertion 53 bp; frameshift		++	0.9	Picketts et al. (1996)
17	Ped 22, case 15	4950	1538	M:T→G; Val→Gly§		+++	11	Picketts et al. (1996)
18	Ped 14, case 5	5163	1609	M:A→G; His→Arg		+++	1.6	Gibbons et al. (1995b)
19	Ped 5, NE	5177	1614	M:T→C; Cys→Arg		++++	>5	Gibbons et al. (1995b)
20	Ped 21, case 13	5287	1650	M:G→T; Lys→Asn		Normal	0.4	Gibbons et al. (1995b)
	Ped 21, case 14	5287	1650	M:G→T; Lys→Asn		Normal	0.6	Gibbons et al. (1995b)
21	Ped 37	5376	1680	M:T→C; Ile→Thr		++++	+	Unpublished
22	III-1	5474	1713	M:C→T; Pro→Ser		Normal	0	Villard et al. (1996b)
23	IV-10	5610–5785		S:deletion 176 bp; frameshift		+++	30	Villard et al. (1996c)
	IV-9	5610–5785		S:deletion 176 bp; frameshift		Normal	13	Villard et al. (1996c)
	IV-16	5610–5785		S:deletion 176 bp; frameshift		Normal	<0.001	Villard et al. (1996c)
24	Ped 54	6294–6359		S:deletion 66 bp; in frame		+	+	Unpublished
25	Ped 23, MEF	6441	2035	M:A→T; Asp→Val		+++	7	Gibbons et al. (1995b)
	Ped 23, MF	6441	2035	M:A→T; Asp→Val		+++	27	Gibbons et al. (1995b)
26	Ped 15, case 6	6554		S:insertion 124 bp; frameshift	+	++	1.4	Picketts et al. (1996)
27	Ped 3, SW	6587	2084	M:T→C; Tyr→His		+++	>5	Gibbons et al. (1995b)
28	JM3,4,IV-1	6729	2131	M:G→A; Arg→Gln		+++	nd	Villard et al. (1996a)
29	Ped 13, case 4	6825	2163	M:A→G; Tyr→Cys	+	+	12	Gibbons et al. (1995b)
30	Ped 17, case 8	7493	2386	N:C→T; Arg→stop	+	++++	0.02	Gibbons et al. (1995b)
	Ped 17, III-1	7493	2386	N:C→T; Arg→stop	+	++++	nd	Gibbons et al. (1995b)
	Ped 38	7493	2386	N:C→T; Arg→stop		++++	v. rare	Unpublished
31	Ped 27, case 1	7499	2388	N:C→T; Glu→stop		++++	0.03	Gibbons et al. (1995b)
	Ped 27, case 2	7499	2388	N:C→T; Glu→stop		++++	nd	Gibbons et al. (1995b)
32	IV-18	7538–7545		S:deletion 8 bp; frameshift		++++	0¶	Ion et al. (1996)
33	Ped 26, case 1	7538–9126		D		++++	1.1	Gibbons et al. (1995b)
	Ped 26, case 2	7538–9126		D		++++	0.03	Gibbons et al. (1995b)
	Ped 26, case 3	7538–9126		D		++++	0.09	Gibbons et al. (1995b)

* Mutations: D, deletion; M, missense; N, nonsense; S, splice site.

† +, mutation demonstrated to have arisen *de novo* within family; GS, gonosomal mosaicism; GL, germline mosaicism.

‡ Genital abnormality ranges from normal; to +, very mild: high-lying testes; to +++, ambiguous genitalia or male pseudohermaphrodite.

§ This previously unpublished relatively conservative amino acid change in a non-conserved location may represent a polymorphism rather than a disease-causing mutation.

¶ 0/5000 red cells had HbH inclusions but α-/β-globin chain ratio = 0.85, 15% below control samples.

nd, not determined.

Table 12.6 Haematological and clinical data on patients with ATMDS.

	Age	Sex	Ethnicity	Splenomegaly	Hb (g/dl)	MCV (fl)	MCH (pg)	%BCB	%HbH	α/β Ratio	Karyotype	Diagnosis	Reference
1	60	M	CA		N/A	N/A	N/A	30	N/A	N/A		Erythroleukaemia	White et al. (1960)
2	46	M	CA		N/A	N/A	N/A	20	N/A	N/A		Erythroleukaemia	White et al. (1960)
3	49	F	CA		N/A	N/A	N/A	1	N/A	N/A		Erythroleukaemia	White et al. (1960)
4	72	M			7.8	93	16	N/A	N/A	N/A		Atypical haemolytic anaemia	Bergren & Sturgeon (1960)
5	74	M			8.7	74	22	N/A	N/A	N/A		Atypical haemolytic anaemia	Bergren & Sturgeon (1960)
6	56	M	CA		N/A	N/A	N/A	N/A	10	N/A		Atypical CML	Beaven et al. (1963)
7	76	M			N/A	N/A	N/A	N/A	N/A	N/A		AML	Labie et al. (1968)
8	70	M	CA	+	6.1	66	15	93	42	N/A	46XY	Erythroleukaemia	Rosenzweig et al. (1968)
9	80	M		−	10.0	97	29	N/A	10	N/A	46XY	Erythroleukaemia	Rosenzweig et al. (1968)
10	73	F	CA	+	4.6	63	15	60	20	0.13		Myeloproliferative disorder	Hamilton et al. (1971)
11	66	M	CA	+	7.7	N/A	N/A	60	N/A	N/A		Erythroleukaemia	Andre et al. (1972)
12	72	M	CA		8.6	N/A	N/A	30	15	N/A		Erythroleukaemia	Beaven et al. (1978)
13	47	M	LE		N/A	71	21	40	20	N/A		Sideroblastic anaemia	Boehme et al. (1978)
14	65	M	CA	−	N/A	80	N/A	50	18	N/A		Sideroblastic anaemia	Boehme et al. (1978)
15	81	M	CA	−	11.3	66	16	90	57	0.07	46XY	Myeloproliferative disorder	Weatherall et al. (1978)
16	84	M	CA	−	6.9	69	19	60	18	0.39		Myeloproliferative disorder	Lindsey et al. (1978)
17	82	M	SP	+	N/A	N/A	N/A	80	27	N/A		Sideroblastic anaemia	Villegas et al. (1979)
18	85	M	SP	+	N/A	N/A	N/A	12	N/A	N/A		Myelodysplasia (RAEB)	Villegas et al. (1979)
19	68	M	CA	+	10.7	59	N/A	80	37	0.05		Myeloproliferative disorder	Veer et al. (1979)
20	59	M	OR	+	10.6	75	26	9	3	0.67		AML	Tanaka et al. (1979)
21	30	M	IN	−	4.0	N/A	N/A	1	N/A	N/A		Myelofibrosis	Dash & Dash (1980)
22	42	M	OR	+	4.3	N/A	N/A	4	2	N/A		Myelofibrosis	Nakatsuji et al. (1980)
23	63	M	OR	−	N/A	78	N/A	66	27	0.1	46XY	Myeloproliferative disorder	Yoo et al. (1980)
24	18	F	OR	+	6.0	N/A	N/A	50	N/A	N/A	46XX	ALL	Kueh (1982)
25	68	M	IT		7.5	66	19	N/A	4	0.43		Sideroblastic anaemia	Massa et al. (1987)
26	61	M	CA	+	5.9	97	21	4	4	0.09	46XY	Myelofibrosis	Higgs et al. (1983b)
27	77	M	CA	−	12.7	69	19	57	20	0.09	46XY	Myeloproliferative disorder	D.R. Higgs, unpublished (JP)
28	78	M	CA	−	9.0	89	29	7	1	0.66		Myeloproliferative disorder	D.R. Higgs, unpublished (AC)
29	86	M	CA		8.8	82	28	14	10	0.29		Sideroblastic anaemia	D.R. Higgs, unpublished (RC)
30	76	M	CA		7.9	N/A	23	N/A	4	N/A		Myelodysplasia	D.R. Higgs, unpublished
31	56	M	CA		8.3	69	N/A	N/A	1	0.53		Sideroblastic anaemia	D.R. Higgs, unpublished
32	65	M	CA		9.7	84	27	N/A	N/A	N/A	46XY	Sideroblastic anaemia post AML	D.R. Higgs, unpublished
33	68	M	CA	+	10.2	59	16	N/A	37	N/A		Sideroblastic anaemia	D.R. Higgs, unpublished

No.	Age	Sex	Ethnicity	Splenomegaly							Karyotype	Diagnosis	Reference
34	72	M			8.9	78	N/A	N/A	33	0.15	46XY	Myelodysplasia (RA)	Anagnou et al. (1983)
35	29	M	OR	−	8.4	98	N/A	34	2	N/A		Sideroblastic anaemia	Tokuda et al. (1984)
36	75	M	CA	−	7.3	59	18	70	27	0.18		Myelodysplasia (RAEBT)	Annino et al. (1984)
37	64	M	CA	−	9.2	76	22	N/A	1	N/A	46XY	Myelodysplasia (RA)	Abbondanzo et al. (1988)
38	56	M	OR	+	6.0	78	24	N/A	N/A	N/A	46XY20q-	Refractory anaemia	Yoshida et al. (1990)
39	74	M	CA	−	8.2	69	21	64	3	N/A		Erythroleukaemia	Bürgi et al. (1992)
40	76	M	CA	−	9.3	84	29	1	N/A	0.47		Myelodysplasia	D.R. Higgs, unpublished (CS)
41	87	F	CA	−	8.2	80	26	20	N/A	0.62		Essential thrombocythaemia	D.R. Higgs, unpublished (MG)
42	72	M	CA	+	11.9	59	17	40	17	0.09	46XY	Myelodysplasia (RA)	D.R. Higgs, unpublished (DW)
43	68	M	CA	−	8.9	91	29	6	N/A	0.6	47XY del20 +8	Myelodysplasia (RA)	D.R. Higgs, unpublished (CW)
44	63	M	CA	+	5.2	N/A	N/A	20	3	N/A	46XY	Myelodysplasia (RA)	D.R. Higgs, unpublished (DB)
45	60	M	CA		5.6	67	10	35	9	0.18	46XY	Myelodysplasia (RA)	D.R. Higgs, unpublished (JP)
46	72	M	CA	−	6.9	80	24	48	8	0.09	46XY	Myelodysplasia (RA)	D.R. Higgs, unpublished (JS)
47	63	M	CA	−	9.0	65	18	N/A	3	N/A	46XY	Myelodysplasia (CMML)	D.R. Higgs, unpublished (WW)
48	73	M	CA	+	8.9	67	N/A	N/A	1	N/A		Myelodysplasia	D.R. Higgs, unpublished (EP)
49	57	M	CA	−	9.7	76	23	25	23	N/A		Myelodysplasia (RA)	D.R. Higgs, unpublished (GL)
50	78	M	CA	−	12.2	85	29	30	2	N/A		Myelodysplasia (RA)	D.R. Higgs, unpublished (AS)
51	60	M	CA	−	10.3	70	23	4	N/A	N/A		Myelodysplasia (RA)	D.R. Higgs, unpublished (LF)
52	78	M	CA	−	11.9	79	23	25	15	0.13		Myelodysplasia (RAEB)	D.R. Higgs, unpublished (HW)
53	75	M	CA	−	7.9	73	23	42	15	N/A		Myelodysplasia (RAEB)	D.R. Higgs, unpublished (FC)
54	83	M	CA	−	11.0	69	19	75	38	0.09		Myelodysplasia (RAEB)	D.R. Higgs, unpublished (AK)
Average	66				8.5	75	22	38	15	0.28			
SD	14				2.15	11	5	27	14	0.22			

M, males; F, females.

Ethnicity: CA, Caucasian; IN, Asian Indian; IT, Italian; LE, Lebanese; OR, Oriental; SP, Spanish.

Splenomegaly was either present (+), absent (−) or not recorded.

ALL, acute lymphoblastic leukaemia; AML, acute myeloid leukaemia; CML, chronic myeloid leukaemia; CMML, chronic myelomonocytic leukaemia; N/A, not available; RA, refractory anaemia; RAEB, refractory anaemia with excess blasts.

These data were compiled by C.F. Craddock (Craddock 1994).

Clinical features

Table 12.6 summarizes the findings in 54 patients with ATMDS, including all cases so far described together with 22 previously unpublished cases studied in our laboratory. The patients are predominantly males (50/54) with a mean age of 66 years at presentation. It is of interest that two of the four females had an atypical underlying haematological disease: one had acute lymphoblastic leukaemia (Kueh 1982); another, (no. 41), developed MDS after treatment for essential thrombocythaemia, whereas most patients with this syndrome have primary MDS.

The predominant clinical features, which are those associated with myelodysplasia, include symptoms of anaemia, an increased proneness to infection, and bleeding due to thrombocytopenia. Some of these patients have high levels of HbH and, as discussed in Chapter 11, may show symptoms of anaemia at relatively high haemoglobin values. About 30% of patients have splenomegaly. Most of them eventually develop acute myeloid leukaemia or refractory cytopenias, as would be expected in a group of patients with MDS.

Haematological findings

Patients are always anaemic at presentation; the mean haematological values for the cases reported in Table 12.6 are: haemoglobin 8.5 g/dl; red-cell count $4.3 \times 10^{12}/1$; MCH 22 pg; and MCV 75 fl. These abnormalities are even more striking when compared with a control population of patients with MDS (Dr D. Oscier, personal communication), who tend to have slightly high MCH values, approximately 31 pg, at presentation (Fig. 12.10). The red-cell diameter width (RDW) was increased in all patients studied, with a mean value of 29.1 microns (normal range 6.7–7.7 microns).

These findings are reflected in the red-cell morphology (Fig. 12.11). The red cells are hypochromic and microcytic and in many cases there is marked anisopoikilocytosis. In some it appears that there are at least two populations of cells, one quite well haemoglobinized and another with 'ghost cells' containing very little haemoglobin (Fig. 12.11).

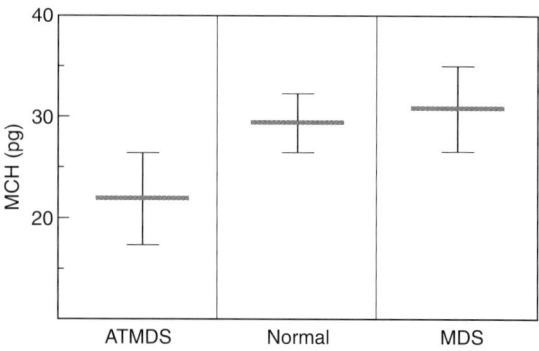

Fig. 12.10 The MCH values in patients with ATMDS, normal individuals and a group of patients with myelodysplasia (MDS). The mean is shown as a thick horizontal bar. 1 SD (ATMDS and MDS) or 2 SD (normal) values are shown as thin vertical lines.

Haemoglobin analysis

All patients with ATMDS have detectable amounts of HbH in the peripheral blood at some stage in the disease, the recorded levels at presentation ranging between 1 and 57% (mean 15%). Often it is not possible to obtain accurate estimations because of previous blood transfusion. In some, trace amounts of Hb Bart's have been found. In the presence of these high-affinity haemoglobins the whole-blood oxygen dissociation curve is shifted to the left (Weatherall *et al.* 1978) (Fig. 12.12).

At presentation, the proportion of red cells containing HbH inclusions after incubation with brilliant cresyl blue varies between 0.5 and 93% (mean 38%). Like the α-/β-globin synthesis ratios, the proportions of HbH and cells containing HbH inclusions vary during the course of the illness.

α-/β-Globin RNA and synthesis ratios

The ratio of α- to β-globin mRNA in the peripheral blood was extremely low in the case illustrated in Fig. 12.12 (Weatherall *et al.* 1978) and was severely reduced in three other cases studied by us (0.06–0.50) (Higgs *et al.* 1983b). The α-/β-globin synthesis ratio was similarly reduced (mean 0.28, range 0.05–0.67) in all 22 patients in which it has been reported. In the most severely affected individuals α-chain synthesis was almost abolished (Fig. 12.13). The α-/β-chain synthesis ratio may vary quite considerably during the course of the disease (Higgs *et al.* 1983b).

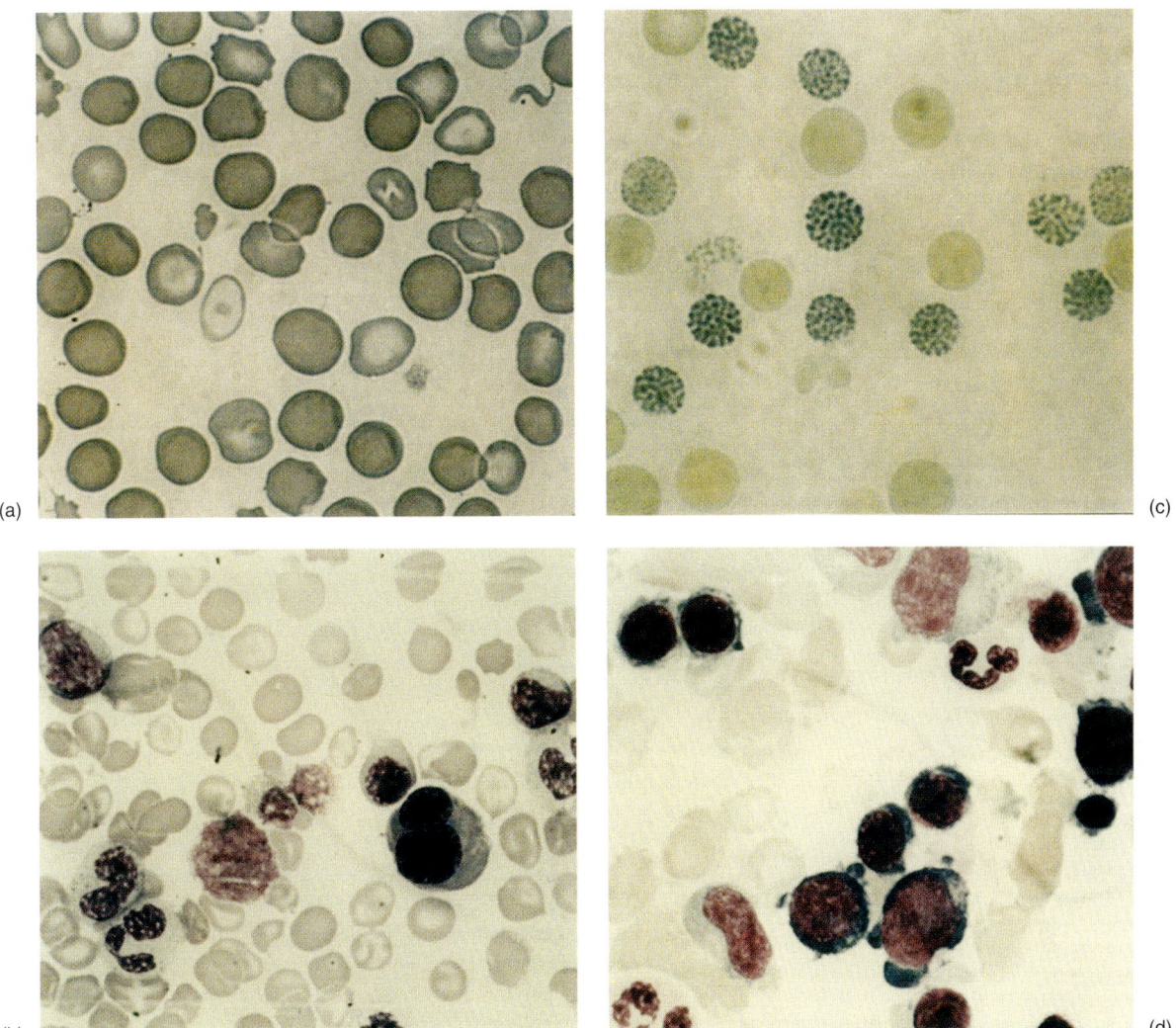

(a)

(c)

(b)

(d)

Fig. 12.11 Peripheral blood film (a) and peripheral blood stained with brilliant cresyl blue (b) from a patient with ATMDS and an α-/β-chain biosynthesis ratio of less than 0.1. Bone-marrow samples from the same patient (c,d) show erythroid expansion with dyserythropoietic features including binuclearity and cytoplasmic vacuolation. The neutrophils appear hypogranular.

Cellular and molecular basis

Some patients with this condition have less than 10% of the normal levels of α-globin mRNA and α-globin synthesis (see Table 12.6 and Fig. 12.13). The values are lower than those encountered in patients with one functional α-globin gene (−−/−α), implying that all four α genes are downregulated. In the case illustrated in Fig. 12.13, cDNAα hybridization to DNA obtained from an erythroid bone-marrow sample showed no evidence for a loss of α-globin genes (Old *et al.* 1977). Structural analysis of the α-globin genes and ~130 kb of their flanking regions on chromosome 16p has revealed no abnormalities in severely affected patients (Higgs *et al.* 1983b; Craddock 1994). Furthermore, provisional analysis of the pattern of methylation appears normal (Anagnou *et al.* 1983; Craddock 1994). Although we have not excluded

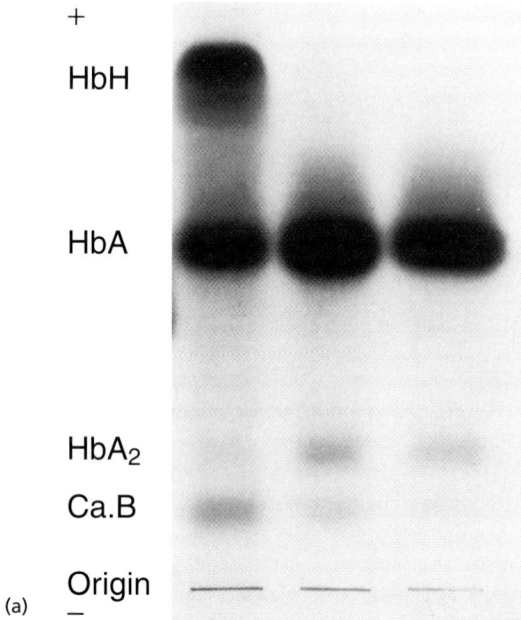

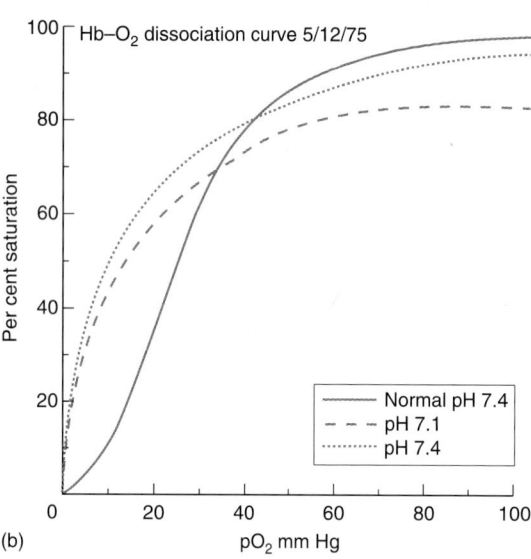

Fig. 12.12 Haemoglobin constitution and function in acquired haemoglobin H disease. (a) Haemoglobin electrophoresis (starch gel, pH 8.5, amido black stain) showing about 40% HbH. (b) Oxygen dissociation curve of whole blood showing marked shift to left. The patient was an 81-year-old male with a myeloproliferative disorder that terminated in leukaemia. From Weatherall *et al.* (1978).

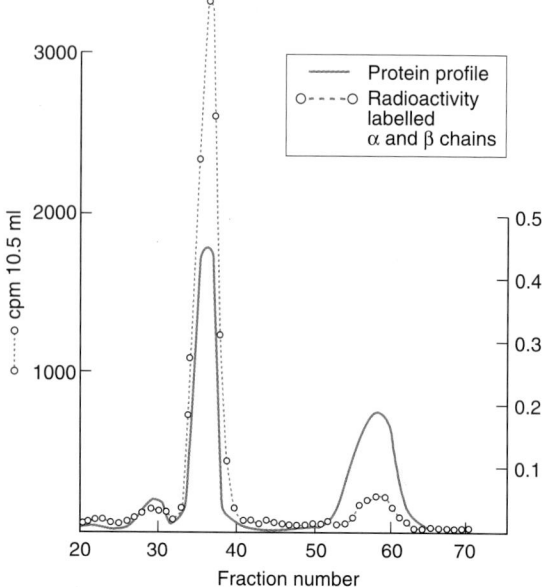

Fig. 12.13 Separation of radioactively labelled α and β chains (o-o) from a patient with ATMDS. The conditions are as solid in Chapter 5. The protein profile is shown as a solid line. The study shows a severely reduced level of α-chain synthesis (the α-globin peak is around fraction 58).

small rearrangements or single nucleotide changes, the presence of two *cis*-acting mutations seems a very unlikely basis for ATMDS. It is more likely therefore that the α genes are downregulated by a *trans*-acting mutation, either in a factor that normally controls α-gene expression or in a gene that exerts a dominant negative effect.

It is possible that in the ATMDS clone there is *trans*-acting defect that completely abolishes α-gene expression. The very low levels of α mRNA and α-chain synthesis (Fig. 12.13) might be the product of a small number of normal haematopoietic clone(s) or MDS clone(s) unaffected by the α-thalassaemia mutation. Clonal evolution in this situation would explain the variations in HbH and α-/β-globin synthesis observed during the course of the disease. Alternatively, the ATMDS mutation might cause variable downregulation of α-globin expression in all cells within a single MDS clone. This would provide a less satisfactory explanation for changes in HbH and globin synthesis during progression of the disease. At present we are unable to distinguish between these two possibilities.

This issue is of importance in designing further experiments to analyse ATMDS. For example, Helder and Deisseroth (1987) made interspecific hybrids between bone marrow from ATMDS patients and APRT-deficient mouse erythroleukaemia (MEL) cells. After selection, such hybrids retained human chromosome 16 derived from the ATMDS patient and it directed normal levels of human α-globin synthesis. While this might provide further evidence that ATMDS results from a *trans*-acting mutation, the interpretation critically depends on whether the human cell that originally fused with the MEL cell could have been from an unaffected clone.

The problem now is to localize and ultimately identify the acquired *trans*-acting abnormality in ATMDS. This would be of great importance to our understanding of α-gene regulation and might also elucidate the molecular pathway to clonal evolution in MDS. Are there any clues to help this search? One of the most striking features of ATMDS is the marked male sex bias not seen in previous studies of MDS (Juneja *et al.* 1983; Noël *et al.* 1993). Superficially, this might suggest involvement of the X chromosome, with only one somatic mutation required to create a null mutation in XY males. However, this argument also applies to females because, in each haemopoietic stem cell, one X chromosome is inactivated by Lyonization. It is interesting that another acquired clonal haematopoietic disorder, paroxysmal nocturnal haemoglobinuria, results from mutations in an X-linked gene and this occurs with equal frequency in males and females. The X-chromosome hypothesis might apply to a gene which escapes X inactivation, so that females have two active copies, and is not present on the Y chromosome, or if there were a high frequency of Y-chromosome loss in the MDS clones.

In the absence of any lead of this kind we are left to search for non-random chromosome abnormalities. To date no consistent chromosome abnormalities have been found in the four ATMDS patients studied in this way. Finally, are there any candidate genes? It would be expected that the general erythroid transcription factors, GATA-1 and NF-E2 for example, would affect α- and β-globin expression equally. However, the ATR-X gene (see earlier) encodes a putative transcriptional regulator that specifically affects α-globin expression. To date, provisional analysis of this gene in several patients has detected no abnormality.

Chapter 13
Thalassaemia intermedia

Introduction

In Chapter 7 we described how the heterozygous states for the β thalassaemias are characterized by a fairly homogeneous clinical and haematological picture. In particular, there is only a mild degree of anaemia, the spleen is not usually palpable, there is no jaundice, and either there is a normal level of HbF or it is only minimally raised. On the other hand, the transfusion-dependent homozygous or compound heterozygous forms of β thalassaemia are associated with severe anaemia, icterus, spleno-megaly and relatively high levels of HbF. However, it has been quite clear since the studies of the Italian workers, Greppi, Rietti and Micheli, in the mid-1920s, that there are forms of thalassaemia of intermediate severity which do not resemble what were later recognized as the heterozygous or homozygous forms of the illness.

La Malattia di Rietti–Greppi–Micheli (see Chapter 1) was characterized by moderate anaemia, jaundice and splenomegaly, a condition much more severe than heterozygous β thalassaemia. Interest-ingly, Wintrobe's first description of a milder form of thalassaemia in the USA was an intermediate form of the illness of this kind (Wintrobe *et al.* 1940). In Marmont and Bianchi's extensive review of the early Italian literature, published in 1948, they point out that there are many patients in Italy with Mediter-ranean anaemia of intermediate severity. Similarly, in their summary of the Italian literature Chini and Valeri (1949) point out that many of the early case reports describe patients with moderately severe anaemia and splenomegaly, a condition which they call the anaemic form of the 'Mediterranean haema-tologic disorder'. Extensive studies of this type of thalassaemia were carried out in the late 1940s by Sil-vestroni and Bianco, who used the descriptive term 'anaemia microcitica costituzionale' (Silvestroni & Bianco 1944–45, 1945, 1948, 1951; Bianco *et al.* 1952). Their papers include many descriptions of patients with thalassaemia with varying degrees of anaemia

and splenomegaly; in retrospect it seems likely that many of these cases represented what was later to be called β thalassaemia intermedia.

In the American and British literature the term 'thalassaemia intermedia' has been used to describe the clinical and haematological findings in patients whose illness is not as severe as thalassaemia major but which is more severe than the carrier state (Stur-geon *et al.* 1955). Over the last 20 years it has become apparent that this clinical picture can result from the interaction of many different thalassaemia alleles, one with another or with those for structural haemo-globin variants. Hence, the term is simply a useful descriptive title for a particular clinical phenotype and has no clear-cut genetic meaning. However, because we are still not at the stage at which we can always describe precisely the genetic interactions which can produce this clinical picture, it seems useful to retain the term.

Because the intermediate forms of thalassaemia are extremely common, and because their patho-physiology and clinical manifestations have been neglected over the years, we have devoted this chapter to summarizing the genetic interactions which can produce this condition, its main features and complications, and what little is known about its pathophysiology and natural history. As will be apparent from Table 13.1, which shows the known genetic interactions which can underlie this form of thalassaemia, many of the conditions that comprise this syndrome are described elsewhere in this book. Hence, this chapter will focus on the intermediate forms of β thalassaemia which, globally, after HbE β thalassaemia are by far the most important and chal-lenging varieties of the condition.

Over recent years several groups have reviewed different aspects of this field (Wainscoat *et al.* 1987; Fiorelli *et al.* 1988; Cao *et al.* 1990; Camaschella & Cappellini 1995; Weatherall & Clegg 1996; Rund *et al.* 1997; Ho *et al.* 1998a).

Table 13.1 Thalassaemia intermedia.

1 *Mild deficit in β-globin production*
Homozygous mild β^+ thalassaemia
Compound heterozygosity for severe β^0 or β^+ and mild β^+ thalassaemia
Interactions of β^0 with 'silent' or 'mild' β thalassaemia
Homozygosity for 'silent' β thalassaemia
2 *Reduced globin imbalance due to co-inheritance of α and β thalassaemia*
Homozygous or compound heterozygous β^0 or β^+ thalassaemia with two or three α-gene deletions
Homozygous or compound heterozygous severe β^0 or β^+ thalassaemia with non-deletion α2-gene mutation
Homozygous or compound heterozygous severe β^+ thalassaemia with one or two α-gene deletions
3 *Severe β thalassaemia with increased capacity for γ-chain synthesis*
Homozygous or compound heterozygous β^0 or β^+ thalassaemia with heterocellular HPFH
Homozygous or compound heterozygous β^0 or β^+ thalassaemia with particular β-globin RFLP haplotype
Mechanism unknown
4 *Deletion forms of δβ thalassaemia and HPFH*
Homozygous $(\delta\beta)^0$ or $(^A\gamma\delta\beta)^0$ thalassaemia
Compound heterozygosity for β^0 or β^+ and $(\delta\beta)^0$ or $(^A\gamma\delta\beta)^0$ thalassaemia
Homozygosity for Hb Lepore (some cases)
Compound heterozygosity for Hb Lepore and β^0 or β^+ thalassaemia (some forms)
Compound heterozygosity for $(\delta\beta)^0$, $^G\gamma\beta^+$ or $^A\gamma\beta^+$ HPFH and β^0 or β^+ thalassaemia
Compound heterozygosity for $(\delta\beta)^0$ thalassaemia and $(\delta\beta)^0$ HPFH
5 *Compound heterozygosity for β or δβ thalassaemia and β-chain structural variants*
Hbs S/, C/, E/β or δβ thalassaemia
Many other rare interactions
6 *Other β-thalassaemia alleles or interactions*
Dominant β thalassaemia
β-Thalassaemia trait associated with ααα- or αααα-gene arrangements
Highly unstable β-globin chain variants

How is thalassaemia intermedia defined?

There is no adequate definition of thalassaemia intermedia and it has an extraordinarily diverse clinical spectrum. As mentioned earlier, the haematological findings in heterozygous β thalassaemia are characterized by a mild degree of anaemia; splenomegaly is very much the exception. Hence, any patient with a haemoglobin level persistently below 9–10 g/dl, particularly if there is associated splenomegaly, falls into the intermediate class of β thalassaemias.

It is at the more severe end of the spectrum that a genuine difficulty in definition arises. Some children go through early life with haemoglobin levels in the 5–6 g/dl range and manage to survive and develop, albeit poorly. Although they are often classified as having thalassaemia intermedia, particularly if they present relatively late, many of them have a miserable childhood and develop gross skeletal deformities. Thus most clinicians feel that they should receive blood transfusions to avoid these distressing complications. Whether they should be classified as having severe thalassaemia intermedia or thalassaemia major is merely a question of semantics.

However, some patients with β thalassaemia have haemoglobin values between 6 and 9 g/dl, and grow and develop reasonably well and reach adult life. Hence it is useful to retain the term 'thalassaemia intermedia' for this type of case. It should be remembered that a patient of this kind may become transfusion dependent if complications such as hypersplenism develop or if the anaemia is exacerbated by other factors such as folic acid deficiency, nutritional deficiency or intercurrent infection. Clearly, the term thalassaemia intermedia can cover a very broad and shifting clinical spectrum, from almost complete health to a condition characterized by severe growth retardation and skeletal deformity requiring transfusion therapy; it is a descriptive diagnosis that can be made only after a considerable period of observation and which often requires revision. We shall return to this problem in Chapter 15.

Genetic mechanisms responsible for the phenotype of β thalassaemia intermedia

As shown in Table 13.1 there are many different interactions and mutations that can give rise to the phenotype of β thalassaemia intermedia. Here we focus on those in which either both or at least one of the thalassaemia alleles involves the β-globin-gene locus. Conditions which produce a similar clinical picture, the δβ thalassaemias and their interactions, and the interactions of β thalassaemia with structural haemoglobin variants for example, are described in Chapters 8 and 9.

The interactions of silent or mild β-thalassaemia alleles

In the current thalassaemia literature it is customary to divide the mild β-thalassaemia alleles, which can interact one with another or with more severe alleles to produce thalassaemia intermedia, into the 'silent' and 'mild' β⁺ thalassaemias. While useful in practice, this is a somewhat artificial classification. Although many of the so-called 'silent' alleles show no haematological changes in heterozygotes, if large numbers are studied it is apparent that at least some of them have slightly reduced mean cell volume (MCV) or mean cell haemoglobin (MCH) values, and slightly elevated HbA_2 levels and α-/β-globin synthesis ratios. However, there is so much overlap with normal values that, for practical purposes, it is reasonable to classify these extremely mild alleles as 'silent', not in the least because, perhaps with the exception of the measurement of globin synthesis, they would not be identified by standard screening methods to detect β-thalassaemia heterozygotes.

On the other hand the 'mild' β⁺-thalassaemia alleles have obvious changes in the red-cell indices and elevated HbA_2 levels. Previously, the silent β thalassaemias have been classified as type 1 normal HbA_2 β thalassaemias. Since we now understand the molecular pathology of many of these conditions, and it is clear that the forms of β thalassaemia with normal HbA_2 levels with typical haematological features of β-thalassaemia trait, which constitute type 2, are usually compound heterozygotes for β and δ thalassaemia, this classification has now outlived its usefulness.

Table 13.2 'Silent' β-thalassaemia alleles.

−92 C→T
−101 C→T
5′ UTR +10 −T
5′ UTR +33 C→G
CAP +1 A→C
IVS2-844 C→G
3′ UTR +6 C→G

Table 13.3 Mild β-thalassaemia alleles.

−90 C→T	−28 A→G (mild in Blacks; severe in Chinese)
−88 C→A	5′ UTR +22 G→A
−88 C→T	CD19 A→G Malay
−87 C→A	CD24 T→A
−87 C→G	CD26 G→A HbE
−87 C→T	CD27 G→T Knossos
	IVS1-6 T→C
−86 C→G	?3′ UTR 47 C→G
−31 A→G	Poly(A) AATAAA→AA**C**AAA
−30 T→A	Poly(A) AATAAA→AAT**U**AA
−30 T→C	Poly(A) AATAAA→AATA**G**A
−29 A→G	Poly(A) AATAAA→AATAA**C**

One of the problems in characterizing these mild forms of β thalassaemia is that many of them have only been recorded as a single case report, usually as part of an interaction with a more severe form of β thalassaemia. The reported mutations that underlie silent and mild forms of β thalassaemia are summarized in Tables 13.2 and 13.3. In the sections that follow we shall review what is known of the phenotypes and interactions for those varieties in which there has been sufficient experience to provide a reasonably reliable picture of the clinical findings in heterozygotes and their various interactions with more severe β-thalassaemia alleles (Table 13.4).

Interactions of silent β thalassaemias

As mentioned earlier, the term 'silent' β thalassaemia is a misnomer. In the few large series that have been reported, heterozygotes have, on average, mild abnormalities of the red-cell indices and/or HbA_2 levels, and imbalanced α-/β-globin synthesis ratios. However, these changes are so small and variable that in any individual case it is quite possible for a carrier to have no significant abnormalities.

Table 13.4 Some interactions of silent, mild and severe β-thalassaemia alleles as the basis for thalassaemia intermedia (TI). Where data are available the severity is classified as mild (MTI) or severe (STI). TI indicates a variable phenotype, or insufficient information. Data from Huisman *et al.* (1997), Ho *et al.* (1998a) and references cited in text.

Mutation	−101 C→T	−92 C→T	−88 C→T	−87 G→G	−87 C→T	−86 C→A	−30 T→C	−29 A→G	5' UTR +10 −T	5' UTR +22 G→A	5' UTR +33 C→G	CAP +1 A→C	CD19 A→G	CD26 G→A*	CD27 G→T	IVS1-6 T→C	IVS2-844 C→G	β term+6 C→G	AATAAA → AATAAG	AATAAA → AACAAA	AATAAA → A−AAA
CD8 −AA										STI					TI	TI					
CD8/9 +G																		STI			
CD15 G→A			TI																		
IVS1-1 G→A											TI	TI									
IVS1-5 G→C											TI	TI/STI									
IVS1-5 G→T	MTI																				
IVS1-110 G→A	MTI	TI		STI						MTI	MTI				TI	STI					
CD36/37 −T	MTI				TI																
CD39 C→T	TI		STI	TI				TI			MTI					STI					
CD41 −C	MTI																				
CD41/42 −TTCT												MTI/STI									
CD44 −C	MTI									MTI					TI	STI					
IVS2-1 G→A							?TI			MTI					TI	MTI					
IVS2-654 C→T	MTI	TI																			STI
IVS2-745 C→G	MTI																MTI				
IVS2-748 C→A																					
IVS2-849 A→G																					

* HbE interactions are described in Chapter 9.

These alleles are so mild that, in the rare cases where homozygotes have been encountered, the condition may be little more severe than β-thalassaemia trait. However, when they are inherited together with severe β-thalassaemia alleles the resulting clinical picture may be one of β thalassaemia intermedia of varying severity. Thus the usual clinical setting in which they are encountered is a family in which there is a patient with β thalassaemia intermedia, one of whose parents appears at first sight to be haematologically normal.

β–101 C→T

This mutation, which occurs in the distal CACCC box, seems to downregulate globin-gene transcription very slightly (Gonzalez-Redondo et al. 1989a). It is fairly widespread among Mediterranean populations and in Israel and Turkey (Ristaldi et al. 1990a; Bianco et al. 1997a,c; Rund et al. 1997). Bianco and her colleagues have presented detailed haematological and haemoglobin synthetic data on a large series of heterozygotes who, in addition, were all shown not to have deletional forms of α thalassaemia. About a third of them had completely normal haematological findings and haemoglobin analyses, whereas the remainder had either a very slightly reduced MCH, a marginally elevated HbA$_2$ in the 3.2–3.5% range, or slight globin imbalance, with α/β ratios of approximately 1.2–1.3. Similar data are reported by Maragoudaki et al. (1999).

The homozygous state has not been characterized. The compound heterozygous states with a variety of different severe β-thalassaemia alleles have been reported. These include: CD39 C→T; IVS1-110 G→A; IVS1-1 G→A; IVS2-745 C→G; CD44 –C; CD36/37 –T; IVS1-5 G→T; and others (Ristaldi et al. 1990a; Bianco et al. 1997c; Rund et al. 1997). Without exception they result in an extremely mild form of β thalassaemia intermedia with steady-state haemoglobin values in the 9–12 g/dl range, a marked reduction in the MCV and MCH, elevated HbA$_2$ levels in the 4.5–6.0% range, HbF values ranging from 10 to 45% with the majority in the 10–20% range, and α-/β+γ-globin synthesis ratios of approximately the same magnitude as those of β-thalassaemia heterozygotes. Approximately two-thirds of these patients had very mild splenomegaly, palpable 2–3 cm below the costal margin.

β CAP +1 A→C

This mutation was first observed in an Asian Indian homozygote who had the clinical phenotype of β-thalassaemia trait (Wong et al. 1987). The heterozygous phenotype is completely silent but interactions with different β-thalassaemia alleles produce the clinical phenotype of β thalassaemia intermedia of varying severity (Ho et al. 1998a). For example, although its interaction with β IVS1-5 G→C produces mild to moderately severe forms, that with β CD41/42 –TTCT results in a severe variety.

β 5′-Untranslated region (UTR) +10 (–T)

This mutation seems to be completely silent in heterozygotes, while the compound heterozygous state with the allele β CD39 C→T is characterized by a mild form of thalassaemia intermedia, with a haemoglobin level of approximately 9.0 g/dl, HbA$_2$ 4.8%, HbF 5.8% and imbalanced globin synthesis (Athanassiadou et al. 1994).

β CAP +33 C→G

This variant is almost silent in the heterozygous state although the HbA$_2$ level may be slightly elevated and the α-/β-globin synthesis ratio varies from 1.5 to 1.8 (Ho et al. 1996c). It has been reported in the compound heterozygous state with several β-thalassaemia alleles, including IVS1-1 G→A and IVS1-110 G→A (Ho et al. 1996c; Traeger-Synodinos et al. 1996). Overall, these interactions are extremely mild, with haemoglobin values ranging from 7 to almost 12 g/dl, hypochromic red cells, elevated HbA$_2$ levels in the 5–7% range, but only slightly elevated HbF values, in the 1–4% range. There is clearly demonstrable globin imbalance. As expected, these interactions appear to be more severe with β^0-thalassaemia alleles.

IVS2-844 C→G

This allele was first described in an Italian family in a patient with an extremely mild form of β thalassaemia intermedia in which the other β-globin allele appeared to be normal (Murru et al. 1991). Heterozygotes show no abnormalities, while homozygotes have the haematological and haemoglobin characteristics of β-thalassaemia trait (Rosatelli et al. 1994). It has been observed in interactions with the splice mutation β IVS2-745 C→G, resulting in a mild form of β thalassaemia intermedia (Rosatelli *et al.*1994), or with β⁰-thalassaemia alleles, resulting in a variable phenotype ranging from severe to extremely mild β thalassaemia intermedia (Bianco *et al.*1997c).

β Termination codon +6 C→G

This mutation seems to be completely silent in heterozygotes but the α-/β-globin synthesis ratio ranges from 1.2 to 1.9 (Jankovic *et al.* 1991; Maragoudaki *et al.* 1998). It has been observed in a compound heterozygote for the β allele IVS1-1 G→A, with the clinical picture of a moderately severe thalassaemia intermedia, a haemoglobin level of 7.7 g/dl, and HbA₂ and HbF levels of 4.7 and 10.0%, respectively. This patient had an occasional requirement for blood transfusion and had mild thalassaemic bone changes. However, other reports of interactions with β⁰- or β⁺-thalassaemia alleles all described mild forms of β thalassaemia intermedia (Maragoudaki *et al.*1998).

From such data as are available, therefore, it appears that the interactions of these silent forms of β thalassaemia with more severe β-thalassaemia alleles always give rise to the phenotype of β thalassaemia intermedia. Overall, it can be expected to be a relatively mild form although, particularly in the case of co-inheritance with β⁰-thalassaemia alleles, the interaction may occasionally result in a disorder at the more severe end of the spectrum.

Interactions of mild β-thalassaemia alleles

As shown in Table 13.3 numerous mild β-thalassaemia alleles have been identified. However, in many cases there are very few published data about their haematological characteristics or about the results of their interactions with other β-thalassaemia alleles.

β –88 C→T

This mutation, which decreases the rate of transcription of the β-globin gene, probably because of decreased binding by transcription factors, is relatively common among Africans and Afro-Americans (Orkin *et al.*1984a; Gonzalez-Redondo *et al.*1988a). Its heterozygous phenotype is typical of β-thalassaemia trait, although compared with more severe β-thalassaemia alleles the MCH, within the

range 23–25 pg, is higher. The homozygous condition is characterized by a relatively mild form of thalassaemia intermedia, with haemoglobin values in the range 9.8–12.3 g/dl, HbA₂ values in the 4–8% range, and surprisingly high levels of HbF for the mild degree of globin imbalance, in the range 40–72%. The high HbA₂ and F values may reflect the inadequate binding of transcription factors to the β-globin-gene promoters, thus freeing them for interaction with the γ and δ promoters; this concept is strengthened by the observation that heterozygotes for this condition appear to have significantly higher levels of HbA₂ than those for more severe β-thalassaemia alleles. This allele is also found on a chromosome with the C→T change (*Xmn* I polymorphism) at ᴳγ –158, which also may contribute to the high HbF response to a mild form of β thalassaemia (see Chapter 10). Its interactions with Hbs S and C is described in Chapter 9; its mildness is further underlined by the relatively high level of HbA in these compound heterozygotes.

There have been a few descriptions of the interaction of this allele with other β-thalassaemia alleles in African or Afro-American populations. In the compound heterozygous state with the other common promoter allele in this ethnic group, β –29 A→G, the phenotype was extremely mild, with a haemoglobin value of 13.3 g/dl, thalassaemic red-cell indices, 7.4% HbA₂ and 57% HbF (Gonzalez-Redondo *et al.* 1988a).

β –87 C→G

This condition has been observed mainly in Mediterranean populations, notably in Italy and Turkey. It also seems to result in less effective binding of transcription factors to the β-globin gene (Treisman *et al.* 1983). The heterozygous phenotype is a typical β-thalassaemia trait, although both the MCV and the MCH appear to overlap with normal values in some cases. The HbA₂ level is in the 4.2–4.5% range, but unfortunately there are insufficient published data to determine whether the HbF is significantly higher than usually found in heterozygotes. The homozygous state was described in a short report by Camaschella *et al.* (1990a). The patient was a 62-year-old male with normal development, mild jaundice and 'moderate' splenomegaly. The skull X-ray was normal. The haemoglobin level was 7.4 g/dl and there was marked hypochromia and microcytosis; the HbA₂ level was 5% and the HbF level 65%. Another homozygote is mentioned by Diaz-Chico *et al.* (1988b); the patient's condition is described as being 'mild', with no transfusion requirements and an HbF value of 31%; no other clinical details are given.

This mutation has been observed in the compound heterozygous state with several different β-thalassaemia alleles, such as CD39 C→T (Rosatelli *et al.* 1989; Meloni *et al.* 1992) and IVS1-110 G→A (Meloni *et al.* 1992; Ho *et al.* 1998a). The best characterized of these interactions are with the codon 39 nonsense mutation (Rosatelli *et al.* 1989). These patients have thalassaemia intermedia with steady-state haemoglobin levels of about 10 g/dl and a remarkably wide variation in fetal haemoglobin values, in the range 25–80%; some have thalassaemic bone changes and most have mild to moderate splenomegaly. They have received sporadic transfusions, usually associated with intercurrent illness.

β–87 C→T

The compound heterozygous state for this mutation and the β-thalassaemia allele IVS1-110 G→A was reported by Kulozik *et al.* (1991b). The patient was a 20-year-old male of German/Italian descent who appeared to have a moderately severe form of β thalassaemia intermedia, as evidenced by marked hepatosplenomegaly and bone changes despite his steady-state haemoglobin level of approximately 9 g/dl. Haemoglobin analysis showed an HbF level of 62.5% and an elevated HbA$_2$ at 5.1%. His mother, who was the carrier of the –87 C→T mutation, was not anaemic and although her red cells were said to be slightly hypochromic and microcytic the MCV was 86 fl while the MCH was 26 pg. She did however, show an elevated HbA$_2$ of 5.5% and a slightly elevated HbF at 3.4%. Thus the findings in this patient are very similar to those described above for the interactions of the β –87 C→G mutation with the IVS1-110 G→A allele.

β–31 A→G

An individual homozygous for this mutation has been reported in a Japanese family (Takihara *et al.* 1986). The heterozygous phenotype is a typical β-thalassaemia trait. The homozygote has a moderately severe form of thalassaemia intermedia with a steady-state haemoglobin level of 7.2 g/dl, red cells with marked microcytosis and hypochromia, an HbA$_2$ value of 5.9% and an HbF level of 14%. No interac-

tions with other thalassaemia alleles have been observed.

β–30 T→A

This mutation has been found in Turkish, Macedonian and Tunisian families (Fei *et al.* 1988b; Fattoum *et al.* 1991). Heterozygotes have typical β-thalassaemia trait. Homozygotes show a mild form of thalassaemia intermedia, with steady-state haemoglobin levels in the 10.0 g/dl range, moderate hypochromia and microcytosis, HbA$_2$ levels of approximately 4%, and HbF levels of 12–14%. These patients have not required blood transfusion. No interactions with other β-thalassaemia alleles have been reported.

β–29 A→G

This is the most common β-thalassaemia mutation in Africans and Afro-Americans. It has been observed in the homozygous state and in the compound heterozygous state together with Hbs S, C, O Arab and N Baltimore (see Chapter 9). Heterozygotes show changes typical of the β-thalassaemia trait, with relatively high HbA$_2$ levels and HbF values which are slightly higher than those of many β-thalassaemia alleles (see Chapter 7). Homozygotes are, by and large, asymptomatic or become anaemic during periods of stress such as intercurrent infection or pregnancy. None have been transfusion dependent, although some show evidence of progressive iron loading (Gonzalez-Redondo *et al.* 1988a,b; Safaya *et al.* 1989). Their steady-state haemoglobin levels are between 10 and 12 g/dl, their blood films show moderate microcytosis and hypochromia, and they all have elevated HbA$_2$ levels, ranging from 3 to 10%, and HbF values in the 50–70% range, with an occasional exception in the 10–15% range (Gonzalez-Redondo *et al.* 1988a). The reasons for the unusually high HbA$_2$ and F values are probably similar to those which we discussed earlier for the –88 C→T allele.

Because the –29 A→G allele is so common in Afro-American populations there have been some opportunities to study its interactions with other β-thalassaemia alleles. Several cases of the compound heterozygous state with β CD24 T→A have been reported (Gonzalez-Redondo *et al.* 1988a). There is very little information about the codon 24 mutation but its interaction with this allele produces a fairly mild form of thalassaemia intermedia, with haemoglobin values ranging from 9 to 13.5 g/dl, typical thalassaemic blood changes, HbA$_2$ values in the 2.6–9.3% range and HbF values in the 24–67% range. These findings suggest that the codon 24 splice mutation may itself be a relatively mild form of β thalassaemia. There is a single case report of compound heterozygosity for this allele and β IVS2-848 C→A, which probably diminishes splicing at the adjacent invariant AG dinucleotide, though not completely. This 48-year-old female was found to have a more severe form of thalassaemia intermedia, with a haemoglobin value of 5.8 g/dl and thalassaemic red-cell changes. Surprisingly, the MCV was 97 fl and the MCH 25 pg. The HbA$_2$ and HbF values were 4.0 and 74.0%, respectively. Very little is known about the IVS2-848 C→A allele, but this interaction suggests that it causes a severe form of β$^+$ thalassaemia.

The β –29 A→G allele has also been observed in a single Chinese homozygote with severe, transfusion-dependent thalassaemia major (Huang *et al.* 1986). It has been suggested that the different phenotype from that observed in black populations may reflect the fact that, in the latter, the mutation is on a chromosome carrying the *Xmn* I ^{G}γ polymorphism while this was not the case in the Chinese patient. It is not clear whether this major phenotypic difference between the two populations can be explained solely by the presence or absence of this particular polymorphism. As we shall see later in this chapter, homozygosity for the *Xmn* I ^{G}γ polymorphism has been implicated in some mild phenotypes associated with β^0 thalassaemia. Hence this suggestion is not entirely improbable; further information about the phenotypic expression of these mild β-thalassaemia alleles in different chromosomal settings is needed before this question can be answered with certainty.

β Codon 19 A*A*C→A*G*C; β19 Asn→Ser, Hb Malay

This substitution, as well as leading to the production of a neutrally charged haemoglobin variant, creates an alternative splice site between codons 17 and 18 and hence decreases the efficiency of the normal donor site at IVS1. It is found mainly in south-east Asians of Malaysian origin. The heterozygous state is characterized by a typical β-thalassaemia trait, although the red-cell indices tend to be higher than those associated with more severe β-thalassaemia alleles. The haematological findings are as follows: haemoglobin 12–16 g/dl; MCV 66–79 fl; MCH 22–

26 pg; HbA$_2$ 3.3–3.8%; HbF not elevated. Homozygotes have a mild form of thalassaemia intermedia characterized by splenomegaly, haemoglobin levels in the 8.5–9 g/dl range, extremely hypochromic, microcytic red cells, HbA$_2$ levels of 5–7% and HbF values of 10–25% (Yang *et al.* 1989; Thein *et al.* 1990b).

The mild forms of β thalassaemia intermedia that result from the interaction of this variant with HbE are described in Chapter 9.

β Codon 26 (GAG→AAG; β26 Glu→Lys, HbE)

The mild thalassaemias associated with the heterozygous and homozygous states for HbE, and the varieties of thalassaemia intermedia which result from its interaction with severe β-thalassaemia alleles, are described in detail in Chapter 9.

β Codon 27 (GCC→TCC; β27 Ala→Ser, Hb Knossos)

This form of silent β thalassaemia results from two different mutations. First, a codon 27 change activates an alternative splice site, resulting in a slight reduction in the quantity of normal β-globin messenger RNA. In addition, however, the δ-globin gene in *cis* has a deletion of a single A in codon 59, leading to premature termination at codon 60, i.e. δ^0 thalassaemia (Fessas *et al.* 1981; Arous *et al.* 1983; Orkin *et al.* 1984b; Olds *et al.* 1991). The δ^0/β^{Knossos} allele appears to be widespread in the Mediterranean and adjacent regions.

The heterozygous state is associated with slightly reduced MCH and MCV values, a low or low-normal HbA$_2$ level, and no increase in HbF. Globin synthesis is balanced. The homozygous state is characterized by mild anaemia, with haemoglobin values in the 9–12 g/dl range, hypochromia and microcytosis with significantly reduced MCV and MCH values, the absence of HbA$_2$ and, in some cases, a slight elevation of HbF, in the 2–4% range. There is imbalanced globin synthesis, with α/β ratios in the 1.5–2.5 range. In one of the reported cases the tip of the spleen was just palpable but in others there has been no detectable splenomegaly or any other clinical features of thalassaemia (Baklouti *et al.* 1986; Olds *et al.* 1991).

The Hb Knossos allele has been found in the compound heterozygous state with several more severe β-thalassaemia alleles, including IVS1-6 T→C, codon 8 –AA, IVS1-110 G→A, IVS1-1 G→A and IVS2-1 G→A (Arous *et al.* 1983; Galacteros *et al.* 1984; Olds *et al.* 1991; Huisman *et al.* 1997; Ho *et al.* 1998a). All these interactions are associated with the clinical picture of a mild to moderate thalassaemia intermedia. In the case of the interaction with the IVS1-110 G→A allele, the disorder has been severe enough to require occasional blood transfusion during intercurrent infection, and splenectomy. The haemoglobin level ranges between 7.5 and 9.5 g/dl, the red cells are markedly hypochromic and microcytic, and HbA$_2$ values range from low normal to 8%. There is a similar broad range of HbF values, ranging from 3.5 to 40%. In the few cases for which globin synthesis data are available there appears to be marked imbalance, with α-/non-α-chain synthesis ratios in the 2–5 range.

One sibship has been reported for a compound heterozygote for this allele and the β IVS1-110 G→A allele (Ho *et al.* 1998a). Although both patients had thalassaemia intermedia there was a considerable phenotypic difference between them. One had never been transfused and had only mild splenomegaly and a steady-state haemoglobin of 8 g/dl; the other had much more marked splenomegaly and a lower steady-state haemoglobin and had required irregular transfusions over several years. Although the major phenotypic difference between these patients was the steady-state level of HbF there was no obvious genetic explanation for this finding.

The interaction with the HbS allele is described in Chapter 9, and with Hb Lepore in Chapter 8.

β IVS1-6 T→C

This splice mutation, sometimes called the Portuguese variant, is one of the commonest forms of mild β thalassaemia and is widespread among Mediterranean populations (Orkin *et al.* 1982a; Tamagnini *et al.* 1983; Wainscoat *et al.* 1983b). There have been extensive studies of the homozygous and heterozygous states and many examples of its interaction with different structural haemoglobin variants (Tamagnini *et al.* 1983; Öner *et al.* 1990; Scerri *et al.* 1993; Efremov *et al.* 1994a; Rund *et al.* 1997; Ho *et al.* 1998a).

In the first description of homozygotes from Portugal they were reported to have a mild to moderate form of thalassaemia intermedia. Many of them had grown and developed normally and although they all had splenomegaly they had rarely required transfusion. These observations were confirmed in a later study of 29 homozygotes from different ethnic groups (Efremov *et al.* 1994a); two-thirds had never been transfused and none had required regular transfusion. On the other hand, in a later report from Israel, Rund and her colleagues described a much more variable clinical phenotype (Rund *et al.* 1997). At one extreme nine patients had baseline haemoglobin levels as high at 10.6 g/dl, none had been splenectomized, and transfusion had either been rare or never been required. Although some had mild thalassaemic bone changes, many had gone through a normal puberty and were fertile. At the other extreme, however, there were nine patients with baseline haemoglobin values of 6–7 g/dl who were transfused either infrequently or regularly, even though they had undergone splenectomy. This group had growth retardation, pronounced bone changes and thalassaemic facies and absent puberty, and required chelation therapy for iron overload. Fifteen homozygotes were described as being of intermediate severity, with haemoglobin levels of 7–8 g/dl, which improved after splenectomy. There have also been reports of severely affected homozygotes from the Lebanon (Chehab *et al.* 1987). Efremov *et al.* (1994a) found that the only feature that could explain the phenotypic diversity was the steady-state HbF level, which, at least in part, could be related to different β-globin restriction-fragment-length polymorphism (RFLP) haplotypes.

The steady-state haemoglobin levels in homozygotes range between 5 and 11 g/dl; there is always marked hypochromia and microcytosis. The HbA$_2$ values are always elevated, in the 4–9% range; the HbF values, while usually in the 15–40% range, may also be much lower, between 5 and 10%.

The heterozygous state for this mutation is characterized by findings typical of heterozygous β thalassaemia, with haemoglobin levels in the 11–13 g/dl range, reduced values for the MCH and MCV, elevated levels of HbA$_2$ averaging approximately 4%, and only a slight elevation of HbF in some cases (Öner *et al.* 1990).

Because this particular mutation is so common there have been many opportunities for studying its interaction with other β-thalassaemia alleles, particularly the more severe forms that are common to the Mediterranean region. Unfortunately, however, many of these reports do not give complete genotypic data, including the state of the α-globin genes, nor are there the kind of detailed clinical data that are required to provide an adequate picture of the natural history and severity of these important interactions. What is clear, however, is that they cover a remarkably broad clinical spectrum (Diaz-Chico *et al.* 1988b; Rund *et al.* 1997; Ho *et al.* 1998a).

The most extensive published experience describes the interactions between this allele and the IVS1-110 G→A and CD39 C→T alleles. Other less common interactions between a wide variety of severe β-thalassaemia alleles are described by Rund *et al.* (1997) and Ho *et al.* (1998a). Overall, it appears that the interactions with β[0]-thalassaemia alleles are more severe and result in a picture at the most severe end of the spectrum of thalassaemia intermedia. On the other hand, interactions with β[+]-thalassaemia mutations are more varied in their phenotype, some of them being described as moderately severe, others mild. However, where the α-globin genes have been studied (Ho *et al.* 1998a), it is clear that the latter interactions are genuinely mild in those cases in which there is also a deletional form of α thalassaemia. Rund *et al.* (1997) also comment on the heterogeneity of these interactions and suggest that they may be further modified by the level of HbF production; in compound heterozygotes of this type there appears to be an inverse relationship between the steady-state level of HbF and the haemoglobin level. It is possible that some of this variability can be related to the presence of the *Xmn* I polymorphism –158 to the [G]γ gene; we shall return to this question later.

Poly(A); AATAAA→AACAAA

A number of mutations involving the poly(A) addition site, which result in their inefficient cleavage and polyadenylation, have been reported (see Chapter 4). From what little is known about their phenotypic expression it appears that they are probably mild alleles. This particular mutation (Orkin *et al.* 1985; Altay *et al.* 1991) is associated with typical β-thalassaemia trait in heterozygotes. Recently, a homozygote has been encountered (Dr J. Old, personal communication). This 35-year-old Indian had suffered no symptoms suggestive of thalassaemia and was found to have pallor and a moderate degree of splenomegaly but no skeletal abnormalities. His steady-state haemoglobin level was 7.3 g/dl with red cells showing marked hypochromia and microcytosis. The HbF and A[2] values were 13.3 and 9.2%, respec-

tively. The findings in his heterozygous relatives were indistinguishable from those of a typical β-thalassaemia trait, with HbA[2] levels of approximately 4%.

When this allele is found in combination with the β[0]-thalassaemia allele, IVS2-1 G→A, there is a moderately severe form of thalassaemia intermedia with steady-state haemoglobin levels ranging from 6.2 to 8.3 g/dl, hypochromic red cells, normal to slightly elevated HbA[2] levels and HbF values between 30 and 50%. So far this mutation has been found in individuals of African and Turkish backgrounds (Altay *et al.* 1991).

Poly(A); AATAAA→AATAAG

This mutation has been found in Kurdish Jewish families (Rund *et al.* 1990, 1991). It interacts with other mild β-thalassaemia alleles, –20 A→C for example, to produce a very mild form of thalassaemia intermedia; none of these patients have required transfusion or splenectomy and they have minimal bone changes (Rund *et al.* 1997). On the other hand, a more severe phenotype is generated when this variant is inherited together with the β[0]-thalassaemia allele.

Poly(A); AATAAA→AATAGA

This mutation, which has only been observed in Malaysia, is associated with an extremely mild interaction with HbE and therefore is probably a mild β-thalassaemia allele (Jankovic *et al.* 1990b). No other interactions are reported.

Poly(A); AATAAA→AATGAA

In heterozygotes this allele is associated with fairly typical thalassaemic red-cell indices and an HbA[2] level ranging between 3.8 and 4.1%. In the compound heterozygous state with the CD29 C→T β-thalassaemia allele, it produces a mild form of thalassaemia intermedia (Jankovic *et al.* 1990b).

Interactions between α and β thalassaemia

After the first report of a patient thought to be heterozygous for both α and β thalassaemia (Fessas 1961) there was considerable speculation about whether the clinical picture of severe β thalassaemia might be modified by the co-inheritance of different α-thalassaemia alleles. First, by the use of careful haematological studies, and later by the addition of globin synthesis analyses, it was possible to define a remarkably heterogeneous collection of clinical syndromes incorporating almost all the theoretical possibilities for different combinations of the α- and β-thalassaemia genes (Pearson 1966; Todd *et al.* 1967; Wasi *et al.* 1969; Kan & Nathan 1970; Knox-Macaulay *et al.* 1972; Bianco *et al.* 1973; Özsoylu *et al.* 1973; Shahid *et al.* 1974; Altay *et al.* 1977a; Bate & Humphries 1977; Loukopoulos *et al.* 1978; Musumeci *et al.* 1978; Furbetta *et al.* 1979; Weatherall *et al.* 1981b).

Despite the difficulties in distinguishing between the different α-thalassaemia alleles by globin synthesis, it was still possible to obtain some valuable information about these interactions. In particular, it became clear that the severe homozygous or compound heterozygous states for β thalassaemia could be significantly ameliorated by the co-inheritance of one or more α-thalassaemia determinants (Kan & Nathan 1970; Musumeci *et al.* 1978; Weatherall *et al.* 1981b). Indeed, it became apparent that these remarkable experiments of nature were living proof, if such were needed by then, that the major pathophysiological factor in the generation of the β-thalassaemia phenotype is imbalanced globin synthesis.

Once it became possible to analyse the α-globin genes directly, we were able to re-study some of these critical families and to show quite unequivocally that the interaction of either deletional or non-deletional forms of α thalassaemia has a beneficial effect on the clinical phenotype of severe β thalassaemia (Weatherall *et al.* 1981b).

The next step was to try to determine the clinical importance of these interactions. This entailed comparing the α-globin genotypes of patients with thalassaemia major or thalassaemia intermedia in different ethnic groups (Furbetta *et al.* 1983; Wainscoat *et al.* 1983a,b; Winichagoon *et al.* 1985; Thein *et al.* 1988a; Galanello *et al.* 1989). Although in some of these studies the β-globin-gene mutations were not defined, overall, they showed that the inheritance of one or more α-thalassaemia alleles has an important effect in modifying the phenotype of severe β^+ thalassaemia, though is less effective in ameliorating the β^0 thalassaemias (Table 13.1).

More recently, a different approach to this problem has been taken. In this case, detailed molecular studies have been carried out in an attempt to define all the known variables involved in generating the phenotype of β thalassaemia intermedia. This has involved studies of the mutations at both the α- and β-globin-gene loci, together with attempts to exclude genetic factors that are involved in an unusually high level of fetal haemoglobin production in β thalassaemia. These extensive, time-consuming and often frustrating analyses have provided further information about the phenotypic effects of the interactions of α and β thalassaemia, although the numbers involved have been relatively small (Camaschella & Cappellini 1995; Rund *et al.* 1997; Ho *et al.* 1998a). It is these data, sporadic studies and the population analyses outlined above that form the basis for our current and rather limited knowledge about the phenotypic effects of these important interactions. Furthermore, it should be emphasized that, despite all this work, the number of examples for any particular genotype are still relatively small and therefore it is often very difficult to make clinically useful generalizations about the likely course of any particular combination of α and β thalassaemia.

β-Thalassaemia trait modified by the co-existence of α thalassaemia

Although these interactions do not result in any clinical disability they are important in the context of both thalassaemia intermedia and population screening for β thalassaemia. In particular, they provide a valuable indicator that there may be α-thalassaemia genes segregating within families with β thalassaemia, and hence that the homozygous and compound heterozygous phenotypes may be modified.

Although there were hints in the literature prior to 1980 that the co-inheritance of α- and β-thalassaemia traits might alter the phenotype of the latter, it was only with the advent of globin-gene mapping that it became possible to study these interactions in detail and to determine the effects of different α-thalassaemia alleles on the phenotype of heterozygous β thalassaemia. In the first study of this type, Kanavakis *et al.* (1982) noted that the co-inheritance of β thalassaemia with homozygous α^+ thalassaemia (–α/–α) had a highly significant effect on the red-cell indices; in the β-thalassaemia heterozygotes with four α genes the mean MCV and MCH were 66.2 and 21.2, respectively, while similar figures for those who were homozygous for α^+ thalassaemia were 76.0 and

24.8, respectively. There was no significant difference in the HbA_2 and F values between the two groups; the HbA_2 values were all elevated in the 5% range. These data correlated well with the α-/β-globin synthesis ratios; the mean value for β-thalassaemia heterozygotes with four α genes was 2.2, and for those with two α genes it was 0.8. There was a significant, though much less marked, increase in the MCV and MCH in β-thalassaemia carriers who were heterozygous for $α^+$ thalassaemia (–α/αα).

Similar data were obtained by Melis *et al.* (1983) and by Rosatelli *et al.* (1984). In eight individuals heterozygous for $β^0$ and $α^+$ thalassaemia the MCV ranged from 77 to 90 fl, and the MCH from 26 to 30 pg. These workers also observed normal MCH and MCV values in two $β^0$-thalassaemia heterozygotes who were also heterozygous for $α^0$ thalassaemia, although they could not exclude co-existent non-deletion α thalassaemia. Interestingly, in the study of Kanavakis *et al.* the two individuals who were heterozygous for β thalassaemia and for $α^+$ thalassaemia with the highest MCH and MCV values were also thought to have co-existent non-deletional forms of α thalassaemia. Kanavakis *et al.* also described four additional individuals who were heterozygous for β thalassaemia and who also had the genotype of HbH disease, i.e. they had both $α^0$ and $α^+$ thalassaemia. Two of the siblings described by Knox-Macaulay *et al.* (1972) probably had this genotype (Fig. 13.2). In these cases the red cells are extremely hypochromic and microcytic with marked reductions in the MCV and MCH; the HbA_2 level is still elevated in the β-thalassaemia range, however. More recently it has been established that heterozygotes for β thalas-

saemia and $α^0$ thalassaemia also have higher MCV and MCH values than those who are heterozygous for either trait alone (Table 13.5 and Fig. 13.1).

These studies indicate that homozygosity for $α^+$ thalassaemia or heterozygosity for $α^0$ thalassaemia together with heterozygous β thalassaemia can result in a normal or almost normal haematological picture; the only clue to the presence of a β-thalassaemia gene is an elevated HbA_2 level. As well as for studying families with α and β thalassaemia these observations

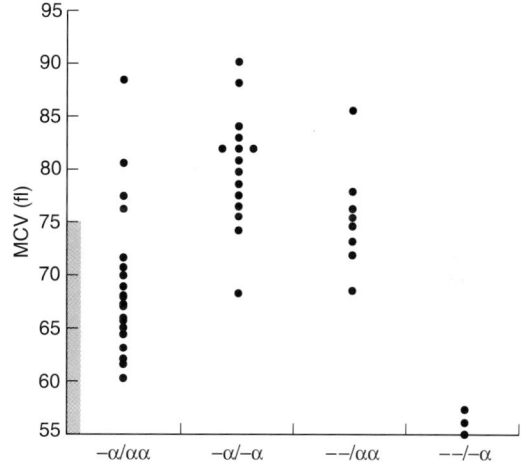

Fig. 13.1 The effect of the co-inheritance of different α-thalassaemia alleles on the mean cell volume of individuals with the β-thalassaemia trait. The shaded box shows the range for the β-thalassaemia trait alone. The different α-thalassaemia alleles found in association with β-thalassaemia trait are indicated below. References in text.

Table 13.5 Haematological findings in β-thalassaemia heterozygotes, related to number of α-globin genes.

Condition	*n*	Hb (g/dl)	MCV (fl)	MCH (pg)	HbA_2 (%)	HbF (%)	α/β ratio
αα/αα	53	12.5 ± 1.2	65 ± 4	21 ± 1	4.9 ± 0.7	1.3 ± 1.1	2.2 ± 0.3
αα/–α	36	13.0 ± 1.4	67 ± 4	22 ± 1	5.2 ± 0.7	1.2 ± 0.3	1.4 ± 0.1
–α/–α	11	13.9 ± 1.1	77 ± 3	25 ± 1	5.1 ± 0.6	1.1 ± 0.7	0.8 ± 0.1
–α/––	6	11.8 ± 0.8	55 ± 3	18 ± 1	4.6 ± 0.2	–	0.5 ± 0.1
ααα/ααα*	7	11.7 ± 1.9	65 ± 5	21 ± 2	5.0 ± 0.9	2.3 ± 1.5	2.1 ± 0.4
	11	9.1 ± 0.9	70 ± 8	21 ± 2	4.9 ± 0.6	4.3 ± 2.1	2.9 ± 0.6
αααα/αααα	3	9.3 ± 0.9	65 ± 3	21 ± 1	4.6 ± 0.3	6.8 ± 2.9	4.0 ± 0.4

* Seven cases presenting with phenotype of thalassaemia trait, 11 presenting as thalassaemia intermedia.
MCH, mean cell haemoglobin; MCV, mean cell volume.
Data from references in text.

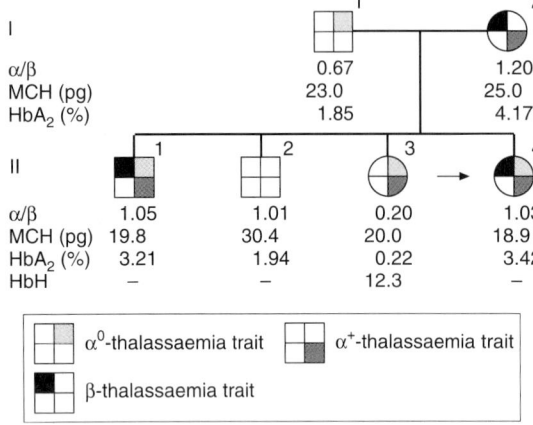

Fig. 13.2 The presumed interaction of α^0 and α^+ thalassaemia with β thalassaemia. Individual II3 has typical HbH disease. Individuals II1 and II4 were originally thought to have both α^0- and β-thalassaemia traits. From what is now known about these interactions it seems more likely that, as shown, they had α^0- and α^+-thalassaemia traits (HbH disease) together with β-thalassaemia trait. Modified from Knox-Macauley *et al.* (1972).

have important implications for population screening, as described in more detail in Chapters 7 and 14. They have never been adequately explained. Kanavakis *et al.* (1982) pointed out that the red cells in β-thalassaemia heterozygotes, with α-/β-globin synthesis ratios of approximately 2/1, are typically hypochromic and microcytic. At the other end of the spectrum, that is, the co-inheritance of β-thalassaemia trait with the genotype of HbH disease, in which three α-globin genes are lost, the red cells are equally or even more hypochromic and microcytic and the α-/β-globin synthesis ratio is almost exactly reversed, i.e. in the region of 0.5. As the globin synthesis ratio approaches unity, with less imbalance if there are two, rather than one, α genes deleted, the red cells become increasingly well haemoglobinized; they are hypochromic in the presence of imbalanced globin production, whether it reflects excess α- or β-chain production. The relative level of HbA$_2$ remains the same, regardless of whether there is balanced or imbalanced globin production although, in absolute terms, the amount of δ chain produced in the hypochromic red cells is smaller.

It is usually assumed that, in heterozygotes, the compensatory increase in β-chain production from the β locus in *trans* to the β-thalassaemia locus is mediated at the transcriptional or translational

levels, although there is no evidence that this is the case. Since these remarkable changes in haemoglobinization of the red cells are observed in β^0-thalassaemia heterozygotes who are also heterozygous for the deletional forms of α^+ thalassaemia, it appears that there is a major increase in β- (and α-) globin production from the normal loci. It follows therefore that when there is unbalanced globin synthesis the normal α- and β-globin-gene loci do not achieve their full capacity for compensating for the defective output of their partners. While this could be mediated at the translational or transcriptional levels, it is also possible that it simply reflects the effect of globin excess on the cell-cycling properties of the erythroid progenitors and hence on the number of terminal divisions that they undergo. Unfortunately, we know nothing about the factors which set the final level of haemoglobin in the red cell; as pointed out by Stohlman (1964) it is not clear whether it is the concentration of haemoglobin that determines the number of terminal cell divisions, or vice versa. It is disappointing that we still have not been able to translate these simple observations about the interactions of the α and β thalassaemias into a better understanding of this fundamental step in erythropoiesis.

Our lack of understanding of the mechanisms involved notwithstanding, the definition of the effects of these interactions on the red-cell indices has extremely important implications for the elucidation of the cause of thalassaemia intermedia, for attempting to determine the prognosis for different forms of thalassaemia in individual families, and for population screening (see Chapters 7 and 14).

The co-inheritance of the homozygous or compound heterozygous state for severe β thalassaemia and different varieties of α thalassaemia

Following the work reviewed earlier, suggesting that inheritance of one or more α-thalassaemia alleles might reduce the severity of the homozygous or compound heterozygous β thalassaemia, a number of studies were carried out to analyse the α-globin genes of patients with thalassaemia intermedia. In five patients with moderately severe β thalassaemia intermedia due to the homozygous or compound heterozygous inheritance of β$^+$ thalassaemia, it was found that three were also heterozygous for α^+ thalassaemia of the deletion type ($-\alpha/\alpha\alpha$), while two appeared to be heterozygous for a non-deletion α^+-

thalassaemia allele (Weatherall *et al.* 1981b). These studies were followed by investigations of groups of patients with thalassaemia major or intermedia of Cypriot, Sardinian or Asian background in order to determine whether there was a significantly increased frequency of different forms of α thalassaemia in the group with disease of intermediate severity (Wainscoat *et al.* 1983a,b; Thein *et al.* 1988a; Galanello *et al.* 1989). The main conclusions were as follows: homozygotes for β^0 thalassaemia who co-inherit the loss of two α-globin genes, usually –α/–α, or a non-deletional form of α^+ thalassaemia involving the α2-globin genes, are more likely to have the clinical phenotype of thalassaemia intermedia than major. On the other hand, β^0-thalassaemia homozygotes who inherit a single α-globin-gene deletion usually have thalassaemia major, albeit with a slightly later clinical presentation. In the case of homozygous or compound heterozygous β^+ thalassaemia, the co-inheritance of the deletion of two α-globin genes is usually associated with a milder clinical phenotype, and this may sometimes be the case if only a single α-globin-gene deletion is inherited. The contrasting effects of the inheritance of a single α-globin-gene deletion with those resulting from the inheritance of a non-deletional α-thalassaemia allele are because the latter causes a greater overall reduction in α-chain production (see Chapters 4, 5 and 11).

Other studies (Antonarakis *et al.* 1988; Oggiano *et al.* 1988; Kulozik *et al.* 1993; Gringras *et al.* 1994; Camaschella & Cappellini 1995) confirmed and expanded these observations. However, the importance of the co-inheritance of α thalassaemia in generating β thalassaemia intermedia varies between different populations. For example, while the co-inheritance of deletional forms of α^+ thalassaemia seems to play a role in the generation of thalassaemia intermedia in Italian patients (Camaschella & Cappellini 1995), it rarely accounts for the mild forms of β thalassaemia in Israel (Rund *et al.* 1997). The latter finding, of course, reflects the relatively low frequency of α thalassaemia in this population.

Relatively few studies that have tried to analyse the role of the α-globin genotype in modifying β thalassaemia have defined the severity of the disease. Ho *et al.* (1998a), in an attempt to address this problem, divided their patients into three groups based on blood transfusion requirement. This approach, while relatively simple, begs the question regarding some of the most important complications of the disease, in particular retarded development, bone deformity,

and so on. However, using these criteria, and with a knowledge of the underlying β-globin-gene mutations, it is clear that there is considerable clinical heterogeneity, even within interactions with α thalassaemia and identical β-thalassaemia genotypes. For example, in patients who were compound heterozygotes, IVS1-6 T→C/IVS1-110 G→A, that is, for a mild and severe β^+-thalassaemia mutation, the co-inheritance of the heterozygous state for α^+ thalassaemia was associated with both mild and moderately severe phenotypes. The co-inheritance of this type of α thalassaemia with homozygosity for the IVS1-110 G→A mutation resulted in a severe form of thalassaemia intermedia. On the other hand, the effect of a single missing α gene on compound heterozygosity for IVS1-5 G→C and the frameshift mutation 8/9 +G, a severe β^+ and a β^0-thalassaemia mutation, resulted in an extremely mild phenotype.

What can be concluded from these limited studies? In the report of Galanello *et al.* (1989), at least as judged by the steady-state haemoglobin levels, the patients described as having β thalassaemia intermedia would, by the criteria used by Ho *et al.* (1998a), be classified as mild. Overall, therefore, there is a reasonable correlation between the inheritance of homozygous β^0 or severe β^+ thalassaemia together with homozygous α^+ thalassaemia and the mildness of the phenotype. On the other hand, the loss of a single α-globin gene has minimal phenotypic effect on homozygosity for β^0 thalassaemia, and an unpredictable effect on compound heterozygosity for β^+ or β^0 or homozygosity for β^+ thalassaemia. As more is learnt about the latter interactions, and about the subtle differences in severity of the β^+ thalassaemias (Kulozik *et al.* 1993), it may be possible to be more precise about the prediction of these clinical phenotypes. It is equally clear that, because of its relative infrequency in many populations, α thalassaemia plays only a modest role in the generation of the intermediate forms of thalassaemia.

Homozygous β^+ or β^0 thalassaemia associated with compound heterozygosity for α^+ and α^0 thalassaemia

There have been a few reports of the occurrence of homozygous β thalassaemia with the genotype of HbH disease in the same individual (Loukopoulos *et al.* 1978; Furbetta *et al.* 1979). We have also studied a family in which three Greek Cypriot siblings are affected in this way.

In the Greek Cypriot patient described by Loukopoulos *et al.* (1978) the combination produced the phenotype of a moderately severe form of β thalassaemia intermedia. Early in life the patient was pale with mild jaundice but had a normal body habitus; there were no bone deformities and sexual development was normal. There was a moderate degree of hepatosplenomegaly. The haemoglobin values ranged between 6 and 8 g/dl, though, curiously, later in life they tended to range between 9 and 10 g/dl. Haemoglobin analysis showed approximately 48% HbA, 40% HbF, 9.6% HbA$_2$ and 2% Hb Bart's; no HbH was demonstrated. The most extraordinary feature about this patient's blood picture was the gross degree of hypochromia and microcytosis, with MCH values in the 8–9 pg range and MCV values in the 41–48 fl range (Fig. 13.3). The α-/β-globin synthesis ratio was greater than unity. We have observed three siblings with almost identical clinical pictures, but with steady-state haemoglobin levels of 5–6 g/dl, despite which growth and development was normal. A splenectomy carried out between the ages of 20 and 30 years resulted in no improvement in the haemoglobin level and was followed by severe thromboembolic complications in two cases.

In the patient reported by Furbetta *et al.* (1979) excellent evidence was presented for the patient being homozygous for β^0 thalassaemia together with

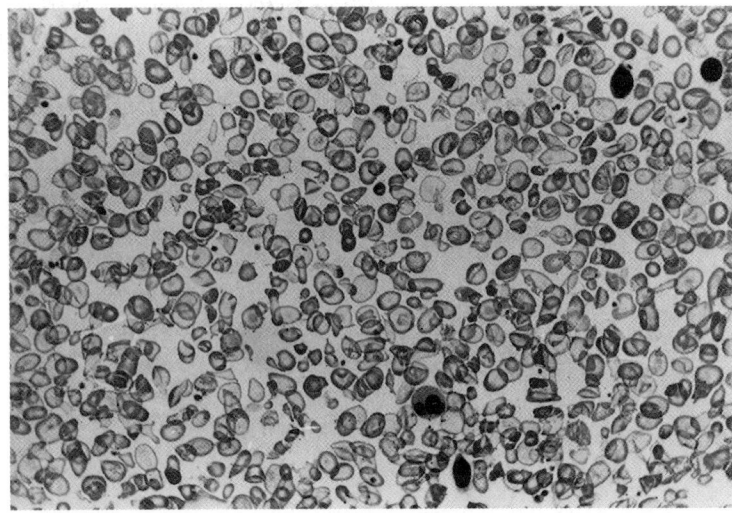

(a)

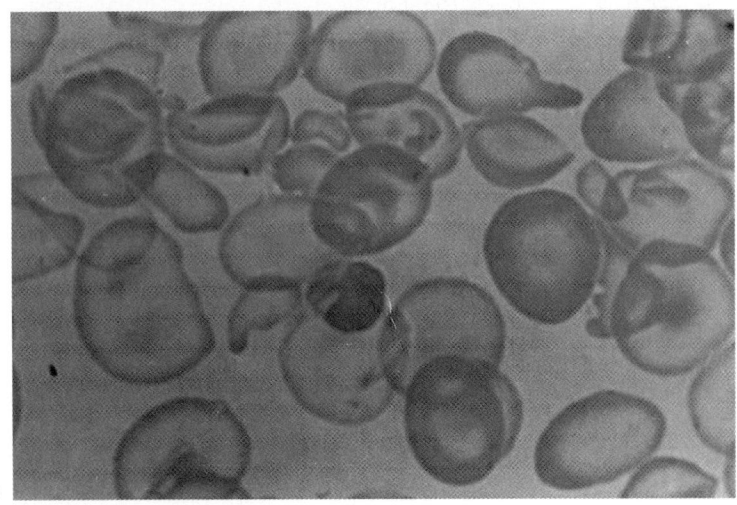

(b)

Fig. 13.3 Grossly hypochromic red cells in a patient homozygous for β thalassaemia who also has the genotype of haemoglobin H disease.

the genotype of HbH disease. At the age of 12 months this child was pale and somewhat growth retarded with splenomegaly and early thalassaemic bone changes. The haemoglobin level was 7.4 g/dl, again with remarkably hypochromic and microcytic red cells. The haemoglobin pattern consisted of Hbs F and A_2, with no HbA; HbA_2 made up 7.5% of the total.

The extremely high HbA_2 values in these patients are of interest. They seem to be a feature of other interactions between α and β thalassaemia. As pointed out in Chapter 5 there is remarkable heterogeneity in the peripheral blood of severe β thalassaemics with respect to the cellular distribution of Hbs F, A and A_2; the HbF-rich population has a low level of HbA_2, and vice versa. It is possible that the unusually high levels of HbA_2 in these particular cases reflect the survival of red-cell populations with relatively high levels of δ-chain production, which do not normally reach the peripheral blood in homozygous β thalassaemia.

The interactions between the α thalassaemias and HbE are described in Chapter 9.

Pathophysiology of the α/β thalassaemias

Although some of the more extreme examples of the interaction of α and β thalassaemia are rare, they represent unique experiments of nature which have told us a great deal about the pathophysiology of thalassaemia in general. In particular, they underline the central importance of globin imbalance in determining the severity of a thalassaemic illness. This principle is illustrated most beautifully in some of these families. For instance, in the study of Knox-Macaulay *et al.* (1972) it was shown that a sibling with HbH disease and two others who were almost certainly heterozygous for $α^0$, $α^+$ and $β^+$ thalassaemia had similar degrees of anaemia and morphological changes of their red cells and, even more interestingly, almost identical abnormalities of membrane function as evidenced by the relative rates of potassium leak. On the other hand, they showed completely different red-cell survival times. Those with relatively balanced globin synthesis had normal red-cell survival while the sibling with HbH disease, and hence unbalanced globin synthesis, had a markedly shortened red-cell survival. Clearly, at least in this family, the functional abnormalities of the membranes of the red cells were of secondary importance

and what determined their survival was globin imbalance and the formation of HbH (Fig. 13.2).

Similarly, the remarkable patient described by Loukopoulos *et al.* (1978), who was homozygous for β thalassaemia together with the genotype of HbH disease, while having grossly hypochromic red cells associated with a severe degree of potassium leakage, had almost normal red-cell survival; iron kinetic studies suggested only a very mild degree of ineffective erythropoiesis. The latter was mirrored by the presence of a myeloid/erythroid ratio in the bone marrow of 0.55, very similar to that observed in the β-thalassaemia trait and much higher than the ratios, in the 0.1 range, which are found in β thalassaemia intermedia. And, as pointed out by Loukopoulos and colleagues, the association of one α-thalassaemia gene with two β-thalassaemia genes seems to be much less effective in altering the overall picture of homozygous β thalassaemia than the addition of one β-thalassaemia gene to the genetic background of HbH disease. This observation is in keeping with the findings that excess α chains are probably more injurious to erythroid precursors and their progeny than excess β chains (see Chapter 5).

The role of haemoglobin F in generating thalassaemia intermedia

In previous editions of this book we discussed the notion that variation in the ability to produce HbF in the postnatal period might be a major factor in the generation of the phenotype of β thalassaemia intermedia. While many threads of evidence pointed in this direction, perhaps the most convincing were reports of patients apparently homozygous for $β^0$ thalassaemia with the clinical course of β thalassaemia intermedia. This picture was observed in many ethnic groups, including Britons (Knox-Macaulay *et al.* 1973), Algerians (Godet *et al.* 1977), Italians (Bianco *et al.* 1977), Arabs (Cividalli *et al.* 1978; Weatherall *et al.* 1981b) and Indians and Pakistanis (Weatherall *et al.* 1981b). In many of these reports the parents of the patients both had elevated HbA_2 levels, though in many cases globin synthesis data were not given and therefore it was not possible to exclude the co-existence of an α-thalassaemia determinant. However, in a few families studied in detail, the α-/β-globin synthesis ratios in the parents of patients of this type were typical of heterozygous β thalassaemia and therefore the co-existence of an α-thalassaemia gene seemed unlikely (Weatherall *et al.* 1981b). Furthermore, although in some of these families, or in others with mild forms of β⁺ thalassaemia intermedia, a determinant for heterocellular hereditary persistence of fetal haemoglobin (HPFH) appeared to be segregating (Knox-Macaulay *et al.* 1973; Cappellini *et al.* 1981; Weatherall *et al.* 1981b), this was not always the case; detailed studies of the fetal haemoglobin of parents or relatives did not always evidence for a second determinant of this type (Weatherall *et al.* 1981b).

Once it became possible to examine the globin-gene clusters directly using DNA technology this problem could be explored in more detail. For example, it was feasible to ask whether the determinants for a greater ability to produce HbF lay within the β-gene cluster, or whether they were outside the cluster or even on other chromosomes. The identification of RFLP haplotypes provided valuable markers across the cluster; if increased facility for producing HbF segregated with a particular haplotype the determinant must lie within the β-globin-gene complex. In addition, questions could be asked about the relationship of particular β-thalassaemia or related mutations to the production of HbF. A wide variety of studies of this kind, combined with structural analyses of the $^{G}\gamma/^{A}\gamma$-chain composition of HbF, have provided some valuable information about the mechanisms that set the level of fetal haemoglobin synthesis in β thalassaemia and have gone some way to accounting for different forms of β thalassaemia intermedia. However, as we shall see, many questions remain unanswered. We have already considered some of these issues in Chapters 5 and 10. Here, we shall summarize the evidence that links increased fetal haemoglobin production to thalassaemia intermedia.

Determinants within the β-globin-gene cluster

In Chapter 10 we reviewed the evidence that varying ability to produce HbF in sickle-cell anaemia is related to particular RFLP haplotypes of the β-globin-gene cluster. At about the same time as this work was being carried out evidence was obtained that the same relationship exists with respect to HbF synthesis in β thalassaemia (Labie *et al.* 1985b; Thein *et al.* 1987b). Some of the data from the extensive studies of Thein *et al.* are summarized in Table 13.6. These focused on the 5′ β haplotype, generated by the following enzymes (using + or – to indicate the presence or absence of a restriction-enzyme cleavage site), in the order 5′ to 3′, as follows: *Hind* II ε, *Hind* III $^{G}\gamma$, *Hind* III $^{A}\gamma$, *Hind* II ψβ, and *Hind* II 3′ ψβ. When large groups of patients with thalassaemia major or thalassaemia intermedia of Asian Indian or Italian backgrounds were compared, it was found that one particular haplotype, –+–++, had a strong association with β thalassaemia intermedia. For example, in the Asian group 14 out of 28 β-globin chromosomes from thalassaemia intermedia patients had this haplotype while it was found in only 10 out of 84 chromosomes from the thalassaemia major groups. The majority of those who were homozygous for this haplotype had a relatively mild clinical course, and in patients with thalassaemia major with this haplotype there was a significant tendency for a late presentation. Furthermore, there was a reasonable relationship between heterozygosity and homozygosity for this haplotype and the absolute level of HbF. But, although there was a trend, the

5′ β haplotype	β thalassaemia major	β thalassaemia intermedia
+––––	52 (61.9%)	10 (35.7%)
+–––– (β⁰ del type)	21 (25.0%)	1 (3.1%)
–+–++	10 (11.4%)	14 (50.0%)
–++–+	1 (12.%)	0 (0%)
++–++	0 (0%)	1 (3.6%)
–+––+	0 (0%)	1 (3.6%)
+––––	0 (0%)	1 (3.6%)
Total	84	28

Table 13.6 Distribution of β-globin haplotypes of Asian patients with homozygous β thalassaemia. (From Thein *et al.* 1987b)

5′ β haplotype: (+) indicates the presence of a restriction enzyme cleavage site and (–) its absence. The order of the sites 5′ to 3′ is as follows: *Hind* II ε, *Hind* III $^{G}\gamma$, *Hind* III $^{A}\gamma$, *Hind* II ψβ and *Hind* II 3′ ψβ.

relationship between the haplotype and HbF levels in heterozygotes was not statistically significant. Similar data were obtained for the Italian populations studied, although because the frequency of this haplotype was much lower the results were less impressive.

A further series of studies showed that this subhaplotype is in linkage disequilibrium with the C→T polymorphism at position –158 in the $^G\gamma$-globin gene, i.e. *Xmn* I(+). This change had been previously associated with increased expression of the $^G\gamma$ gene in patients with sickle-cell anaemia or β thalassaemia of diverse origins (Gilman & Huisman 1985; Harano *et al.* 1985; Labie *et al.* 1985b). Taken together, these studies suggested that homozygosity or heterozygosity for the $^G\gamma$ *Xmn* I(+) polymorphism might play an important role in underlying the milder forms of homozygous β⁰ thalassaemia in Afro-Asian populations, though less in Italians. Later studies in Sardinia gave essentially similar findings (Galanello *et al.* 1989). Out of 61 patients homozygous for β⁰ thalassaemia who were also homozygous or heterozygous for the Mediterranean haplotype IX, which contains the –+–++ 5′ subhaplotype, 56 showed the phenotype of thalassaemia intermedia, while only five manifested thalassaemia major. Interestingly, in this population this haplotype is linked to a particular β⁰-thalassaemia allele, namely the frameshift (–1 bp) at codon 6 (Galanello *et al.* 1989). It appears therefore that the homozygous state for the $^G\gamma$ *Xmn* I(+) site may be sufficient to ameliorate the clinical picture of homozygous β thalassaemia, regardless of the type of β-thalassaemia mutation, that is, β⁰ or β⁺. Further experience suggests that heterozygosity for this site has a more limited effect, restricted to β⁺ rather than β⁰ thalassaemia.

These conclusions were validated in later comparisons of patients with thalassaemia major and intermedia (Camaschella *et al.* 1995; Ho *et al.* 1998a). In the study of Ho *et al.* (1998a) it was clear that there is a strong association of the $^G\gamma$ *Xmn* I(+) polymorphism with the β⁰-thalassaemia IVS1-1 G→T mutation in Asian Indians. Overall, homozygotes for this mutation have a slightly milder disease than other forms of β⁰ thalassaemia. This is manifest by a later onset of transfusion requirements, though many of them subsequently become transfusion dependent in later life. Of the seven patients homozygous for this mutation who had the clinical phenotype of thalassaemia intermedia, two fell into the mild category,

two into the moderately affected, and three into the severe category. In the 16 patients in this study with thalassaemia intermedia who were homozygous for β⁰ thalassaemia due to a number of different alleles, nine had mild disease, seven of whom were $^G\gamma$ *Xmn* I(+) homozygotes, compared with four of seven patients in the severe group. As discussed in Chapter 10, although there is no direct evidence, it is believed that the *Xmn* I(+) polymorphism in the promoter region of the $^G\gamma$ gene is associated with an increased capacity for fetal haemoglobin production in conditions of erythroid 'stress'. It is clear from these limited data that homozygosity for this polymorphism may sometimes be associated with a milder clinical course in homozygous or compound heterozygous β thalassaemia.

These observations leave many questions unanswered. It is not absolutely certain that these haplotype associations reflect the action of the $^G\gamma$ *Xmn* I polymorphism; they could be marking another region in the β-globin-gene cluster that is related to an increased propensity for fetal haemoglobin production. Furthermore, it is not clear why there is such phenotypic heterogeneity among patients who carry this polymorphism. As discussed in Chapter 10, it is clear that different chromosomes which carry the *Xmn* I site change are associated with widely differing levels of fetal haemoglobin production in patients with sickle-cell anaemia. As also described in Chapter 10 a great deal of work has gone into trying to define other polymorphisms or other structural changes in the β-globin-gene cluster that may be associated with increased fetal haemoglobin synthesis, either in the steady state or related to stress (Labie & Elion 1996; Steinberg 1996). So far no other candidates have been found. Thus apart from the deletional and non-deletional forms of HPFH, and occasional cases of γ-globin-gene triplications or quadruplication (Yang *et al.* 1986), there is currently no definite evidence for regions other than $^G\gamma$ –158 C→T (*Xmn* I polymorphism) that play a major role in elevating γ-chain synthesis in β thalassaemia intermedia.

β-Thalassaemia mutations and haemoglobin F production

Overall, there are very few β-thalassaemia mutations which, by themselves, seem to play a role in elevating the HbF level to a sufficient degree to produce a milder phenotype. This appears to occur in the case of the rare forms due to partial or complete deletions of the β-globin gene and may be of relevance in the particular mild phenotypes associated with point mutations involving the β-globin-gene promoters.

Deletional forms of β thalassaemia

At least 17 different β-thalassaemia alleles have been described which are characterized by a partial or complete deletion of the β-globin gene (see Chapter 4). These do not include the longer deletions of the β-globin-gene cluster that give rise to εγδβ thalassaemia, but are simply those which are restricted to the β-globin gene itself. Particularly if they involve the β-globin-gene promoter region, they tend to be associated with unusually high levels of HbA$_2$ and significantly increased levels of HbF in heterozygotes (Thein 1993; Huisman *et al.* 1997). As described in Chapter 10, it is thought that the absence of the β-globin-gene promoters causes upregulation of the δ and γ genes through freeing particular DNA binding proteins which may be present in rate-limiting quantities.

The only common deletional form of β thalassaemia is that associated with the loss of 619 bp at the 3′ end of the β-globin gene, which occurs frequently in northern India. This is a severe, transfusion-dependent disorder. This may well be because it spares the β-globin-gene promoters. On the other hand, the so-called Dutch deletion, which removes the entire β-globin gene and part of the region between the β and δ genes, has a completely different homozygous phenotype (Schokker *et al.* 1966; Gilman *et al.* 1984). In the family described by Schokker *et al.* two homozygotes were asymptomatic except for occasional bouts of jaundice. They had marked radiological abnormalities of the skeleton, however. Their haemoglobin levels were 12.1 and 14.3 g/dl, respectively, and the morphological changes of their red cells were typical of thalassaemia intermedia. Haemoglobin analysis revealed only Hbs F and A$_2$, with no HbA. The heterozygotes in this family had HbA$_2$ values ranging between 5 and 7% and all had HbF values in the 6–10% range. A similar mildly affected homozygote, of Indian extraction, was reported by Craig *et al.* (1992). In this case the underlying deletion was slightly shorter, 10 329 bp, but it had a similar 5′ extension into the region between the δ- and β-globin genes to the Dutch deletion. Again, the homozygote

had a mild form of β thalassaemia intermedia with a steady-state haemoglobin level of 8.8 g/dl; the haemoglobin consisted of 98% HbF and 2.0% HbA$_2$. All the heterozygotes in this family had HbF levels in the 3–5% range and unusually high levels of HbA$_2$.

Clearly, at least some of these deletional forms of β thalassaemia are associated with an extremely mild phenotype in their homozygous states. Whether this reflects the removal of the β promoters, or whether there are other important regulatory regions for γ-chain production in the region between the δ- and β-globin genes, a question which we discussed in relationship to Hb Lepore in Chapter 8, remains to be seen.

Point mutations of the β-globin gene

There is indirect evidence that certain point mutations that underlie β thalassaemia may also be involved in producing an unusually effective fetal haemoglobin response. As pointed out in Chapter 5, one of the main mechanisms for the elevation of fetal haemoglobin in β thalassaemia is cell selection. It follows therefore that this should be greater in those forms that are associated with the most severe globin imbalance; in the milder forms of β thalassaemia, with relatively high levels of β-chain production, there should be much less selection of red-cell precursors that synthesize γ chains and therefore lower levels of HbF. This expectation is well illustrated in the mild form of β thalassaemia due to the IVS1-6 T→C mutation, in which homozygotes have thalassaemia intermedia with levels of HbF in the 10–20% range. On the other hand, as mentioned earlier in this chapter, and as discussed in Chapter 10, the promoter mutations of the β-globin genes, which, in the homozygous state, are also associated with very mild forms of thalassaemia intermedia, are characterized by much higher levels of HbF production. This is usually reflected as 50% or more of HbF, and since the steady-state haemoglobin value is 2–3 g/dl higher than homozygotes for the IVS1-6 mutation, it is clear that the absolute amount of HbF produced is remarkably high, despite the mildness of these β-thalassaemia mutations.

In previous editions of this book, in which we analysed in detail all the homozygous and compound heterozygous states for β thalassaemia in Afro-American populations, we were puzzled by the remarkably high levels of fetal haemoglobin in such mild forms of the disease. This did not seem to be a population-specific characteristic since the same responses were not observed in sickle-cell anaemia. The answer is now clear; nearly all these cases were undoubtedly homozygotes or compound heterozygotes for promoter mutations. It appears therefore that, even in the presence of a very mild β-thalassaemia allele, if it also tends to increase the likelihood of γ-chain production, possibly in this case because of the involvement of the β-globin-gene promoter, the final level of HbF production may be quite high, despite only a moderate degree of globin imbalance. However, the pathophysiology of these consistent findings is still not entirely clear.

One of the problems in determining the reasons for the extremely high levels of HbF in association with mild homozygous or compound heterozygous β thalassaemia in patients of African origin is that, in many instances, the mutation occurs on a chromosome with the $^G\gamma$ *Xmn* I(+) polymorphism which, as we have seen, appears to carry the propensity for increased fetal haemoglobin production. In the study of Gonzalez-Redondo *et al.* (1988a) one of their patients who was homozygous for the β –88 C→T promoter mutation was also homozygous for a haplotype which does not have the $^G\gamma$ *Xmn* I(+) polymorphism, yet this 23-year-old male still had a steady-state haemoglobin of 11.0 g/dl, with 56.6% fetal haemoglobin. Three of the patients with the lowest fetal haemoglobin values in this study were also heterozygous for the deletional form of α thalassaemia, which may also modify the level of HbF. The homozygous state for the –87 C→G form of β⁺ thalassaemia, reported by Camaschella *et al.* (1990a), found in a 62-year-old transfusion-independent patient with mild thalassaemia intermedia, was associated with a steady-state haemoglobin level of 9.4 g/dl and 65% fetal haemoglobin. In this case the patient was found to be homozygous for a β-globin-cluster RFLP haplotype that does not have the $^G\gamma$ *Xmn* I(+) polymorphism, and hence the authors suggest that the extremely high level of fetal haemoglobin production is more likely to be related to the β-globin-gene promoter mutation.

Taken altogether, and considering that heterozygotes for the promoter gene mutations tend to have a slightly higher level of fetal haemoglobin than those for other forms of β thalassaemia, these observations suggest that at least part of the unusual elevation of fetal haemoglobin in these mild forms of β thalassaemia is related to the underlying β-thalassaemia mutation.

Homozygous or compound heterozygous β thalassaemia with heterocellular HPFH

As mentioned in Chapter 10, there is very good genetic evidence that certain forms of heterocellular HPFH can interact with β thalassaemia or the sickle-cell gene to raise the level of HbF above that usually seen in the traits for these conditions. There have been relatively few opportunities to study the interaction of these determinants with the homozygous or compound heterozygous states for β thalassaemia, but such evidence that exists suggests that they may have the capacity to considerably ameliorate these conditions. It should be remembered, however, that until the molecular basis for these forms of heterocellular HPFH is determined these interactions have to be assumed, based on a careful family study. The key features are a milder phenotype of what is usually a severe form of β thalassaemia together with higher than usual levels of HbF in the parents and the observation that one or more of the unaffected relatives also have significant elevations of HbF. There have only been a few reports of patients and families which meet these criteria.

In the family reported by Cappellini *et al.* (1981) the proband was a 52-year-old male who had never had symptoms ascribable to thalassaemia except for slight jaundice during intercurrent infections. Radiological examination of his bones was normal. His haemoglobin level ranged between 11.6 and 12.4 g/dl and he had typical thalassaemic red-cell changes. Haemoglobin analysis showed 97.2% HbF, the remainder being HbA₂. Among his children, grandchildren and lateral relatives there were β-thalassaemia heterozygotes with unusually high HbF levels and otherwise normal individuals with elevated levels of HbF in the 1–2% range. A subsequent genetic analysis of an extended pedigree indicated that this determinant for HPFH is not linked to the β-globin-gene cluster (Gianni *et al.* 1983). It appears therefore that in this family a β⁰-thalassaemia homozygote almost certainly inherited at least one genetic determinant for heterocellular HPFH and hence presented with the phenotype of an extremely mild β thalassaemia intermedia.

In the family reported by Thein and Weatherall (1989) the propositus was a 33-year-old Asian Indian male who presented at the age of 18 years with mild anaemia and jaundice. For reasons which are not absolutely clear he underwent splenectomy, after which his steady-state haemoglobin level was 12.1 g/dl with a typical thalassaemic blood picture. Globin synthesis analysis showed no β-chain production and an α-/γ-chain synthesis ratio of 2.86. Studies of several generations of this large family revealed heterozygotes with unusually high levels of HbF in some cases, together with otherwise normal individuals with raised levels of HbF. Later genetic analyses of an extended family pedigree showed that the determinant for elevated HbF is not linked to the β-gene cluster or the X chromosome but that it is on chromosome 6 (Craig *et al.* 1996) (for further discussion of this family see Chapter 10).

Another approach to this problem was reported by Ho *et al.* (1998a). As part of a large study of the molecular basis of thalassaemia intermedia eight sibling pairs were identified with this condition. Unexpectedly, there was considerable difference in the severity of the disease between siblings in seven pairs, despite the fact that these patients had identical β-thalassaemia mutations and, except for one family, intact α-globin genes. The major difference between them, and the only finding that could account for the varying severity of their disease, was the steady-state HbF level, the differences between siblings ranging from 1 g/dl to as much as 8–9 g/dl. In three of the seven families it was possible to identify a heterocellular HPFH determinant. In this study, in addition to these seven sibships, co-inheritance of an HPFH determinant was implicated in a further six patients, five homozygous for β^0 thalassaemia and one for a severe form of β^+ thalassaemia. Despite the absence or severe deficit of β chains, these patients were only mildly affected, and able to maintain haemoglobin levels, almost all of which was fetal in type, of 9–13 g/dl. In all these patients other factors such as the upstream polymorphisms of the $^G\gamma$-globin gene were excluded as a cause of the unusually high level of HbF.

If, as appears from many of these pedigrees, a single dose of a gene for heterocellular HPFH can have this remarkable ameliorating effect on severe β thalassaemia it is difficult to understand how this is achieved. In the heterozygous state, either alone or together with β thalassaemia, the augmentation of fetal haemoglobin production is extremely small. Yet when it interacts in severely affected homozygotes or compound heterozygotes the determinant appears to have the effect of raising the fetal haemoglobin by several g/dl. Although there is enough evidence to point to these interactions being an important cause of thalassaemia intermedia, an understanding of how the increased HbF production is mediated will have to await the isolation of the genes involved.

Heterozygous β thalassaemia with the phenotype of thalassaemia intermedia

There are two main mechanisms whereby heterozygous β thalassaemia can be associated with the phenotype of β thalassaemia intermedia (Table 13.1). First, there are cases in which β thalassaemia is complicated by the inheritance of chromosomes carrying more than the usual number of α-globin genes. Second, there are particular β-globin-gene mutations which, because they produce products with unusual properties, give rise to severe phenotypes in heterozygotes. The latter are now called the dominant β thalassaemias.

Heterozygous β thalassaemia with increased numbers of α-globin genes

In earlier chapters we described how unequal crossing over between the linked α-globin genes on chromosome 16 may generate chromosomes with single or triplicated α-globin genes. The triplicated arrangement is found in most populations, indicating that this type of event is relatively common. There have been a few frequency studies. In most cases it occurs at no higher than about 1% of the population; however, we have recently observed the ααα arrangements in just over 3% of the Sri Lankan population. Both triplicated and quadruplicated α-globin-gene arrangements seem to have very little effect in otherwise normal individuals but, when inherited with a single β-thalassaemia allele, there appears to be sufficient globin imbalance to produce a family of β thalassaemias, all of which are more severe than the heterozygous state for β thalassaemia alone.

Heterozygous β thalassaemia with ααα/αα

There are extensive published data on the phenotypic consequences of this interaction (Galanello *et al.* 1983c; Kanavakis *et al.* 1983; Sampietro *et al.* 1983; Kulozik *et al.* 1987b; Camaschella *et al.* 1987a, 1995; Bianco *et al.* 1997c; Rund *et al.* 1997; Ho *et al.* 1998a). It results in a variable phenotype. At one end of the spectrum it is little different from the β-thalassaemia trait alone, although the HbF values tend to be slightly higher. On the other hand, some individuals have a picture of mild thalassaemia intermedia with haemoglobin values ranging from 8 to 10 g/dl and splenomegaly from 2 to 5 cm below the costal margin. In some cases this has necessitated splenectomy. This broad clinical spectrum is well exemplified in the 31 cases reported in detail by Bianco *et al.* (1997c). Eight would have been classified as having the β-thalassaemia trait, 16 a very mild form of β thalassaemia intermedia, and seven a more severe form of the latter, requiring splenectomy. In this study the associated β-thalassaemia alleles were characterized and there was no obvious association with the phenotype although in most cases they were β^0-thalassaemia mutations. The reasons for this clinical diversity are not clear.

Homozygous β thalassaemia with ααα/αα

In the study of Kanavakis *et al.* (1983) there were five β-thalassaemia homozygotes in the family studies which involved triplicated α-globin-gene arrangements. In four out of five of these patients the phenotype was that of an unexpectedly mild form of β thalassaemia intermedia. While this result has to be interpreted with caution, particularly since these families were ascertained during a study of patients with thalassaemia intermedia, there were no other factors found in these families which would ameliorate the severity of β thalassaemia. The authors speculate that there may be some forms of triplicated α-globin genes in which one or more of the genes are non-functional and hence are associated with a phenotype of non-deletional α thalassaemia. A triplicated α-gene arrangement behaving as an α-thalassaemia allele was encountered in Saudi Arabia by Pressley (1980), who described a family in which a mother and two offspring with ααα/αα had HbH disease. In this population this condition usually results from homozygosity for a non-deletional form of α thalassaemia and it appears that the triplicated α-gene haplotype in this family behaves identically to the ($\alpha\alpha^T$) haplotype. It is possible therefore that there is heterogeneity of the expression of the tripli-

cated α-globin-gene arrangement and, in some cases, it could behave as an α-thalassaemia allele.

A word of caution is necessary, however. To our knowledge there have been no further reports of triplicated α-globin-gene arrangements behaving as α-thalassaemia alleles and these studies were carried out before it was possible to sequence the α- or β-globin genes. Furthermore, they were based on a study of thalassaemia intermedia so the population sample would have been biased. Clearly, further information about this intriguing possibility is required.

Heterozygous β thalassaemia with ααα/ααα

The homozygous state for the triplicated α-globin-gene arrangement in association with heterozygous β thalassaemia has been observed mainly in Mediterranean populations (Galanello *et al.* 1983c; Thein *et al.* 1984a; Oron *et al.* 1994; Traeger-Synodinos *et al.* 1996; Bianco *et al.* 1997c; Ho *et al.* 1998a). Most of these patients have been heterozygous for β^0- or severe β^+-thalassaemia mutations. In all cases the clinical picture has been a moderate to severe form of thalassaemia intermedia, with haemoglobin values in the 6–9 g/dl range, moderate splenomegaly and, in some cases, bone changes and growth retardation. Interestingly, despite these relatively severe phenotypes, and presumably a marked degree of globin imbalance, high levels of HbF seem to be unusual; in most series they have ranged between 2 and 10%.

Heterozygous β thalassaemia associated with αααα/αα

As might be expected, the inheritance of six α-globin genes together with heterozygous β thalassaemia has much the same phenotype whether it is the homozygous inheritance of the triplicated α-globin gene or the compound heterozygous inheritance of the quadruplicated and normal α-globin-gene complement (Thompson *et al.* 1989). This genotype is associated with the phenotype of a mild to moderate form of thalassaemia intermedia, with haemoglobin values in the 7–9 g/dl range and splenomegaly of 3–4 cm (Beris *et al.* 1999). Surprisingly, in one of the patients reported by Bianco *et al.* (1997c), the spleen was said not to be palpable despite a steady-state haemoglobin value of 7.5 g/dl.

Dominant β thalassaemia associated with αααα/αα

In the one reported case of this interaction (Thein *et al.* 1990a) the patient had a severe form of thalassaemia intermedia and became transfusion dependent in adult life. Presumably this reflects the more severe effect of the particular β-thalassaemia allele (see next section) together with the unusual degree of imbalanced globin synthesis.

Dominant forms of β thalassaemia

Early reports

In 1973 an unusual form of β thalassaemia was identified in an Irish family, several members of which had moderate anaemia, intermittent jaundice, splenomegaly, marked thalassaemic changes of their red cells and intense erythroid hyperplasia together with morphological abnormalities of the red-cell precursors in the bone marrow (Weatherall *et al.* 1973). Many of the latter, and the nucleated red cells in the peripheral blood of two family members who had been splenectomized, showed inclusion bodies similar to those seen in the severe forms of β thalassaemia. The disorder was transmitted in an autosomal dominant fashion. Similar clinical features associated with inclusions in the normoblasts and peripheral red cells after splenectomy were observed in a Swiss French family by Stamatoyannopoulos *et al.* (1974), who proposed the term 'inclusion body β thalassaemia' for this condition. However, since inclusions of this type are a well recognized feature of all the more severe forms of β thalassaemia, it became customary to call it 'dominant β thalassaemia'.

As more families were described, and methods became available for studying its molecular pathology, some interesting insights were obtained into how what is usually a recessively inherited disorder can change to a dominant one. Using β-globin RFLP linkage analysis it was found that these disorders segregate with the β-globin gene, suggesting that they are due to mutations at or near this locus (Thein *et al.* 1990a). Subsequently, sequence analyses of the β-globin genes demonstrated that, while they are quite heterogeneous at the molecular level, many of them seem to involve mutations of exon 3 of the β-globin gene. These include frameshifts, premature chain termination (nonsense) mutations and complex

rearrangements which lead to the synthesis of truncated or elongated and highly unstable β-globin-gene products (Beris *et al.* 1988; Fei *et al.* 1989b; Kazazian *et al.* 1989; Thein *et al.* 1990a; Kazazian *et al.* 1992). The different mutations that underlie the dominant β thalassaemias are described in detail in Chapter 4.

Mechanism of the dominant β-thalassaemia phenotype

By comparing the lengths of the abnormal gene products due to nonsense or frameshift mutations in the β-globin gene it has been possible to develop a hypothesis to explain why most heterozygous forms of β thalassaemia are mild, while those due to mutations involving predominantly exon 3 are more severe (Thein *et al.* 1990a) (discussed in detail in Chapter 4). Nonsense or frameshift mutations that would produce truncated β chains up to about 72 residues in length are usually associated with a mild phenotype in heterozygotes. It is now believed, however, that the mRNAs associated with these mutations are not transported to the cytoplasm, and hence no gene product is made. On the other hand mRNAs with mutations in exon 3 are transported and translated normally. They produce long, unstable products; it is likely that the associated phenotypes reflect their haem-binding properties and instability. Those with only 72 residues or less cannot bind haem whereas those truncated to residue 120 or longer should bind haem since only helix H of the β chain is missing. Furthermore, such haem-containing products should have some secondary structure and hence be less susceptible to proteolytic degradation. The lack of helix H, which would expose one of the hydrophobic patches of helix G and those of helices E and F, would also lead to aggregation. It was suggested therefore that the large inclusions in the red-cell progenitors of these patients consists of aggregates of precipitated β-chain products, possibly together with excess α chains (Thein *et al.* 1990a), a prediction which was later confirmed (Ho *et al.* 1997).

These conditions, unlike the unstable haemoglobin disorders, in which intact haemoglobin molecules precipitate in the red cells during their lifespan and cause a haemolytic anaemia, are characterized by ineffective erythropoiesis due to the early precipitation of these unstable β-globin products together with α chains in the red-cell precursors. Although not studied formally, it seems likely that the mechanism

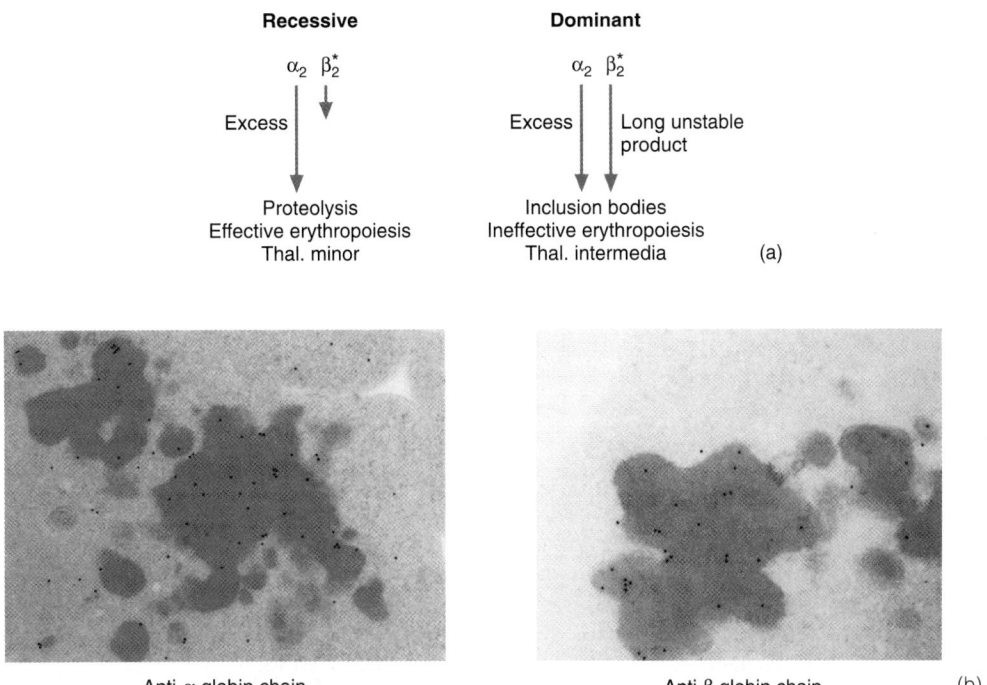

Fig. 13.4 A comparison of the molecular pathology of recessive and dominant β thalassaemia. (a) A schematic representation showing how the small excess of α chains does not cause severe ineffective erythropoiesis in the recessive forms of β-thalassaemia trait, whereas the production of long unstable products together with excess α chains results in the formation of inclusion bodies and ineffective erythropoiesis in the dominant forms. (b) Electron-microscopic appearances of inclusion bodies in dominant β thalassaemia labelled with anti-α- and anti-β-chain antibodies showing that, unlike the inclusions in the recessive forms of β thalassaemia (see Fig. 7.15, Chapter 7), the inclusions contain both α and β globin. *Indicates β thalassaemia mutation.

of destruction of red-cell precursors is broadly similar to those described in Chapter 5 for the α and β thalassaemias (Fig. 13.4).

Mechanisms underlying phenotypic diversity

Some of these disorders are very much milder than others and, at one end of the spectrum, they differ very little from the standard forms of heterozygous β thalassaemia. In fact there is a spectrum of heterozygous conditions due to defective β-globin-chain production. At one end, there are those which are associated with no β-globin synthesis, or a very low output of β chains. These conditions are associated with the usual picture of β-thalassaemia trait. Then there are the dominant β thalassaemias, in which highly unstable gene products have enough secondary structure to form dimers which may aggregate one with another, form inclusions and damage the red-cell precursors, causing ineffective erythropoiesis. Finally, at the other end of the spectrum, there are the unstable β-haemoglobin disorders in which viable tetramers are formed which survive their passage through the bone marrow and which only precipitate in the peripheral blood, and hence which result in a haemolytic anaemia.

One of the difficulties in relating genotypes to phenotypes in this family of diseases is the lack of good haematological data that accompany many of the reports of their molecular characterization. For example, in many cases said not to show red-cell inclusions the bone marrows were not examined and the patients had intact spleens; since inclusions are rarely seen in the peripheral blood in patients with β thalassaemia with intact spleens, and they can only be generated in the case of unstable haemoglobin disorders, without this information it is impossible to say whether there is early precipitation of globin.

However, allowing for difficulties of this kind, it is likely that the account of the pathophysiology of these conditions outlined above is an oversimplification of an extremely complex problem. For example, Hb Chesterfield (β28 Leu→Arg) appears to be associated with a mixed picture of ineffective erythropoiesis and haemolysis (Thein *et al.* 1991). This mutation is in exon 2. Other substitutions of β28, Leu→Pro in the case of Hb Geneva for example, give rise to the phenotype of a severe haemolytic anaemia with Heinz bodies in the erythrocytes, typical of an unstable haemoglobin disorder (Sansone *et al.* 1967). Similarly the substitution β28 Leu→Gln (Hb St Louis) also produces a haemolytic anaemia rather than a thalassaemic phenotype (Thillet *et al.* 1976). These two substitutions must result in the production of a partially viable tetramer. These observations make it particularly difficult to understand why Hb Chesterfield is associated with a dominant thalassaemic phenotype. Perhaps the abnormal β chains are so unstable that very few viable tetramers are made and hence they form aggregates with resultant damage to the red-cell precursors. These discrepancies underline the extreme subtlety of the behaviour of these abnormal β chains with respect to whether they are subject to immediate proteolysis, survive long enough to form aggregations on the red-cell membrane, or are able to produce a haemoglobin tetramer, albeit an unstable one.

Another curious feature of these conditions is that, although the degree of anaemia may be in the same range as that found with other forms of β thalassaemia intermedia, with only a few exceptions the level of HbF is rarely elevated above the 2–5% range. In most cases the HbA_2 level is elevated but this is also observed with unstable β-chain variants. Although where careful globin synthesis studies have been carried out there is usually imbalanced synthesis, with an excess of α chains and an expanded pool of free α chains (Weatherall *et al.* 1973), this is of a similar magnitude to that found in β-thalassaemia trait. These observations, together with the relatively low level of HbF, reflecting relative lack of preferential survival of precursors that synthesize more γ chain, may be a further indication that the primary pathophysiological defect in these conditions is not so much imbalanced globin synthesis as the deleterious effects of the early precipitation of abnormal β

globin with its resultant damage to the membranes of the red-cell precursors.

Genotype/phenotype relationships in thalassaemia intermedia

Given the remarkable number of different genetic interactions that can produce the clinical phenotype of β thalassaemia intermedia (Fig. 13.5) it is not surprising that this is an extremely heterogeneous condition. Unfortunately, there are no series of any one interaction of sufficient magnitude to determine how much of the clinical heterogeneity seen in this disorder is genetic in origin. In order to carry out a study of this kind it would be necessary to compare the clinical phenotypes of patients of similar ages, ideally who had or who had not been splenectomized and who could be observed in a steady state over a reasonably long period. It would also be essential for them to be folate replete and, as far as possible, to ensure that other acquired factors which might modify the phenotype were excluded.

The problem of distinguishing between genetic and acquired or environmental factors which may modify the phenotype of β thalassaemia, particularly in its intermediate forms, is one which is still relevant to the entire abnormal haemoglobin field and, for that matter, to all the monogenic diseases. Since there are virtually no twin or sibling pair studies we have very little information about the relative roles of nature and nurture in determining the phenotypes for any of the globin disorders. In this context, Ho *et al.* (1998a) described the findings in eight sibships with β thalassaemia intermedia. Obviously they had the same β-globin genotypes and in only one case was there a single-deletion form of α^+ thalassaemia. In fact there were considerable differences between their phenotypes. As mentioned earlier, the only factor which seemed to account for this discrepancy was the steady-state level of HbF, which could, in some but not all cases, be related to the co-existence of a gene for heterocellular HPFH. This wide clinical heterogeneity within this carefully controlled group of patients underlines the problems of trying to relate genotype to phenotype in thalassaemia intermedia and how it is only possible to provide an approximate prognostic picture of the likely clinical course for any particular genetic interaction.

It is against this background of extreme complexity

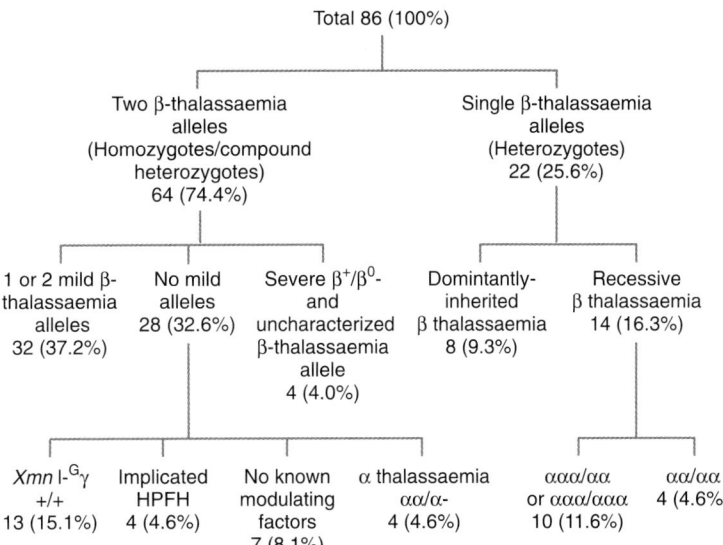

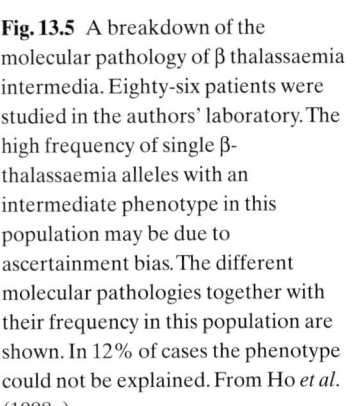

Fig. 13.5 A breakdown of the molecular pathology of β thalassaemia intermedia. Eighty-six patients were studied in the authors' laboratory. The high frequency of single β-thalassaemia alleles with an intermediate phenotype in this population may be due to ascertainment bias. The different molecular pathologies together with their frequency in this population are shown. In 12% of cases the phenotype could not be explained. From Ho *et al.* (1998a).

and lack of knowledge about many of the factors which can modify the phenotype that we have to discuss the clinical manifestations of its intermediate forms.

Clinical features

In this section we shall discuss the main clinical features of β thalassaemia intermedia. It would have been helpful to be able to describe these manifestations against the background of a clinical classification of the severity of this heterogeneous disorder. Unfortunately, however, this has not been possible, not least because, as mentioned earlier, the phenotype tends to change with age in many cases.

Ho *et al.* (1998a) attempted to grade the severity of the disease according to age at presentation, haemoglobin value at presentation and in the steady state, age of first transfusion and frequency of transfusion, presence of splenomegaly/hepatomegaly, bone changes and growth, and overall clinical status. In the event, it was only possible to evolve a simpler classification based on the steady-state haemoglobin level: 'mild', if a haemoglobin value of greater than 7.5 g/dl could be maintained without transfusion, the transfusion frequency was less than once every 2 years, or less than 6-monthly if transfusion was started after the age of 10 years; and 'severe', if transfusion requirements began at the age of 4 years or above with a frequency between 6 weeks and 4

months, or between 3 and 4 months if transfusion requirements commenced before the age of 4 years. Those with transfusion requirements between these extremes were classified as 'moderately' affected. A rather complex clinical classification of this type is useful for comparing genotypes with phenotypes, but only provided that the patients are iron and folate replete and do not show major discrepancies with respect to age and spleen size. But in practice there is so much individual variation between the haemoglobin level and other important clinical features, and between patients of apparently identical genotypes, that such an approach is of limited value.

Early clinical descriptions

As mentioned earlier, it seems likely that many of the case reports of the Rietti–Greppi–Micheli syndrome in the early Italian literature were example of β thalassaemia intermedia of varying severity. Excellent clinical descriptions of this condition are to be found in the papers of Silvestroni, Bianco and their coworkers (Silvestroni & Bianco 1944–45, 1945, 1951; Bianco *et al.* 1952). Much of the early Italian literature, together with further reports of cases of what are almost certainly β thalassaemia intermedia, were reviewed by Marmont and Bianchi (1948). Later series included those of Gabuzda *et al.* (1963), Pearson (1964), Erlandson *et al.* (1964a), Bannerman *et al.* (1967), Aksoy (1970), Aksoy *et al.* (1978a),

Bianco *et al.* (1977), Gallo *et al.* (1979) and Pippard *et al.* (1982b). The extensive literature on β thalassaemia in African and Afro-American populations, outlined in previous editions of this book, also contains some excellent clinical descriptions of the milder forms of β thalassaemia intermedia (Scott *et al.* 1962; Heller *et al.* 1966; Friedman *et al.* 1972; Braverman *et al.* 1973; Charache *et al.* 1974; Friedman *et al.* 1974; Schroeder *et al.* 1974; Ahern *et al.* 1975; Kreimer-Birnbaum *et al.* 1975; Willcox 1975).

Unfortunately, the clinical descriptions of this disorder of more recent years have been less complete and this is one of the major reasons why it is so difficult to relate genotype to phenotype (Wainscoat *et al.* 1987; Fiorelli *et al.* 1988; Cao *et al.* 1990; Camaschella & Cappellini 1995; Weatherall & Clegg 1996; Rund *et al.* 1997; Ho *et al.* 1998a). In the sections that follow we shall try to put together a picture of this condition, based on a mixture of information gleaned from these early papers, the more limited recent publications that relate the disease to its genotype at the molecular level, and some personal observations which attempt to combine the two approaches.

Age at diagnosis

The age of presentation remains one of the most useful indicators of the likely course of homozygous or compound heterozygous β thalassaemia. Kattamis *et al.* (1975), in a series of 54 severely affected β thalassaemics, noted that the mean age of presentation was 13.1 months, with a range from 2 to 36 months. However, in comparing 121 severely affected β-thalassaemic children with 37 who had β thalassaemia intermedia, Modell and Berdoukas (1984) noted that 60% of the severely affected patients presented in the first year, 29% in the second year and only 9% later. On the other hand only 11% of patients with thalassaemia intermedia presented in the first year, while 30% presented in the second year and 59% later than the second year. Although the age of presentation will depend on many factors, including the socioeconomic environment in which children are brought up, we have been struck by how late many children with the intermediate forms of thalassaemia present, even if they run a relatively severe course.

The late onset of presentation in thalassaemia intermedia is observed even in the case of β^0-thalassaemia homozygosity (Cao 1988). In a series of 34 patients of this type it was found that those who were to be transfusion dependent presented at a mean age of 8.5±9.1 months, while those who were to remain independent of transfusion presented at a mean age of 17.4±11.8 months. Interestingly, the presenting haemoglobin levels were not significantly different. All these patients were homozygous for the common β CD39 C→T nonsense mutation.

A curious feature of the study of Modell and Berdoukas (1984) was that, although the reticulocyte count showed little difference between babies who had thalassaemia major compared with intermedia, the bilirubin levels during the early years of life were significantly higher in those with thalassaemia intermedia. This is difficult to explain; Modell and Berdoukas suggest that, because bone-marrow erythroblasts may mature further and generate more haemoglobin in thalassaemia intermedia, the higher level of bilirubin may reflect the relative increase in haemoglobin catabolism.

Course during early years of life

There are few good published data on the haemoglobin levels over the first few years of life. Although some children maintain a steady-state haemoglobin value which seems to vary little during the early years of life, others do not. While it is believed that a falling haemoglobin over the first few years may reflect increasing hypersplenism (Modell & Berdoukas 1984), it is not clear whether this is so in all cases. From our own experience many children with the intermediate forms of thalassaemia do not reach a steady-state haemoglobin for several years and it is very important not to reach a conclusion about whether this will be a mild or severe form of the condition without a relatively long period of observation.

Clinical features

The clinical manifestations of β thalassaemia intermedia are extremely variable. In some cases the disorder presents early in life with anaemia, while in others it may not appear until later due to a complication such as hypersplenism. Many patients have been found to have this disorder on routine clinical examination. Growth and development may be normal or there may be some retardation as occurs in homozygous β thalassaemia. The major symptoms in early childhood are anaemia and mild jaundice. There is nearly always some degree of splenomegaly and often hepatomegaly. The bone changes are extremely variable and range from almost none at all to severe skeletal deformity identical to that observed in poorly managed homozygous β thalassaemia.

Some babies who have presented relatively late with haemoglobin values in the 6–7 g/dl range, or lower, are clearly destined for transfusion from the beginning. When observed over a few months there is failure to thrive, listlessness, proneness to infection and a poor appetite. From developmental studies over a short period it is clear that these infants are not putting on weight or growing and developing normally, and hence they should be considered to have thalassaemia major, and treated accordingly.

The course for those infants who, despite their relatively low haemoglobin levels, are fully active and thriving is usually one of a chronic, well compensated anaemia which may be exacerbated during periods of infection or folate deficiency or, most commonly, by increasing hypersplenism.

While patients with this condition may require no blood transfusions, or occasional transfusion during periods of exacerbation of their anaemia, there is increasing evidence that β thalassaemia intermedia is a condition associated with many distressing clinical complications.

Complications

Hypersplenism

Increasing splenomegaly leading to hypersplenism is a relatively common feature of β thalassaemia intermedia. In most of the larger series cited above, a significant proportion of the patients had undergone splenectomy for worsening of their anaemia, thrombocytopenia or neutropenia. There is frequently a history of the patient becoming transfusion dependent and then having a splenectomy after which they did not require further transfusion. The mechanism and pathophysiology of the splenomegaly and hypersplenism are the same as described earlier for homozygous β thalassaemia (see Chapters 5 and 7).

Iron loading

Curiously, although patients with thalassaemia intermedia have an expanded bone-marrow mass and increased iron absorption, reports of iron loading in transfusion-independent or rarely transfused

patients have, until recently, been rare. Bannerman *et al.* (1967) described a 41-year-old Sicilian with β thalassaemia intermedia who had gross iron loading with associated cardiac failure, diabetes mellitus, hypopituitarism and porphyrinuria. However, Erlandson *et al.* (1964a) did not consider that iron loading was a major problem in this disorder, although no details of her patients' iron status are given. In a study from the authors' laboratory (Pippard *et al.* 1979) the degree of iron loading in 15 patients with β thalassaemia intermedia was examined. There was a highly significant increase in plasma ferritin levels with age and the majority of the patients over 20 years old in the series had totally saturated iron binding capacities (Fig. 13.6). Liver biopsies of three of the older patients showed excessive iron deposition associated with portal cirrhosis in each case (Fig. 13.7). Since many of these patients had received little or no blood it was assumed that the iron must have been derived from increased absorption and this was found to be the case (Tables 13.7 and 13.8). In an extension of these studies it was found that the steady-state haemoglobin level was a poor guide to the risk of iron overload. However, the extent of erythroid hyperplasia, judged by ferrokinetic studies or, more simply, by analysis of the erythroid/myeloid ratio after bone-marrow aspiration, was more useful in predicting both the rate of iron loading and the need for iron chelation therapy (Pippard & Weatherall 1984).

Later studies, though disappointingly few, tend to confirm these observations. Pootrakul *et al.* (1981b) described increasing ferritin levels in patients with HbE thalassaemia and suggested that the rate of iron loading might be more rapid after splenectomy (see

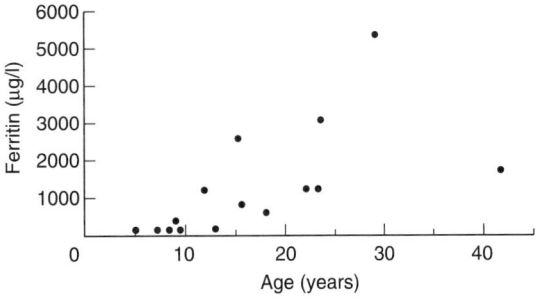

Fig. 13.6 The relationship between age and serum ferritin levels in a group of patients with β thalassaemia intermedia. From Pippard *et al.* (1979).

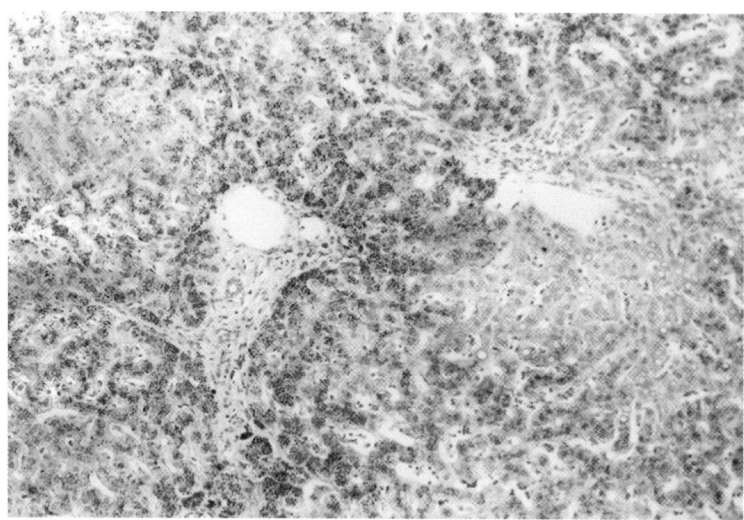

Fig. 13.7 A section of liver showing early iron loading in a patient with β thalassaemia intermedia (Perl's stain ×300).

Table 13.7 Iron absorption and data on iron status in 15 patients with thalassaemia intermedia. From Pippard *et al.* (1979).

| | | | | % ^{59}Fe absorption | | | |
Patient number	Age (years)	Previous transfusions (units)	Serum iron (μmol/l)	Total iron binding capacity (μmol/l)	Ferritin (μg/l)	5 mg Fe^{++}	Labelled meal
1	4	0	30.5	49.5	139	—	—
2	7	0	18.5	51.0	197	28	31
3	8	2	18.5	42.0	117	35	—
4	9	0	23.0	51.0	146	53	54
5	9	40	38.0	38.0	399	88	—
6	12	25	47.5	48.0	277	69	—
7	13	0	29.0	37.5	211	47	—
8	15	10	16.0	39.0	2270	17	—
9	16	0	25.5	37.5	703	—	—
10	18	4	45.5	51.0	679	85	26
11	23	6*	37.0	43.5	1120	73	—
12	23	48	40.0	48.0	1240	78	—
13	24	25	36.0	48.0	3099	76	45
14	30	40	27.5	30.0	5200	37	—
15	42	15	42.0	48.0	1590	89	—

*For 4 years had venesections, one unit every 2 weeks.

Chapter 9). Cossu *et al.* (1981), in a small series of patients with thalassaemia intermedia, reported an increasing ferritin level with age associated with an increased amount of urinary iron excreted in response to desferrioxamine. Buonanno *et al.* (1984) observed increasing serum ferritin levels with age and, from the results of liver biopsies, reported that there was histological evidence of liver damage before the serum ferritin values became markedly elevated. In a more extensive series of 38 adult

patients with β thalassaemia intermedia Fiorelli *et al.* (1990) attempted to evaluate the factors that might be responsible for the observed heterogeneity of their iron status. The level of transferrin saturation, serum ferritin and desferrioxamine-induced urinary iron excretion were spread over a wide range and did not correlate with age or steady-state haemoglobin levels. In this study significant differences in the degree of iron loading were observed between patients who had undergone splenectomy compared

Table 13.8 Iron balance in five patients with thalassaemia intermedia (Pippard *et al*. 1979).

Patient number*	Iron (mg in 24 h)				% retention of food iron†	% retention of $^{59}Fe^{++}$ food iron
	Food	Stool	Urine	Balance		
2	10.6	4.7	0.2	+5.7	56	31
4	10.2	2.8	0.2	+7.2	73	54
8‡	11.7	8.7	0.4	+2.6	26	—
11	23.7	14.5	0.6	+8.6	39	—
13‡	15.4	7.1	0.6	+7.7	54	45

* Numbers refer to patients shown in Table 13.7.

† $\text{Retention} = \left(\dfrac{\text{Food Fe} - \text{Stool Fe}}{\text{Food Fe}} \right) \times 100$

‡ Food intake estimated from food tables for those patients, who were also on ascorbate supplements during the iron balance period.

with those with intact spleens; the iron burden was considerably greater in the splenectomized group. Overall, a considerable proportion of patients showed evidence of significant iron overload.

In a study from Turkey Gumruk *et al*. (1992) were not able to demonstrate increased iron absorption in a group of children with β thalassaemia intermedia and concluded that the serum ferritin values were not high enough to necessitate chelation therapy. However, the mean age of their patients was 13.4±7.5 years. Apart from the iron absorption results these findings are not surprising, since the earlier work of Pippard *et al*. (1979) showed quite clearly that iron accumulation occurred much more slowly in thalassaemia intermedia than in thalassaemia major and that significantly elevated serum ferritin values were unusual over the first 15 years of life (see Fig. 13.6).

Pootrakul *et al*. (1988) found that there was a reasonably close agreement between the degree of erythroid hyperplasia and the rate of iron loading in patients with HbE thalassaemia and other forms of thalassaemia intermedia. There have been several reports suggesting that there may be progressive liver damage. Frigerio *et al*. (1984) noticed a reasonable correlation between the serum ferritin and *N*-acetyl-β-D-glucosaminidase levels in patients with β thalassaemia intermedia. These changes were thought to reflect enhanced lysosomal fragility due to iron damage.

While these data are still limited they leave little doubt that severe iron loading, which we shall see later is from the gastrointestinal tract, is a common feature of β thalassaemia intermedia. This can undoubtedly lead to liver damage and cirrhosis and to other complications of iron overload. It is also clear that serum ferritin values, though they provide an overall guide to the rate of iron loading, do not provide really useful information about when the associated manifestations of liver damage will occur. Clearly more information is needed about this important topic.

Endocrine function

There have been very few reports of endocrine deficiency consequent on iron loading in thalassaemia intermedia. In the patient studied by Bannerman *et al*. (1967) there were severe diabetes mellitus and hypopituitarism. McIntosh (1976b) described a woman with thalassaemia intermedia and multiple endocrine deficiencies; replacement therapy was followed by a normal pregnancy. Interestingly, many of the larger series contain a significant number of patients with diabetes mellitus (Erlandson *et al*. 1964a; Pippard *et al*. 1982b). Of the 15 patients reported by Pippard *et al*. one was frankly diabetic and three showed a reduced first-phase insulin response associated with high-normal fasting plasma glucose concentrations during standard glucose tolerance tests, findings which suggest that they had an impairment of pancreatic β-cell function. Similar results were obtained in three out of 11 patients with thalassaemia intermedia studied by De Sanctis *et al*. (1986). There are very few data on the function of the other endocrine glands. Bannerman and colleagues' patient had unequivocal hypopituitarism. In our own series (Pippard *et al.* 1982b) tests of adrenal, pituitary and thyroid function were relatively normal except that two individuals showed a subnormal luteinizing hormone response to stimulation with luteinizing hormone-release hormone (LHRH). Plasma prolactin levels were all within normal limits.

In several series of patients with β thalassaemia intermedia there was a history of normal puberty and menarche although the latter was sometimes delayed (Erlandson *et al.* 1964a; Pippard *et al.* 1982b). These observations suggest that, unlike inadequately chelated, transfusion-dependent homozygous β thalassaemics, many patients with β thalassaemia intermedia have relatively normal endocrine function up to and beyond puberty. However, when they reach the third or fourth decades there appears to be a significant incidence of diabetes mellitus, and other minor endocrine deficiencies occur. Clearly, we require much more information about these changes in older patients.

Interestingly, Jensen *et al.* (1997) suggest that, even within a population of patients with transfusion-dependent forms of β^0 or β^+ thalassaemia, the severity of the disease in relationship to endocrine function and glucose tolerance may be modified by the co-existence of α thalassaemia or by the presence of less severe β-thalassaemia alleles.

Cardiac complications

Because in the absence of regular blood transfusion the rate of iron loading is much slower in β thalassaemia intermedia than in thalassaemia major, it would be expected that, if cardiac complications occur at all, they would only appear in adult life. Although there have been single case reports of cardiac failure in this disorder in patients aged between 25 and 40 (Bannerman *et al.* 1967; Mancuso *et al.* 1985), and the patient described by Mancuso *et al.* seemed to respond to intense treatment with desferrioxamine, there have been few systematic studies of cardiac function.

Fiorelli *et al.* (1988) provided some information about the cardiac status on 18 of their patients with thalassaemia intermedia in Italy. All had cardiomegaly and systolic flow murmurs compatible with the degree of anaemia. Their ECGs showed some modifications of the QRS complexes, compatible with ventricular hypertrophy. No consistent abnormalities of rhythm or conduction were observed. In five of the 18 patients, echocardiograph analysis showed enlarged diastolic dimensions and some rather non-specific functional alterations. In 15 patients studied in our own centre, echocardiographic analysis showed essentially similar changes; three of 15 patients had enlarged diastolic dimensions. However, both the ejection fractions and fractional shortening were normal in all cases. Holter monitoring over a 24-h period showed that six out of seven patients studied had some non-specific abnormalities including periods of bradycardia, tachycardia and supraventricular extrasystoles. All these patients were adults with elevated serum ferritin levels and, in some cases, liver iron values (Pippard *et al.* 1982b).

Olivieri *et al.* (1992d) reported studies on a 29-year-old Italian male who, though he had not received transfusions after the age of 5 years, nevertheless presented with hepatomegaly, abnormal liver function tests, an elevated serum ferritin level and marked iron loading of the liver as judged by liver biopsy and quantitative magnetic resonance imaging (MRI) of the liver. This patient was treated with the oral chelating agent deferiprone (L1). Before treatment he showed an abnormal resting electrocardiogram with atrial bigeminy, which reverted to sinus rhythm during exercise. The left ventricular ejection fraction was 60% at rest with no increase at peak exercise. Mild right ventricular dilatation, and abnormalities in diastolic function were also observed. After treatment, the resting left ventricular ejection fraction remained normal with a normal increase on exercise. The abnormalities of ventricular diastolic function did not change during treatment except for improvement in the atrial contribution, 14% before treatment as compared with 17% afterwards. Although these are relatively mild changes the fact that they changed after treatment suggests that there were some functional cardiac anomalies secondary to iron loading. Unfortunately, there are no series of adult patients with β thalassaemia intermedia studied by sequential cardiac investigations and therefore we have no knowledge about the number of patients who might be at risk for developing cardiac disease in adult life. This important question needs further investigation.

In discussing the pathophysiology of HbE thalassaemia in Chapter 9, we referred to the syndrome of pulmonary hypertension and right-heart failure, particularly in patients who had undergone splenectomy. This complication has also been described in β thalassaemia intermedia (Aessopos *et al.* 1995). These workers analysed seven patients who presented with congestive cardiac failure and pulmonary hypertension. All but one had undergone splenectomy. In each case there was dilatation of the main pulmonary artery and cardiac enlargement, signs of right ventricular hypertrophy on the ECG, and a dilated right ventricle, with good left ventricular function as judged by echocardiography. Right-heart catheterization showed a markedly raised pulmonary pressure with increased pulmonary vascular resistance. The pulmonary capillary wedge pressure was in the normal range. The authors conclude that the pulmonary hypertension in these patients is almost certainly related to their β thalassaemia although, as in the case of HbE β thalassaemia, the precise mechanisms remain to be determined. The possible aetiology of right-heart failure in β thalassaemia is discussed further in Chapters 5, 7 and 9.

Gallstones

A high incidence of pigment stones, sometimes associated with biliary colic and cholecystitis, has been a feature of all the series of patients with β thalassaemia intermedia (Erlandson *et al.* 1964a; Gallo *et al.* 1979; Fiorelli *et al.* 1988; Goldfarb *et al.* 1990). Many patients are chronically jaundiced, probably due to a combination of ineffective erythropoiesis and haemolysis. It appears that persistent hyperbilirubinaemia, and the formation of pigment stones, is one of the commonest complications.

Folic acid deficiency

There are many well documented cases of folate deficiency (Erlandson *et al.* 1964a; Bannerman *et al.* 1967; Pippard *et al.* 1982b). It may cause worsening of the anaemia and megaloblastic erythropoiesis. The degree of anaemia may be profound. Three patients reported by Modell and Berdoukas (1984) presented in heart failure with haemoglobin values of 3.7, 4.1 and 3.1 g/dl, respectively. After treatment with folic acid the haemoglobin level rose in each case to 9.0 g/dl or more.

Skeletal deformities and bone and joint disease

Some patients with β thalassaemia intermedia develop severe skeletal deformities, very similar to those seen in thalassaemia major (Fig. 13.8) (see Chapter 7). There is also an increased frequency of fractures following minor trauma, particularly in older patients. There are other distressing bone and joint complications about which less has been written. In their study of 'thalassaemic osteoarthropathy' Gratwick *et al.* (1978) described a curious form of periarticular disease in patients with either thalassaemia major or intermedia. It was characterized by dull aching pains in the ankles which were exacerbated by weight bearing and relieved by rest. There was no evidence of inflammatory disease of the joints. Radiological changes included widening of the medullary spaces, thin cortices with coarse trabeculation, and evidence of microfractures. Histological analysis confirmed the presence of the latter and showed osteomalacia and increased osteoblastic and osteoclastic surface areas with iron depositions in the calcification front and cement lines.

We have observed this complication in several patients; X-rays of one of them are shown in Fig. 13.9. This 29-year-old Cypriot woman developed severe pain in her ankles 2 years before the period of study. An arthrodesis had been performed on her right ankle with relief of pain, but following the operation she walked on long crutches for 3 months and subsequently developed severe and incapacitating pain and limitation of movement of both shoulders associated with a severe destructive arthropathy. In our early series of 15 patients with β thalassaemia intermedia (Pippard *et al.* 1982b) three others experienced intermittent joint pains, a symptom which was not associated with the gross radiological changes seen in the Cypriot woman.

Another complication secondary to severe bone disease was reported by Korovessis *et al.* (1990). They described four female patients who developed secondary acetabular protrusion, possibly the result of rarefaction of the pelvis due to bone-marrow hyperplasia. They pointed out that this was the first report of non-traumatic acetabular protrusion in patients with thalassaemia. In an extensive study, which included bone biopsy and electron-microscopic analysis of biopsy specimens of the synovial membrane of patients with thalassaemia intermedia, a number of morphological changes were demonstrated, including iron deposition and impairment of the vessels of the microcirculatory bed (Musaev *et al.* 1991).

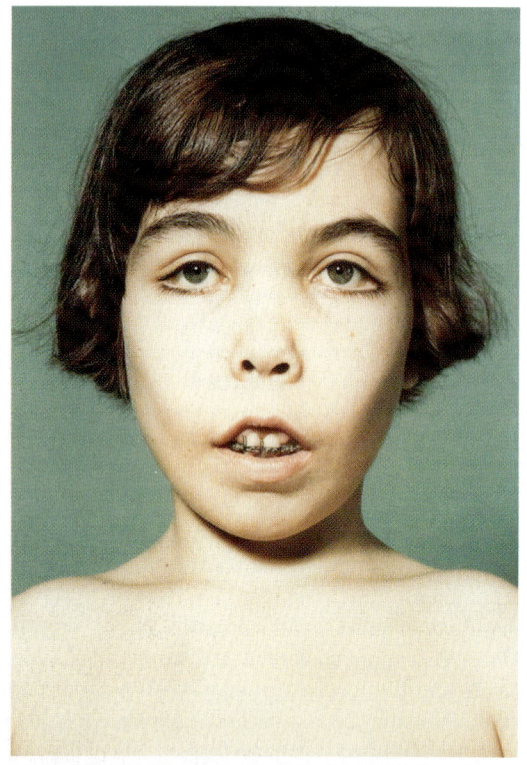

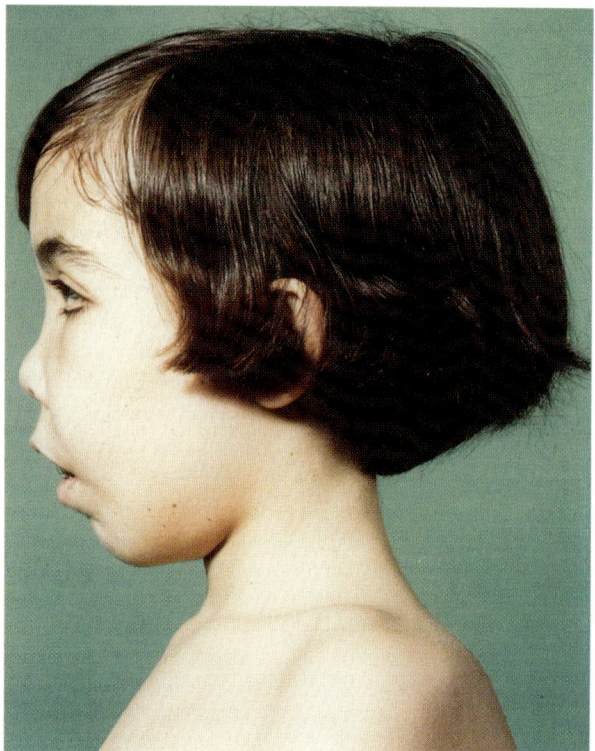

(a)

(b)

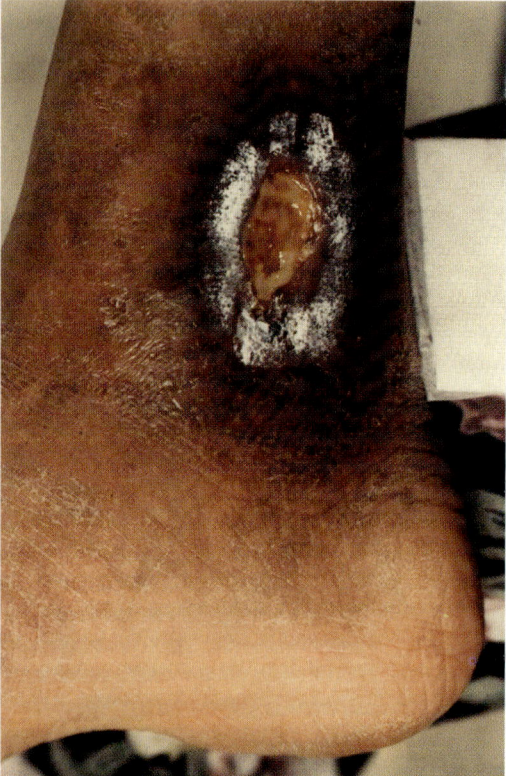

(c)

Fig. 13.8 Clinical features of severe β thalassaemia intermedia. (a,b) Facial appearances; (c) chronic leg ulcer.

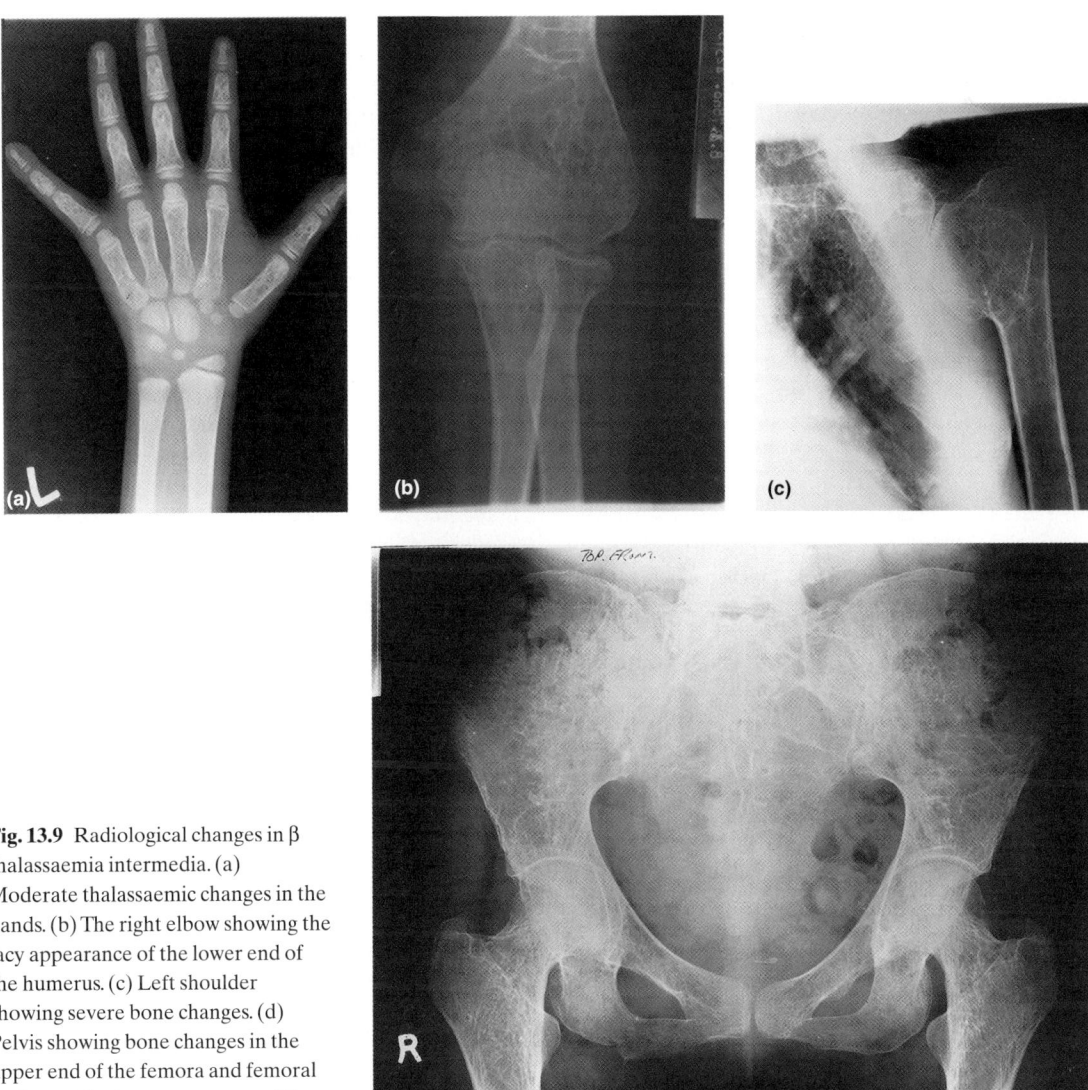

Fig. 13.9 Radiological changes in β thalassaemia intermedia. (a) Moderate thalassaemic changes in the hands. (b) The right elbow showing the lacy appearance of the lower end of the humerus. (c) Left shoulder showing severe bone changes. (d) Pelvis showing bone changes in the upper end of the femora and femoral necks and the lacy appearance of the pelvic bones.

Although these data are sparse, it is apparent that bone disease in thalassaemia intermedia may be extremely severe, particularly in older patients. It does not simply involve the usual skeletal changes observed in under-transfused patients with β thalassaemia major, but also includes distressing forms of osteoarthropathy, which presumably reflect gross thinning of the bones over a long period of time. This neglected topic needs much more extensive evaluation.

Finally, as well as localized pain round bones and joints, patients with thalassaemia intermedia may have quite severe generalized bone pain. This symptom is highlighted by Modell and Berdoukas (1984) and we have observed it in a number of our own patients. The mechanism is not known.

Extramedullary erythropoiesis

The production of tumour masses composed of extramedullary erythropoietic tissue is a well documented feature of β thalassaemia intermedia (Erlandson *et al.* 1964a; Ben-Bassat *et al.* 1977; Genovese *et al.* 1979; Pippard *et al.* 1982b; Yu *et al.* 1991; Alam *et al.* 1997). We were surprised to find that these large tumour masses were not always correlated with gross radiological changes of the skeleton. The commonest site is in the paraspinal region (Fig. 13.10) but in one of our patients there were associated pleural masses. Alam *et al.* (1997) provide a valuable summary of the radiological characteristics of these lesions. Although they do not usually cause any symptoms, Bate and Humphries (1977) described a patient with severe β thalassaemia intermedia who developed spinal cord compression associated with extramedullary haemopoietic tissue. Although uncommon, there have been several reports of this

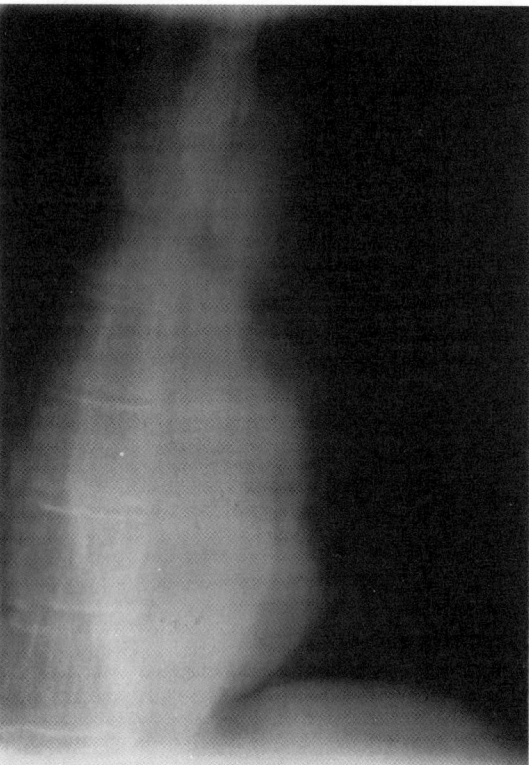

Fig. 13.10 A mass of extramedullary erythropoietic tissue in the posterior mediastinum of a patient with β thalassaemia intermedia.

complication (David & Balusubramaniam 1983; Cardia *et al.* 1994) and one example of a cauda equina lesion (Mancuso *et al.* 1993). Though haemorrhage from extramedullary haemopoietic tissue must be rare, a case of massive haemothorax has been documented (Smith *et al.* 1988).

These extramedullary haemopoietic masses may cause considerable diagnostic problems, particularly if they present in unusual sites. We discussed the way in which they may simulate a cerebral tumour in patients with HbE β thalassaemia in Chapter 9. Sproat *et al.* (1991) describe the problems posed by a patient who presented with a painful presacral mass in which the diagnosis could only be confirmed by a needle biopsy guided by computed tomography (CT). Occasionally, extramedullary haematopoietic tissue may aggregate at the anterior end of the ribs, producing a particularly curious deformity (Rao *et al.* 1989).

From the limited published experience it appears that it is usual to diagnose this complication by conventional radiology (Alam *et al.* 1997). In a study of masses of extramedullary haemopoietic tissue in three patients, one of whom had thalassaemia intermedia, Papavasiliou *et al.* (1990) found a good correlation between the radiological or CT appearances of the masses and MRI analysis. They produce a low-intensity signal, similar to that of the adjacent marrow of the thoracic spine, and are surrounded by a characteristic high-intensity signal rim attributed to a surrounding layer of fat. The latter finding has been confirmed by Martin *et al.* (1990). In another study, a group of patients underwent total body CT; the volume of the foci of ectopic erythropoiesis was calculated by an algorithm. There was a good correlation between the level of serum transferrin receptors and the volume of the ectopic erythropoietic masses (Sergiacomi *et al.* 1993).

Hitherto, it has been thought that the appearance of extramedullary erythropoietic masses is a relatively rare complication. In an attempt to determine the frequency, 29 adult patients were subjected to total body CT analysis. Ectopic erythropoiesis, located mainly in the paravertebral gutters in the thorax, was detectable in 65.5% of the patients. There seemed to be a good relationship between the development of this tissue and an early age of presentation, the necessity for splenectomy and the presence of high levels of fetal haemoglobin (Dore *et al.* 1992).

It appears that some of these extramedullary lesions may undergo fatty transformation with time or if the haemoglobin level is raised, by splenectomy for example (Martin *et al.* 1990).

Infection

In Chapter 5 we summarized the evidence that children with β thalassaemia are unusually prone to infection, and discussed the limited information about the underlying mechanisms. We returned to this theme in Chapters 7 and 9 when we discussed the role of infection in severe, transfusion-dependent forms of β thalassaemia and HbE β thalassaemia. It is not clear whether patients with other forms of β thalassaemia intermedia are particularly susceptible to infection although this seems likely. Infective episodes were a common feature in the series of Erlandson *et al.* (1964a), Pearson (1964), Gallo *et al.* (1979), Pippard *et al.* (1982b) and Mela *et al.* (1988). It is quite clear from these reports that infection may be associated with a marked fall in haemoglobin level and this seems to be the commonest indication for blood transfusion.

There are few data regarding the overall patterns of infection in thalassaemia intermedia. However, it is clear that specific infections which are common in the β thalassaemias occur in this condition. For example, there are a number of well documented cases of severe *Yersinia* infections associated with the administration of desferrioxamine (Kelly *et al.* 1987; de Mazzoleni *et al.* 1991), and aplastic or hypoplastic episodes associated with parvovirus infection have been recorded (Brownell *et al.* 1986). It appears that patients who have been transfused are, like others with transfusion-dependent forms of β thalassaemia, prone to hepatitis B and C (Mela *et al.* 1988). But, although a number of studies have been carried out to search for an immune basis for increased susceptibility to infection (Guglielmo *et al.* 1984), no consistent abnormalities have been found. The observation of increased serum levels of interleukin 8 in patients with thalassaemia major and intermedia may reflect hyperactivity of thalassaemic macrophages in relationship to chronic haemolysis (Dore *et al.* 1995).

Hyperuricaemia and gout

Although in several reported series some patients with β thalassaemia intermedia had elevated uric acid levels, secondary gout seems to be an uncommon complication (Gratwick *et al.* 1978; Pippard *et al.* 1982b).

Leg ulcers

The occurrence of chronic ulcers, usually just above the medial malleolus, was reported in the early Italian literature and has been documented in more recent series (Gallo *et al.* 1979; Gimmon *et al.* 1982; Modell & Berdoukas 1984; Fiorelli *et al.* 1988; Camaschella & Cappellini 1995). We have seen this complication quite frequently in Cypriot patients with thalassaemia intermedia in the UK (Fig. 13.8). Its relationship to the rheological properties of the red cells is discussed by Gimmon *et al.* (1982).

Pregnancy

A detailed account of a single pregnancy was described by Walker *et al.* (1969). The patient, with typical thalassaemia intermedia, became profoundly anaemic after becoming pregnant and required transfusions to prevent the development of cardiac failure. She was delivered at 37 weeks by Caesarean section and a further transfusion was given immediately postpartum. The infant was healthy.

Later series confirmed that pregnancy may be associated with severe, sometimes life-threatening anaemia (Afifi 1974; Dolfin *et al.* 1983). Among the 24 Egyptian women reported by Alifi, there was a 50% fetal loss among those who were untransfused, compared with a 'normal fetal wastage' among those maintained at a haemoglobin in excess of 9 g/dl throughout pregnancy.

Thromboembolic disease

In Chapters 5 and 7 we discussed the increasing suspicion that many forms of β thalassaemia may be associated with a hypercoagulable state and an increased proneness to thrombotic episodes. We also pointed out that, while this may be the case, there are very limited data about the frequency of this complication; the β thalassaemia intermedia literature is equally uninformative.

In their review of thromboembolic events in β thalassaemia, Borgna-Pignatti *et al.* (1998a) identified 32 patients with this complication out of a total 735 subjects, of whom 683 had thalassaemia major and 52 thalassaemia intermedia, corresponding to an incidence of 3.95 and 9.61%, respectively. The spectrum and distribution of thrombotic episodes described in this study are discussed in detail in Chapter 7. In the five thrombotic episodes encountered in patients with thalassaemia intermedia there appeared to be no particular associated risk factors, with the possible exception of chronic liver disease.

Apart from this report there are only a few isolated case reports of severe thrombotic disease, particularly after splenectomy. For example, Skarsgard *et al.* (1993) described three patients, one of whom had thalassaemia intermedia, who presented with abdominal pain, nausea and fever approximately 1–2 weeks postsplenectomy. Abdominal Doppler ultrasound and/or CT showed an intraluminal filling defect with partial obstruction to flow in one main branch of the portal vein, splenic vein thrombosis with complete occlusion of the main portal and proximal superior mesenteric veins, and a complete thrombosis of the splenic vein. It should be pointed out, however, that in this report there were two other patients who developed the same complications who had different blood disorders. However, with the exception of HbE β thalassaemia, which was discussed in Chapter 9, there have been no other reports of thrombotic complications in patients with thalassaemia intermedia.

On the other hand, recent studies indicate that, like patients with β thalassaemia major, those with thalassaemia intermedia may have a chronic hypercoagulable state associated with platelet activation which correlates with red-cell anionic phospholipid exposure (Ruf *et al.* 1997). In short, it appears that prethrombotic changes, described in Chapters 5 and 7 as being associated with the severe forms of β thalassaemia, are also demonstrable in patients with thalassaemia intermedia. But, until more clinical information is available, it is impossible to make any judgements about the clinical relevance of these laboratory findings. Similarly, it is not clear how they relate to reports of the occurrence of recurrent priapism following splenectomy for this condition (Macchia *et al.* 1990; Dore *et al.* 1991).

Haematological findings

There is a variable degree of anaemia, with haemoglobin values in the 5–10 g/dl range. The red-cell indices are typically thalassaemic with low MCH and MCV values. In splenectomized patients we have observed higher MCH values than would be expected from the appearances of the peripheral blood film. However, this may reflect the presence of large numbers of small distorted cells which are not counted in the electronic cell counter. The peripheral blood film shows major abnormalities in the shape and size of the red cells, indistinguishable from those of transfusion-dependent β thalassaemia. There are always some nucleated red cells in the peripheral blood and, following splenectomy, they may reach very high levels. Except in the presence of hypersplenism the white-cell count and platelet counts are usually normal. The reticulocyte count is elevated and, in some forms of β thalassaemia intermedia, on staining with methyl violet, nucleated red cells show ragged inclusion bodies, similar to those observed in homozygous β thalassaemia.

Bone-marrow examination shows marked erythroid hyperplasia and, again, many of the red-cell precursors contain inclusion bodies. The morphological changes are the same as those in transfusion-dependent β thalassaemia.

Red-cell survival, ferrokinetics and erythrokinetics

Red-cell survival studies have been reported in two series of patients with β thalassaemia intermedia (Erlandson *et al.* 1964a; Gallo *et al.* 1979). In the earlier report there was a moderate reduction in red-cell survival time while in the more recent study there was considerable shortening, with ^{51}Cr $T_{1/2}$ values ranging from 10 to 16 days.

As mentioned earlier there is a marked increase in iron absorption from the gastrointestinal tract (Heinrich *et al.* 1973; De Alarcon *et al.* 1979; Pippard *et al.* 1979; Pippard & Weatherall 1984). The results of iron absorption and balance analyses carried out on five patients in the authors' laboratory are shown in Tables 13.7 and 13.8. They were all in a positive balance of between 2.6 and 8.6 mg Fe per day. Using a sophisticated iron kinetic-based measure of erythropoiesis, Cavill *et al.* (1978) studied two patients who had not received transfusion for 5 years. They found that the marrow iron turnover was approximately six times normal but that most of this increased activity was ineffective; the mean red-cell production rates were 0.86 and 2.22×10^6 cells per litre of blood per second, respectively, as compared with a normal value of 0.51×10^6. These findings indicate a fairly extreme degree of ineffective erythropoiesis. Similar results were reported by Najean *et al.* (1985). Barosi *et al.* (1987) found that erythropoietic activity was invariably related to haemoglobin levels and correlated with the level of HbF. In an extensive series of studies Pootrakul *et al.* (1988) observed ineffective erythropoiesis and marked expansion of the erythroid mass, the extent of which correlated with the degree of increased iron loading.

More recently the estimation of the serum transferrin receptor level has been used to determine the degree of erythroid expansion in different forms of thalassaemia. In a study by Dore *et al.* (1996) of untransfused subjects with a steady-state haemoglobin level of 9.6 g/dl the mean basal transferrin receptor level was 30.3 as compared with 12.8 in a series of age-matched healthy controls. These observations suggest a highly significant increase in the size of the erythron. Interestingly, the response of the serum transferrin level to erythropoietin was quite inconsistent, a topic to which we shall return in the next section.

Erythropoietin response

There have been several studies of serum erythropoietin (Epo) levels in β thalassaemia intermedia (Dore *et al.* 1993; Camaschella *et al.* 1996; Nisli *et al.* 1997). Dore and colleagues found that the mean level of serum Epo was significantly higher than in normal controls and the levels were lower in transfusion-dependent subjects. In untransfused patients there was an inverse relationship between serum Epo values and the haemoglobin level. These results were confirmed by Nisli and colleagues, who also observed that if transfusion-dependent patients with thalassaemia major were studied at the same haemoglobin concentrations as those with thalassaemia intermedia the mean serum Epo level was significantly higher in the former group.

Camaschella and her colleagues found more variation in the Epo levels. Six patients showed inappropriately low Epo levels and, even excluding these cases, there was no clear relationship between the haemoglobin levels and those of erythropoietin or transferrin receptors. These workers also found that in two groups of patients with similar haemoglobin levels, but low or high levels of HbF, the latter group have higher serum Epo values. Curiously, no difference in the serum transferrin receptor levels were observed between the two groups. These findings are surprising; *higher* levels of Epo might be expected to occur in those with more HbF, because of its greater oxygen affinity. Furthermore, this should have been reflected by a higher erythroid mass as determined by the level of transferrin receptors. The authors conclude that the relationship between anaemia, the level of HbF and the erythroid mass in thalassaemia intermedia is more complex than expected! This should not surprise us. As we saw in earlier chapters, the relationship between the erythropoietin response and the degree of anaemia is inconsistent in most forms of β thalassaemia as compared with other forms of anaemia. The reasons for this discrepancy remain to be determined.

Mechanisms of red-cell destruction

In Chapter 5 we considered the effects of globin imbalance on the survival of red-cell precursors and mature red cells in α and β thalassaemia. It seems likely that the mechanisms of damage to the red cells and their precursors are similar across the spectrum of the β thalassaemias (Schrier 1997). In short, it appears that it reflects excess α-chain production, the effects of inclusion body formation, the interaction of α chains with the various components of the red-cell membrane, and the deleterious effects of the degradation products of excess haemoglobin subunits, notably haem, haemin and iron.

In the red-cell precursors, haem, haemichromes and iron components of α globins serve as foci for the generation of reactive oxygen species that result in the partial oxidation of band 4.1, and for a decrease of the spectrin/band 3 ratio. In the red cells the formation of membrane-bound haemichrome creates a copolymer of macromolecular dimensions which promotes clustering of band 3 in the membrane. These clusters are opsonized with autologous IgG complement and hence removed by macrophages. In addition, band 4.1 is partially oxidized. These changes are aggravated by excess iron accumulation and the generation of oxygen free radicals, with subsequent damage to several membrane components, including lipids and protein, as well as intracellular organelles such as mitochondria and lysosomes.

Much of the work that has yielded these concepts has been carried out on the cells of patients with β thalassaemia intermedia (Shinar *et al.* 1989; Advani *et al.* 1992b; Scott *et al.* 1992; Mannu *et al.* 1995); the changes in calcium homeostasis in thalassaemic cells, described in Chapter 5, were defined in the cells of similarly affected patients (Bookchin *et al.* 1988). Shaeffer (1988) has demonstrated that the ATP-dependent proteolysis of excess α chains in β thalassaemia intermedia is ubiquitin dependent.

In magnetic resonance spectroscopy analyses of the red cells of patients with β thalassaemia intermedia compared with those of heterozygous β thalassaemics and normals, it was found that there were similar concentrations of ATP and 2,3-diphosphoglycerate in the three groups. However, the profile of glucose metabolism was quite different in the red cells of patients with β thalassaemia intermedia; there was a threefold faster rate of glucose metabolism, which was thought to reflect increased activity of the pentose phosphate pathway, possibly as a consequence of the elevated oxidative state of the red cells (Ting *et al.* 1994).

It appears therefore that the major pathways to red-cell damage are similar in all forms of β thalassaemia and that, ultimately, it is the magnitude and properties of the excess α chains that are the major factors which determine the survival of the red-cell precursors and their progeny. Since, for one reason or another, the level of globin imbalance is usually less in β thalassaemia intermedia than in the more severe forms of the disease, it follows that, overall, the degree of disordered erythropoiesis and peripheral red-cell destruction is less marked.

Haemoglobin constitution

Considering the extraordinarily diverse genotypes that may underlie the phenotype of thalassaemia intermedia it is not surprising that it is characterized by a wide range of different haemoglobin constitutions. Indeed, there is no one pattern that could be called typical. For this reason, it is only possible to make a few generalizations based on the different genetic interactions outlined in Table 13.1.

In the thalassaemia intermedias that result from the homozygous state for mild β⁺-thalassaemia mutations the level of HbF tends to be low compared with other types of β thalassaemia that result from the interaction of two alleles. This is exemplified in the homozygous state for the common Mediterranean mutation, IVS1-6 T→C, in which the fetal haemoglobin level tends to be in the region of 20% of the total, though there is considerable scatter (Efremov *et al.*

1988). As pointed out earlier, the exceptions to this rule are the homozygous or compound heterozygous states for promoter mutations of the β-globin gene. In this case there tends to be an unexpectedly high level of fetal haemoglobin, usually in excess of 50% of the total (Gonzalez-Redondo *et al.* 1988a). In both these disorders homozygotes have, as a rule, increased levels of HbA₂. In homozygotes for β⁰ thalassaemia intermedia the haemoglobin is made up almost entirely of the fetal variety and the HbA₂ level is usually in the normal range (Thein *et al.* 1988a).

These forms of β⁰ thalassaemia intermedia, such as the Dutch variety, which are due to deletions of the 5′ end of the β-globin gene, are often associated with unusually high levels of Hbs F and A₂ in heterozygotes (Thein 1993).

In the interactions between the homozygous or compound heterozygous state for β⁺ or β⁰ thalassaemia in association with the heterozygous states for α⁺ or α⁰ thalassaemia the haemoglobin pattern does not seem to alter from that found with the β-thalassaemia mutations alone. On the other hand, the interaction between these forms of β thalassaemia and the genotype of HbH disease produces a quite different haemoglobin pattern. In this case, while the amounts of Hbs A and F do not differ significantly from those seen in homozygous or compound heterozygous β⁺ or β⁰ thalassaemia, there is an unusually high level of HbA₂ and traces of Hb Bart's can be demonstrated (Loukopoulos *et al.* 1978; Furbetta *et al.* 1979; our unpublished observations).

The haemoglobin findings in individuals with different dominant forms of β thalassaemia are summarized in Table 13.9. Overall, they have levels of HbF in the 3–5% range; their HbA₂ level, while usually elevated, has been almost normal in a few well documented cases.

Haemoglobin synthesis

Several studies have reported α-/non-α-globin synthesis ratios in patients with β thalassaemia intermedia (Bianco *et al.* 1977; Gallo *et al.* 1979; Pippard *et al.* 1982b). They were all carried out before the days when it was possible to determine the underlying mutations and therefore it is impossible to relate these data to more recent work of the molecular pathology of β thalassaemia intermedia. Over recent years it has not been customary to measure globin synthesis ratios in these conditions and therefore

		Hb (g/dl)	MCH (pg)	MCV (fl)	Retics (%)	HbF (%)	HbA₂ (%)	Inc	Phenotype
CD28 T→G (Leu→Arg)	Chesterfield	7–9	30	87	10	3.4	4.0	+(PB)	Transfusion dependent. Splenectomy
CD32 T→G (Leu→Glu)	Medicine Lake	7.8		73	19	6.8	3.4	Nil in PB	Transfusion dependent.
CD98 G→A (Val→Met)									Splenomegaly ++
CD60 T→A (Val→Leu)	Cagliari	6–12	21–35	73–96	15–50	8–16	4.6	+(PB)	Splenectomy. Sporadic transfusion postsplenectomy
CD106 T→G (Leu→Arg)	Terre Haute	4.7–7.4	26	75–93	14	12	2.6	+(PB)	Splenectomy. Transfusion dependent ↑
CD110 T→C (Leu→Pro)	Showa-Yakushiji	7.6–9.8	18–20	56–60	2.4–4	1.3–2.0	5.2	?	
CD114 T→C (Leu→Pro)	Durham NC/Brescia	6–12		72	?	6–7	3.3–5.0	+	Splenectomy. Sporadic transfusions
CD115 C→A (Ala→Asp)	Hradec Kralove	9.6	28	91	↑(?)	4.0	4.2	+	Splenomegaly
		9.8	25	79		13.0	4.0	+	Age 8 months
CD127 A→C (Gln→Pro)	Houston	8–9	21	67	↑	24	4.7	−	Splenectomy
		8.7		80	8	10	5.7	+	Transfusion. Splenectomy
CD127 A→G (Gln→Arg)	Dieppe	7.5		83		18	N		Splenectomized
CD30-31 +CGG (+Arg)	−	9.9	23	79	9.9	1.9	4.9	+	Splenectomized
CD32-34 −GGT (−Val)	Korea	7.0	17	61	4–7	3.6	5.3	Nil (PB)	Splenomegaly (mild)
CD108-112 −12bp	−	10.4		61	12	2.3	4.4	?	
CD124-126 +CCA	−	7–9				<1	5.0		Splenomegaly (mild)
CD127-128 −AGG	Gunma	11.3	20	65	?	3.4	4.3	?	Splenomegaly (moderate)
CD134-137 −12+6	−	10.4	21	79		3.5	4.0	+	Splenomegaly (moderate)
		10.6	21	75	?	2.2	4.8	+	Splenomegaly (severe)
		12.6	24	76	?		5.4	+	Severe→variable. Splenectomy
CD121 G→T (Glu→Term)	−	9–10	18–22	60–6	2–12	2.4–3.9	3.8–4.8	+	Severe→variable. Splenectomy
CD127 C→T (Gln→Term)	−	9.0	24	77	8	4.0	4.2	+	
		10.6	20	65		0.9	4.4		
		11.6	20	62		1.0	5.0		
IVS2-2,3+11,−2	−	9.5	19	60	4.0	3.0	5.3	?	Splenomegaly (moderate)
IVS2-4,5 −AG	−	7.3–11.4	21–24	64–78	2–20	0.8–7.0	3.5–7.0	+(PB)	Splenomegaly in some
CD94+TG	Agnana	6.6	25	70		10	2.2	+	Bone changes. Transfusion. Died aged 27
CD100−CTT, +TCTGAGAACTT	−	9.6		80	3.7	18	2.9	Nil (PB)	Mild thalassaemia intermedia
CD109 −G	Manhattan	8.5	22	67	1.2		4.5	Nil	*Splenectomized
CD114 −CT+G	Geneva	9.5	27	81	36*	2.4	3.6	+	*Splenectomized
		11.6	26	77	42*	1.6			
		10.6	22	70	4.6	3.6	4.0		
		10.5	21	68	5.8	1.6	3.3		
With HbE thalassaemia									
CD103 −A	Makabe	9.1	33	101		12.9	3.7	+	Two sibs died. Splenectomy
CD123-5-ACCCCACC	Khon Kaen	5–8			1–3	3.0			Severe
CD124 −A									Severe. Transfusion dependent
CD125 −A									Splenomegaly (moderate)
CD126 −T	Vercelli	9.0		77		10.8	3.5	+	Splenomegaly (moderate)
Thalassaemia major in homozygote, severe thalassaemia intermedia with HbE									
CD126-131 −17bp	Westdale	11.0	34	95	9.0	3.7	4.1	+	Splenectomy. Iron loading
CD128-129 −4,+5,−11	−	11.8	25	80	2.0	1.3	3.9	+	Splenectomy. Iron loading
		10.7	35	103	19.0	1.4	4.0	+	Splenectomy. Iron loading

MCH, mean cell haemoglobin; MCV, mean cell volume; PB, peripheral blood; Retics, reticulocytes. Main references in Table 4.6, Chapter 4.

there are very few data about the relative degrees of globin imbalance associated with different genotypes. In the earlier studies cited above it was clear that there is relatively less globin imbalance in thalassaemia intermedia compared with transfusion-dependent forms of the disease. Data relating to dominant forms of β thalassaemia are discussed earlier in this chapter.

Other biochemical abnormalities

Apart from a persistent elevation in the bilirubin and serum lactic dehydrogenase levels, there are no consistent biochemical abnormalities which are typical of this condition. Data on serum iron, ferritin and uric acid levels were presented earlier in this chapter.

Clinical features peculiar to the dominant forms of β thalassaemia

This group of patients may sometimes present with a different kind of clinical picture from that observed in other forms of β thalassaemia intermedia. In fact, there have been very few detailed clinical descriptions of these patients followed over a long period of time. However, where this information is available, as evidenced by the first cases to be described (Weatherall *et al*. 1973; Stamatoyannopoulos *et al*. 1974), it is

clear that clinicians must be aware of some of the unexpected complications that may be encountered in what may be, at first sight, a relatively mild disease.

In the three siblings described by Weatherall *et al*. (1973) the apparent mildness of the disease, with steady-state haemoglobin levels in the 10–11 g/dl range, gave no indication of its potential severity. Apart from some tiredness and intermittent jaundice they had no complaints early in their lives until complications of the disease resulted in a wide variety of clinical problems. The only abnormal physical findings were intermittent scleral icterus and moderate splenomegaly; the spleens were palpable between 2 and 4 cm below the costal margin. This apparently mild phenotype was associated with striking morphological abnormalities of the red cells (Fig. 13.11) and intense erythroid hyperplasia of the bone marrow, with some features suggestive of a congenital dyserythropoietic anaemia. On light microscopy, and after staining the marrow with methyl violet, many of the red-cell precursors were shown to contain large inclusions. The electron-microscopic appearances of these inclusions are shown in Fig. 13.11.

There is no doubt that these patients absorbed increased amounts of iron and in one, who died from the complications of cirrhosis and diabetes, an autopsy showed severe iron loading, liver damage with fibrosis and widespread vascular disease resulting from diabetes.

These patients had a normal haemoglobin

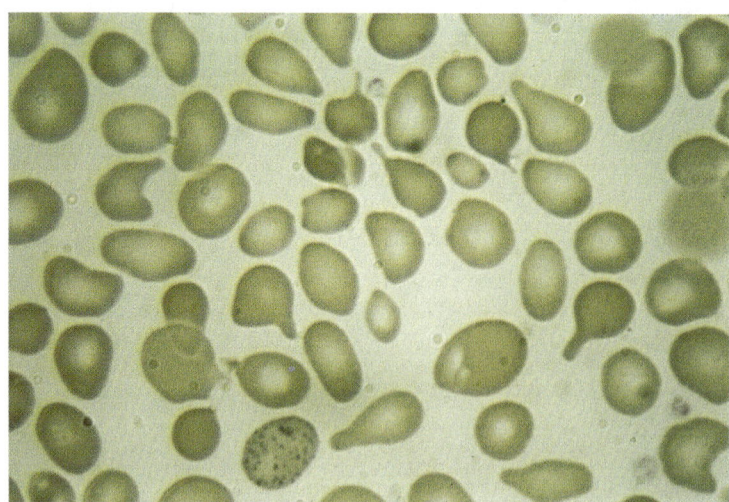

(a)

Fig. 13.11 The peripheral blood picture in dominant β thalassaemia. (a) Red cells showing gross anisopoikilocytosis and basophilic stippling. *Continued.*

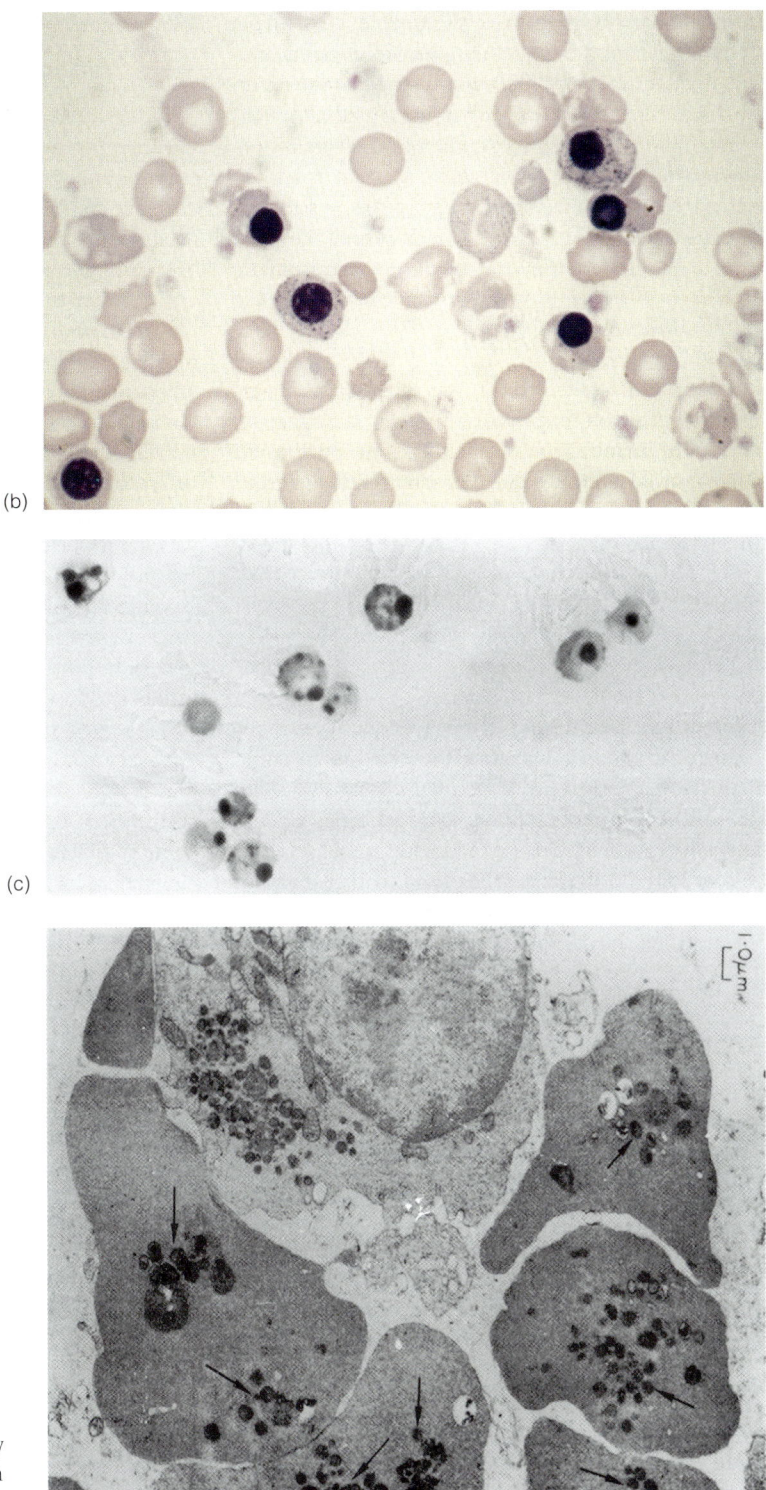

Fig. 13.11 *Continued.* (b) Peripheral blood after splenectomy. (c) Methyl violet stain of blood after splenectomy showing inclusion bodies. (d) Electron micrograph of a red-cell precursor showing diffuse red-cell inclusions. From Weatherall *et al.* (1973).

electrophoresis pattern with slightly elevated values of HbF and moderately, though unequivocally, elevated values of HbA_2. Extensive studies showed no evidence for the presence of an unstable haemoglobin. Globin synthesis, in both the marrow and blood, showed an α/non-α ratio similar to that found in heterozygous β thalassaemia, and it was possible to demonstrate a pool of free α chains in both the bone marrow and the peripheral blood. Detailed kinetic studies of β-globin synthesis revealed no evidence of an unstable haemoglobin variant. Preliminary peptide mapping of the inclusion bodies revealed both α and β chains and this was later confirmed by immuno-electron microscopy (Ho *et al.* 1997). A variety of metabolic studies carried out on the red cells showed abnormalities of electrolyte flux and osmotic fragility, similar to those observed in the β-thalassaemia trait.

It is very important to realize therefore that, although these patients may be only mildly anaemic, they iron-load over many years and they may develop severe tissue damage as evidenced by cirrhosis and diabetes.

Although the studies were less detailed, later reports of patients with dominant β thalassaemia describe many of these features. As shown in Table 13.9, some have been slightly more anaemic, but the striking feature is dyserythropoiesis with inclusion bodies in red-cell precursors and, like other forms of β thalassaemia, only in the peripheral blood after splenectomy. It is also clear that some of these conditions are milder, without severe dyserythropoiesis, and closer to the clinical phenotype of heterozygous β thalassaemia. In others, a haemolytic component seems to predominate over dyserythropoiesis. Presumably, these changes reflect the relative stability of the abnormal β-chain products; these issues were discussed in detail earlier in this chapter and in Chapter 4.

In short, dominant β thalassaemia reflects a family of conditions ranging from severe dyserythropoiesis, splenomegaly and the picture of thalassaemia intermedia, through milder phenotypes of thalassaemia minor, to more florid haemolytic anaemias of a similar kind to those reported for some structural β-globin-chain variants. Their apparently mild phenotypes may lull clinicians into a state of false security; in many cases there may be progressive and potentially life-threatening iron loading.

Population variation in the different forms of thalassaemia intermedia

From our rather limited understanding of the molecular pathology of the intermediate forms of β thalassaemia, it is only possible to make some fairly general statements about the occurrence of its different forms in particular population groups. As mentioned in Chapter 6, only some 20 alleles account for the great majority of all β-thalassaemia determinants. Each population has its own particular varieties of thalassaemia and, as shown in Fig. 13.12, most populations only have one or at most two mild β-thalassaemia alleles. Since, overall, the co-inheritance of α thalassaemia tends to modify the genotype of the interactions of the more severe β-thalassaemia alleles, it is clear that in populations where the two forms of thalassaemia occur together at a high frequency there will be many opportunities for their co-inheritance. Less is known about the distribution of the putative genes that are involved in increasing γ-chain production in the β thalassaemias, except that the $^{G}\gamma$ –158 C →T (*Xmn* I) polymorphism is widespread throughout most parts of the world.

Perhaps the most striking observation that has come from the determination of the world distribution of thalassaemia mutations is the very high frequency of promoter mutations in Africa. This may reflect the evolutionary consequences of there being two different types of alleles at the same locus, which may provide protection against malaria. In Africa the sickle-cell mutation offers a greater degree of protection than β thalassaemia. Furthermore, the compound heterozygous state, sickle-cell β thalassaemia, is a severe disorder except in those cases that are due to the interaction of the β-globin promoter mutations with the sickle-cell gene. In this setting, therefore, these mild β-thalassaemia mutations may have flourished at the expense of more severe ones. But, whatever the mechanism, there is no doubt that β thalassaemia in Africans tends to be of the mild, intermediate variety because of the high frequency of the β-globin-gene promoter mutations.

In the Mediterranean region and the Middle East there is only one common mild β-thalassaemia allele, IVS1-6 T→C. This is spread rather unevenly, being more prevalent in the Portuguese populations, less common in Greece and the Mediterranean islands, and occurring again at a higher fre-

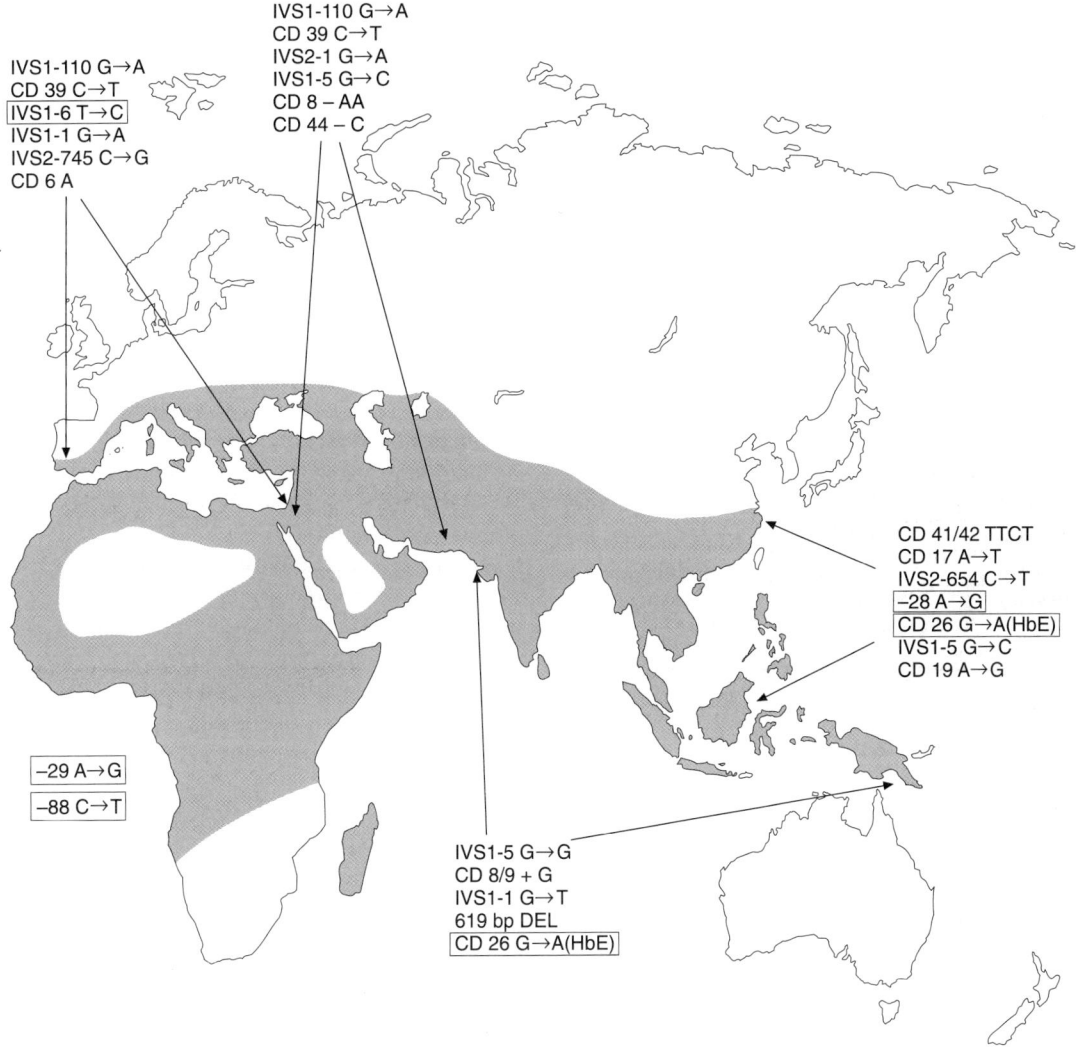

IVS1-110 G→A
CD 39 C→T
IVS2-1 G→A
IVS1-5 G→C
CD 8 – AA
CD 44 – C

IVS1-110 G→A
CD 39 C→T
IVS1-6 T→C
IVS1-1 G→A
IVS2-745 C→G
CD 6 A

CD 41/42 TTCT
CD 17 A→T
IVS2-654 C→T
–28 A→G
CD 26 G→A(HbE)
IVS1-5 G→C
CD 19 A→G

–29 A→G
–88 C→T

IVS1-5 G→G
CD 8/9 + G
IVS1-1 G→T
619 bp DEL
CD 26 G→A(HbE)

Fig. 13.12 World distribution of mild β-thalassaemia alleles. The milder alleles are boxed. Most populations only have one or two mild alleles, the exception being West Africa, where the majority of the alleles are of the mild variety.

quency in Israel. Thus it plays a variable role in generating the phenotype of β thalassaemia intermedia in these regions, and the role of the different α-thalassaemia alleles may be as, or even more, important.

Throughout the eastern half of the Indian subcontinent, Burma and south-east Asia, by far the most important mild thalassaemia allele is HbE. This is responsible for the great majority of cases of β thalassaemia intermedia in these populations although the –28 A→G mutation also occurs fairly frequently.

Since α thalassaemia is particularly common in parts of south-east Asia this also plays a major role in modifying the β thalassaemias in these populations.

Finally, it is clear that in parts of Saudi Arabia and India there is a β-globin-gene haplotype which is associated with an unusually high level of fetal haemoglobin production, both in sickle-cell anaemia and in β thalassaemia. In Chapters 4 and 10 we discussed the question of whether this simply reflects the C→T polymorphism at $^{G}\gamma$ –158 and came to the conclusion that this is not the whole story and that other factors must be involved. Apart from this, we know very little about the world distribution of other genetic factors that are involved in increased α-globin synthesis in the β thalassaemias and related disorders.

Postscript

Over recent years considerable progress has been made towards defining the different genetic interactions that underlie the clinical syndrome of thalassaemia intermedia. Clearly, the major modifiers of the β-thalassaemia phenotype are the co-inheritance of α thalassaemia and a genetically determined ability to increase the output of fetal haemoglobin in adult life. While the localization and identity of the genes that are involved in increased γ-chain production remain to be elucidated, it is clear that several are involved. Furthermore, it is still not absolutely clear whether there are other important genetic modifying factors involved which have not yet been identified. Although variation in the rates of proteolysis of excess α chains has often been suggested (see Chapter 5), there is no hard evidence that this is the case. And, at the time of writing, there are

no other obvious candidate genes to be explored. From such limited sibling-pair data as are available, it appears unlikely that there is another major genetic component to unravel, since most of the heterogeneity between sibships with identical β-globin-gene haplotypes can be related to variation in fetal haemoglobin production. However, it would be dangerous to leave things here and we must continue to search for other genetic factors involved in the heterogeneity of β thalassaemia.

While we have made some genuine progress towards an understanding of the molecular basis for the intermediate phenotype, we have badly neglected its clinical features. We still know very little about the natural history of the disease and of its complications in older patients. In particular, there are very limited data about the rates of iron loading and of its complications, and virtually nothing is known about the pathogenesis and potential complications of the bone disease which is undoubtedly a serious problem for at least some older patients. As described in Chapter 15, these uncertainties about the clinical course and pathophysiology combine to make the optimal type of management one of the major challenges for the thalassaemia field in the future.

Part 4
Diagnosis and management
of thalassaemia

Contributors:
J.M. Old
Nancy F. Olivieri
Swee Lay Thein

Chapter 14
Avoidance and population control

Introduction

As described elsewhere in this book and in several recent reviews (Weatherall & Clegg 1996; Weatherall 1998b), the thalassaemias will assume a major health problem in the new millennium because of the changing demography of disease in many countries. As populations become richer, and standards of nutrition and public health improve, there is a fall in childhood mortality, that is, in the number of deaths that occur during the first 5 years of life. Figures published in 1993 by the World Bank indicate that, with the exception of sub-Saharan Africa, there has been a remarkable decline in childhood mortality throughout the developing world over the last 30 years. Hence, increasing numbers of babies with serious genetic diseases like thalassaemia now survive the early months of life and present for treatment. Throughout the Middle East, the Indian subcontinent and south-east Asia, many thousands of children with thalassaemia will be born each year, most of whom will now live long enough to require treatment.

The consequences of changes of this kind were graphically illustrated in Cyprus, a country that underwent this kind of demographic transition shortly after the Second World War. Thalassaemia was not identified in Cyprus until 1944, when, after a major malaria eradication programme and accompanying improvements in public health measures, it became clear that among the children on the island there was a common form of anaemia which was not due to infection (Fawdry 1944). By the early 1970s it was estimated that, if no steps were taken to control the disease, in about 40 years' time the blood required to treat all the severely affected children would amount to 78'000 units per annum, 40% of the population would be donors, and the total cost to the health services would equal or exceed the island's health budget (WHO 1983; Modell & Berdoukas 1984).

In recent projections of the changing patterns of disease burden for the new millennium, compiled by the World Bank and WHO and assessed in DALYs (disability-adjusted life years), 'congenital anomalies' rank 13th for the disease burden for demographically developed countries (*World Development Report*, World Bank 1993). Thalassaemia and the other major haemoglobinopathies were not included in these tables because it was felt that insufficient is known about their frequency in different populations (Dr Christopher Murray, personal communication). Unfortunately, this is true and, as pointed out in Chapter 6, work over recent years has focused on the molecular pathology of the disease rather than its frequency and distribution among different populations.

Despite these uncertainties there are at least some indications of the magnitude of the problem that will be faced in some parts of the world, south-east Asia for example. By 1969 it was known that there were more than 60 varieties of thalassaemia in Thailand and that there were over a quarter of a million symptomatic children in the population (Wasi *et al.* 1969). More recently it has been estimated that, over the next 30 years, approximately 100'000 new cases of HbE β thalassaemia alone will be added to the Thai population; if the World Bank's estimate of a population increase in that country between 1991 and 2025 of 57 to close to 100 million is correct, this figure may be a gross underestimate. In Indonesia, in which the Bank estimates a population increase from 180 to close to 300 million, the situation will be even more serious. In a preliminary survey of approximately 15 of the island populations it has been estimated that, if all the homozygous β thalassaemics and about half of the patients with HbE β thalassaemia are given regular transfusions, approximately 1.25 million units of blood will be needed each year (unpublished observations). And from what little is known of the gene frequencies for these diseases in other parts of south-east Asia and the Indian subcontinent, taken together with the World Bank estimates for population increases, it is clear that there will be a massive expansion of the populations of children requiring expensive treatment for thalassaemia.

This problem has been addressed by a number of WHO Working Parties (WHO 1983, 1985, 1987, 1989a, 1994), much of the work of which is summarized in an excellent review by Angastiniotis and Modell (1998). Based on the limited amount of gene frequency data available to them it was concluded that, world-wide, there may be something in the order of 269 million carriers for the important haemoglobin disorders, the bulk of which live in south-east Asia, where the thalassaemias are most common, with Africa coming next with its very high frequency of sickling disorders. It was further estimated that approximately 365'000 infants are born each year with major haemoglobin disorders. Because of the limited information about gene frequencies these are probably minimal estimates: taken together with the World Bank's estimates of the future increase in size of populations, the greatest of which are likely to occur in high-frequency regions for thalassaemia (Fig. 14.1), the position may change considerably over the next 20 years. Much will depend on birth rates, which tend to fall as countries become richer. But, however these figures are looked at, there is no doubt that this new millennium will see a major increase in the frequency of babies born with severe forms of thalassaemia.

It was the realization of the enormous burden on health resources that would be posed by the thalassaemias that, in the 1970s, led a number of Mediterranean countries and some of the industrialized Western countries with large immigrant populations to think about how thalassaemia might be controlled at the population level. Their experience over the last 20 years has provided a valuable baseline for future planning for its control in the larger mainland populations of the Middle East, Indian subcontinent and south-east Asia.

Strictly speaking, we should talk about 'avoiding' rather than 'preventing' genetic diseases like thalassaemia. There is no way we can prevent genetic disease; mutations occur all the time and inherited disorders are simply the scars that we carry from evolution working through mutation and natural selection to make us what we are. If we wish to avoid recessive genetic diseases like the thalassaemias we have to identify carriers in the community and provide them with appropriate genetic counselling. There are several different options available to them.

They might wish to avoid marrying a similarly affected person. Alternatively, if two carriers marry they could avoid having children altogether, adopt, have children in the hope that they will be fortunate enough not to have a severely affected child, or undergo prenatal diagnosis with termination of those pregnancies in which the fetus has received a thalassaemia gene from both of them.

In this chapter we shall discuss the mechanisms and logistics of screening and counselling and describe the methods that can be used for prenatal diagnosis and how effective they are. But before we do so we thought it important to introduce this topic by a brief discussion of some of the ethical and pastoral issues that have to be considered before embarking on this type of programme.

Are programmes for the control of thalassaemia justified? The ethical issues

In the period during which ideas about population screening and prenatal diagnosis for the control of thalassaemia have evolved there has been increasing concern about the ethical issues arising from the 'new genetics'; fears which are voiced in an extensive literature to which we shall refer in later sections. Yet despite the fact that the term 'new genetics' stemmed directly from the discovery of a restriction-fragment-length DNA polymorphism in linkage disequilibrium with the sickle-cell gene, and the concept that genetic variability of this type might be used to map the human genome to facilitate the pinpointing of genes for different diseases, the haemoglobin disorders do not figure highly in these writings. Rather, most of these ethical discussions focus on monogenic diseases and multigenic disorders which are common in richer Western societies. When the haemoglobinopathies are discussed it is usually in the context of the problems and dangers of stigmatization in immigrant populations. But, because the thalassaemias and other common haemoglobin disorders occur widely and in such diverse ethnic groups, the ethical issues that relate to programmes for their avoidance are, in fact, much more complex and multifaceted.

Eugenic concerns

The reasons for the increasing public concern over modern molecular genetics are not always easy to

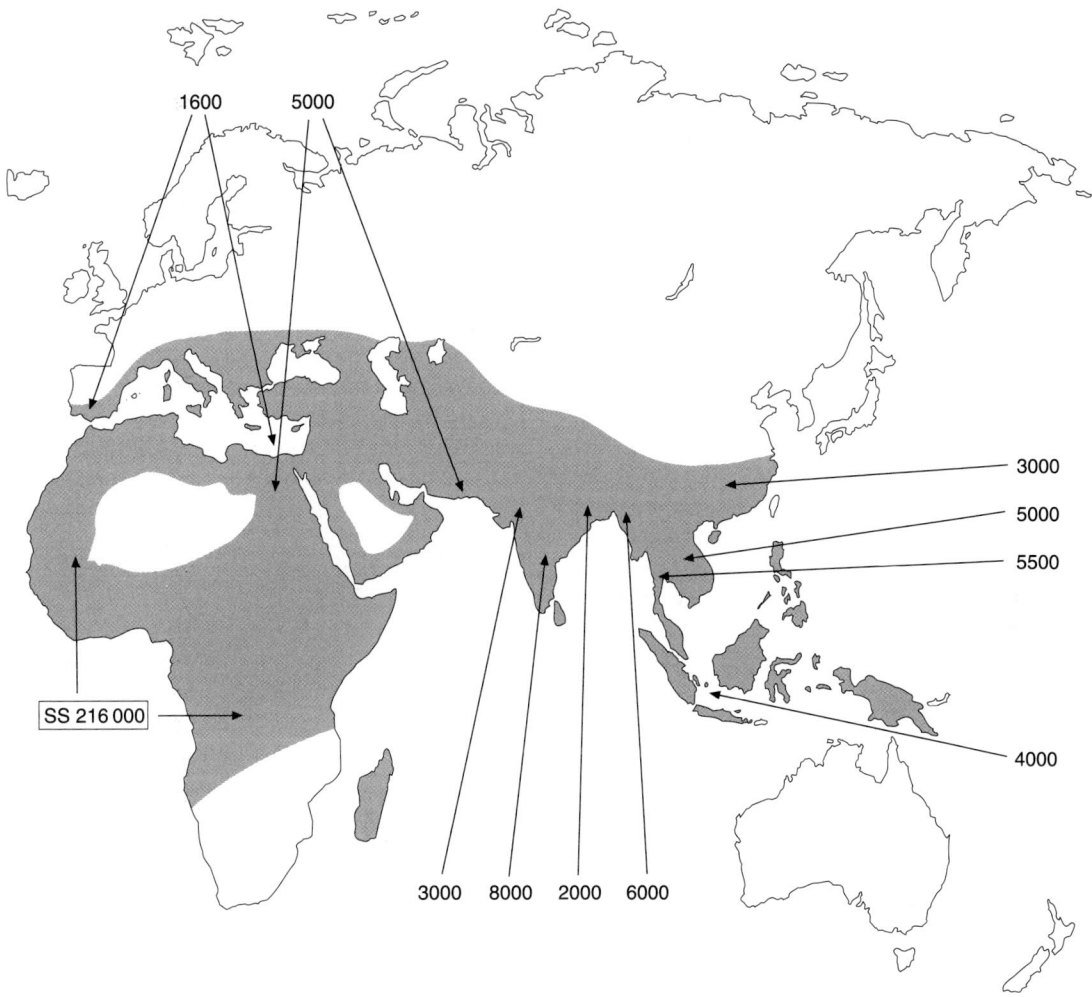

Fig. 14.1 Some estimated annual numbers of new births of thalassaemia or sickle-cell anaemia. All the figures shown are for severe forms of thalassaemia except for those for Africa, which refer to sickle-cell anaemia. These data are taken from some of the WHO estimations referenced in the text and from the authors' unpublished studies. They do not give any indication of the total problem that will be posed by thalassaemia and the sickling disorders, but simply highlight some gross approximations for certain high-frequency areas.

define. Our increasing ability to isolate genes and the potentials of genetic manipulation have made society uneasy. Where might this facility to meddle with our genetic make-up take us? Many of these fears are based on the fear of eugenics, a movement started at the end of the nineteenth century in Great Britain by Francis Galton. Galton invented the word, which literally means 'well born', to describe the improvement of the human species by selective breeding. He collected pedigrees which purported to show how a

variety of 'desirable' traits appear to segregate within families, those of eminent statesmen for example. He believed therefore that such people should be encouraged to breed, while those who were less gifted or fortunate should be discouraged. This movement caught on for a time in many countries. In the United States, under the auspices of John D. Rockefeller, Charles Davenport established the Eugenics Record Office in Cold Spring Harbor, to which young men and women came for courses for training in human heredity and field research techniques. Once indoctrinated, they were sent off into the community with a 'trait book'. The information that they collected was returned to the Eugenics Record Office and duly catalogued. By 1914 at least 30 states had enacted new marriage laws, which restricted marriage among the unfit of various categories. The first State Sterilization Act was passed as early as 1907, and over the next 10 years similar laws were enacted by 15 or more states. In 1924 an act based on eugenic principles was passed and signed into law by President Coolidge, who, when Vice-President, had declared 'America must be kept American. Biological laws show . . . that Nordics deteriorate when mixed with other races.' By the end of the first half of the last century the eugenics movement was active in many countries and had taken many different forms (Adams 1990).

By the end of World War II, and with the dissemination of the news of the atrocities carried out in Germany in the cause of eugenics, the movement tended to peter out. However, those who have shown concern about the more recent developments in medical genetics, particularly population screening and prenatal diagnosis, have used the rather emotive term 'the new eugenics' to describe these activities (discussed by Kevles 1985). It is beyond the scope of this book to discuss this concept in detail. However, since the thalassaemias are the only disorders for which there has been a global effort to introduce programmes for the avoidance of a genetic disease, it is important that we review briefly some of these concerns and discuss what we are attempting to achieve in the context of the ethical frameworks which have been drawn up to safeguard activities of this kind.

Is it right to avoid genetic diseases by screening and prenatal diagnosis?

To what extent, if at all, is it right to avoid genetic disease? The extreme view is, of course, that under no circumstances should parents be allowed to decide to avoid or terminate a pregnancy in which the baby has a serious genetic handicap. Rather, society should look after these children, many of whom, it is said, can lead happy and fulfilled lives if properly cared for. Arguments of this type are not confined to those who have had no experience of dealing with sick children, but are often voiced by patients with thalassaemia

who have received good medical care and who live in a society which can afford it. Indeed, it would be surprising if these attitudes were not common among patients, doctors and thoughtful members of society, regardless of whether they are based on religious or humanistic beliefs. After all, doctors are trained to preserve life, and to many the idea of terminating a pregnancy on medical grounds is an anathema. On the other hand, equally caring physicians and colleagues maintain that, if we have the knowledge, parents with the potential for having a genetically abnormal child should be allowed to decide what kind of children they wish to bring into the world. Has society the right to deny them the choice if medical progress has made it possible?

Some of those who believe that termination of pregnancy for genetic disability is wrong take their case to the extreme. Surely, they argue, physical disability is not always a bad thing. Some of our greatest creative artists suffered in this way. Is it right to terminate a pregnancy and risk losing a Beethoven? Appleyard (1993) has emphasized how irrational these arguments can become. He quotes from G.K. Chesterton, an author who had an intense fear of the eugenics movement: 'Keats died young; but he had more pleasure in a minute than eugenecists get in a month.' Appleyard points out that a genius with tuberculosis is a phenomenon we like to feel is beyond any rational balancing of probabilities, and that it is natural therefore to imagine that an aborted fetus or a pregnancy prevented by genetic counselling might have become a Keats or an Einstein. He is right, of course: we are all irrational at times, but arguments along these lines do not help us in a serious debate about the global control of genetic disease.

Religious beliefs

Since the thalassaemias occur in such widely diverse ethnic groups, one of the major issues in thinking about mechanisms for their control must be the attitude of different religions to activities like screening and prenatal diagnosis. This is a difficult and sensitive topic, not least because what appears to be the official teaching of a particular religion is often interpreted quite differently by those who practise it. Of the various branches of Christianity, the Roman Catholic Church's formal position is very clear; there should be no interference with a pregnancy, whatever the reason. The attitude of different branches of Christianity to these questions have been well exemplified in Cyprus and Sardinia (Cao & Rosatelli 1993). When screening and prenatal diagnosis were being established in Cyprus, the Orthodox Church contributed greatly to their overall success by encouraging premarital carrier screening and developing formal education programmes in the school curricula. In contrast, in Sardinia, the Roman Catholic Church assumed what Cao and Rosatelli describe as 'an uninterested attitude' towards a similar campaign. Presumably much the same must be happening in other parts of Italy. For example, new cases of β thalassaemia are now extremely unusual in Ferrara, almost entirely due to a control programme which was instituted some 20 years ago. Since the Roman Catholic Church has not changed its views on the control of genetic disease this state of affairs presumably reflects both a 'laissez-faire' attitude on the part of the Church and the emergence of an increasingly secular society.

Although it is widely believed that Islam does not permit any form of interference with the natural course of events it appears that this may not be the case (El-Hashemite *et al.* 1997). The Muslim jurisconsults, both Sunni and She'at, have agreed that, if genetic tests prove definitely that a fetus is affected by serious disease which will keep a baby disabled after birth, abortion is permissible and lawful. More specifically, they stipulate that a pregnancy can only be terminated before the time of 'breathing the soul', that is, before 120 days' gestation. However, as pointed out by Salihu (1997), the situation is not quite as straightforward as this. Working in Cameroon he found that it is extremely difficult to convince a Muslim population with a high illiteracy rate that Islamic jurisconsults in Western capitals have found that it is permissible to condone the termination of pregnancy. These people tend to believe only what their local imams (that is, Muslim leaders) tell them, and follow it to the letter. Certainly, in the experience of Salihu, most of them are strongly against termination of any form of life, regardless of its relationship to the breathing of the soul.

Recently, Ghanei *et al.* (1997) have reported on their experiences of population screening in the Isfahan province of Iran, a largely Islamic country. Over 100000 individuals preparing for marriage were screened for β-thalassaemia trait and at-risk couples were referred for further consultation. After the project had been running for 3 years the proportion of high-risk couples initially deciding not to marry was 90% and no new cases of thalassaemia were detected in the children of the population which was screened.' This remarkable outcome raises some important issues which require further investigation. For example, the authors write: 'those couples where both members had the trait who wanted to marry would have to register their marriage and perform the religious ceremony in another area outside the district of Isfahan.' This was because the clergymen and marriage offices had agreed not to register such couples (due to the high risk of birth of a child with major thalassaemia and the prohibition of abortion and the risks associated with illegal abortion). In the discussion of this paper the authors suggest that the high rate of those choosing not to marry, 90% compared with less than 10% in Cyprus, may be related to the Iranian custom of there being no long-term relationships between couples before marriage. However, while this may be the case, it is not absolutely clear from this paper how much pressure was brought to bear on these couples not to marry; the fact that they could not marry in their own province if they were both carriers must surely have had a major effect on their decision.

The experiences in countries which have large Buddhist populations are reviewed by Wasi and Fucharoen (1995). They describe the situation as it exists in Thailand and also touch briefly on Sri Lanka, a country in which one of the present authors has had considerable experience. The form of Buddhism in these populations, Theravada, has the same root. The first Buddhist precept is to refrain from killing. But, although many Buddhists equate abortion with killing human beings, the Thai population in general do not adhere strictly to this precept as it relates to abortion, but for medical purposes. Indeed, Thai law permits abortion only when continuation of the pregnancy might be life-threatening to the mother; there is no provision for or discussion about the condition of the fetus. Despite this, prenatal diagnosis for thalassaemia is established, so far largely for couples who have had previously affected children. However, there continues to be a debate on the ethical issues involved; some Thai doctors do not accept that termination of pregnancy is consistent with the Buddhist faith. On the other hand Wasi and Fucharoen quote one distinguished Buddhist scholar who had a child with thalassaemia as advocating prenatal diagnosis and selective abortion. In Sri Lanka the Buddhist precepts are more strictly interpreted and prenatal diagnosis is not allowed. However, this may reflect a complex interplay between politicians and monks, rather than public inclination. The whole question is still under discussion, however. The Hindu faiths seem to have a similar approach to these questions. Overall, however, it appears that these two religions accept prenatal diagnosis under some circumstances and this raises tensions in populations in which where there is a mix of Buddhist, Hindu and Islamic religions.

At the present time, therefore, it appears that many of the world's religions are still struggling to define their attitudes to genetic diagnosis and termination of pregnancy, but, even when they do, their teachings may take a long time to percolate down to the population, particularly in societies with high illiteracy rates. Wasi and Fucharoen (1995) note that patients from strictly Muslim societies often come to Thailand or other countries where prenatal diagnosis is permissible. It appears that, just as is the case in Roman Catholic Italy, parents of thalassaemic children from Islamic countries, particularly if they are well informed, are increasingly seeking out this kind of service.

In many societies it is now generally accepted that prenatal diagnosis followed by termination of pregnancies for a severe disease like β thalassaemia is an acceptable option if the parents wish it. Even in these populations there will, of course, be those who do not think that it is right, based on religious or other arguments. The position in other parts of the world is more complex, and continually shifting.

Dysgenic effects

One of the major concerns about any form of medical intervention for genetic disease is the possibility that it will result in an increase in the size of the pool of abnormal genes in a population. This is a very complex issue, which is discussed in detail by Bodmer and Cavalli-Sforza (1976) and more recently in a thoughtful paper by Modell and Kuliev (1989).

There are many factors which have to be taken into account when considering future changes in frequency for the different forms of thalassaemia. As pointed out in Chapter 6, there is now very strong evidence that the high frequency of the α thalassaemias has been maintained because of resistance of those

with milder forms of the disease to *Plasmodium vivax* and *P. falciparum* malaria, and, although there are fewer data, it seems very likely that the β thalassaemias and HbE have come under the same selective pressure. Thus before we even consider the effects of direct medical intervention for the treatment or avoidance of thalassaemia it is important to remember that malaria eradication programmes will undoubtedly have a major, if slow, effect on the frequency of the thalassaemias in the future. And even here there are uncertainties because at the present time these programmes are failing, partly due to neglect but also due to the emergence of resistant strains of parasites and their mosquito vectors. But, assuming that it is possible to slowly eradicate malaria, Bodmer and Cavalli-Sforza point out that, in populations where thalassaemia has an incidence of about 1%, this figure would be halved in five generations, and halved again in five more generations if the selective force of malaria were removed. It follows that any potential dysgenic effects due to medical interventions directed against thalassaemia are likely to be counterbalanced, at least to some degree, if malaria eradication programmes become more successful again in the future (Fig. 14.2).

When considering the possible dysgenic effects of programmes for carrier detection and prenatal diagnosis of the thalassaemias, a number of other complex issues have to be taken into account. There is no doubt that in some communities families that have had offspring with serious genetic diseases tend to have large numbers of children in order to ensure that they have sufficient normal ones to care for their older relatives and to act as breadwinners. It is usually held that, if all pregnancies carrying severely affected infants are aborted, the gene frequency for the particular disorder will increase in the population. This is because homozygotes are replaced by healthy individuals, two-thirds of whom are heterozygous and hence will pass on their genes. But, as pointed out by Modell *et al.* (1997), this assumes that couples undergoing prenatal diagnosis will attain the population norm for their final family size. Such evidence as there is suggests that this may not be the case; studies in Cyprus, for example, showed that approximately 25% of the decrease in thalassaemic births is due to limited reproduction.

Overall then, the changes in the size of the thalassaemia gene pool that might follow interventions of this kind are likely to be extremely small. The situa-

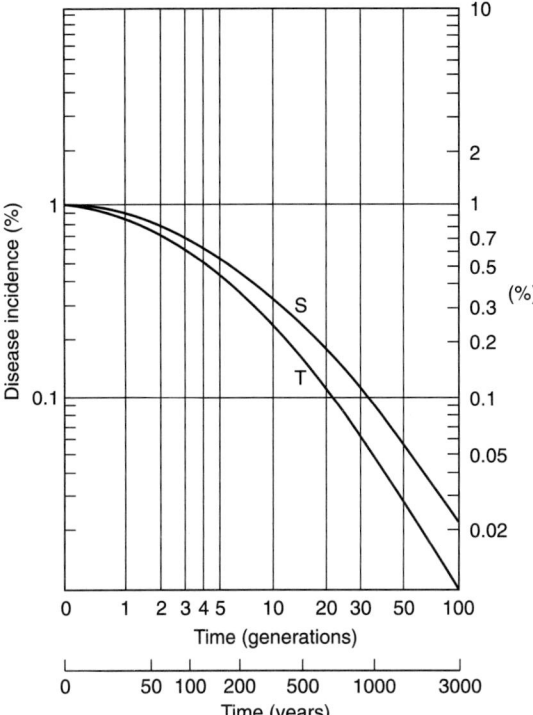

Fig. 14.2 Theoretical fall in incidence of sickle-cell anaemia (S) and thalassaemia (T) following malaria control. From Bodmer and Cavalli-Sforza (1976).

tion is summed up by Bodmer and Cavalli-Sforza (1976) as follows:

> It would seem therefore that the dysgenic effect of medicine is not a real threat. By the time it may have a clearly perceptible global effect, 200 or 300 years from now—when the incidence of severe genetic disease may have doubled on average—our descendants almost certainly will have discovered simple methods of therapy, unless our civilization will have been destroyed by its own lack of wisdom!

An ethical basis for developing screening and prenatal diagnosis programmes

Western medical practice is founded on four ethical principles: autonomy, that is, a patient's right to make their own choices; non-maleficence, the avoidance of harm; beneficience, or doing good; and justice, which requires doctors to act fairly with their patients. In practice, an analysis of a particular ethical problem is based on three interconnected sets of arguments (O'Neill 1991). The duty-based approach simply follows the history and tradition of the medical profession and the norms which are laid down for it by its professional bodies, the General Medical Council in the UK for example. The second principle involves the rights-based approach, which has it that the autonomy of the individual patient is paramount; they have an absolute right to determine their own destiny even in circumstances in which others may judge that the proposed action may be against their best interest. Finally, there is the utilitarianist approach, based on the 'greatest happiness principle', first enunciated by Jeremy Bentham and John Stuart Mill. This was a school of philosophy that weighed actions in terms of consequences; something is right if it promotes good consequences and wrong if it promotes bad ones. In a medical setting this is particularly relevant to the imposition of burdens on individuals for the benefit of others.

Based on these broad principles, and with specific problems of population screening and prenatal diagnosis in mind, a number of bodies have set out useful ethical frameworks on which to develop programmes of this type (Council for International Organizations of Medical Sciences 1991; European Commission 1991; American Association for the Advancement of Science 1992; Nuffield Council on Bioethics 1993; Advisory Committee on Genetic Testing 1997). While the principles set out by some of these working groups and committees are of considerable value for some Western societies, it is quite clear that each country will, within the overall blanket of international practice, have to develop guidelines which are relevant to its particular social and religious beliefs and norms.

Most of the guidelines which have been established are based on the same general principles. There is an overwhelming consensus that adequately informed consent must be a requirement for all genetic screening programmes. It follows that, if it is to be genuinely 'informed' consent, any screening programme must be preceded and backed up by an education programme for the population at large, with the provision of detailed but simply understood information for individual patients and their families. This is best delivered in both written and oral forms. When informed consent cannot be obtained, particularly in the case of children, their parents should act for them. In the case of adults where this is not possible, the mentally subnormal for example, screening should not be carried out unless it is to the clear benefit of the family. The second and equally important recommendation is that screening programmes must be accompanied by adequate counselling for all those who are being screened. Furthermore, counselling must be available at all stages of the screening process.

In disclosing the outcome of screening it is regarded as axiomatic that individuals should be fully informed, not just about the particular result but of all its implications for both themselves and their families. In addition, accepted standards of confidentiality of all medical information must be followed as far as possible. When genetic screening reveals information that may have serious implications for the relatives of those who have been screened it is essential that counsellors explain why this should be communicated to other family members; they should always try to persuade the individual to allow the disclosure of this information. In the UK both the law and professional guidelines provide for exceptional circumstances, particularly when an individual cannot be persuaded to inform family members with a legitimate right to know. In such cases an individual's desire for confidentially may be overridden. But this decision can only be made case by case.

The question of whether it is necessary to disclose carrier status for the thalassaemias prior to employment rarely arises. As regards insurance, in many countries it has been recommended that insurance companies should adhere to their current policy of not requiring any genetic tests as a prerequisite for obtaining insurance. This question is under discussion, however. In the UK the advice of an expert committee to continue along these lines was turned down by the government. We have been involved in at least two cases in which patients with β-thalassaemia trait have had their insurance policies loaded, an occurrence that indicates the extraordinary ignorance about this condition on the part of insurance companies, certainly in countries in which the thalassaemias are not particularly common.

These relatively simple and common-sense guidelines are adhered to in most Western and Mediterranean populations. However, premarital screening for thalassaemia is required by law in northern Cyprus, and in China rigorous requirements for couples with a family history of genetic disease are

at an advanced stage of discussion. Whether the consensus of the international community will persuade the Chinese government to change its mind remains to be seen. These trends are worrying because they seem to remove one of the essential premises on which the ethics of medical practice have evolved, that is, the principle of individual freedom. However, this question may become extremely complicated, even in populations in which prenatal testing is not mandatory. For example, when the uptake of prenatal diagnosis is very high, families that opt to continue to have affected children may find themselves stigmatized by their societies. It is essential to carefully monitor these issues within particular populations.

Readers who wish to learn more about the ethical issues and other concerns about population screening and prenatal diagnosis, particularly as they relate to notions about the resurgence of eugenics, are referred to a number of monographs on this subject, all of which are directed at general readers (Kevles & Hood 1992; Jones 1993; Wilkie 1993; Bodmer & McKie 1994).

Screening

Although screening programmes for β thalassaemia have been well established in some countries for over 20 years, and a great deal of experience has been gained, there are still formidable difficulties to be overcome, particularly when considering approaches to screening large rural populations in the less developed countries.

Under what circumstances is a screening programme of value?

The criteria to be considered before setting up a screening programme for β thalassaemia are set out in detail in a report of a WHO Working Party (1994). Clearly it must be preceded by an estimation of the gene frequency for thalassaemia in the particular population. Since, as discussed in Chapter 6, the distribution of the disease may be extremely patchy, even in small countries, or it may be confined to certain immigrant groups, it is very important to try to obtain an adequate overall spectrum of its frequency, and only to develop screening programmes if they are likely to be cost-effective.

The WHO Working Group recommend that in

developed countries carrier screening, counselling and prenatal diagnosis services should be provided as part of the general health-care programme, whatever the frequency of the disorders. Currently, there is a wide range of variability in the effectiveness of programmes of this type. Perhaps the gold standard is the Montreal thalassaemia screening programme, developed as part of a broader service for genetic disease, which was initiated by Scriver and his colleagues (Scriver *et al.* 1984; Wilkie 1993; Mitchell *et al.* 1996). Experiences with a similar programme, though with a different approach to case finding, are reported by Rowley *et al.* (1985, 1990). However, such programmes, particularly if expanded to encompass larger populations, must be backed up by properly organized screening programmes and a well developed policy by those who provide health services. Modell *et al.* (1997), in an audit carried out in the UK, have shown how variation in the adequacy of screening and counselling services in different parts of the country and in different ethnic groups can result in a very wide range of outcomes. While some health authorities in the UK run adequate screening programmes, others do not and this is clearly reflected in the frequency of new cases of β thalassaemia in the population.

The decision as to whether to develop a screening programme in less developed countries is more complicated. The WHO Working Party concluded that the need for a national control programme only begins to be considered when the infant mortality has fallen to the range of 20–40/1000, a level at which many infants with β thalassaemia survive. The need for the development of a screening programme then depends on a number of factors, particularly the birth rate of affected infants. The WHO suggest that if this exceeds 0.1/1000 there is a strong case for developing a programme. However, many other factors have to be taken into account, notably the level of development of the infrastructure of the health provision system and the type of health care, that is, whether there is a government-based health service or whether care is mainly organized by the private sector. In the latter case the establishment of screening programmes is much more difficult.

Who should be screened?

Genetic screening may be retrospective or prospective. Retrospective screening, that is, testing and

giving advice to a couple who have already had an affected child, is ineffective and has relatively little influence on the birth rate of new cases of thalassaemia. Prospective screening can either be done in the antenatal clinic or at an earlier stage. While screening in the antenatal clinic is carried out in many countries it has the disadvantage that women are already pregnant and have the added burden of decision placed on them. Furthermore, many women present too late in pregnancy to allow many options. Hence, many countries in which there is a particularly high frequency of β thalassaemia have opted to try to develop screening programmes in the community so that carriers may be given both the time and information on which to plan the future of their families.

Some of the most advanced population screening programmes have been developed in Montreal, Sardinia, Greece and Cyprus. Experiences from the Montreal programme suggest that the most effective way to develop a national screening programme is through schools, directed at students in the 14–18 years range, on a voluntary basis (Mitchell *et al.* 1996; Capua 1998). Using a programme of this type, with a participation rate varying between 70 and 80%, between 1980 and 1992 over 25'000 students were screened and nearly 700 carriers were detected. The Montreal programme, which is firmly based on the ethical principles outlined earlier in this chapter, seems to have been successful largely because of the excellent educational programme that accompanies it. The incidence rate of newly diagnosed cases of β thalassaemia has fallen by 90% since its inception. An account of the management of the educational and clinical sessions involved in this programme is given by Capua (1998).

The remarkably successful screening programme in Sardinia is described by Cao and Rosatelli (1993) and Cao (1994). This has involved a major public education programme. It has been estimated that most of the spouses were well informed about β thalassaemia via the mass media (approximately 44% of the population), general practitioners (31%) and obstetricians (23%). Similar public education programmes have been established in Cyprus, where an annual thalassaemia week is organized and magazines and numerous pamphlets are issued. Meetings between physicians, particularly paediatricians and obstetricians, family planning associations, nurses and social workers appear to have been an important part of these education programmes. Similarly, the use of information booklets, which include details on how and when to be tested for thalassaemia, have been made available at various centres, including marriage register offices, doctors' surgeries and family planning clinics. In both Greece and Cyprus formal education on inherited anaemias has been introduced into the school curricula. In Cyprus and Italy programmes directed at adolescent school children have also been established (see Angastiniotis & Hadjiminas 1981; Bianco *et al.* 1985).

Establishing a screening strategy

Although there are disadvantages, as described earlier, the establishment of a screening programme for pregnant women when they first present for antenatal care, together with offering testing for partners of carriers so detected, is probably the linchpin of most screening programmes. Even if a successful community screening programme is established it will require an antenatal component of this type, both as a backup and for confirmation of individuals identified in the community programme. It requires a major education campaign for obstetricians, nurses and midwives, and for haematologists or others who carry out the laboratory work.

Certainly in high-frequency regions one or other forms of population screening should be developed at the same time. Both these approaches may be augmented with what is sometimes called 'cascade screening', that is, the study of as many relatives as possible of carriers who have been ascertained, either in the community or in the antenatal clinic.

Finally, the question is often raised as to whether these forms of screening should be augmented by a neonatal screening programme. This is not particularly effective in the case of the thalassaemias. However, it is an important part of the haemoglobinopathy programme in populations in which the sickle-cell gene is common. The diagnosis of sickle-cell disease or sickle-cell β thalassaemia should be made as soon after birth as possible because of the importance of the early administration of prophylactic penicillin and immunization against infection (see next chapter).

Methods for screening

A general approach to screening for the different forms of thalassaemia is considered in Chapter 16. Whatever variety of thalassaemia is being screened the principles are the same. The initial screen is based on changes in the red cells and is followed up by one or more confirmatory tests which analyse the haemoglobin constitution.

The initial screen

By far the best screening method for the different carrier forms of thalassaemia is the measurement of the red-cell indices, that is, the mean cell volume (MCV) and mean cell haemoglobin (MCH). Unfortunately, at least in terms of cost, reliable measurements of red-cell indices require the use of electronic cell counters. It is not possible to count red cells sufficiently accurately in any other way and without a precise red-cell count the indices are completely unreliable. A number of studies have analysed the values for the MCH and MCV below which it is essential to carry out confirmatory tests for thalassaemia. It is now generally accepted that blood samples with an MCH below 27 pg or an MCV below 76–77 fl should be investigated further (Scriver *et al.* 1984; Rowley *et al.* 1985; WHO 1985, 1994). As described in Chapter 7, a recent study directed at the analysis of the sensitivity of this approach to the diagnosis of β thalassaemia in pregnancy suggested that, although it may involve a larger number of confirmatory HbA_2 estimations, cut-off values for the MCV and MCH of 80 fl and 27 pg, respectively, would detect virtually all affected women (Weatherall and Letsky 2000). While this is certainly true for the majority of the severe thalassaemia alleles, except when co-inherited with α thalassaemia, as described in Chapters 7 and 13, there is a wide spectrum of MCV and MCH values associated with the mild β-thalassaemia alleles; some typical values are illustrated in Chapter 7. This may be another reason for raising the discriminatory levels to those suggested by Weatherall and Letsky (2000).

Alternative approaches to the initial screen

As described in Chapter 1 Silvestroni and Bianco and their colleagues in Rome developed a single-tube osmotic-fragility screen as a simple approach to carrying out thalassaemia screening in large populations. While this has undoubtedly been a valuable tool it is not easy to standardize. In a more recent description and critique of the method its value was again promoted (Kattamis *et al.* 1981a). These authors give very precise instructions and the conditions required to make this test useful in clinical practice. However, it does give false negatives as well as positives and any country contemplating setting up a screening programme for β thalassaemia should think very carefully before using this approach. After all, electronic cell counters are becoming cheaper, servicing is available in most parts of the world, and the cost of missing the diagnosis, not to mention the potentially tragic consequences for individual families, is such that the osmotic-fragility approach cannot be recommended. This question is discussed further in Chapter 16.

Recently, Escuredo *et al.* (2000) have found that β-thalassaemia carriers and heterozygotes and homozygotes for HbE have reduced levels of red-cell pyrimidine-5′-nucleotidase activity. There is no overlap with normal levels and the results are not modified by iron deficiency. Preliminary studies suggest that the level of the enzyme is not decreased to a diagnostic level in the different carrier states for α thalassaemia. The precise role of this new assay is not yet established. It undoubtedly has the potential for simplification and automation and it may be possible to link it to a colour change reaction. This will depend on whether it can be exploited commercially and, ultimately, on the cost of any standardized diagnostic kit which could be produced.

Further investigations after the initial screen

Samples with reduced MCH or MCV values should be studied further. The first step is to measure the HbA$_2$ level. The HbA$_2$ values in β-thalassaemia trait are discussed in detail in Chapter 7. Clearly, they will differ slightly depending on the method used but most of the techniques that are described in Chapter 16 give a cut-off figure of about 3.5%, above which the diagnosis of β-thalassaemia trait is almost always secure. The major problem in screening programmes is what to do about values of HbA$_2$ in the 'no-man's land' of 3–3.5%. This problem is also discussed in Chapter 7. Because a high proportion of these cases turn out to be forms of mild β thalassaemia, or interactions between α and β thalassaemia, the answer is to investigate them further. It should be emphasized that, although early studies suggested that iron deficiency might be capable of reducing the HbA$_2$ level

in β-thalassaemia trait into the normal range, subsequent experience has indicated that this almost never happens (Galanello *et al.* 1981).

At this stage in the screening process normal samples and those with a clear-cut diagnosis of β-thalassaemia trait will have been identified. The next problem is what to do with samples with a reduced MCH and MCV but with normal HbA$_2$ levels. This usually reflects either iron deficiency, different forms of α thalassaemia or, less commonly, β thalassaemia with a normal HbA$_2$ level. Although a wide variety of mathematical treatments have been used to distinguish iron deficiency from thalassaemia trait, none have become widely used in clinical practice (see Chapter 16). At this stage, therefore, it is important to measure the serum iron or ferritin levels and, if iron deficiency is found, to give a course of treatment with iron and then measure the red-cell indices again. Incidentally, it should be emphasized that, if iron deficiency is severe enough to reduce the red-cell indices to those typical of β-thalassaemia trait, the haemoglobin level is usually considerably lower than that observed in β-thalassaemia carriers.

In individuals with normal HbA$_2$ levels and thalassaemic red-cell indices in whom iron deficiency has been excluded the next step is to attempt to exclude α thalassaemia or normal HbA$_2$ β thalassaemia. Here, the ethnic background of the patient may be extremely helpful. Alpha$^+$ thalassaemia is widespread in individuals of African descent, some Middle East populations and, to a lesser extent, in those from the Indian subcontinent. Apart from iron deficiency the commonest cause of microcytosis with a normal HbA$_2$ level in these populations is the homozygous state for α$^+$ thalassaemia. Because α^0 thalassaemia is so uncommon this is harmless in these populations. Hence it is usually not necessary to pursue the diagnosis further. However, in south-east Asian and some Mediterranean populations α^0 thalassaemia is common and in its heterozygous state the red-cell indices are similar to those of β-thalassaemia trait though, of course, the HbA$_2$ level is normal. This is an important diagnosis to establish because of the potential results of its interaction with other α^0-thalassaemia carriers or with α$^+$-thalassaemia heterozygotes (see Chapters 4 and 11). The only way that this can be done with certainty is by DNA analysis and therefore in populations in which α^0 thalassaemia is common it is important to set up at least one central laboratory that is able to carry out procedures of this kind.

Finally, in any screening programme there will be a small number of cases in which there are thalassaemic indices, there is no evidence for iron deficiency, and both β-thalassaemia trait and either the heterozygous state for α^0 thalassaemia or the homozygous state for α^+ thalassaemia have been excluded. In these cases it is important to try to exclude the various forms of normal HbA_2 β thalassaemia. Practical approaches to this problem, and to trying to define the cause for cases in which the HbA_2 level is marginally elevated, are described in detail in Chapter 7.

It cannot be emphasized too strongly that all the techniques used in screening, both haematological and those involving haemoglobin analysis, must be the subject of frequent standardization, audit and quality control. And, however the laboratory services that back up screening programmes are organized, it is essential that reference laboratories are established which are carrying out these procedures daily and in which the results are being constantly monitored. From experience in the UK it is clear that laboratories that only occasionally have to carry out estimations such as HbA_2 levels tend to produce quite unreliable results.

Communicating the results; counselling

As mentioned earlier, one of the ground rules of clinical genetics is that no screening or other forms of genetic diagnostic programmes are established without first making sure that adequate facilities are available for transmitting the results and for detailed counselling about their meaning and any actions that need to follow. Like all genetic disease, thalassaemia is complex; the more that is learnt about the interactions of its different varieties the more difficult it becomes to transmit the meaning of results to patients and their families, or to those who have been discovered to be carriers in population surveys.

A counselling programme is best organized in something of a hierarchical pyramid. First, there must be national centres in which there are genuine experts in the field. Normally these will be paediatricians, paediatric haematologists or 'adult' haematologists. Occasionally, specialists in other fields may develop this expertise; their clinical background does not really matter provided they are properly trained.

While in smaller populations, the Mediterranean islands for example, one thalassaemia centre may be sufficient, in larger countries more than one is usually required. It is essential that these centres interact well with each other. One of the problems of the thalassaemia field is that patients with the disease now grow up and at some time there may be a break in continuity of care between paediatricians and haematologists who look after adults. Ideally, thalassaemia centres should take on responsibility for the entire lives of their patients.

The next level in the hierarchy is the hospitals and other medical centres within the community, which either have to interpret the results of antenatal screening and take action or, when there is uncertainty, ask for help from the centres. This means that the first step in the education programme is to ensure that there is at least some understanding of the disease in this second tier.

The third level, and one that is absolutely vital for countries which are planning screening programmes, is the community counsellor and nurse. Once adequate numbers of trained workers of this kind are available the bulk of individuals who are ascertained on screening programmes or in antenatal clinics can be counselled by them. With the help of simple pamphlets and publications they must explain to the carriers the nature of the disease, the consequences of having children with another carrier, and the options that are open to them. Similar information must be given to women who have been found to be carriers in antenatal screening programmes and every effort must be made to bring in their partner for screening. At that time, when a woman is in the early stages of pregnancy, counselling has to be particularly sensitive, especially if the discovery of the thalassaemia trait is made for the first time.

After counselling, carriers who do not yet have a partner should be given simple written information with a clear record of their diagnosis. In countries with multiracial immigrant populations it is vital that both the counselling and the information is passed on in the patient's own language, particularly if they are not proficient in the language of the country in which they are living. In all forms of counselling, whether it is in the community or in the antenatal clinic, the ethical principles outlined earlier in this chapter must be adhered to.

It is very difficult to give hard and fast rules for the number of counsellors required and indeed there are few published data. A Working Party of the WHO has attempted to address this problem and some figures derived from the experiences of Sardinia, Cyprus, Greece and the UK are provided in its published proceedings (WHO 1994).

To what extent should genetic counselling attempt to distinguish between the likely clinical course of the different forms of β thalassaemia?

The question of whether counselling and decisions about prenatal diagnosis of thalassaemia should involve discussions about the likely outcome of particular interactions has not received a great deal of attention or discussion. Kollia *et al.* (1990) briefly addressed this problem and came to the conclusion that the state of the art for predicting the milder forms of β thalassaemia, that is, the β thalassaemia intermedias, has not yet reached the stage when it can be applied in clinical practice. This question is considered in detail in Chapter 13. Overall, work that has been published on this particular problem since 1990 still emphasizes the complexities of trying to predict phenotypes from genotypes in β thalassaemia. While the promoter mutations which are so common in African populations are usually mild there may be exceptions. And certainly the mild β-thalassaemia allele which is so common in Mediterranean populations, IVS1-6 T→C, shows remarkable phenotypic diversity in some populations, notably those of Israel. There seems little doubt that the δβ thalassaemias and many of their interactions are extremely mild but the symptomatic forms of α thalassaemia, notably HbH disease, also show wide phenotypic diversity. It is even more difficult to predict the outcome of some of the interactions between α and β thalassaemia. However, it is true to say that, overall, we have a reasonable idea about the likely degree of severity of different molecular forms of thalassaemia, while not being able to predict the clinical outcome with certainty in any individual case, at least not yet.

In the report by Kollia *et al.* (1990) they describe how they asked a large number of medical and paramedical staff whether they would accept having children with different forms of thalassaemia intermedia; the unanimous answer was no. The authors concluded therefore that prenatal diagnosis should not be denied selectively to couples at risk for thalassaemia intermedia. There are, however, obvious dangers in carrying out a survey of this kind, particularly involving medical staff, who, it is feared, might not express views that are typical of society as a whole!

One of the difficulties with this particular question is that we do not yet know much about the natural history of many forms of thalassaemia intermedia. This is particularly relevant to the problem of HbE β thalassaemia, which will pose a major public health problem in parts of Asia in the new millennium (see Chapter 9). Because of these uncertainties a number of our colleagues have expressed the view that we should not include these subtleties in our counselling of patients at risk for any form of thalassaemia, but should simply go ahead with prenatal diagnosis programmes, treating all forms of thalassaemia alike.

We believe that this rather indiscriminate approach to the prenatal diagnosis of thalassaemia is a dangerous path to follow, and one that is difficult to defend on ethical grounds. Clearly we must continue to strive better to understand the factors that modify the thalassaemic phenotype. But in the meantime it seems only right to include in our counselling an honest description of what is known about the milder forms of the illness, how they may interact and what the likely outcome will be in any particular case. We already know enough about the phenotypes of some of the interactions to be able to give a reasonable estimation of the clinical course, and provided that we are completely open and tell parents that there are always exceptions to these rules it seems only appropriate that they should take part in this difficult decision-making. At least we have some inkling about the factors that modify the thalassaemic phenotype; the widescale application of prenatal diagnosis to sickle-cell anaemia, in which we still know so little about the mechanisms that underlie the remarkable clinical heterogeneity, seems to us to be premature.

The outcomes of screening programmes

Currently we know relatively little about the efficacy of community screening programmes for thalassaemia and related disorders. In particular there is very limited knowledge about their effect on the choice of marital partners or about decisions regarding having children. The first exercise of this kind that was carried out in the USA, for screening for the sickling disorders, is a perfect example of how not to set up a 'service' of this kind. There was no attempt at an adequate education programme about the nature of the disease and the programme was not supported by provisions for genetic counselling. In several states laws were passed which made screening mandatory without any attempt at education and counselling. The result was large-scale public anxiety, stigmatism, job and health insurance discrimination and many other undesirable effects; virtually nothing was achieved. In contrast, the Montreal thalassaemia screening programme, which was developed on the back of very considerable experience in developing community programmes for screening for other genetic disorders, seems to have been remarkably successful (Mitchell *et al.* 1996; Capua 1998). In 1993, a survey of 720 high-school participants indicated that 99–100% of them wished to be tested and to receive both the results and counselling. Interestingly, prenatal diagnosis for thalassaemia became available in Quebec in the mid-1970s. During the period that the population programme has been running 32 couples have sought prenatal diagnosis, of whom 24 originated from the screening programme. By 1998 virtually all prenatal diagnosis referrals originated from this programme. Albeit on a relatively small scale, this shows how successful a population-based screening programme can be if it is backed up by adequate education and counselling.

Cao and Rosatelli (1993) have reviewed some of the results of the education and screening programmes in the Mediterranean island populations and part of the Italian mainland. It is clear from the figures from these countries, and from the studies of Modell and colleagues in Great Britain (Modell *et al.* 1984), that where these programmes are successful the uptake of prenatal diagnosis is extremely high, over 90% in Sardinia for example. But, as shown quite clearly in the UK, there is a major discrepancy between the uptake of prenatal diagnosis between population groups which have had access to adequate counselling and screening programmes and those in which these services have not been adequately provided (Modell *et al.* 1984, 1997, 2000).

The outcome of the first screening programme in Iran, reported recently by Ghanei *et al.* (1997), was discussed earlier. Of 100 000 cases screened in the Isfahan province over 90% of couples at risk decided not to marry and have children. During the period 1991–1995 this resulted in a fall of new cases born each year from approximately 30 to 6.

Cost–benefit considerations

The problems of the costs of avoidance and treatment of the thalassaemias were discussed by a Working Group of the WHO in 1994 and more recently by Modell and Kuliev (1998). Although a number of crude attempts have been made at cost–benefit analyses, and the Montreal programmes have been studied in detail in this respect, it is very difficult to draw many conclusions about this difficult question. However, it is quite clear from these discussions that, particularly in view of the increasing numbers of patients with different forms of thalassaemia who will survive to require treatment in the future, the results of most cost analyses have strongly supported the provision of prenatal diagnosis within health services. Not only do they reduce the number of affected children born, but they also increase the availability of treatment for those who already exist. However, as pointed out by the WHO Group, this type of statement is rather simplistic; it seems to imply that prenatal diagnosis is an alternative to patient management, rather than a complementary aspect of a control programme. It is also necessary to use cost analyses sensitively, at the same time taking into account aspects other than finance when considering prevention programmes. Particularly important advantages of these programmes also include the benefits of a better-educated population, informed choice for couples at risk, the birth of healthy infants or of affected ones who are accepted by their parents and society, and the replacement of affected fetuses with healthy infants (WHO 1994). Some of these issues are discussed in detail by Drummond (1980).

The choices for a couple at risk; the role of the counsellor

The options for couples at risk for having thalassaemic children, summarized in Table 14.1, are quite limited. While the nature of thalassaemia and the options open to carriers can be explained by trained counsellors quite adequately, when the final decision-making is required, particularly if it involves prenatal diagnosis, it is better if the counsellor is medically qualified, or at least is fully conversant with genetic

Table 14.1 Options for couples at risk for having a child with a severe form of thalassaemia.

Avoid pregnancy
Adoption
Risk having an affected child
Prenatal diagnosis: termination if fetus is affected
Pre-implantation diagnosis
Use of egg or sperm donor with normal globin genotype

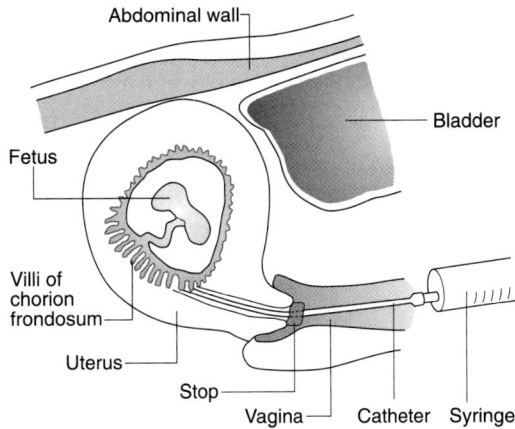

Fig. 14.3 Chorionic villus sampling.

counselling and has a thorough knowledge of thalassaemia in all its aspects. It is vital that adequate time is given for this interview and, if possible, the couple are able to go away and come back for a second visit after an adequate interval for thought. As mentioned earlier, it is important to touch on every aspect of thalassaemia, including the variable clinical course in particular cases. It may be helpful to introduce potential parents to a well run thalassaemia clinic and to let them discuss their doubts and problems with parents, and meet patients. In many countries thalassaemia support groups have been established to help patients and their parents and it may be helpful for potential parents to be introduced to these societies during their decision-making.

As is the case for all genetic diseases, counselling potential parents in making these difficult decisions requires extreme sensitivity. As mentioned at the beginning of this chapter, one of the central ethical issues that underlies all screening programmes and decisions about reproduction is individual choice. But 'neutral' counselling can be extremely difficult. Not infrequently the counsellor is asked the difficult question 'what would you do if you were us?' The counsellor must go through all the pros and cons of the particular course again, to make sure they are completely understood. But it may also be necessary to venture an opinion, not least to help share the burden of guilt which some parents feel if they are moving towards the decision to undergo prenatal diagnosis with possible termination of the pregnancy. This extremely delicate issue can only be dealt with by counsellors who know the field well and have had long experience of dealing with parents in this unfortunate situation.

Prenatal diagnosis

In Chapter 1 we discussed how, in the early 1970s, studies of haemoglobin patterns during fetal development combined with the development of methods for *in vitro* estimation of the rates of globin synthesis led to the first attempts at prenatal diagnosis of the thalassaemias. It was first achieved in 1974 following the development of a safe approach to fetal blood sampling. Despite the technical difficulties involved, this method was used successfully for the prenatal diagnosis of α and β thalassaemia and the sickling disorders in many countries, including the USA, Greece, Cyprus, Italy and the UK (WHO 1985). However, it has now been largely replaced in the majority of diagnostic centres by fetal DNA analysis.

Prenatal diagnosis by direct mutation identification was originally developed using DNA from amniotic fluid cells early in the second trimester, but, when it became possible to obtain DNA by chorionic villus sampling (CVS) late in the first trimester, this soon became the method of choice (Fig. 14.3). However, the methods of DNA analysis, in particular Southern blotting combined with the linkage analysis of restriction-fragment-length polymorphisms (RFLPs) or the hybridization of oligonucleotide probes, were complex and time consuming, and prenatal diagnosis programmes were restricted to a few specialized centres until the advent of the polymerase chain reaction (PCR).

The development of diagnostic methods based on PCR revolutionized the process of mutation screening and most thalassaemia mutations can now be diagnosed in the laboratory in 1 day, enabling prenatal diagnosis to be carried out rapidly, simply and cheaply in nearly every case. The remainder of this chapter is devoted to a description of the major advances which have led to this remarkable achievement, and to a summary of the DNA analysis technology and diagnostic strategy currently in use in the authors' laboratory. For readers who wish to explore this topic in more detail, several extensive reviews are available (Alter 1984; Weatherall *et al.* 1985; Old *et al.* 1989; Weatherall 1991; Cao & Rosatelli 1993; Embury 1995; Old 1996a).

Fetal blood sampling and analysis of fetal globin production

Fetal blood sampling

Early studies indicated that there might be small amounts of HbA in the blood of young fetuses (Walker & Turnbull 1955; Huehns *et al.* 1964b). As methods for analysing globin synthesis were developed it became clear that β-globin synthesis constitutes about 7% of haemoglobin production at 5 weeks and increases to approximately 11% at 20 weeks. These observations suggested that if small blood samples could be obtained from fetuses of between 10 and 20 weeks' gestation, and subjected to globin synthesis techniques developed by Clegg *et al.* (1965) and Weatherall *et al.* (1965), it might be possible to diagnose homozygous β thalassaemia *in utero*.

The first approach to fetal blood sampling involved the aspiration of blood from the placenta under ultrasound guidance (Kan *et al.* 1974a). Although this method was reasonably successful, it yielded a sample consisting of a mixture of fetal and maternal cells. It was therefore necessary to determine the relative contributions of each using a Coulter Channelyser; in many cases multiple samples were required until an adequate number of fetal cells were obtained. Several methods for enriching the yield of fetal cells were developed, the most useful being the Orskov procedure, based on the principle that only adult cells contain carbonic anhydrase and lyse in the presence of NH_4Cl and NH_4HCO_3 (Alter *et al.* 1979a).

The later development of direct fetal blood sampling by fetoscopy yielded pure fetal blood samples (Hobbins *et al.* 1974; Rodeck 1980). Blood was originally obtained from fetal vessels on the chorionic plate, but better results followed when it was drawn directly from the umbilical vein at the placental insertion of the cord. In skilled hands this procedure regularly yielded a sample containing 100% fetal cells. The final modification of this approach was the development of cordocentesis. This technique provides pure fetal blood by puncture of the umbilical cord using ultrasound guidance without the need for the direct visualization required for fetoscopy.

Globin synthesis

Measurement of the relative rates of fetal globin synthesis is essential. This is achieved by incubating the fetal blood cells with [^{3}H] leucine, separating the globins by CM-cellulose chromatography, and determining the amount of radioactivity incorporated into each type of globin (see Chapters 5 and 16). For the diagnosis of β thalassaemia, the ratio of β- to γ-chain production is determined (Fig. 14.4). In a normal fetus β-chain synthesis is approximately 10% of that of γ chains, giving a β/γ ratio of approximately 0.1. A fetus with β-thalassaemia trait synthesizes about half the normal amount of β globin, giving a β/γ ratio of approximately 0.06. A fetus with β thalassaemia major makes either no β globin (if homozygous for $β^0$ thalassaemia) or only a trace amount (if homozygous for $β^+$ thalassaemia), and, in both such cases, the β/γ ratio is usually below 0.025. However, in the case of milder $β^+$-thalassaemia mutations, it may be difficult to distinguish a $β^+$-thalassaemia homozygote or compound heterozygote from a heterozygote. In fact, cases in which a fetus with $β^+$ thalassaemia major yields a β/γ ratio above the cut-off value, and is therefore diagnosed as a heterozygote, are the main sources of error with this technique.

The chosen cut-off point between heterozygotes and homozygotes is slightly different in each centre performing this technique, and has to be determined locally because it depends on the types of $β^+$-thalassaemia mutations found in a particular region and the technical niceties of the protocol adopted by the laboratory, such as the method used for determining the baselines of the chromatographic peaks.

Other important haemoglobinopathies can be diagnosed by this technique. The homozygous state for $α^0$ thalassaemia (Hb Bart's hydrops fetalis syndrome) is characterized by absence of α-globin synthesis. Structural haemoglobin variants can be detected, provided that the charge of the mutant

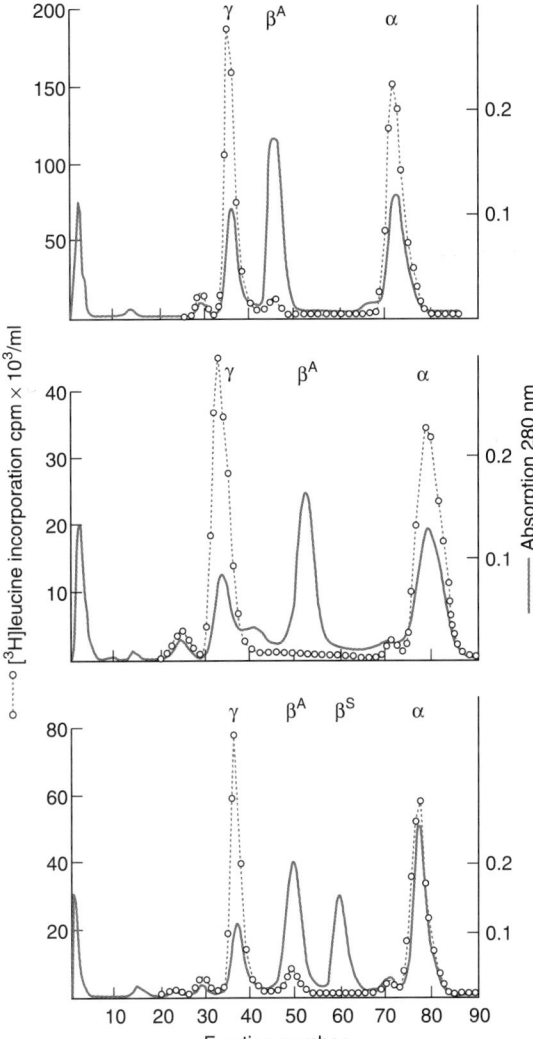

Fig. 14.4 Prenatal detection of haemoglobin disorders by fetal blood sampling and radiolabelling of globin. The globin was separated by CM-cellulose chromatography (see Chapter 5). The protein profile is shown by a continuous line and the radioactive profile by a broken line. Top, normal fetal blood (unlabelled adult globin has been added to demonstrate the position of elution of the adult β chains). Middle, blood from a fetus with β⁰ thalassaemia showing no β-chain production; adult blood has been added to show where radioactive β chains would have eluted. Bottom, a normal profile in a fetus at risk for carrying the sickle-cell trait or disease. Unlabelled blood from a person with sickle-cell trait has been added to show the position of elution of the βˢ chains, were any present.

globin is different from that of β globin (Fig. 14.4); under standard conditions for globin fractionation, abnormal globins elute in characteristically different positions from βᴬ globin. In this way, Hbs S, E, C, Oᴬʳᵃᵇ and Lepore can be identified in fetal life.

Related methods

Although prenatal diagnosis from CM-cellulose column chromatography gives very reproducible results, it is relatively expensive and slow. Many centres involved in prenatal diagnosis must process large numbers of samples in a short time; this requirement led to the development of a number of alternative approaches to separating globins or haemoglobins, such as high-performance liquid chromatography, which provides an answer in hours. Simple polyacrylamide gel electrophoresis or isoelectric focusing of haemoglobin tetramers can also be used. A detailed description of these and other methods, including the separation of haemoglobins by Bio-Rex column chromatography, can be found in the review of Alter (1989).

Results

Prenatal diagnosis of thalassaemia by fetal blood sampling was adopted widely in many countries and proved very successful, despite the complexity of the methodology. Indeed, during the period from June 1974 to December 1989, for which a registry of cases tested world-wide was maintained by Alter, more than 20 centres performed a total of 13·921 diagnoses, of which the great majority were for β thalassaemia (Table 14.2). Homozygous (or compound heterozygous) pregnancies were diagnosed in 24.9% of cases and there were 63 recorded errors (0.5% of cases). In all there were 408 fetal losses, representing 3.1% of all attempts. These data clearly show that the fetal loss and diagnostic error rates improved dramatically over the final period of the registry (1986–89), due largely to the introduction of cordocentesis, a procedure which routinely provided pure fetal blood samples and allowed a move to the simpler, machine-based analytic techniques of high-performance liquid chromatography and isoelectric focusing (Table 14.3). These results show that prenatal diagnosis of thalassaemia by fetal blood sampling is remarkably successful and, in experienced hands, is relatively safe and reliable.

The value of this approach is highlighted when the data from a single prenatal diagnosis laboratory are examined (the results published for the Athens centre from 1977 to 1989 (Loukopoulos *et al.* 1990), for example Table 14.4). In more than 4000 cases of second-trimester prenatal diagnoses of thalassaemia, referred from all over Greece, the number of 'homozygotes' diagnosed was 25.4%, very close to the theoretical 25% figure. This suggests that there must have been very few cases that were incorrectly diagnosed as affected. The number of false-negative diagnoses gradually diminished with increasing experience, as did the number of obstetric complications,

with the fetal loss rate settling at around 2.5%. The diagnostic error rate was less than 1%, a level of accuracy to which the later move to DNA analysis had to aspire.

Prenatal diagnosis by DNA analysis

DNA analysis was applied to prenatal diagnosis in the late 1970s and early 1980s, first using amniotic fluid cell DNA and, later, chorionic villus DNA. However, fetal blood sampling remained popular throughout the 1980s because of the complex and sophisticated nature of the DNA analysis techniques, which required hybridization of radioactive gene probes. It was not until the advent of the polymerase chain reaction and the subsequent development of simple and rapid diagnostic techniques for prenatal diagnosis of haemoglobinopathies that many centres, including those in Cyprus and Greece, switched over to DNA analysis. By December 1989, more than 6000 fetal DNA diagnoses had been recorded by the prenatal diagnosis registry (Alter 1990) and the use of fetal blood sampling was rapidly declining. However, it still remains a useful option when DNA studies are uninformative or are not performed in the first trimester of pregnancy, as illustrated by the recent report of a successful series of prenatal diagnoses of thalassaemia in India by anion-exchange high-performance liquid chromatography (HPLC) of cord blood (Rao *et al.* 1997).

Table 14.2 Haemoglobinopathies diagnosed by fetal blood sampling, June 1974 to December 1989. Data from Alter (1990).

Disorder	Number of cases reported
β Thalassaemia	12 383
δβ Thalassaemia	24
α Thalassaemia	22
α Thalassaemia/β thalassaemia	14
HbE/β thalassaemia	46
Hb Lepore/β thalassaemia	52
Sickle-cell anaemia	508
HbS/β thalassaemia	227
HbS/HbC	9
HbS/HbO[Arab]	6
Total	13 921

Table 14.3 Fetal blood testing for haemoglobinopathies, June 1974 to December 1989. From Alter (1990).

	1974–1985	1986–1989	Total	
Cases at risk	7955	5336	13 291	(100%)
Affected cases	2036	1273	3309	(24.9%)
Fetal losses	303	105	408	(3.1%)
Diagnostic errors	46	17	63	(0.5%)
Sampling methods				
Aspiration	2175	69	2244	(17.3%)
Fetoscopy	5445	1236	6681	(51.5%)
Cordocentesis	11	4031	4042	(31.2%)
Analytical methods				
CM-cellulose chromatography	7455	2805	10 206	(77.2%)
High-performance liquid chromatography	500	2210	2710	(20.4%)
Isoelectric focusing	0	321	321	(2.4%)

Table 14.4 Fetal blood testing for haemoglobinopathies in Greece, 1977–1989. From Loukopoulos *et al.* (1990).

	1977	1978	1979	1980	1981	1982	1983	1984	1985	1986	1987	1988	1989	Total
Fetal blood studies (n)	14	90	132	209	295	354	405	454	424	473	484	470	407	4211
Cases diagnosed to have thalassaemia major														
n	1	24	25	48	95	110	106	103	123	122	111	101	99	1068
%	7.1	26.7	18.9	23.0	32.3	31.0	26.2	22.7	29.0	25.8	23.0	21.5	24.3	25.36
False diagnoses														
False negative	1	1	3	3	2	1	2	0	0	1	0	1	1	16
False positive (probable)	0	0	0	2	1	0	0	0	0	0	0	1	0	4
Obstetric complications														
Failures to obtain sample	0	2	8	5	4	1	1	4	4	3	1	—	—	33
Fetal losses directly associated with the procedure	4	10	7	10	9	9	8	10	12	4	6	6	4	99*

* Approximately 2.5% of total procedures.

Second-trimester diagnosis using amniotic fibroblast DNA

Amniocentesis offered a safer option than fetal blood sampling because the fetal loss rate is only around 0.5% above the spontaneous mid-trimester figure. At 16–20 weeks' gestation a 20-ml amniotic fluid sample contains just sufficient fetal cells to provide enough DNA for analysis; an aliquot may be cultured to provide additional DNA within 2 weeks, if required. Thus it was clearly desirable to develop techniques for prenatal diagnosis using amniotic fluid cells rather than fetal blood cells as soon as techniques for diagnosing globin-gene mutations were available.

The first group of globin-gene mutations to be characterized at the molecular level were the major gene deletions, using the technique of molecular hybridization. In 1976 Kan *et al.* studied a fetus at risk for α thalassaemia and were able to show that it had α-thalassaemia trait. Gene mapping by Southern blot analysis was developed soon after, and homozygous α^0 thalassaemia and $(\delta\beta)^0$ thalassaemia were diagnosed successfully by restriction endonuclease analysis of amniotic fluid cell DNA (Orkin *et al.* 1978; Dozy *et al.* 1979a). The first report of a restriction endonuclease polymorphism existing in linkage disequilibrium to a gene mutation, the restriction enzyme *Hpa* I and the sickle-cell mutation (Kan & Dozy 1978b), quickly led to the application of this linked polymorphic DNA marker for the prenatal diagnosis of sickle-cell disease (Kan & Dozy 1978a) and, as more polymorphisms were discovered, to the diagnosis of β thalassaemia (Boehm *et al.* 1983) by the same approach. By 1982, 175 cases of amniocyte DNA diagnosis had been reported to the prenatal diagnosis registry, without any diagnostic errors (Alter 1984), confirming the reliability of linkage analysis for the diagnosis of genetic disorders.

However, this approach, like fetal blood sampling, is restricted to the second trimester of pregnancy. The development of a method of obtaining fetal tissue at 8–12 weeks' gestation by the aspiration or biopsy of chorionic villi provided the next major advance in the field. Chorionic villus sampling (CVS) quickly replaced amniocentesis as the source of fetal DNA for prenatal diagnosis, and by December 1989 a total of 4581 CVS compared with 1222 amniocyte DNA diagnoses had been recorded by the registry (Alter 1990).

First-trimester diagnosis using chorionic villus DNA

The history of the development of CVS was reviewed by Rodeck and Morsman (1983). First used in China to obtain tissue for fetal sexing, it was adapted for genetic diagnosis in the embryo in the late 1960s (Hahnerman & Mohr 1968).

Chorionic villus sampling

The chorion is composed of an outer layer, or trophoblast, an inner mesodermal layer and fetal blood vessels, which supply the villi and extend all over the gestation sac until the end of the second month of pregnancy (Fig. 14.3). As development proceeds, continuing growth of the gestation sac causes thinning of the decidua capsularis until, by 14 weeks, the extraplacental chorion is almost denuded of villi.

CVS can be carried out by either the transcervical or transabdominal routes, both under ultrasound guidance (Fig. 14.3). While much of the early experience was gained with the transcervical approach (Ward *et al.* 1983) the later development of transabdominal sampling (Smidt-Jensen *et al.* 1986; Brambati *et al.* 1991) had the advantage that it could be used up to 14-15 weeks' gestation (Brambati *et al.* 1991).

Complications

There were early concerns about the safety, for both the mother and fetus, of this potentially invasive approach. Because of the spontaneous loss of pregnancies in the first trimester, several trials were required to determine whether CVS would be associated with a greater rate of fetal loss than amniocentesis. In 1989 the first report of the Canadian Collaborative CVS–Amniocentesis Clinical Trial Group, which compared CVS with amniocentesis, indicated that there was no difference in maternal morbidity between the groups, while there were 7.6% of fetal losses in the CVS group and 7.0% in the amniocentesis group. Mean birth weights for each week of gestation were similar in both groups. Later studies confirmed these findings and showed that the rate of fetal loss was no different whether the transcervical or transabdominal approach was used (Jackson *et al.* 1992). The likelihood of maternal bleeding is approximately 7% and 20% with the

transabdominal and vaginal routes, respectively; in neither case has this been associated with maternal mortality (Jackson *et al.* 1990b) or fetal loss (Jackson *et al.* 1986).

Concerns have been expressed about the possibility of an increased frequency of limb-reduction defects in the fetus if CVS is performed between 55 and 66 days' gestation (Firth *et al.* 1994). In a series of 289 pregnancies, Firth and colleagues identified five infants with severe limb abnormalities following early transabdominal CVS. Although additional cases had been reported, it seems likely that these defects occur in no more than 6 per 1000 CVS, only slightly higher than is observed in pregnancies that have not undergone this procedure (Froster-Iskenius & Baird 1989; Jackson *et al.* 1991). Since there is some evidence that these limb deformities tend to occur when CVS is done in the 9th week or before, most obstetricians now wait until 10–11 weeks' gestation to minimize the risk.

Yield of DNA

Chorionic villus sampling usually provides 5–25 mg of tissue, from which approximately 5 μg DNA/mg can be extracted (Jackson *et al.* 1990b). In fact, Old *et al.* (1986b) found that the yield of DNA from CVS varied from 2 to 100 μg, with an average of about 20 μg. There was a good linear relationship between yield of DNA and the weight of chorion biopsy tissue, as shown in Fig. 14.5.

Early results

The first successful prenatal diagnoses of β thalassaemia and sickle-cell anaemia following CVS were reported by Old *et al.* (1982b). This approach was soon taken up by other centres and further reports of successful diagnosis of sickle-cell anaemia (Goossens *et al.* 1983) and of β thalassaemia (Rosatelli *et al.* 1985) were reported. In 1986, Old *et al.* (1986a) published their experience of over 200 first-trimester diagnoses for haemoglobin disorders, including 133 cases at risk for β thalassaemia and 55 for sickle-cell anaemia. A successful diagnosis was made in all but one case, an error due to plasmid contamination. There were two failures due to insufficient material, but a diagnosis was made subsequently by amniocentesis.

The development of first-trimester prenatal diagnosis for thalassaemia was a major step forward. It is much more acceptable to women than methods which can only be used in later pregnancy; they have not had so long to become adapted to the fact that they are carrying a living being and, if termination is required, it is much easier. Hence, over recent years CVS has become the method of choice for prenatal diagnosis, with amniocentesis as a backup for women who present too late for this procedure. In addition, however, there has been a steady improvement in the technology of DNA analysis, which has had the added advantage of improving both the speed and accuracy of prenatal diagnosis. In the sections that follow we shall outline these advances before summarizing the most effective current approaches toward fetal DNA analysis.

Evaluation of methods used to analyse fetal DNA

The thalassaemias and sickle-cell disorders have been used as prototype monogenic diseases in the

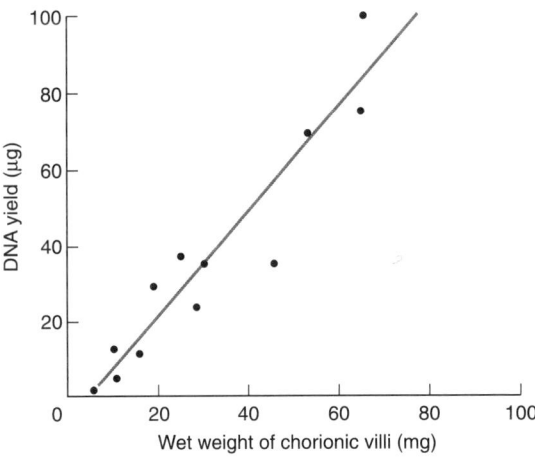

Fig. 14.5 The relationship between the weight of chorionic villus material and DNA yield.

development of prenatal diagnostic methods for the last 20 years. Consequently many different methods of DNA analysis have been employed. The current techniques for identifying globin-gene mutations are described in Chapter 16. Here we shall outline the development of DNA analysis for prenatal diagnosis and describe the methods currently used in our laboratory.

By December 1989 there were 29 diagnostic centres world-wide performing prenatal diagnosis for the haemoglobinopathies by DNA analysis; the methods used are listed in Table 14.5. By that time PCR-based techniques were still in the early days of development and had only been applied in 21% of cases. The majority were based on Southern blotting and utilized either RFLP linkage, deletion mapping, restriction-enzyme analysis or allele-specific oligonucleotide hybridization.

Restriction-fragment-length polymorphism linkage analysis

The RFLPs in the globin-gene cluster are described in Chapter 2. Their discovery led to the first DNA-based method to be widely exploited for prenatal diagnosis. One of the first RFLPs to be reported, an *Hpa* I polymorphism 3′ to the β-globin gene, was observed to be strongly associated with the sickle-cell (βS) gene in West Africans (Kan & Dozy 1978b). It was found to exist in linkage disequilibrium with 70% of Afro-American sickle-cell genes and thus homozygous inheritance could be excluded in 70% of pregnancies at risk for sickle-cell anaemia (Kan & Dozy 1978a) (Fig. 14.6). The first RFLP to be found in linkage disequilibrium to a β-thalassaemia gene was a *Bam* HI polymorphism associated with the common β⁰-thalassaemia mutation CD39 C→T in Sardinia (Kan *et al.* 1980). This polymorphism occurred in all Sardinian β⁰-thalassaemia alleles but was observed in only two-thirds of normal β-globin-gene alleles. Therefore its absence in fetal DNA reflects the pres-

Table 14.5 Methods of fetal DNA testing for haemoglobinopathies, June 1974 to December 1989. From Alter (1990).

Method	Total	%
Restriction-fragment-length polymorphism linkage analysis	689	21.5
Deletion mapping	375	11.7
Restriction-enzyme analysis	854	26.6
Allele-specific hybridization	615	19.2
Polymerase chain reaction methods	674	21.1

Direct Analysis: *Bgl* II

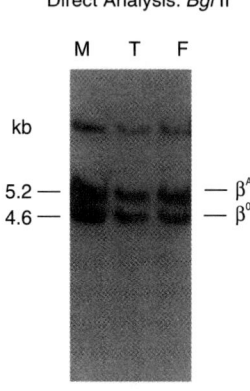

β⁰ thalassaemia

Linkage Analysis: *Hpa* I

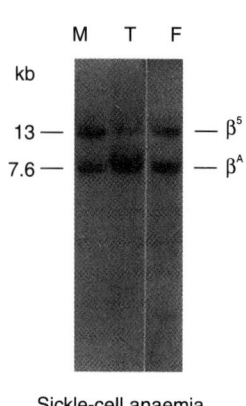

Sickle-cell anaemia

Fig. 14.6 Prenatal diagnosis by fetal DNA analysis using Southern blotting. On the left is shown the prenatal diagnosis of β^0 thalassaemia due to a 619-bp deletion at the 3' end of the β-globin gene. The enzyme *Bgl* II normally cuts on either side of the β-globin gene to produce a 5.2-kb fragment. When this deletion is present a 4.6-kb fragment is generated. In this case both the parents (M and F) and the fetus (T) were heterozygotes. On the right is shown the prenatal diagnosis of sickle-cell disease using the *Hpa* I polymorphism which is in linkage disequilibrium with the sickle-cell mutation, as described in the text. Again, both the parents and fetus are heterozygotes.

ence of a normal β gene and excludes this particular β-thalassaemia gene. Another useful RFLP for the prenatal diagnosis of β thalassaemia in Mediterranean populations was found by Wainscoat *et al.* (1984a). An *Ava* II site was absent in over 50% of chromosomes carrying β thalassaemia, yet missing in only 4 out of 120 chromosomes carrying a normal β-globin gene. This marked association of the *Ava* II site polymorphism with thalassaemia greatly improved the feasibility of prenatal diagnosis in the Cypriot population. However, polymorphisms associated with particular mutations turned out to be very rare, and their linkage to a particular mutation was not always absolute.

As described in Chapter 2, a number of polymorphic restriction enzyme sites were discovered in the β-globin-gene cluster by Antonarakis *et al.* (1982) and were found to exist on individual chromosomes in a non-random pattern called a haplotype. Although within any particular population group it was shown that particular β-thalassaemia mutations were linked to specific haplotypes (Orkin *et al.* 1982a), the same haplotypes occurred in normal individuals in the same population and thus the association could not be used for prenatal diagnosis. However, because of the variety of haplotypes found in any particular population, they could be used for prenatal diagnosis through linkage to specific β-globin genes by family studies (Old *et al.* 1984).

The way in which RFLP linkage analysis by a family study is used for prenatal diagnosis is outlined in Fig. 14.7. The idea is to study the parents and any previously born children or other relatives using

several restriction enzymes and appropriate gene probes to see if an RFLP can be found on the chromosome carrying the mutant gene in each parent. If so, and if the fetus is homozygous for the particular RFLP, then it must also be homozygous for the particular mutation. Obviously there are a number of permutations that can be added to this general approach, but however it is done it is essential to obtain information about the chromosomal location of the RFLP in relationship to the β-thalassaemia gene.

The problem with this method is that, to establish a useful linkage, a previously born child or other family members are required, and hence a considerable amount of time-consuming laboratory work must be done before a diagnosis can be made. Furthermore, the frequency of different RFLP markers varies between different ethnic groups. For example, studies in Britain suggest that this approach for the prenatal diagnosis of β thalassaemia would only be feasible in about four-fifths of Cypriot and Asian families (Old *et al.* 1989).

Deletion mapping

Major gene deletions or rearrangements of the globin genes were the first mutations to be identified directly by restriction-enzyme mapping. Large gene deletions can be diagnosed either by the disappearance of a particular restriction-enzyme fragment on a Southern blot, or by the appearance of a new fragment containing one or both of the breakpoint ends of the deletion. The disorders that were detected in

Fig. 14.7 The principles of restriction-fragment-length polymorphism linkage analysis for prenatal diagnosis. The abnormal gene (A) and its normal allele (N) are shown on the parental chromosomes (both parents are heterozygous). There is a polymorphic site P on one chromosome and a gene M for which a probe is available. Depending on the presence or absence of this site a 10-kb or 7-kb fraction is obtained with the appropriate enzyme. Thus the resulting gene map from heterozygous parents shows two bands, 10˙kb and 7˙kb. A family study shows that a previously affected child only has the 10-kb fraction, indicating that the abnormal allele (A) is on the chromosome with the polymorphism (+). Since the fetus shows the same pattern it must also be homozygous for the defect.

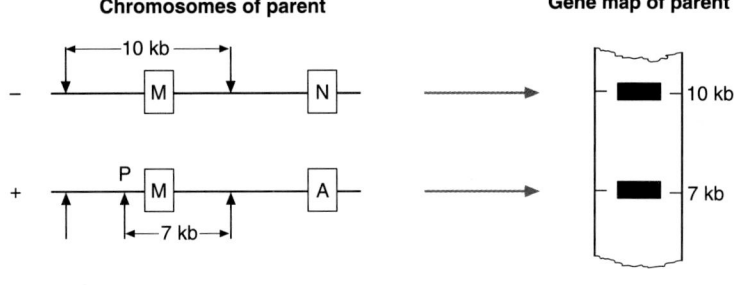

this way for prenatal diagnosis included the α^0 thalassaemias, the Indian form of β^0 thalassaemia due to a 619-bp deletion at the 3′ end of the β-globin gene (Fig. 14.6), the δβ thalassaemias and Hb Lepore (Alter 1984).

Once the sequences of the α- and β-globin-gene clusters were determined, the breakpoints of many of these deletions could be determined accurately. This allowed the design of suitable primers complementary to the breakpoint end sequences which can be used for prenatal diagnosis of deletion mutations by the technique of gap PCR, that is, amplification across the gap to produce a characteristic abnormal PCR fragment (see later section). However, the breakpoint sequences of some of the rarer deletions have yet to be determined and Southern blot analysis remains the only diagnostic method for their identification (Old 1996a).

Restriction-enzyme analysis

This was the first direct method for the detection of point mutations to be used for prenatal diagnosis and again the sickle-cell gene was the first target. Several groups observed that the sickle-cell mutation, an AT

change in codon 6 of the β-globin gene, alters a DNA sequence normally recognized and cleaved by three different restriction enzymes, *Dde* I, *Mnl* I and *Mst* II (Geever *et al.* 1981; Chang & Kan 1982; Orkin *et al.* 1982c). For technical reasons *Mst* II proved the most useful and was widely used for prenatal diagnosis until PCR techniques were introduced, when, for technical reasons again, the enzyme *Dde* I proved to be more suitable (Old *et al.* 1989). However, although this approach is one of the most useful methods for the prenatal diagnosis of sickle-cell anaemia, it turned out to be of little value for thalassaemia. Only a few uncommon β-thalassaemia mutations create or abolish restriction-enzyme sites; the need for a general method for the direct detection of all the β-thalassaemia mutations led to the development of the technique known as allele-specific oligonucleotide (ASO) hybridization .

Allele-specific oligonucleotide hybridization

The DNA probes used for deletion and gene mapping studies were too long to detect single base changes of the kind that cause many forms of thalassaemia. However, once it became possible to synthesize short DNA fragments *in vitro*, it was found that oligonucleotides of 19 bases long could be used as DNA probes to hybridize to homologous but not heterologous DNA sequences, even those with a single base difference (Wallace *et al.* 1981; Conner *et al.* 1983). Wallace's group showed that these synthetic probes, when radioactively labelled to a very high specific activity, could be used to distinguish a normal β-globin gene from a $β^S$ gene after hybridization to restriction-enzyme-digested genomic DNA on a Southern blot. This was the first time that DNA probes had been used to diagnose a genetic disease resulting from a point mutation.

Similar oligonucleotide probes were made to detect several common β-thalassaemia mutations (Orkin *et al.* 1983a; Pirastu *et al.* 1983a; Rosatelli *et al.* 1985; Thein *et al.* 1985) and were used successfully for the prenatal diagnosis of β thalassaemia. However, although in the theory the technique held great promise because it could be applied in any family in which the specific point mutation was known, many technical difficulties were encountered which prevented its widespread adoption for prenatal diagnosis. For example, the hybridization and washing conditions were absolutely critical to discriminate between normal and abnormal sequences, and a probe of very high specific activity was required. It was not until the discovery of PCR that this technique achieved its true potential. By using amplified DNA instead of digested genomic DNA, the hybridization and washing conditions became less critical, and non-radioactive labels could be used to provide a simple colorimetric assay.

Polymerase chain reaction (PCR)-based methods

The PCR permits the primer-mediated enzymatic amplification of target sequences in genomic DNA, resulting in the exponential increase of at least one millionfold of the DNA sequence of interest. This scale of amplification makes detection of a DNA sequence easier, quicker and cheaper than by any of the Southern blot analysis methods.

In their original description of PCR, Saiki *et al.* (1985) showed it was possible to detect the sickle-cell mutation in amplified β-globin-gene sequences by using radioactively labelled oligonucleotide probes hybridized in solution to the amplification product fixed on to a nylon filter in the form of dots (dot blotting). The β-globin genotype could be deter-

mined in this way in less than 1 day, and on samples of less than 0.1 µg of DNA. The same group soon simplified the process by using a thermostable DNA polymerase, and by carrying out the reaction in thermal cyclers (Saiki *et al.* 1988). It was quickly adopted by diagnostic laboratories for the identification of β-thalassaemia mutations and for prenatal diagnosis of β thalassaemia. By December 1989, a total of 674 prenatal diagnoses had been performed world-wide for β thalassaemia and sickle-cell disease (Table 14.5).

However, this application of PCR was restricted mainly to experienced diagnostic laboratories in the USA and Europe, and it was not until the development of non-radioactive PCR techniques that prenatal diagnosis programmes began to be established in new laboratories in developing countries. The next advance was the development of ASO hybridization probes covalently labelled with horseradish peroxidase (Saiki *et al.* 1988). Using dot-blotted, amplified β-globin-gene sequences, the hybridized probes could be detected with a simple colorimetric assay. This approach was not widely adopted, however, mainly because of the complexity of linking the horseradish peroxidase to the probes and the drawback of having to diagnose multiple β-thalassaemia mutations, one at a time, by dot-blot hybridization.

The amplification refractory mutation system

A simpler method for the identification of β-thalassaemia mutations was developed by Old *et al.* (1990) based on the amplification refractory mutation system (ARMS), first described by Newton *et al.* (1989) (Fig. 14.8). This utilizes the principle of allele-specific priming of the PCR, in which a primer will only permit amplification to take place when it perfectly matches the target DNA sequence at the 3′ terminal nucleotide. ARMS primers can be designed to signal the presence of any point mutation or normal DNA sequence at that position, and thus they can be used to detect normal, heterozygous and homozygous mutant sequences in the target DNA without the need for radionuclides. They were first developed for the prenatal diagnosis of β thalassaemia in the Asian Indian and Cypriot populations in the UK by Old *et al.* (1990). Subsequently ARMS primers were made for all the common β-thalassaemia mutations (Old 1996a); ARMS is

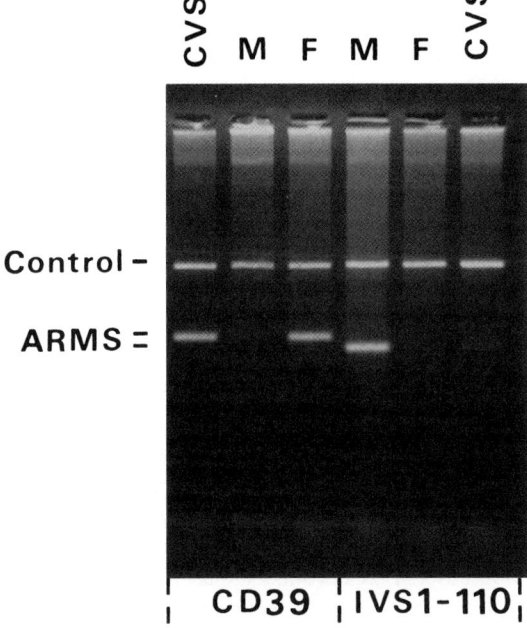

Fig. 14.8 Prenatal diagnosis from analysis of chorionic villus DNA. This shows a prenatal diagnosis using ARMS, as described in the text. In this case one parent has the common Mediterranean CD39 C→T mutation, the other the IVS1-110 G→A mutation. The fetus (CVS) is, like the father (F), heterozygous for the CD39 mutation, while the mother (M) is heterozygous for the IVS1-110 mutation.

Table 14.6 Details of some DNA analysis-based prenatal diagnosis services in developing countries. From Petrou and Modell (1995).

Country	Year started	No. of cases to mid-1995
Thailand	1985	288
Turkey	1992	79
Lebanon	1993	18
Iran	1993	108
India		
New Delhi	1992	300
Bombay	1994	118
Pakistan	1994	75
Nigeria	1994	40

currently the main approach for prenatal diagnosis in the UK for β thalassaemia, HbE β thalassaemia and the sickling disorders (Modell *et al.* 1997). The technique quickly spread to other diagnostic laboratories and was incorporated into their prenatal diagnosis programmes alongside other PCR-based diagnostic methods, particularly ASO hybridization, with good results. In a direct comparison of ARMS and ASO, Tan *et al.* (1994) concluded the ARMS method was simpler, more rapid and much cheaper than ASO for prenatal diagnosis in nine Singapore couples at risk for six different β-thalassaemia mutations. The ARMS method is also established in India and Pakistan, making the development of a prenatal diagnosis programme based on DNA analysis realistic for the first time. A list of prenatal diagnosis programmes started in some developing countries is presented in Table 14.6.

Reverse dot blotting

The ARMS method satisfies the main practical requirements for the prenatal diagnosis of known β-thalassaemia mutations, including speed, cost, convenience and the facility to test for multiple mutations simultaneously. Recently, reverse dot blotting, another PCR-based technique, has been developed, which also meets these requirements and holds much promise for the future. In this method, originally described by Maggio *et al.* (1993), probes for the specific mutations are fixed to a nylon filter and then hybridized together in one reaction to labelled, amplified genomic DNA. This permits a large number of mutations to be screened in a single hybridization step. It is estimated by Cai *et al.* (1994) that, by using strips containing probes to detect the most common mutations in Asians, Afro-Americans and Mediterraneans, it should be possible to obtain a 95% world-wide coverage of thalassaemia mutations by this approach. It is amenable to standardization, and a kit for the detection of seven Mediterranean β thalassaemias is now commercially available. This approach has been used for the prenatal diagnosis of β thalassaemia in Thailand, China and Sicily (Giambona *et al.* 1995; Sutcharitchan *et al.* 1995; Xu *et al.* 1996).

Gap PCR

Gene deletions can be detected by amplification across the breakpoints, a technique known as gap PCR (see also Chapter 16). For the small number of β-thalassaemia deletions of under 1 kb in size, the primer pair spans both breakpoint ends and generates two products, the smaller fragment arising from the deletion allele. For example, the pair of control primers used in the ARMS analysis also spans the 619-bp deletion β-thalassaemia gene, resulting in fragments of 861 bp (normal allele) and 242 bp (β-thalassaemia allele). For larger deletions, such as those causing Hb Lepore, δβ thalassaemia and α^0 thalassaemia, the distance between the breakpoints is too large for amplification of the normal allele with flanking primers and thus it must be amplified using primers spanning just one of the breakpoints. The technique requires the characterization of both breakpoints by DNA sequencing and currently can only be used for the Hb Lepore deletion, six δβ thalassaemia deletions and three α^0-thalassaemia deletions (see Chapters 4 and 11). Prenatal diagnosis of the other known δβ-thalassaemia and α^0-thalassaemia deletions still has to be carried out by Southern blot analysis.

Current strategies for prenatal diagnosis

Given this plethora of technology, what is the best approach to establishing a prenatal diagnosis programme? If adequate screening and counselling programmes have been established, as outlined earlier in this chapter, the majority of families referred for prenatal diagnosis will have already been adequately investigated as regards their haemoglobin genotype. However, it must never be assumed that the results of these investigations are correct and it cannot be emphasized too strongly that, before embarking on any form of prenatal diagnosis, it is vital to double-check the parents for evidence of an important form of thalassaemia or structural haemoglobin variant. There have been a number of unfortunate cases in which this was not done and where an error occurred. Thus, it is vital that any laboratory that carries out sophisticated DNA testing as part of a prenatal diagnosis programme is also able to carry out reliable genotyping of the parents' blood.

The second important prerequisite is to develop a clear line of communication and a mechanism for the transportation of material with the obstetrician who is carrying out the CVS or any other approach to obtaining fetal material. It is important to know, well ahead of time when samples are arriving, if there is more than one patient to be studied, so that adequate precautions for labelling of samples are taken; and whether the material has been checked under the

light microscope to ensure, as far as possible, that it is of fetal origin. It is also vital to be aware of any problems that were encountered while fetal material was being obtained.

General strategy

The major methods for the analysis of fetal DNA are outlined in Table 14.7. Although each laboratory must carry out preliminary studies utilizing a number of these approaches in order to find out which is best suited to its needs, it is clear that one form of ASO hybridization or ARMS currently forms the linchpin for the diagnosis of the bulk of thalassaemias after CVS. It may well be that in some cases reverse dot blotting may prove more simple. The laboratory also needs to become proficient at gap PCR and in carrying out RFLP linkage analysis in some cases. To provide a comprehensive service, at least one central laboratory in each country should be able to sequence globin genes for those rare cases in which there is clear-cut phenotypic evidence of β thalassaemia in the parents, but mutations cannot be identified.

But whatever the technique that is used for fetal DNA diagnosis it is essential to confirm the initial findings, either by repeating the particular analysis using the same method, or by a different approach.

As we shall see, one of the commonest causes of error in fetal DNA diagnosis is the contamination of the CVS with maternal tissue. Where possible, each sample should be analysed to exclude this complication. There are a number of methods available and these are discussed in a later section.

As we have already suggested, each laboratory must work out for itself which are the best techniques and approaches for their particular population. In the account which follows we describe our own approach to identifying the different mutations in fetal DNA. Cao and Rosatelli (1993) also give a detailed account of their methods, based on experiences of a large number of prenatal diagnoses carried out in Sardinia over many years.

β Thalassaemia

It is now clear that only approximately 20 different mutations account for the majority of β thalassaemia alleles in all at-risk populations (reviewed in Chapter 6 and by Huisman 1990 and Flint *et al.* 1993a, 1998). The mutations are regionally specific and each population has a few common mutations together with a

Table 14.7 Current strategies for fetal DNA diagnosis.

Disorder	Approach	Mutation detection
α^0 Thalassaemia	Southern blot PCR	Probes: α genes, ζ genes, LO* Across breakpoints

β Thalassaemia	PCR	(1) Direct: ASO dot blot
		      ARMS analysis
		      Restriction enzymes
		      Across breakpoints
		(2) Indirect: RFLP linkage
		      Heteroduplex analysis
		(3) DNA sequencing

$\delta\beta$ Thalassaemia	PCR Southern blot	Across breakpoints Probes: γ gene
Hb Lepore	PCR	Across breakpoints
HbS	PCR	(1) *Dde* I digestion (2) ARMS analysis (3) ASO dot blot
HbC	PCR	(1) ARMS analysis (2) ASO dot blot
HbE	PCR	(1) ARMS analysis (2) ASO dot blot (3) *Mnl* I digestion
HbD Punjab	PCR	*Eco*R I digestion
HbO Arab	PCR	*Eco*R I digestion

*LO is a probe located downstream from the ζ-globin gene (see Chapter 16).
ASO, allele-specific oligonucleotide; PCR, polymerase chain reaction.

variable number of rare ones. The strategy for identifying β-thalassaemia mutations depends on knowing the spectrum of common and rare mutations in the ethnic group of the individual being screened. Usually the common ones are investigated simultaneously using ASO dot blot or ARMS primers. For example, this strategy will identify the mutation in more than 80% of cases in the Asian Indian population in the UK (Old *et al.* 1990); further screening for previously identified rare mutations will characterize another 15% of cases (Varawalla *et al.* 1991a). Mutations which remain unidentified are then sought by the application of a non-specific detection method to localize them, heteroduplex analysis by denaturing gradient gel electrophoresis for example, followed by direct sequencing of the amplified gene sequence (Varawalla *et al.* 1991b).

Similar strategies have been reported by Rosatelli *et al.* (1992b) and Cao and Rosatelli (1993) for the Sardinian population, using dot-blot hybridization combined with DNA sequencing. They found that eight common mutations were observed in 93% of individuals with β-thalassaemia trait, and nine rare ones in a further 6% of cases. Therefore a two-step procedure, molecular screening by testing for the common mutations first, and then, if necessary, for rare ones, permits prenatal diagnosis for almost all couples at risk for β thalassaemia in a very short period of time.

α Thalassaemia

Because of the associated maternal complications, particularly toxaemia of pregnancy and difficulties associated with delivery of a hydropic infant and an enlarged, friable placenta, and the distress caused by the delivery of a dead baby, prenatal diagnosis is being widely applied for couples at risk for having a baby homozygous for α^0 thalassaemia. Since HbH disease is usually a relatively mild condition, associated with a good quality of life, prenatal diagnosis for this condition is not usually considered. However, it is becoming increasingly clear that there are severe forms of this condition and, as more is learnt about the molecular basis, there may be subsets of families with this condition that may wish to be considered for prenatal diagnosis. The different syndromes of HbH disease associated with mental retardation (see Chapter 12), particularly the X-linked form, can be identified in the fetus now that the gene involved has been identified. Prenatal diagnosis for this condition is being requested with increasing frequency.

PCR techniques can be used to diagnose the three most common types of α^0-thalassaemia deletions: the south-east Asian, $--^{SEA}$ (Chang *et al.* 1991; Bowden *et al.* 1992) and the two Mediterranean, $--^{MED}$ and $-(\alpha)^{20.5}$ (Bowden *et al.* 1992), as well as other less common variants such as $--^{THAI}$ and $--^{FIL}$ (Liu *et al.* 2000). Amplification across the deletion (gap PCR) offers a quick method for identification of α^0 thalassaemia (Winichagoon *et al.* 1995) but requires careful application because of the high sensitivity of PCR and other technical reasons. Amplification of sequences in the α-globin-gene cluster is technically more difficult than that of the β-globin-gene cluster, and requires more stringent conditions because of its higher GC content; Ko *et al.* (1997b) have reported four cases of amplification failure in PCR-based prenatal diagnosis in 180 cases of α^0 thalassaemia. In two, amplification of the normal sequence failed, resulting in the incorrect diagnosis of an affected homozygote, and in the others PCR failed to generate a mutant sequence, resulting in a misdiagnosis of a 'normal homozygote'; in the two cases wrongly diagnosed as affected, Southern blotting revealed heterozygous α^0 thalassaemia and termination of pregnancy was not performed.

Experience in our laboratory has also shown that some primer pairs are unreliable, resulting occasionally in unpredictable reaction failures, and Southern blot analysis is at present the standard diagnostic test for both screening and prenatal diagnosis of α^0 thalassaemia, although improved PCR-basedmethods are currently under development. Restriction-enzyme analysis of genomic DNA, using a combination of digests and probes in one test, permits the detection-of all the α-thalassaemia deletion genes, including those which cannot yet be diagnosed by PCR (Old 1996a). In addition, this approach provides diagnostic information on triple and quadruple α-gene loci, which, when co-inherited with β-thalassaemia trait, can result in thalassaemia intermedia (see Chapter 13).

Rare forms of thalassaemia and structural haemoglobin variants

As part of a comprehensive prenatal diagnosis programme it is important to have techniques available for fetal DNA analysis which encompass the rare forms of thalassaemia and the important structural haemoglobin variants which may interact with β thalassaemia to produce a severe disease, particularly Hbs S and E. The most commonly used methods for their identification are summarized in Table 14.7, and the methods are given in more detail in Chapter 16. The question of whether the various interactions of these variants with more severe forms of thalassaemia, which, overall, tend to give milder clinical phenotypes, should be considered for prenatal diagnosis was discussed earlier in this chapter.

Reliability of fetal DNA analysis

With the introduction of first-trimester diagnosis by CVS, an important question which had to be answered was whether the reliability of fetal DNA diagnosis was as good as or better than globin synthesis. By December 1989, Alter (1990) was able to collect data on 6324 prenatal diagnoses performed by DNA analysis, which revealed that there had been 29 diagnostic errors world-wide, giving an error rate of 0.5%, a figure that was almost identical to that recorded for fetal blood analysis.

By 1990 there was a definite shift towards DNA analysis because of its apparent reliability and lower fetal loss rate, and, most importantly, because it could be carried out by CVS in the first trimester. In the UK, early diagnosis by a mutation-specific PCR analysis has been possible for all couples at risk at three diagnostic centres since 1990. A national audit of the UK prenatal diagnosis results for the first 20 years, from 1974 to 1994, by Modell *et al.* (1997), revealed 22 recorded diagnostic errors (1.1%), seven as the result of the misreferral of a prenatal genotype and 15 due to technical problems associated with the diagnostic techniques (Table 14.8). There were eight misdiagnoses by globin synthesis (1.6%), five by Southern blot analysis (1.0%) and two by PCR (0.2%). It appears therefore that the accuracy of prenatal diagnosis has improved with each new technical development.

The PCR-based techniques now provide a quick

Table 14.8 Diagnostic errors and laboratory methods for prenatal diagnosis (PND) of haemoglobinopathies in the UK (1974–94).

Diagnostic methods	Total PNDs	Errors No.	Errors (%)	Misdiagnosis	Consequences
Globin synthesis	517	8	(1.55)	*Borderline results for β thalassaemia* 2 fetuses with thalassaemia major were diagnosed as trait 3 fetuses with thalassaemia trait were diagnosed as major *Human errors* 1 misinterpretation of results 1 crossover of samples affecting 2 pregnancies	2 children with thalassaemia major were born; 1 died of iron overload aged 16 years 2 unaffected pregnancies were aborted One couple continued an 'affected' pregnancy, but the child had thalassaemia trait 1 thalassaemia major child born; successful bone-marrow transplant 1 unaffected pregnancy was aborted 1 thalassaemia major child born: died after bone-marrow transplant
Southern blotting	583	5	(0.86)	1 plasmid contamination (α thalassaemia) 1 partial digestion with a restriction enzyme 1 maternal DNA contamination 2 erroneous linkage assignments (same case)	1 stillbirth of infant with hydrops fetalis 1 thalassaemia major child 1 fetus predicted to be AS was AA at birth 1 fetus diagnosed normal, had thalassaemia trait at birth 1 fetus diagnosed with thalassaemia trait, had thalassaemia major at birth
PCR	968	2	(0.21)	1 partial digestion with a restriction enzyme 1 non-paternity	1 fetus diagnosed as carrier was normal at birth 1 fetus diagnosed as affected, had thalassaemia trait at birth
Total	2068	22	(1.06)		

and relatively simple method for prenatal diagnosis of β thalassaemia and sickle-cell disease and are being employed in an increasing number of diagnostic centres in developing countries (Gorakshakar *et al.* 1997; Saxena *et al.* 1998). They have proved to be reliable and extremely accurate, provided careful attention is paid to prevent the coamplification of maternal sequences, the most important precaution being the careful removal of any maternal decidua from chorionic villi by microscopic dissection (Petrou *et al.* 1990). No misdiagnoses were reported in a total of 457 first-trimester diagnoses for β thalassaemia in the Italian population by dot-blot analysis (Rosatelli *et al.* 1992c). For sickle-cell disease, one misdiagnosis occurred in a programme of 500 prenatal diagnoses in the USA, most probably as a result of contamination of an amniotic fluid sample with maternal blood (Wang *et al.* 1994). However, for α^0 thalassaemia, seven misdiagnoses due to maternal DNA contamination of CVS DNA were reported in 180 cases (3.8%) of prenatal diagnosis by gap PCR (Ko *et al.* 1997b).

Thus contamination of fetal tissue with maternal cells is a constant risk for PCR-based DNA analysis and a number of precautions should be undertaken to limit the incidence of diagnostic error. They include the use of a limited number of amplification cycles, analysis in duplicate by a different molecular approach, analysis of DNA prepared from single villus fronds, and amplification of a highly informative DNA polymorphism to monitor for the presence of maternal contamination (Bhavnani *et al.* 1994).

Another potential source of error with PCR diagnoses is a so-called 'allele drop-out', that is, the failure to amplify one of the two target DNA alleles. This problem is mainly associated with prenatal diagnosis of α^0 thalassaemia, as reported by Ko *et al.* (1997b), but may occur with the amplification of any gene sequence when the hybridization of a primer or probe is compromised by an unexpected change in the target DNA sequence (Chan *et al.* 1993).

Population and psychosocial consequences of prenatal diagnosis

While we have made enormous progress in the technology of prenatal diagnosis we know far less about

its effects on society and about the psychological and other stresses that it might induce.

Modell *et al.* (1980), in an important early study of the effects of prenatal diagnosis on reproductive behaviour of families at risk for thalassaemia, found that, at least in the UK, knowledge of the risk of this disease led them to stop having children and to seek termination of the majority of any pregnancies which did occur, most of which were accidental. On the other hand, the introduction of prenatal diagnosis permitted the resumption of nearly normal reproduction by at-risk families with, of course, fewer than 30% of pregnancies being terminated for thalassaemia major. While these observations may well pertain to many richer countries they are unlikely to be so relevant to parts of the developing world. Here, the natural tendency is to have large families if children are born with congenital malformation or genetic disease. With improving social conditions there is always a tendency for family sizes to become smaller and it is quite likely that a similar pattern to that observed by Modell and colleagues in England would be observed eventually. But, in truth, very little is known about the effect of the introduction of prenatal diagnosis programmes on the overall birth rate in affected families.

The medical care of patients who have undergone prenatal diagnosis does not, of course, end after the termination of the pregnancy. Many women go through a period of depression and guilt and require considerable support. Of course, similar emotions may be experienced by those who give birth to their child with a severe form of thalassaemia, a problem which also seems to occur in populations in which the majority of mothers undergo prenatal diagnosis (Professor Antonio Cao, personal communication).

We badly need more information about the psychosocial aspects of screening and prenatal diagnosis, not just in richer Western societies but in other parts of the world and in different social and religious settings. Further discussion of the various approaches that are being taken to investigate this important problem are summarized in a review by Green and Statham (1996).

Overall effects of prenatal diagnosis programmes

The overall results of prenatal diagnosis programmes

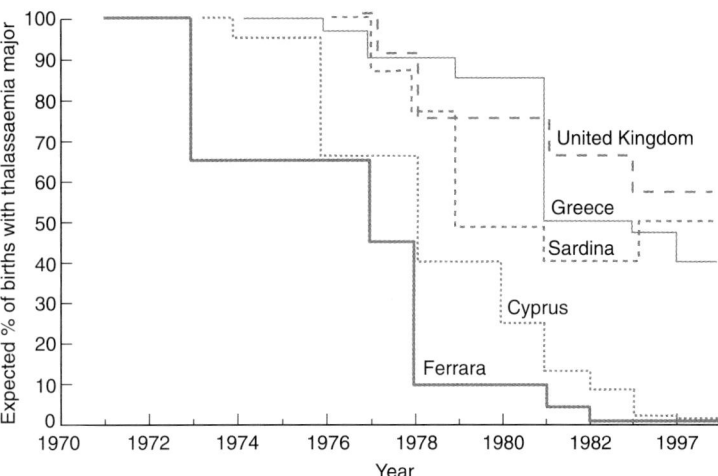

Fig. 14.9 Decline in the severe forms of thalassaemia in different populations during the period just after the first introduction of prenatal diagnosis. During the early part of this period prenatal diagnosis was carried out by fetal blood sampling and globin synthesis. DNA diagnosis was introduced in the late 1970s and became the main approach during the 1980s. Adapted from Modell & Bulyshenkov (1988) Distribution and control of some genetic disorders. *World Health Statistics Quart.* **41**, 21.

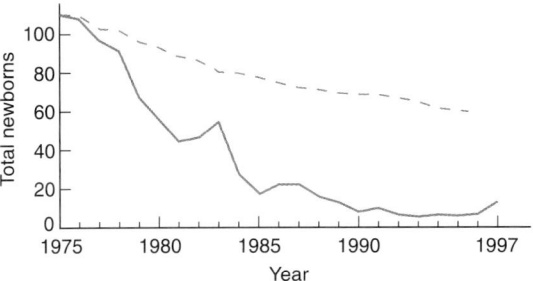

Fig. 14.10 Fall of birth rates of babies with severe β thalassaemia in Sardinia. The broken line shows the predicted numbers of newborns had no control programme been introduced; the continuous line shows the actual numbers. The ordinate values are absolute numbers of children affected by thalassaemia major. Adapted from Cao *et al.* (1998).

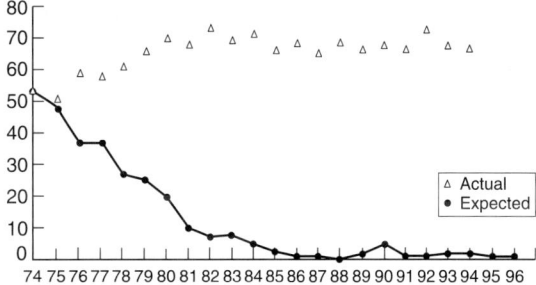

Fig. 14.11 The effects of the prenatal diagnosis programme in Cyprus. The dotted line shows the expected number of births had the programme not been started, and the continuous line shows the actual number of new births. The ordinate values are the number of births of thalassaemic children each year. Adapted from Angastiniotis and Modell (1998).

have been discussed recently by Modell and Kuliev (1998) and the effect on the birth rate of new cases of β thalassaemia for selected countries is summarized in Figs 14.9–14.11. The most remarkable results have been obtained in Cyprus and Sardinia, where the frequency of births of affected babies has dropped quite dramatically over the period since screening and prenatal diagnosis was introduced. As shown in Fig. 14.10, in Sardinia there was a brief interruption in the otherwise steady fall in the birth rate of affected infants between 1981 and 1983 and this was due to temporary withdrawal of funding for community education. There has been a small increase in the last

year or two again and this has been ascribed to the belief by some families that more definitive forms of treatment are in the offing. The rather indifferent results shown for the UK in Fig. 14.9 are discussed by Modell and Kuliev (1998). It appears that only a small proportion of the babies born with severe forms of thalassaemia in the UK were the result of informed parental choice, and approximately 80% were due simply to lack of adequate information or, possibly, varying religious beliefs and practices.

Taken at face value these results reflect a remarkable success for a public health programme directed at the control of a serious genetic disease. Obviously it is much easier to achieve a result of this type in small island populations or in smaller countries and it will be much more difficult to translate them into similarly successful programmes in the large mainland populations of the Indian subcontinent and southeast Asia. Earlier in this chapter we discussed the remarkable reduction in the births of new cases of β thalassaemia reported from Iran, where genetic counselling was followed by the decision not to marry in 90% of cases. This is an even more remarkable result. However, it will be very important to keep a very close watch on all these programmes with particular respect to ensuring that families are not being pressurized into these critical reproductive decisions. This pressure can come from many different sources; some of them are not obvious at first sight. While the pressures of the state and religious leaders are easier to define, the more subtle pressures put on families where it has become the norm to terminate pregnancies which are likely to result in serious forms of thalassaemia may be equally strong. The thalassaemia field has led the way into the era of prenatal diagnosis by DNA analysis. For this reason it is all the more important that it continues to monitor the psychological and pastoral aspects of the control of genetic disease extremely carefully in the future.

Recent developments in prenatal diagnosis

The ability to amplify DNA from a single fetal cell has led to the development of alternative methods for prenatal diagnosis. The sensitivity of PCR to detect mutations is greatly enhanced by the technique of nested PCR. In short, in the first reaction a pair of primers is used to amplify a short DNA region encompassing the mutation, after which a small aliquot of the product is reamplified with an internal set of nested primers in a second round of PCR. Globin-gene mutations can be detected in the PCR product by various methods, such as ASO dot blotting, heteroduplex analysis or restriction-enzyme digestion. This technique has stimulated research directed at prenatal diagnosis by the analysis of fetal cells in maternal blood and preimplantation diagnosis.

Fetal cells in maternal blood

Fetal cells have long been known to be present in the

maternal circulation and they provide an attractive, non-invasive approach to prenatal diagnosis. Although much research using immunological methods and cell sorting has been directed at enriching fetal lymphocytes, trophoblasts or erythroblasts, sufficient for fetal DNA analysis (Simpson & Elias 1994), by itself this approach has so far failed to provide a population of cells of sufficient purity for single gene analysis, and until recently the analysis of fetal genotypes in this way could only be used for the prenatal diagnosis of thalassaemia in women whose partners carried a different mutation, as reported in the diagnosis of Hb Lepore using maternal peripheral blood (Camaschella *et al.* 1990b).

The recent development of methods to isolate cells by micromanipulation promises to facilitate the analysis of fetal genes at the single cell level (Takabayashi *et al.* 1995). Indeed, this approach has already been used successfully for the prenatal diagnosis of sickle-cell anaemia and β thalassaemia (Cheung *et al.* 1996). To achieve this end Cheung and colleagues first separated the mononuclear cells from 18 ml of maternal blood by centrifugation on a step Ficoll-hypaque gradient. The enriched mononuclear cells were incubated with anti-CD71 (transferrin receptor) antibodies coupled with magnetic beads, and then enriched further by magnetic cell sorting. Finally, the cells were smeared on a slide, stained with anti-ζ-globin antibodies to identify fetal erythroblasts (approximately 20 cells), and individual fetal cells were plucked from the slide by microdissection. The authors pooled the isolated cells for PCR in order to minimize the technical problem of allele drop-out. Thus the goal of using fetal cells from maternal blood as a definitive prenatal diagnostic procedure has now been realized, although a great deal more work is required to determine the reliability of the technique.

Preimplantation diagnosis

Preimplantation diagnosis has the advantage over all the other methods of prenatal diagnosis that, by selection of only those oocytes identified by DNA analysis as unaffected for replacement in the uterus, the mother avoids the possibility of having to terminate an affected pregnancy. Two approaches are in the process of development, the analysis of single cells biopsied from cleaving stages or the removal and analysis of the two polar bodies extruded during the maturation of the oocyte (Delhanty 1994; Handyside & Delahunty 1997). Both sampling methods have been found to be subject to the problem of allele drop-out and this resulted in two misdiagnoses of cystic fibrosis following preimplantation diagnosis (Ray & Handyside 1996). However, this problem is now being overcome by the simultaneous analysis of other maternal and paternal polymorphic markers and the sequential analysis of both polar bodies, only using oocytes for which, because of a recombinational event, the first polar body contains both the normal and mutant gene and the second polar body contains the mutant gene, and hence which must contain the normal allele. The pregnancy rate for fertile couples undergoing preimplantation diagnosis appears to be about 30%, only slightly higher than the normal *in vitro* fertilization rate of 23%, and thus the procedure will be most suitable for those couples at risk with a bad obstetric history of prenatal diagnosis and termination of pregnancy. Preimplantation diagnosis of β thalassaemia by polar body analysis is currently being applied by Y. Verlinsky's group in Cyprus, resulting in a number of continuing pregnancies (Kuliev *et al.* 1998, 1999).

Avoidance versus treatment in the future

The development of methods for screening and prenatal diagnosis, first by fetal blood sampling and globin synthesis and later by DNA analysis, is a telling example of the rapid transfer of technologies from the research laboratory to the field, and the reduction in the number of new births with thalassaemia in many countries is a remarkable achievement. Since it is unlikely that cheap and effective ways of treating or curing the important forms of thalassaemia will appear on the horizon in the immediate future, these programmes will remain an important part of thalassaemia control in the richer countries; just how successful they will be in the large rural populations of the developing countries remains to be seen. Clearly, it would be better if methods were to become available for avoiding termination of pregnancy, and it is important to carry out further work on preimplantation diagnosis. However, whether it will become effective and cheap enough to be applied on a large scale remains to be seen.

Given the costs of the alternatives, and the likelihood that it will be a long time before better forms of treatment for thalassaemia are developed, those countries in which the disease will be such a major problem in this new millennium will have to seriously consider whether avoidance programmes of this type are appropriate for their societies. There are still many practical issues to be addressed but there is no doubt that screening and avoidance for genetic diseases like thalassaemia are now well established and a genuine option for their control.

Chapter 15
Management and prognosis

Introduction

In introducing this chapter in our previous edition we were not optimistic:

> With each successive edition of this book we have been struck by the remarkable advances in our understanding of the pathophysiology and molecular biology of thalassaemia. Despite this spectacular progress we have approached the chapter on management in our usual state of trepidation. This stems from the unfortunate fact that the clinical spin-off from the technological advances that have enabled us to reach our present understanding of the thalassaemia syndromes has been relatively small. Indeed, it is true to say that there have been no fundamental advances in the management of these conditions over the last eight years.

It is now possible to write about the management and prognosis of the thalassaemias with much more enthusiasm. While it is still true that our early hopes that an understanding of the molecular mechanisms that underlie these diseases might lead to a definitive cure by gene therapy have so far turned out to be unfounded, and many more years of research and development are required before they will come to fruition, there is no doubt that the management of the thalassaemias has improved out of all recognition over recent years. In particular, there is now unequivocal evidence that children who are managed appropriately with regular blood transfusion and adequate chelation therapy are surviving to adult life in good health and, increasingly, are able to lead relatively normal lives and have families of their own (Fig. 15.1). Furthermore, there has been sufficient experience of bone-marrow transplantation for it to be clear that, in selected cases and with appropriate donors, it can cure the disease. Hence there is a much more positive attitude among those responsible for its clinical management, and a feeling among research workers that, sooner or later, it

will be possible to correct the underlying molecular pathology.

In this chapter we review the management of the severe forms of β thalassaemia and then discuss the treatment of other forms of the disease. Although most of our personal experience in the treatment of these disorders has been in the setting of richer countries with well established, if often maligned, government health services, throughout this discussion we shall try to keep in mind the needs of the developing countries in which the thalassaemias are likely to pose an increasing public health problem in the new millennium.

General management

When the diagnosis of transfusion-dependent thalassaemia is made early in life the patient and the family are destined for a lifelong association with their physicians and hospitals. As with the management of any chronic illness, it is vital for the clinician to get off on the right foot with both the patient and their relatives. Hence, when the disease is suspected, an infant should be referred to a centre with a special knowledge and interest in these disorders. In this way it should be possible to obtain a firm diagnosis and to provide the parents with a clear picture of the child's future. There is nothing worse than for them to receive a series of half-truths and vague generalizations at the beginning of what is, for even the most balanced of families, an extremely traumatic experience.

The first two questions which are always raised in managing thalassaemia are: when can the diagnosis be established with certainty, and when should treatment be initiated?

Diagnosis and initiation of treatment

It was pointed out in Chapter 7 that the majority of transfusion-dependent thalassaemics present with severe anaemia during the first year of life. If a baby presents later than this the possibility of the diagnosis

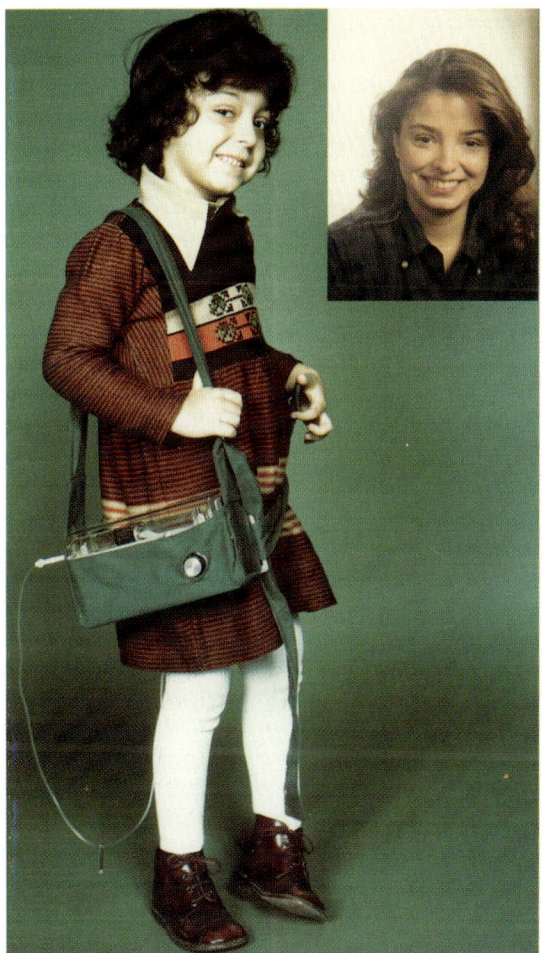

Fig. 15.1 Successful management of β thalassaemia with transfusion and chelation therapy. This patient was one of the first to be treated by overnight infusions of desferrioxamine (Pippard *et al.* 1978a,b). This technique was developed because it was realized that it would not be practical for children to wear clockwork pumps as shown in this figure (left). The inset on the right shows the same patient at the age of 28 years. She has grown and developed quite normally, is married and has a successful career as a lawyer.

of thalassaemia intermedia should be seriously considered. However, many infants with milder forms of thalassaemia also present within the first year and therefore it is essential to wait to determine the steady-state haemoglobin level, and to assess whether it is compatible with normal development or

whether regular transfusion will be required. Unless this is done there is a danger of starting an infant with thalassaemia intermedia on a life of unnecessary treatment.

There is another very important problem related to the haemoglobin level at presentation. Quite often babies with different forms of thalassaemia present to the hospital with severe anaemia during a period of an intercurrent illness, particularly infection. After establishing a diagnosis it is often necessary to transfuse these babies to a safer haemoglobin level. However, it is vital to then observe them over a reasonable period to try to find out what their steady-state haemoglobin level really is. It is quite clear, when tracing histories and trying to establish why children with thalassaemia were started on regular blood transfusion, that it was often during an episode like this, after which it was simply assumed that the infant would be transfusion dependent in the long term. Unfortunately, many patients with thalassaemia have started a life of unnecessary transfusion in this way; once started it may be difficult to stop, even though they are able to sustain a haemoglobin level compatible with adequate development.

During this critical waiting period before the decision to start a transfusion regimen is made, the infant should be seen regularly to assess its level of activity, feeding, growth and spleen size. The decision to commence blood transfusion should be made on information of this kind, and not on the steady-state haemoglobin alone.

It is also important to carry out the appropriate diagnostic laboratory tests before the first transfusion is given. The haematological findings and changes in the haemoglobin pattern, together with the times that these are established in infancy, are discussed in Chapter 7. Assuming that the infant may require regular transfusion in the future it is also important to carry out a full blood-group genotype at this time.

Early interviews with the parents

In the first interviews with the parents it is important to tell them precisely why regular blood counts are being done, but to avoid becoming involved in a discussion of long-term management until the decision whether or not to transfuse has been made. When a well designed policy for the future has been established, the parents should be given a detailed explanation of the nature of thalassaemia and of the likely course for their child.

An early attempt should be made to try to explain the genetic implications of the diagnosis of thalassaemia. This should be done in language appropriate to the level of education and intelligence of the particular parents. There is still a stigma attached to genetic disease, and feelings of guilt are often engendered in the parents. The concept of 'mutations' and the fact that all of us carry a certain number of 'bad genes' can be explained in simple lay language, and the reasons for the high frequency of the thalassaemia genes in certain populations can be communicated in the same way. If the infant is the first affected family member it is appropriate to provide advice about future family planning and to outline the possibility of prenatal diagnosis if this is available in the community. All these facets should be dealt with in considerable detail at the first few meetings.

Our own approach and advice to parents at early interviews goes along the following lines. We explain that the child is unable to produce sufficient red cells and that for this reason they will have to be maintained by regular transfusion. We explain that this can be carried out on a short-stay outpatient basis or on a single overnight visit every 3–4 weeks, and that if this is done regularly the child's early growth and development will be satisfactory. Indeed, there is no reason why the infant should not grow and develop like any normal youngster. We then give a completely frank explanation of the potential problems and hazards of blood transfusion, particularly as related to iron overload. We discuss in detail the use of chelating agents. We then point out that it is now possible to maintain these children in iron balance and that, although the techniques are cumbersome and sometimes painful, if they manage their infant in this way it will have every chance of long-term survival, with a good quality of life. It is absolutely essential to give this degree of encouragement at an early stage.

At the end of the early interviews the parents are usually rather shattered by the events and it is at subsequent interviews that many of their questions are framed. For this reason it is essential that the same clinician takes on the long-term management and that parents are not shunted from doctor to doctor in busy hospital outpatient departments.

It is also important that families should be well briefed as to the dangers inherent in having a chronically sick child. Arrangements must be made for both parents to help in the management of the child and where possible to share the duties of bringing the child to hospital for check-ups and transfusion. We have found that it is often possible to gain the support of employers and hence to arrange time off work for this purpose. If the total burden falls on one parent they may become pathologically close to the affected child and tend to neglect their other children and their partner. At worst this results in a broken marriage and lack of the family stability so vital for the thalassaemic child.

Thalassaemic infants and children are best looked after by a clinician who has a special expertise in blood disorders and good laboratory support. The primary clinician should be a haematologist with particular knowledge of the disease, working together with a team of paediatricians, other specialists and well trained nurses. It is better for the same clinician to follow the care of these patients right through adolescence into adult life; they should not be 'handed over' at puberty. It is also extremely helpful if a social worker with a special knowledge of the problems of thalassaemia is attached to clinics looking after these patients. Regular home visits during the early years of the illness and liaison with other social services and the family doctor can be extremely useful in supporting the family.

Many communities in which there is a high incidence of the disease have formed thalassaemia societies similar to those associated with other chronic diseases of childhood, cystic fibrosis for example. Many parents find these helpful in that it immediately becomes apparent that they are not unique, and they can benefit from the experiences of other parents and from information which is provided by well run societies of this type. It is essential, however, that the medical advice to groups of this kind is of the highest calibre and that sensational news of new treatments and similar untried 'advances' are put into proper perspective for parents who are desperately anxious to hear of any progress in the field.

Symptomatic treatment

The main basis of treatment for all forms of severe thalassaemia is blood transfusion. This is combined with good all-round general medical care, the judicious use of splenectomy in a proportion of cases, the provision of chelating agents and the early management of complications, particularly infection. In the sections which follow we shall deal with the problem of the transfusion-dependent β-thalassaemic child. In later sections we shall deal with specific problems relating to such disorders as thalassaemia intermedia, the α thalassaemias and the common conditions resulting from the interaction of β thalassaemia with structural haemoglobin variants.

Blood transfusion

The determination of the optimal transfusion regimen for a thalassaemic child has probably been the single most important advance in the management of the disorder over the last 30 years. The story of how our present thinking about the correct approach to blood transfusion in thalassaemia evolved from the pioneering work of Wolman and colleagues in Philadelphia is outlined in Chapter 1, together with an account of the studies of later workers who built on these beginnings. In this section we shall describe current practice and some of the problems which may be encountered in establishing transfusion services for thalassaemic children in the developing countries.

When to transfuse

In Chapter 7, and earlier in this chapter, we emphasized the importance of not embarking on a transfusion regimen too early and, particularly in infants who have presented during infection, of establishing a steady-state haemoglobin level. Children with haemoglobin values below 6–7 g/dl should be observed very carefully at regular intervals, with particular respect to their activity, growth and development, spleen size and any suggestion of early skeletal changes. Any infant who is showing deleterious effects of anaemia of this kind, which would include most of those with haemoglobin values much below 6–7 g/dl, will require transfusion. As mentioned earlier, to prevent allosensitization to important blood-group antigens, the patient's full blood-group genotype should be established before the institution of transfusion therapy.

Type of blood product

Because of the dangers of transfusion reactions there is no place for the use of whole blood or untreated packed red blood cells. In order to avoid leucocyte sensitization, leucocytes should be removed from the blood to be transfused, either by washing with saline or by the use of filters which remove the majority of leucocytes from banked blood (Meryman 1989). There are a variety of different types of filter available. Some are designed to filter blood in the blood bank before delivery to the ward; others, which are easier to use but rather more expensive, are used to filter the blood while it is being administered to the patient. Most standard filters will allow no more than two units of blood to be transfused, though for young patients one-unit filters are now available. The use of frozen red cells, while this process almost entirely depletes the preparations of leucocytes, is extremely costly and cumbersome and is not available in many centres. Furthermore, freshly filtered blood offers the additional advantage of having a higher level of 2,3-diphosphoglycerate, and hence more effective oxygen-carrying properties; it has been shown that frozen cells are defective in this respect (Correra *et al.* 1984; Piomelli 1993).

There have been a number of attempts made to separate cells according to their age by density centrifugation with the objective of extending the intervals between transfusion and reducing the body iron load (Piomelli *et al.* 1978; Propper *et al.* 1980). In discussing this approach Propper and colleagues suggested that the least dense fraction of red cells isolated after centrifugation has a mean age of approximately 12 days and hence would be expected to have a life expectancy of approximately 108±12 days. This must be compared with the life expectancy of a conventional unit of blood, with a red-cell survival of approximately 60 days. Propper and colleagues also suggested that it might be possible to transfuse a patient using a cell separator, removing the lowest layer of old, dense cells at the same time as the young cells are given. In this way it would be theoretically possible to achieve a high-level transfusion regimen with a daily positive iron balance of no more than 2–5 mg. Certainly, early studies confirmed that a modest extension of the transfusion interval could be obtained by the use of neocytes (Cohen *et al.* 1984b). Later work, which used a simpler modification of the preparative method

(Simon *et al.* 1989), confirmed these findings (Kevy *et al.* 1988).

A more recent study has shown that the reduction in total annual transfusional iron load during neocyte transfusions varies widely, from less than 10% to more than 25% (Spanos *et al.* 1996). Cost–benefit analysis of neocyte transfusion remains complicated; the undoubted benefits of reduced iron administration are accompanied by an increased requirement for units of blood, and up to a fivefold increase in the cost of preparation over those of standard red-cell concentrates (Collins *et al.* 1994).

How much blood and how often?

These important questions are reviewed by Piomelli (1993). The objective of a transfusion regimen is to correct the anaemia and clinical manifestations of the disease and to suppress the patient's endogenous erythropoiesis. From a physiological point of view therefore, the more often transfusion can be given the better. In practice, it is necessary to compromise; in most centres patients are transfused every 3–4 weeks with 10–15 ml/kg of packed red cells. Sometimes there are situations in which it is necessary to transfuse larger amounts of blood at longer intervals, particularly when patients have to travel great distances for their treatment, but this practice could result in a greater iron load (Piomelli *et al.* 1985).

It is generally advised that the transfusion rate should not exceed 4–5 ml/kg/h, so as to avoid sudden perturbations of blood volume. This is satisfactory for patients who are otherwise well, but in those with cardiac insufficiency the transfusion intervals should be reduced to once a week, and the rate of transfusion should be no more than 2 ml/kg/h or even lower. As in all forms of anaemia, patients who are showing signs of cardiac failure should be given diuretics along with the transfusion.

At every transfusion session it is essential to weigh the child, measure the pretransfusion haemoglobin level, measure and record the size of the spleen and, where possible, to obtain a post-transfusion haemoglobin value. It is extremely helpful to chart a graphic record to visualize the course of transfusion therapy.

At what level should the haemoglobin be maintained?

The optimal baseline haemoglobin level at which a patient with severe thalassaemia should be maintained has been a matter of controversy for many years. The origins of the argument, reviewed by Piomelli (1993), range round the concept that, once a patient's blood volume has been replenished, the amount necessary to maintain a higher baseline haemoglobin level should be the same as for a lower one. Piomelli points out that at the beginning of transfusion therapy, particularly in very young patients or in those who have been maintained at a very low haemoglobin level, there is a substantial reduction in plasma volume and hence it may appear that the amount of blood required to maintain a higher level of haemoglobin is similar to that necessary to achieve a lower baseline (Propper *et al.* 1980). However, once homeostasis is achieved a difference may become apparent. In practice, this has not always been the case, however. Some workers found that, after transfusing patients to levels of 14 g/dl or higher, the haemoglobin level could be maintained at this value without increasing the overall amount of blood administered above that required to maintain a lower level (see Propper *et al.* 1980), while others found that increased amounts of blood were required to maintain higher haemoglobin levels (Modell & Berdoukas 1984; Piomelli 1993). However, as pointed out by Piomelli the important goal is not the maintenance of an average haemoglobin, but rather a constant baseline. It was suggested by Piomelli *et al.* (1985) that a baseline haemoglobin level of 10.5 g/dl is adequate to correct the anaemia to a point at which endogenous erythropoiesis is suppressed, and that it is quite unnecessary to maintain a higher level.

Recently, an analysis of 10 years of administration of a 'moderate' transfusion regimen, that is, a mean pretransfusion haemoglobin level which did not exceed 9.5 g/dl, suggested that the resulting reduction in body iron loading, at least as estimated by the serum ferritin concentration, was associated with a no more than threefold increase in marrow activity and a lower incidence of endocrine and cardiac complications (Cazzola *et al.* 1997).

These observations suggest that children with severe β thalassaemia should be maintained on a transfusion regimen in which their pretransfusion haemoglobin levels do not drop below 9.5 g/dl. There seems little place for the older 'high' transfusion programmes, which attempted to maintain pretransfusion haemoglobin levels much closer to normal. It is very important to assess the annual blood requirements in order to predict the onset of hypersplenism (see later section).

Has the minimal safe haemoglobin level to be maintained by transfusion been established?

As we have seen, it is clear that to establish the required baseline haemoglobin level for transfusion-dependent children depends on striking a balance between the minimal amount of blood that is required, and hence the minimal possible iron load (and cost), while at the same time suppressing endogenous erythropoiesis and providing sufficient oxygenation for normal growth and development and, in addition, preventing skeletal deformity. Judging by the bone-marrow turnover studies reported by Cazzola *et al.* (1997) a baseline level of 9.5 g/dl may be getting fairly close to the critical level below which development may be compromised. However, as discussed in Chapters 9 and 13, some patients with thalassaemia intermedia grow and develop quite adequately at steady-state haemoglobin levels below 9.5 g/dl. Thus, while it may be a useful rule of thumb to maintain transfusion-dependent children at this level, a great deal more work needs to be done to try to define the factors other than the haemoglobin level that determine the rates of growth and development at lower haemoglobin levels, particularly in the 7–9 g/dl range so commonly observed in thalassaemia intermedia. This question is particularly relevant to the developing countries, where increasing demands on limited transfusion services will cause a major problem in the future.

Dangers of transfusion

The major dangers of transfusion are blood-borne infection and transfusion reactions.

Blood-borne infection

The more common blood-borne infections were discussed in detail in Chapter 7. To prevent hepatitis B infection, donor blood should be tested for hepatitis surface antigen and antibody and for hepatitis B core antibody. Hepatitis B vaccination should be administered to all patients who are hepatitis B-virus negative or who lack demonstrable antibodies. Booster vaccination is recommended when the antibody titre is lower than 10 IU/l, usually about 5 years after vaccination. Donor blood should also be screened for hepatitis C virus (HCV) and human immunodeficiency virus (HIV). All chronically transfused patients should be tested yearly for HCV and for HIV. It is also important to check the patient's cytomegalovirus (CMV) status before regular transfusion is embarked on, particularly in those who may be considered for bone-marrow transplantation. If negative for CMV antibody, patients should ideally be given CMV-negative blood.

Transfusion reactions

The commonest reactions result from sensitivity to leucocytes or plasma proteins. They tend to occur after several years of transfusion, and are characterized by a modest rise in temperature, sometimes accompanied by flushing and shivering. When this occurs the transfusion may be temporarily suspended and the patient given an antihistamine or an antipyretic agent. Occasionally these reactions are more severe and are associated with rashes or facial oedema and, again, the transfusion should be stopped and hydrocortisone administered.

Multi-transfused patients may develop antibodies, usually against some of the rarer blood groups. They should be investigated in a centre with expertise in blood-group serology and attempts made to find compatible units of blood.

It should always be borne in mind that a patient who develops pyrexia and tachycardia associated with a blood transfusion could have received an incompatible unit of blood or one that is infected. Although these complications are, mercifully, rare they must always be considered. In either case the transfusion must be stopped immediately and blood taken from the patient for further investigation for a cross-matching error.

The main aim of treatment after an incompatible transfusion is to maintain the urine output in excess of 100 ml per hour, together with a normal systemic blood pressure until the reaction subsides. A saline or dextrose infusion is usually adequate for this purpose, though occasionally, when the urine output declines, a forced mannitol diuresis may be used to good effect. Fresh frozen plasma may be given if coagulation factors are being consumed.

If there is any possibility that the blood was infected the remainder should be sent for Gram staining and both aerobic and anaerobic culture. Appropriate antibiotics should be administered together with adequate fluid replacement, and the patient managed in an intensive care unit, with facilities for renal dialysis.

Special hazards in tropical countries

Because of the increased frequency of both viral hepatitis and HIV infection it is particularly important to develop donor screening programmes. The problem of blood-borne malarial infection was considered in Chapter 7. Where donor screening is not feasible it is very important to examine the blood for malarial parasites in any child who develops a pyrexial illness after a transfusion. Since drug resistance is widespread it is essential that clinics which run transfusion programmes in tropical countries are aware of the pattern of local drug sensitivity to antimalarials so that appropriate treatment can be given (see later section).

Iron chelation therapy

As discussed in Chapter 7, without regular chelation therapy to control iron accumulation, transfusion-dependent children with severe forms of thalassaemia die during the second decade of life. The rather long and chequered history of how desferrioxamine (Desferal®) was first introduced, the initial disappointments, and the later realization that, if administered appropriately, it could control iron accumulation, was outlined in Chapter 1. It is now clear that, in patients who are compliant, the effective administration of this agent is able to extend survival indefinitely and to dramatically improve the quality of life.

Pharmacology of desferrioxamine (DF)

Early studies on the pharmacology of DF were reviewed by Keberle (1964) and by Waxman and Brown (1969). Its pharmacological properties are discussed by Hershko and Weatherall (1988). It is a member of the hydroxamic acid class of iron chela-

tors and is produced by the organism *Streptomyces pilosus*. Its three hydroxamic acid groups form six coordination ligands with ferric iron with a very high affinity (stability constant of 10^{31}). The chelate, ferrioxamine, is excreted in the urine, to which it gives a red coloration, although up to 50% of the iron chelated in response to DF may appear in the faeces (Cumming *et al.* 1969). The half-life of DF in the circulation is only about 75 min. Although patients with iron overload may have massive iron stores, most of this is unavailable for chelation; at any given time only a small pool is chelatable and it seems likely that the latter is only slowly refilled from the stores; during the period of refilling there is very little iron available for chelation and this, combined with the short half-life of DF in the circulation, probably explains the suboptimal response to intramuscular bolus injections of the drug.

Unfortunately, DF is poorly absorbed from the gastrointestinal tract (Callender & Weatherall 1980) and rapidly metabolized in the plasma (Summers *et al.* 1979). Hence it has to be given by prolonged, parenteral infusion during which time the plasma concentration reaches a plateau at about 12 h (see Hershko & Weatherall 1988). The sources that are chelatable by DF were reviewed by Hershko and Weatherall (1988) and Brittenham *et al.* (1994). Iron bound by DF is rendered virtually inactive, and hence the drug can prevent or reverse the effects of free-radical formation and lipid peroxidation (Bacon *et al.* 1983; Morehouse *et al.* 1984; Link & Pinson 1985; O'Connell *et al.* 1985).

The evolution of methods for the administration of desferrioxamine

The early studies that led to the introduction and further development of DF as a chelating agent are outlined in Chapter 1. The major advance followed the development of its administration by prolonged subcutaneous infusion (Hussain *et al.* 1976; Propper *et al.* 1976, 1977). It was found more practical to carry out these infusions overnight and, because the same amount of iron can be removed by increasing the dose of DF as by increasing the infusion time, infusions could be limited to no longer than 12 h (Pippard *et al.* 1978b) (Fig. 15.2). These observations, and the discovery that, in addition to a substantial increase in the urinary output of iron, a considerable amount was

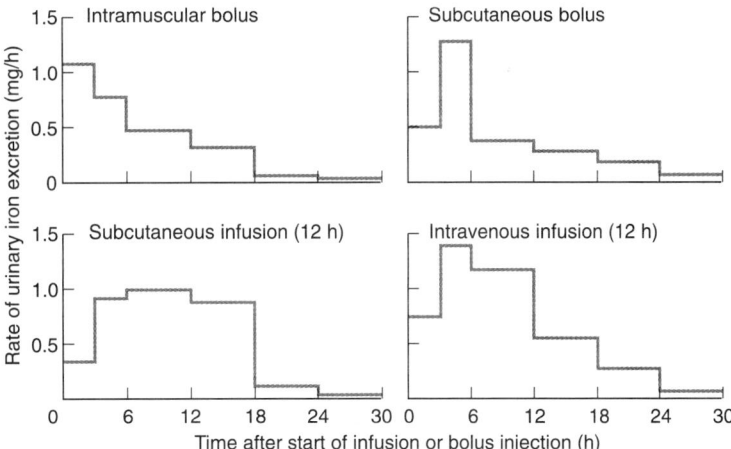

Fig. 15.2 The urinary output after the administration of desferrioxamine by different routes in children homozygous for β thalassaemia. From Pippard *et al.* (1978b).

excreted through the bowel (Pippard *et al.* 1982a), together with the finding that the amount of iron removed could be augmented by ascorbate repletion (Modell & Beck 1974; O'Brien 1974; Nienhuis *et al.* 1976; Hussain *et al.* 1977; Propper *et al.* 1977; Pippard *et al.* 1978b), made it possible to design regimens of nightly subcutaneous DF infusions using portable ambulatory pumps (Hussain *et al.* 1976; Propper *et al.* 1977; Pippard *et al.* 1978b). Although there have been further modifications of this approach to the administration of DF, described later in this section, this method is still the major therapeutic linchpin on which the modern management of transfusion-dependent thalassaemia is based.

Evidence of the clinical effectiveness of desferrioxamine

There are several factors which suggest that DF is an extremely effective agent for the prevention of iron overload in β thalassaemia. First, net negative iron balance is feasible over a long period; adequate therapy has led to survival curves that approximate to those of the normal population (Brittenham *et al.* 1994; Olivieri *et al.* 1994b; Gabutti & Piga 1996; Olivieri & Brittenham 1997). Second, it is clear that it may be possible to reverse some, though probably not all, the complications of iron overload (Gabutti & Piga 1996; Olivieri & Brittenham 1997). Finally, even in patients who are unable or unwilling to administer nightly subcutaneous DF it is possible to develop protocols for alternate means of administration. Fur-

thermore, because of the rarity of genuine allergic reactions to the drug, there are very few patients who cannot tolerate it.

In the sections which follow we shall briefly outline some of the evidence that supports the beneficial effects of DF on organ function in transfusion-dependent patients with β thalassaemia.

The heart

The cardiac complications of iron loading were described in Chapter 7. Since cardiac failure was the major cause of death in thalassaemia before adequate chelation regimes were established it was particularly important to assess the effectiveness of DF in preventing this complication. Early suspicions that survival might be prolonged by the adequate use of DF have been confirmed by two studies, both of over 10 years' duration, which have demonstrated quite unequivocally that the effective long-term use of the drug is associated with long-term survival free of the cardiac complications of iron overload (Brittenham *et al.* 1994; Olivieri *et al.* 1994b). In addition, these studies identified the magnitude of the body iron burden as the principal determinant of the clinical outcome. In one, which used serum ferritin to evaluate iron load, over the period of follow-up most patients with serum ferritin concentrations less than 2500 μg/l had an estimated cardiac disease-free survival of 91% after 15 years. On the other hand, most of those in whom most serum ferritin concentrations had exceeded 2500 μg/l had an estimated cardiac disease-free survival after 15 years of less than 20% (Fig. 15.3a). In the other study, the relationship between the total amount of iron administered by transfusion, the cumulative use of DF and the magnitude of the body iron burden, as determined by measurements of hepatic iron stores, was assessed. Using a threshold for transfusional iron load reflected by a hepatic storage iron concentration of about 80 μmol iron/g liver, wet weight (about 15 mg iron/g liver, dry weight), patients were classified as having received ineffective or effective chelation therapy. Ineffective therapy was associated with the greatest risk of clinical complications and early death; the probability of survival to at least the age of 25 years was only 32% among patients above the threshold. In contrast, effective chelation protected against cardiac disease and early death as well as diabetes; importantly, no deaths had occurred among patients below the threshold (Fig. 15.3b).

Borgna-Pignatti *et al.* (1998b) observed similar trends in an Italian population born between 1960 and 1987. Overall, the probability of survival to the age of 20 years was 89%. Cardiac failure was seen in 6.4% of patients and dysrhythmias in 5%. Heart disease was the leading cause of death, and the prevalence of this complication at the age of 15 years had declined from 5% in the cohort born in the years 1970–1984 to 2% in those born between 1980 and 1984. Despite some problems arising from the lower age in the second cohort, these data, taken together, also suggest a favourable impact of chelation therapy on the incidence of cardiac disease in the younger group (Fig. 15.4).

Liver disease

As mentioned in Chapter 1 and earlier in this chapter, the observation that, even using what would now be considered to be inadequate doses of DF, progressive fibrosis might be arrested was the major incentive to the re-evaluation of chelation therapy in the early and mid-1970s (Barry *et al.* 1974). As judged by a reduction in liver iron concentration, improvement in liver function tests and arrest of hepatic fibrosis, there is now substantial evidence for the beneficial effects of the administration of DF on iron loading of the liver (Barry *et al.* 1974; Cohen *et al.* 1984a; Aldouri *et al.* 1987). High-dose DF administered intravenously has been reported to achieve some benefits even in patients with massively

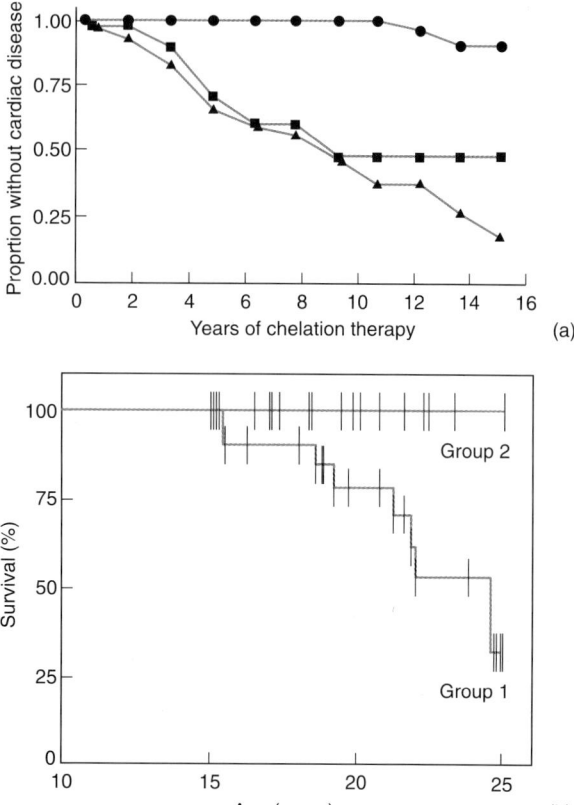

Fig. 15.3 Survival data related to effectiveness of iron chelation therapy in β thalassaemia. (a) Survival without cardiac disease according to the proportion of serum ferritin measurements >2500 ng/ml. The circles show cardiac disease-free survival among patients in whom less than 33% of ferritin measurements exceeded 2500 ng/ml. Squares show survival among those in whom 33–67% of ferritin measurements exceeded 2500 ng/ml. Triangles show survival among those in whom more than 60% of ferritin measurements exceeded 2500 ng/ml. From Olivieri *et al.* (1994). (b) Survival related to hepatic iron concentration. Group 1 is assessed as having effective chelation therapy, group 2 ineffective. Based on hepatic iron concentrations as discussed in the text and as shown in Fig. 7.8, Chapter 7. From Brittenham *et al.* (1994).

elevated hepatic iron concentrations (Cohen *et al.* 1989b).

The importance of adequate iron chelation in patients with heavy iron loads of the liver who are being treated for hepatitis C is discussed later in this chapter.

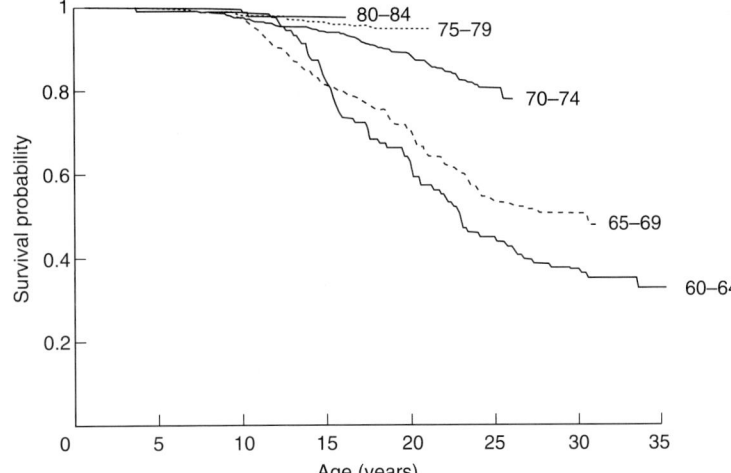

Fig. 15.4 Survival probability (%) as of January 1996 of thalassaemic patients born in Italy between 1960 and 1984. Kindly prepared for the authors by Dr Borgna-Pignatti.

Endocrine function

The consequences of iron loading of the endocrine glands were discussed in Chapters 5 and 7. The impact that iron chelation therapy has had on endocrine function and growth is still under evaluation. Many of the studies that examined this question have only reported short periods of observation on treatment and have also been complicated by the relatively advanced age at the start of DF therapy and the short duration, or inadequate compliance with subcutaneous DF administration (Borgna-Pignatti *et al.* 1985; Sklar *et al.* 1987; Maurer *et al.* 1988; Kwan *et al.* 1995; Rodda *et al.* 1995; Roth *et al.* 1997). Overall, at least as estimated by serum ferritin values, the most recent data suggest that adequate chelation therapy has some beneficial effect on growth, development and sexual maturation, probably the most significant indicators of endocrine function (Bronspeigel-Weintrob *et al.* 1990; Grundy *et al.* 1994; Italian working Group on Endocrine Complications in Non-endocrine Diseases 1995; Papadimas *et al.* 1996; Jensen *et al.* 1997). However, the findings are not entirely consistent. For example, Gabutti and Piga (1996) found that in patients born after 1977, and maintained with a serum ferritin level below 2000μg/l, pubertal development was normal in 73% of girls and 58% of boys. On the other hand, in another series of Italian patients born between 1960 and 1987, hypogonadism was noted in 55% of 578 patients who had reached

puberty (Borgna-Pignatti *et al.* 1998b). However, Bronspeigel-Weintrob *et al.* (1990) found a good correlation between the age of commencing chelation therapy and sexual development and growth; those who started before the age of 10 years fared better than those who started later.

In discussing the disappointingly high frequency of retarded sexual function in thalassaemic patients, even if maintained on adequate chelation therapy (see Chapter 7), we suggested that the anterior pituitary may be unusually susceptible over time to iron-induced damage and, unlike the heart and liver, the consequences of iron deposition within gonadotropes may be irreversible.

Further work is required to answer these difficult questions. This must entail the measurement of body iron burden by measuring the hepatic iron concentration; Dr N.F. Olivieri *et al.* (unpublished) have preliminary data that suggest that levels of between 9 and 13 mg/g liver, dry weight, may be associated with a high risk of the development of pituitary failure. Further work is required to assess both the body iron burden and anterior pituitary function in patients followed from infancy.

Diabetes mellitus

Adequate chelation therapy appears to reduce the likelihood of the development of pancreatic damage and diabetes mellitus (Brittenham *et al.* 1994).

The reversal of iron-induced organ dysfunction

Several reports have suggested that intensive DF therapy can reverse iron-induced cardiac and liver dysfunction (Freeman *et al.* 1983; Marcus *et al.* 1984; Rahko *et al.* 1986; Aldouri *et al.* 1990). We shall discuss the practical applications later in this chapter.

What is the optimal body iron level in patients with β thalassaemia major?

Because the magnitude of body iron burden is the principal determinant of the clinical outcome, its control is the prime goal of iron chelation therapy. A level must be achieved which will both minimize the risk of adverse effects from the iron chelating agent and yet, at the same time, prevent the complications of iron overload. As discussed later, there appears to be a good relationship between the dose of DF and the risk of adverse reactions. Hence, therapy directed towards maintaining a normal body iron, corresponding to a hepatic iron level of about 1–9 μm iron/g liver, wet weight, or about 0.2–1.6 mg iron/g liver, dry weight, might reduce the likelihood of complications of iron overload yet greatly increase the probability of dose-related drug toxicity.

In the absence of any data from prospective clinical trials to answer this important question, guidance about the risk of complications associated with lower levels of body iron have had to be derived from clinical experience with hereditary haemochromatosis (HH). In this condition, iron overload is the result of ineffective regulation of iron absorption. Minor iron loading develops in about one-quarter of heterozygotes, but their body iron stores do not increase beyond about two to four times the upper limit of normal (Cartwright *et al.* 1979). In contrast, homozygotes, who develop much greater iron burdens, have an increased risk of cardiac disease, hepatic fibrosis, diabetes mellitus, endocrine abnormalities and, indeed, every complication of iron overload. Just as in the case of thalassaemia, in HH the greater the body iron excess, the higher the risk of adverse consequences.

Despite the complex factors that modify the toxic manifestations of iron overload, discussed in Chapter 7, these considerations suggest that a conservative goal for iron chelation therapy in patients with thalassaemia major is to maintain an 'optimal' body iron

corresponding to hepatic storage iron concentrations of about 18–38 μm iron/g liver, wet weight, or about 3.2–7 mg iron/g liver, dry weight, that is, in the range found in heterozygotes for HH. As discussed below, the risk of DF toxicity associated with body iron levels within this range is probably minor but it is almost certainly increased at lower body iron burdens. Patients with higher liver iron concentrations, up to about 80 μm iron/g liver, wet weight, or about 15 mg iron/g liver, dry weight, are considered to be at increased risk of hepatic fibrosis, diabetes mellitus and other complications and need more intensive iron chelation therapy. Those with yet higher body iron burdens are recognized as having a greatly increased risk of cardiac disease and early death, and are candidates for continuous intravenous ambulatory DF therapy (see below). These ranges are shown graphically in Fig. 7.8, Chapter 7.

The relationship of serum ferritin levels to optimal body iron loads is discussed below.

Practical aspects of chelation therapy with desferrioxamine (Table 15.1)

Initiation of therapy

Uncertainties exist about the optimal age to start chelation therapy. Reports of abnormal linear growth and metaphyseal dysplasia in children treated with intensive regimens of DF before the age of 3 years (De Virgiliis *et al.* 1988; Piga *et al.* 1988; Olivieri *et al.* 1992c; Rodda *et al.* 1995) have led to recommendations for starting later (Rodda *et al.* 1995). On the other hand, as discussed in Chapter 7, early hepatic biopsies have revealed moderate to severe iron overload at an early age. Furthermore, elevated hepatic iron concentrations associated with fibrosis, not always evidenced by determinations of serum ferritin levels or abnormal liver function tests, have been observed in transfused children of less than 3 years of age (Berkovitch *et al.* 1993; Angelucci *et al.* 1995a; Saxon *et al.* 1997). Another factor to be taken into consideration is data suggesting that early chelation therapy may reduce the frequency of failure of growth and sexual maturation (Olivieri *et al.* 1990a).

Clearly, therefore, the time of the initiation of therapy cannot be determined on absolutely sound grounds (Olivieri & Brittenham 1997). Very recent data emerging from prospective studies of young children aged 1–2 years, following the start of transfusions but before the initiation of chelation therapy, suggest that there are very variable tissue iron concentrations and degrees of tissue damage during this period (Saxon *et al.* 1997). We recommend therefore that, ideally, hepatic iron concentrations should be measured after approximately 1 year of regular transfusion. Iron chelation therapy is indicated in patients whose hepatic iron concentrations exceed 7 mg/g liver, dry weight. The initial dose should depend on the hepatic iron concentration, but if a liver biopsy is not possible at the start of therapy, treatment with subcutaneous DF, not exceeding 25–35 mg/kg body weight/24 h, should be initiated approximately 1 year after the start of regular transfusion. The basis for this recommendation, and a titration scheme which offers effective chelation, while attempting to circumvent drug toxicity, is discussed below and in Table 15.1. We shall return to the dose regimens for DF in patients who are already iron loaded or have symptoms of organ dysfunction in a later section.

Modes of administration

Most patients and their parents find it most convenient to administer DF by means of an overnight infusion with the rate set to empty the syringe in 8–12 h. A variety of small portable syringe-driver pumps or disposable infusers are available. The drug is infused through a disposable 'butterfly' set with a fine (25 g) needle, which can be sited anywhere on the body, although most patients prefer the abdomen, thigh or upper arm. It is most important to follow a careful aseptic technique while setting up the infusion and the dose of DF must be diluted to a maximum concentration of 1 g/5 ml. At the end of the infusion there may be a small, tender nodule that normally takes 1–3 days to resorb although occasionally larger and longer-lasting swellings occur. It is usually possible to maintain iron balance with an infusion given four to five nights each week, with a rest at the weekends. The management of local reactions to the drug is considered later.

Ascorbate

As described in Chapter 5 and earlier in the present

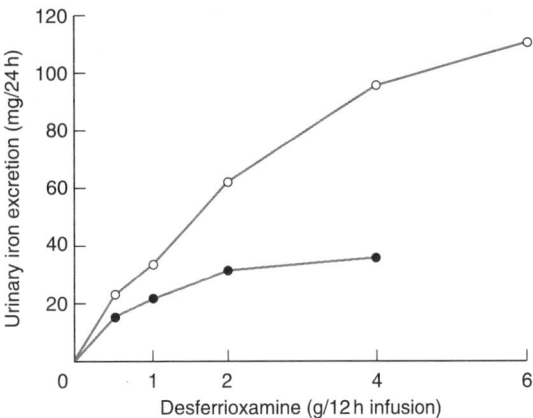

Fig. 15.5 The effect of ascorbic acid on urinary iron excretion after the administration of desferrioxamine. The closed circles show the course of excretion before administering ascorbate and the open circles the course after ascorbate treatment. From Pippard *et al.* (1978b).

chapter, ascorbate deficiency is common in patients with β thalassaemia and there is excellent evidence that the efficacy of DF is improved by the administration of ascorbate (Chapman *et al.* 1982). It is not clear whether the increased rate of iron excretion observed during co-administration of ascorbate (Fig. 15.5) is due to the drug's action in the cellular compartment alone or in both cells and plasma. One potential mechanism by which ascorbate might increase the rate of iron loss is by facilitating the chelation of non-transferrin-bound plasma iron (see Chapter 5) by DF. On the other hand, ascorbate-induced expansion of this pool has the potential to enhance free-radical formation and to aggravate the toxicity of iron (Nienhuis 1981). For this reason some authors discourage the use of ascorbate for the potentiation of the action of DF (Fosburg & Nathan 1990). One approach is to measure the tissue ascorbate concentration and, if this is reduced, to administer ascorbic acid on the same day as the infusion of DF. In practice, most patients receive up to 100 mg ascorbate on the day of the infusion, approximately 30 min–1 h before it is started. This seems to be a reasonable compromise and as far as we know it has not led to any side-effects. Given the current lack of evidence about the risks of ascorbate-related iron toxicity, this rather ad hoc approach is the best that can be recommended.

Table 15.1 Management of iron chelating therapy in thalassaemia. Adapted from Olivieri & Brittenham (1997).

Time-point	Assessment	Comment	Results	Treatment recommendations
At start of therapy	Liver biopsy under U/S guidance with quantitative liver iron, histology, PCR for hepatitis C RNA	Should be obtained after approx. 1 year of regular transfusion	HIC <3.2 mg/g dry weight	Defer chelation; reassess HIC in 6 months
	Radiographs of cartilage in wrists, knees, thoracolumbosacral spine; bone age	Should be reviewed by paediatric radiologist and endocrinologist with experience in toxicity of DF	HIC ≥3.2 mg/g dry weight	Initiate DF at 25 mg/kg/night × 5 nights/week
	Standing and sitting heights			
	Serum ferritin, Fe, and TIBC			
	Serum ALT			
	Hepatitis screen			
	WBC ascorbate concentration			If WBC ascorbate low, administer vitamin C po 100 mg/night during DF infusion
Yearly, before age 5 years	Liver biopsy under U/S guidance; assessment as above		HIC <3.2 mg/g dry weight	Discontinue DF; reassess HIC in 6 months
			HIC ≥3.2 but <7 mg/g dry weight	Continue DF at 25 mg/kg/night × 5 nights/week
			HIC ≥7 mg/g dry weight	Increase DF to 35 mg/kg/night × 6–7 nights/week
	Radiographs as above	Same as above	If severe spinal or metaphyseal changes present, reduce DF to 25 mg/kg/night × 4 nights/wk even if HIC ≥7 mg/g dry weight Reassess in 6 months	
	Serum ferritin, Fe, and TIBC			
	Serum ALT			
	Hepatitis screen			
	WBC ascorbate concentration			If WBC ascorbate low, administer vitamin C po 100 mg/night during DF infusion

Every 18 months, from age 5–10 years	Liver biopsy under U/S guidance with quantitative HIC, histology, PCR for hepatitis C RNA	HIC <3.2 mg/g dry weight HIC ≥3.2 but <7 mg/g dry weight HIC ≥7 but <15 mg/g weight HIC ≥15 mg/g dry weight	Discontinue DF; reassess HIC in 6 months Maintain DF at 40 mg/kg/night×5 nights/wk Maintain DF at 40 mg/kg/night×6–7 nights/wk Maintain DF at 40–50 mg/kg/night ×7 nights/wk
	Radiographs as above Standing and sitting heights	Same as above	Titrate DF as above
	Serum ferritin, Fe, and TIBC Serum ALT Hepatitis screen WBC ascorbate concentration	If abnormal, reassess HIC promptly	If WBC ascorbate low, administer vitamin C po 100 mg/night during DF infusion
Every 18 months, after 10 years	Liver Bx under U/S guidance; assessments as above	HIC ≥3.2 mg/g dry weight HIC ≥3.2 but <7 mg/g dry weight HIC ≥7 but <15 mg/g weight HIC ≥15 mg/g dry weight	Discontinue DF; reassess HIC in 6 months Maintain DF at 40 mg/kg/night×5 nights/wk Maintain DF at 40 mg/kg/night×6–7 nights/wk Maintain DF at 50 mg/kg/night×7 nights/wk
	Radiographs as above Standing and sitting heights	Same as above	Titrated DF as above
	Serum ferritin, Fe, and TIBC Serum ALT Hepatitis screen WBC ascorbate concentration	If abnormal, reassess HIC promptly	If WBC ascorbate low, administer vitamin C po 100 mg/night during DF infusion

ALT, alanine aminotransferase; BX, biopsy; DF, desferrioxamine; HIC, hepatic iron concentration; PCR, polymerase chain reaction; po, orally; TIBC, total iron binding capacity; U/S, ultrasound; WBC, white blood cells.

Table 15.2 Assessment of body iron burden in thalassaemia. Adapted from Olivieri and Brittenham (1997).

Test	Organ	Comments
Indirect		Most tests widely available
Serum/plasma ferritin concentration		Non-invasive
		Lacks sensitivity and specificity
		Poorly correlated with hepatic iron concentration in individual patients
Serum transferrin saturation		Lacks sensitivity
Tests of 24-h desferrioxamine-induced urinary iron excretion		Less than half of outpatient aliquots collected correctly
		Ratio of stool/urine iron variable; poorly correlated with hepatic iron concentration
Imaging of tissue iron		
Computed tomography	Liver	Variable correlation with hepatic iron concentration reported
Magnetic resonance	Liver	Variable correlations with hepatic iron concentration reported
		Treatment-induced changes confirmed by liver biopsy
	Heart	Only method available to image cardiac iron stores; changes observed during chelating therapy are consistent with reduction in cardiac iron
	Anterior pituitary	Only method available to image pituitary iron; signal moderately well correlated with pituitary reserve
Evaluation of organ function		Most tests lack sensitivity and specificity; may identify established organ dysfunction
Direct		Most tests not widely available
Cardiac iron quantification: biopsy		Imprecise due to inhomogeneous distribution of cardiac iron
Hepatic iron quantification: biopsy		Reference method; provides direct assessment of body iron burden, severity of fibrosis and inflammation
		Safe when performed with ultrasound guidance
Superconducting susceptometry (SQUID)		Non-invasive; excellent correlation with biopsy-determined hepatic iron

Monitoring progress; the assessment of body iron burden

Current methods for assessing the body iron burden were discussed in Chapter 7 and have been reviewed in detail by Olivieri and Brittenham (1997) (Table 15.2). While it is the practice of many centres that look after children with β thalassaemia to rely on serum ferritin levels, and to try to maintain values of less than 2000 μg/l, as discussed in Chapters 5 and 7 and reviewed by Olivieri and Brittenham (1997) this approach has limited precision. Because of the wide scatter of liver iron concentrations with ferritin levels in the region of 2000 μg/l it is quite possible to have dangerously high body iron burdens with serum ferritin values that appear to be in the 'safe' range. Similarly, there is the danger of inducing DF toxicity in patients with serum ferritin values of

500–1000 μg/l. For these reasons we believe that the regular estimation of liver iron levels is, currently, the best approach to following the progress of children receiving chelation therapy.

Of the many reasons why clinicians seem loath to follow this approach, the perceived dangers of liver biopsy are probably the most important. For example, in a series of 6379 adults with a variety of conditions two deaths were recorded and intraperitoneal haemorrhage requiring blood transfusion occurred in 40 cases (Sherlock *et al.* 1985). In contrast, in a study of children with thalassaemia a 0.5% rate of major complications was reported, including bleeding and biliary peritonitis; there were no fatalities (Angelucci *et al.* 1995).

In a study in Toronto, the centre with the most experience of liver biopsies in thalassaemic children, 198 percutaneous biopsies in 105 regularly transfused children were analysed (Saxon *et al.* 1997). The children, with a mean age of 10.9±4.8 (range 1.4–18.4) years, were observed over 30 consecutive months. A total of 55 patients underwent two biopsies; 19 patients underwent three. Before all procedures the international normalized prothrombin ratio (INR), platelet counts and clotting function were assessed as adequate (INR less than 1.3, platelet count greater than 100×10^9/l). Conscious sedation was achieved with midazolam, 0.1–0.2 mg/kg body weight given intravenously, and intravenous pethedine, 1 mg/kg, was administered 5–10 min before the procedure. All biopsies were performed under ultrasound guidance by one of two radiologists, using an 18-gauge Angiomed needle (Bard, Canada); up to three passes per procedure were obtained. The children were admitted for the biopsy on the day of transfusion, observed for 6 h while the transfusion was administered, and discharged home in the late afternoon. Immediately after the biopsy the specimen was frozen at –70°C without further treatment; quantification of hepatic iron was carried out at one centre and samples for histological assessment were prepared from the fresh biopsy specimens. No complications were observed and there was no increase in admission time. All biopsies were adequate (0.6 mg dry weight) for quantification of hepatic iron. It appears therefore that in centres which are carrying out this procedure regularly it is safe. However, it requires expertise and experience on the part of the operator and those who are involved in the ultrasound guidance.

If measurement of the hepatic iron concentration is not feasible, and access to SQUID (see Chapter 7) is not possible, the serum ferritin level has to be used to attempt to maintain the body iron level in the optimal range. As discussed earlier, a serum ferritin level of above 2500 μg/l may be used as a threshold value to identify patients at an increased risk of cardiac disease and early death (see Olivieri *et al.* 1994b). The concentrations corresponding to the optimal range for hepatic iron, shown in Fig. 7.8, Chapter 7, are less clearly defined. Preliminary analysis of studies of a large number of adults with thalassaemia major after more than 15 years of DF therapy has suggested that very rigorous control of body iron burden, as suggested by maintenance of serum ferritin concentrations under 1000 μg/l, is associated with a very low incidence of iron-induced complications. On the other hand, as mentioned earlier, iron-related morbidity may increase significantly with even slightly less effective iron chelation therapy (Lai *et al.* 1995).

Another approach to monitoring progress by the serum ferritin level is to calculate a 'toxicity' index, defined as the mean daily dose of DF (mg/kg) divided by the serum ferritin concentration (μg/l), estimated every 6 months; it should not exceed 0.025 (Porter *et al.* 1989b).

Desferrioxamine toxicity

Local cutaneous reactions

These are by far the most commonly observed adverse effects, and may sometimes be quite difficult to manage. Irregular absorption from the site of injection may account for pain and formation of lumps under the skin; hypertonicity of the solution may increase their frequency but they are observed even with adequate dilution of DF. Itching and weal formation are also common. The reason for these side-effects is not always clear; sometimes they appear to result from contaminants in particular batches of the drug. Poor injection technique may also be a factor.

Severe sensitivity reactions; desferrioxamine allergy

Rarely, patients may have more severe, generalized sensitivity reactions to DF. These reactions must be very uncommon. Modell and Berdoukas (1984) were only able to find two cases out of 200 in the UK in which patients had developed reactions of this type, and were only able to quote one patient in Italy and two from the USA. The reactions take the form of acute episodes characterized by wheezing, tachypnoea, tachycardia, hypertension and, occasionally, coma. Although this points to an allergic mechanism, evidence supporting an immunological basis for this is lacking, while a direct, immunoglobulin-E-dependent activation of dermal mast cells by DF has been demonstrated (Shalit *et al.* 1991). These severe reactions may be managed effectively using rapid intravenous desensitization similar to protocols recommended for penicillin allergy (Miller *et al.* 1981; Bousquet *et al.* 1983; Lombardo *et al.* 1996a).

Chronic systemic side-effects

The majority of serious toxic effects of DF are observed in patients who are receiving doses in excess of 50 mg/kg body weight, or in those on smaller doses in the presence of very modestly elevated body iron burdens (De Virgiliis *et al.* 1988; Porter & Huehns 1989).

Ocular manifestations include cataracts and retinal damage. Several patients with cataracts have been reported (Waxman & Brown 1969; Modell 1979; Davies *et al.* 1983). The condition usually improves after stopping the drug, which can be safely restarted at a lower dose after 2–3 weeks or when symptomatic recovery is complete (Porter & Huehns 1989). Overall, this seems to be a mild complication in that none of the reported patients have had visual loss associated with the opacities of their lens. Retinal damage was first reported by Davies *et al.* (1983) in two patients who were receiving a very high dose of DF intravenously. The retinal changes were associated with an inability to see in dim light and impaired peripheral vision. The visual acuity was normal, with a normal visually evoked response (VER), but there was peripheral field loss with bilateral annular scotomata. On stopping the drug the retinal changes improved although some visual field loss remained. Retinal signs have now been described in detail by a number of authors (Borgna-Pignatti *et al.* 1984b; Olivieri *et al.* 1986; Freedman *et al.* 1989). Most of these reports described night-blindness, annular field loss together with electro-oculogram (EOG), Granzfield electroretinogram (ERG) and VER abnormalities. Fundal pigmentation has been a feature, which does not regress on stopping DF. Some degree of optic atrophy has also been observed, in one case leading to blindness (Olivieri *et al.* 1986). The fact that some of these symptoms may resolve, there may be partial regression of signs on stopping DF, and that they are particularly likely to occur in patients with low body iron loads, suggests that these changes are undoubtedly due to the drug.

Given the importance of DF for survival in thalassaemia, it is difficult to know how to manage these complications. It has been suggested that if they are symptomless and there are only minor electrophysiological changes the drug can be continued, though with great caution; in symptomatic cases this is clearly not advisable (Porter & Huehns 1989). What little is known about the mechanisms of retinal damage, and

its relationship to the pathogenesis of retinitis pigmentosa, to which it bears some resemblance, is discussed by Porter and Huehns (1989).

Ototoxicity is another important complication of DF therapy. It was first noticed by Marsh *et al.* (1981) and there were further reports by Guerin *et al.* (1985). Olivieri *et al.* (1986) and Freedman *et al.* (1989) studied a total of 89 patients receiving DF; 13 had symptomatic high-frequency hearing loss and another eight were asymptomatic but had abnormal audiometry. The major risk factors for ototoxicity were the dosage of DF, a low body iron burden and the patient's age. These observations have been confirmed more recently (Porter *et al.* 1988; Wonke *et al.* 1989).

Again, management is difficult. In patients who are symptomatic, or who have abnormal audiometry, it is very important to reduce the dose of DF and, if the body iron burden is low as judged by liver iron or serum ferritin levels, the dosage should be reduced even further. If, despite this, the patient's audiometry continues to deteriorate the drug must be stopped.

One of the major concerns of DF therapy in young children is its effect on linear growth, often associated with evidence of cartilaginous dysplasia of the long bones and spine (Piga *et al.* 1988; Brill *et al.* 1991; Olivieri *et al.* 1992c; Orzincolo *et al.* 1992; Hartkamp *et al.* 1993; Sher *et al.* 1993; Hatori *et al.* 1995; Olivieri *et al.* 1995a; Rodda *et al.* 1995) (Fig. 15.6). These complications may result in short stature, primarily related to disproportionate truncal growth and loss of sitting height, probably due to the effect of DF on spinal cartilage. Some patients complain of back pain. The radiological changes of the spine are shown in Fig. 15.6.

Because of these distressing complications it has been suggested that it is better to start DF early in life, using reduced doses to balance between risk and benefit. This practice is supported by studies of children who received low-dose DF (15–35 mg/kg/night) from the age of 3 years, all of whom had normal sitting heights, standing heights and spinal X-rays. In contrast, in a second cohort, in which DF was administered at standard doses (50 mg/kg) from an equally early age and had induced a comparable reduction in body iron burden, the mean sitting height was markedly abnormal and X-ray abnormalities were frequently observed (Olivieri *et al.* 1995a). These data suggest that abnormal linear growth is probably a

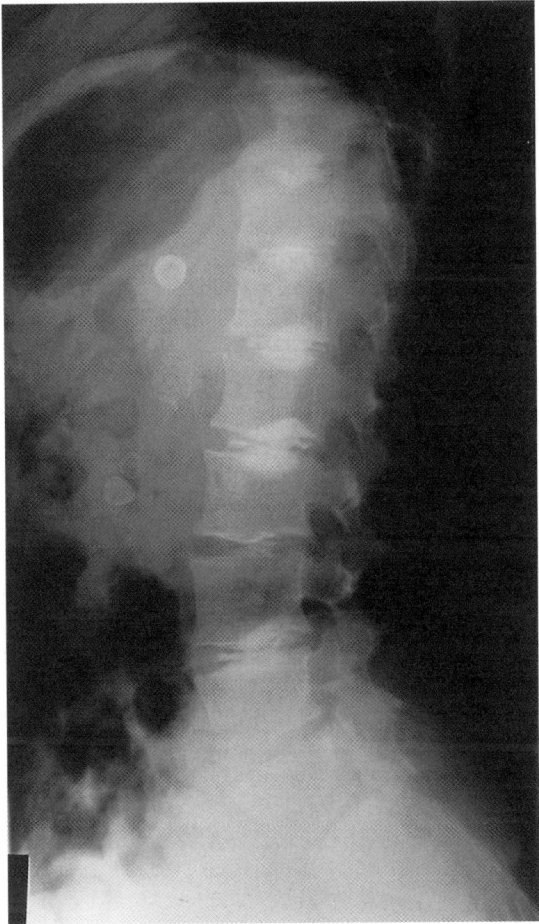

Fig. 15.6 Changes in the spine induced by desferrioxamine. This X-ray is from a 26-year-old patient who received intensive chelation treatment from early childhood. There is striking calcification of the intervertebral discs together with a dysplastic appearance of the spine, with irregularity and undulation of the vertebral end-plates, short pedicles, narrow disc spaces and a narrowed interpedicular distance. We are grateful to Dr David Lindsell for reviewing these X-rays.

direct toxic effect of prolonged administration of higher doses of DF, unrelated to changes in body iron. Furthermore, because improvement in growth of patients with spinal abnormalities has not been observed, even following the reduction of the dosage of DF, it is clearly important to prevent this type of drug toxicity.

Other, and much less common, side-effects ascribed to DF have included loss of consciousness (Blake *et al.* 1985) or acute aphasia with visual loss (Dickerhoff 1987).

The increased susceptibility to infection in patients receiving DF, in particular due to *Yersinia* spp., was discussed in Chapter 7. It has also been suggested that patients receiving this drug may be more prone to infection with *Pneumocystis carinii* (Kouides *et al.* 1988), mucormycosis (invasive zygomycosis) (Boelaert *et al.* 1987) and other agents. On the other hand, it has been reported that the progression of HIV infection towards the advanced stages of the disease may be significantly slower in patients receiving doses of DF exceeding 40 mg/kg/day (Costagliola *et al.* 1992).

There have been occasional reports of an acute pulmonary syndrome during the administration of relatively high doses of DF. This consists of restrictive dysfunction, interstitial infiltrates on chest X-ray and alveolar damage with fibrosis on lung biopsy (Castriota Scanderbeg *et al.* 1990; Freedman *et al.* 1990; Tenenbein *et al.* 1992).

Other miscellaneous effects, including potential zinc and copper deficiency, thrombocytopenia, nausea and vomiting, and renal toxicity are reviewed by Porter and Huehns (1989).

A practical approach to monitoring for DF toxicity is shown in Table 15.3.

The use of desferrioxamine in pregnancy

Concerns about the teratogenicity of DF are based on studies in which effects on bone formation were demonstrated when doses of approximately five times the maximum human dose were administered to pregnant mice. At least 40 patients have been reported to have received DF during several weeks or months of gestation and, to date, no toxic or teratogenic effects have been observed. Only 11 have been documented to have used the drug in the early stages of pregnancy (Singer & Vichinsky 1999). These authors suggest that DF may be used in pregnancy, especially during the second and third trimester. Although a safe general principle is to avoid any drugs in pregnancy that are not absolutely necessary, concern has been raised that if DF is abandoned during the entire pregnancy, tissue iron accumulation could worsen, possibly aggravated by increased transfusion requirements as a result of the pregnancy. Of course the fetus and placenta will deviate approximately 800 mg of iron from the mother but this only

Table 15.3 Monitoring of desferrioxamine-related toxicity. Adapted from Olivieri & Brittenham (1997).

Toxicity	Investigations	Frequency	Alteration in therapy
High-frequency sensorineural hearing loss	Audiogram	Yearly; if patient symptomatic, immediate reassessment	Interrupt DF immediately; directly assess body iron burden; discontinue DF×6 months if HIC 3.2–7 mg/g dry weight tissue; repeat audiogram every 3 months until normal or stable; adjust DF to HIC as per Table 15.1
Retinal abnormalities	Retinal examination	Yearly; if patient symptomatic, immediate reassessment	Interrupt DF immediately; directly assess body iron burden; discontinue DF×6 months if HIC 3.2–7 mg/g dry weight tissue; review every 3 months until normal or stable; adjust DF to HIC as per Table 15.1
Metaphyseal and spinal abnormalities	X-rays of wrists, knees, thoraco-lumbar-sacral spine; bone age of wrist	Yearly	Reduce DF to 25 mg/kg/day × 4/wk; directly assess body iron burden; discontinue DF×6 months if HIC ≤ 3 mg/g dry weight tissue; reassess HIC after 6 months; adjust DF to HIC as per Table 15.1
Decline in height velocity and/or sitting height	Determination of sitting and standing heights	Twice yearly	Reduce DF to 25 mg/kg/day × 4/wk; directly assess body iron burden; discontinue DF×6 months if HIC ≤ 3 mg/g dry weight tissue; reassess HIC after 6 months; adjust DF to HIC as per Table 15.1; regular (6-monthly) assessment by paediatric endocrinologist

DF, desferrioxamine; HIC, hepatic iron concentration.

represents 4 units of blood. Given our current state of knowledge we still feel that DF should be avoided in pregnancy, wherever possible. This should certainly be the case in women in whom regular surveillance has shown that they have body iron loads that, as judged by the hepatic iron concentration, are at a safe level (see previous section) shortly before the pregnancy. If this is not the case, and if regular transfusion throughout pregnancy is required, the drug might be used with caution after the first trimester.

Use of desferrioxamine to rescue patients with severe iron loading and organ damage

As discussed earlier, there is limited evidence that there may be some improvement in both liver and cardiac function in patients who are heavily iron loaded and in whom there is evidence of defective organ function. These patients are most easily managed by the administration of DF intravenously through implantable venous ports, although they need to pay scrupulous attention to the care of access sites and require regular visits for surveillance by experienced medical personnel. There are a number of intravenous delivery systems available includ-

ing Port-a-Cath or Hickman lines. Because of the dangers of high-dose DF administration it is recommended that the drug is given by continuous infusion at a dose of up to 50 mg/kg/day (Davis & Porter 2000).

Alternatives to subcutaneous infusions

Regimens of continuous ambulatory intravenous desferrioxamine infused through implantable subcutaneous ports, in which the infusion site cannot be manipulated by the patient, overcome the disadvantages of drug preparation and self-administration, eliminate the irritation associated with subcutaneous infusions, and improve compliance (Olivieri *et al.* 1992a). This system requires that the site is changed weekly by medical personnel at a clinic visit. Those unwilling to visit the clinic frequently, and those for whom standard pumps are unwieldy, may benefit from new systems in which the desired concentrations of continuous subcutaneous or intravenous desferrioxamine can be infused using a lightweight, disposable, silent balloon infuser (Baxter), which exerts continuous pressure without a battery or other mechanical device (Araujo *et al.* 1996; Lombardo *et al.* 1996b).

Prevention of desferrioxamine toxicity

Clearly, DF is a relatively safe drug which has transformed the prognosis for transfusion-dependent patients with β thalassaemia. With our increasing understanding of its use it is now possible to administer the drug with minimal likelihood of side-effects. It is clear that these are most likely to occur at low body iron burdens and therefore, as discussed earlier, it is important to evaluate the hepatic iron concentration at regular intervals. If for any reason this is not possible it should be monitored by a serum ferritin estimation and the dosage of DF should be monitored by the use of a toxicity index, as described earlier in this chapter. Patients should also have regular assessments of their height and weight, plotted on standard percentile charts (Tanner & Whitehouse 1976), expert examination of their eyes and hearing, and radiological examination of their bones. An approach to the long-term management of a child receiving DF is outlined in Table 15.3.

Finally, it should be remembered that compliance is still the major difficulty in managing patients on DF (Piga *et al.* 1987; Olivieri & Brittenham 1997). It may be improved by intensive social and psychological support (Piga *et al.* 1987; Zani *et al.* 1995).

Alternative chelating agents

Because of the considerable expense and inconvenience of DF therapy there has been a major effort directed towards developing other chelating agents which, ideally, would be active when given orally.

It is beyond the scope of this chapter to discuss this topic in detail. Readers who are interested in learning about the problems that have been encountered, particularly the complex chemistry of potential oral chelating drugs, are referred to the reviews of Porter *et al.* (1989a) and Porter (1996).

The other parenterally administered chelating agent that received extensive evaluation in the period while DF was being developed was diethylene triamino-pentaacetic acid (DTPA). Sephton-Smith (1964) showed that this agent was at least as effective and sometimes more so than DF in inducing iron excretion when administered intravenously. Unfortunately, it turned out that it is not as specific as DF for iron and caused a significant increase in the excretion of other metals, notably magnesium (Muller-Eberhard *et al.* 1963). Furthermore, other toxic effects

were encountered (Fairbanks *et al.* 1963). Although if administered at the same time as transfusion DTPA was usually well tolerated, it caused an unacceptably high frequency of rigors, fever, nausea, vomiting, diarrhoea, pruritus and muscle cramps (Barry *et al.* 1974). Modell (1979) found that DTPA can be given by subcutaneous infusion provided that it is diluted before administration. Wonke *et al.* (1989) have recommended its use, with zinc supplementation, for treating patients with DF-induced auditory complications.

Over recent years several orally active iron chelators have been evaluated. The compounds *N,N'*-bis(2-hydroxybenzoyl) ethylenediamine, *N,N'*-diacetic acid (HBED), the arylhydrazone pyridoxal isonicotinoyl hydrazone (PIH), and the di-ethyl hydroxypyridinone CP94 have all been subjected to limited clinical trials (Brittenham 1990; Porter *et al.* 1991; Grady *et al.* 1993; Porter 1996). However, these drugs are not under clinical development at the present time.

Deferiprone

The only orally active iron chelator to reach extended clinical trials is 1,2-dimethyl-3-hydroxypyridin-4-one (deferiprone; L1) (Hider *et al.* 1982).

Pharmacology

The pharmacology of L1 is reviewed by Olivieri and Brittenham (1997). The drug forms a neutral 3/1 chelator/ferric iron complex at pH 7.4. It may mobilize iron from ferritin, haemosiderin, lactoferrin and diferric transferrin. Animal studies have reported widely variable efficacy in iron chelation. In transfused patients with thalassaemia major 75 mg L1/kg body weight induces urinary iron excretion approximately equivalent to that achieved with 30–40 mg DF/kg. However, because faecal iron excretion induced by L1 is much less than that induced by DF, the short-term efficacy of L1 is inferior to that of DF.

Effectiveness of deferiprone

The effectiveness of deferiprone was initially evaluated using the serum ferritin concentration (Kontoghiorghes *et al.* 1990; Olivieri *et al.* 1990a; Tondury *et al.* 1990; Agarwal *et al.* 1992; Al-Refaie *et al.* 1995). The earlier studies reported no sustained decrease in serum ferritin concentration over 1–15 months of deferiprone treatment (Agarwal *et al.* 1990; Kontoghiorghes *et al.* 1990; Tondury *et al.* 1990). Subsequently, however, there were two reports of a significant reduction of serum ferritin concentration in patients with thalassaemia, the most substantial decrease occurring in those whose prestudy ferritin concentrations exceeded 5000 µg/l (Agarwal *et al.* 1992; Al-Refaie *et al.* 1992). A reduction in hepatic iron stores by deferiprone was first demonstrated in a patient with thalassaemia intermedia (Olivieri *et al.* 1992d); subsequently, a favourable effect of deferiprone on tissue iron concentration was reported in thalassaemia major (Olivieri *et al.* 1995b). Although support for both a long-term, open-label study and a randomized trial of deferiprone and DF was terminated prematurely by the corporate sponsor in 1996, follow-up of hepatic storage iron concentrations in both cohorts provided information about the long-term effectiveness of deferiprone in thalassaemia major. In one-third of patients in the long-term treatment cohort of deferiprone-treated patients (Olivieri *et al.* 1995b) hepatic iron stabilized at, or increased to, concentrations which place patients at risk for cardiac disease and early death (Brittenham *et al.* 1994). Changes in compliance did not account for the ineffectiveness of long-term deferiprone treatment (Olivieri 1996a).

In the only randomized trial of deferiprone and DF, 38 of 51 patients remained on study at termination; a final hepatic iron concentration was obtained in 37 patients. After 33 months, the hepatic iron level of the DF-treated patients had not changed significantly from baseline, while in deferiprone-treated patients it increased approximately 100% over baseline. Compliance with deferiprone, measured with computerized bottles, was significantly better than with desferrioxamine (Olivieri 1996a). These results, supported by the findings of another report, in which the hepatic iron of liver biopsies obtained after an extended period of deferiprone therapy exceeded the threshold for cardiac disease and early death in 50% of patients (Hoffbrand *et al.* 1998), raise concerns that long-term therapy with deferiprone may not provide adequate control of body iron in a substantial proportion of patients with thalassaemia major, findings which were further substantiated by Tondury *et al.* (1998). Experience of the combined use of DF and deferiprone is so far limited to a small pilot study (Wonke *et al.* 1998b).

Toxicity

During limited toxicity studies of deferiprone in rodents, adrenal hypertrophy, gonadal and thymic atrophy, bone-marrow atrophy and pancytopenia, growth retardation and embryotoxicity were observed (see Brittenham 1992; Berdoukas *et al.* 1993; Olivieri & Brittenham 1997). The first adverse effects to be observed in humans included arthralgia, neutropenia and agranulocytosis (Hoffbrand 1996; Olivieri & Brittenham 1997). Preliminary results of a multicentre safety trial of deferiprone were reported by Cohen *et al.* (1998). The original designers of the trial were able to recruit 187 patients, who were unable or unwilling to use DF, from four centres; 162 patients completed 1 year of therapy. Patients with a history of neutropenia or chronic active hepatitis wer excluded. Nine subjects developed neutropenia, and one agranulocytosis. Other reasons for discontinuing the drug included nausea, voluntary withdrawal, high liver enzymes, a low platelet count, fatigue and depression. The ALT levels rose within 3 months of therapy in a high proportion of cases. Other side-effects included arthralgia, which occurred in 6% of cases, and nausea or vomiting which occurred in 24%. In this study therefore the incidence of haematological toxicity attributable to L1 therapy was 7.4% over 1 year of treatment, even in these carefully monitored patients. Equally worrying was the rise in liver enzymes; ALT levels increased to twice the baseline value on at least one measurement in 48% of subjects. Liver biopsies were not carried out in patients in this study.

Chronic co-administration of iron dextran and 1,2-diethyl-3-hydroxypyridin-4-one, a closely related hydroxypyridinone, results in increased iron accumulation in the liver and heart, worsening of hepatic fibrosis and development of cardiac fibrosis in gerbils (Carthew *et al.* 1994). In guinea-pigs, chronic administration of deferiprone was associated with hepatic, myocardial and musculoskeletal necrosis, in the absence of iron overload (Wong *et al.* 1997). In the Toronto long-term treatment cohort a retrospective review indicated that deferiprone treatment was, unexpectedly, associated with progression of hepatic fibrosis (Olivieri *et al.* 1998a). The estimated median time to progression of fibrosis for the entire cohort exceeded 3 years. While several authors subsequently claimed that they did not observe progressive liver fibrosis in patients treated with deferiprone, these studies were either uncontrolled (Hoffbrand *et al.*

1998), or of too short a duration, compared with the median time to fibrosis of 3.2 years in the Toronto study, to be comparable (Stella *et al.* 1998; Tondury *et al.* 1998).

In view of the possibility that fibrosis can be induced by deferiprone, it is particularly important to determine whether this agent might cause cardiac toxicity. In studies of the efficacy of deferiprone and DF in the reversal of iron-induced damage to cell organelles in cultured rat heart cells *in vitro*, at relatively high concentrations both chelators were equally effective. On the other hand, at low concentrations similar to those obtained *in vivo*, deferiprone and related compounds were less effective than DF (reviewed by Olivieri & Brittenham 1997). As mentioned earlier, there is good experimental evidence that compounds closely related to deferiprone can cause cardiac fibrosis in experimental animals. Unfortunately, there are very limited data on the possible cardiotoxic effects of the drug in humans. In one well documented patient, the only one so far reported to have undergone cardiac biopsy during L1 therapy, acute congestive cardiac failure developed after deferiprone therapy had been administered for 3–5 years; cardiac biopsy showed extensive fibrosis. These findings are of concern, particularly since the hepatic iron level in this patient had been maintained within concentrations associated with a reduced risk for cardiac disease (Olivieri *et al.* 1998c).

The role of deferiprone in the management of thalassaemia remains uncertain, therefore. This should not surprise us; DF went through an equally long and tortuous period of development and it was many years before the optimal method of administration was determined, and even longer before its full spectrum of side-effects became apparent. Since liver fibrosis in thalassaemia may be caused by many factors, including iron and hepatitis, uncontrolled, long-term observational studies of the drug, even if they include liver biopsy, may not unmask potential fibrotic complications. Hence, before deferiprone can be recommended for general clinical use, further evaluation of long-term effectiveness and toxicity in prospective, randomized, controlled clinical trials will be necessary (Olivieri & Brittenham 1997; Pippard & Weatherall 2000).

Splenectomy

Splenectomy has been performed on patients with thalassaemia major for almost as long as the disease has been recognized (see Penberthy & Cooley 1935). The early literature is reviewed by Bouroncle and Doan (1964). Over the years a large and rather confusing literature grew up around this subject but, by and large, most series seemed to conclude that a proportion of children with severe forms of thalassaemia had a reduction in transfusion requirements after the operation, though it was not always sustained (Lichtman *et al.* 1953; Smith *et al.* 1955; Reemsta & Elliot 1956; Smith *et al.* 1960; Bouroncle & Doan 1964; Engelhard *et al.* 1975; Montouri *et al.* 1975; Modell 1977). When more effective transfusion regimens were introduced it was suggested that children maintained at adequate haemoglobin levels have smaller spleens and a lower incidence of hypersplenism (O'Brien *et al.* 1972; Necheles *et al.* 1974; Piomelli *et al.* 1974; Modell 1977).

This important question was addressed again by Modell and Berdoukas (1984). They observed a small group of patients over the first 6 years of life, when hypersplenism most often develops. In order to assess its magnitude they utilized a transfusion quotient, the rationale of which is outlined in a later section. They concluded that those children who had been maintained on the highest transfusion programmes were least hypersplenic. More recently it has become clear that children maintained from early life on an adequate transfusion regimen rarely have significant hypersplenism (Olivieri & Brittenham 1997; Viens *et al.* 1998). Furthermore, in the study of Viens *et al.* (1998) splenectomy seemed to offer no advantage regarding growth, iron loading or allo-immunization in patients of this kind.

Another long-standing question about splenectomy is whether it has deleterious effects on iron metabolism and, in particular, whether it increases the rate of iron loading. This is based on the belief that the spleen serves both as a scavenger by increasing red-cell destruction and iron redistribution, and as a storage depot by sequestering released iron in a potentially non-toxic pool. However, in one of the few studies that address this question adequately, Risdon *et al.* (1975) observed no difference between splenectomized and non-splenectomized patients with regard to liver pathology.

Another important question that had to be addressed when considering the role of splenectomy was whether it is possible, by moving from a low to a high transfusion regimen, to halt the progression of hypersplenism. This problem was the subject of a study of seven non-splenectomized patients by Modell and Berdoukas (1984). Although the change to a high transfusion programme appeared to halt the progression of hypersplenism, in no case did the increased annual blood requirement return to the normal range. From these limited data it does not appear as though it is possible to completely reverse hypersplenism and that, although its speed of progression may be retarded, patients who have developed this complication at one time or another are always likely to require more blood than the theoretical norm for their body weight.

Since many children, particularly in the developing countries, are still maintained on a suboptimal blood transfusion programme, it is clear that there will still be a role for this operation, at least for the foreseeable future.

In the sections which follow we shall discuss the assessment of patients for splenectomy first, and then review the hazards of the operation. We shall confine the discussion to splenectomy in patients who are receiving regular blood transfusions; we shall return to the problem of splenectomy in thalassaemia intermedia later in the chapter.

Assessment for splenectomy

The assessment of whether a patient will benefit from splenectomy can be made either on clinical grounds or from the results of sophisticated splenic function tests, or both. In the previous edition of this book we discussed the growing battery of investigations of splenic function, which involve assessment of the red-cell survival and sites of destruction, measurements of the size of the red-cell pool in the spleen and attempts to estimate the amount of splenic erythropoiesis. In the event, these time-consuming investigations have only been carried out in centres with a special interest in the pathophysiology of the spleen, and have played very little role in the assessment of thalassaemic patients for splenectomy. As further experience has been gained it has become clear that, in practice, the most useful way to assess splenic function in transfusion-dependent patients is by a careful assessment of their blood requirements over time.

The size of the spleen, alone, is rarely a clear-cut indication for splenectomy. Although it has been suggested that it is unusual to observe hypersplenism

unless the spleen is palpable at more than about 6 cm below the costal margin (Modell & Berdoukas 1984), and very large spleens are associated with an increased plasma volume as well as a large red-cell pool, size alone is not usually a sufficient basis on which a decision for splenectomy should be made. If a very large spleen is causing considerable physical discomfort, and particularly if it is associated with pancytopenia, these factors alone may be sufficient to warrant its removal. But in the majority of cases it is essential to obtain evidence that the hypersplenism is reflected in an increased transfusion requirement.

The first studies which attempted to assess the degree of hypersplenism in transfusion-dependent β thalassaemics were carried out by Modell and colleagues (Modell & Matthews 1976; Modell 1977; Modell & Berdoukas 1984). By measuring the pre- and post-transfusion haemoglobin levels, the mean haemoglobin level over a year was calculated; that is, the average of the mean pre- and post-transfusion haemoglobin values. In this way it was possible to derive a curve for the rate of haemoglobin fall between transfusions and hence to calculate the annual blood requirements to maintain a particular haemoglobin level (see Chapter 7). It turned out that, in the case of splenectomized thalassaemic children, the annual blood requirement was somewhere in the range 150–300 ml/kg, depending on whether the child was on a moderate or high transfusion regimen. However, this relationship did not hold for unsplenectomized patients, whose blood consumption turned out to be anywhere between 200 and 1200 ml/kg/year. Furthermore, it was calculated that if a thalassaemic patient's observed blood consumption is divided by the expected consumption the figure is almost always greater than unity in unsplenectomized patients. From these data Modell and colleagues developed a 'transfusion quotient', which expressed the increase in blood requirements over that expected due to the activity of the spleen. They suggested that if there is more than a 50% increase in consumption, that is, a transfusion quotient of two or more, there is significant hypersplenism and splenectomy should reduce the level of blood consumption to somewhere near the standard curve. It was also found that there is a poor relationship between blood consumption and the results of ^{51}Cr red-cell survival and it was concluded that this investigation is of little value in assessing the degree of hypersplenism.

These studies were an important contribution to our understanding of the role of the spleen in thalassaemia and in the natural history of the evolution of hypersplenism. At the same time as these data were being collected similar work suggested that if the transfusion requirement exceeds 200–250 ml of packed red cells/kg/year, at a minimum haemoglobin level of 10 g/dl, splenectomy is likely to be beneficial (Cohen *et al.* 1980; Graziano *et al.* 1981). As we shall see later, both these approaches to the assessment of transfusion-dependent patients for splenectomy, which are based on the same principle, have turned out to be a useful guide in practice as to whether a patient is likely to have an adequate response to splenectomy. Hence it is important to maintain very careful records from the beginning of a transfusion regimen. If the haemoglobin level is being maintained in the range that is recommended earlier in this chapter, an increase in the transfusion requirement exceeding 200 ml of packed cells/kg/year provides reasonable evidence that a child will benefit from removal of the spleen.

Results of splenectomy

Because patients were not always maintained on what would now be considered to be adequate transfusion regimens, or because of the heterogeneity of the populations studied, early reports on the results of splenectomy for severe forms of β thalassaemia were difficult to evaluate. Overall, however, at least some patients seemed to benefit, though the length of follow-up was rarely sufficient to establish whether the improvement was sustained (Smith *et al.* 1960; Engelhard *et al.* 1975).

Later studies suggested that, if the criteria that are defined in the previous section are adhered to when assessing patients for splenectomy, the results are encouraging. In a series of 58 patients subjected to splenectomy because their transfusion requirements were 50% or more above their theoretical norm, Modell (1977) reported that there was a reduction to the theoretical level in all but three cases, all of whom had been maintained on a low transfusion regime. Further follow-up data on this series were reported by Modell and Berdoukas (1984). It appeared that the reduced blood requirement had been maintained in the majority of patients who had been kept on a high transfusion regimen and that the small number

in whom it had not had succumbed to other complications of thalassaemia. These findings were substantiated by several other studies that were initiated at about the same time. It was found that if splenectomy had been carried out in children whose red-cell requirements exceeded 200 ml/kg/year, and if they had been maintained at an average haemoglobin value of 10 g/dl subsequently, there was a reduction in blood requirements in almost every case (Piomelli *et al.* 1985; Cohen *et al.* 1989a). Even more encouragingly, it appeared that the reduction in blood requirements to something approaching the predicted 200 ml of red cells/kg/year remained stable over many years (Cohen *et al.* 1989a).

It should be emphasized that most of these studies have been carried out in centres in which it has been possible to maintain children at an adequate haemoglobin level and to manage other complications of the disease successfully over a long period. If this is not possible, and particularly if children are not transfused adequately, the results of splenectomy are far less impressive. We shall return to this question in the next section when we consider the complications of splenectomy.

Complications

In competent hands, splenectomy is a safe operation. Even when there is massive splenomegaly, splenic infarcts are very unusual and therefore the spleen does not become adherent to the peritoneal surfaces, as is the case with splenomegaly due to neoplastic disorders. There is a small risk of postoperative infection, particularly related to subphrenic collections of blood, and the usual dangers of wound infection. Provided the children are adequately transfused very few of them seem to develop particularly high platelet counts in the period immediately after splenectomy and the risk of thrombotic disease in the immediate postoperative period appears to be very small.

Infection

Without doubt the major complication of splenectomy is severe and sometimes overwhelming infection. This is not confined to patients with thalassaemia and occurs after splenectomy for a variety of indications (Erikson *et al.* 1968). The possible mechanisms are discussed in Chapter 5. There have been many well documented reports of severe and over-whelming infection in children with β thalassaemia who have had their spleens removed (Penberthy & Cooley 1935; Lichtman *et al.* 1953; Glenn *et al.* 1954; Clement & Taffel 1955; Gofstein & Gellis 1956; Reemsta & Elliot 1956; Smith *et al.* 1957; Mainzer & O'Connor 1958; Wolff *et al.* 1960; Smith *et al.* 1962, 1964; Wasi 1972; Engelhard *et al.* 1975; Modell 1977). Although it was thought that postsplenectomy infection is more severe in the early years of life (Wahidijat *et al.* 1972), and this is probably the case, an analysis of the ages at which infection occurs in thalassaemic children shows a broad scatter (Engelhard *et al.* 1975; Modell 1977). It should be emphasized that the increased proneness to infection covers most systemic infections and is not restricted to overwhelming septicaemia (Modell & Berdoukas 1984).

Splenectomized children are particularly prone to serious and sometimes overwhelming infection due to *Streptococcus pneumoniae*, *Haemophilus influen-zae* and *Neisseria meningitidis*. Because removal of the spleen may reduce the primary immune response to encapsulated organisms, and because of the evidence that severe and overwhelming infections are commoner in the early years of life, it is customary to delay the operation until children are aged 5 years or more. There is some evidence that those who are maintained on an adequate transfusion regimen are at less risk of postsplenectomy infection.

Although earlier studies (Smith *et al.* 1962, 1964) suggested that there may be an increased incidence of recurrent attacks of pericarditis in thalassaemic children who have had their spleens removed, this relationship remains controversial and difficult to assess. It was not observed in the relatively small series reported by Modell and Berdoukas (1984). This question was discussed in Chapter 7.

Overall, the pattern of postsplenectomy infection seems to be similar in different populations (reviewed by Modell & Berdoukas 1984). The lack of information about the perceived risk of severe malaria in splenectomized patients was discussed in Chapter 7. Surprisingly, there are no published data on the risks to splenectomized children in countries where malaria is still endemic, or in those in which there is an increasing frequency of drug-resistant malaria.

Iron loading

Although, as mentioned earlier, it had been suggested that the spleen may act as a storage depot by sequestering iron in a potentially non-toxic pool (Witzleben & Wyatt 1961; Berry & Marshall 1967; Okon *et al.* 1976), there has never been any good evidence that splenectomy has a deleterious effect on the rate of accumulation of iron. As also discussed earlier, Risdon *et al.* (1975) were unable to demonstrate any difference between splenectomized and non-splenectomized patients with regard to liver pathology at similar body iron burdens. It is currently believed that the excess iron resulting from increased blood requirements consequent on hypersplenism is much more important than the loss of a potential iron store. We shall return briefly to this question when we discuss the problems of splenectomy in thalassaemia intermedia.

Thrombotic complications

The increased propensity to thromboembolic complications in thalassaemic children was discussed in Chapters 5 and 7. Except for the problem of pulmonary thrombotic complications in patients with HbE β thalassaemia and other forms of thalassaemia intermedia, to which we shall return later, there is only limited evidence that children who have undergone splenectomy and been maintained at an adequate haemoglobin level have a greater risk of thrombotic complications in the long term than those who have been splenectomized for other conditions. However, it is only in recent years that this aspect of thalassaemia has received much attention.

In a recent multicentre review from Italy, Borgna-Pignatti *et al.* (1998b) observed 27 thromboembolic episodes in 683 patients with β thalassaemia major. Interestingly, 13 of these patients had been splenectomized and their mean haemoglobin level had been maintained at 11.7 g/dl (range 9–14 g/dl). This study also confirmed the likelihood of thromboembolic disease in patients with thalassaemia intermedia maintained at a lower steady-state haemoglobin level. Unfortunately, however, the overall number of patients who had undergone splenectomy in this large series is not given and hence it is not possible to assess the risk of thromboembolic disease that can be ascribed to splenectomy. Thus, apart from some of the anecdotal reports of postsplenectomy thromboembolic disease cited in Chapters 5 and 7, it is not clear whether there is an excess risk of thrombotic disease in β-thalassaemic patients who have been adequately transfused after surgery.

We shall return to the question of the risk of thrombosis in those whose postsplenectomy haemoglobin levels are maintained at a lower level when we discuss the management of thalassaemia intermedia.

Progressive hepatic enlargement

It has been the impression of clinicians with considerable experience of splenectomy in thalassaemic patients that it may be followed by progressive hepatic enlargement, together with an increase in transfusion requirement. This complication was described in a series of patients who had been maintained on a low transfusion regime in a report from Israel by Engelhard *et al.* (1975). It is also documented by Modell and Berdoukas (1984), who observed a syndrome characterized by increased blood requirement, gross, soft hepatomegaly, and stunting of growth in six out of 14 splenectomized patients from Cyprus, maintained at a mean haemoglobin level of 7 g/dl. In each case the spleen had been removed more than 5 years previously. We have observed the same clinical picture in patients with HbE β thalassaemia in Sri Lanka, in some of whom the liver was enlarged up to 15 cm below the costal margin.

The one thing that these reports have in common is the relatively low steady-state haemoglobin levels in the years following splenectomy. Modell and Berdoukas suggested that the hepatomegaly may reflect the trapping of abnormal thalassaemic cells in a large hepatic pool, causing engorgement and hypertrophy. Apart from the hepatic sequestration crises of sickle-cell anaemia (see Chapters 2 and 9) we know of no evidence that this type of pathology can occur. It seemed possible that the hepatomegaly reflects intensive extramedullary haemopoiesis as a response to continued anaemia. Recently, we have had the opportunity to examine several liver biopsies from patients with this clinical picture who have undergone splenectomy for HbE β thalassaemia. The predominant finding is, indeed, very extensive erythropoiesis, particularly involving the hepatic sinusoids. Thus, although there may be other causes of hepatic enlargement in patients of this type, it

seems very likely that, in the absence of the spleen, there is a major shift to the liver as an organ of extramedullary erythropoiesis.

Haematological sequelae

As mentioned earlier, where it has been studied the red-cell survival appears to increase after splenectomy. The peripheral blood films of patients who are maintained at a relatively low haemoglobin level show the remarkable changes in red-cell morphology which are described in detail in Chapter 7. There is an increase in the number of nucleated red cells, many of which show typical inclusion bodies consisting of precipitated α chains. Persistent thrombocytosis is unusual except in patients who are maintained at a low haemoglobin level. There may be a moderate leucocytosis although the differential count is usually normal.

Practical implications

As we have seen, any child with transfusion requirements in excess of 200 ml red cells/kg/year should be considered for splenectomy. The operation should be carried out at the child's ideal haemoglobin level to minimize postoperative thrombocytosis. The possibility of subphrenic collections and thrombotic complications should be minimized by early mobilization and breathing exercises.

The major issue is how to reduce the possibility of infection. Patients should be immunized before the operation with polyvalent pneumococcal, meningococcal and *H. influenzae* vaccines. It is now customary to also give prophylactic oral penicillin daily to avoid colonization of strains not covered by the vaccines, particularly in young children. Since there are no adequate trial data it is difficult to decide whether to continue penicillin prophylaxis when splenectomized patients grow older. For this reason practices vary; it is currently our policy to maintain it indefinitely.

It is equally important to warn patients and their families about the risks of infection after splenectomy. Many countries now supply a card or other documentation that states that the patient has undergone splenectomy, which they should carry with them at all times. Since pneumococcal septicaemia may kill within hours it is also important to warn patients' primary-care physicians of this risk and to advise that if they become acutely ill they receive a large, parenteral dose of penicillin before being moved to hospital.

For those rare patients who develop thrombotic complications the first-line treatment is with heparin, followed by warfarin or a similar agent, together with the use of antiplatelet agents. Since from what little information is available on this complication it appears that if there has been a thrombotic episode it may recur, these patients should be maintained on anticoagulant therapy and antiplatelet agents.

Alternatives to splenectomy

Because of the risks of infection following splenectomy, particularly in young children, alternative approaches to the management of hypersplenism have been explored. These include partial splenectomy and splenic embolism.

Partial splenectomy

There have been several reports of the use of partial splenectomy for the management of thalassaemia major (Kheradpir & Albouyeh 1985; de Montalembert *et al.* 1990). In the series of de Montalembert *et al.* the operation was performed on 30 patients with β thalassaemia major with a follow-up period of 1–4 years. Although the results were initially quite encouraging, recurrence of hypersplenism occurred in nine of the 24 patients, necessitating a complete splenectomy. The authors conclude that this operation should be restricted to children under the age of 5 years, who have the greatest risk of overwhelming postsplenectomy infection. However, since these episodes can be largely prevented by adequate measures, the place for this procedure must be very limited.

Splenic embolization and related procedures

As another approach to reducing the degree of hypersplenism, partial splenic embolization (Politis *et al.* 1987) or partial vascular disconnection of the spleen (Revillon & Girot 1985) has been proposed. Although these are interesting alternatives, because of the lack of control over the end result, and because there are now effective means of prevention of postsplenectomy infection, it seems unlikely that these methods will be used widely in the future.

Prophylactic cholecystectomy during splenectomy

It was suggested by Feretis *et al.* (1985) that, because of the increased frequency of gallstones and gallbladder disease in patients with β thalassaemia, it might be appropriate to carry out a prophylactic cholecystectomy at the same time as splenectomy. In a controlled study these authors found that the procedure was not associated with increased postoperative morbidity. However, it seems unlikely that cholecystectomy is indicated in patients with β thalassaemia major who are to be maintained at a relatively high haemoglobin level and hence in whom the bone marrow is suppressed, making the production of pigment stones much less likely. Clearly, the biliary tract should always be carefully assessed at surgery but in the absence of disease there seems little place for prophylactic cholecystectomy, certainly in transfusion-dependent children.

Other aspects of symptomatic treatment

Delayed development and endocrine deficiency

The difficult problem of growth retardation and failure of sexual development in transfusion-dependent patients with β thalassaemia was discussed in Chapter 7. It was emphasized that delayed growth may have many different causes and that delayed sexual maturation is primarily the result of central hypogonadism with secondary sex steroid deficiency. As was pointed out in Chapter 7, and discussed earlier in this chapter, it seems likely that once the iron-mediated damage is done there is very little chance of it being reversed. It is vital to investigate patients with disturbances of growth and development extremely thoroughly to rule out non-endocrine causes, particularly the toxic effects of DF. Once this has been done it is important to obtain the help of those with expertise in the endocrinological investigation and management of children or young adults.

Overall, there are limited published data on the results of the management of growth retardation and failure of sexual development. Hitherto, it has usually been the practice to institute therapy with androgen or oestrogen replacement, although even this apparently straightforward treatment can be fraught with difficulties (see Vullo *et al.* 1990). However, it is still used in many centres. Over recent years, and with increasing evidence that both growth failure and lack of sexual development may reflect iron-mediated damage to the hypothalamic/pituitary/gonadal axis, attempts have been made towards a more physiological approach to hormone replacement. For example, pulsatile gonadotrophin-releasing hormone (GnRH) infusions have been used in an attempt to induce puberty (Chatterjee *et al.* 1988, 1993a). More recently Chatterjee and Katz (2000) have found that those patients with severe organ damage due to iron load are apulsatile with respect to their gonadotrophin profiles and are likely to have irreversible damage to the hypothalamic/pituitary axis. On the other hand those with less severe iron load seem to have potentially reversible hypogonadotrophic hypogonadism. Wonke *et al.* (1998a) have described a regimen for the management of genuine growth-hormone insufficiency using recombinant growth hormone (rhGH), self-administered by daily subcutaneous dosages of 0.6–0.9 IU/kg body weight/week. Based on growth velocity increments their patients can be divided into responders, partial responders and non-responders. The same authors also describe a protocol for defining growth-hormone resistance by measuring levels of IgF1 and IgF-BP3 (see Chapter 7) in the serum. Principles of management of the resistant cases are based on the use of increasingly large doses of rhGH.

Clearly it is too early to evaluate the applicability of these more sophisticated approaches to the management of growth retardation and hypogonadism to the thalassaemic population at large. But what is clear is that, once iron-related damage to the hypothalamic/pituitary axis has occurred, it may be very difficult to help many patients. This is further evidence, if any were needed, of the importance of extremely careful management of iron chelation during the critical early years of puberty.

The management of diabetes, thyroid and hypothyroid deficiency is more straightforward, and simply involves standard replacement therapy.

Cardiac disease

The clinical features and investigation of cardiac disease in iron-loaded patients with β thalassaemia were discussed in Chapter 7. The principles of management are to remove iron by intensive chelation therapy by the intravenous route, as described earlier in this chapter, and to manage the symptoms of failure with the judicious use of diuretics, digoxin, inotropes and agents that reduce afterload.

The extent to which patients with established cardiac disease can be rescued by intensive intravenous chelation therapy is not absolutely clear; in some reports the length of follow-up after initial improvement was too short to assess the full efficacy of this form of treatment. However, there have been sufficient reports of the reversal, or partial reversal, of cardiac dysfunction in iron-loaded patients who have received intensive intravenous DF therapy to suggest that this form of therapy is well worth a trial in any patient who presents with this distressing complication (Freeman *et al.* 1983; Marcus *et al.* 1984; Rahko *et al.* 1986; Aldouri *et al.* 1990).

There has been one report of a successful combined heart and liver transplant in a patient with thalassaemia major with advanced cardiac and hepatic disease (Olivieri *et al.* 1994a).

Bone disease

The complex mechanisms that underlie bone disease in β thalassaemia were discussed in Chapter 7. In inadequately transfused patients the main approach to therapy is to establish the patient on a standard transfusion regimen as outlined earlier in this chapter. The prevention and management of bone disease resulting from DF toxicity are also discussed earlier in this chapter. The major difficulty arises in the forms of osteoporosis which seem to result mainly from hypogonadism. Osteoporosis is a progressive condition and, since its treatment is unsatisfactory, prevention and early diagnosis are particularly important.

All symptomatic thalassaemic patients should have regular estimations of their bone density and those who are osteopenic should be treated with oral calcium and vitamin D supplementation, advised to take active exercise and told not to smoke. Those in whom there is unequivocal evidence of hypogonadism should be treated by hormone replacement therapy. Although biphosphonates are under evaluation for the management of osteoporosis their role in thalassaemic patients remains to be determined (Wonke 1998).

Vitamin supplementation

The value of ascorbic acid in iron chelation therapy was discussed earlier in this chapter.

In Chapter 7, we reviewed the question of folate requirements in patients with β thalassaemia major. Undoubtedly, patients who are maintained at a relatively low haemoglobin level should be maintained on folate supplements. Those that are treated with an adequate transfusion regime, and in whom the bone marrow is relatively depressed, probably do not require folate supplementation. However, since even these patients have some increase of bone-marrow activity, and the folate content of diets varies so widely, we believe that all patients with severe forms of β thalassaemia should receive folate supplementation. This is particularly important at times when there are increased folate requirements, during intercurrent illnesses and, in particular, pregnancy.

The role of vitamin E in the pathophysiology of the thalassaemic red cell was discussed in Chapters 5 and 7. A number of studies have tried to assess the possibility of increasing red-cell survival by the use of vitamin E supplementation. Overall, these studies proved to be disappointing (see, for example, Rachmilewitz *et al.* 1979) and, certainly in the well transfused patient, there is no evidence that vitamin E has any therapeutic role.

Infection

It is beyond the scope of this section to cover every form of infection which may affect thalassaemic patients. We have already discussed the prevention of postsplenectomy infection and focus here on a few life-threatening situations.

Severe postsplenectomy infection

Streptococcus pneumoniae remains the commonest cause of overwhelming infection in patients who have undergone splenectomy. The onset of symptoms may be extremely rapid and patients may collapse and become moribund within a few hours. After a blood culture has been taken these patients should receive maximum body weight-related doses of crystalline penicillin, by either the intravenous or intramuscular routes. While penicillin-insensitive pneumococci are rarely encountered in the richer

countries, this is not the case in the developing world. Hence, although a lack of response to penicillin may indicate that the infection is due to another organism, in some countries the possibility of penicillin resistance has to be considered. There is still considerable uncertainty about how to manage patients with septicaemia due to penicillin-resistant pneumococci. Because there are different grades of insensitivity it is suggested that large doses of penicillin should still be administered, but if this fails a third-generation cephalosporin such as ceftriaxone is usually the next choice of antibiotic. It should be remembered, however, that neither penicillin nor the cephalosporins can be used for the treatment of pneumococcal meningitis and in this case the first-line drug is probably vancomycin.

Not all severe, life-threatening infections in debilitated thalassaemic patients or in those who have undergone splenectomy are pneumococcal in origin. Where there are any doubts, or where there is a lack of response to therapy directed at the pneumococcus, it is wiser to begin a regimen similar to that which would be used to cover any serious infection in a compromised host. There are several well validated regimens, either the combination of an antipseudomonal penicillin with an aminoglycoside, piperacillin with gentamycin for example, or the use of a single, extended spectrum cephalosporin such as ceftazidine. The latter has the added advantage that it may be effective against penicillin-resistant pneumococci.

Infections due to Yersinia

As mentioned in Chapters 5 and 7, patients who are receiving DF may occasionally develop severe infections due to *Yersinia enterocolitica* or related species. They usually present with severe abdominal pain and diarrhoea, vomiting, fever and sore throat and the disease can rapidly progress. This infection should be suspected in any patient receiving DF who presents with this clinical picture. The drug should be stopped and stools cultured for *Yersinia* spp. Empirical treatment should commence immediately with either an aminoglycoside or co-trimoxazole at full body weight dosage. The clinical manifestations and management of this complication are the subject of a comprehensive review by Adamkiewicz *et al.* (1998).

Blood-borne infections

As mentioned earlier in this chapter, in many populations there is a relatively high frequency of blood-borne viral infections, particularly hepatitis B and C. Unfortunately, infections with HIV are also becoming commoner. Since both hepatitis B virus (HBV) and hepatitis C virus (HCV) can induce chronic active hepatitis, leading to cirrhosis and a relatively high incidence of hepatic carcinoma, the prevention and treatment of these disorders have become a major part of the management of thalassaemia. Their prevention was described earlier in this chapter. Here we shall consider briefly the management of established cases.

It has been estimated that there are probably 300 million people in the world chronically infected with HBV, the highest prevalence being in tropical Africa, Central and South America, China, Japan and Indonesia. The persistence of the virus and the development of chronic active hepatitis after the acute phase vary considerably, depending on the age of the patient; from 2 years onwards the infection only persists in approximately 2–5% of cases. The diagnosis of the acute phase involves the identification of HBs, that is, the surface antigen, in the serum. This also is found in the chronic phase and the two are distinguished by the additional presence of high-titre IgM anti-HBc (core antigen) in the acute phase. Patients with chronic hepatitis B are initially HBe-antigen positive, although eventually this is cleared and antibody appears in the serum. In many cases the appearance of anti-HBe is associated with the control of viraemia and resolution of the hepatitis; the continued production of HBs antigen depends on the presence of viral DNA integrated into cellular DNA sequences. The diagnosis of chronic active hepatitis is made by liver biopsy.

Hepatitis C usually produces a mild form of hepatitis without jaundice. However, 50% of patients develop chronic infection and hepatitis, 20% of whom develop cirrhosis with a risk of hepatocellular carcinoma. The presence of persistent viraemia is determined by polymerase chain reaction amplification of HCV-RNA from the serum. Again, the diagnosis of chronic active hepatitis depends on the appearances on liver biopsy.

The management of post-transfusion hepatitis is both expensive and not entirely satisfactory (Telfer

et al. 1997; Wonke *et al.* 1998a). In the case of hepatitis B the administration of α interferon has been shown to cause transient inhibition of viral replication and, in 40% of cases, treatment for at least 6 months produces permanent inhibition with conversion from HBe antigen to antibody, followed several years later by clearance of HBs antigen. Patients with high concentrations of transaminases and severe chronic active hepatitis on biopsy are most likely to respond. In the case of hepatitis C, α interferon in doses in the range 3–5 MU three times weekly for 6–12 months normalizes transaminase levels in 50–80% of cases but, unfortunately, about half these patients relapse. Long-term control is obtained in about 25–40% of thalassaemic patients (Di Marco *et al.* 1997; Wonke *et al.* 1998a). The use of longer-term treatment and trials of ribavirin, either alone or combined with α interferon, are still under evaluation (Telfer *et al.* 1997). Preliminary results suggest that ribavirin given as a single agent is ineffective, but when combined with α interferon the results are much more promising.

There are a number of important issues to be considered in the management of hepatitis C in thalassaemic children. As mentioned earlier in this chapter, there is increasing evidence that iron loading of the liver tends to increase the severity of this condition and therefore it is very important to establish the hepatic iron concentration, which should be done at the time of the first liver biopsy, and to treat patients who have increased levels of iron with vigorous chelation therapy. The drug regimens for hepatitis C are associated with a variety of side-effects. Patients receiving α interferon may suffer from pyrexia, rigors, fatigue, depression, marrow suppression and weight loss. Furthermore, this drug may induce hypothyroidism; patients who are heavily iron loaded may already have some thyroid dysfunction. Hence it is very important to monitor thyroid function while on therapy. Ribavirin may cause a haemolytic anaemia or a variety of skin eruptions. Taking into account these unwanted reactions, together with the cost of these agents, it is clear that the treatment of this condition raises a number of important issues, particularly for poorer countries. Furthermore, it is clear that we do not know enough about its natural history to be certain that it always requires treatment, particularly if it is contracted very early in life (Jonas 1999). The hepatitis C field is a rapidly changing scene and clinicians are advised to consult the current natural history and trial literature before embarking on treatment.

Unfortunately, human immunodeficiency virus (HIV) infection and acquired immunodeficiency syndrome (AIDS) are becoming increasingly prevalent in many of the developing countries in which thalassaemia is common. The dangers and approaches to the prevention of infection by blood products were considered earlier in this chapter. Accounts of the particular problems of HIV in the developing countries are given by the WHO (1994) and by Gilks (1995). There are particular difficulties in the diagnosis as the result of the cost of HIV antibody testing and difficulties in the maintenance of quality control. Although very little has been published about the patterns of AIDS in thalassaemic children (see Chapter 7) there is no reason to believe that it will not produce the same types of problems that are seen throughout the developing world. These include presentation with acute and chronic respiratory infection, a gastrointestinal syndrome associated with chronic diarrhoea and weight loss, generalized lymphadenopathy, a high frequency of extremely aggressive forms of tuberculosis, repeated pneumococcal infections and systemic salmonellosis. The prevention and treatment of AIDS are a constantly changing scene. There is increasing evidence that the use of antiviral agents such as zidovudine, didanosine and zalcitabine both retard the development of AIDS in seropositive individuals and prolong life in established cases. Currently, combination therapy using several antiviral agents has shown distinct promise although the cost of this type of regimen may preclude its use in many of the poorer countries.

Malaria may be contracted either by a bite from an infected mosquito or from infected blood. Although donor screening is carried out widely in many tropical countries transfusion-borne infections still occur. Because of the frightening recrudescence of drug-resistant malaria in many parts of the world it seems likely that this will become an increasing problem for thalassaemic patients in tropical countries in the future. Indeed, because of global warming malaria may re-occur in countries where it has not existed for many hundreds of years. Again, it is beyond our scope to cover this in detail and it has been the subject of several extensive reviews (Bradley *et al.* 1995). Here we shall discuss a few aspects which are particularly relevant to patients with thalassaemia.

In many countries, donor or other forms of screening for malaria, if they are practised at all, are not totally reliable and in areas of high endemicity blood-borne malaria infection is still quite common. In these populations it is wiser to give prophylactic antimalarials appropriate to the local sensitivity of the parasite to patients who are receiving blood transfusion, or at least to keep them under extremely careful observation for several weeks after the transfusion; paradoxically, the incubation time is longer, up to 12 days, for transfusion-borne infections than following a mosquito bite. Unfortunately, malaria control programmes have broken down completely in many countries where there is a high frequency of thalassaemia. Although attempts at vector control are being made, together with early treatment and regular assessment, these measures are unlikely to have a major effect for some years to come. Similarly, there is no guarantee that vaccines will become available. Hence, it is important that children with thalassaemia take all the simple measures that are possible to prevent being infected. These include avoiding exposure to mosquito bites in the evening, the use of bed nets, and, in parts of the world where the transmission rate is sufficiently high, malaria prophylactics.

Malaria should be suspected in any thalassaemic child in an at-risk population who develops unexplained fever and chills. Severe malaria due to *Plasmodium falciparum* infection, particularly if it involves the brain, is a major medical emergency. It should be remembered that although this form of malaria is frequently associated with high levels of parasites in the peripheral blood this is not always the case. As well as leading to coma, with all the associated complications of the unconscious patient, the severe forms of malaria are complicated by profound anaemia, disturbances of fluid and electrolyte balance, progressive renal failure, metabolic acidosis, pulmonary oedema, hypotension, hypoglycaemia and bleeding disorders. Because of widespread chloroquine resistance the first-line drug for severe malaria is quinine, although even quinine resistance is being encountered. The only agent for which resistance has not yet been reported is artemisinin (qinghaosu), the active ingredient of the Chinese herb *Artemisia annua*. Clinicians in countries in which malaria is common (and, because of increased international travel, even where it is not) must keep themselves constantly informed about regional variations in drug resistance.

It is important to emphasize that very little work has been done on the role of antimalarial prophylaxis in the management of thalassaemia in countries in which the disease is prevalent, or in which there appears to be a recrudescence. Because of the current pattern of drug resistance this will be a particularly important issue in the next few years.

Skeletal and dental deformity

The severe skeletal deformities which were such a problem in this disease in the past are not usually encountered in children maintained on adequate blood transfusion regimens. However, in populations in which this is not possible, recurrent fractures are a common occurrence and healing is often slow and delayed. The fracture should be treated in the usual way and if possible an appropriate transfusion regimen initiated (see later section). Similarly, the orthodontic problems which were so common in the past (Asbell 1964) and the gross facial deformities which were described in graphic detail by Jurkiewicz *et al.* (1969) are now seen much less frequently. The complications which arise from deformities of the skull, such as deafness and sinus obstruction, were discussed in Chapter 7; they too are prevented by adequate transfusion.

Haemorrhagic and thrombotic complications

As discussed in Chapters 5 and 7, haemorrhagic complications, such as recurrent nose bleeding, which was seen so commonly in the past, are no longer a major feature of thalassaemic children who are maintained on adequate transfusion regimens. Indeed, apart from rare cases of thrombocytopenia due to hypersplenism, or liver failure due to iron loading or chronic active hepatitis, a bleeding tendency is very unusual.

As also discussed in Chapters 5 and 7, although there is increasing evidence that patients with thalassaemia are at risk from thrombotic complications due to a hypercoagulable state, this does not seem to be a feature of children who are maintained at an adequate haemoglobin level, presumably because of the

suppression of endogenous red-cell production. We shall return to the management of these complications in a later section which deals with some of the problems particular to thalassaemia intermedia.

Psychosocial aspects

The psychosocial aspects of the severe forms of thalassaemia have been receiving increasing attention over recent years. In their monograph on the management of thalassaemia Modell and Berdoukas (1984) describe their experience in caring for patients in the Cypriot community in London and discuss the emotional problems of the children and their parents after the diagnosis has first been made and subsequently throughout childhood. They also describe the totally different problems of the adolescent. One of the difficulties with this field is, of course, that the particular psychosocial problems vary enormously between different countries and between different environments and social groups within countries. Thus it is difficult to offer anything but a few broad generalizations about this subject. These are based on our own experiences and on the small literature that exists so far (Cazzetta 1990; Georganda 1990; Masera *et al.* 1990; Nash 1990; Tsiantis 1990; Klein *et al.* 1998; Weissman *et al.* 1998). This subject is also discussed in a report of a Working Party of the WHO (1990). Readers who wish to understand the sensitive and complex relationships between doctors and patients with thalassaemia are strongly advised to read David Nathan's *Genes, Blood and Courage* (Nathan 1995).

Methodology

So far the methodology for studying the psychosocial aspects of thalassaemia has been derived from the standard approaches of the social sciences (WHO 1990). Because of the growing concern about this problem the WHO undertook a large multicentre study in 1995 to evaluate the psychosocial aspects of thalassaemia and sickle-cell anaemia. Because it was found that the questionnaires used by the WHO were either inappropriate or rather cumbersome a more suitable programme was developed by Ratip (quoted by Klein *et al.* 1998). This attempts to define the major psychosocial burdens but also puts them into perspective as seen through the very different eyes of patients and parents. A study carried out on the Toronto thalassaemic population using this approach showed just how important it is not to generalize about psychosocial problems based on studies in any one group of patients or their relatives. For example, they found that the clinical and psychosocial burden was not correlated for parents and children, parents' perceptions of their child's psychological burden correlate well while the child is young but not when the child reaches adulthood, the psychological burden felt by children is affected by that felt by their parents and vice versa, and, while the overall burden is similarly perceived by children and their parents, the value placed on its individual aspects may differ considerably between family members.

Infancy and early childhood

Most of the problems of this phase of development focus round the adaptation of the family to the fact that they have a chronically ill child and the child's initial reaction to therapy. Parents may need extremely careful counselling for a whole variety of untoward reactions towards the knowledge that their child will require lifelong therapy. There is often considerable guilt entailed, a complete lack of understanding of the 'ill luck' aspects of genetic disease, and a considerable amount of anger as to why this has happened to them in particular. As well as skilful counselling it is at this stage that it may be useful for families to join thalassaemia societies to meet other parents and to come to realize that they are not alone and to share their problems with those who have been through them before.

Later childhood and school-days

By this time the parents are usually reasonably well adapted to their children's problems. However, one of the most difficult transitions for a child with chronic disease is from the relative seclusion of their home environment and that of their immediate friends to the wider stresses of school and the outside world. At this stage the child needs a lot of support and the school must be thoroughly informed about the nature of the illness and the fact that the child should be able to lead a completely normal life together with their fellow students. Despite a therapeutic team's best efforts, however, some children develop severe behavioural and emotional problems at this stage which require expert assessment and treatment. An approach to assessing these children, based on the pioneering studies of Michael Rutter in London, is described by Tsiantis (1990). It is particularly helpful at this stage to try to unravel the relationships of the child with its parents and to uncover the problems of overprotective behaviour or, at the other end of the spectrum, excessive pressure on a child through too many demands.

Adolescence

Adolescence offers a particular challenge to many patients with chronic diseases such as thalassaemia. It is the period when they become naturally angry and start to question every aspect of their lot, including their treatment, social relationships and thoughts of the future. It is a particularly difficult time for those who develop any form of hypogonadism and, as well as their physical treatment, they need strong and sympathetic support by clinicians and backup staff with experience of the particular problems of this stage of life. Whether this needs a specially designed adolescent facility is far from clear, but what it essential is adequate continuity of emotional support between childhood and adult life, and thalassaemia centres should be organized such that there is no break of continuity in medical staff.

Comment

Over recent years there has been an increasing realization among medical educationalists in the richer countries that some of the pastoral skills of patient care have been lost during the period of the development of high technology medical practice. Attempts are being made to redress this situation by an increasing emphasis on communication skills, better clinical method and other aspects of good doctoring. Nowhere are these attributes more valuable than in the management of patients with chronic illnesses like thalassaemia. These patients are extremely demanding of time and they must be managed by a team which includes clinicians who genuinely understand the disease, backed up by social workers and nurses who are able to take over some of the pastoral role of the management of these patients. Because many of them have to come to hospital regularly the thalassaemia centre often has to take over the role of the primary-care clinician and to look after every aspect of care, clinical, psychological and pastoral.

Given the rather limited knowledge that we have of the psychological aspects of chronic illnesses and their management, and the fact that these problems vary enormously between different ethnic groups, it is very difficult to provide more guidance than the simple suggestions that we have outlined in the previous sections. This is a field where a great deal of work needs to be done. In sitting in thalassaemia clinics in some of the poorer countries we have been very struck by the extraordinary diversity of attitude to disease in different countries. In some, a chronic disease like thalassaemia is seen as a stigma and these children are excluded from the community. We need to know much more about these cultural differences and how they are translated to immigrant populations in other countries. In short, our knowledge of the total effect of chronic illness on a patient's life is extremely limited.

Thalassaemia societies and associations

There is no doubt that support societies for patients and their parents with different forms of thalassaemia are an enormous help, and do much to cover the deficiencies of medical practitioners in the management of these diseases. However, they must be well organized and well informed. Their medical advisers must keep them up to date but they must avoid the temptation of telling families what they want to hear rather than the real facts, however unpleasant they may be. Similarly, it is very important that these societies, as they grow in size and influence, must not try and pressure the medical profession into using untested forms of treatment, however attractive they may appear. At their best, these societies are of enormous value to thalassaemic patients but only if they are constantly in touch with those who can provide them with an objective and scientifically based view of current practice. The addresses of the international and national societies are given in the Appendix, p. 821.

Bone-marrow transplantation

Background

Bone-marrow transplantation (BMT) from HLA-

identical siblings has been an established form of treatment for neoplastic disorders of the bone marrow, and some non-malignant conditions, for many years. The first successful transplantation for a patient with β thalassaemia was carried out by Thomas *et al.* (1982). The patient, a 14-month-old child who had never received a blood transfusion, is still alive and well and is, in effect, the longest surviving patient who has been cured of thalassaemia. As pointed out by Giardini (1997), at the same time, a 14-year-old thalassaemic patient who had already received 150 red-cell transfusions, received a bone-marrow transplant in Pesaro, but this was followed by recurrence of the patient's thalassaemia after the graft had been rejected.

Since these pioneering studies extensive experience has been gained of marrow transplantation for patients with β thalassaemia. By 1997 over 1000 transplants had been performed at three centres in Italy (Argiolu *et al.* 1997; Di Bartolomeo *et al.* 1997; Galimberti *et al.* 1997). In addition this form of therapy was taken up in other centres around the world and, although the numbers were much smaller, a considerable amount of experience of this approach has been obtained (Vellodi *et al.* 1994; Walters & Thomas 1994; Clift & Johnson 1997; Roberts *et al.* 1997a). In reviewing the reasons for the steady improvement in the results of bone-marrow transplantation Giardini (1997) suggests that, as well as increasing experience, the major factors have been the establishment of more effective pretransplant regimens, the introduction of cyclosporin, more effective treatment of cytomegalovirus infection, improved aseptic techniques and a better understanding of the use of systemic antibiotic therapy.

In assessing the current role of marrow transplantation for the treatment of thalassaemia we have relied mainly on the Italian experience since it is far greater than that of other centres throughout the world. It is summarized extensively in a review by Lucarelli *et al.* (1995).

Overall results

During their early analyses of bone-marrow transplantation for thalassaemia the Pesaro group found a number of factors which appeared to influence the outcome (Lucarelli *et al.* 1990, 1991). Thus, in assessing the overall results, it is useful to classify them using the criteria of Lucarelli and colleagues.

Patient subclasses

Based on a history of the adequacy of iron chelation therapy, the presence of liver fibrosis, and whether or not patients have hepatomegaly, the Pesaro group have classified patients into three classes: class 1 has a history of adequate iron chelation and has neither liver fibrosis nor hepatomegaly; class 2 is characterized by having either hepatomegaly or liver fibrosis; class 3 has both complications.

Results in relationship to prior classification
(Fig. 15.7)

Among class 1 children who have undergone transplantation early in the course of their disease,

disease-free survival is assessed at 90–93%, with a risk of mortality related to the procedure of 3–4% (Lucarelli *et al*. 1993, 1995). Comparable results have been reported from other centres in this low-risk group of patients (Argiolu *et al*. 1997; Di Bartolomeo *et al*. 1997). For class 2 patients, which form the intermediate-risk group, the survival and disease-free survival rates are 86% and 82%, respectively. For what is considered to be the high-risk group, that is, class 3, the survival and disease-free survival rates are 62 and 51%, respectively (Lucarelli *et al*. 1996).

In the early experience of the Italian group the patients were mainly transplanted during the first few years of life. Later, they reported on the results of an older group, aged greater than 16 years, where the survival rate and disease-free survival rates were

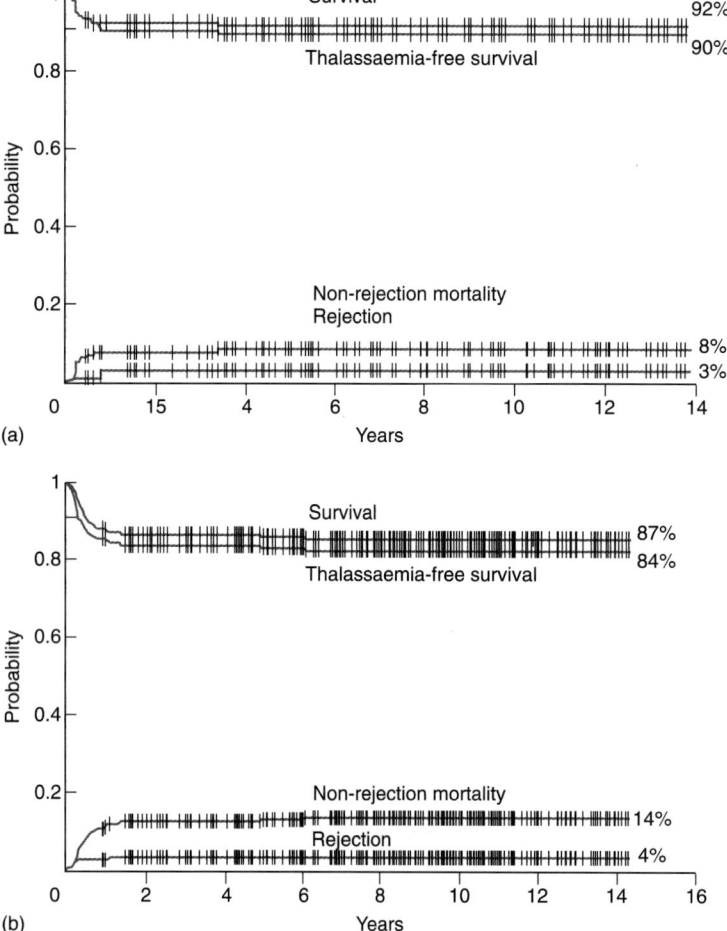

Fig. 15.7 Survival after bone-marrow transplantation in the three classes of patients based on different prognostic risk factors as described in the text. (a) 126 class 1 patients; (b) 297 class 2 patients; (c) 143 class 3 patients aged less than 17 years; (d) 109 adults, aged over 16 years. These figures were kindly prepared for the authors by Professor Guido Lucarelli.

65% and 63%, respectively (Lucarelli *et al.* 1992, 1995).

Complications

Apart from the major complications that occur in the immediate post-transplant period, most of which relate to infection or rejection, the major problems, as with all forms of bone-marrow transplantation, is the development of acute or chronic graft-versus-host disease (GVHD).

Graft-versus-host disease

In a review of the frequency and risk factors for GVHD, Gaziev *et al.* (1997a) reported that the overall frequency of mild to severe grades of acute GVHD ranged between 13 and 27%. Important risk factors seem to be a patient age of less than 4 years, male sex, whether prophylaxis has been attempted with cyclosporin and methyl prednisolone or with methotrexate and methyl prednisolone, elevated alanine aminotransferase levels, and seropositivity for herpes viruses. The probabilities of developing moderate to severe chronic GVHD were 8% and 2%, respectively. Risk factors for the latter appeared to be a previous acute episode, female sex, the use of allo-immune donors for male patients, and the same relationship to drug prophylaxis as for the acute form.

It appears that the most significant risks associated with BMT are concentrated within the first year. The Pesaro group have followed up some of their patients

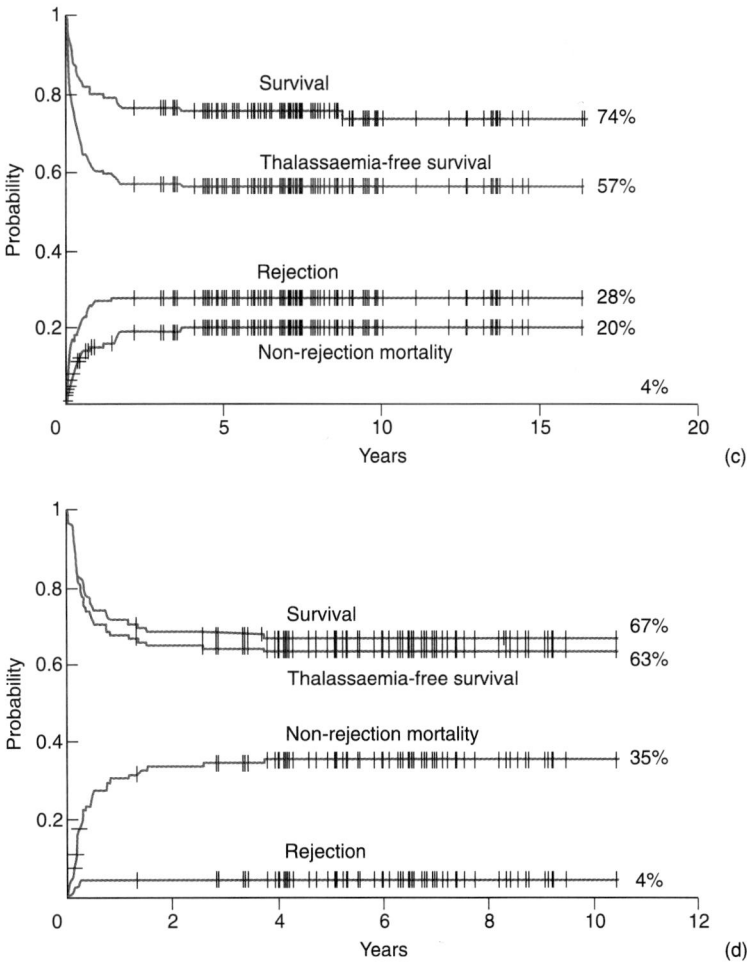

Fig. 15.7 *Continued.*

for over 15 years. The majority of them appear to be well and have shown normal pubertal development and growth patterns (De Sanctis *et al.* 1997). A small number have had to remain on long-term immuno-suppressive therapy due to a chronic GVHD.

Drug toxicity

Apart from the inevitable myelosuppressive proper-ties of the drugs involved in bone-marrow transplan-tation, the major difficulty that has been experienced is the unpredictability of the pharmacological pro-perties of busulphan, used in most preparative re-gimens. It appears that hyperabsorption is associated with hepatic veno-occlusive disease, while a reduced rate of absorption may lead to rejection and re-currence of a thalassaemic blood picture. A variety of approaches have been proposed to obtain better control of busulphan levels during induction (Shulman & Hinterberger 1992).

Mixed chimerism

Although this phenomenon does not seem to have a deleterious effect on the course of patients who have received bone-marrow transplantation, there is no question that if they are studied in detail approxi-mately 10% of them show mixed chimerism, that is, both normal and thalassaemic cell populations in the peripheral blood. It appears that attempts to reduce the dose of either busulphan or cyclophosphamide in the conditioning regimen are associated with higher rates of chimerism. Furthermore, there appears to be a higher frequency of rejection within the first 2 years after transplantation if chimerism is present. On the other hand some patients with dual cell populations in their peripheral blood seem to have survived in good health for well over 2 years, suggesting that the co-existence of both donor and host cells may be a reflection that mutual tolerance has been induced (Andreani *et al.* 1996).

Long-term risk of malignant disease

So far the longest follow-up of patients after marrow transplantation is between 15 and 20 years. There does not appear to have been a case of haematologi-cal malignancy, although the number of patients followed for the appropriate length of time is still rel-atively small (Gaziev *et al.* 1997b).

The use of unrelated, phenotypically matched donors

This difficult topic, as it relates to marrow trans-plantation in thalassaemia, is reviewed by Giardini (1997). While there have been a few successful marrow transplantations of this type (La Nasa *et al.* 1997) there is still too little experience to be able to draw any useful conclusions. It is a subject of a number of pilot studies in several countries.

The management of pre-existing complications of thalassaemia after bone-marrow transplantation

Patients who have undergone BMT for β thalas-saemia who already are iron loaded before the proce-dure may require further treatment, despite the fact that their rate of iron loading should, theoretically, return to normal (Lucarelli *et al.* 1993; Muretto *et al.* 1994). Experiences of the use of DF after transplanta-tion, reported by Giardini *et al.* (1995) and Angelucci *et al.* (1997), suggested that it might be more effective to reduce the body iron after transplantation by the use of regular phlebotomy, in a similar way to that used in patients with hereditary haemochromatosis. Mariotti *et al.* (1997) have reported preliminary data that suggest that there may be improvement in cardiac function in heavily iron-loaded patients by regular phlebotomy. Preliminary studies have also been reported on the use of α-interferon therapy for chronic non-A non-B hepatitis after bone-marrow transplantation for thalassaemia, with encouraging results.

Although there is increasing experience of manag-ing these complications in thalassaemic patients who have undergone marrow transplantation, it requires them to be subjected to further long courses of rela-tively unpleasant treatment. Particularly in view of the trauma associated with the transplantation itself, and the better results that are obtained if the proce-dure is done early in life, before these complications have arisen, the case for making an early decision as to whether to proceed to transplantation becomes all the more pressing.

The present place for bone-marrow transplantation in thalassaemia

The use of BMT in thalassaemia has not been without its controversies. They revolve mainly round some rather complex ethical issues and uncertainties about the overall results in centres other than those like Pesaro, where a very large experience of the procedure has been gained (Lucarelli & Weatherall 1991; Weatherall 1992; Roberts 1994; Giardini 1995). The central problem, though complex, is easily stated. Is it right to subject a baby or young child to a procedure which still has a small but significant mortality rate, and a not inconsiderable morbidity, when, in countries which are rich enough to be able to offer this procedure, these patients can be maintained indefinitely in good health by adequate transfusion and chelation therapy? And can we be confident that there is no long-term risk of secondary malignancies of the bone marrow in children treated in this way? The answer to the second question will not be clear for some time, although it is beginning to look as though the risk must be very small.

Given the greatly improved results in experienced hands, the question of marrow transplantation must now be the subject of very careful discussion between the clinician and the family of a patient who is diagnosed as having β thalassaemia for the first time. The Italian workers have undoubtedly shown that BMT, performed early and in patients who have not yet developed complications, is a genuine therapeutic option for the treatment of this disease and, even for older patients, is still a possibility if they find that they are not able to tolerate the rigours of symptomatic treatment. The ethical issues are still difficult, however, particularly since the decisions have to be made by parents on behalf of their children, and before they are fully aware of the rigours of caring for a child for many years and the problems that they will encounter during the symptomatic management of thalassaemia.

The other problem which has clouded these issues is the inability of some marrow transplant centres to reproduce the excellence of the results reported by the Pesaro group. This may well simply reflect relative lack of experience. Other centres are now finding that, with increasing experience, their results are matching those of the Italian group (Dr Irene Roberts, personal communication). But it is quite clear that this procedure should not be embarked on by any centre unless it is likely to attract a large patient population and to be able to gain considerable experience of the procedure. However, there is little doubt from the pioneering studies of Lucarelli and colleagues, and from the increasing experience of

other countries, that BMT is now a genuine option for children with β thalassaemia, and one that must be discussed openly and with a clear explanation of the pros and cons, at an early stage after the diagnosis is made.

Practical implications

It is beyond our scope to discuss the practical and financial problems of establishing a bone-marrow transplantation centre for thalassaemia. Similarly, we shall not enlarge on the outline presented earlier of the various conditioning regimens and approaches to managing graft-versus-host disease and other complications. Anyone who is considering setting up a marrow transplant programme should spend time in an established centre, become familiar with the state of the art approaches to the procedure and its follow-up, and only proceed if it is clear that sufficient cases are going to be treated each year for adequate experience to be obtained. There is no place for treating the 'occasional case' and transplantation must be carried out in a properly designed and staffed centre.

Peripheral blood stem cells in bone-marrow transplantation

There is a great deal of interest at the time of writing about the possibility of using peripheral blood stem cells for marrow transplantation. In the haemoglobinopathy field there has been particular focus on the possibility of using cord blood stem cells. This subject has been reviewed recently by Gluckman *et al.* (1999). In discussing the limited world-wide experience of cord blood stem-cell bone-marrow transplantation, particularly that of the Eurocord Consortium (Miniero *et al.* 1999), Gluckman *et al.* point out that only five out of 10 patients for which detailed data are available showed engraftments. Obviously it is too early to draw conclusions, although the authors suggest that at the present time cord blood transplantation should be reserved for younger patients in order to increase the dose of cells infused. Currently, there is no case for the use of cord blood transplantation from unrelated donors. Clearly, it is too early to try to anticipate the role of this new approach, particularly given the current success rates for conventional bone-marrow transplantation.

Therapeutic problems of particular varieties of thalassaemia

Thalassaemia intermedia

In the previous edition of this book, we discussed the limited information that was available about the appropriate way to manage patients with the intermediate forms of β thalassaemia, and stressed that nearly every aspect required further careful study. It is sad to reflect that, 20 years on, it is necessary to repeat this plea. Furthermore, it has become apparent that this is not an insignificant problem. Globally, HbE β thalassaemia, which typifies many of the problems of the assessment and management of the intermediate forms of β thalassaemia, is one of the commonest forms of the disease.

In this section we shall review briefly what is known about the management of the intermediate forms of β thalassaemia and highlight those areas in which further work is urgently required.

Assessment and management over the early years of life

At the beginning of this chapter we outlined the early management of patients with β thalassaemia and pointed out how important it is not to commence a transfusion regimen before carefully assessing the steady-state haemoglobin level and general well-being of the baby. We also emphasized that the key factors at this critical stage of development are the level of the infant's activity, feeding and, in particular, the rate of growth and development. This approach remains the only way of assessing the early course of β thalassaemia intermedia and of determining whether it is safe for an infant to remain untransfused, or whether a long-term transfusion regimen should be embarked on.

The role of accurate genotyping

In Chapter 13 we described what is known about genotype/phenotype relationships in the intermediate forms of β thalassaemia, and similar issues were discussed as they relate to HbE β thalassaemia in Chapter 9. In short, it is clear that although certain genotypes are often associated with a mild course, there is still considerable clinical variation

within each particular interaction. Perhaps the only exception is the homozygous or compound heterozygous state for the promoter mutations which are particularly common in African populations. But for the remainder, and this includes the common IVS1-6 T→C mutation in the Mediterranean populations, the clinical phenotypes are so heterogeneous as to make accurate prediction of the course of the illness in any particular patient very unreliable.

Further assessment during early development

Once the decision not to transfuse a baby with a potential intermediate form of β thalassaemia has been made they should be kept under extremely careful surveillance during the early years of life. It cannot be emphasized too strongly that the decision to change to a transfusion regimen should not be made on the basis of the steady-state haemoglobin level alone. As well as assessment of activity and rates of growth and development it is essential to monitor the skeleton for early signs of bone deformity involving the face. Again this has to be done on clinical grounds; there are no other guidelines to help the clinician. If, during early childhood, there appears to be a genuine falling off in growth velocity, evidence from the child's lifestyle that its activity is being curtailed by anaemia, or early changes in bone structure, it may be necessary to establish a transfusion regimen identical to that described earlier for patients with the major forms of β thalassaemia. If, on the other hand, growth and development are adequate and there are no early bone changes, these children should be kept under careful surveillance and complications should be treated as and when they arise.

Hypersplenism

Although most of the published reviews on thalassaemia intermedia emphasize the high frequency of hypersplenism (Pippard *et al.* 1982b; Modell & Berdoukas 1984; Wainscoat *et al.* 1987; Fiorelli *et al.* 1988; Camaschella & Cappellini 1995) there are very few data on series of sufficient size to determine whether splenectomy is of genuine benefit. Of the 26 patients reviewed by Pippard *et al.* (1982b) 16 had undergone splenectomy at a mean age of 12 years, for worsening anaemia. In seven, this appeared to have removed the need for regular transfusions. Two further patients, aged 8 and 16 years, were later transfused because of increasing anaemia and bone deformity; in neither case was there a sustained increase in the steady-state haemoglobin level. Although Modell and Berdoukas (1984) suggested that splenectomy generally restores the haemoglobin level to its highest previous value, data were only provided for a single patient. In the series of 18 patients described by Fiorelli *et al.* (1988), eight were splenectomized 'for increasing splenomegaly leading to hypersplenism' at a mean age of 14 years; in only two did the operation prevent the need for subsequent blood transfusion. Although Camaschella and Cappellini (1995) recommend splenectomy for a falling haemoglobin level, no data are presented or references cited. As far as we know there are no published data on folate-replete patients whose steady-state haemoglobin level has been observed for a relatively long period, on whom splenectomy was carried out, and for whom an adequate follow-up study was pursued.

A study of four patients pre- and postsplenectomy by Blendis *et al.* (1974) and a presplenectomy study by the present authors both indicated that there was major pooling of the red cells in the spleen of patients with thalassaemia intermedia. Splenectomy in these cases resulted in a significantly higher steady-state haemoglobin than before the operation.

It is against this background of lack of data and ignorance that we have to assess the most appropriate way to identify and manage hypersplenism in this condition. As pointed out by Modell and Berdoukas (1984) it is quite common to observe a steady fall in the mean annual haemoglobin level associated with progressive splenomegaly in patients with thalassaemia intermedia over the age of 2 years. But, as these authors emphasize, the effects of hypersplenism may be more subtle than this. There may be further compensatory hypertrophy of the bone marrow, leading to general malaise and defective growth and development, even though the haemoglobin level may not change dramatically. These suggestions are supported by the small study of Blendis *et al.* (1974), who observed a significant reduction in the degree of ineffective erythropoiesis after splenectomy in three out of the five patients studied. In assessing patients with thalassaemia intermedia for splenectomy it is absolutely vital to make sure that they are folate replete, as judged by serum and red-cell folate analyses. If this is the case, and there is pro-

gressive enlargement associated with either a fall in the steady-state haemoglobin level observed for at least a year, or a falling off in the rates of growth with or without associated general symptoms of anaemia or malaise, splenectomy should be considered. From the limited data that are available it seems likely that the fall in haemoglobin may be arrested or there may be a restoration of the growth curves towards the normal pattern, even if the haemoglobin level does not rise. It is useful to monitor the state of the bone marrow after surgery by regular measurements of the nucleated red-cell count or circulating transferrin receptor levels. The potential problem of an increased risk of thromboembolic disease is discussed in a later section.

Considering the complications of splenectomy, particularly the increased proneness to infection and thromboembolism, splenectomy should certainly not be embarked on without an extremely careful period of observation. We desperately need more data to determine the genuine value of this procedure; clearly, the postoperative haemoglobin level is only one of many parameters that have to be considered. And, as mentioned earlier in this chapter, we need much better documentation of the frequency and significance of the 'large liver syndrome' which seems to follow splenectomy, particularly in patients with thalassaemia intermedia in whom the postoperative haemoglobin level remains relatively low.

Extramedullary haemopoiesis

The frequent occurrence of extramedullary haemopoietic tumour masses and some of the complications that they may cause were discussed in detail in Chapter 13. Although this complication may occur in any form of thalassaemia intermedia the most experience of its clinical manifestations and complications has been obtained in patients with HbE β thalassaemia, particularly in Thailand. When these masses are found on a routine chest X-ray and are asymptomatic nothing is required beyond occasional surveillance. However, those that present with spinal cord compression or with symptoms similar to a cerebral tumour require urgent treatment. In reviewing 12 cases of this kind Issaragrisil *et al.* (1981) pointed out that, although these tumour masses regress when patients are started on a transfusion regimen to maintain the haemoglobin level in excess of 9–10 g/dl, this

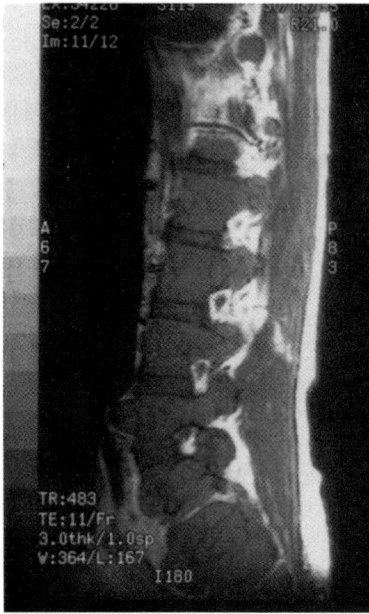 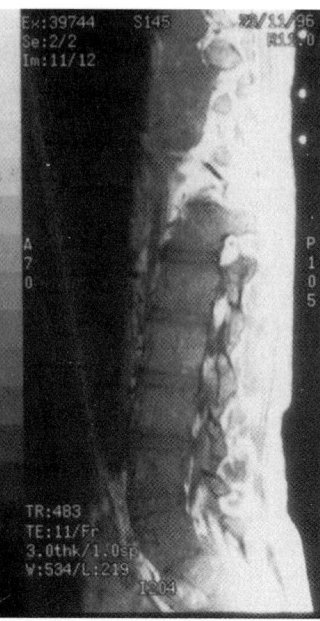

Fig. 15.8 Resolution of extramedullary haemopoiesis with hydroxyurea therapy. MRI showing: left, anterolateral mass with signal intensity similar to that of bone marrow; right, after treatment. From Saxon *et al.* (1998).

process may be too slow to manage those who present with neurological complications. The Thai authors observed very rapid resolution of these lesions following X-ray therapy and recommend this as standard treatment for this complication. They suggest that if a patient presents with spinal cord compression X-rays should be carried out to rule out a fracture and, if possible, myelography should be performed to confirm that the cord is compressed and to determine the level of the lesion. Exploratory laminectomy is rarely required. Once having established the diagnosis a dose of 2000–3000 rads should be administered as soon as possible.

Recently, Saxon *et al.* (1998), using magnetic resonance imaging, have demonstrated a striking reduction in a spinal haemopoietic mass in a patient treated with increasing doses of hydroxyurea (Fig. 15.8). This treatment produced a modest rise in both the fetal haemoglobin and steady-state haemoglobin levels, but probably insufficient to cause a reduction in the red-cell mass. Thus it seems possible that hydroxyurea may have a direct effect on these extramedullary tumour masses and, at least as judged by this case report, may offer a safe and effective approach to their management. Because of the potential hazards of deep X-ray therapy it may be sensible to use hydroxyurea as first-line manage-

ment in this condition and restrict X-ray therapy for those who do not respond, or in whom the response is too slow in the face of progressive neurological damage.

Iron loading

The mechanisms and factors which determine the increased rate of iron loading in patients with thalassaemia intermedia were discussed in Chapter 13. The body iron status of every patient with thalassaemia intermedia should be assessed at regular intervals, as described earlier in this chapter for transfusion-dependent patients. While serum ferritin values may be a useful guide, for those that are elevated much above 800 µg/l a liver biopsy should be carried out, with careful assessment of the histology and concentration of iron. The long-term objective should be to maintain safe body iron levels, as defined earlier in this chapter.

The prevention and management of iron loading in patients with thalassaemia intermedia were discussed by Cossu *et al.* (1981) and Pippard *et al.* (1982b). The use of dietary manipulation to reduce the rate of iron loading remains unproven and if, after a suitable period of observation, it is clear that the rate of iron loading has exceeded, or is likely to exceed, acceptable levels a regimen of iron chelation therapy should be instituted.

Cossu *et al.* (1981) showed that, by using subcutaneous infusions of DF under the same conditions as described earlier in this chapter for transfusion-dependent patients, it was possible to produce a negative iron balance and to reduce the serum ferritin levels. They suggested that the frequency of dosage should be worked out for each individual patient and that once a safe body iron level had been established it should be possible to continue on an intermittent treatment of this type, tailored to the patient's particular needs. We have found that, once the iron load has been reduced to a safe level, it can be controlled by a bolus injection of DF, either weekly or at longer intervals.

In the study of Pippard *et al.* (1982b), a 23-year-old male was reported who had undergone venesection at 2-week intervals for 4 years, with the removal of an estimated 12 g of iron. As far as we know there have been no other reports of this approach to the management of iron loading in thalassaemia intermedia and it was only possible in this patient because of a well sustained haemoglobin level. Further studies along these lines seem warranted, though they will have to include assessments of the effect of venesection on the degree of erythroid expansion.

Leg ulcers

As described in Chapter 13, leg ulcers seem to be particularly common in patients with thalassaemia intermedia. Because nothing is known of their aetiology it is difficult to offer sensible advice about their management. Small ulcers usually heal with simple measures, which include pressure dressings and, where possible, elevation of the leg and rest. Since it seems possible that, at least in part, they may reflect the abnormal rheology of thalassaemic blood, possibly combined with the relative hypoxia resulting from a reduced haemoglobin level, the most logical approach to the management of ulcers which do not heal should be a period of transfusion. However, there have been no controlled studies using this approach, and because of the associated hazards and problems of stopping transfusion, this should be reserved for particularly resistant cases. Interestingly, long-standing leg ulcers have been noted to heal during the administration of arginine butyrate in an attempt to raise the fetal haemoglobin level (see later section). It will be interesting to see whether further studies confirm this interesting observation. The case reports of healing ulcers following the application or injection of growth factors (Voskaridou *et al.* 1999) also need further verification.

Bone and joint complications

The severe skeletal deformities with changes in the skull and facial bones which are well documented in β thalassaemia intermedia are undoubtedly the result of marrow expansion and can be prevented by blood transfusion. An important question is whether, once established, these changes can be reversed to any extent by starting a transfusion regimen in a hitherto untransfused patient who has been maintained at a relatively low haemoglobin level. Although some remodelling may occur in young children, as they grow older the extent is unpredictable and for this reason it is extremely important to try and prevent this complication by extremely careful monitoring of the facial appearance, growth and development during the early course of the disease.

The problems that accompany the widespread osteoporosis and periarticular disease that are so common in thalassaemia intermedia were discussed in detail in Chapter 13. It is also pointed out in Chapter 7, and earlier in this chapter, that there is increasing evidence that osteoporosis is common in patients with thalassaemia major who have been maintained on adequate transfusion regimens. Hence if the pathophysiology is similar in the major and intermediate forms of thalassaemia, and this is by no means certain, the bone changes cannot be entirely explained by marrow expansion. While it is customary to start patients with thalassaemia intermedia with severe bone pain or pathological fractures on a transfusion regimen there is no definite evidence that this is helpful and clinical trials on this important question are urgently needed. Given our current lack of knowledge about this problem, it seems reasonable to treat patients with symptomatic bone disease with oral calcium and vitamin D supplementation, to encourage exercises and, as in the case of the transfusion-dependent patients, if there is evidence of hypogonadism to provide hormone replacement therapy. Currently, there are a number of studies examining the use of inhibitors of bone resorption, notably biphosphonates, in patients with transfusion-dependent β thalassaemia who have developed osteoporosis. As far as we know there has been no experience of the use of this agent in patients with thalassaemia intermedia.

Gallstones

As mentioned in Chapter 13 pigment stones are extremely common in patients with thalassaemia intermedia and are frequently associated with attacks of biliary colic or cholecystitis. Patients who suffer this complication require cholecystectomy.

Infection

From the limited data that are available there is no evidence that the pattern of infection is any different in thalassaemia intermedia from that in thalassaemia major. The guidelines outlined earlier in this chapter should be followed for the treatment of infective episodes, remembering that these are often associated with a profound fall in the haemoglobin level and hence patients with thalassaemia intermedia who develop infections should be observed extremely carefully in hospital.

Folate deficiency

As described in Chapter 13 this is a particularly common feature of thalassaemia intermedia. Patients should be maintained on regular folate supplements and folate deficiency should be suspected if there is a fall in the haemoglobin level.

Thrombotic complications

As described in Chapter 13 there is increasing evidence that patients with β thalassaemia intermedia have a hypercoagulable state, although as we pointed out, the evidence that this frequently leads to thrombotic episodes is still limited. Major thrombotic episodes, particularly postsplenectomy, should be treated initially with heparin followed by an anticoagulant such as warfarin to maintain the prothrombin time in the therapeutic range. If this episode has not followed a precipitating event, surgery or a long period of immobilization for example, it may be wiser to maintain the patient on long-term anticoagulant therapy, although there are insufficient data to be sure about the likelihood of a recurrent episode.

The syndrome of progressive right-heart failure and hypoxaemia in patients with HbE β thalassaemia who have undergone splenectomy was discussed in detail in Chapter 9. Based on the assumption that some of these changes might reflect abnormal platelet aggregation in the pulmonary arterial circulation two studies of the effect of aspirin on the hypoxaemia in this condition have been undertaken (Fucharoen *et al.* 1981b; Israngkura *et al.* 1988). Unfortunately, there has been no follow-up of these studies reported and, as mentioned in Chapters 5 and 9, the frequency of right-heart failure secondary to pulmonary arterial disease is still not known. Until more work has been carried out, with a follow-up of patients with this condition, we can only suggest that, if it is encountered, treatment is instituted with antiplatelet drugs, and/or attempts to reduce the platelet count by either transfusion or the use of hydroxyurea, together with appropriate measures for the symptomatic treatment of heart failure.

Unrelated medical conditions

Patients with thalassaemia intermedia may, of course, suffer from diseases unrelated to thalassaemia. These are managed in the usual way and rarely have any effect on the cause of the genetic disease. One complication we have encountered is chronic renal failure, which may exacerbate the anaemia. We have cared for one patient of this type who, eventually, had a renal transplant. Erythropoietin production from the transplanted kidney was adequate, and there was no significant difference between the steady-state haemoglobin levels before the onset of renal failure and after surgery.

The α thalassaemias

The haemoglobin Bart's hydrops fetalis syndrome

The clinical picture, maternal complications and methods of early diagnosis of this condition are described in Chapter 11. Because of the high frequency of associated congenital abnormalities and maternal complications during pregnancy, in many countries in which there is a high frequency of α^0 thalassaemia the potential for this condition is considered to be an important indication for prenatal screening and diagnosis. However, as described in Chapter 11, several infants with this condition have now survived after receiving early transfusion and supportive treatment during the neonatal period. In some cases congenital malformations or delayed postnatal neurological development has been reported (Beaudry *et al.* 1986; Bianchi *et al.* 1986; Carr *et al.* 1995). In contrast, the development of other infants, in whom the risk of hydrops fetalis had been established before birth, and transfusion had been established either prenatally or soon after birth, has been reported as normal. All the reported cases of this type have subsequently required a regimen of regular transfusion and iron chelation therapy, similar to that for patients with β thalassaemia. They are listed in Chapter 11.

As discussed in Chapter 11, it seems very likely that babies with this disorder become hypoxic very early during fetal development. It is not clear whether this is the cause of the associated fetal abnormalities. Furthermore, although many of the latter can be determined by ultrasound examination this is not always possible. Therefore the management of this condition in parents who particularly wish the pregnancy to continue is fraught with difficulties. However, it does appear as though some infants who are given early, intrauterine transfusion may be able to survive and develop normally, though they are, of course, transfusion dependent. However, if parents do wish these babies to be rescued, it must be done with the clear knowledge that there is a significant risk of associated congenital abnormality, and that even with the earliest possible intrauterine transfusion it is unlikely that these can be avoided. All these complex issues, and the risk of a difficult pregnancy, must be discussed in great detail and on more than one occasion with parents who have to make this very difficult decision.

The question of intrauterine stem-cell therapy is considered later.

Haemoglobin H disease

As described in Chapter 11, the majority of patients with HbH disease go through life with a reasonable haemoglobin level and only become anaemic at times of stress, such as infection or after receiving oxidant drugs. They should be warned of the risk of drugs of this type and maintained on folate supplementation.

Some patients with this disorder appear to develop hypersplenism as they get older and this may be associated with worsening of the anaemia. Early reports showed some enthusiasm for splenectomy (Gouttas *et al.* 1955; Minnich *et al.* 1958; Lie-Injo & de V. Hart 1963; Wasi *et al.* 1969) and, when measured, red-cell survival studies indicated an increased ^{51}Cr half-life after the operation (Woodrow *et al.* 1964). In the series described by Wasi *et al.*, which concerned 50 patients who had been splenectomized, it was reported that the haemoglobin level was raised on average by 2–3 g/dl. However, Wasi *et al.* (1974) point out that the haemoglobin level tends to fluctuate considerably in patients with this condition. For this reason, in the last edition of this book we questioned the value of splenectomy except in patients who had particularly large spleens and were becoming progressively anaemic. As mentioned in Chapter 11, it is also important when assessing patients of this type to try to obtain a reasonably accurate estimate of the level of HbH in the blood. As we pointed out, HbH is physiologically useless and patients who have relatively large amounts, in excess of 20% of the total haemoglobin, may be more incapacitated than their steady-state haemoglobin suggests. Unfortunately, however, these patients have to be assessed on an individual basis; there have been no extensive series of splenectomies reported since the early papers, and clinicians have only this small and anecdotal experience to guide them.

Another reason for reluctance to carry out splenectomy unless absolutely necessary is the rare, but serious, complication of migrating thrombophlebitis and deep venous thrombotic disease, which was described in detail in Chapter 11. We have now seen two deaths from this condition and, following the early report from Hong Kong of similar cases by Tso *et al.* (1982), further examples have been observed in their Chinese population. Because of the bad prognosis for this complication we believe that, despite the paucity of data, patients who develop this curious syndrome should be maintained on anticoagulants and antiplatelet drugs indefinitely.

In short, given the paucity of evidence and the undoubted risk involved, we believe that the rarer symptomatic forms of HbH disease should be managed by regular transfusion using the same approach as that for β thalassaemia major. There may be an occasional place for splenectomy but it should be avoided where possible, and, if it is carried out, patients should be monitored very carefully for any evidence of venous thrombotic disease.

Sickle-cell thalassaemia

As discussed in Chapter 9, patients with sickle-cell β^0 thalassaemia, or sickle-cell β^+ thalassaemia in which the β-thalassaemia allele is of the severe variety, may have a clinical picture indistinguishable from that of those with sickle-cell anaemia. It is beyond our scope to deal with every aspect of the management of the sickling disorders and we shall briefly mention only those that have particular clinical importance. Readers who wish to study this subject in greater detail are referred to reviews and monographs which deal with the management of this condition more fully (Serjeant 1992; Bunn 1997; Ballas 1998; Dover & Platt 1998).

Prevention of infection

Since infection is the major cause of mortality and morbidity at all ages in patients with sickling disorders it is vital to make the diagnosis as early as possible. Ideally, babies of 'at-risk' parents should be screened at birth, when it is possible to diagnose sickle-cell β^0 thalassaemia with certainty based on the absence of HbA in the cord blood; the diagnosis of sickle-cell β^+ thalassaemia can usually be made by the second or third month (Serjeant 1992). Once the diagnosis is established the family should be educated about the importance of the early detection and management of infection. Prophylactic penicillin should be given to all children younger than 5 years of age and they should receive pneumococcal, *H. influenzae* and hepatitis B vaccines. They should also receive prophylactic folic acid at a dose of 1 mg daily.

The steady state

Most patients with sickle-cell anaemia or the severe forms of sickle-cell β thalassaemia adapt well to their relatively low haemoglobin levels and no special treatment is required. They should have regular ophthalmological examinations from school age onwards and these should be repeated every few years unless a sickling retinopathy is discovered, when follow-up should be more frequent, with fluoroscein angiography to assess the speed of evolution of the retinal lesions.

The management of crises

The different forms of acute exacerbation of the sickling disorders, called crises, were described in Chapters 2 and 9. Their management is reviewed in detail by Okpala (1998), Golden *et al.* (1998) and Ballas (1997).

Mild *painful crises* may be managed at home with first-line analgesics such as aspirin or paracetamol together with adequate fluids. But, because the pain can be so severe, all but the particularly mild forms of painful crisis should be treated in hospital with careful observation and adequate analgesia. It is important to search for a precipitating factor such as infection although very frequently this is not found. The basis of treatment is adequate hydration, analgesia and very careful clinical and haematological surveillance (Okpala 1998). First-line analgesics may be inadequate and it may be necessary to administer diamorphine by slow, titrated intravenous infusion. If this is necessary, it is very important that the patient should remain under close observation, with regular monitoring of respiration and blood gases. The haemoglobin level and reticulocyte count should be estimated at least daily but, unless there is a fall in the haemoglobin level or evidence of an impending aplastic crisis as reflected by a drop in the reticulocyte count, transfusion is not required. These episodes usually settle in 2 or 3 days. Details of other regimens, including approaches to self-management, are reviewed by Ballas (1997).

Among the more serious forms of crises, those which are associated with rapid sequestration of sickle cells in particular organs are particularly life threatening. Since the spleen regresses and becomes fibrotic after the first few years of life, the *splenic sequestration* crisis is confined to infancy (Serjeant 1992). It is characterized by the rapid onset of the symptoms and signs of severe anaemia associated with progressive increase in the size of the spleen, often over a few hours. Since infants can sequester a high proportion of their red cells in the spleen in these episodes they may become profoundly anaemic. Mothers should be taught to palpate the spleen and to bring the baby to hospital if it appears to be enlarging. This condition requires urgent blood transfusion and, since it tends to recur, should probably be followed by splenectomy. *Hepatic sequestration* crises tend to occur in older patients and are characterized by rapid enlargement of the liver with a fall in haemoglobin level. They also require urgent transfusion to a safe haemoglobin value. The most serious form of sequestration crisis in older patients is the *lung syndrome* (Golden *et al.* 1998). This is characterized by dyspnoea and chest pain and the presence of pulmonary infiltrates, and may be very difficult to distinguish from pneumonia. Patients with these symptoms should be kept under very close observation with regular blood gas and haematological estimations. A falling Po_2, particularly if it is associated with a falling platelet count and haemoglobin level, is very suggestive of the evolution of a lung crisis. These patients require monitoring on an intensive care unit and should undergo urgent exchange transfusion or, if the initial haemoglobin is low, should receive red cells sufficient to raise their haemoglobin level to a value at which the number of sickleable cells is less than 30% of the total. We shall return to the question of whether it is always necessary to carry out exchange transfusions in this situation. It should be remembered that a chest infection or, rarely, a fat embolus can simulate a pulmonary sequestration episode. If there is any doubt about infection, antibiotics should not be withheld.

The other serious complication, which is well documented in sickle-cell β thalassaemia as well as in sickle-cell anaemia, is *neurological involvement and stroke*. As described in Chapter 9, this often follows curious hypertrophic changes in the carotid circulation, which can be anticipated by regular Doppler examination, or from microaneurysms developing round regions of infarction. This condition requires urgent treatment with transfusion. Originally it was believed that it was always necessary to lower the number of sickleable cells below 30% by exchange transfusion in patients who are not severely anaemic, but recent clinical trials (Vichinsky *et al.* 1995) have suggested that this may not be necessary; the same result may be obtained by hypertransfusion. The same principle may also apply to other complications inducing the chest syndrome. After an episode of this type children should be maintained on transfusion indefinitely.

During an *aplastic crisis* there may be a profound fall in haemoglobin level associated with a reticulocytopenia. Since this condition is most often due to par-

vovirus infection it may affect more than one family member. It requires urgent treatment by blood transfusion.

Recurrent priapism is also observed in patients with sickle-cell β thalassaemia. It has been found that nearly two-thirds of major episodes are preceded by 'stuttering' attacks and it has been suggested that effective therapy at this stage may reduce the risk of sustaining a major attack (see Serjeant 1992). Preliminary, though still unsubstantiated, data suggest that stilboestrol, 5 mg daily, may be effective in preventing a major event in those who have had minor episodes. Fully developed priapism is a serious complication because, if not rapidly relieved, it frequently leads to permanent impotence. It has been suggested that conservative treatment should be restricted to 24 h at the most. During this time the patient should be hydrated, given adequate analgesia and exchange transfused. If there is no improvement after these measures surgery should not be delayed. The most efficient procedure is a cavernosus spongiosum shunt, a relatively minor procedure that produces a very good cosmetic result. Anticoagulants have shown little value in clinical trials (reviewed by Serjeant 1992). Recent studies, reviewed by Okpala (1998), indicate that α-adrenergic stimulants such as etileforme, injected locally, may be effective. Further information is required.

Chronic complications

The management of leg ulcers is unsatisfactory. Clinical trials have shown that transfusion does not speed the rate of healing and skin grafting does not always give good results. Most heal with bed rest and simple debridement, although relapses are common.

Small vessel disease leading to aseptic necrosis of the femoral heads may require total hip replacement. Unfortunately the results are variable and unpredictable and, currently, it is not understood why the failure rate is so high. For this reason simple measures like analgesia and weight restriction should be persisted with as long as possible. Sickle-cell retinopathy, which probably also results from small vessel disease consequent on sickling, may require laser treatment if it is progressive.

Recurrent haematuria is a worrying symptom for the patient, although it nearly always settles and there is no evidence that any form of treatment shortens the period of bleeding. Terminal renal failure, which occurs in older patients with sickling disorders, should be managed as any other form of renal insufficiency; several studies have now shown that renal transplantation is possible (reviewed by Serjeant 1992).

The prevention of crises and other complications

Until recently the only way of preventing crises in sickle-cell anaemia was by long-term transfusion to maintain the patient's haemoglobin level at approximately 10 g/dl and hence to suppress endogenous erythropoiesis. This is still the best approach to treating children who have had neurological complications or patients who are having painful crises at sufficiently short intervals to make life intolerable. As mentioned earlier, it was originally thought that it was necessary to partially exchange transfuse patients of this type, and to carefully maintain the number of sickleable cells below 30%, a theoretical figure derived from a blood viscosity study. Recent clinical trials suggest that it is safe to transfuse patients to this haemoglobin level without prior exchange transfusion (Vichinsky *et al.* 1995). In addition, a multicentre study has shown that it is possible to prevent strokes by transfusing children who have abnormal findings on transcranial Doppler ultrasonography of their carotid and cranial arterial systems (Adams *et al.* 1998).

Recently, another approach has been shown to reduce the frequency of painful crises and, incidentally, the acute chest syndrome. A double-blind, randomized, placebo-controlled study of the administration of hydroxyurea to adult patients with sickle-cell anaemia showed that there was a highly significant reduction in the number of painful crises, blood transfusions required and episodes of the chest syndrome (Charache *et al.* 1995, 1996). It is not clear whether this result reflects the modest increase in fetal haemoglobin production in these patients, a reduced white-cell count, alteration in the degree of hydration of the red cells or, indeed, a combination of these factors. But this is the first time that any form of treatment has been shown to reduce painful crises in a properly designed trial. The drug has been licensed for use in adult patients with sickle-cell anaemia in the USA and it has also been shown to be effective when given to children. Until more is known about the very long-term side-effects, if any, its use in children should be limited to those with a particularly

severe clinical course. We shall return to this topic later in this chapter.

Bone-marrow transplantation

There is far less experience with marrow transplantation for the sickling disorders than for β thalassaemia. Indeed, because of the unpredictable course of both sickle-cell anaemia and sickle-cell β^0 thalassaemia, many clinicians feel that it is premature to begin large-scale transplantation for these conditions. Hence, the early series have usually included patients who are older than those in whom the best results are obtained in β thalassaemia, and who already have a history of complications from their disease. For example Walters *et al.* (1996) give detailed information about bone-marrow transplantation in 23 patients with sickle-cell disease; two died and the procedure did not stop the progression of central nervous system involvement in patients who had had a stroke before the transplantation. Given our current state of knowledge and experience we would advise great caution before submitting young children with sickle-cell β thalassaemia to marrow transplantation. The factors which are known to modify the clinical course of this condition were summarized in detail in Chapter 9. But, as we pointed out, even the clinical course of sickle-cell β^0 thalassaemia is not predictable and, currently, we have no way of knowing which patients will develop severe complications of the disease.

Experimental therapy

There are several promising areas of research which, at the time this book goes to press, are sufficiently advanced to suggest that they may play an important role in the treatment of these conditions in the future. It is beyond our scope to cover all this work in detail, and we shall simply outline the current state of development of those potential lines of treatment which seem of most promise. They are summarized in Table 15.4.

The reactivation or stimulation of fetal haemoglobin production

As outlined throughout this book, and as discussed in detail in Chapters 5, 9, 10 and 13, there is abundant evidence that patients with the more serious forms of

Table 15.4 Selected approaches to the future treatment of the thalassaemias. References in text.

Gene manipulation
Reactivation/augmentation of HbF production
Selective suppression of α-globin production

Gene therapy
Viral or retroviral transfer
Liposome-mediated transfer
Receptor-mediated transfer
Targeted gene transfer
Artificial chromosomes
Suppressor RNAs
Ribozymal modification of mRNA

Stem-cell biology for transplantation and/or gene therapy
Human peripheral blood stem cells
Human embryonic stem cells

β thalassaemia who produce unusually high levels of HbF tend to have a milder disease. The reasons are quite clear. Any patient whose red-cell precursors produce relatively more γ chains will be at an advantage, simply because γ chains bind α chains to produce HbF, so reducing the degree of globin imbalance. Although HbF has certain disadvantages as an oxygen carrier, notably its left-shifted oxygen dissociation curve, it is still quite adequate for the needs of extrauterine life. For this reason there has been a major interest in discovering ways of either augmenting or reactivating γ-chain production. Since all the evidence suggests that babies with β thalassaemia switch from γ- to β-chain production at the normal time, and that the high levels of HbF in their peripheral blood are largely a reflection of cell selection and bone-marrow hypertrophy, possibly set against a genetic predisposition to produce more or fewer γ chains, what we are talking about in most cases is the reactivation of γ-chain production.

This research field has attracted a very large literature over recent years. Here we can only summarize the modest advances that have been made. Those who wish to study this topic in more detail are referred to several recent reviews, which will direct them to much of the published experimental data in this field (Olivieri 1996b; Jane & Cunningham 1998; Olivieri & Weatherall 1998; Swank & Stamatoyannopoulos 1998; Bunn 1999). The regulation of the switch from fetal to adult haemoglobin production is discussed in detail in Chapter 2.

Background

The notion that it might be possible to reactivate fetal haemoglobin production after it has been completely switched off came from observations of transient increases in the level of HbF in patients recovering after treatment with cytotoxic agents for leukaemia (Sheridan *et al.* 1976), following marrow transplantation (Alter *et al.* 1976c), or in animals after phlebotomy or the administration of erythropoietin (DeSimone *et al.* 1982; Al-Khatti *et al.* 1987). Similarly, it was found that, in sheep, HbC, which is normally only expressed transiently during the perinatal period, can be induced in adult animals by phlebotomy or exposure to acute hypoxia, both of which stimulate erythropoietin secretion (Benz *et al.* 1978).

These observations suggested that rapid erythroid regeneration may be one mechanism by which it is possible to stimulate or reactivate HbF production. The most vigorously cycling cells are mature erythroblasts and late erythroid progenitors. Since S-stage-cytotoxic drugs kill cycling cells and result in a reduction in the pools of more mature erythroid progenitors, this is followed by rapid, compensatory erythroid cell regeneration. It was found that in both anaemic monkeys and patients with sickle-cell anaemia the S-stage-specific drug, hydroxyurea, was capable of causing a modest elevation in fetal haemoglobin production (Letvin *et al.* 1984; Platt *et al.* 1984). A similar result was obtained in baboons using cytoarabinoside (Papayannopoulou *et al.* 1984).

While these early studies utilized rapid erythroid regeneration as an approach to stimulating HbF production, others focused on agents which might directly stimulate γ-chain production. The first drug of this type to be explored was 5-azacytidine, a potentially potent inducer of fetal haemoglobin synthesis, possibly by acting through demethylation of regulatory sequences in the β-globin-gene locus and, at the same time, inducing rapid erythroid regeneration. While the use of this agent selectively increased γ-chain synthesis in a patient with β thalassaemia, and had some effect on its production in a small number of patients with sickle-cell anaemia (Charache *et al.* 1983; Ley *et al.* 1983), it proved too toxic for further clinical trials.

In 1985, while investigating the reason for the delay in the switch from adult to fetal haemoglobin in the infants of diabetic mothers, Perrine and her colleagues (Perrine *et al.* 1985) found that this effect was mediated by butyrate, a four-carbon fatty acid. Infusion of this agent into sheep fetuses was subsequently shown to cause a delay in the switch from γ- to β-globin production (Perrine *et al.* 1988). Subsequently, arginine butyrate was administered intravenously to a patient homozygous for Hb Lepore; this was followed by a dramatic response with a major rise in both the haemoglobin and HbF values (Perrine *et al.* 1993). What little has been determined subsequently about the mechanisms of action of the butyrate compounds is reviewed by Swank and Stamatoyannopoulos (1998).

These early studies generated a large number of clinical trials for the treatment of both sickle-cell anaemia and β thalassaemia using agents that would stimulate fetal haemoglobin production, either by promoting rapid erythroid regeneration or by reactivating the γ-globin genes directly.

Clinical studies of the augmentation of fetal haemoglobin production

It is impossible for us to review and give references for every clinical trial that has been carried out with the object of stimulating fetal haemoglobin production. Those that were carried out up to 1995 are reviewed by Olivieri (1996b) and more recent trials are summarized by Olivieri and Weatherall (1998), Swank and Stamatoyannopoulos (1998) and Bunn (1999).

As mentioned earlier, a large-scale controlled trial of the use of hydroxyurea in adult patients with sickle-cell anaemia resulted in an approximate doubling of the mean level of HbF and F cells; the HbF rose from a baseline of approximately 5 to an average of 9% (Charache *et al.* 1996). There was a broad scatter in HbF levels in the treated group and in some cases the rise was much greater. More recently it has been found that the same effect can be obtained in children (Ferster *et al.* 1996; Jayabose *et al.* 1996; Scott *et al.* 1996).

In studies in which hydroxyurea has been administered to patients with different forms of β thalassaemia, there have only been minimal responses in haemoglobin or HbF levels (Hajjar & Pearson 1994; Huang *et al.* 1994; Bachir *et al.* 1995; Cohen *et al.* 1995; Zeng *et al.* 1995; Fucharoen *et al.* 1996).

Because of reports of a suboptimal erythropoietin response to anaemia in β thalassaemia (see Chapter 5), and because of the early work in animals that showed that a rapid erythroid expansion may favour HbF production, there have been several studies to assess the effects of recombinant erythropoietin in thalassaemia or sickle-cell anaemia, either alone or in combination with hydroxyurea (Goldberg *et al.* 1990; Rachmilewitz *et al.* 1991; Olivieri *et al.* 1992b; Rodgers *et al.* 1993; Loukopoulos *et al.* 1995). The results have been variable and, overall, the increase in haemoglobin and HbF has been unremarkable, although it is interesting that in the patients with sickle-cell β thalassaemia studied by Loukopoulos *et al.* (1995) considerable clinical benefit appears to have been observed.

The administration of butyrate compounds has also been associated with varying responses. In the initial study, quoted above, there was a quite dramatic response to arginine butyrate in a patient who was homozygous for Hb Lepore and who could not be transfused because of blood-group sensitization. Because of difficulties in the long-term treatment with this agent this patient was treated over a long period with a combination of sodium phenylbutyrate and, later, hydroxyurea. She had a dramatic response to this combination of drugs, with a total rise of haemoglobin to 10–11 g/dl, reflecting an increase of HbF of approximately 5 g/dl. She has remained non-transfusion dependent and well for over 5 years (Olivieri *et al.* 1997). Interestingly, her younger brother has had an equally dramatic response to a combination of sodium phenylbutyrate and hydroxyurea (Fig. 15.9). One other patient, in this case a compound heterozygote for Hb Lepore and β thalassaemia, showed a good response to hydroxyurea alone, with a rise in the haemoglobin of 4 g/dl (Rigano *et al.* 1997). However, in a further study involving arginine butyrate involving 10 patients with different types of β thalassaemia, only modest, or no, changes in the haemoglobin or HbF levels were noted (Sher *et al.* 1995). In a pilot study of 11 patients with β thalassaemia treated with oral sodium phenylbutyrate, four showed a rise in total HbF of approximately 1 g/dl (Collins *et al.* 1995); the same agent also produced a modest rise in HbF in some patients with sickle-cell anaemia (Dover *et al.* 1994). There have been some reports of the efficacy of pulsed doses of butyrate in patients with sickle-cell anaemia and thalassaemia (Faller & Perrine 1995), and, recently, more detailed results of this approach have been published (Atweh *et al.* 1999). These authors describe a regimen

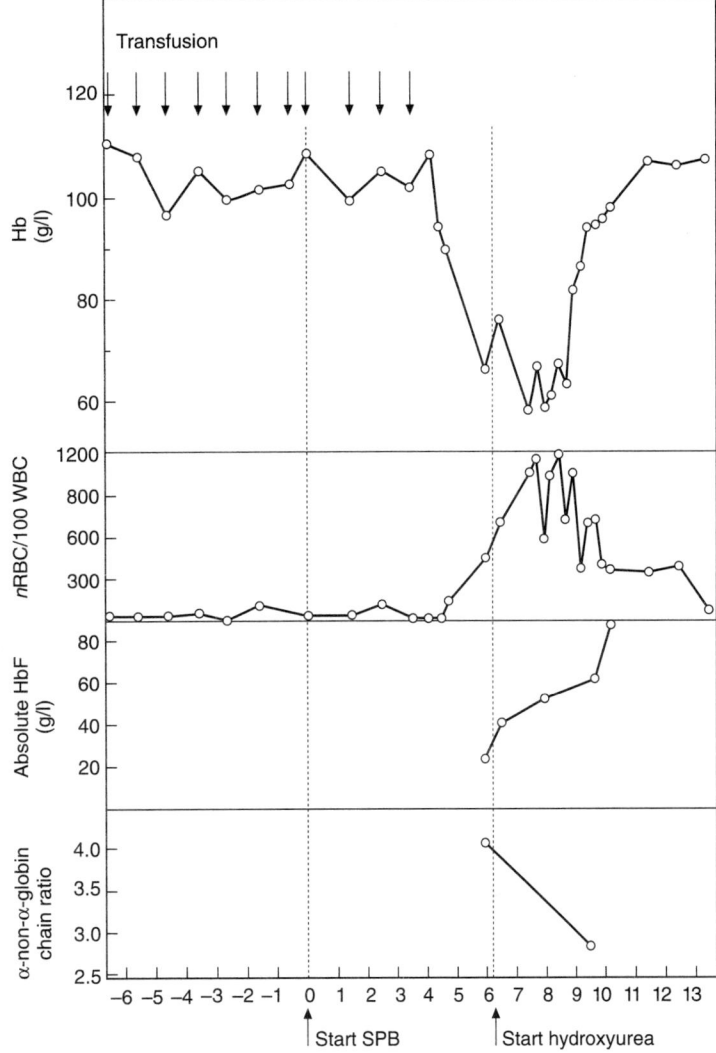

Fig. 15.9 Pharmacological manipulation of fetal haemoglobin production. The patient was a transfusion-dependent homozygote for Hb Lepore Washington/Boston. The arrows indicate blood transfusions. Treatment was started with sodium phenylbutyrate (SPB) and later hydroxyurea was added. There was a rise in the absolute amount of HbF of approximately 5 g/dl and the child remains transfusion independent 4 years later. From Olivieri *et al.* (1997).

in which arginine butyrate was infused through a central venous line over 8–12 h for 4 days, followed by 10–24 days' rest. This pulse regimen induced fetal haemoglobin gene expression in nine of 11 patients; the mean HbF in this group increased from 7.2 to 21.0% after a mean duration of 29.9 weeks. There was a modest rise in the total haemoglobin level which was just significant. There did not appear to be any major side-effects. But, unlike the hydroxyurea trial mentioned earlier, it is not known whether this form of therapy resulted in any improvement in the clinical features of sickle-cell disease.

The future

This long and painstaking saga in thalassaemia and sickle-cell anaemia research has taught us one thing for certain; it is undoubtedly possible under certain circumstances to stimulate or reactivate HbF synthesis after birth. The results of the adult sickle-cell anaemia/hydroxyurea trial are extremely encouraging and the patients reported by Olivieri *et al.* (1997) have been virtually cured of their disease over a long period of follow-up. But, for the rest, the results of the trials directed at different forms of β thalassaemia have been rather disappointing to date. Furthermore, myelotoxic agents have the long-term potential for generating haematological malignancies; butyrate is, though relatively non-toxic, difficult to administer; and erythropoietin is extremely expensive and has to be given in relatively large doses with all the associated concerns about further marrow expansion and the potential dangers of raising the steady-state haemoglobin in patients with sickling disorders.

However, the position may well be rather similar to how it was in the field of leukaemia treatment in its early days. Single agents were both toxic and relatively ineffective, and it was only when the ideal combinations were worked out, by carefully designed clinical trials, that the disease came under control. Since there are no other obvious approaches to stimulating fetal haemoglobin production on the horizon, the next step is to attempt to find out why some patients respond better than others, possibly by analysing the associated molecular lesions, and to try to discover combinations of these agents which are more effective. As should have been clear from the discussion of thalassaemia intermedia in Chapter 13, an increase in the haemoglobin level of 1–2 g might make all the difference between symptomatic disease and good health in this group of patients.

Another, though longer-term approach to augmenting fetal haemoglobin production lies in defining the *trans*-acting loci which are involved in the generation of heterocellular hereditary persistence of fetal haemoglobin. While it is a long shot, it is possible that some of these factors are the products of loci that are involved in the regulation of HbF production. Their characterization would offer a totally different pharmacological approach to the control of HbF production. There are, in addition, other ways in which this might be achieved but this would require some form of genetic manipulation, a topic which we shall consider in the following section. Finally, an approach which is being explored by several groups follows the well-trodden road of medicinal chemistry; hundreds of compounds are being screened using *in vitro* assay systems in the hope that one of them might have the properties of stimulating HbF production.

In utero *haematopoietic stem-cell transplantation*

This different approach to stem-cell transplantation is based on the concept that in early gestation the fetus is immunologically immature and tolerant to foreign antigen and, in theory at least, it should be possible to engraft allogeneic or xenogeneic cells without the need for immunosuppression or ablation of the bone marrow. Since it is possible to identify the important forms of thalassaemia early during gestation these disorders were an obvious target for early attempts at this new form of therapy. So far, the results have been extremely disappointing.

Recent experience in *in utero* stem-cell transplantation has been reviewed by Flake and Zanjani (1999). So far five attempts have been made at intrauterine stem-cell therapy for β thalassaemia; there were two intrauterine deaths, including one septic abortion, and the others have shown no evidence of engraftment. Similarly, of three attempts for the Hb Bart's hydrops syndrome, one pregnancy was terminated at 24 weeks because of lack of peripheral donor cell expression, one showed no evidence of engraftment, and the other, though alive at 1 year and showing microchimerism, is fully transfusion dependent. The sources of stem cells in these cases were either fetal liver or paternal CD34-enriched populations.

These results are extremely disappointing and suggest that many of the early premises on which this approach were based will have to be revised. We shall discuss the ethical issues involved in this kind of experimental treatment at the end of the chapter.

Somatic cell gene therapy

As outlined in Chapter 1, in the early days of the elucidation of the molecular pathology of the thalassaemias it was assumed that this knowledge would soon lead to methods for the definitive cure of these diseases by genetic manipulation. Gene therapy, it appeared, was just round the corner. In retrospect, it is easy to see why this thinking was naïve. If patients were not to be treated repeatedly, the target cell for gene therapy would have to be the haemopoietic stem cell, an elusive entity which was impossible to identify and which was known to constitute only a very small proportion of bone-marrow cells. There was also the problem of finding a vector which would transfer normal globin genes into haemopoietic stem cells, where they would have to express themselves at the high level required to correct either α or β thalassaemia over a long period. And, as if all this were not enough, very little was known about the regulatory regions of the globin genes that would be needed for their appropriate expression in their new home. At the time of writing at least some of these problems are closer to solution, but there is still a long way to go before somatic cell gene therapy for thalassaemia becomes a reality.

Over the last 15 years a great deal has been written about gene therapy, including its history; it must be the only field of medicine which has had its past enshrined before it has successfully treated one patient! It is a constantly changing field and all we can do here is outline some of the principles involved, together with some of the approaches that are being taken towards successful transfer of the globin genes. Readers who want to pursue this subject further will find the basic principles set out in a very readable fashion in two edited monographs (Lever & Goodfellow 1995; Lemoine & Cooper 1996).

General approaches to gene therapy

There are two main approaches to gene therapy. First, any cells other than germ cells might have their genetic make-up altered. Somatic cell gene therapy of this kind would change an individual's genetic constitution only during their lifetime and would not affect their children; it would be no different in principle from any form of organ transplantation. Alternatively, germline gene therapy would entail injecting 'foreign' genes into fertilized eggs; the inserted genes would be distributed among somatic and germ cells and hence would be transmitted to future generations. For a variety of ethical and technical reasons current research in most countries is restricted by law to somatic cell gene therapy.

Ideally, gene therapy would emulate transplantation surgery, that is, removing a gene carrying a mutation and replacing it with a normal one. Another way of achieving the same end, gene correction, would entail the specific alteration of a mutated sequence using nature's way of exchanging genetic material, that is, by site-directed recombination.

Because of the technical difficulties of these approaches, much current research in gene therapy is directed towards gene augmentation, that is, intro-

ducing a gene into cells in a way that will allow it to produce sufficient of its product to compensate for the lack of expression of its defective counterpart. Because most of the thalassaemias are recessive disorders they are well suited to correction in this way. It will not, however, be of value for dominantly inherited disorders in which abnormal gene products interfere with cellular function.

Another approach which is being explored is to leave the defective gene alone and attempt to alter its mRNA product.

Requirements for gene therapy

The requirements for gene therapy are easily stated but extremely difficult to fulfil. First, it is necessary to isolate a particular gene together with its regulatory sequences. Second, it must be possible to obtain sufficient numbers of cells into which the gene is to be inserted and to find an effective way of returning them to the patient. Third, there must be an efficient mechanism for inserting the gene into the target cells. And, finally, the inserted gene must produce sufficient amounts of its product over a reasonable length of time, and the procedure must not have any deleterious effects on the genome of the recipient cell.

Regulation

When thinking about gene therapy it is useful to categorize genes into two classes. There are housekeeping genes, that is, genes that are expressed in most tissues at all stages of development and which do not require precise regulation. Alternatively, there are genes like the globin genes that are tissue specific in their expression, developmentally regulated, and which require very tight control over the levels of their products.

As described in detail in Chapter 2, the main regulatory regions for the α- and β-globin-gene clusters have been identified. However, even here there are problems because when constructs containing these regulatory regions together with the appropriate human genes are inserted into mice they are not always stable and rearrangements may take place. Furthermore, it is not yet possible to obtain high-level expression of the α-globin genes. Thus, although the problems of regulation and the type of construct that will be required for gene therapy are known in outline, more work is required before it will be possible to be confident that everything needed for long-term, stable, high-level expression has been identified (Higgs *et al.* 1998).

Approaches to gene transfer

DNA can be conveyed into cells in a variety of ways. There are several physical methods, including calcium phosphate or cation lipid mediated, or electroporation; that is, inserting the DNA in a powerful electric field. Unfortunately, these approaches are too inefficient to transfect sufficient numbers of target cells.

Because they integrate their DNA into the gene of their hosts, much research in gene transfer has focused on retroviral vectors; that is, retroviruses from which many of the viral genes have been removed or altered so that no viral proteins are made in the cells which they infect (Miller 1990; Sadelain 1997). Viral replication functions are provided by 'packaging' cells that contain helper viruses that produce all the viral proteins that are required, but which themselves have been disabled so that they are unable to produce infectious viruses (Fig. 15.10). The main advantage of these vectors is the high efficiency

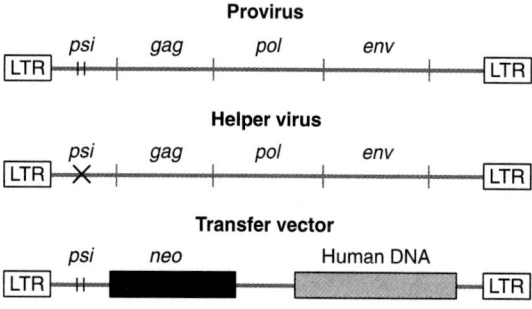

Fig. 15.10 A simplified model retrovirus vector for gene transfer. The provirus, shown above, is modified by the replacement of the *gag, pol* and *env* genes by the gene that is to be transferred, often together with a selectable marker, in this case *neo*, a gene for neomycin resistance. Packaging is mediated by a helper virus which retains the viral genes but in which the packaging sequence, psi, is removed, so rendering it unable to package its own proteins. env, glycoproteins of viral envelope; gag, structural proteins of viral capsid; LTR, long terminal repeats; pol, reverse transcriptase.

of gene transfer in replicating cells. On the other hand it is difficult to insert large pieces into them, and most retroviruses are unable to infect non-dividing cells. Furthermore, integration is random and there is a danger of unwanted side-effects, insertional mutagenesis for example.

Despite these problems a number of workers in the late 1980s showed that tissue-specific expression of a retrovirally encoded human β-globin gene could be obtained in murine bone-marrow chimeras (Karlsson *et al.* 1988; Miller *et al.* 1988a; Dzierzak *et al.* 1998). Unfortunately, these studies were bedevilled by low levels of gene transfer and expression, and enthusiasm for this approach waned. However, with the discovery of the β-globin locus-control region and the advantage of a deletion in the second intron of the β-globin gene, together with improved knowledge of the regulation of the Moloney murine leukaemia virus vector, considerable improvements in globin-gene transfer were obtained (Miller *et al.* 1988a; Sadelain *et al.* 1995) and it was possible to increase viral titres and to improve the efficiency of transfection. For example, in transduced murine erythroleukaemia (MEL) cells bearing single-copy vectors, human β-globin expression was induced to 70–80% of that of the endogenous mouse β-globin gene (Leboulch *et al.* 1994; Sadelain *et al.* 1995). However, further studies indicated that transcription was not dependent on the integration site and was heavily affected by flanking chromatin.

Similar high levels of expression were also obtained using adeno-associated virus (AAV) vectors, although in this case about half the MEL cell clones showed a rearranged vector (Einerhand *et al.* 1995). However, these experiments did establish quite unequivocally that the incorporation of elements of the β-globin locus-control region (LCR) increased *trans*-gene expression in virally transduced cells. On the other hand, they suggested that the modification of the size of the LCR in this system makes it function more like a classical enhancer rather than conferring position-independent expression. Further details of some of these problems are discussed in a review by Sadelain (1997). Recently, the introduction of lentivirus vectors and the further modification of the β globin/LCR constructs have resulted in major improvements in the expression of human β globin in mice with β thalassaemia (reviewed by Bodine 2000).

Other types of vectors are also being explored. For example, the possibility of transferring and maintaining DNA by the use of extrachromosomal elements is a distinct possibility. Such elements are formed after fusion of mouse cells with a yeast artificial chromosome (YAC) containing a human gene. Unfortunately, they segregate poorly during cell division and are lost from the cells. But recent progress in defining the sequences required for both centromere and telomere function in mammalian cells may, in the long term, make it possible to construct mammalian artificial chromosomes for gene therapy.

Targeted sequences have been introduced into cells by physical methods and, under appropriate conditions, homologous recombination can be obtained with specific sequences (Shesely *et al.* 1991). However, this approach, which in many ways is ideal, is far too inefficient to be practical at the current state of its development.

Target cells

Because of the very low number of target cells in the bone marrow, most of which are non-cycling, a variety of new approaches have been explored to try to tackle this fundamental barrier to gene therapy. The wide variety of methods which are being employed to try to alter the cycling properties of these cells are reviewed by Sadelain (1997). It is now clear that they are extremely heterogeneous with respect to their level of expression of the amphotropic receptor required for transduction by retroviral vectors. The cloning of these receptors will enable the study of factors which may be used to enhance their surface expression (Cosset & Russell 1996). There is also considerable interest in the use of peripheral blood stem cells as targets for gene transfer. Attention is focusing on particular subsets, including CD34+ cells and their various subgroups, although whether these populations can retain long-term haemopoietic potential remains to be determined.

Transplantation strategies

As pointed out by Sadelain (1997), when it actually comes to attempting to replace bone-marrow cells transfected with normal globin genes for the treatment of thalassaemia, it will be necessary to develop a programme which allows competitive repopulation of the genetically modified cells; in the case of β thalassaemia such a competitive advantage would be imparted to cells expressing high levels of normal β globin. While this is true there would be no advantage to earlier progenitors carrying normal β-globin genes, nor would it apply to sickle-cell anaemia. Thus it may be necessary to confer an advantage on the graft through incorporating a drug resistance gene, for methotrexate for example, into a second transcription unit, the other encoding the β-globin gene. The problems of chimerism and transplant biology are discussed in detail by Blau (1998) and the possibility of the generation of haemopoietic progenitors from human embryonic stem (ES) cells, which would be a major step forward, is discussed by Keller and Snodgrass (1999)

The current status of all these aspects of gene therapy for thalassaemia is reviewed by Persons and Nienhuis (2000).

Other approaches to genetic manipulation for the treatment of thalassaemia

Other novel approaches directed towards the therapy of the thalassaemias are summarized in Table 15.5. They include various ways of improving gene replacement by homologous recombination, or targeted mutagenesis as a way of repairing defective genes.

Another approach to repairing the defect in thalassaemia would be to aim to restore normal splicing in cases of splicing mutations (Dominski & Kole 1993). Here the idea is to develop 2′-*O*-methylribo-oligonucleotides complementary to mutated β-globin-gene pre-mRNAs and in this way to reverse the aberrant splicing. Other approaches to the same end are also being investigated. For example, Lan *et al.* (1998) described a new way of correcting the molecular defect in sickle-cell anaemia which combines the double benefit of deleting the sickle-cell mutation and, potentially, augmenting fetal haemoglobin levels in the red cells. Essentially, the experiment was carried out as follows. A source of nucleated red-cell precursors was obtained from erythroid colonies and then a *trans*-splicing group 1 ribozyme was used to alter the mutant β-globin-gene transcript in these cells. Lan *et al.* created a ribozyme that was able to convert the β^S-globin transcript to RNAs encoding γ globin. This approach is reviewed in detail by

Weatherall (1998a). As pointed out in this commentary, although this ingenious experiment worked well in cultured cells, the jump to an *in vivo* approach to gene correction therapy will require a great deal more work.

When will gene therapy be feasible for the treatment of thalassaemia?

This field has been very active over recent years. It is generally believed that gene therapy will be successful for short-term gains such as the treatment of cancer or vascular disease before it is possible to correct genetic diseases. Although there has been genuine progress, it seems likely that we shall have to wait for many years before it can be applied for the treatment of thalassaemia. One of the prerequisites of all ethical committees that deal with this field is that the prognosis of the disease can be predicted with some accuracy, and that other forms of treatment are inadequate. Both these issues will have to be debated very clearly before the first trials of gene therapy for thalassaemia. And there will have to be extensive studies in experimental animals before moving to trials on humans. There are still considerable uncertainties about the safety of any of the current approaches to gene therapy; this will be a major issue, particularly considering the other forms of treatment that are available for thalassaemia. Much will depend on whether it is possible to improve the results of bone-marrow transplantation from non-related donors and, if this is possible, the relative costs of this procedure compared with somatic cell gene therapy. We are a long way off from having to make these difficult decisions, but all the signs are that sooner or later we shall have to.

Ethical issues relating to experimental forms of treatment

Clearly, new forms of experimental treatment must be attempted or there will be no progress in the thalassaemia field. However, as the results of symptomatic treatment and bone-marrow transplantation for the thalassaemias continue to improve, and prenatal diagnosis becomes even safer and more accurate, parents will have a number of very clear-cut options about the future planning of families with potential thalassaemic children. And it is,

of course, the parents who must make the final decisions about whether to allow their unborn infants or affected children to undergo these experimental procedures.

In most countries any form of somatic gene therapy requires the agreement of a detailed protocol by a national regulatory body. Any completely new experimental treatment should come under equally careful scrutiny.

One of the major tasks which faces any regulatory body or ethics committee in examining experimental protocols is a risk–benefit analysis. In the case of inherited diseases for which there are no forms of treatment this may be relatively easy. But, for diseases like thalassaemia for which much can be done already, the situation becomes more complicated. As mentioned in the previous section, there will have to be very strong evidence from animal experimentation that any approach to somatic cell gene therapy for thalassaemia carries a good chance of success and minimal risk. Recently there have been a number of deaths due to attempts at gene therapy for monogenic disease, and much more will have to be learnt about the safety of gene transfer vectors, particularly their immune properties and the possibility of the induction of neoplasms, and, indeed, every aspect of the procedure.

In discussing risk–benefit in the case of intrauterine stem-cell therapy Flake and Zanjani (1999) suggest that at the present time the risks appear to be small relative to potential benefits. It is difficult to see how the authors arrived at this conclusion in the case of the α and β thalassaemias, given the abysmal results to date. It is also frightening to observe that, both in their paper and in recent discussions about the possibility of intrauterine gene therapy for α thalassaemia, in no case is the high frequency of associated fetal abnormalities mentioned.

There is a genuine danger that technology is moving too quickly in some areas of modern medicine. Overall, most countries have, after a long debate, made some sensible recommendations as to the criteria needed before somatic cell gene therapy is embarked on. It is vital that the same types of public discussion and control are set in place for every form of experimental therapy. The recent publications about the possibility of intrauterine somatic cell gene therapy for α thalassaemia suggest that there may be a major communication gap between the technologists who wish to apply these approaches and clinicians who have a broad knowledge and experience of the diseases that will form the basis for these experiments. It is vital therefore that those that have responsibility for the care of patients with thalassaemia embark on a broad-ranging discussion with their families, biomedical scientists and the public at large before setting off into these unknown territories.

Chapter 16
The laboratory diagnosis of the thalassaemias

Since the last edition of this book there have been major technical advances in the identification of the abnormal haemoglobin disorders and the thalassaemias. However, a diagnosis of these conditions that is sufficiently accurate for most clinical purposes, except prenatal detection, can usually be established from a detailed personal and family history, and a complete clinical and haematological examination of the patient and members of their family, together with a few simple studies of their haemoglobin constitution.

Over recent years the evolution of fully automated high-performance liquid chromatography (HPLC) (Bissé & Wieland 1988; Galanello *et al.* 1995; Riou *et al.* 1997; Wild & Stephens 1997) has led to substantial improvements in the speed, accuracy and reproducibility of qualitative and quantitative haemoglobin analysis. However, these systems have limitations, and most of them are expensive and their use can only be justified in reference centres in which there is a high throughput of samples. Similarly, although many of the molecular diagnostic techniques are now available in the form of kits, these are also costly and require considerable experience in their day-to-day use. Hence we believe that these approaches, together with globin synthesis analysis, which is still extremely valuable as a preliminary approach to identifying thalassaemia-like disorders with normal HbA_2 levels, should be restricted to reference laboratories which are carrying out large numbers of investigations and so can become aware of the pitfalls of these different approaches.

In this chapter we shall discuss the differential diagnosis of the different forms of thalassaemia and describe some of the techniques which are of particular value in hospital laboratories and reference centres. Strategies for carrier screening and population studies are described in detail in Chapter 14. It is beyond our scope to cover every practical aspect of the diagnosis of the thalassaemias. For more detailed coverage of other haematological and haemoglobin analytical techniques the reader is advised to consult

one of the monographs which deal with these topics in greater detail (Schmidt & Huisman 1974; Dacie & Lewis 1975; Lehmann & Kynoch 1976; Huisman & Jonxis 1977; Chanarin 1989). There are several laboratory manuals on general techniques of DNA analysis (Mathew 1991).

General diagnostic approaches and differential diagnosis of the thalassaemias

Patients homozygous for β or δβ thalassaemia or with HbH disease usually present with the symptoms of the disease, whereas carriers for α or β thalassaemia are usually found during examination of the relatives of more severely affected patients, as part of screening programmes or during the investigation of mild, iron-refractory hypochromic anaemias.

The homozygous and compound heterozygous states for β thalassaemia

Diagnosis

These conditions usually present in early life and the severity of the anaemia, ethnic background of the patient and associated physical findings of enlargement of the spleen and liver and early bone changes are helpful clues to the diagnosis (see Chapter 7 for a full discussion).

There is nearly always a severe degree of anaemia and the mean cell volume (MCV) and mean cell haemoglobin (MCH) values are usually reduced, although because of the marked variation in shape and size of the red cells it is difficult to obtain accurate red-cell indices, particularly after splenectomy. The reticulocyte count, although elevated, is low relative to the degree of anaemia. If the patient has been splenectomized the peripheral blood should be incubated with methyl violet to demonstrate α-chain inclusions in the normoblasts and red cells. They can be found in the red-cell precursors in the bone marrow in all cases of homozygous β thalassaemia, though it is not usually necessary to carry out a bone-marrow examination as part of the initial work-up.

Having established that the haematological changes are typical of β thalassaemia the next step is to determine the level of HbF. This will be significantly elevated in nearly every case of severe β thalassaemia unless a large blood transfusion has been administered immediately before the analysis. The complete absence of HbA indicates homozygous β^0 thalassaemia, while the diagnosis of β^+ thalassaemia is suggested by the finding of small amounts of HbA. A word of caution is necessary here, however. Transfused blood survives for a surprisingly long period in many patients with β thalassaemia; by the use of methods which are described later in this chapter for identifying cells which contain either HbF or HbA we have observed a considerable population of transfused red cells in the peripheral blood for periods exceeding 3 months. Haemoglobin A_2 analysis is of no diagnostic help but it is important to carry out qualitative haemoglobin electrophoresis, using cellulose acetate, citrate agar or isoelectric focusing, to rule out structural variants such as the Lepore haemoglobins.

These simple investigations will serve to diagnose the vast majority of homozygous β thalassaemics and may allow their classification into β^+ or β^0 thalassaemia. In situations where the patient has been heavily transfused globin synthesis studies or DNA analysis will distinguish β^0 from β^+ thalassaemia.

The diagnosis is confirmed by the finding of heterozygous β thalassaemia in both parents.

Differential diagnosis (see also Chapter 7)

There are very few conditions which cause genuine difficulty in the diagnosis of the severe forms of β thalassaemia. The presence of anaemia from early in life, with the associated red-cell abnormalities and high levels of HbF, is unique to the β thalassaemias. The other anaemias of early life, such as severe nutritional anaemia, congenital haemolytic anaemia due to red-cell enzyme defects and the congenital aplastic anaemias, all have completely different haematological pictures. Similarly, conditions associated with high levels of HbF, such as juvenile chronic myeloid leukaemia and some of the congenital aplastic anaemias, can be distinguished easily by the associated white-cell and platelet changes. We have seen several cases of congenital sideroblastic anaemia misdiagnosed as β thalassaemia, particularly if the patient has been transfused heavily before an adequate diagnosis has been made. The haematological picture is quite different and the bone marrow in β thalassaemia does not show the marked morphological abnormalities of the red-cell precursors that are observed in the different classes of congenital dyserythropoietic anaemia.

Homozygous δβ thalassaemia, haemoglobin Lepore thalassaemia and hereditary persistence of fetal haemoglobin

Homozygous δβ thalassaemia is diagnosed by the finding of typical thalassaemic red-cell changes associated with 100% HbF and the absence of both Hbs A_2 and A. In the past, the distinction between the $(^A\gamma\delta\beta)^0$ and $(\delta\beta)^0$ forms was made by amino acid analysis of the cyanogen bromide cleaved peptide, γCB3 (Huisman & Jonxis 1977; Clegg *et al.* 1979), or by electrophoresis of globin under conditions that separate the $^G\gamma$ and $^A\gamma$ chains (Alter 1979; Alter *et al.* 1980). Currently, however, it is simpler to establish a molecular diagnosis by Southern blot analysis or by using one of the polymerase chain reaction (PCR)-based techniques (see later section). The homozygous and compound heterozygous states for Hb Lepore are easily identified by the severity of the anaemia and the finding of variable amounts of Hb Lepore on haemoglobin electrophoresis.

The distinction of homozygous δβ thalassaemia from homozygous hereditary persistence of fetal haemoglobin (HPFH) may be difficult. In the former there is usually splenomegaly, a moderate degree of anaemia and more globin imbalance than in the homozygous state for HPFH. The red cells also tend to be more hypochromic and microcytic in homozygous δβ thalassaemia. Compound heterozygotes for HPFH and β thalassaemia are usually asymptomatic or mildly anaemic; the proportions of Hbs A and F are dependent on the type of β-thalassaemia and HPFH mutations. On the other hand, considerable variation has been observed in the clinical phenotypes of δβ-thalassaemia/β-thalassaemia compound heterozygotes, ranging from a mild anaemia to thalassaemia major; they tend to be more severely affected than δβ-thalassaemia homozygotes. It is often easier to distinguish these conditions in related carriers by analysis of the haematological changes and intercellular distribution of HbF.

Differential diagnosis

The differential diagnosis for the δβ thalassaemias, the Hb Lepore thalassaemias and HPFH follows the same lines as that for the β thalassaemias.

Heterozygous β or δβ thalassaemia

As for the homozygous states, the heterozygous carriers of β thalassaemia are identified by careful haematological studies followed by electrophoretic analysis of haemoglobin.

The blood film shows morphological changes of the red cells including hypochromia, microcytosis, anisochromia and anisopoikilocytosis in most cases. By far the most useful investigation in screening for heterozygous β or δβ thalassaemia is to determine the MCV and MCH. Details of the ranges and their discriminatory values are given in Chapter 14. It is very unusual to find a β- or δβ-thalassaemia carrier with a normal MCH and MCV value except in the presence of co-existent α-thalassaemia trait (see below).

Once it has been established that there are thalassaemic red-cell indices, the HbA_2 level should be measured, by either quantitative cellulose acetate electrophoresis, column chromatography or HPLC. It is also important to carry out qualitative haemoglobin electrophoresis on cellulose acetate or isoelectric focusing (IEF) to identify structural variants like Hb Lepore. Haemoglobin F estimation is of interest but not of any great diagnostic value except in persons in which the HbA_2 level is normal. In such cases a chemical estimation of the level of HbF should be carried out to determine whether the patient is a δβ-thalassaemia carrier. If the HbF level is in the 5–20% range it is helpful to determine the intercellular distribution to distinguish between HPFH and δβ thalassaemia.

It is rarely necessary to assess globin synthesis for the diagnosis of heterozygous β thalassaemia if the HbA_2 is elevated. However, it should be remembered that a person with many of the characteristics of heterozygous β thalassaemia can also carry an α-thalassaemia gene. This should be suspected if the MCV and MCH values are close to normal (see Chapter 13). The diagnosis can be confirmed by family studies and DNA analysis.

It should be remembered that the HbA_2 level may be moderately elevated if an individual has both the sickle-cell trait and α-thalassaemia trait. In this situation, the HbA_2 may be in the 3.5–4.0% range. The relative increase in this case is a post-translational phenomenon due to a greater affinity of α for δ chains compared with $β^S$ chains, which is accentuated by limiting amounts of α chains (see Chapter 11). The simplest way of obtaining a correct diagnosis is to quantify the HbS level. In uncomplicated sickle-cell trait, it is less than 40% of the total haemoglobin. Co-existing α-thalassaemia trait reduces the level of HbS whereas co-existing β-thalassaemia trait results in a level of HbS of more than 60% of the total haemoglobin. Again, the diagnosis can be confirmed by family studies, which demonstrate the segregation of the two traits.

Some β thalassaemias are associated with normal levels of Hbs A_2 and F in the heterozygous state, accompanied by minimal reduction in the MCV and MCH values (the so-called 'silent β thalassaemia', see Chapters 4, 7 and 13). The homozygous states for these conditions are characterized by a mild form of thalassaemia intermedia with elevated HbF levels in the 10–30% range and elevated HbA_2 levels. As discussed in Chapters 4 and 13, globin synthesis studies in heterozygotes usually show slightly unbalanced synthesis ratios.

Distinction of β- and δβ-thalassaemia traits from iron deficiency

In practice the commonest problem that is encountered in the diagnosis of the β-thalassaemia carrier states is their distinction from iron-deficiency anaemia. This should rarely pose a problem if the haematological findings are carefully examined. To produce MCH and MCV values as low as those found typically in β-thalassaemia carriers, iron deficiency is usually associated with a much lower haemoglobin level than that found in association with these traits. However, occasionally the distinction can be more difficult. The measurements of the serum iron and total iron binding capacity (TIBC) are usually sufficient to distinguish between the two. The serum ferritin level is also a valuable guide to iron deficiency. It should be remembered that iron deficiency is often found together with β-thalassaemia trait; the effect on the HbA_2 level was discussed in Chapter 7.

Because electronic cell counters are now used to

screen for thalassaemia, there has been much interest in determining whether it is possible to develop mathematical models which will discriminate between iron-deficiency anaemia and β thalassaemia from the red-cell indices. Various formulae based on the blood count have been devised (Mentzer 1973; England & Fraser 1979). We feel that, while these are interesting theoretical studies, the simple analytical techniques required to measure HbA_2 levels must now be available to any laboratory which has the resources to own an electronic cell counter. Furthermore, the various discriminatory functions are not completely reliable and are not applicable to children, pregnant women or patients with polycythaemia complicated by iron deficiency, and will only predict the correct diagnosis in 80–90% of patients (d'Onofrio *et al.* 1992). We recommend that all individuals with thalassaemia-like red-cell indices should have their HbA_2 level determined.

The problem of the significance of 'borderline' levels of HbA_2, in the 3.2–3.5% range, is discussed in Chapter 7.

Haemoglobin H disease

Haemoglobin H disease is characterized by anaemia accompanied by typical thalassaemic changes of the red cells in which HbH inclusions can be generated (see Chapter 11). The diagnosis should be confirmed by haemoglobin electrophoresis; HbH can be demonstrated by electrophoresis on cellulose acetate or starch gel either at alkaline pH or, uniquely, at neutral or acid pH. Haemoglobin electrophoresis on cellulose acetate at alkaline pH shows an abnormal band anodal to HbA comprising 1–40% of the total Hb. Haemoglobin A_2 levels are usually reduced. If one of the α-chain termination mutants such as Constant Spring is involved it can be demonstrated by starch gel or cellulose acetate electrophoresis, or IEF (see Chapter 11).

The haemoglobin Bart's hydrops syndrome

This condition, which is described in detail in Chapter 11, usually offers no diagnostic problems. While the clinical findings may resemble other causes of hydrops fetalis, the typical thalassaemic blood changes with a marked normoblastaemia together with the finding of up to 80% Hb Bart's are found in no other condition.

α-Thalassaemia carrier states

The diagnostic problems involved in identifying the different α-thalassaemia carrier states and the homozygous states for α^+ thalassaemia were discussed in detail in Chapter 11. In summary, the heterozygous states for the deletion (–α/αα) and non-deletion ($\alpha^T\alpha/\alpha\alpha$) forms of α thalassaemia usually show minimal haematological changes and no abnormalities of the haemoglobin pattern. In some, but not all, cases there is an elevated level of Hb Bart's in the 1–3% range in the neonatal period. The heterozygous states for α^0 thalassaemia (––/αα), and the homozygous states for α^+ thalassaemia (–α/–α) are characterized by significantly reduced levels of the MCV and MCH together with hypochromic red cells. There are no changes in the haemoglobin pattern in adult life but in the neonatal period from 5 to 10% Hb Bart's is found. The latter conditions can also be identified by globin synthesis; the α-/β-chain ratios are discussed in Chapter 11. However, the ratios are the same in the two forms of α thalassaemia and therefore although this approach identifies the condition as a type of α thalassaemia it does not allow a definitive diagnosis. Similarly, and as discussed in Chapter 11, there may be a few cells with HbH inclusion bodies, particularly in heterozygotes for α^0 thalassaemia, but their absence does not exclude the diagnosis. In short, the only definite way of identifying the different α-thalassaemia carrier states and homozygous states for α^+ thalassaemia is by DNA analysis (see later section).

An approach to the laboratory diagnosis of the thalassaemias

The diagnosis of thalassaemia may be required either because a patient presents with a clinical picture which raised suspicions or as part of a programme of carrier screening. The general approach to the laboratory diagnosis of these conditions, outlined in Table 16.1 and Fig. 16.1, is the same regardless of the way in which the disorder first presents. It entails three distinct phases. First, there is the primary screen, which is based on haematological changes. This is followed by a secondary screen which involves HbA_2 and, sometimes, HbF estimations, followed by haemoglobin electrophoresis to identify any structural haemoglobin variants. It may also involve some further haematological studies to identify particular types of

Table 16.1 Laboratory diagnosis of the thalassaemias (abbreviations are defined in the text).

Primary screen
Automated blood cell counter. Hb, MCH, MCV

Secondary screen
Haemoglobin A_2 estimation
    Cellulose acetate; micro-column chromatography; HPLC
Haemoglobin F estimation
    Alkali denaturation
Identification of abnormal haemoglobins; haemoglobin
        electrophoresis
    Cellulose acetate; citrate agar; starch gel; IEF
Demonstration of inclusion bodies
    Methyl violet; brilliant cresyl blue
Globin synthesis
Intercellular distribution of HbF

Definitive diagnosis
α Thalassaemia
    Deletions: GAP PCR; Southern blotting
    Non-deletional forms: PCR; DGGE; SSCA + sequencing
β Thalassaemia
    PCR/ASO; dot blot; reverse dot blot; ARMS;
        PCR/restriction-enzyme DGGE
δβ Thalassaemia; hereditary persistence of fetal
        haemoglobin
    Southern blotting; GAP PCR
Haemoglobin variants
    Restriction enzymes; ARMS-PCR; sequencing

inclusion bodies in the red cells and, sometimes, globin synthesis. At this stage it is possible to make an adequate diagnosis of many of the different forms of thalassaemia, but in many cases it is necessary to go one step further, that is, to obtain a definitive diagnosis. This entails the identification of the underlying mutation, or mutations, by DNA analysis.

The primary screen

The primary screen for all forms of thalassaemia involves an accurate blood count, ideally carried out on a well calibrated electronic cell counter which will provide accurate red-cell indices. In the symptomatic forms of thalassaemia this should always be followed by a careful examination of a stained blood film.

We discussed carrier screening in detail in Chapter 14. We concluded that individuals with hypochromic, microcytic red-cell indices, that is, with MCH values below 27 pg or MCV values below 80 fl, should be investigated further. We also mentioned the question

of whether a primary screen for carriers could be carried out using a single-tube osmotic fragility test, a particularly attractive option when expense might preclude the possibility of electronic red-cell counting (Silvestroni & Bianco 1959). The effectiveness of this approach has been evaluated using 0.36% saline instead of the more commonly used 0.32% saline solutions (Kattamis *et al.* 1981a) or glycerine saline (Gottfried & Robertson 1974; Flatz & Flatz 1980). It has also been the subject of a series of more recent papers from India, which describe the reliability of what the workers call NESTROFT (naked-eye single-tube red-cell osmotic fragility test) (Raghaven *et al.* 1991; Gomber *et al.* 1997; Manglani *et al.* 1997; Thool *et al.* 1998). In the most recent of these papers, Thool *et al.* (1998) suggest that using a 0.36% buffered saline NESTROFT gives almost 100% positive diagnoses and has a negative prediction value of about 83%, with a sensitivity of 95.2%. Of course, false-positive tests do not really matter and the major concern is false-negative tests. In all these studies the frequency of false negatives was quite low but undoubtedly some carriers were missed. Furthermore, they represent studies done as part of a research programme and there is still uncertainty about the robustness of this approach in day-to-day clinical use. But, while further studies need to be carried out, and osmotic fragility screening may be useful for population studies, we strongly recommend that laboratories that are screening for β thalassaemia carry out the initial screen using red-cell indices obtained from electronic cell counting.

The secondary screen

In symptomatic patients who are anaemic with thalassaemic changes of their red cells, the secondary screen simply involves haemoglobin electrophoresis to search for HbH and to rule out any other structural haemoglobin variants, and a chemical estimation of the level of HbF, which will be raised in almost all forms of β thalassaemia. The HbA_2 level is of little diagnostic help in the more severe forms of thalassaemia. These simple investigations will be sufficient to provide a diagnosis in the vast majority of cases.

Asymptomatic individuals with hypochromic microcytic red-cell indices, i.e. with MCH values below 27 pg or MCV values below 80 fl, should be investigated for thalassaemia trait. Further investiga-

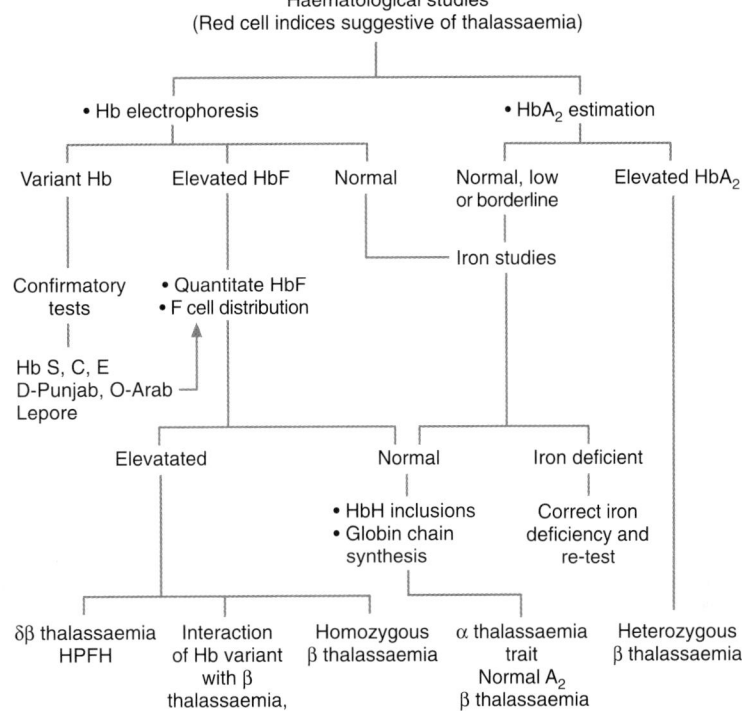

Haematological studies
(Red cell indices suggestive of thalassaemia)

• Hb electrophoresis

• HbA$_2$ estimation

Variant Hb   Elevated HbF   Normal

Normal, low   Elevated HbA$_2$
or borderline

Iron studies

Confirmatory
tests

• Quantitate HbF
• F cell distribution

Hb S, C, E
D-Punjab, O-Arab
Lepore

Elevatated   Normal   Iron deficient

• HbH inclusions   Correct iron
• Globin chain   deficiency and
synthesis   re-test

δβ thalassaemia   Interaction   Homozygous   α thalassaemia   Heterozygous
HPFH   of Hb variant   β thalassaemia   trait   β thalassaemia
with β   Normal A$_2$
thalassaemia,   β thalassaemia
δβ, HPFH

Fig. 16.1 A simplified flow chart showing the major steps in the diagnosis of the different forms of thalassaemia. Family studies should be carried out whenever possible. The precise identification of the molecular pathology always requires DNA analysis. • indicates basic investigations required for the diagnosis of the thalassaemias.

tions should include haemoglobin electrophoresis on cellulose acetate at alkaline pH (pH 8.2–8.6), which enables the provisional identification of Hbs A, F, S/G/D, A$_2$/C/E/O Arab, H, Lepore and a number of less common haemoglobin variants. Good electrophoretic techniques should demonstrate HbF levels of >2% and a split HbA$_2$ band, which is useful in differentiating an α-chain from a β-chain variant. The secondary screen must also include an estimation of the HbA$_2$ level.

An increased HbA$_2$ level, i.e. >3.7%, together with hypochromic microcytic red cells is diagnostic of heterozygous β thalassaemia. Haemoglobin A$_2$ values of <3.2% are usually considered to be normal, while those between 3.2% and 3.7% (borderline) should be interpreted with care (see Chapter 7). After those individuals with elevated HbA$_2$ values have been defined, a group will remain who have thalassaemic red-cell indices with normal, low or borderline HbA$_2$ levels. It is important to exclude iron deficiency, since iron deficiency severe enough to cause mild anaemia can produce falsely low HbA$_2$ levels. If iron deficiency is suspected it should be corrected and the

HbA$_2$ estimation repeated. Some of those who are iron replete with low or normal HbA$_2$ levels will have elevated HbF levels, indicating that they are heterozygous for δβ thalassaemia. Of the remainder, the majority will be α^0-thalassaemia carriers or α$^+$-thalassaemia homozygotes, or heterozygotes for the forms of β thalassaemia with normal HbA$_2$ values (see Chapter 7). Individuals with α^0-thalassaemia trait may have a few red cells with HbH inclusions but their absence does not exclude α thalassaemia. It is possible to distinguish α-thalassaemia carriers from heterozygotes for normal HbA$_2$ β thalassaemia by globin synthesis studies.

If the HbF level is elevated, as suggested by cellulose acetate electrophoresis, it should be quantified. It is helpful to examine the intercellular distribution by the Kleihauer method or by the more sensitive technique of immunofluorescence using an anti-γ-chain antibody.

The intercellular distribution of HbF is determined to differentiate HPFH from δβ thalassaemia—in individuals with HPFH it is homogeneous, or pancellular (with the exception of heterocellular HPFH), whereas an uneven or heterocellular F-cell distribution is typical of heterozygous δβ thalassaemia. However, with better understanding of the molecular basis of these disorders, this distinction has become less useful. It appears that the intercellular distribution is a reflection of the overall numbers of red cells containing HbF and the sensitivity of the technique used to stain for it. Thus, a heterocellular distribution with the acid elution method of Kleihauer may become pancellular with the more sensitive immunofluorescence assay. Modest increases of HbF levels (1–4%) with a heterocellular distribution in otherwise normal individuals with normal haematology fall into the group of conditions referred to as 'heterocellular' HPFH (see Chapter 10).

Haemoglobin electrophoresis on cellulose acetate at alkaline pH should distinguish most of the common haemoglobin variants; additional investigations that may be useful in the identification of the less common ones include electrophoresis on citrate agar at acid pH and isoelectric focusing. The β thalassaemias, δβ thalassaemias and HPFH may be coinherited with any of the common haemoglobin variants, producing a spectrum of genetic interactions. A guideline to interpreting them is shown in Table 16.2, but family studies should always be carried out.

Definitive diagnosis

The definitive diagnosis of the thalassaemias involves determination of the underlying mutations through DNA analysis. Some of the methods used in our laboratory are outlined later in this chapter.

Laboratory methods

Preparation of haemoglobin solution for electrophoresis

Blood can be collected into any of the standard anticoagulants. Packed red cells are washed three times with 3–5 volumes of 0.9% saline and then lysed with 1–1.5 volumes of distilled water and 0.4 volumes of CCl_4. The mixture is shaken in a centrifuge tube either by hand for not less than 4 min or by a vortex mixer for 30 s. The mixture is then centrifuged at 3000 g for 20 min. At this stage the clear supernatant haemoglobin solution is carefully pipetted off and is ready for haemoglobin electrophoresis.

Where samples are being examined for small amounts of HbH or unstable haemoglobin it is probably better to avoid shaking with organic solvents and, after washing the cells, to lyse them with a minimum of 4 volumes of distilled water and to separate the cellular debris by high-speed centrifugation (e.g. 18 000 g for 20 min at 4°C).

Although we find that distilled water is quite satisfactory for most purposes, lysates can also be prepared by the addition of 1.5 volumes of 5 mM phosphate and 0.5 mM EDTA solution to the washed red blood cells. After allowing the samples to stand for a few minutes, 0.1 volume of 9% saline is added and the mixture is centrifuged at 4°C. Lysates prepared in this way may be stored at –20°C for up to 4 weeks; they can be stored at –70°C indefinitely.

Red-cell lysates can be kept at 4°C without deterioration for periods of up to 7–10 days. If they are to be stored for longer times it is better to dialyse them against 0.05 M sodium phosphate buffer, pH 7.2, for 24 h at 4°C. The dialysed lysate can be stored indefinitely at –70°C. In most cases the haemoglobin can be kept as oxyhaemoglobin although the carbonmonoxy form is more stable. The latter is particularly useful for preserving HbH but is not suitable for HbF analysis. Haemoglobin solutions that have been kept for any length of time may become oxidized, with the production of variable amounts of methaemoglobin. The latter produces additional bands on electrophoresis but this problem can be overcome by the addition of potassium cyanide to the haemoglobin solution since cyanmethaemoglobin has the same charge as oxyhaemoglobin. This is achieved by adding a drop of 1% solution of potassium cyanide to 1–2 ml of red-cell lysate.

It is possible to post whole blood for haemoglobin analysis provided that shipment only takes 24–48 h. Another useful form of transportation is in the form of washed red cells which have been treated with carbon monoxide. Ideally, samples should be maintained on ice for transportation but washed cells are usually satisfactory if maintained at ambient temperature for periods of up to a week.

Qualitative cellulose acetate electrophoresis

Cellulose acetate electrophoresis is rapid and simple and we find that it is an extremely useful technique for preliminary analysis of haemoglobin variants. There are a variety of commercially available tanks

Table 16.2 Some characteristic findings in the genetic interactions between β thalassaemia, δβ thalassaemia or hereditary persistence of fetal haemoglobin (A) and the common β-chain variants (B).

(A)

Thalassaemia type	Homozygote	Heterozygote
β^0 thalassaemia	Thalassaemia major: HbF 98%; HbA$_2$ 2%; no HbA	Thalassaemia minor: HbA$_2$ 3.7–7.0%; HbF 1–3%; α/β 2.0
β^+ thalassaemia (severe)	Thalassaemia major: HbF 70–95%; HbA$_2$ 2%; trace of HbA	Thalassaemia minor: HbA$_2$ 3.7–7.0%; HbF 1–3%; α/β 2.0
Mild β^+ thalassaemia	Thalassaemia intermedia to thalassaemia major: HbF 20–80%; HbA$_2$ 2–5%	Thalassaemia minor: HbA$_2$ 3.5–7.0%; α/β 1.5–2.0
'Silent' β thalassaemia	Asymptomatic to mild thalassaemia intermedia: HbF 10–30%; HbA$_2$ 2–5%	Usually 'silent': HbA$_2$ 3.3–3.5%; α/β 1.2–1.5
Normal HbA$_2$ β^+ or β^0 thalassaemia	Thalassaemia major: HbA$_2$ absent to trace; HbF 95–100%; HbA absent to trace	Thalassaemia minor: HbA$_2$ normal; HbF 1–3%; α/β 2.0
Deletion HPFH	Asymptomatic; normal to increased Hb levels with mildly hypochromic microcytic red blood cells; HbF 100%; α/γ ~ 1.5	Mild anaemia; normal RBC indices; HbA$_2$ normal; F-cell distribution–pancellular
Non-deletion HPFH	Asymptomatic; normal Hb levels with normal red blood cell indices; HbF 20–40%; HbA$_2$ 1–1.5%; α/non-α ~ 1.2	Normal to mild anaemia; borderline red blood cell indices; HbA$_2$ normal; F-cell distribution–pancellular
δβ thalassaemia	Mild anaemia to thalassaemia major: hypochromic microcytic red blood cells; HbF 100%; α/γ 2.5–5.0	Mild anaemia; hypochromic microcytic red blood cells: HbA$_2$ normal; HbF 5–20%; F-cell distribution–heterocellular
Hb Lepore	Severe thalassaemia intermedia to thalassaemia major: HbF 80%; Hb Lepore 20%	Thalassaemia minor: Hb Lepore 8–20%; HbF 2–4%

(B)

	Homozygote	Heterozygote
HbS/β^0 thalassaemia	Sickle-cell anaemia	HbS 75–100%; HbF 0–20%; HbA$_2$ 4–6%; no HbA
HbS/β^+ thalassaemia (severe type)	Sickle-cell anaemia	HbS 50–80%; HbF 0–20%; HbA 10–30%; HbA$_2$ 4–6%
HbS/β^+ thalassaemia (mild type)	Sickle-cell trait	HbS 50–65%; HbA ~ 25%; HbA$_2$ 4–6%; HbF ~ 5%
HbE/β^0 thalassaemia	Thalassaemia intermedia to thalassaemia major	HbE 30–40%; no HbA, rest HbF
HbE/β^+ thalassaemia	Thalassaemia intermedia to thalassaemia major	HbE 50–70%; HbF 15–30%; HbA trace to 10%

and trays for this purpose. The Mylar-backed plates, which are supplied by Helena Company, Beaumont, Texas, on which eight samples can be run simultaneously and loaded with a simple mechanical applicator, are very simple to use. Several plates can be analysed simultaneously at a relatively low cost. Because of their adaptability for both qualitative and quantitative work, we also use Shandon Model U77 electrophoretic tanks. These have the advantage that they are designed to take different-sized cellulose acetate strips and can be used for simple analytical studies or for quantification of HbA$_2$ or various other haemoglobin fractions.

In practice we use cellulose acetate electrophoresis

for rapid screening for haemoglobin variants or increased levels of HbF, and for the demonstration of Hbs Bart's and H.

Buffer systems

A Tris–EDTA–borate system, pH 7.9, is used for screening for haemoglobin variants and a phosphate system, pH 6.5, is used for separation of Hbs H and Bart's.

Tris–EDTA–borate system (pH 7.9)
Tris (hydroxymethyl) aminomethane 5.1 g, EDTA (acid) 0.3 g, boric acid 6.4 g, dissolved in 1 l distilled water.

Phosphate system (pH 6.5)
Potassium di-hydrogen phosphate (KH_2PO_4) 3.11 g, disodium hydrogen phosphate (Na_2HPO_4 $2H_2O$) 1.87 g, dissolved in 1 l distilled water.

Method

Cellulose acetate strips measuring 25 mm × 120 mm (Shandon, Celogram) are soaked in the appropriate buffer and gently blotted. The strips are placed in the Shandon electrophoretic tank and secured at each end by a double layer of Whatman no. 3 filter-paper. One to two μl of an 8–10 g/100 ml solution of haemoglobin is applied in a short (1-cm) line midway between the centre of the strip and its cathodal end. After the samples have soaked into the strip the haemoglobins are separated using a current of about 5 mA (about 220 V) across the strip.

Agar gel electrophoresis

Agar gel electrophoresis can be carried out using commercial kits, in shallow trays or on individual microscope slides.

Buffer system (citrate, pH 5.9)

Sodium citrate 147 g is dissolved in 600 ml of water and titrated to pH 5.9 with 50% citric acid. The total volume is then made up to 1 l with distilled water. This stock buffer is diluted to 1/10.

Commercial kits

Premixed reagents for citrate buffer can be obtained from Helena Laboratories, or from Isolab Inc.

Slide method

For analysis on microscope slides 1 g Difco agar in 100 ml of buffer containing 1 drop of 5% KCN is heated in boiling water until the agar has melted. Then 1.5 ml of the solution is deposited evenly on the microscope slide, which can then be kept for several days at 4°C. Red-cell lysates to be analysed are applied from the tip of a round toothpick and about 50–100 V are delivered for about 30–45 min. The slides can be stained with the following: bromophenol blue, 100 mg dissolved in 1 l distilled water containing 10 ml glacial acetic acid. The stain is poured off the slides after about 20–30 min and the slides are then washed with distilled water.

Larger-scale analysis on perspex trays

First 2 g of agar is dissolved in 200 ml of citrate buffer, pH 5.9, and heated until the agar has completely dissolved. The molten agar is poured into trays 25 cm × 30 cm × 0.1 cm and allowed to cool in a draught-free area. Haemoglobin solutions of at least 10 g/100 ml are applied to the centre of the gel by means of pieces of Whatman no. 3 (1 cm × 0.5 cm) filter paper. Filter-paper wicks are placed on the surface of the agar at each end and allowed to dip into electrode chambers containing at least 2 l of citrate buffer. As soon as the haemoglobin has migrated into the gel the pieces of filter-paper are removed with fine-pointed forceps and the whole gel is sprayed with a plastic spray (Krylon, no. 130L) to prevent drying during electrophoresis. Alternatively, a thin sheet of cellophane may be placed over the gel. Better separation of haemoglobin fractions is obtained if, after 3–4 h, the agar gel tray and buffer tank electrodes are reversed. After a further 3–4 h the plastic spray is peeled off and the gel immersed in bromophenol blue for 5–10 min. After staining (using bromophenol blue, as for the slide method, while still on the electrophoretic tray), the gel is placed in a shallow trough of distilled water so that it is just immersed. A piece of waxed paper is then gently pushed between the agar gel and tray until the gel has floated clear on to the paper. The gel and paper are allowed to dry with weights at several points round the edge of the paper supporting a protective sheet of glass, which is elevated about 1–3 cm above the agar gel. In this way permanent preparations can be obtained.

Estimation of haemoglobin A₂ and other variants

Haemoglobin A_2 levels can be estimated visually by paper or starch gel electrophoresis but in the authors' experience this is not satisfactory and some form of quantitative method is required. These include electrophoresis on cellular acetate or column chromatography. The various advantages and disadvantages of these different approaches have been analysed in detail by Schmidt *et al.* (1975), Efremov (1977), Brosious *et al.* (1978) and Schmidt and Brosious (1979).

Electrophoresis

The simplest method is cellulose acetate electrophoresis and the following modification of the method of Marengo-Rowe (1965) has been found to give excellent results: cellulose acetate strips measuring 25 mm × 120 mm (Shandon, Celogram) are soaked in a Tris–EDTA–borate buffer, pH 8.9 (Tris (hydroxymethyl) aminomethane 14.4 g, EDTA (acid) 1.5 g, boric acid 0.9 g, distilled water to 1 l) and gently blotted. The strips are placed in a Shandon electrophoretic tank (Shandon Model U77) and secured at each end by a double layer of Whatman no. 3 filter-paper. 10 μl of 8–10 g/100 ml solution of haemoglobin is applied in a short (2-cm) line midway between the centre of the strip and its cathodal end. After the samples have soaked into the strip, HbA and A_2 are separated completely in 2 h using a current of 5 mA (about 220 V) across the strip. The HbA and A_2 zones are cut out and eluted in 15 and 1.5 ml of buffer, respectively. After 30 min (to ensure total elution) the optical density at 415 nm is determined and the level of HbA_2 calculated from the formula:

$$\frac{OD_{415\,nm}HbA_2 \times 100}{10 \times \left(OD_{415\,nm}HbA\right) + OD_{415\,nm}HbA_2}$$

It has been found that, under these conditions, HbA_2 values ranging from 0.3 to 7.5% give optical densities within a range which follows Beer's law for oxyhaemoglobin solutions at this wavelength. Forty estimations on a single sample gave a range of 2.28–2.88 (SD 0.22%). The distribution of HbA_2 levels in 200 healthy individuals obtained by this technique ranged from 1.5 to 3.5% (mean 2.48) (Weatherall *et al.* 1971). Prolonged storage has little effect on HbA_2 values determined in this way.

For the determination of Hbs A and C or S in heterozygotes, or similar estimations on other mixtures of haemoglobin variants, the same cellulose acetate electrophoretic system can be used, but for this purpose 2 μl of haemolysate is applied to cellulose strips measuring 25 mm × 180 mm. Better separation of the major components is obtained using buffer systems described for qualitative cellulose acetate electrophoresis. Haemoglobins A and S are eluted in 3 ml and HbA_2 in 1.5 ml. Storage experiments have indicated that the accurate quantification of HbS can only be achieved in haemolysates which have been prepared for less than 7 days. After this time there is progressive reduction in the relative amount of HbS in samples stored at 4°C or frozen.

Amounts of Hbs H and Bart's as low as 0.5% of the total haemoglobin can be accurately determined by cellulose acetate electrophoresis using either a Tris–EDTA–borate or phosphate buffer system, pH 7.9 and 6.5, respectively, as described above. After separation the fractions are eluted to 2-ml volumes of buffer and their $OD_{415\,nm}$ determined.

Column chromatography

Haemoglobin A_2 levels may be estimated by DEAE-cellulose chromatography at room temperature. Commercial microcolumns are produced by Helena Laboratories or Isolab, but they require careful quality control to obtain consistent results.

Haemoglobin A_2 estimations may also be carried out in this way using disposable Pasteur pipettes (0.5 cm × 6 cm). The tapered end of the pipette is loosely packed with cotton, and the pipette is placed vertically inside a test-tube. The column and cotton plug are moistened with 0.05 M Tris–HCl buffer, pH 8.5, and the column is then packed with a slurry consisting of a suspension of DE52 DEAE cellulose. Once the column has settled excess buffer is removed from the top and a sample of three drops of red-cell lysate (see previous section), diluted with seven drops of 0.05 M Tris–HCl buffer, pH 8.5, is applied to the top of the column. After the sample has entered the column the walls are rinsed with the same buffer, which is allowed to flow into the absorbent. A simple reservoir is then attached to the top of the pipette by a suitable piece of plastic tubing on the stem of a simple filter funnel. All the effluent that has been collected thus far in the test-tube is discarded. The first 6–8 ml of effluent is collected in a 10-ml volumetric flask and the volume is adjusted to 10 ml with distilled water. This effluent contains HbA_2. When all the HbA_2 has completely eluted, the buffer in the reservoir is changed to 0.05 M Tris–HCl buffer, pH 7.0. The first 5–10 ml of effluent, which contains the remaining haemoglobins, is collected in a 25-ml volumetric flask and diluted to 25 ml. The optical densities of the two samples are then read at 415 nm using the Tris buffer as a blank calculated as follows:

The percentage of HbA_2 is

$$\frac{OD\ HbA_2}{(OD\ \text{in remaining } Hb \times 2.5) + OD\ HbA_2} \times 100 = \%\ HbA_2$$

Starch gel electrophoresis

Although starch gel electrophoresis is used less commonly now that more rapid methods are available it is still extremely valuable for defining minor fractions or studying the non-haemoglobin proteins of the red cell (Fig. 16.2). Starch gel electrophoresis can employ either a vertical or a horizontal system (Smithies 1959). There are now a variety of vertical starch gel trays on the market, all of which have a set of removable teeth incorporated into the base. When removed these produce a series of wells in the starch for insertion of the sample. The advantage of the vertical system is that more sample can be loaded and minor components studied in greater detail. Furthermore the degree of resolution is higher than in the horizontal system. On the other hand most of the vertical starch gel trays require a considerable quantity of starch and are therefore expensive to run for routine purposes. A horizontal system is cheaper and gives adequate resolution. A horizontal starch gel tray can be easily constructed from perspex. The size is not critical and depends on the number of samples to be studied, but a tray measuring 15 cm × 15 cm × 0.5 cm will be found to be adequate for most purposes. For routine haemoglobin electrophoresis the Tris–EDTA–borate system, pH 8.65, gives satisfac-

tory results. For separation of Hbs Bart's and H a phosphate buffer system, pH 7.0, gives the best resolution. For the study of minor components and isozyme patterns the discontinuous system of Poulik (1957) is useful although gels made with this buffer tend to be more friable than those made with the Tris–EDTA–borate system. Starch gel electrophoresis can be adapted for globin separation using the 6 M urea barbital system described by Chernoff and Pettit (1964).

Buffer systems

Different systems are available. The continuous and discontinuous systems are equally good for routine use.

Tris–EDTA–borate system (pH 8.6, 0.08 M) (Boyer et al. 1963a) 0.9 M Tris (hydroxymethyl) aminomethane, 0.5 M boric acid, 0.02 M EDTA (acid). The stock buffer is diluted 1/20 for making gels, 1/5 for the anodal chamber and 1/7 for the cathodal chamber.

Discontinuous Tris–citrate system (pH 8.5, 0.04 M) (Poulik 1957) 45.9 g Tris (hydroxymethyl) aminomethane, 5.0 g citric acid, 5 l distilled water for the gel buffer, while the chamber buffers are made as follows: 92.5 g boric acid, 25.0 ml 10 N sodium hydroxide, 5 l distilled water.

Phosphate system (pH 6.5–7.1, 0.005 M (Gammack et al. 1961) This is the best buffer system for demonstrating small amounts of Hb Bart's and H. 0.04 M disodium hydrogen phosphate is titrated to pH 7.1 with orthophosphoric acid. For preparation of gels 40 ml of the resultant buffer is diluted with 300 ml distilled water. The undiluted buffer is used for the electrode chambers. The separation usually takes about 4 h.

Method

Starch (Connaught Laboratories or similar brand of hydrolysed starch) is mixed with the appropriate amount of buffer so as to produce enough molten starch to just overfill the tray. The maker's instructions should be followed regarding the amount of starch to be used, although this is usually 9–12 g/100 ml buffer and varies slightly between different lots. The starch, suspended in the appropriate buffer, is thoroughly shaken in 1-l Erlenmeyer flasks and

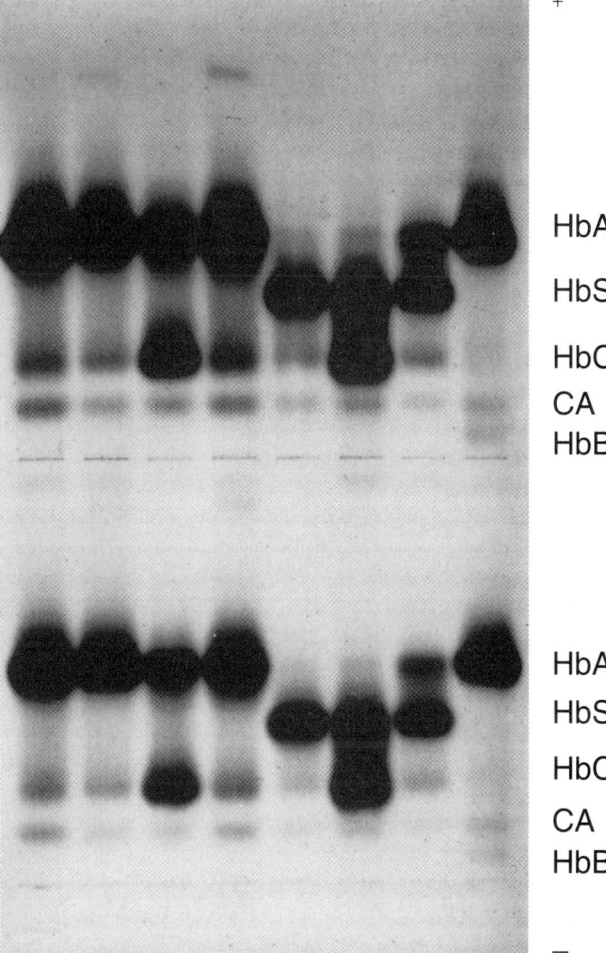

+

HbA
HbS
HbC
CA
HbB$_2$

HbA
HbS
HbC
CA
HbB$_2$

−

Fig. 16.2 Vertical starch gel electrophoresis, pH 8.5, amido black stain, showing a variety of haemoglobin variants. Left to right: 1 and 2, normal adult; 3, HbC trait; 4, β-thalassaemia trait; 5, sickle-cell anaemia; 6, HbSC disease; 7, sickle-cell β thalassaemia; 8, an adult with a δ-chain variant (HbB$_2$). The figure shows a duplicate analysis on a tray which will carry 16 samples. The non-haem protein which migrates behind HbA$_2$ is the major red-cell carbonic anhydrase (CA).

then heated to boiling with continuous shaking until a translucent gel appears. The flask is then degassed under vacuum until all the large bubbles have been dispersed and a uniform mixture containing small bubbles is obtained. Excessive degassing results in a dry gel and poor migration. The molten gel is then poured into the appropriate tray, after which a pre-heated glass plate is placed over the gel, the excess being allowed to run over the sides. Excessive pressure on the gel should be avoided since thin gels tend to crack or pull away from the sides of the mould on cooling.

After cooling the tray is turned over and the bars containing the teeth removed, so producing a series of wells into which the haemoglobin solution is introduced with Pasteur pipettes. For routine work the best resolution is obtained with solutions of about 2–4 g/100 ml; the minor components are better visualized with more concentrated haemolysates. The samples are kept in place by sealing with just-molten pure petroleum jelly and in the vertical system the gels are set upright, after unscrewing the ends, in suitable buffer chambers. Contact at the upper end is obtained by a wick of double- or triple-thickness Whatman no. 3 filter-paper placed over the end of the gel, while the lower end of the gel stands immersed in the chamber buffer. The duration of electrophoresis is variable depending on the buffer system and voltage. The Tris–EDTA–borate and Tris–citrate–borate systems are run for about 12–18 h with a current of about 25 mA across the gel (4 V/cm) while good resolution can be obtained with the phosphate system in 2–4 h with a similar current. Where possible the electrophoresis should be performed at 4°C.

If the horizontal system is used trays can be obtained commercially which, like those for the vertical system, incorporate teeth within the base. In that case the method of sample loading is the same as that for the vertical gels. However, simple inexpensive trays can easily be made from plastic and the samples applied on small pieces of Whatman no. 3 filter-paper, which are soaked in haemolysate and inserted into the gel with the aid of a razor-blade or flat knife.

Gel slicing and staining

After the electrophoretic runs gels are removed from the tray and placed on a clean, smooth bench surface. Horizontal slicing can be achieved either with a specially devised slicer designed after a cheese cutter or using a sharp flat blade. After slicing, the gels are placed with the cut surface uppermost in suitable trays or plastic boxes and stained. For staining the following solution is made up: glacial acetic acid 200 ml; methanol 900 ml; distilled water 900 ml. A stain is prepared by dissolving 0.4 g amido black in 500 ml of this solution. It is poured over the starch gel and left until each of the major haemoglobin fractions is darkly stained. It is then poured off and can be used again. The gel is washed with several changes of the glacial acetic acid/methanol/distilled water mixture until the background is clear. Gels treated in this way can be kept in cellophane wraps indefinitely (Fig. 16.2).

Isoelectric focusing (IEF)

Generally, IEF produces a separation of haemoglobins similar to that by electrophoresis on cellulose acetate membranes but the bands are sharper and the resolution of some haemoglobins is better. IEF is not usually required for secondary screening but is a useful supplement to cellulose acetate electrophoresis in reference centres where there is a large throughput of samples. Precast agar gels are commercially available. We use the 'Isolab system', which allows the differentiation between Hbs A, F, S, C, D Punjab but does not differentiate between Hbs G Philadelphia and Lepore, or between Hbs E, A_2 and O Arab. An increased percentage of HbA_2 may be visible but this technique is not reliable for the quantification of HbA_2.

IEF is a valuable technique to differentiate Hb Bart's from other 'fast' variants such as Hbs J and N in umbilical cord blood samples. It is also useful for screening dried blood samples spotted on membranes (such as Guthrie cards) because interference from methaemoglobin, which can prevent adequate resolution of the haemoglobin bands on electrophoresis, is reduced. Figure 16.3 shows an IEF gel with various haemoglobin variants.

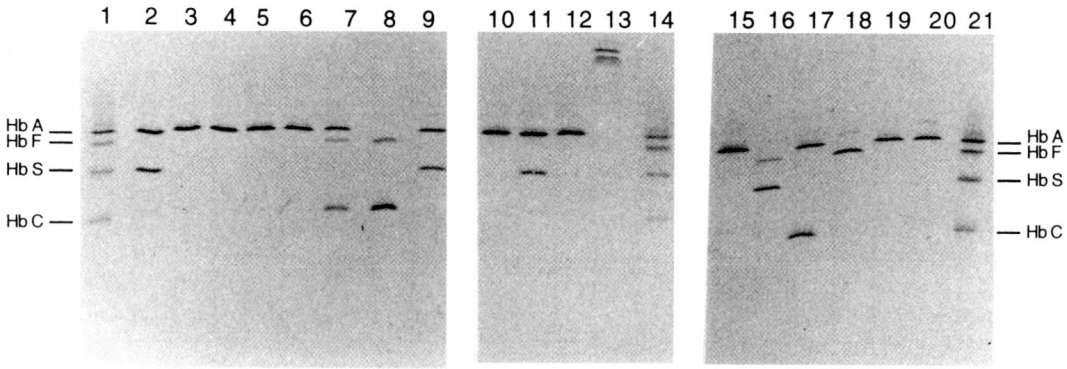

Fig. 16.3 Haemoglobin analysis by isoelectric focusing. Separation of normal haemoglobin and variants by isoelectric focusing (IEF) using precast agar plates (Isolab Inc., Akran, USA). Lanes 1, 14 and 21 show the standard control sample (Hbs A, F, S and C) used in this system. The various genotypes detected by IEF are represented as follows: lane 2, A/S with increased HbA_2 level; lanes 3–6, normal A/A; lane 7, A/E with increased HbF level; lane 8, E/E with increased HbF; lane 9, A/S; lane 10, normal A/A; lane 11, A/S; lane 12, normal A/A; lane 13, Hb Bart's with no HbA or HbF; lane 15, normal A/A; lane 16, S/S with increased HbF; lane 17, A/C; lane 18, fetal blood, all HbF, no HbA; lanes 19 and 20, normal AA.

High-performance liquid chromatography (HPLC)

The introduction and evolution of automated HPLC systems has brought a radical change in the identification and quantification of haemoglobin variants. Several automated HPLC systems are commercially available; they are expensive to buy and, for an evaluation of the different systems, the reader is advised to consult the reports of Galanello *et al.* (1995), Waters *et al.* (1996), Bain and Phelan (1997), Wild and Stephens (1997) and Riou *et al.* (1997).

We use the Bio-Rad Variant and the 'β thal short program' to screen and quantify the levels of Hbs A_2, F, S and C. There are limitations to this system. Since Hbs Lepore and E are co-eluted with HbA_2, a precise quantification of these haemoglobin variants is not possible; they should be thought of if the sample gives an HbA_2 level of more than 10%, which is most unusual in β-thalassaemia carriers. There may also be a false increase of HbA_2 levels in HbS carriers due to co-elution of minor components with HbA_2 (thought to be due to post-translational modifications of HbS). Haemoglobins H (β_4) and Bart's (γ_4) may be detected, but not quantitatively because they are eluted prior to the start of the integration. This system is not reliable for measuring low levels of HbF.

Automated HPLC systems give accurate and reproducible HbA_2 estimations (except when certain haemoglobin variants are present) but the peak shape, baseline and resolution should always be checked before using the computed peak areas.

Haemoglobin H inclusions

Haemoglobin H inclusions can be generated *in vitro* by the redox action of certain dyes. They are found in HbH disease, and sometimes in α^0-thalassaemia carriers and in the Hb Bart's hydrops fetalis syndrome. They must be distinguished from the preformed single HbH inclusions found in the blood of splenectomized patients with HbH disease. Due to batch variation of the dyes, any new batch should always be checked with a positive control.

Blood (preferably anticoagulated with EDTA and used within 24 h of venesection) is incubated with 1% brilliant cresyl blue (in 0.9% NaCl) at room temperature (or better at 37°C) for 4 h. One part of blood is incubated with two parts of dye and a normal control should always be included. Blood films are made, allowed to air dry and examined under oil immersion.

Haemoglobin H inclusions are distinguished by the 'golf ball' appearance of the cells. Typical inclusions are found in 30–100% of the red cells in HbH disease. As mentioned above they may also be found in a few red cells (1/1000 to 1/10000) of individuals with α^0-thalassaemia trait, but their absence does not exclude the diagnosis.

α-Chain inclusions

Alpha-chain inclusions can be seen in the cells of homozygous β thalassaemics or of patients with thalassaemia intermedia. In non-splenectomized persons they can only be found in the red-cell precursors in the bone marrow, but after splenectomy they can be seen in nucleated red cells in peripheral blood and in non-nucleated cells.

Equal parts of blood and 1% solution of methyl violet in 0.9% NaCl are mixed and incubated at room temperature for periods ranging from 30 min to 2 h. Blood films are made and allowed to dry and examined under oil immersion. The preformed Heinz bodies can also be easily seen using wet preparations under a cover slip.

Determination of the relative amount of haemoglobin F

No one technique is entirely satisfactory for the determination of the level of HbF. In practice we find that for accurate determination of relatively low levels the 2-min alkali denaturation technique of Betke *et al.* (1959) as slightly modified in our own laboratory (Pembrey *et al.* 1972) gives highly reproducible results over the range 0.5–50%. The original 1-min alkali denaturation test of Singer *et al.* (1951) is quick and useful but it tends to give slightly high values in the low range, i.e. below 5% HbF, and like the 2-min method of Betke *et al.* (1959) is inaccurate in the higher ranges. Probably the most useful of the alkali denaturation methods for work in the higher ranges of HbF, i.e. in excess of 50% of the total haemoglobin, is the method of Jonxis and Visser (1956). If very accurate estimations of the level of HbF are required, particularly in the high ranges, a variety of chromatographic techniques are available; these are reviewed by Huisman and Jonxis (1977).

Method of Singer et al. (1951)

Haemoglobin solutions are prepared as for haemoglobin electrophoresis (see below). 3.2 ml of 0.083 N sodium or potassium hydroxide (pH 12.7) are pipetted into a test-tube at room temperature. 0.2 ml of the haemoglobin solution, at a concentration of approximately 10 g/100 ml, is pipetted into the alkali, the mixture agitated vigorously and a stopwatch started. After exactly 1 min, 6.6 ml of acidified 50% saturated ammonium sulphate (50% saturated ammonium sulphate, 800 ml; 10 N HCl, 2 ml) is added and after further vigorous shaking the mixture is filtered. The amount of alkali-resistant haemoglobin is estimated by comparing the optical density (540 nm) of the filtrate with a standard made by adding 0.2 ml of the original haemoglobin solution to 4.8 ml of 0.04% (v/v) ammonia solution. This gives a standard equivalent to 100% haemoglobin. The comparison of standard and control may also be made in a colorimeter with an Ilford 625 filter. Whichever method is used for determining the concentration of haemoglobin it is usually necessary to dilute the standard 1/5 or 1/10 so as to compare the optical densities in approximately the same range. The normal adult range using this method is 0.8–2.5% of alkali-resistant haemoglobin.

Modification of the method of Betke et al. (1959)

The following modification of this method has been found to give highly reproducible values for alkali-resistant haemoglobin in the range 0.5–50% (Pembrey *et al.* 1972).

0.6 ml of a red-cell lysate (approximately 8.0 g/100 ml) is added to 10.0 ml of Drabkin's solution (KCN 0.05 g, K_3FeCN_6 0.20 g, distilled water to 1 l). The dilute haemoglobin solution obtained in this way is used for both test and standard. 0.2 ml of 1.2 N sodium hydroxide is added to 2.8 ml of the haemoglobin solution and the mixture is gently agitated for 2 min. 2.0 ml of saturated ammonium sulphate is then added and, after shaking, the mixture is allowed to stand for at least 5 min before it is filtered through a double layer of Whatman no. 6 filter-paper. The whole procedure is carried out at room temperature. A blank is prepared as follows: cyanmethaemoglobin solution 1.4 ml, distilled water 1.6 ml and saturated ammonium sulphate 2.0 ml. The best results are obtained if the optical density of both test and blank are read at 415 nm. To achieve this it is necessary to dilute the blank 1/10. The percentage fetal haemoglobin is calculated as follows:

$$\frac{OD_{415\,nm} \text{ of test} \times 100}{OD_{415\,nm} \text{ of standard} \times 20}$$

It is most important to ensure that the filtrate is fully clarified, and if necessary it should be refiltered before the optical density is determined.

Estimation of haemoglobin F by HPLC or electrophoresis

Although HbF can be separated from other haemoglobins by HPLC we have found that this method gives unreliable results with HbF levels of less than 5%. This approach can be modified to separate the $^G\gamma$ from the $^A\gamma$ chains. Other electrophoretic methods such as IEF also allow the clear separation of HbF but, again, they are not suitable for measuring low levels.

The normal adult range is 0.2–0.8% alkali-resistant haemoglobin.

The acid elution technique for the intercellular distribution of haemoglobin F (Kleihauer et al. 1957)

The method is based on the principle that HbF is relatively stable at low pH whereas HbA is denatured under these conditions. Blood films are exposed to a low pH buffer, washed and stained. The HbF-containing cells appear deeply stained whereas the cells which contain HbA appear as 'ghosts'.

Reagents

The following agents and stains are required.
(a) Citric acid–phosphate buffer pH 3.3.
   Solution A (0.1 M).
   Dissolve 21.01 g of citric acid monohydrate in 1000 ml of distilled water.
   Solution B (0.2 M).
   Dissolve 35.60 g Na_2HPO_4 in 1000 ml of distilled water.
   Combine 73.4 ml of Solution A with 26.6 of Solution B to give a buffer of pH 3.3; check pH and correct if necessary.
(b) Ethanol: 80 vol%.

Stains

(a) 0.1% of erythrosin in water.

(b) Ehrlich's acid haematoxylin. Dissolve 4.0 g of crystalline haematoxylin in 200 ml 95 vol% ethanol and add 8 ml 10% sodium iodate. Add to this solution 200 ml of water and boil the mixture. After cooling, add 200 ml of glycerine, 6.0 g of aluminium sulphate and 200 ml of glacial acetic acid. Allow solution to stand for at least 14 days.

Method

Thin smears are prepared from capillary blood or venous blood collected into anticoagulants such as heparin, oxalate, citrate or EDTA. Smears are air dried for between 10 and 60 min, fixed in 80 vol% ethanol for 5 min at 20–22°C, rinsed with tap water and air dried. Films are then immersed in the citrate phosphate buffer for 5 min at 37°C and gently agitated for 1 to 3 min. Slides are rinsed with tap water, dried and stained with Ehrlich's acid haematoxylin for 3 min, rinsed with water and dried again. They are counterstained with erythrosin for 3 min. After a final rinse, films are dried and examined under ordinary light microscopy without oil immersion.

Haemoglobin F-containing cells are densely stained with erythrosin, HbA-containing cells appear as ghost cells, while intermediate cells are stained more or less pink. Reticulocytes containing HbA may appear as intermediate cells and/or may show intracellular granulation. Inclusion bodies (Heinz bodies, precipitated α chains or β chains) are seen in eluted cells as compact inclusions of different sizes. Haemoglobin A is eluted regardless of whether it is oxyhaemoglobin, methaemoglobin, cyanmethaemoglobin, reduced haemoglobin or carboxylhaemoglobin.

The analysis of the intercellular distribution of HbF in δβ thalassaemia or HPFH is sometimes helped by raising the pH of the buffer to 3.4.

Immunological detection of haemoglobin F

Production of monoclonal antibody against the γ chain of HbF has greatly improved the detection and quantification of small amounts of HbF in haemolysate as well as within intact red cells. The radial immunodiffusion method for measurement of HbF in haemolysate is simple, but rapid determination of HbF is not feasible. Monoclonal anti-γ-chain antibody can be used to detect erythrocytes containing HbF (F cells) in fixed blood smears after immunofluorescence staining (Wood *et al.* 1975), or by fluorescence-activated cell sorting (FACS) after labelling of the intracellular HbF (Thorpe *et al.* 1994).

A protocol routinely used in our laboratory for the detection of small amounts of HbF in intact red cells is carried out in the following way. The monoclonal antibody against the γ chain of HbF ($\alpha_2\gamma_2$) is a gift from Professor Peter Beverley. Staining is performed on blood smears prepared from whole EDTA blood. It is very important to ensure that the glass slides are grease-free and that only 1-2 μl whole blood is used, so that only one-cell-thick smears are produced. Blood can be stored up to a week prior to making the smears, but it is preferable to prepare them from fresh blood before haemolysis has occurred. Once prepared, air-dried smears can be stored in tissue-paper at room temperature for long periods. (We have successfully stained blood smears that are up to 5 years old.) 'Old' slides need a longer incubation in trypsin; as long as 40 min may be necessary. It is advisable to carry out a time course on a control slide prior to the study. A frequently encountered problem is lysis of the cells, especially after trypsinization, and this is usually due to the incorrect pH of the calcium chloride. We have recently found that trypsin tablets (available from the Sigma Chemical Company) are simple to use and reliable.

This method is a very good alternative to F-cell estimation by FACS and extremely valuable if there is no access to a FACS scan apparatus. Figure 16.4 shows the F-cell distribution in various conditions associated with increased HbF levels.

Materials

The following are prepared.

Cleaned microscope slides. Use prewashed and precleaned slides from BDH: Superfrost (Cat. no. 406/0169/02). Clean slides with acetone followed by ethanol and allow to air dry for at least 1 h.

Prepare 4–5 very thin smears, one-cell thick, per individual using 1–2 μl of fresh blood on the cleaned slides. Allow smears to dry for at least 2 days or, for the best result, for more than 1 week.

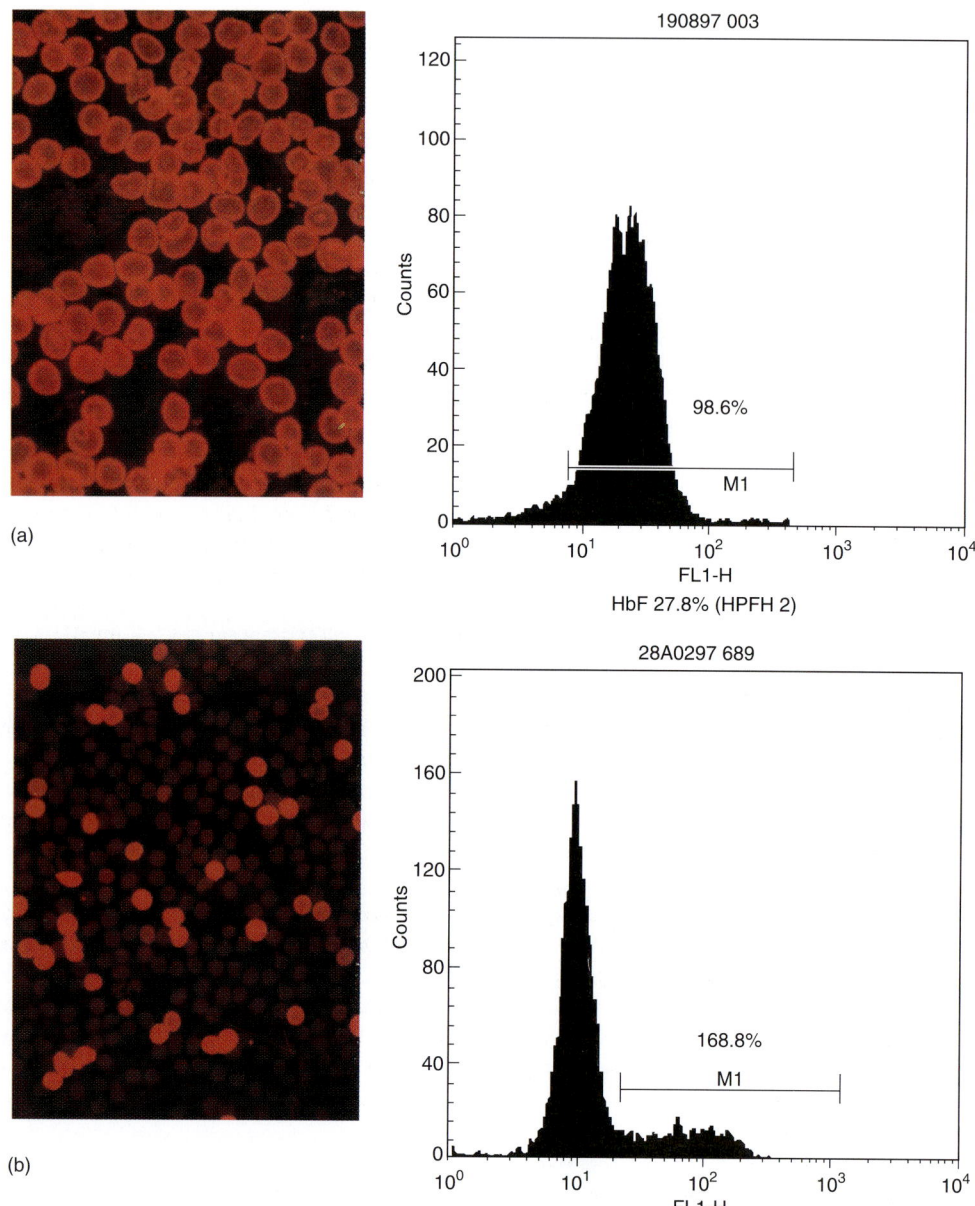

Fig. 16.4 F-cell estimation by (left) staining and (right) fluorescence-activated cell sorting (FACS). (a) A heterozygote for hereditary persistence of fetal haemoglobin (HPFH 2). (b) Heterocellular HPFH. M1; gate width for normal cell population.

Acetone/ethanol/methanol (6/2/2 v/v)

Phosphate-buffered saline (PBS) Sigma P-4417

Trypsin solution. 0.1% trypsin in 0.1% calcium chloride ($CaCl_2$) at pH 7.8. Prepare 10 ml solution (10 mg of trypsin (ICN; Cat. no. 150213) + 10 mg $CaCl_2$ + 10 ml distilled water) and store at –20°C in 1-ml aliquots. Alternatively, use trypsin tablets (Sigma; Cat. no. T-7168). Dissolve one tablet in 1 ml deionized water, store at –20°C in 10-µl aliquots. Before use, make up to 500 µl (i.e. add 490 µl) with deionized water.

Prewarm to 37°C before use. *Note*: pH of CaCl$_2$ is very important.

Anti-monoclonal antibody. Undiluted supernatant.

Tetramethylrodamine isothiocyanate (TRITC) conjugate antimouse IgG (Sigma T-6653). Store frozen in 10-µl aliquots. Working solution: dilute 1/32 in PBS.

Humidity chamber. Moist tissue in plastic chamber.

Glycerol/PBS (1/1v/v) or *antifade Vectashield*, mounting medium for fluorescence (Vector; Cat. no. H-1000).

Method

The following steps should be followed.

1 Mark on the smear a small area of approximately 5 mm diameter using a diamond cutter.

2 Fix smears in acetone/ethanol/methanol fixative for 20 min. Air dry for 2 min (do not overdry).

3 Rehydrate in PBS for 5 min (use plenty of PBS in a large glass container) and then rinse very briefly in distilled water. Air dry.

4 Cover the circled area with 8 µl *prewarmed* (37°C) trypsin solution and incubate at 37°C for 15 min in humidity chamber. *Note*: time of trypsinization varies with age of slides but generally 15 min is sufficient.

5 Wash in PBS for 5 min with gentle agitation and rinse in distilled water. Air dry.

6 Cover trypsinized area with 5–10 µl anti-γ antibody, incubate at 37°C in humidity chamber for 30–40 min.

7 Wash as before and air dry.

8 Cover circled area with 5–10 µl fluorescent antimouse IgG and incubate at 37°C for 20–30 min in the humidity chamber.

9 Wash as before with PBS, rinse in distilled water, air dry.

10 Mount in glycerol/PBS or antifade.

We generally count ~1000 red cells, which corresponds to four to five high-power fields. The number of fields, of course, depends on the density of cells. Hence, it is very important to master the art of making thin blood smears.

Determination of proportion of F cells by fluorescence-activated cell sorting (FACS)

Materials

The following are required.

4% PBS/formaldehyde. For 10 ml, add
1 ml of '40% formaldehyde stock';
1 ml 10×PBS; and
8 ml of deionized water
NB: Formaldehyde is sold as 40%; '40% formaldehyde stock' is thus 16% formaldehyde and final fixative is actually 1.6% PBS/formaldehyde.

Ice bucket at –15°C to –20°C. Fill a quarter of the ice bucket with dry ice. Make a mix of 9/10 wet ice and 1/10 NaCl and add to the dry ice. Use a thermometer and do not just estimate temperature.

Precooled acetone. Keep in ice bucket at –15°C to –20°C.

Precooled acetone/water (50/50). Keep in ice bucket at –15°C to –20°C.

10% albumin. Make from 35% solution, Bovine Fraction V; Sigma A-8918.

Anti-γ-globin-chain antibody. Dilute antibody (neat supernatant) with 10% albumin (1/1) before use.

FITC conjugate. Antimouse IgG (whole molecule, absorbed with human serum proteins); Sigma No. F-2012. Store in 50-µl aliquots at –20°C. Before use, add 1 ml PBS and 1 ml albumin 10% to 50-µl aliquot.

PBS. (Sigma phosphate-buffered saline tablets; Sigma P-4417.)

Fixation and permeabilization of erythrocytes

Attention to details of timing and temperature of the acetone and acetone/water steps are very important; inadequate fixation with over-permeabilization will lead to lysis of the red cells, while under-permeabilization will result in poor staining. The following steps should be followed.

1 Wash 80–100 µl blood (collected in EDTA) three

times with PBS, for 2 min at 1500 r.p.m. in microfuge at room temperature.

2 Fix the red cells by adding 40 µl packed red cells to 1 ml 4% PBS/formaldehyde. Gently vortex and leave for 20 min at room temperature.

3 Pellet the red cells by centrifuging at very low speed (1500 r.p.m.) for 2 min at room temperature, remove most of the supernatant and resuspend the cell pellet by gentle vortexing.

4 Transfer all the red cells to a 10-ml polypropylene Falcon tube containing 3 ml of acetone/water (50/50) precooled at −15°C and *incubate for 2 min at 5°C*.

5 Pellet the cells again by centrifuging for 2 min at 1000 r.p.m. at 4°C, remove supernatant and resuspend pellet by gentle vortexing. Add 3 ml of acetone precooled at −15°C and *incubate for 5 min at 5°C*.

6 Repellet the cells by centrifuging for 4 min, 1000 r.p.m. at 4°C, remove supernatant and resuspend pellet by gentle vortexing. Add 3 ml of acetone/water 50/50 precooled at −15°C and *incubate for 2 min at 5°C*.

7 Repellet the cells by centrifugation for 2 min at 1000 r.p.m. at 4°C, remove supernatant and resuspend pellet by gentle vortexing.

8 Set the centrifuge at 20°C and wash the cells in 10 ml PBS at room temperature.

Immunostaining of erythrocytes

The following steps are followed:

1 Pellet the cells by centrifugation at 1000 r.p.m. for 2 min at 20°C. Remove the supernatant and incubate the pellet for 20 min with 60 µl diluted anti-γ antibody at room temperature, with gentle agitation.

2 Wash with 10 ml PBS at room temperature as before and incubate the pellet for 20 min with 60 µl diluted FITC antimouse IgG at room temperature, with gentle agitation.

3 Wash the cells with 10 ml PBS at room temperature, as before, and resuspend the pellet in 2–3 ml PBS for analysis by flow cytometry.

If the sample is not used immediately, store at 4°C in the dark.

Measurement of α-/β-globin synthesis ratios

As mentioned earlier, routine haematological and haemoglobin electrophoresis studies may not always suffice to characterize adequately some of the thalas-saemia disorders, particularly the α-thalassaemia carrier states or the interactions of α and β thalassaemia.

The methods used in our laboratory for measuring rates of globin synthesis are little changed from those that were described in the original publications in the mid- and late 1960s, except for the addition of a few minor modifications to conditions to suit specific purposes (Clegg *et al.* 1965, 1966, 1968a; Clegg 1983). One significant improvement, however, is the introduction of a technique for the removal of white cells from peripheral blood samples (Beutler *et al.* 1976) prior to incubation with radioactive amino acids. This is particularly useful for samples with low reticulocyte counts, where background contamination from white-cell proteins can cause serious problems with the accurate determination of α-/β-globin synthesis ratios.

Reagents

All chemicals should be analytical reagent (AR) grade whenever possible.

α Cellulose. SIGMA C-8002.

Microcrystalline cellulose. Sigma cell type 50 S-5504.

Reticulocyte saline (RS). 0.13 M NaCl, 0.005 M KCl, 0.0074 M $MgCl_2.6H_2O$.

^3H-leucine. L-4,5-^{3}H-leucine (Amersham) 50 Ci/mM in aqueous solution containing 2% ethanol.

Incubation mixture (IM)

The mixture is made up as follows:

1 54 ml amino acid mixture, made up in RS;
2 2.7 ml 0.25 M $MgCl_2$ with 10% glucose, made up in RS;
3 27 ml 0.164 M Tris HCl pH 7.75 made up in H_2O;
4 21.6 ml 0.01 M trisodium citrate, made up in dialysed group AB plasma; and
5 32 ml 0.01 M $NaHCO_3$, made up in dialysed AB plasma.

Dialysed plasma
AB plasma dialysed exhaustively at 4°C against multiple changes of RS.

Amino acid mixture

Amino acids (10×concentration): weight in mg dissolved in final 100 ml H_2O.

Alanine	178
Arginine	87
Aspartic acid	379
Asparagine	264
Glycine	398
Glutamine	1169
Histidine	372
Isoleucine	39
Lysine	263
Methionine	45
Phenylalanine	264
Proline	161
Serine	173
Threonine	202
Tryptophan	61
Tyrosine	145
Cysteine	48

To be diluted 1/10 before use. Check pH and adjust if necessary to 7.75 with NaOH. If a labelled amino acid other than leucine is used, omit the unlabelled amino acid from this mixture and replace with leucine (1312 mg).

The final incubation mixture can be sterilized by filtration, first through a glass-fibre filter and then through a 0.22-μm pore-size Millipore filter and stored frozen at –20°C.

Incubation of reticulocyte-rich peripheral blood cells and preparation of globin

Ten to 20 ml of peripheral blood in heparin is centrifuged at about $3000\,g$ at 4°C for 10 min and the plasma removed. As much as possible of the buffy coat (white cells that have spun up to the plasma–red-cell interface) are removed with a wooden stick. The blood is then washed three times in reticulocyte saline (RS) at 4°C and in between each wash more buffy coat is removed. Finally the cells are suspended in RS and spun hard at 35 500 r.p.m. in a Beckman SW40 rotor at 4°C for 30 min to enrich the reticulocyte fraction. The top 700 μl (0.7 ml) reticulocyte-rich fraction is removed and added to 50 ml RS.

While the red cells are being washed a slurry of 3 parts α cellulose and 1 part microcrystalline cellu-lose in 30 ml RS is allowed to swell for 10 min before being poured into a plugged 10-ml syringe to make a 3–4-ml column. The red-cell suspension is layered on to the top of the column and washed in with more RS. The eluate contains mature red cells and reticulocytes, but not white cells, which remain bound to the cellulose.

The eluted cells are recovered by centrifugation at $3000\,g$ at 4°C, suspended in 1.3 ml of incubation mixture (IM), and 0.075 ml of a solution of ferrous ammonium sulphate (10 mg/10 ml RS) is added. This cell suspension is preincubated for 10 min at 37°C in a shaking water bath to start the metabolism of the cells, after which 200 μCi ^{3}H-leucine are added, and the incubation is continued for 60 min. The incubation is stopped by the addition of an excess of cold (4°C) RS and the cells are washed three times in ice-cold RS. After the final wash the supernatant is removed and globin prepared from the cells. The cell pellet is lysed in 3 ml distilled water and the lysate is dropped into 20 volumes of acid–acetone containing a few μl of mercaptoethanol (2% conc. HCl in acetone) at –20°C, and the mixture allowed to stand at –20°C for 20 min for full globin precipitation. (A sufficient excess of acid–acetone over sample and low temperature of precipitation are important. Failure to observe these points may result in globin which is unsatisfactory for subsequent chromatography.)

The globin precipitate is washed four times in acetone at –20°C, using only gentle spins (15, 20, 25 and 30 s sequentially) at the centrifugation steps, as compacting the precipitate will prevent adequate removal of the acid–acetone. Finally, the globin is washed in ether, pelleted by centrifugation for 35 s and allowed to air dry. It may be stored at –20°C.

Chromatographic separation of globin

An 8 M urea solution (freshly prepared from AR reagent—the solution should not be heated) is filtered through Whatman no. 3 paper and made 0.05 M in 2-mercaptoethanol and sufficient Na_2HPO_4 added to establish the required initial Na^+ concentration (see below). The pH is then adjusted to the required value with 20% H_3PO_4. This solution is the *starting buffer* (SB).

A CM 23 carboxymethyl cellulose slurry (2.5 g in

50 ml SB) is prepared and poured into a 1.5 cm × 25-cm column to give a bed height of about 15–20 cm. The column is washed at a flow rate of 0.5 ml/min with SB for about 1 h. In the meantime the globin sample (15–60 mg) is dissolved in 2 ml of SB and dialysed for 1 h against two changes of 50 ml SB. The dialysed sample is then applied to the column and washed in with 2–3 ml SB. SB is then pumped through the column at 0.5 ml/min for 30–40 min to allow unbound material (non-haem proteins, membrane proteins, residual haem derivatives, etc.) to elute from the column before the gradient is started. Fractions (5 ml) are collected and the absorbance of the effluent is monitored at 280 nm.

For most purposes a linear Na^+ ion gradient, made by mixing 200 ml SB with 200 ml *limit buffer* is satisfactory, but in certain circumstances this can be modified. We have found, for example, that an exponential gradient made in a three-chamber apparatus is especially useful for extended γ-/β-chain separations and bone-marrow incubations.

Radioactivity is determined by counting aliquots of the collected fractions in an appropriate scintillant. It is usually best to add some water to prevent urea precipitation. For routine purposes we use 0.4 ml sample, 0.1 ml H_2O and 5 ml emulsifier scintillant (Packard 299). Specific activities are determined by dialysing the contents of the peak tubes against three 12-h changes of 0.5% HCOOH, measuring the 280-nm absorbance and counting a known volume. Corrections are made for the differences in absorbance of α, β and γ chains. We use the values originally given by Schwartz *et al.* (1969): α 0.56; β 0.84; γ 1.12.

After plotting out the radioactivity profile the total counts in each globin peak can be determined by adding the counts for the appropriate tubes, after subtracting the background counts. This method is more reliable than pooling tubes from peaks, measuring the volume and then counting an aliquot, since inspection of the radioactivity profile can often indicate problems that may have arisen during chromatography.

Buffer conditions

Normal separations: starting buffer (200 ml) 0.008 M Na_2HPO_4, pH 6.4; limit buffer (200 ml) 0.034 M Na_2HPO_4, pH 6.4. For extended γ/β separations use three gradient chambers with the first two containing starting buffer and the third limit buffer. Starting buffer (2 × 200 ml) 0.012 M Na_2HPO_4, pH 6.0; limit buffer (200 ml) 0.040 M Na_2HPO_4, pH 6.0.

The CM-cellulose system can be used over a wide range of pH and salt concentrations and we strongly urge anyone trying these methods for the first time to experiment to establish the optimum conditions for their own particular circumstances. Attention should also be paid to the accuracy of the pH of the starting buffer.

The interpretation of the results of globin synthesis using this approach are discussed in detail in Chapter 5.

Other methods for measuring globin synthesis

Several other chromatographic or electrophoretic approaches to globin synthesis have been described, largely directed at prenatal diagnosis in the pre-DNA period (see Alter 1989). Although they give a quantitative assessment of globin production, because it is not possible to obtain specific activity data, their use is limited.

DNA analysis

Some of the numerous techniques of DNA analysis that have been developed to diagnose the various globin-gene mutations and deletions are reviewed in the following section. In most cases there are several methods available for the diagnosis of any one particular mutation and the practical details of the methods described here are simply the ones we have had most experience of in our laboratory, and those which have given us reliable results over the years.

α Thalassaemia

The α-thalassaemia alleles consist of either deletion mutations in and around the globin-gene cluster or point mutations within one of the two globin genes. The deletion breakpoints of four of the most common deletions have now been sequenced and these alleles can now be diagnosed by the polymerase chain reaction (PCR) using the technique sometimes known as gap PCR. The other deletion alleles have to be diagnosed by Southern blot analysis and this approach remains in use in many laboratories for the molecular diagnosis of α thalassaemia because of its ability to diagnose all alleles in one test.

PCR for deletion mutations

The five most common α^0-thalassaemia deletion genes, the $--^{FIL}$, $--^{MED}$, $-(\alpha)^{20.5}$, $--^{THAI}$ and the $--^{SEA}$ alleles, can be diagnosed by a PCR-based technique called gap PCR (Bowden *et al.* 1992; Dodé *et al.* 1993; Baysal & Huisman 1994; Ko & Li 1999; Liu *et al.* 2000) (Table 16.3). Gap PCR is the simplest of amplification techniques, using two primers complementary to the sense and antisense strand of the DNA regions flanking the deletion. Amplified product is obtained only from the thalassaemia deletion allele as the primers are too far apart to amplify successfully the normal DNA sequence. Therefore the normal allele (α) is detected by amplifying the DNA sequences spanning one of the breakpoints, using a primer complementary to the deleted sequence. The two common α^+-thalassaemia deletions, $-\alpha^{3.7}$ and $-\alpha^{4.2}$, can also be detected by PCR methods (Dodé *et al.* 1993; Baysal &

Huisman 1994; Liu *et al.* 2000) but none of the published protocols are yet sufficiently robust for them to be recommended as the *sole* diagnostic approach.

PCR for point mutations

The non-deletion α^+-thalassaemia mutations can be identified by PCR using the technique of selective amplification of the α-globin genes (Molchanova *et al.* 1994b). Each gene's amplified product is then analysed for the appropriate known mutation or sequenced to identify new ones. Several of the non-deletion mutations alter a restriction-enzyme site and may be analysed for restriction-enzyme digestion, in a similar manner to that reported for the mutation creating the variant Hb Constant Spring (Ko *et al.* 1993b). In theory any other technique for the direct detection of point mutations, such as allele-specific oligonucleotide hybridization or allele-

Table 16.3 Thalassaemia deletion mutations which have been diagnosed by gap PCR.

Disorder	Deletion mutation	Reference
α^0 thalassaemia	$--^{SEA}$	Molchanova *et al.* (1994b)
	$--^{MED}$	Molchanova *et al.* (1994b)
	$-(\alpha)^{20.5}$	Molchanova *et al.* (1994b)
	$--^{FIL}$	Ko & Li (1999)
	$--^{THAI}$	Liu *et al.* (2000)
α^+ thalassaemia	$-\alpha^{3.7}$	Baysal & Huisman (1994)
	$-\alpha^{4.2}$	Baysal & Huisman (1994)
β^0 thalassaemia	290-bp deletion	Faa *et al.* (1992)
	532-bp deletion	Waye *et al.* (1991)
	619-bp deletion	Old *et al.* (1990)
	1393-bp deletion	Thein *et al.* (1989)
	1605-bp deletion	Dimovski *et al.* (1993)
	3.5-kb deletion	Lynch *et al.* (1991)
	10.3-kb deletion	Craig *et al.* (1992)
	45-kb deletion	Waye *et al.* (1994b)
Hb Lepore	Hb Lepore	Craig *et al.* (1994)
$(\delta\beta)^0$ thalassaemia	Spanish	Craig *et al.* (1994)
	Sicilian	Craig *et al.* (1994)
	Vietnamese	Craig *et al.* (1994)
	Macedonian/Turkish	Craig *et al.* (1994)
$(^A\gamma\delta\beta)^0$ thalassaemia	Indian	Craig *et al.* (1994)
	Chinese	Craig *et al.* (1994)
HPFH	HPFH 1	Craig *et al.* (1994)
	HPFH 2	Craig *et al.* (1994)
	HPFH 3	Craig *et al.* (1994)

specific priming, may be used for the diagnosis of non-deletion α^+-thalassaemia. However, the only strategy reported to date for the diagnosis of all the known point mutations involves the combined application of the indirect detection methods of denaturing gradient gel electrophoresis (DGGE) and single-strand conformation analysis (SSCA), followed by direct DNA sequencing (Harteveld *et al.* 1996b).

Southern blot analysis

All of the common α-thalassaemia deletion mutations plus the triple and quadruple gene alleles can be diagnosed routinely by Southern blot analysis using a combination of restriction enzyme digests and gene probes. A list of the characteristic abnormal restriction fragments which are used in our laboratory for diagnostic purposes is presented in Table 16.4. A *Bam*H I digest hybridized to an α-globin-gene probe is used to identify the single, double, triple and quadruple α-globin-gene alleles and it also provides a diagnostic test for the Mediterranean α^0-thalassaemia deletion gene $-(\alpha)^{20.5}$. A *Bam*H I digest hybridized to a ζ-globin-gene probe provides a diagnostic test for the $--^{SEA}$ α^0-thalassaemia allele and, similarly, a *Bgl* II digest hybridized to a ζ-globin-gene probe is used to identify the $--^{MED}$ allele. Diagnosis of most of the α-thalassaemia alleles requires the interpretation of the results from two different enzyme digests and probe hybridizations, usually a *Bam*H I/α-probe blot and a *Bgl* II/ζ-probe blot. This is because several alleles have similar-sized abnormal *Bgl* II/ζ-probe fragments, and some have similar sizes to normal gene fragments. For example both the $-\alpha^{3.7}$ and $\alpha\alpha\alpha$ alleles yield a 16-kb *Bgl* II/ζ fragment, the $-\alpha^{4.2}$, $--^{SA}$ and $--^{BRIT}$ alleles yield similar-sized 7–8-kb *Bgl* II/ζ fragments, and the $--^{SEA}$ allele yields fragments which can be confused with a 10.5-kb normal fragment. A combination of *Bam*H I and *Bgl* II digestions (Fig. 16.5) can be used for the diagnosis of all the common α-thalassaemia deletion genes

Table 16.4 The diagnosis of thalassaemia and other alleles by Southern blotting.

| Allele | Restriction enzyme/gene probe | | | | |
	*Bam*H I/α	*Bgl* II/α	*Bam*H I/ζ	*Bgl* II/ζ	*Sst* I/LO
$\alpha\alpha$	14	12.6 7.4	10–11.3 5.9	12.6 or 5.2 10–11.3	5.0
$\alpha\alpha\alpha$	<u>18</u>	12.6 7.4	10–11.3 5.9	12.6 or <u>13</u> 10–11.3	5.0
$\alpha\alpha\alpha\alpha$	<u>22</u>	12.6 7.4	10–11.3 5.9	12.6 or <u>20</u> 10–11.3	5.0
$-\alpha^{3.7}$	<u>10.3</u>	<u>16</u>	10–11.3 5.9	<u>16</u> 10–11.3	5.0
$-\alpha^{4.2}$	<u>9.8</u>	<u>8.0</u> 7.4	10–11.3 5.9	10–11.3 <u>8.0</u>	5.0
$-(\alpha)^{20.5}$	<u>4.0</u>	<u>10.8</u>	5.9	<u>10.8</u>	5.0
$--^{MED}$	None	None	5.9	<u>13.9</u>	5.0
$--^{SEA}$	None	None	<u>20</u> 5.9	<u>10.5</u>	5.0
$--^{SA}$	None	None	5.9	<u>7.0</u>	5.0
$--^{BRIT}$	None	None	5.9	<u>7.5</u>	5.0
$--^{THAI}$	None	None	None	None	<u>8.0</u>
$--^{FIL}$	None	None	None	None	<u>7.4</u>

Fragment sizes are given in kilobase pairs. Characteristic abnormal fragments are underlined.

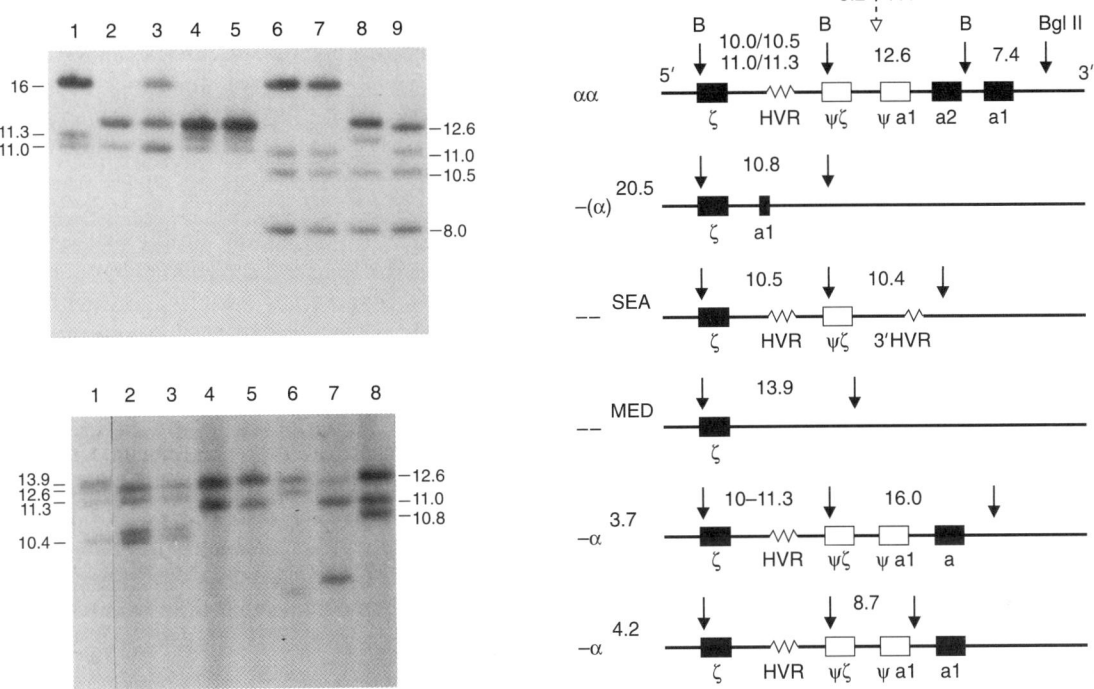

Fig. 16.5 Two Southern blots showing *Bgl* II-digested DNA from persons with normal and α-thalassaemia alleles hybridized to a ζ-globin-gene probe, together with maps illustrating positions of the *Bgl* II sites. The genotypes and approximate band sizes in kilobase pairs (in parentheses) for each DNA track are:
Upper blot: 1, $-\alpha^{3.7}/-\alpha^{3.7}$ (16/11.3/11.0); 2, αα/αα (12.6/11.0); 3: $-\alpha^{3.7}/\alpha\alpha$ (16/12.6/11.0); 4, αα/αα (12.6/11.3/11.0); 5, αα/αα (12.6/11.3/11.0); 6, $-\alpha^{3.7}/-\alpha^{4.2}$ (16/11.0/10.5/8.0); 7, $-\alpha^{3.7}/-\alpha^{4.2}$ (16/11.0/10.5/8.0); 8, $-\alpha^{4.2}/\alpha\alpha$ (12.6/11.3/10.5/8.0); 9, $-\alpha^{4.2}/\alpha\alpha$ (12.6/11.0/10.5/8.0).
Lower blot: 1, $--^{MED}/\alpha\alpha$ (13.9/12.6/11.3/10.4); 2, $--^{SEA}/\alpha\alpha$ (12.6/11.3/10.5/10.4); 3, $--^{SEA}/\alpha\alpha$ (12.6/11.3/10.5/10.4); 4, αα/αα (12.6/10.5); 5, αα/αα (12.6/10.5); 6, $--^{BRIT}/\alpha\alpha$ (12.6/11.3/7.5); 7, $-\alpha^{4.2}/\alpha\alpha$ (12.6/11.0/8.0); 8, $-(\alpha)^{20.5}/\alpha\alpha$ (12.6/11.0/10.8).
The inter-ζ-gene hypervariable region gives rise to normal DNA fragments of variable band sizes. There are four common *Bgl* II band sizes (10.0, 10.5, 11.0 and 11.3 kb), one per chromosome. A duplicated ζ-globin-gene allele gives two bands per chromosome. The ψζ gene contains two small variable regions, which give rise to occasional variation in the size of the 12.6-kb *Bgl* II fragment. There is a polymorphic *Bgl* II site, which, when present, reduces the 12.6-kb and $-\alpha^{3.7}$ 16-kb fragments to a 5.2-kb fragment. The polymorphic site is usually linked to a 10.5-kb normal fragment.

except for the $--^{THAI}$ and $--^{FIL}$ deletions. These two alleles are diagnosed using an *Sst* I digest hybridized to a DNA probe (named LO) located down-stream from the ζ-globin gene (Fischel-Ghodsian *et al.* 1988).

β Thalassaemia

Although about 200 different β-thalassaemia mutations have been characterized, analysis of the fre-

quency of the mutations in most at-risk populations have shown that only approximately 20 occur at a frequency of 1% or greater and thus account for the majority of the mutations world-wide (Huisman 1990) (see Chapter 6). All of the mutations are regionally specific and the spectrum of mutations for individual populations has now been determined; each has been found to have just a few common mutations together with a larger and more variable number of rare ones.

The strategy for identifying β-thalassaemia mutations in most diagnostic laboratories depends on knowing the spectrum of common and rare mutations in the ethnic group of the individual being screened. Usually the common ones are analysed first using a PCR technique which allows the detection of multiple mutations simultaneously. This approach will identify the mutation in more than 90% of cases and then a further screening for the possible rare mutation will identify the defect in most of the remaining cases. Mutations remaining unidentified after this second screening are characterized by direct DNA sequence analysis, usually following the localization of the site of the mutation by the application of a non-specific detection method such as DGGE. Although a bewildering variety of PCR techniques have been described for the diagnosis of point mutations, most diagnostic laboratories are using one or more of the techniques described below.

PCR: allele-specific oligonucleotides

The hybridization of allele-specific oligonucleotide (ASO) probes to amplified genomic DNA bound to a nylon membrane in the form of dots was the first PCR method to be developed. The method is based on the use of two oligonucleotide probes for each mutation, one complementary to the mutant DNA sequence and the other complementary to the normal gene sequence at the same position. The probes are usually 5′ end-labelled with either ^{32}P-labelled deoxynucleoside triphosphates, biotin or horseradish peroxidase. The genotype of the DNA sample is determined by the presence or absence of the hybridization signal of both the mutation-specific and normal probe. The technique has been applied in many laboratories with great success, especially for populations with just one common mutation and a small number of rare ones, such as Sardinia (Ristaldi *et al.* 1989). However, when screening for a large number of different mutations the method becomes limited by the need for separate hybridization and washing steps for each mutation.

To overcome the problem of screening for multiple mutations, a method of reverse dot blotting has been developed in which the roles of the oligonucleotide probe and the amplified genomic DNA are reversed (Saiki *et al.* 1989). Unlabelled oligonucleotide probes complementary to the mutant and normal DNA

sequences are fixed to a nylon membrane strip in the form of dots or slots. Amplified genomic DNA, labelled by either the use of end-labelled primers or the internal incorporation of biotinylated dUTP, is then hybridized to the filter. This procedure allows multiple mutations to be tested for in one hybridization reaction. It has been applied to the diagnosis of β-thalassaemia mutations in Mediterraneans (Maggio *et al.* 1993), Afro-Americans (Sutcharitchan *et al.* 1995) and Thais (Newton *et al.* 1989), using a two-step procedure with one nylon strip for the common mutations and another for the less common ones.

PCR: primer-specific amplification

A number of different methods have been developed based on the principle of primer-specific amplification, which is that a perfectly matched PCR primer is much more efficient in annealing and directing primer extension than a mismatched one. With the method known as the amplification refractory mutation system (ARMS) (Newton *et al.* 1989), the target DNA is amplified using a common primer and either of two allele-specific primers, one complementary to the mutation to be detected (β-thalassaemia primer) and the other complementary to normal DNA at the same position in the sequence (normal primer). A second pair of primers complementary to a different part of the β-globin gene is included in the PCR to amplify a fragment simultaneously in order to control the amplification step of the procedure. The method provides a quick screening method which does not require any form of labelling, as the amplified products are visualized simply by agarose gel electrophoresis and ethidium bromide staining, as is described in detail in the next section. Details of the mutation-specific and normal-sequence-specific primers used in our laboratory to diagnose the common β-thalassaemia mutations are presented in Tables 16.5 and 16.6. More than one mutation may be screened for at the same time in a single PCR reaction (multiplexing), provided the ARMS primers are coupled with the same common primer (Tan *et al.* 1994). Fluorescent labelling of the common primer allows the sizing of the amplification products on an automated DNA fragment analyser (Zschocke & Graham 1995).

If the normal and mutant ARMS primers for a spe-

Table 16.5 Primer sequences used for the detection of the common β-thalassaemia mutations by the allele-specific priming technique.

Mutation	Oligonucleotide sequence	Second primer	Product size (bp)
–88 (C→T)	TCACTTAGACCTCACCCTGTGGAGCCTCAT	A	684
–87 (C→G)	CACTTAGACCTCACCCTGTGGAGCCACCCG	A	683
–30(T→A)	GCAGGGAGGGCAGGAGCCAGGGCTGGGGAA	A	626
–29 (A→G)	CAGGGAGGGCAGGAGCCAGGGCTGGGTATG	A	625
–28 (A→G)	AGGGAGGGCAGGAGCCAGGGCTGGGCTTAG	A	624
CAP +1 (A→G)	ATAAGTCAGGGCAGAGCCATCTATTGGTTC	A	597
CD5 (–CT)	TCAAACAGACACCATGGTGCACCTGAGTCG	A	528
CD6 (–A)	CCCACAGGGCAGTAACGGCAGACTTCTGCC	B	207
CD8 (–AA)	ACACCATGGTGCACCTGACTCCTGAGCAGG	A	520
CD8/9 (+G)	CCTTGCCCCACAGGGCAGTAACGGCACACC	B	225
CD15 (G→A)	TGAGGAGAAGTCTGCCGTTACTGCCCAGTA	A	500
CD16 (–C)	TCACCACCAACTTCATCCACGTTCACGTTC	B	238
CD17 (A→T)	CTCACCACCAACTTCAGCCACGTTCAGCTA	B	239
CD24 (T→A)	CTTGATACCAACCTGCCCAGGGCCTCTCCT	B	262
CD39 (C→T)	CAGATCCCCAAAGGACTCAAAGAACCTGTA	B	436
CD41/42 (–TCTT)	GAGTGGACAGATCCCCAAAGGACTCAACCT	B	439
CD71–72 (+A)	CATGGCAAGAAAGTGCTCGGTGCCTTTAAG	C	241
IVS1-1 (G→A)	TTAAACCTGTCTTGTAACCTTGATACCGAT	B	281
IVS1-1 (G→T)	TTAAACCTGTCTTGTAACCTTGATACCGAAA	B	281
IVS1-5 (G→C)	CTCCTTAAACCTGTCTTGTAACCTTGTTAG	B	285
IVS1-6 (T→C)	TCTCCTTAAACCTGTCTTGTAACCTTCATG	B	286
IVS1-110 (G→A)	ACCAGCAGCCTAAGGGTGGGAAAATAGAGT	B	419
IVS2-1 (G→A)	AAGAAAACATCAAGGGTCCCATAGACTGAT	B	634
IVS2-654 (C→T)	GAATAACAGTGATAATTTCTGGGTTAACGT*	D	829
IVS2-745 (C→G)	TCATATTGCTAATAGCAGCTACAATCGAGG*	D	738
βˢCD6 (A→T)	CCCACAGGGCAGTAACGGCAGACTTCTGCA	B	207
βᶜCD6 (G→A)	CCACAGGGCAGTAACGGCAGACTTCTCGTT	B	206
βᴱCD26 (G→A)	TAACCTTGATACCAACCTGCCCAGGGCGTT	B	236

The above primers are coupled as indicated with primers A, B, C or D:
A   CCCCTTCCTATGACATGAACTTAA;
B   ACCTCACCCTGTGGAGCCAC;
C   TTCGTCTGTTTCCCATTCTAAACT; or
D   GAGTCAAGGCTGAGAGATGCAGGA.
The control primers used for all the above mutation-specific ARMS primers except the two marked * are primers D plus E: CAATGTATCATGCCTCTTTGCACC. For IVS2-654 (C→T) and IVS2-745 (C→G), the ᴳγ-*Hind* III restriction-fragment-length polymorphism (RFLP) primers (Table 16.6) are used as control primers.

cific mutation are coamplified in the same reaction they compete with each other to amplify the target sequence. This technique is called competitive oligonucleotide priming (COP) and requires the two ARMS primers to be labelled differently. Fluorescent labels permit a diagnosis to be made by means of a colour complementation assay (Chehab & Kan 1989). A variation of this method is simply to use ARMS primers that differ in length and thus a diagnosis can made by analysis of the two product sizes.

This technique, called mutagenetically separated polymerase chain reaction (MS-PCR), has been applied to the prenatal diagnosis of thalassaemia in Taiwan (Chang *et al.* 1995a).

PCR: restriction-enzyme analysis

More than 40 β-thalassaemia mutations are known to create or abolish a restriction endonuclease site (Table 16.7). The majority of these can be

Table 16.6 Primer sequences used for the detection of the normal DNA sequence by the allele-specific priming technique.

Mutation	Oligonucleotide sequence	Second primer	Product size (bp)
–87 (C→G)	CACTTAGACCTCACCCTGTGGAGCCACCCCA	A	683
CD5 (–CT)	CAAACAGACACCATGGTGCACCTGACTCCT	A	528
CD8 (–AA)	ACACCATGGTGCACCTGACTCCTGAGCAGA	A	520
CD8/9 (+G)	CCTTGCCCCACAGGGCAGTAACGGCACACT	B	225
CD15 (G→A)	TGAGGAGAAGTCTGCCGTTACTGCCCAGTA	A	500
CD39 (C→T)	TTAGGCTGCTGGTGGTCTACCCTTGGTCCC	A	299
CD41/42 (–TCTT)	GAGTGGACAGATCCCCAAAGGACTCAAAGA	B	439
IVS1-1 (G→A)	TTAAACCTGTCTTGTAACCTTGATACCCAC	B	281
IVS1-1 (G→T)	GATGAAGTTGGTGGTGAGGCCCTGGGTAGG	A	455
IVS1-5 (G→C)	CTCCTTAAACCTGTCTTGTAACCTTGTTAC	B	285
IVS1-6 (T→C)	AGTTGGTGGTGAGGCCCTGGGCAGGTTGGT	A	449
IVS1-110 (G→A)	ACCAGCAGCCTAAGGGTGGGAAAATACACC	B	419
IVS2-1 (G→A)	AAGAAAACATCAAGGGTCCCATAGACTGAC	B	634
IVS2-654 (C→T)	GAATAACAGTGATAATTTCTGGGTTAACGC	D	829
IVS2-745 (C→G)	TCATATTGCTAATAGCAGCTACAATCGAGC	D	738
β^SCD6 (A→T)	AACAGACACCATGGTGCACCTGACTCGTGA	A	527
β^ECD26 (G→A)	TAACCTTGATACCAACCTGCCCAGGGCGTC	B	236

See Table 16.5 footnote for details of primers A–D and control primers.

detected quickly by restriction endonuclease analysis of amplified DNA. The presence or absence of the enzyme recognition site is determined from the pattern of digested fragments after agarose or poly-acrylamide gel electrophoresis. As a screening method, this approach is limited by the small fraction of thalassaemia mutations that affect a restriction-enzyme site and also because some of the restriction enzymes involved are very expensive to purchase.

Mutations which do not naturally create or abolish restriction sites may be diagnosed by the technique of amplification-created restriction sites (ACRS). This method uses primers that are designed to insert new bases into the amplified product in order to create a restriction-enzyme recognition site adjacent to the mutation sequence. This permits known mutations that normally do not alter a recognition site to be detected by restriction-enzyme digestion of the PCR product. This technique has been applied to the detection of Mediterranean β-thalassaemia muta-tions (Lindeman *et al.* 1991).

Gap PCR

Deletion mutations in the globin-gene sequence may be detected by PCR using two primers complemen-tary to the sense and antisense strand in the DNA regions which flank the deletion (Faa *et al.* 1992). For large deletions, amplified product using flanking primers is obtained only from the deletion allele as the distance between the two primers is too great to amplify normal DNA. In such cases the normal allele may be detected by amplifying sequences spanning one of the breakpoints, using a primer complemen-tary to the deleted sequence and one complementary to flanking DNA (Waye *et al.* 1994b). As well as dele-tion thalassaemia, the deletions in the globin-gene cluster which result in Hb Lepore and a number of δβ-thalassaemia and HPFH mutations can be diag-nosed by this method (Table 16.4) (Craig *et al.* 1994). The diagnosis of the Indian $(^A\gamma\delta\beta)^0$-thalassaemia deletion is shown in Fig. 16.6.

PCR methods for unknown mutations

A number of techniques have been applied for the detection of thalassaemia mutations without prior knowledge of the molecular defect. The most widely used of these methods is denaturing gradient-gel electrophoresis (DGGE), which allows the separa-tion of DNA fragments differing by a single base change according to their melting properties (Losekoot *et al.* 1991b). Another approach is by heteroduplex analysis using non-denaturing gel electrophoresis. Unique heteroduplex patterns can

Table 16.7 β-Thalassaemia mutations detectable by restriction-enzyme digestion of amplified product.

Position	Mutation	Ethnic group	Affected site
–88	C→T	African/Asian Indian	+*Fok* I
–87	C→G	Mediterranean	–*Avr* II
–87	C→T	Italian	–*Avr* II
–87	C→A	African/Yugoslavian	–*Avr* II
–86	C→G	Lebanese	–*Avr* II
–86	C→A	Italian	–*Avr* II
–29	A→G	African/Chinese	+*Nla* III
+43 to +40	–AAAC	Chinese	+*Dde* I
Initiation CD	T→C	Yugoslavian	–*Nco* I
Initiation CD	T→G	Chinese	–*Nco* l
Initiation CD	A→G	Japanese	–*Nco* I
CD5	–CT	Mediterranean	–*Dde* I
CD6	–A	Mediterranean	–*Dde* I
CD15	–T	Asian Indian	+*Bgl* I
CD17	A→T	Chinese	+*Mae* I
CD26	G→T	Thai	–*Mnl* I
CD26	G→A	South-east Asian (HbE)	–*Mnl* I
CD27	G→T	Mediterranean (Hb Knossos)	–*Sau*96 I
CD29	C→T	Lebanese	–*Bsp*M I
CD30	G→C	Tunisian/African	–*Bsp*M I
CD30	G→A	Bulgarian	–*Bsp*M I
IVS1-1	G→A	Mediterranean	–*Bsp*M I
IVS1-1	G→T	Asian Indian/Chinese	–*Bsp*M I
IVS1-2	T→G	Tunisian	–*Bsp*M I
IVS1-2	T→C	African	–*Bsp*M I
IVS1-2	T→A	Algerian	–*Bsp*M I
IVS1-5	G→A	Mediterranean	+*Eco*R V
IVS1-6	T→C	Mediterranean	+*Sfa*N I
IVS1-116	T→G	Mediterranean	+*Mae* I
IVS1-130	G→C	Turkish	–*Dde* I
IVS1-130	G→A	Egyptian	–*Dde* I
CD35	C→A	Thai	–*Acc* I
CD37	G→A	Saudi Arabian	–*Ava* II
CD38/39	–C	Czechoslovakian	–*Ava* II
CD37/8/9	–GACCCAG	Turkish	–*Ava* II
CD39	C→T	Mediterranean	+*Mae* I
CD43	G→T	Chinese	–*Hinf* I
CD47	+A	Surinamese	–*Xho* I
CD61	A→T	African	–*Hph* I
CD74/75	–C	Turkish	–*Hae* III
CD121	G→T	Polish, French, Japanese	–*Eco*R I
IVS2-I	G→A	Mediterranean	–*Hph* I
IVS2-4,5	–AG	Portuguese	–*Hph* I
IVS2-745	C→G	Mediterranean	+*Rsa* I

be generated for each mutation by annealing an amplified target DNA fragment with an amplified heteroduplex generator molecule, a synthetic oligonucleotide of about 130 bases in length containing deliberate sequence changes or identifiers at known mutation positions (Savage *et al.* 1995). Other methods, such as mismatch cleavage (CMC), single-stranded conformational polymorphism (SSCP) analysis and protein truncation test, are also good ways of detecting unknown mutations but they have not been applied to the haemoglobinopathies.

The above techniques simply pinpoint the presence of a mutation or DNA polymorphism in the amplified target sequence. Sequencing of the am-

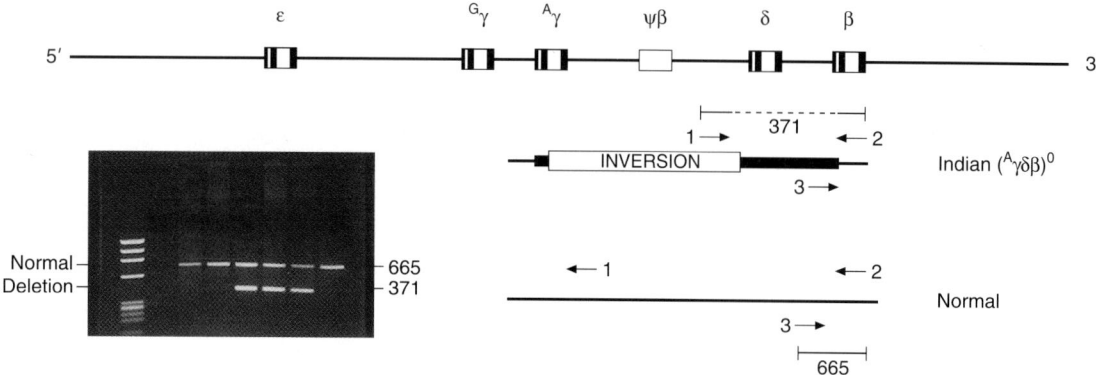

Fig. 16.6 The diagnosis of the Indian $(^A\gamma\delta\beta)^0$-thalassaemia inversion deletion by gap PCR. The amplification products after gel electrophoresis and ethidium bromide staining are shown from six persons with suspected $(^A\gamma\delta\beta)^0$ thalassaemia. The results show that three are heterozygous for the deletion. The diagram shows the positions of the two primers (2 and 3) which generate the deletion-specific product (371 bp) and the two primers (1 and 2) that generate a normal DNA-specific product (665 bp). Primer 1 is complementary to the inverted sequence of the deletion and thus faces in the opposite direction when annealed to the normal DNA sequence. Hence it cannot generate a normal fragment with primer 2. Primer 3 is complementary to the deleted sequence; it cannot generate a mutation-specific product with primer 2.

plified product is then required to identify the localized mutation. This can now be done very efficiently using an automated DNA sequencing machine utilizing fluorescence detection technology. The specialized equipment required for this technique is currently very expensive, but, as the more efficient second-generation machines are developed, the cost will come down and direct DNA sequencing will probably become the primary method of mutation detection.

Once a rare mutation has been identified by DNA sequencing, the DNA sample can be used as a control to develop ASO or ARMS primers for its detection in further cases. With this approach we have developed ARMS primers to detect a large number of mutations for use in our laboratory, and this technique is described in greater detail below.

β-Globin-gene haplotype analysis

At least 18 restriction-fragment-length polymorphisms (RFLPs) have been characterized within the β-globin-gene cluster (Kazazian & Boehm 1988). However, most of these RFLP sites are non-randomly associated with each other and thus they combine to produce just a handful of haplotypes (Antonarakis *et al.* 1982). In particular they form a 5′ cluster which is 5′ to the δ gene and a 3′ cluster

which extends downstream from the globin gene. In between is a 9-kb stretch of DNA containing a relative hotspot for meiotic recombination. The recombination between the two clusters has been calculated to be approximately one in 350 meioses (Chakravarti *et al.* 1984). Hybridization studies have shown that each thalassaemia mutation is strongly associated with just one or two haplotypes (Orkin *et al.* 1982a), probably because of their recent origin compared with the haplotypes (Flint *et al.* 1998), and thus haplotype analysis has been used to study the origins of identical mutations found in different ethnic groups.

The β-globin-gene cluster haplotype normally consists of five RFLPs located in the 5′ cluster (*Hind* II/ε gene; *Hind* III/$^G\gamma$ gene; *Hind* III/$^A\gamma$ gene; *Hind* II/3ψβ; and *Hind* II/5ψβ) and two RFLPs in the 3′ cluster (*Ava* II/β gene; *Bam*H I/β gene) (Old *et al.* 1984). Although originally analysed by Southern blotting, all the RFLPs except the *Bam*H I polymorphism can be easily detected by PCR, as illustrated in Fig. 16.7. The method is described in detail in the laboratory methods section and the primer sequences together with the sizes of the fragments generated are listed in Table 16.8. The *Bam*H I RFLP is located within an L1 repetitive element creating amplification problems and a *Hinf* I RFLP located just 3′ to the β-globin gene is used instead, because these two

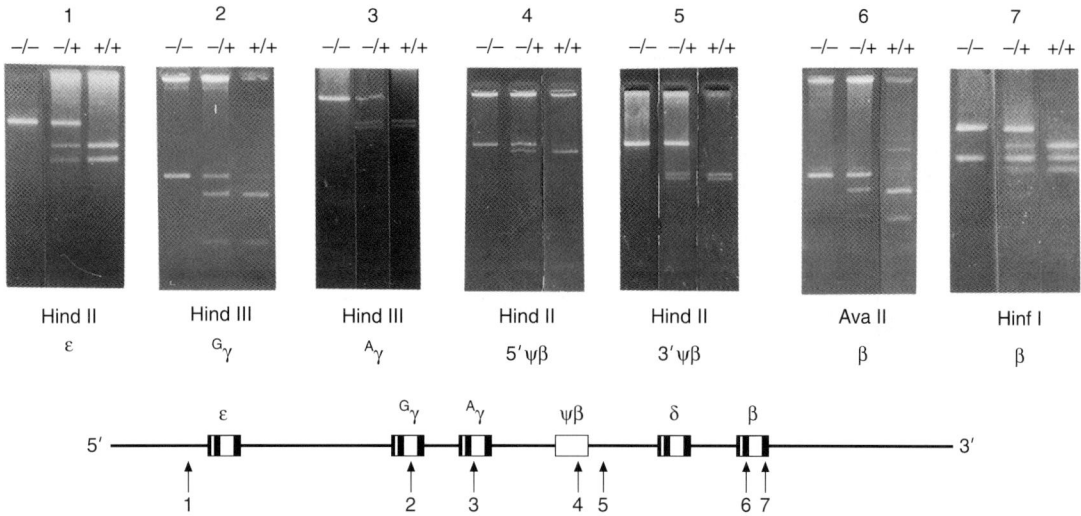

Fig. 16.7 PCR analysis of the seven β-globin-gene RFLPs which make up the standard β-globin-gene haplotype. Each gel shows the digestion products of amplified DNA from patients homozygous for the absence of the RFLP site (–/–), heterozygous for the presence of the site (–/+) and homozygous for the presence of the site (+/+), using the primers listed in Table 16.8. The approximate location of each RFLP site is shown underneath the gel pictures.

RFLPs have been found to exist in linkage disequilibrium (Semenza *et al.* 1989).

Three other RFLPs are included in Table 16.8. An *Ava* II RFLP in the gene is extremely useful in haplotype analysis of Mediterranean β-thalassaemia heterozygotes. The (–) allele for this RFLP is frequently found on chromosomes carrying the IVS1-110 G→A mutation while it is very rare on normal β-globin chromosomes (Wainscoat *et al.* 1984a) and thus it is a very useful informative marker for individuals heterozygous for this mutation. The *Rsa* I RFLP located just 5′ to the β-globin gene is useful for linkage analysis because it appears to be unlinked to either the 5′ cluster or the 3′ cluster RFLPs and thus may be informative when the 5′ haplotype and the 3′ haplotype are not. Finally the ᴳγ-*Xmn* I RFLP, created by the non-deletion HPFH C→T mutation at position –158, is included because of its use in the analysis of sickle-cell gene haplotypes and in individuals with thalassaemia intermedia.

δβ Thalassaemia, haemoglobin Lepore and hereditary persistence of fetal haemoglobin

The δβ thalassaemia, Hb Lepore and HPFH deletion mutations were characterized originally by restriction-enzyme mapping and Southern blotting. Consequently each deletion mutation may be diagnosed by the identification of characteristic abnormal DNA fragments which span the breakpoint of the deletion. Selection of the right restriction-enzyme digest and gene probe depends upon identifying the ethnic origin of the individual to be studied and characterization of the phenotype in the heterozygous state. A similar strategy is required for PCR-based diagnosis by GAP PCR, which can now be applied for Hb Lepore (Camaschella *et al.* 1990b) and eight thalassaemia and HPFH deletion mutations, for which both breakpoint DNA sequences have been characterized (Craig *et al.* 1994), as described in Table 16.3 and illustrated in Fig. 16.6. The practical details of this technique are described in a later section.

Haemoglobin variants

More than 700 haemoglobin variants have been described to date, of which the clinically most important ones requiring routine diagnosis are HbS, HbC, HbE, HbD Punjab and HbO Arab. The mutations for these five abnormal haemoglobins can be

Table 16.8 Primers used for the analysis of β-globin-gene cluster restriction-fragment-length polymorphisms (RFLPs).

RFLP and primers: 5' primer 3' primer	Product size (bp)	Coordinates on GenBank sequence U01317	Absence of site (bp)	Presence of site (bp)	Annealing temperature (°C)
Hind II/ε	760		760	315	55
5'TCTCTGTTTGATGACAAATTC		18652–18672		445	
5'AGTCATTGGTCAAGGCTGACC		19391–19411			
Xmn I/Gγ	657		657	455	55
5'AACTGTTGCTTTATAGGATTTT		33862–33883		202	
5'AGGAGCTTATTGATAACCTCAGAC		34495–34518			
Hind III/Gγ	326		326	235	65
5'AGTGCTGCAAGAAGAACAACTACC		35677–35700		91	
5'CTCTGCATCATGGGCAGTGAGCTC		35981–36004			
Hind III/Aγ	635		635	327	65
5'ATGCTGCTAATGCTTCATTAC		40357–40377		308	
5'TCATGTGTGATCTCTCAGCAG		40971–40991			
Hind II/5'ωβ	795		795	691	55
5'TCCTATCCATTACTGTTCCTTGAA		46686–46709		104	
5'ATTGTCTTATTCTAGAGACGATTT		47457–47480			
Ava II/ωβ	795		795	440	55
Sequence as for Hind 5' RFLP		46686–46709		355	
		47457–47480			
Hind II/3'ωβ	913		913	479	55
5'GTACTCATACTTTAAGTCCTAACT		49559–49582		434	
5'TAAGCAAGATTATTTCTGGTCTCT		50448–50471			
Rsa I/β	1200		411	330	55
5'AGACATAATTTATTAGCATGCATG		61504–61527	plus constant	81	
			fragments	plus 694	
5'CCCCTTCCTATGACATGAACTTAA		62680–62703	of 694 & 695	& 695	
Ava II/β	328		328	228	65
5'GTGGTCTACCCTTGGACCCAGAGG		62416–62439		100	
5'TTCGTCTGTTTCCCATTCTAAACT		62720–62743			
Hinf I/β	474		320	213	55
5'GGAGGTTAAAGTTTTGCTATGCTGTAT		63974–64001	plus constant	107	
5'GGGCCTATGATAGGGTAAT		64429–64447	fragment		
			of 154	& 154	

identified by a variety of techniques, as described below. The majority of the other abnormal variants have never been sequenced at the DNA level, and, although the mutations can be presumed from the amino acid change in most cases, DNA sequencing is required to confirm the nucleotide change before other diagnostic methods can be developed for screening purposes.

Haemoglobin S

The sickle-cell mutation has been diagnosed by a wide variety of DNA analysis techniques because it has been used as a prototype for the development of almost every new diagnostic method. Two different PCR techniques are currently used for prenatal diagnosis in our laboratory and both are described in a later section. The methods used are ARMS-PCR

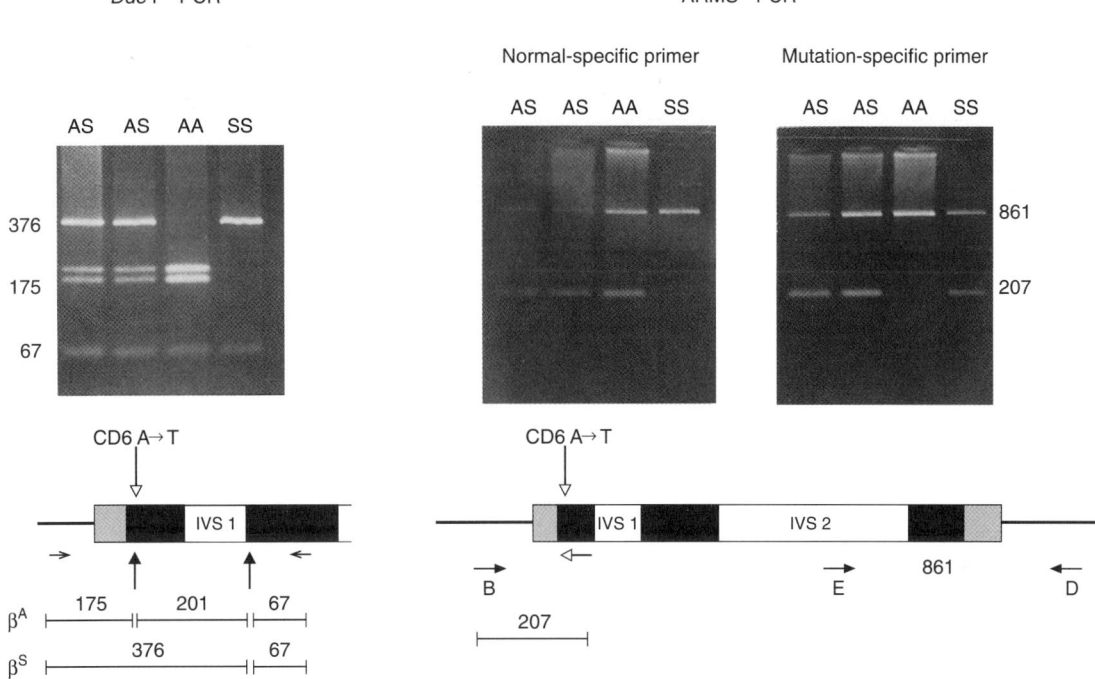

Fig. 16.8 The diagnosis of the sickle-cell anaemia mutation by two direct detection methods. The left-hand diagram shows a diagnosis by *Dde* I digestion of amplified DNA; the right-hand diagram shows a diagnosis by ARMS-PCR. Maps depict the location of the PCR primers used (as listed in Tables 16.5, 16.6 and 16.8) and the sites of the *Dde* I sites with respect to the β^S-gene mutation at codon 6. The DNA samples shown in each gel are the same: lane 1, AS genotype; lane 2, AS genotype; lane 3, AA genotype; lane 4, SS genotype.

and restriction endonuclease digestion, as shown in Fig. 16.8.

HbS (β6 Glu→Val) is caused by an A→T substitution in the second nucleotide of the 6th codon of the β-globin gene. The mutation destroys the recognition site for three restriction enzymes, *Mnl* I, *Dde* I and *Mst* II. The latter is now unavailable commercially and an isoschizomer such as *Cvn* I, *Oxa*N I or *Sau* I has to be used instead. *Mst* II was the enzyme of choice for detection of the β^S allele by Southern blot analysis (Orkin *et al.* 1982c) because it cuts infrequently around the globin gene, producing large DNA fragments. However, this is not a problem if the analysis is done by PCR and the cheaper enzyme *Dde* I may be used (Old *et al.* 1989). *Dde* I is a frequent cutter and several constant sites can be included in the amplified β-gene fragment to act as a control for the complete digestion of the amplified product. The

primer sequences currently used in our laboratory are present in Table 16.9. The β^S mutation can also be detected by a variety of other PCR-based techniques such as ASO/dot blotting or the ARMS method. The primer sequences for the latter method are included in Table 16.5.

Haemoglobin C

The HbC (β6 Glu→Lys) mutation, a G→A substitution at codon 6, also occurs inside the recognition sites for *Mnl* I, *Dde* I and *Mst* II. However it does not abolish the site for *Dde* I or *Mst* II because the mutation affects a non-specific nucleotide in the recognition sequence. Thus *Dde* I or *Mst* II cannot be used to detect the β^C mutation and another method such as ASO hybridization to amplified DNA or the allele-specific priming technique must be used. The primer sequences used for the ARMS method are included in Table 16.5.

Haemoglobins D Punjab and O Arab

The mutations giving rise to the abnormal variants HbD Punjab (β121 Glu→Gln) and HbO Arab (β121 Glu→Lys) both abolish an *Eco*R I site at codon 121 (Trent *et al.* 1984a) and their detection is carried out very simply by amplification of a fragment containing the site and digesting with *Eco*R I. As there are no other *Eco*R I sites within several kilobases of the globin-gene site, care should be taken to always run appropriate control DNA samples. The primer sequences used for this approach are listed in Table 16.9.

Haemoglobin E

The HbE mutation, a G→A mutation at codon 26, abolishes an *Mnl* I site and may be diagnosed by PCR and restriction enzyme analysis (Thein *et al.* 1987a). The primer sequences for this approach are listed in Table 16.8. The point mutation may also be diagnosed by the use of ASO probes or ARMS primers. The

primer sequences for the latter technique are listed in Tables 16.5 and 16.6.

Laboratory methods

Direct detection of β-thalassaemia mutations by the ARMS technique

The allele-specific priming technique known as the amplification refractory mutation system (ARMS) was developed as a quick, simple and inexpensive method for the prenatal diagnosis of β thalassaemia (Old *et al.* 1990; Old 1996b). For prenatal diagnosis two primers must be designed that will generate specific amplification products, one with the mutant allele and the other with the normal sequence. The nucleotide at the 3' terminus of each primer is complementary to the base in the respective target sequence at the site of the mutation. In addition, a deliberate mismatch to the target sequence is included at the second, third or fourth base from the 3' end. This enhances the specificity of the primer since all 3' terminal mismatches on their own (except for C-C, G-A and A-A) will allow some extension of the primer and thus generate non-specific amplifica-

Table 16.9 Oligonucleotide primers for the detection of β^S, β^E, β^D Punjab and β^O Arab mutations by restriction-enzyme (RE) digestion.

Mutation and affected RE site	Primer sequence 5'–3'	Annealing temperature (°C)	Product size (bp)	Absence of site (bp)	Presence of site (bp)
β^S CD6 (A→T)	ACCTCACCCTGTGGAGCCAC	65	443	386	201
(loses *Dde* I site)	GAGTGGACAGATCCCCAAAGGACTCAAGGA	65		67	175
β^E CD26 (G→A)	ACCTCACCCTGTGGAGCCAC	65	443	231	171
(loses *Mnl* I site)	GAGTGGACAGATCCCCAAAGGACTCAAGGA			89	89
				56	60
				35	35
				33	33
β^D Punjab	CAATGTATCATGCCTCTTTGCACC	65	861	861	552
CD121 (G→C)	GAGTCAAGGCTGAGAGATGCAGGA	65			309
(loses *Eco*R I site)					
β^O Arab	CAATGTATCATGCCTCTTTGCACC	65	861	861	552
CD121 (G→A)	GAGTCAAGGCTGAGAGATGCAGGA	65			309
(loses *Eco*R I site)					

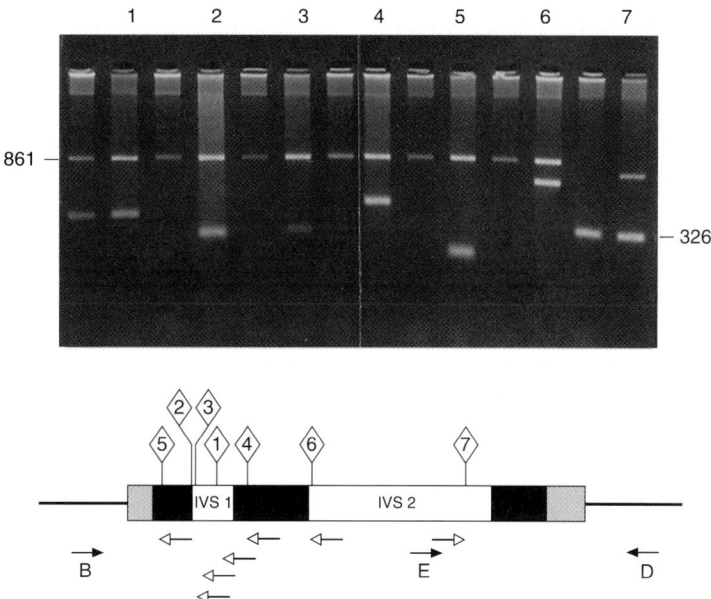

Fig. 16.9 The screening of a DNA sample for seven common Mediterranean β-thalassaemia mutations by ARMS-PCR. The diagram shows the β-globin gene and the positions of the seven mutations: 1, IVS1-110 G→A; 2, IVS1-1 G→A; 3, IVS1-6 T→C; 4, CD39 C→T; 5, CD6−A; 6, IVS2-1 G→A; 7, IVS2-745 C→G. The gel shows the amplification products from DNA of a β-thalassaemia heterozygote and products generated by control DNAs, run in pairs for each mutation screened as numbered above. The results show that the individual carries the mutation IVS1-110 G→A. For mutations 1–6, the control primers D and E produced an 861-bp fragment. However for mutation 7, IVS2-1 G→A, the *Hind* III/ᴳγ-gene RFLP primers were used, giving a control band of 326 bp. The primers used are listed in Table 16.5.

tion product (Kwok *et al.* 1990). The mutation-specific ARMS primers for the most common β-thalassaemia mutations and β-globin variants are listed in Table 16.5. All are the same length (30 mers) so that all can be used at one annealing temperature (65°C) enabling multiple mutations to be screened for simultaneously. Primers for the specific detection of the corresponding normal alleles are listed in Table 16.6. These are required for prenatal diagnosis in cases where both partners of a couple at risk for β thalassaemia carry the same mutation. Normal ARMS primers must be tested with DNA from an individual homozygous for the particular mutation before diagnostic use in order to check that the primer works correctly.

Each ARMS primer requires a second primer to generate the allele-specific product and, in addition, two control primers must be included in the PCR reaction in order to generate an unrelated product

that indicates that the reaction mixture was set up properly and everything is working correctly. The DNA sample is amplified with each mutant ARMS primer in a separate amplification reaction and the products are visualized after electrophoresis. Figure 16.9 illustrates screening of a sample for seven Mediterranean thalassaemia mutations at one time. A control DNA known to carry each mutation was also amplified for comparison and run beside the unknown sample in each case. The unknown DNA sample produced an amplified product with only the IVS1-110 G→A mutant primer (first track). For couples of Cypriot origin, this mutation is usually screened for first because it is so common and then, if it is not found, all the others are screened for simultaneously afterwards. Similarly, for Asian Indian couples, the four most common mutations IVS1-5 G→C, IVS1-1 G→A, CD8/9 +G and CD41/42 −TCTT (Varawalla *et al.* 1991b) are screened for first.

The 619-bp deletion gene is also detected by the ARMS test, as the control pair of primers is designed to span the deletion, which generates a characteristic 242-bp fragment in place of the normal 861-bp fragment (Old *et al.* 1990). The DNA from an individual doubly heterozygous for the 619-bp deletion and, say, the IVS1-5 mutation will produce three bands: the 861-bp fragment from the IVS1-5-allele, an IVS1-5 specific fragment of 285 bp from the mutant IVS1-5 ARMS primer and the 242-bp fragment.

Reagents

The reagents required are listed as follows.

1 The PCR buffer used is the standard Perkin–Elmer buffer: 50 mM KCl, 10 mM Tris–HCl (pH 8.3 at room temperature), 1.5 mM $MgCl_2$, 100 μg/ml gelatin. A 10× buffer can be prepared by adding together 0.5 ml 1 M Tris–HCl, pH 8.3, 1.25 ml 2 M KCl, 75 μl 1 M $MgCl_2$, 5 mg gelatin and 3.275 ml distilled water. The 10× buffer is heated at 37°C until the gelatin dissolves and is then frozen in aliquots.

2 Stock deoxynucleotide mixture: 1.25 mM each dNTP. Add together 50 μl of a 100-mM solution of each dNTP and 3.8 ml of distilled water. The 1.25 mM dNTP stock should be stored at –20°C in 0.8-ml aliquots.

3 Ready-made 100-mM dNTP solutions are now easily obtainable commercially (e.g. from Roche Diagnostics Limited, Lewes, UK), although purists may still wish to make up their own stocks from dNTP salts (which are less expensive) as follows: Dissolve to approx. 200 mM, neutralize carefully with 0.05 M Tris base to a pH of 7.0 by checking droplets on pH paper, read the optical density of a diluted aliquot at the correct wavelength (259 nm: A; 253 nm: G; 271 nm: C; 260 nm: T), calculate the concentration from the extinction coefficient (for a 1-cm path length: 1.54×10^4: A; 1.37×10^4: G; 9.1×10^3: C; 7.4×10^3: T), and finally adjust to 100 mM with distilled water.

4 PCR reaction mixture stock solution (4 ml). Add together 0.5 ml 10× PCR buffer, 0.8 ml 1.25 mM dNTP stock solution and 2.7 ml distilled water.

5 Dilute aliquots of primer stock solutions to make working solutions at a concentration of 1 OD U/ml. Our primers are synthesized commercially (OSWEL DNA service, Southampton, UK) and are HPLC purified. The primers are stored at –20°C.

6 *Taq* DNA polymerase: AmpliTaq (Perkin-Elmer

UK, Applied Biosystems Division, Warrington, UK) is the gold standard but cheaper thermostable DNA polymerases may be used successfully (e.g. Advanced Biotechnologies, Leatherhead, UK).

7 ARMS primers should be 30 or more oligonucleotides long in order to use a high annealing temperature of 65°C for the prevention of non-specific amplified products. The mutation-specific primer has its 3′ terminal base complementary to the mutation, the normal specific primer should be complementary to the corresponding normal sequence. If the 3′ terminal mismatch is a strong one then a weak additional mismatch is engineered at either the second, third or fourth nucleotide from the 3′ end. If the 3′ terminal mismatch is a weak one, then a strong mismatch should be added to increase the specificity of the ARMS reaction. Strong ones are C-C, G-A and A-A mismatches, weak ones are T-T, T-C, T-G, G-G and A-C mismatches.

8 The common and control primers should also be 30 bases long and selected to have a G+C content of approximately 50%. It is important to ensure that there are no known mutations or polymorphic DNA sequences located in the DNA sequences chosen for any of the primers. Any such occurrence is liable to reduce the effectiveness of the primer and may lead to an erroneous result. The size of the control product should be such that it runs well away from the expected ARMS products.

9 Both positive and negative control DNAs for each mutation being screened for must always be amplified and run on the gel alongside the test samples. Primers designed to detect the normal DNA sequence at the site of a mutation must be tested using control DNA from an individual homozygous for the mutation in question.

Method

The standard PCR conditions recommended by Perkin-Elmer for their 'AmpliTaq' enzyme can be used. These are: 10 mM Tris–HCl, pH 8.3, 50 mM KCl, 1.5 mM $MgCl_2$, 0.01% gelatin, 0.2 μM each primer, and 200 μM each of dATP, dCTP, dGTP and dTTP. The reaction volume can be scaled down from the recommended 100 μl to just 25 μl, which then requires only 0.5 units of 'AmpliTaq' enzyme and 0.1–0.5 μg of genomic DNA to complete the reaction. The method is as follows:

1 Set up the reaction mixture as follows using a

dedicated set of automatic pipettes which are never used for handling the amplified product:

2 Pipette 20 µl of the PCR reaction mixture stock solution into a 0.5-ml Eppendorf tube.

3 Add 1 µl of each control primer, 1 µl of the common primer, and 1 µl of the appropriate ARMS primers.

4 Add 0.5 units of 'AmpliTaq' enzyme. This is supplied at a concentration of 5 U/µl and therefore only 0.1 µl is required. This is difficult to estimate and therefore it is best to make a dilute solution of enzyme at a concentration of 0.5 U/µl using distilled water.

5 If the same four primers are being used in every tube (for example when screening a number of DNA samples for one mutation), then all four primers and enzyme can be mixed together (1 µl each primer and 0.1 µl U enzyme per tube) and then 4.1 µl of primer/enzyme mixture can be added to each tube.

6 Add 1 µl DNA solution (at approx. 0.1–0.5 mg/ml).

7 Add 25 µl light paraffin oil.

8 Place the tubes in a PCR machine and program for 25 cycles at:

    94°C for 1 min
    65°C for 1 min
    72°C for 1.5 min

with a final extension period of 3 min at 72°C after the last cycle.

9 The annealing temperature of 65°C is appropriate for primers of 30 nucleotides in length. No initial denaturation step is necessary before the programme of 25 cycles unless the target DNA is GC rich.

10 Remove the tubes from the PCR machine and pipette 5 µl of ficoll/bromophenol blue dye (15%/0.05%) into each tube.

11 Vortex the mixture to incorporate the blue dye and spin for 5 s in a microfuge.

12 Remove a 20-µl aliquot of the blue aqueous mixture underneath the paraffin oil layer, and load into the well of submerged agarose minigel. For most purposes a 3% agarose gel is used, made up of 1.5% agarose and 1.5% NuSieve agarose (FMC Bio-Products, Kent, UK, marketed through Flowgen). For the separation of small DNA fragments very similar in size, increase the percentage agarose gel to 4% (3% NuSieve/1% agarose) or even 4.5% (3.5% NuSieve/1% agarose).

13 After electrophoresis at 100 V for approximately 45 min in standard Tris–acetate buffer, the gel is stained in ethidium bromide solution (0.5 g/ml) and photographed on a UV transilluminator (312 nm), using an electronic camera system or a Polaroid CU-5 instant camera fitted with an orange filter (e.g. Wratten 22 A).

Interpretation of results

The relationship of fragment intensities should be constant for all DNA samples of the same genotype. Any deviation from the expected pattern of band intensities should be treated as suspect (e.g. a trace of maternal DNA contamination in a fetal DNA sample or a false-positive ARMS-PCR result) and the sample retested.

Pitfalls

As mentioned, sometimes an ARMS primer may produce a positive signal that is less intense relative to the control fragment than expected. If the same faint band is observed in the negative control sample, the signal is probably a false-positive result occurring either when there has been a subtle change of reaction conditions or if the ARMS primer has started to lose its specificity. The latter has occurred occasionally with the stock primer solutions and possibly results from some degradation of the 3′ end of the oligonucleotide, in which case the primer needs to be resynthesized.

Negative results

No amplification product from the control primers may result from the DNA samples being too dilute (reprecipitate in a smaller volume), the DNA being too concentrated (try a 1/10 dilution) or the DNA containing impurities (re-extract with phenol/chloroform).

Restriction endonuclease digestion of PCR product

This is a simple and reliable technique for the diagnosis of point mutations, insertions or deletions which result in the creation or abolition of a restriction endonuclease site. Primers are designed to span the recognition site and produce easily identifiable fragments after digestion and electrophoresis of the products in an agarose gel. A mixture of 1.5%

agarose and 1.5% NuSieve agarose will give good separation of fragments in most cases but for good resolution of very small fragments of 100 bp or less a 4% gel in the ratio of 1% agarose/3% NuSieve may be used.

This technique is routinely applied in our laboratory for the diagnosis of the abnormal variants HbS, HbD Punjab and HbO Arab. It is useful for confirming the diagnosis of β-thalassaemia mutations where possible and for confirmation of a prenatal diagnosis of thalassaemia by linkage analysis of single RFLPs or globin haplotypes. RFLPs can often be used for prenatal diagnosis of thalassaemia in the rare cases where one or both of the mutations remain unidentified after screening using a direct detection method such as ARMS. The technique can also enable the prenatal diagnosis of uncharacterized δβ-thalassaemia deletion mutations through the apparent non-Mendelian inheritance of RFLPs (due to the hemizygosity created by the inheritance of deleted sequences on one chromosome).

Method

The procedure is as follows:

1 Set up a total reaction volume of 25 µl as described for the ARMS-PCR test except for the addition of only two primers as specified for the RFLP under study.

2 Place the tubes in a PCR machine and program for 30 cycles at:

94°C for 1 min
55°C or 65°C for 1 min (see Tables 16.6 and 16.7)
72°C for 1.5 min

with a final extension period of 3 min at 72°C after the last cycle.

3 Remove tubes from the PCR machine and add 5–10 units of the appropriate restriction enzyme plus 2 µl of the recommended 10× concentration restriction-enzyme buffer.

4 Incubate at 37°C for a minimum of 1 h.

5 Add 5 µl of blue dye, mix and spin.

6 Load sample on to an agarose gel made of 1.5% agarose and 1.5% NuSieve GTG agarose, and electrophorese, stain and photograph as described for ARMS-PCR.

Gap PCR

Gap PCR is the simplest of PCR techniques in theory but in practice is one of the more troublesome methods to perfect because of the different stringent amplification conditions required for each deletion-specific primer pair. It is used routinely in our laboratory for the diagnosis of the large deletions in the β-globin-gene cluster listed in Table 16.3. However, for the α-thalassaemia deletion mutations, gap PCR is used for screening purposes but never for prenatal diagnosis without confirmation of the diagnosed genotype by Southern blot analysis, for reasons outlined in the section on prenatal diagnosis.

Method

The procedure is as follows:

1 Adjust the reaction mixture to a final volume of 22 µl in a 0.5-ml tube with the following components, as required:

1 µl genomic DNA (100 ng/l)
1 µl forward primer—flanking sequence (10 pmol/l)
1 µl reverse primer—flanking sequence (10 pmol/l)
1 µl primer—deleted sequence (10 pmol/l)
1 µl primer—inverted sequence (10 pmol/l)
2.5 µl 1.25 mM (dNTP mixture)
2.3 µl of the 10× concentration PCR buffer recommended for the primers
Sterile distilled H_2O to a final volume of 22 µl.

2 Overlay with 25 µl mineral oil.

3 Prepare enzyme mixture:

0.2 µl reaction buffer (10× concentration)
0.1 µl AmpliTaq (5 U/l)
2.7 µl sterile distilled H_2O to a final volume of 3 µl.

4 Mix enzyme mixture and hold on ice.

5 Place reaction mixtures in thermal cycler and perform one cycle as follows, adding 3 µl of the enzyme mix after 2 min of the 94°C denaturation step:

4 min at 94°C
1 min at 55–65°C (as recommended)
1.5 min at 72°C.

6 Continue for 33 cycles with the following steps per cycle:

1 min at 94°C

1 min at 55–65°C (as recommended)
1.5 min at 72°C.
7 Finish with one cycle as follows:
1 min at 94°C
1 min at 55–65°C (as recommended)
10 min at 72°C.
8 Hold at 15°C until gel electrophoresis.
9 Remove tubes from thermal cycler and add 5 μl of

blue dye (15% ficoll/0.05% bromophenol blue). Mix and centrifuge.

10 Load a 20-μl aliquot on to a 1–3% agarose gel (depending on expected fragment sizes) and electrophorese at 100 V for 45 min in Tris–borate–EDTA (TBE) buffer (89 mM Tris, 89 mM boric acid, 10 mM EDTA, pH 8.0). Stain and photograph as described for ARMS-PCR.

Part 5
The future

The future

Just as was the case 100 years ago, as medical practice moved uneasily into the twentieth century, it faces the new millennium in what some commentators have described as a state of total disarray. Not for the first time, history seems to be repeating itself.

In the latter half of the nineteenth century and the beginning of the twentieth century remarkable discoveries in the developing fields of infectious disease and immunology had raised hopes for the early control of the major infectious killers that were decimating large populations. For example, in March 1892 at a meeting of the Berlin Physiological Society Robert Koch announced the discovery of the organism that causes tuberculosis. The news of this work rapidly spread throughout the world and leader writers for the London and New York Times wrote that Koch's discovery would soon lead to a treatment for tuberculosis, perhaps along the lines of Pasteur's successful vaccines. During this period the costs of medical care were increasing and rapidly becoming beyond the means of all but the richer members of Western societies. And as time went on and the fruits of the new developments in medical research seemed to be having little effect on the diseases of the time there was increasing public disillusionment with doctors. In his long preface to the play *The Doctor's Dilemma*, first produced in 1906, Bernard Shaw castigated every aspect of medical research and practice, focusing on the disastrous attempts to treat tuberculosis and the conspiratorial aspects of the professions, medicine in particular.

Nothing changes. Today there is growing cynicism about the likely clinical value of the remarkable developments in molecular and cell biology of the last 20 years. Vast populations live in poverty and without access to the most basic medical care, and none of the richer Western countries have been able to cope with the spiralling costs of health care.

When we consider the future of the thalassaemia field we have to place it in the context of these problems. If history has taught us anything it is that developments in the basic science laboratory often take a long time to bear fruit in the clinic; it was over 70 years from the discovery of the tubercle bacillus to the announcement of a definitive cure for tuberculosis. Similarly, we shall have to consider how we are going to finance the costs of exciting new therapeutic developments; even in richer countries they will have to compete with the spiralling costs of health care as the numbers of their aged populations increase, while in the case of the developing countries, where the thalassaemias reach their highest frequencies, they will have to take second place behind the provision of basic health care.

It is against the background of these doubts and uncertainties that the future of the thalassaemia field must be assessed.

Priorities for thalassaemia research

If for no other reason the compilation of a new edition of this book has been a valuable exercise for the authors in that it has highlighted some of the major gaps in our knowledge about the thalassaemias. In particular, it has emphasized how, by focusing on the molecular aspects of these diseases over recent years, we have tended to neglect some of the less glamorous aspects of the field which, nevertheless, are of critical importance for the future of our patients.

As pointed out in Chapters 6 and 14, major demographic changes in the pattern of disease following improvements in nutrition, hygiene and basic medical care have produced a state of affairs in many developing countries in which children with thalassaemia who would previously have died of infection or malnutrition in the first few years of life are now surviving to present for diagnosis and treatment. Because we have neglected to carry out extensive population surveys in our haste to define the molecular pathology of the disease in different populations, we only have the flimsiest of ideas about the true burden of the disease in many countries. The fields of international health demography and health-care economics are becoming very sophisticated and, if we are to make the case for adequate services for the diagnosis and care of thalassaemic patients, both to governments of individual countries and to the major international health agencies, we need much better information about the frequency and distribution of the different forms of thalassaemia. We are fortunate in the thalassaemia field because the carrier states for the different forms of the disease can all be identified by relatively cheap haematological tests and therefore we do not have to rely on the more expensive forms of screening at the DNA level. However, there is still room for improvement in both the simplicity and accuracy of our current screening procedures.

The second aspect of the field that we still have not explored adequately is the relationship between the genotype and phenotype and the reasons for the remarkable heterogeneity of all the thalassaemias. Haemoglobin E β thalassaemia is a prime example. As we saw in Chapter 9, this disease will affect hundreds of thousands of children throughout the Indian subcontinent and south-east Asia in the future, yet we still know very little about its natural history and the reasons for its remarkable clinical diversity. Without this information it is very difficult to make sensible recommendations about how it should best be managed. We still have much to learn about the reasons for the heterogeneity of other forms of thalassaemia, information which is badly needed if we are to extend our screening and prenatal diagnosis programmes and provide parents with adequate counselling.

The next problem is how we are going to control thalassaemia, particularly in poorer countries where it is going to become so common in the immediate future. Decisions will have to be made about whether to develop screening and prenatal diagnosis programmes and how these may be adapted to the individual needs of particular countries. It is no use waiting for further developments in the basic biological sciences to provide a definitive cure for the thalassaemias by gene therapy. Similarly, we have no way of knowing how long it will be before it is possible to carry out bone-marrow transplantation or some form of stem-cell therapy using unrelated donors. These things may happen, but even when they do they may be prohibitively expensive, at least for the foreseeable future. Therefore we have to maximize our current technology to tide us through what may be a very long wait before better forms of treatment become available. This will require obtaining better data about the frequency and health burden that will be posed by the thalassaemias so that individual governments, helped by international health agencies, can be persuaded to provide the funding to develop screening programmes together with centres for prenatal diagnosis and treatment.

Again because of uncertainties about when more definitive methods of therapy will become available, we need to maximize our current methods of symptomatic treatment with particular respect to optimizing transfusion regimens and developing simpler, cheaper and more effective chelating agents.

Finally, we must further encourage work towards a more definitive cure for the thalassaemias, particularly in the richer countries, which can afford this kind of research yet which may be more interested in diseases that are more relevant to their own populations. We must try to persuade Western governments and their pharmaceutical companies that the needs of the developing countries are of increasing relevance and importance.

Screening and diagnostics

The whole process of genetic screening will be transformed by the technological developments which will follow the Human Genome Project. Remarkable advances in miniaturization technology are making it possible to develop microchips which will encompass large numbers of human mutations and which will enable rapid screening of large populations. Thus, while it is important that we continue to look for cheaper and more accurate haematological or biochemical ways to screen for the common forms of thalassaemia, we should, at the same time, continue to explore this new technology. For example, it is possible that, as the costs of these new approaches fall, as they inevitably will, it may be feasible for one or two laboratories in each high-frequency country to provide services for population screening which are cheaper and more effective than the use of simple approaches carried out in many different hospitals or centres throughout these countries. Indeed, even using technology which is already developed, high-performance liquid chromatography for example, it may be cheaper and more cost effective to provide this type of equipment for one or two central laboratories and to develop ways of transporting samples for screening rather than to establish more widespread screening programmes. The economics and logistics of these approaches need urgent study. It will surely be to the long-term advantage of the companies that manufacture this equipment to join forces with some of the countries of south-east Asia to help them develop pilot studies of this kind.

At the present time the developing countries in which the thalassaemias will present a major health burden in the future are receiving confusing advice about how best to plan for the future. What is urgently needed are some adequate pilot studies to find out which technology would best suit individual populations for screening and counselling, followed by advice from health demographers and planners about the most cost-effective and efficient way to proceed. In this context the major international agencies such as the World Health Organization and World Bank could be of enormous help. But they, in turn, need advice about the importance of these diseases in the future. Currently, there is little evidence that they have understood the increasing burden on scarce health-care resources that these diseases will pose in the future.

Control

As outlined in Chapter 14, every country in which the thalassaemias will become a major problem in the future will have to decide how they wish to control the disease. If they decide to develop a screening and prenatal diagnosis programme they have the experience of the remarkably successful ventures in some of the Mediterranean countries on which to model their plans. If, on the other hand, for religious or other reasons they wish to try to evolve programmes of premarital screening and avoiding marriages between carriers, they would be well advised to develop small pilot programmes in well defined communities to see whether this approach is likely to be successful. As pointed out in Chapter 14, there is very little experience of this way of controlling genetic disease to date. Finally, if countries decide not to develop programmes for the control of the disease, but to treat it when it occurs, they will, based on good population data, have to work out the economics and how to develop their clinical services appropriately.

These are all difficult decisions but none of them can be made without adequate knowledge of the likely burden of the disease based on good population screening data.

Symptomatic treatment

The remarkable success story of the way in which transfusion-dependent thalassaemic children can grow and develop normally if adequately transfused and chelated tends to dominate every discussion about the symptomatic management of thalassaemia. Thus it is assumed that adequate management requires that the haemoglobin level is maintained such that endogenous haemopoiesis is almost entirely shut off. Currently this means that the pretransfusion haemoglobin level should not be allowed to fall below 9.5 g/dl. As discussed in Chapter 15, there is good evidence that children maintained in this way will grow and develop normally provided they receive adequate chelation therapy.

If this approach becomes the gold standard for the management of every form of thalassaemia in the future it means that hundreds of thousands of children with the intermediate forms of β thalassaemia, HbE β thalassaemia for example, will receive regular transfusion. The burden which this will impose for a country like Indonesia was discussed in Chapter 14. But is it really necessary to maintain this level of haemoglobin in all these patients? We are learning that many patients with HbE β thalassaemia grow and develop normally, without skeletal deformity or other unpleasant manifestations of the disease, at much lower steady-state haemoglobin levels. If we are to use our limited resources to best advantage we must try and understand more about the other factors which determine the rates of growth and development in relationship to the haemoglobin level. There is a great deal of important work to do on this neglected aspect of the management of thalassaemia.

The case for developing cheaper and more effective chelating agents remains as strong as ever. As well as patients who are transfusion dependent it is clear that many of those with the intermediate forms of β thalassaemia develop iron loading through increased intestinal absorption and will require chelation therapy, albeit less frequently than those who are transfusion dependent. Although because of its efficacy and low toxicity desferrioxamine has been a remarkable success story, it remains expensive and because of the way it has to be administered will always be associated with difficulties of compliance. Not least because other therapeutic indications for chelation therapy have not appeared, the pharmaceutical industry has been slow to develop more effective oral chelating agents. Here again some encouragement and financial help from the international health agencies would be extremely valuable.

As further potential oral chelating agents become available it is vital that they are adequately tested, both in animals and by properly designed clinical trials, before they become generally available. The story of the current uncertainties about the value and safety of deferiprone, outlined in Chapter 15, should be a constant reminder of the importance of the critical study of any new oral chelation agents. They must be evaluated adequately, and it is vital that the international and national support societies do not pressure clinicians into the premature use of these agents, however well meaning their motives may be.

Finally, since it is becoming clear that even well chelated children develop endocrine damage, further work is needed to try to determine how this might be avoided and the optimal way in which it should be managed. The same principles apply to the increasing problem of metabolic bone disease.

The other major help that could be given to the developing countries by the international health agencies working through their governments is in the funding and organization of improved transfusion services. Blood-borne infections will remain a major problem for many countries for the foreseeable future; the current predictions for the world distribution of HIV infection and the frightening increase in drug-resistant malaria are constant reminders, if any were needed, that this problem will be with us for a long time to come.

Definitive treatment

The search for more definitive forms of treatment for the thalassaemias will be pursued in two major directions. First, it will follow fields of haematology which are endeavouring to find ways of improving marrow transplantation between unrelated and unmatched donors and, at the same time trying to learn how better to isolate and purify stem cells for their use in transplantation. It is likely that there will be major progress in these fields in the near future.

Progress is likely to be slower in the field of somatic cell gene therapy. But patients with thalassaemia and their clinicians should not be too dispirited if they do not see a great deal of work going on focused directly at somatic cell gene therapy for thalassaemia. It is now clear that the first successes for gene therapy are likely to be those that are aimed at short-term gene expression for the management of cancer and vascular disease. For correcting genetic disease we are likely to see the earliest definitive results in disorders like haemophilia or some of the inherited immune deficiencies, in which a relatively low level of gene expression is all that is required to correct the disease. While this work is under way a great deal more will be learnt about the safety and effectiveness of different gene transfer vectors. In the meantime the globin research field has still a considerable amount to learn about the factors that are required for tight regulation of the globin genes. The correction of thalassaemia requires high-level, finely regulated gene expression and, as mentioned in Chapter 2, although a great deal has been learnt about this process there are still some major gaps in our knowledge. However, as stem-cell biology improves, better gene transfer vectors become available and more is learnt about the sequences that are required for long-term, stable expression of the β-globin genes, it should be possible to make some genuine progress in somatic cell gene therapy. But this is likely to be still some time away and even when it is possible it may be an extremely expensive procedure.

Given these difficulties, the most attractive way forward for major research efforts into the management of thalassaemia for the immediate future may be in learning better how to stimulate fetal haemoglobin synthesis. While this may be very difficult in the case of the severe, transfusion-dependent forms of the disease it does not seem beyond the bounds of possibility that it may be possible to raise the fetal haemoglobin output by 1 or 2 g/dl, which would be sufficient to greatly improve the phenotype of the intermediate forms of β thalassaemia, particularly HbE β thalassaemia. While it is disappointing that, despite the enormous effort that has been made, we still don't understand the regulation of the switch from fetal to adult haemoglobin, we have learnt some very encouraging facts from this type of research. The characterization of the molecular basis for many forms of hereditary persistence of fetal haemoglobin has told us that the adult red cell seems to have most of the regulatory machinery required for fetal haemoglobin synthesis. The fact that in the $^G\gamma$ or $^A\gamma\beta^+$ forms of this condition a simple point mutation in the γ-globin-gene promoter is enough to allow the persistence of high levels of γ-chain production is even more encouraging. It suggests that the relative amounts of γ- and β-chain production in adults is in dynamic equilibrium, presumably directed one way or the other by the levels of particular regulatory molecules. It is clear that certain perturbations of erythropoiesis tend to favour the expression of the γ-globin genes and that this effect can be produced by a variety of drugs. Taken together, these facts are extremely encouraging and suggest that it may be possible to improve our current rather primitive efforts at stimulating γ-globin synthesis after birth.

It appears, therefore, that we can look forward to the future for our patients with thalassaemia with a good degree of optimism. The haemoglobin field led the development of molecular medicine, and information obtained from the analysis of the human globin genes at the molecular level was applied remarkably quickly to their prenatal detection in the clinic. The next stage, the use of this information for the treatment of the disease, was bound to take longer. But there are hints of the directions which might be most productive in this respect in the future. In the meantime there is much to do to maximize what can be done for the control and management of thalassaemic patients. We must emphasize again that, if writing this new edition of our monograph has told us anything, it is that we have tended to neglect some of the basic clinical questions posed by the thalassaemias over recent years in our haste to study them at the molecular level. It is essential that we go back to clinical basics and tackle these problems now so that as more definitive approaches to treatment become available we really understand some of the major factors which are involved in determining the clinical variability of this extraordinarily diverse group of diseases.

References

Aasland, R., Gibson, T.J. & Stewart, A.F. (1995) The PHD finger: implications for chromatin-mediated transcriptional regulation. *Trends Biol. Sci.* **20**, 56.

Abbondanzo, S.L., Anagnou, N.P. & Sacher, R.A. (1988) Myelodysplastic syndrome with acquired hemoglobin H disease. *Am. J. Clin. Pathol.* **89**, 401.

Abdalla, S.H., Corrah, P.T. & Higgs, D.R. (1989) α-Thalassaemia in The Gambia. *Trans. Roy. Soc. Trop. Med. Hyg.* **83**, 420.

Abels, J., Michiels, J.J., Giordano, P.C. *et al.* (1996) A *de novo* deletion causing εγδβ-thalassaemia in a Dutch patient. *Acta Haematol.* **96**, 108.

Abraham, E.C., Walker, D., Gravely, M. & Huisman, T.H.J. (1975) Minor hemoglobins in sickle cell anemia, β-thalassemia: a study of red cell fractions isolated by density gradient centrifugation. *Biochem. Med.* **11**, 56.

Abramson, R.K., Rucknagel, D.L., Shreffler, D.C. & Saave, J.J. (1970) Homozygous Hb J Tongariki: evidence for only one alpha chain structural locus in Melanesians. *Science* **169**, 194.

Abreu de Miani, M.S. & Peñalver, J.A. (1983) Incidencia de portadores beta-talasémicos y de deficientes de la glucosa-6-fosfato dehidrogenasa eritrocítica (G6PD) en el área del Gran Buenos Aires. *Sangre*, **28**, 537.

Abuelo, D.N., Forman, E.N. & Rubin, L.P. (1997) Limb defects and congenital anomalies of the genitalia in an infant with homozygous α-thalassaemia. *Am. J. Med. Genet.* **68**, 158.

Abu-Sin, A., Felice, A.E., Gravely, M.E. *et al.* (1979) Hb P-Nilotic in association with β-thalassemia: *cis*-mutation of a hemoglobin β^A chain regulatory determinant. *J. Lab. Clin. Med.* **93**, 973.

Acquaye, C.T.A., Oldham, J.H. & Konotey-Ahulu, F.I.D. (1977) Blood donor homozygous for hereditary persistence of fetal haemoglobin. *Lancet* **i**, 796.

Adachi, K., Surrey, S., Temery, H. *et al.* (1993) Hb Shelby [beta131 (H9)Gln→Lys] in association with Hb S [beta 6(A3)Glu→Val]: characterization, stability and effects on Hb S polymerization. *Hemoglobin* **17**, 329.

Adamkiewicz, T.V., Berkovitch, M., Krishnan, C., Polsinelli, K., Kermack, D. & Olivieri, N.F. (1998) *Yersinia enterocolitica* and beta thalassemia: a report of 15 years' experience. *Clin. Infect. Dis.* **27**, 1367.

Adams, W.H. (1974) A survey for haemoglobinopathies in Nepal. *Trans. Roy. Soc. Trop. Med. Hyg.* **68**, 392.

Adams, M.B (ed.) (1990) *The Wellborn Science: Eugenics in Germany, France, Brazil and Russia.* Oxford University Press, Oxford.

Adams, J.G. III & Coleman, M.B. (1990) Structural hemoglobin variants that produce the phenotype of thalassemia. *Sem. Hematol.* **27**, 229.

Adams, J.G. III, Steinberg, M.H., Newman, M.V., Morrison, W.T., Benz, E.J. & Iyer, R. (1981) β-Thalassemia present in *cis* to a new β-chain structural variant, Hb Vicksburg [β75(E19)Leu→O]. *Proc. Natl Acad. Sci. USA* **78**, 469.

Adams, J.G. III, Morrison, W.T. & Steinberg, M.H. (1982) Double crossover within a human gene. *Science* **218**, 241.

Adams, J.G. III, Coleman, M.B., Hayes, J., Morrison, W.T. & Steinberg, M.H. (1985) Modulation of fetal hemoglobin synthesis by iron deficiency. *N. Eng. J. Med.* **313**, 1402.

Adams, J.G. III, Steinberg, M.H. & Kazazian, H.H.J. (1990) Isolation and characterization of the translation product of a β-globin gene nonsense mutation (β121GAA→TAA). *Br. J. Haematol.* **75**, 561.

Adams, R.J., Kutlar, A., McKie, V. *et al.* (1994) Alpha thalassemia and stroke risk in sickle cell anemia. *Am. J. Hematol.* **45**, 279.

Adams, R.J., McKie, V.C., Hsu, L. *et al.* (1998) Prevention of a first stroke by transfusions in children with sickle cell anemia and abnormal results on transcranial Doppler ultrasonography. *N. Eng. J. Med.* **333**, 5.

Adamson, J.W. (1975) Familial polycythemia. *Sem. Hematol.* **12**, 383.

Adekile, A.D. (1997) Historical and anthropological correlates of β^S haplotypes and α- and β-thalassemia alleles in the Arabian Peninsula. *Hemoglobin* **21**, 281.

Adekile, A.D. & Haider, M.Z. (1996) Morbidity, β^S haplotype and α-globin gene patterns among sickle cell anemia patients in Kuwait. *Acta Haematol.* **96**, 150.

Advani, R., Rubin, E., Mohandas, N. & Schrier, S.L. (1992a) Oxidative red blood cell membrane injury in the pathophysiology of severe mouse beta-thalassemia. *Blood* **79**, 1064.

Advani, R., Sorenson, S., Shinar, E., Lande, W., Rachmilewitz, E. & Schrier, S.L. (1992b) Characterization and comparison of the red blood cell membrane damage in severe human alpha- and beta-thalassemia. *Blood* **79**, 1058.

Advisory Committee on Genetic Testing (1997) *Code of Practice and Guidance on Human Genetic Testing Services Supplied Direct to the Public.* Department of Health, London.

Aessopos, A., Voskaridou, E., Kavouklis, E. *et al.* (1994) Angioid streaks in sickle-thalassemia. *Am. J. Ophthalmol.* **117**, 589.

Aessopos, A., Stamatelos, G., Skoumas, V., Vassilopoulos, G., Mantzourani, M. & Loukopoulos, D. (1995) Pulmonary hypertension and right heart failure in patients with β-thalassemia intermedia. *Chest* **107**, 50.

Afifi, A.M. (1974) High transfusion regime in the management of reproductive wastage and maternal complications of pregnancy in thalassaemia major. *Acta Haematol.* **52**, 331.

Agarwal, M.B., Viswanathan, C., Ramananthan, J. *et al.* (1990) Oral iron chelation with L1. *Lancet* **335**, 601.

Agarwal, M.B., Gupte, S.S., Viswanathan, C. *et al.* (1992) Long-term assessment of efficacy and safety of L1, an oral iron chelator, in transfusion-dependent thalassaemia: Indian trial. *Br. J. Haematol.* **82**, 460.

Agarwal, S., Gulati, R. & Singh, K. (1997) Hemoglobin E-beta thalassemia in Uttar Pradesh. *Indian Ped.* **34**, 287.

Ager, J.A.M. & Lehmann, H. (1958) Observations on some 'fast' haemoglobins: K, J, N and Bart's. *Br. Med. J.* **i**, 929.

Ahern, E.J., Ahern, V.N., Jones, R.T. & Brimhall, B. (1972) Hemoglobin Lepore Washington in two Jamaican families: interaction with beta chain variants. *Blood* **40**, 246.

Ahern, E., Herbert, R., McIver, C., Ahern, V., Wardle, J. & Seakins, M. (1975) Beta-thalassaemia of clinical significance in adult Jamaican Negroes. *Br. J. Haematol.* **30**, 197.

Ahmed, S., Petrou, M. & Saleem, M. (1996) Molecular genetics of β-thalassaemia in Pakistan: a basis for prenatal diagnosis. *Br. J. Haematol.* **94**, 476.

Ajmani, M., Sharma, A., Talukder, G. & Bhattacharya, D.K. (1976) Beta-thalassaemia trait in West Bengal—a methodological study. *Curr. Sci.* **45**, 461.

Aksoy, M. (1959) Abnormal haemoglobins in Turkey. In: *Abnormal Haemoglobins—A Symposium* (eds J. H. P. Jonxis & J. F. Delafresnaye), p. 216. Blackwell Scientific Publications, Oxford.

Aksoy, M. (1963) The first observation of homozygous hemoglobin S-alpha thalassemia disease and two types of sickle cell disease: (a) sickle cell-alpha thalassemia disease (b) sickle cell-beta thalassemia disease. *Blood* **22**, 757.

Aksoy, M. (1970) Thalassaemia intermedia: a genetic study in 11 patients. *J. Med. Genet.* **7**, 47.

Aksoy, M. (1991) The history of beta-thalassemia in Turkey. *Turkish J. Pediatr.* **33**, 195.

Aksoy, M. & Erdem, S. (1968a) Combination of hereditary elliptocytosis and heterozygous beta-thalassaemia: a family study. *J. Med. Genet.* **5**, 298.

Aksoy, M. & Erdem, S. (1968b) The combination of hereditary spherocytosis and heterozygous beta-thalassaemia. A family study. *Acta Haematol. (Basel)* **39**, 183.

Aksoy, M. & Erdem, S. (1968c) Haemoglobin H disease. Study of an Eti-Turk family. *Acta Genet.* **18**, 12.

Aksoy, M. & Lehmann, H. (1957) Sickle-cell-thalassaemia disease in South Turkey. *Br. Med. J.* **i**, 734.

Aksoy, M., Egribozlu, A. & Alpustun, H. (1961) The thalassaemia syndromes. I. Thalassaemia minor with large amount of foetal haemoglobin. Study of a family. *Acta Haematol.* **25**, 136.

Aksoy, M., Cetingil, A.I., Kocabalkan, N. *et al.* (1963) Thalassemia-hemoglobin E disease in Turkey, with hypersplenism in one case. *Am. J. Med.* **34**, 851.

Aksoy, M., Camili, N., Dincol, K., Erdem, S. & Dincol, G. (1973) On the problem of 'rib-within-a-rib' appearance in thalassemia intermedia. *Radiol. Clin. Biol.* **42**, 126.

Aksoy, M., Erdem, S. & Dincol, G. (1974) Delta beta-thalassaemia in two Turkish families. *J. Med. Genet.* **11**, 337.

Aksoy, M., Erdem, S. & Dincol, G. (1975) β-Thalassaemia with normal levels of hemoglobins F and A₂. Simple heterozygous and homozygous forms and doubly heterozygous state with β-thalassaemia with increased hemoglobin A₂. Study in seven families. In: *Proceedings of the International Instanbul Symposium on Abnormal Hemoglobins and Thalassemia*, p. 289. TBTAK, Ankara.

Aksoy, M., Dincol, G. & Erdem, S. (1978a) Different types of beta-thalassaemia intermedia. *Acta Haematol. (Basel)* **59**, 178.

Aksoy, M., Tahsinoglu, M., Erdem, S. & Dincol, G. (1978b) Myelofibrosis in a case of Hb E-β+ thalassemia. *New Istanbul Contrib. Clin. Sci.* **12**, 279.

Aksoy, M., Kutlar, A., Kutlar, F. *et al.* (1984) Hb Beograd-β⁰ thalassemia in a Turkish family from Yugoslavia. *Hemoglobin* **8**, 417.

Aksoy, M., Kutlar, A., Kutlar, F., Dinçol, G., Erdem, S. & Bastesbihçi, S. (1985) Survey on haemoglobin variants, β thalassaemia, glucose-6-phosphate dehydrogenase deficiency, and haptoglobin types in Turks from Western Thrace. *J. Med. Genet.* **22**, 288.

Alam, R., Padmanabhan, K. & Rao, H. (1997) Paravertebral mass in a patient with thalassemia intermedia. *Chest* **112**, 265.

Alberti, R., Maruzzi, G.M., Marinucci, M., Bruni, E. & Tentori, L. (1975) Haemoglobin Hasharon in a north Italian community. *J. Med. Genet.* **12**, 294.

Alberti, R., Tentori, L., Martinucci, M. & Borghesi, V. (1978) Hb A₂-Adria (δ51 Pro yield Arg (D2): a new δ-chain variant found in association with β-thalassaemia. *Hemoglobin* **2**, 171.

Alberts, B., Bray, D., Lewis, J., Raff, M., Roberts, K. & Watson, J.B. (1994) *The Molecular Biology of the Cell*. Garland, New York and London.

Albitar, M., Peschle, C. & Liebhaber, S.A. (1989) Theta, zeta and epsilon globin messenger RNAs are expressed in adults. *Blood* **74**, 629.

Albitar, M., Katsumata, M. & Liebhaber, S.A. (1991) Human α-globin genes demonstrate autonomous developmental regulation in transgenic mice. *Mol. Cell. Biol.* **11**, 3786.

Aldouri, M.A., Wonke, B., Hoffbrand, A.V. *et al.* (1987) Iron state and hepatic disease in patients with thalassaemia major treated with long term subcutaneous desferrioxamine. *J. Clin. Pathol.* **40**, 1352.

Aldouri, M.A., Wonke, B., Hoffbrand, A.V. *et al.* (1990) High incidence of cardiomyopathy in beta-thalassaemia patients receiving regular transfusion and iron chelation: reversal by intensified chelation. *Acta Haematol.* **84**, 113.

Ali, M.A.M. & McBride, J.A. (1973) Globin synthesis in haemoglobin Lepore trait. *Br. J. Haematol.* **25**, 284.

Ali, M.A.M., Quinlan, A. & Wong, S.C. (1980) Identification of hemoglobin E by isopropanol solubility test. *Clin. Biochem.* **13**, 146.

Aljurf, M., Ma, L., Angelucci, E. *et al.* (1996) Abnormal assembly of membrane proteins in erythroid progenitors of patients with beta-thalassaemia major. *Blood* **87**, 2049.

Al-Khatti, A., Veith, R.A., Papayannopoulou, T., Fritsch, E.F., Goldwasser, E. & Stamatoyannopoulos, G. (1987) Stimulation of fetal hemoglobin synthesis by erythropoietin in baboons. *N. Eng. J. Med.* **317**, 415.

Allamanis, J. (1955) Paper electrophoresis of serum proteins in Cooley's anaemia and sickle cell anaemia. *Acta Paediatr.* **44**, 122.

Allen, S.J., O'Donnell, A., Alexander, N.D.E. *et al.* (1997) α+-Thalassaemia protects children against disease caused by other infections as well as malaria. *Proc. Natl Acad. Sci. USA* **94**, 14736.

Allison, A.C. (1954) Protection afforded by sickle-cell trait against subtertian malarial infection. *Br. Med. J.* **i**, 290.

Allison, A.C. (1964) Polymorphism and natural selection in human populations. *Cold Spring Harbor Sympos. Quant. Biol.* **29**, 137.

Allison, A.C. (1965) Population genetics of abnormal haemoglobins and glucose-6-phosphate dehydrogenase deficiency. In: *Abnormal Haemoglobins in Africa* (ed. J. H. P. Jonxis), p. 365. Blackwell Scientific Publications, Oxford.

Aloia, J.F., Ostuni, J.A., Yeh, J.K. & Zaino, E.C. (1982) Combined vitamin D parathyroid defect in thalassemia major. *Arch. Intern. Med.* **142**, 831.

Al-Refaie, F.N., Wonke, B., Hoffbrand, A.V., Wickens, D.G., Nortey, P. & Kontoghiorghes, G.J. (1992) Efficacy and possible adverse effects of the oral iron chelator 1,2-dimethyl-3-hydroxypyrid-4-one (L1) in thalassaemia major. *Blood* **80**, 592.

Al-Refaie, F.N., Hershko, C., Hoffbrand, A.V. *et al.* (1995) Results of long-term deferiprone (L1) therapy. A report by the International Study Group on Oral Iron Chelators. *Br. J. Haematol.* **91**, 224.

Altay, C., Huisman, T.H.J. & Schroeder, W.A. (1976–77) Another form of hereditary persistence of fetal hemoglobin (the Atlanta type)? *Hemoglobin* **1**, 125.

Altay, C., Say, B., Yetgin, S. & Huisman, T.H.J. (1977a) α-Thalassemia and β-thalassemia in a Turkish family. *Am. J. Hematol.* **2**, 1.

Altay, C., Schroeder, W.A. & Huisman, T.H.J. (1977b) The ᴳγ-δβ-thalassemia and $^G\gamma$-β^0-HPFH conditions in combination with β-thalassemia and Hb S. *Am. J. Hematol.* **3**, 1.

Altay, C., Kutlar, A., Wilson, J.B., Webber, B.B. & Huisman, T.H.J. (1987) Hb P-Nilotic or $\alpha_2(\beta\delta)_2$ in a Turkish family. *Hemoglobin* **11**, 395.

Altay, C., Gurgey, A., Öner, R., Kutlar, A., Kutlar, F. & Huisman, T.H.J. (1991) A mild thalassemia major resulting from a compound heterozygosity for the IVS-II-1 (G-A) mutation and the rare T-C mutation at the polyadenylation site. *Hemoglobin* **15**, 327.

Alter, B.P. (1979) The $^G\gamma{:}^A\gamma$ composition of fetal hemoglobin in fetuses and newborns. *Blood* **54**, 1158.

Alter, B.P. (1984) Advances in the prenatal diagnosis of hematologic diseases. *Blood* **64**, 329.

Alter, B.P. (1989) Examination of fetal blood for haemoglobinopathies. In: *Methods in Haematology: Perinatal Haematology* (ed. B.P. Alter), p. 13. Churchill Livingstone, Edinburgh.

Alter, B.P. (1990) Antenatal diagnosis. Summary of results. *Ann. N.Y. Acad. Sci.* **612**, 237.

Alter, B.P. & Nathan, D.G. (1978) Antenatal diagnosis of haematological disorders—1978. *Clin. Haematol.* **7**, 19.

Alter, B.P., Friedman, S., Hobbins, J.C. *et al.* (1976a) Prenatal diagnosis of sickle-cell anemia and alpha G-Philadelphia. Study of a fetus at risk for Hb S/β thalassemia. *N. Eng. J. Med.* **294**, 1040.

Alter, B.P., Modell, C.B., Fairweather, D. *et al.* (1976b) Prenatal diagnosis of hemoglobinopathies. A review of 15 cases. *N. Eng. J. Med.* **295**, 1437.

Alter, B.P., Rappeport, J.M., Huisman, T.H.J., Schroeder, W.A. & Nathan, D.G. (1976c) Fetal erythropoiesis following bone marrow transplantation. *Blood* **48**, 843.

Alter, B.P., Metzger, J.B., Yock, P.G., Rothchild, S.B. & Dover, G.J. (1979a) Selective hemolysis of adult red blood cells: an aid to prenatal diagnosis of hemoglobinopathies. *Blood* **53**, 279.

Alter, B.P., Orkin, S.H. & Nathan, D.G. (1979b) Prenatal diagnosis of the hemoglobinopathies. In: *Laboratory Investigation of Fetal Disease* (ed. A. J. Barson), p. 337. Wright and Sons Ltd, London.

Alter, B.P., Goff, S.C., Efremov, G.D., Gravely, M.E. & Huisman, T.H.J. (1980) Globin chain electrophoresis: a new approach to the determination of the $^G\gamma/^A\gamma$ ratio in fetal haemoglobin and to studies of globin synthesis. *Br. J. Haematol.* **44**, 527.

Amegnizin, K.P.E., Pagnier, J., Wajcman, H., Lapoumeroulie, C. & Labie, D. (1979) Hb J Lome β59 (E3) Lys→Asn associated with HPFH in a Togolese family. *Hemoglobin* **3**, 87.

Ameri, M.R., Aleboiuyeh, M., Ziai, M. & Conn, R.B. (1975) Hypertriglyceridemia in homozygous beta thalassemia. *J. Pediatr.* **87**, 1002.

American Association for the Advancement of Science (1992) *The Genome, Ethics and the Law: Issues in Genetic Testing.* AAAS, Washington DC.

Amin, A.B., Pandya, N.L., Diwin, P.P. *et al.* (1979) A comparison of the homozygous states for $^G\gamma$ and $^G\gamma^A\gamma$ $\delta\beta$ thalassaemia. *Br. J. Haematol.* **43**, 537.

Amselem, S., Nunes, V., Vidaud, M. *et al.* (1988) Determination of the spectrum of β-thalassemia genes in Spain by use of dot-blot analysis of amplified β-globin DNA. *Am. J. Hum. Genet.* **43**, 95.

Anagnou, N.P., Ley, T.J., Chesbro, B. *et al.* (1983) Acquired α-thalassemia in preleukemia is due to decreased expression of all four α-globin genes. *Proc. Natl Acad. Sci. USA* **80**, 6051.

Anagnou, N.P., Papayannopoulou, T., Stamatoyannopoulos, G. & Nienhuis, A.W. (1985) Structurally diverse molecular deletions in the β-globin gene cluster exhibit an identical phenotype on interaction with the β^S-gene. *Blood* **65**, 1254.

Anagnou, N.P., Papayannopoulou, T., Nienhuis, A.W. & Stamatoyannopoulos, G. (1988) Molecular characterization of a novel form of $(^A\gamma\delta\beta)^0$-thalassaemia deletion with a 3' breakpoint close to those of HPFH-3 and HPFH-4: insights for a common regulatory mechanism. *Nucl. Acids Res.* **16**, 6057.

Anagnou, N.P., Perez-Stable, C., Gelinas, R. *et al.* (1995) Sequences located 3' to the breakpoint of the hereditary persistence of fetal hemoglobin-3 deletion exhibit enhancer activity and can modify the developmental expression of the human fetal $^A\gamma$-globin gene in transgenic mice. *J. Biol. Chem.* **270**, 10256.

Anapliotou, M.L., Kastanias, I.T., Psara, P., Evangelou, E.A., Liparaki, M. & Dimitriou, P. (1995) The contribution of hypogonadism to the development of osteoporosis in thalassaemia major: new therapeutic approaches. *Clin. Endocrinol.* **42**, 279.

Anderson, W.F. & Fletcher, J.C. (1980) Gene therapy in human beings: when is it ethical to begin. *N. Eng. J. Med.* **303**, 1293.

Anderson, B.B., Mollin, D.L., Modell, C.B. & Perry, G.M. (1975) Red-cell metabolism of pyridoxine in sideroblastic anaemia and thalassaemia. In: *Iron Metabolism and Its Disorders* (ed. H.E.A. Kief), p. 241. Excerpta Medica, Amsterdam.

Anderson, B.B., Perry, G.M., Modell, C.B., Child, J.A. & Mollin, D.L. (1979) Abnormal red cell metabolism of pyridoxine associated with β-thalassaemia. *Br. J. Haematol.* **41**, 497.

Anderson, K.P., Lloyd, J.A., Ponce, E., Crable, S.C., Neumann, J.C. & Lingrel, J.B. (1993) Regulated expression of the human β globin gene in transgenic mice requires an upstream globin or nonglobin promoter. *Mol. Cell. Biol.* **4**, 1077.

Andre, R., Najman, A., Duhamel, G. *et al.* (1972) Erythro-leucémie avec hémoglobine H acquise et anomalies des antigènes erythrocytaires. *Nouv. Rev. Fr. Hematol.* **12**, 29.

Andre, M., Bergmann, P., Ferster, A., Toppet, M. & Fondu, P. (1991) Serum immunoreactive erythropoietin level: a new parameter for monitoring transfusion management of thalassaemia. *Nouv. Rev. Fr. Hematol.* **33**, 299.

Andreani, M., Manna, M., Lucarelli, G. *et al.* (1996) Persistence of mixed chimerism in patients transplanted for the treatment of thalassemia. *Blood* **87**, 3494.

Andrews, N.C., Erdjument-Bromage, H., Davidson, M.B., Tempst, P. & Orkin, S.H. (1993a) Erythroid transcription factor NF/E2 is a haematopoietic-specific basic-leucine zipper protein. *Nature* **362**, 722.

Andrews, N.C., Kotkow, K.J., Ney, P.A., Erdjument-Bromage, H., Tempst, P. & Orkin, S.H. (1993b) The ubiquitous subunit of erythroid transcription factor NF-E2 is a small basic-leucine zipper protein related to the v-*maf* oncogene. *Proc. Natl Acad. Sci. USA* **90**, 11488.

Angastiniotis, M.A. & Hadjiminas, M.G. (1981) Prevention of thalassaemia in Cyprus. *Lancet* **1**, 369.

Angastiniotis, M. & Modell, B. (1998) Global epidemiology of hemoglobin disorders. *Ann. N.Y. Acad. Sci.* **850**, 251.

Angelini, V. (1937) Primi risultati di richerche ematologiche nei familiari di ammalati di anemia di Cooley. *Min. Med.* **28**, 331.

Angelucci, E., Baronciani, D., Lucarelli, G. *et al.* (1993) Liver iron overload and liver fibrosis in thalassemia. *Bone Marrow Transplant.* **1**, 29.

Angelucci, E., Baronciani, D., Lucarelli, G. *et al.* (1995) Needle liver biopsy in thalassaemia: analyses of diagnostic accuracy and safety in 1184 consecutive biopsies. *Br. J. Haematol.* **89**, 757.

Angelucci, E., Ripalti, M., Baronciani, D. *et al.* (1997) Phlebotomy to reduce iron overload in patients cured of thalassemia by marrow transplantation. *Bone Marrow Transplant.* **19** (Suppl. 2), 123.

Angelucci, E., Brittenham, G.M., Mclaren, C.E. *et al.* (2000) Hepatic iron concentration and total body iron stores in thalassaemia major. *N. Eng. J. Med.* **343**, 327.

Angles-Cano, E., Robles-Arrendondo, I., Ferrer, V., Gonzalez-Constandse, R. & Ortiz-Trejo, J.F. (1977) Talasemia alfa (hemoglobinopatía H) en una familia mestiza mexicana. *Sangre* **22**, 366.

Anneren, G. & Gustavson, K.-H. (1984) Partial trisomy 3q (3q25→qter) syndrome in two siblings. *Acta Paediatr. Scand.* **73**, 281.

Annino, L., Di Giovanni, S., Tentori, L. Jr *et al.* (1984). Acquired hemoglobin H disease in a case of refractory anemia with excess of blasts (RAEB) evolving into acute nonlymphoid leukemia. *Acta Haematol.* **72**, 41.

Anoussakis, C., Alexiou, D., Abatxis, D. & Bechrakis, G. (1977) Endocrinological investigation of pituitary gonadal axis in thalassaemia major. *Acta Paediatr. Scand.* **66**, 49.

Antonarakis, S.E., Boehm, C.D., Giardina, P.V.J. & Kazazian, H.H. (1982) Non random association of polymorphic restriction sites in the β-globin gene complex. *Proc. Natl Acad. Sci. USA* **79**, 137.

Antonarakis, S.E., Orkin, S.H., Cheng, T.-C. *et al.* (1984) β-Thalassemia in American blacks: novel mutations in the TATA box and IVS-2 acceptor splice site. *Proc. Natl Acad. Sci. USA* **81**, 1154.

Antonarakis, S.E., Kang, J., Lam, V.M.S., Tam, J.W.O. & Li, A.M.C. (1988) Molecular characterization of β-globin gene mutations in patients with β-thalassemia intermedia in South China. *Br. J. Haematol.* **70**, 357.

Antoniou, M. & Grosveld, F. (1990) The β-globin dominant control region interacts differently with distal and proximal promoter elements. *Genes Dev.* **4**, 1007.

Antoniou, M., deBoer, E., Habets, G. & Grosveld, F. (1988) The human β-globin gene contains multiple regulatory regions: identification of one promoter and two downstream enhancers. *EMBO J.* **7**, 377.

Anuwatanakulchia, M., Pootrakul, P., Thuvasethakul, P. & Wasi, P. (1984) Non-transferrin plasma iron in β-thalassaemia/Hb E and haemoglobin H diseases. *Scand. J. Haematol.* **32**, 153.

Appleyard, B. (1993) Our plunge in the gene pool. *The Independent* May 12th.

Araujo, A., Kosaryan, M., MacDowell, A. *et al.* (1996) A novel delivery system for continuous desferrioxamine infusion in transfusional iron overload. *Br. J. Haematol.* **93**, 835.

Arcasoy, A. & Çavdar, A. (1978) Electrophoretically detectable abnormal haemoglobins in a healthy Turkish population. *New Istanbul Contrib. Clin. Sci.* **12**, 258.

Arcasoy, M.O. & Gallagher, P.G. (1995) Hematologic disorders and nonimmune hydrops fetalis. *Sem. Perinatol.* **19**, 502.

Arcasoy, A., Çavdar, A., Cin, S. *et al.* (1987) Effects of zinc supplementation on linear growth in beta thalassemia (a new approach). *Am. J. Hematol.* **24**, 127.

Arcasoy, M.O., Romana, M., Fabry, M.E., Skarpidi, E., Nagel, R.L. & Forget, B.G. (1997) High levels of human γ-globin gene expression in adult mice carrying a transgene of deletion-type hereditary persistence of fetal hemoglobin. *Mol. Cell. Biol.* **17**, 2076.

Arends, T. (1984) Epidemiologia de las bariantes hemoglobinicas Venezuela. *Gac. Med. Caracas*, **92**, 189.

Arends, T., Garlin, G., Guevara, J.M. *et al.* (1985) Hemoglobin Hofu associated with beta 0-thalassemia. *Acta Haematol.* **73**, 51.

Argiolu, F., Sanna, M.A., Addari, M.C. *et al.* (1997) Bone marrow transplantation in thalassemia: the experience of Cagliari. *Bone Marrow Transplant.* **19** (Suppl. 2), 65.

Arjona, S.N., Eloy-Garcia, J.M., Gu, L.H., Smetanina, N.S. & Huisman, T.H.J. (1996) The dominant β-thalassaemia in a Spanish family is due to a frameshift that introduces an extra CGG codon (= arginine) at the 5′ end of the second exon. *Br. J. Haematol.* **93**, 841.

Arnett, E.N., Nienhuis, A.W., Henry, W.L., Ferrans, V.J., Redwood, D.R. & Roberts, W.C. (1975) Massive myocardial hemosiderosis: a structure–function conference at the National Heart and Lung Institute. *Am. Heart J.* **90**, 777.

Arnone, A. (1972) X-ray diffraction study of binding of 2,3 diphosphoglycerate to human deoxyhaemoglobin. *Nature* **237**, 146.

Arous, N., Galacteros, F., Fessas, P. *et al.* (1983) Structural study of hemoglobin Knossos, β27(B9)Ala→Ser. A new abnormal hemoglobin present as a silent β-thalassemia. *FEBS Lett.* **147**, 247.

Arribalzaga, K., Ricard, M.P., Carreño, D.L. *et al.* (1996) Hb J-Baltimore [β16(A13)Gly→Asp] associated with β⁺-thalassemia in a Spanish family. *Hemoglobin* **20**, 79.

Asano, H., Li, X.S. & Stamatoyannopoulos, G. (1999) FKLF, a novel Krüppel-like factor that activates human embryonic and fetal β-like globin genes. *Mol. Cell. Biol.* **19**, 3571.

Asbell, M.B. (1964) Orthodontic aspects of Cooley's anemia. *Ann. N. Y. Acad. Sci.* **119**, 662.

Ascenzi, A. & Silvestroni, E. (1957) Étude anatomo-clinique d'un cas de maladia microdrépanocytique. *Acta Haematol. (Basel)* **18**, 205.

Aschauer, H., Sanguamsermsri, T. & Braunitzer, G. (1981) Human embryonic haemoglobins. The primary structure of the zeta chains. *Hoppe Seylers Z. Physiol. Chem.* **362**, 1159.

Ashiotis, T., Zachariadis, Z., Sofroniadou, K., Loukopoulos, D. & Stamatoyannopoulos, G. (1973) Thalassaemia in Cyprus. *Br. Med. J.* **2**, 38.

Astaldi, G., Tolentino, P. & Sacchetti, G. (1951) La talassemia (Morbo di Cooley e forme affini). *Biblioteca 'Haematologica'*, p. XII. Pavia.

Astaldi, G., Rondanelli, E.G., Bernadelli, E. & Strosselli, E. (1954) An abnormal substance present in the erythroblasts of thalassaemia major. Cytochemical investigations. *Acta Haematol.* **12**, 145.

Aswapokee, N., Aswapokee, P., Fucharoen, S. & Wasi, P. (1988a) A study of infective episodes in patients with β-thalassaemia/Hb E disease in Thailand. *Birth Defects* **23**, 513.

Aswapokee, P., Aswapokee, N., Fucharoen, S., Sukroongreung, S. & Wasi, P. (1988b) Severe infection in thalassemia: a prospective study. *Birth Defects* **23**, 521.

Atalay, E.Ö., Çirakoglu, B., Dincolç, G. *et al.* (1993) Regional distributions of β-thalassemia mutations in Turkey. *Int. J. Hematol.* **57**, 207.

Athanassiadou, A., Papachatzopoulou, A., Zoumbos, N., Maniatis, G. & Gibbs, R. (1994) A novel β-thalassaemia mutation in the 5′ untranslated region of the β-globin gene. *Br. J. Haematol.* **88**, 307.

Atwater, J., Schwartz, I.R., Erslev, A.J., Montgomery, T.L. & Tocantins, L.M. (1960) Sickling of erythrocytes in a patient with thalassemia hemoglobin-I disease. *N. Eng. J. Med.* **263**, 1215.

Atwater, J., Schwartz, E. & Gabuzda, T.G. (1970) Hemoglobin Jα in an Italian-American family: lack of interaction with beta-thalassemia. In: *XII International Congress of Haematology*, p. 233. J.F. Lehmanns-Verlag Munchen, Munich.

Atweh, G.F. & Forget, B.G. (1987) Clinical and molecular correlations in the sickle/β⁺-thalassemia syndrome. *Am. J. Hematol.* **24**, 31.

Atweh, G.F., Anagnou, N.P., Forget, B.G. & Kaufman, R.E. (1985) β thalassemia resulting from a single nucleotide substitution in an acceptor splice site. *Nucl. Acids Res.* **13**, 777.

Atweh, G.F., Zhu, D.-E. & Forget, B.G. (1986) A novel basis for δβ-thalassemia in a Chinese family. *Blood* **68**, 1108.

Atweh, G.F., Wong, C.R., Reed, R. *et al.* (1987a) A new mutation in IVS-I of the human β-globin gene causing β-thalassaemia due to abnormal splicing. *Blood* **70**, 147.

Atweh, G.F., Zhu, X.-X., Brickner, H.W., Dowling, C.H., Kazazian, H.H. & Forget, B.G. (1987b) The β-globin gene on the Chinese δβ-thalassemia chromosome carries a promoter mutation. *Blood* **70**, 1470.

Atweh, G.F., Brickner, H.E., Zhu, X.X., Kazazian, H.H. & Forget, B.G. (1988) A new amber mutation in a β-thalassaemia gene with non-measurable levels of mutant mRNA *in vivo. J. Clin. Invest.* **82**, 557.

Atweh, G.F., Sutton, M., Nassif, I. *et al.* (1999) Sustained induction of fetal hemoglobin by pulse butyrate therapy in sickle cell disease. *Blood* **93**, 1790.

Aulehla-Scholz, C., Basaran, S., Agaoglu, L. *et al.* (1990) Molecular basis of β-thalassemia in Turkey: detection of rare mutations by direct sequencing. *Hum. Genet.* **84**, 195.

Aung-Than-Batu & Hla-Pe, U. (1971) Haemoglobinopathies in Burma I. The incidence of haemoglobin E. *Trop. Geogr. Med.* **23**, 15.

Aung-Than-Batu, Khin-Kyi-Nyunt & Hla-Pe, U. (1968) The thalassemias in Burma. *Union of Burma J. Life Sci.* **1**, 241.

Aung-Than-Batu, Hla-Pe, U. & Khin-Kyi-Nyunt (1971) Haemoglobin H disease. *Trop. Geogr. Med.* **23**, 15.

Ausavarungnirun, R., Winichagoon, P., Fucharoen, S., Epstein, N. & Simkins, R. (1998) Detection of ζ-globin chains in the cord blood by ELISA (Enzyme-Linked Immunosorbent Assay): rapid screening for α-thalassemia-1 (southeast Asian type). *Am. J. Hematol.* **57**, 283.

Avissar, N., Inbal, A., Rabizadeh, E., Shaklai, M. & Shaklai, N. (1984) Interaction of spectrin with hemin disaggregates spectrin association. *Biochem. In.* **8**, 113.

Ayala, S., Colomer, D., Pujades, A. & Aymerich, M. & Vives Corrons, J.L. (1996) Haemoglobin Lleida: a new α$_2$-globin variant (12 bp deletion) with mild thalassaemic phenotype. *Br. J. Haematol.* **94**, 639.

Ayala, S., Colomer, D., Aymerich, M., Abella, E. & Vives Corrons, J.L. (1997) First description of a frameshift mutation in the α$_1$-globin gene associated with α-thalassaemia. *Br. J. Haematol.* **98**, 47.

Ayala, S., Colomer, D., Gelpi, J.L. & Vives Corrons, J.L. (1998) α-Thalassemia due to a single codon deletion in the α$_1$-globin gene. Computational structural analysis of the new α-chain variant (Hb Clinic). *Hum. Mutat.* **11**, 412.

Bacalo, A., Kivity, S., Heno, N., Greif, J. & Topilsky, M. (1992) Blood transfusion and lung function in children with thalassemia major. *Chest* **101**, 362.

Bachir, D., Drame, M., Lee, K., Portos, J.-L. & Galacteros, F. (1995) Clinical effects of hydroxyurea in thalassemia intermedia patients. In: *Sickle Cell Disease and Thalassemia: New Trends in Therapy* (eds Y. Beuzard, B. Lubin & J. Rosa), p. 195. Colloque INSERM, Paris.

Bacon, B.R., Tavil, A.S., Brittenham, G.M., Park, C.H. & Recknagel, R.O. (1983) Hepatic lipid peroxidation *in vivo* in rats with chronic iron overload. *J. Clin. Invest.* **71**, 429.

Badens, C., Thuret, I., Michel, G. *et al.* (1996) Novel and unusual deletion-insertion thalassemic mutation in exon 1 of the β-globin gene. *Hum. Mutat.* **8**, 89.

Badens, C., Jassim, N., Martini, N., Mattei, J.F., Elion, J. & Lena-Russo, D. (1999) Characterization of a new polymorphism, IVS-I-108(T→C), and a new β-thalassemia mutation -27(A→T), discovered in the course of a prenatal diagnosis. *Hemoglobin* **23**, 339.

Badr, F.M., Lorkin, P.A. & Lehmann, H. (1973) Haemoglobin P-Nilotic containing a β-δ-chain. *Nature New Biol.* **242**, 107.

Baglioni, C. (1962) The fusion of two peptide chains in hemoglobin Lepore and its interpretation as a genetic deletion. *Proc. Natl Acad. Sci. USA* **48**, 1880.

Baglioni, C. (1963) A child homozygous for persistence of foetal haemoglobin. *Nature* **198**, 1177.

Baglioni, C. (1965) Abnormal human hemoglobins. X. A study of hemoglobin Lepore (Boston). *Biochim. Biophys. Acta* **97**, 37.

Baglioni, C. & Campana, T. (1967) α Chain and globin: intermediates in the synthesis of rabbit globin. *Eur. J. Biochem.* **2**, 480.

Baglioni, C. & Ingram, V.M. (1961) Abnormal human haemoglobins. V. Chemical investigation of haemoglobins A, G, C, X from one individual. *Biochim. Biophys. Acta* **48**, 253.

Baglioni, C., Colombo, B. & Jacobs-Lorena, M. (1969) Chain termination: a test for a possible explanation of thalassemia. *Ann. N. Y. Acad. Sci.* **165**, 212.

Bahl, V.K., Malhotra, O.P., Kumar, D. *et al.* (1992) Noninvasive assessment of systolic and diastolic left ventricular function in patients with chronic severe anemia: a combined M-mode, two-dimensional, and Doppler echocardiographic study. *Am. Heart J.* **124**, 1516.

Baiget, M. & Gimferrer, E. (1986) Geographical distribution of hemoglobin variants in Spain. In: *Hemoglobin Variants in Human Populations* (ed. W. P. Winter), p. 141. CRC Press, Boca Raton, Florida.

Baiget, M., Gimferrer, E., Fernandez, I. *et al.* (1983) Spanish delta-beta-thalassemia: hematological studies and composition of the gamma-chains in ten homozygous patients. *Acta Haematol.* **70**, 341.

Bailey, I.S. & Prankerd, T.A.J. (1958) Studies in thalassaemia. *Br. J. Haematol.* **4**, 150.

Bain, B.J. & Phelan, L. (1997) *An Evaluation of the Primus Corporation CLC 330TM Primus Variant System 99 (PVS99)*. Medical Devices Agency, London.

Baine, R.M., Wright, J.M. & Wilkinson, R.M. (1979) Hb G Waimanalo (α64 Asp→Asn) in a child with homozygous β-thalassemia. *Hemoglobin* **3**, 293.

Baird, B., Driscoll, C., Schreiner, H. *et al.* (1981a) A nucleotide change at a splice in the human β-globin gene is associated with β^0-thalassemia. *Proc. Natl Acad. Sci. USA* **78**, 4218.

Baird, M., Schreiner, H., Driscoll, C. & Bank, A. (1981b) Localization of the site of recombination in formation of the Lepore Boston globin gene. *J. Clin. Invest.* **68**, 560.

Baker, D.H. (1964) Roentgen manifestations of Cooley's anemia. *Ann. N. Y. Acad. Sci.* **119**, 641.

Bakioglu, I., Kutlar, A. & Huisman, T.H.J. (1986) Differences between the levels of ^{G}γ chain in the fetal hemoglobin in two types of hereditary persistence of fetal hemoglobin are linked with a variation in the DNA sequence. *Biochem. Genet.* **24**, 149.

Baklouti, F., Dorleac, E., Morle, L. *et al.* (1986) Homozygous hemoglobin Knossos (α$_2$β$_2$27(B9) Ala→Ser): a new variety of β$^+$ thalassemia intermedia associated with δ^0 thalassemia. *Blood* **67**, 957.

Baklouti, F., Francina, A., Dorleac, E. *et al.* (1987) Association in *cis* of beta$^+$-thalassemia and hemoglobin S. *Am. J. Hematol.* **26**, 237.

Baklouti, F., Ouazana, R., Gonnet, C., Lapillonne, A., Delaunay, J. & Godet, J. (1989) β$^+$-Thalassemia in *cis* of a sickle cell gene: occurrence of a promoter mutation on a β^S chromosome. *Blood* **74**, 1817.

Baldwin, J. (1980a) Structure and cooperativity of haemoglobin. *Trends Biol. Sci.* **5**, 224.

Baldwin, J.M. (1980b) The structure of human carbon monoxy-haemoglobin at 2.7 Å resolution. *J. Mol. Biol.* **136**, 103.

Ballart, I.J., Estevez, M.E., Sen, L. *et al.* (1986) Progressive dysfunction of monocytes associated with iron overload and age in patients with thalassemia major. *Blood* **67**, 105.

Ballas, S.K. (1997) Management of sickle pain. *Curr. Opin. Hematol.* **4**, 104.

Ballas, S.K. (1998) Sickle cell disease: clinical management. *Clin. Haematol.* **11**, 185.

Ballas, S.K., Atwater, J. & Norris, D.G. (1977) The interaction of β⁰ thalassemia with hemoglobin D Punjab: a study of globin chain synthesis in an Indian family. *Hemoglobin* **1**, 697.

Ballas, S.K., Fei, Y.J. & Huisman, T.H.J. (1989a) ζ- and θ1-globin gene deletions located on the same chromosome. *Br. J. Haematol.* **73**, 429.

Ballas, S.K., Talacki, C.A., Rao, V.M. & Steiner, R.M. (1989b) The prevalence of avascular necrosis in sickle cell anemia: correlation with α-thalassemia. *Hemoglobin* **13**, 649.

Balta, G., Brickner, H.E., Takegawa, S. *et al.* (1994) The increased expression of the ᴳγ and ᴬγ globin genes associated with a mutation in the ᴬγ enhancer. *Blood* **83**, 3727.

Baltimore, D. (1970) RNA-dependent polymerase in virions of RNA tumor viruses. *Nature* **226**, 1209.

Bank, A. & Marks, P.A. (1966) Excess α chain synthesis relative to β chain synthesis in thalassaemia major and minor. *Nature* **212**, 1198.

Bank, A. & O'Donnell, J.V. (1969) Intracellular loss of free-α chains in β thalassaemia. *Nature* **222**, 295.

Bank, A., Dow, L.W., Farace, M.G., O'Donnell, J.V., Ford, S. & Natta, C. (1973) Changes in globin synthesis with erythroid cell maturation in sickle thalassemia. *Blood* **41**, 353.

Bannerman, R.M. (1961) *Thalassemia. A Survey of Some Aspects.* Grune and Stratton, New York and London.

Bannerman, R.M. (1964) Iron absorption in thalassaemia. *Br. J. Haematol.* **10**, 490.

Bannerman, R.M. & Callender, S.T. (1961a) Iron absorption in thalassaemia. [Cited by Bannerman, R.M. (1961)]

Bannerman, R.M. & Callender, S.T. (1961b) Thalassaemia in Britain. *Br. Med. J.* **ii**, 1288.

Bannerman, R.M. & Renwick, J.H. (1962) The hereditary elliptocytosis. Clinical and linkage data. *Ann. Hum. Genet. (London)* **26**, 23.

Bannerman, R.M., Grinstein, M. & Moore, C.V. (1959) Haemoglobin synthesis in thalassaemia; *in vitro* studies. *Br. J. Haematol.* **5**, 102.

Bannerman, R.M., Keusch, G., Kreimer-Birnbaum, M., Vance, V.K. & Vaughan, S. (1967) Thalassemia intermedia, with iron overload, cardiac failure, diabetes mellitus, hypopituitarism and porphyrinuria. *Am. J. Med.* **42**, 476.

Baralle, F.E. (1977) Complete nucleotide sequence of the 5′ noncoding region of human α and β globin mRNA. *Cell* **12**, 1085.

Baralle, F.E., Shoulders, C.C. & Proudfoot, N.J. (1980) The primary structure of the human ε-globin gene. *Cell* **21**, 621.

Barbour, V.M., Tufarelli, C., Sharpe, J.A. *et al.* (2000) α-Thalassemia resulting from a negative chromosomal position effect. *Blood* **96**, 806.

Bargellesi, A., Pontremoli, S. & Conconi, F. (1967) Absence of beta globin synthesis and excess alpha globin synthesis in homozygous β thalassemia. *Eur. J. Biochem.* **1**, 73.

Bargellesi, A., Pontremoli, S., Menini, C. & Conconi, F. (1968) Excess of alpha globin synthesis in homozygous beta-thalassemia and its removal from the red blood cell cytoplasm. *Eur. J. Biochem.* **3**, 364.

Barkawi, M., Bashir, N. & Sharif, L. (1991) Sickle cell-thalassemia in a Jordanian family. *Trop. Geogr. Med.* **43**, 94.

Barker, J.E. & Wandersee, N.J. (1999) Thrombosis in heritable hemolytic disorders. *Curr. Opin. Hematol.* **6**, 71.

Barkham, P. & Adinolfi, M. (1962) Observations of the high foetal haemoglobin gene and its interaction with the thalassaemia gene. *J. Clin. Pathol.* **15**, 350.

Barkham, P., Stevenson, M.E. & Pinker, G. (1964) Haemoglobin Lepore trait: an analysis of the abnormal haemoglobin. *Br. J. Haematol.* **10**, 437.

Barnabus, J. & Muller, C.J. (1962) Haemoglobin Lepore (Hollandia). *Nature* **194**, 931.

Barnicot, N.A., Allison, A.C., Blumberg, B.S., Deliyannis, G., Krimbas, C. & Ballas, A. (1963) Haemoglobin types in Greek populations. *Ann. Hum. Genet. (London)* **26**, 229.

Barosi, G., Mascaretti, L., Borgna-Pignatti, C. *et al.* (1987) The relationship between erythropoiesis, foetal haemoglobin and clinical manifestations in thalassaemia intermedia. *Haematologica* **72**, 421.

Barrai, I., Rosito, A., Cappellozza, G. *et al.* (1984) Beta-thalassaemia in the Po Delta: selection, geography, and population structure. *Am. J. Hum. Genet.* **36**, 1121.

Barrios, N.J., Kirkpatrick, D.V., Lohmann, D., McMullen, C.C., Wilson, W. & Humbert, J.R. (1991) Spleen function in children with sickle β⁺ thalassemia. *J. Natl Med. Assoc.* **83**, 819.

Barry, M., Flynn, D.N., Letsky, E.A. & Risdon, R.A. (1974) Longterm chelation therapy in thalassaemia major: effect on liver iron concentration, liver histology and clinical progress. *Br. Med. J.* **i**, 16.

Basak, A.N., Özçelik, H., Özer, A. *et al.* (1992a) The molecular basis of β-thalassemia in Turkey. *Hum. Genet.* **89**, 315.

Basak, A.N., Özer, A., Özçelik, H., Kirdar, B. & Gürgey, A. (1992b) A novel frameshift mutation: deletion of C in codons 74/75 of the β-globin gene causes β⁰-thalassemia in a Turkish patient. *Hemoglobin* **16**, 309.

Basak, A.N., Özer, A., Kirdar, B. & Akar, N. (1993) A novel 13 bp deletion in the 3′UTR of the β-globin gene causes β-thalassemia in a Turkish patient. *Hemoglobin* **17**, 551.

Baserga, A. (1958) Fernando Rietti and hemolytic jaundice with increased globular resistance. *Scientia Medica Italica* **7**, 221.

Baserga, S.J. & Benz, E.J. Jr (1988) Nonsense mutations in the human β-globin gene affect mRNA metabolism. *Proc. Natl Acad. Sci. USA* **85**, 2056.

Bashir, N., Barkawi, M. & Sharif, L. (1992a) Sickle cell/β-thalassemia in North Jordan. *J. Trop. Pediatr.* **38**, 196.

Bashir, N., Barkawi, M., Sharif, L., Momani, A. & Gharaibeh, N. (1992b) Prevalence of hemoglobinopathies in North Jordan. *Trop. Geogr. Med.* **44**, 122.

Basset, P., Beuzard, Y., Garel, M.C. & Rosa, J. (1978) Isoelectric focusing of human hemoglobin; its application to screening, to the characterization of 70 variants, and to the study of modified fractions of normal hemoglobins. *Blood* **51**, 971.

Bate, C.M. (1975) Thalassaemia in Cyprus. *Proc. Roy Soc. Med.* **68**, 514.

Bate, C.M. & Humphries, G. (1977) Alpha-beta thalassaemia. *Lancet* **i**, 1031.

Baty, J.M., Blackfan, K.D. & Diamond, L.K. (1932) Blood studies in infants and in children. I. Erythroblastic anemia; a clinical and pathologic study. *Am. J. Dis. Child.* **43**, 667.

Bauer, C., Ludwig, I. & Ludwig, M. (1968) Different effects of 2,3-diphosphoglycerate and adenosine triphosphate on the oxygen affinity of adult and foetal human haemoglobin. *Life Sci.* **7**, 1339.

Baughan, M.A., Paglia, D.E., Schneider, A.S. & Valentine, W.N. (1968) An unusual haematological syndrome with pyruvate-kinase deficiency and thalassaemia minor in the kindreds. *Acta Haematol.* **39**, 345.

Bauknecht, T., Betteken, F. & Vogel, W. (1976) Trisomy 4p due to a paternal t (4p–; 16p+) translocation. *Hum. Genet.* **34**, 227.

Baumes, R.M. (1972) Abnormal hemoglobins: double heterozygote hemoglobin C-thalassemia. Two cases in a Moroccan family. *Moroc. Med.* **52**, 222.

Bauminger, E.R., Cohen, S.G., Ofer, S. & Rachmilewitz, E.A. (1980) Quantitative studies of ferritin iron in red blood cells of thalassemia, sickle cell anemia and hemoglobin Hammersmith using Mössbauer spectroscopy. *Proc. Natl Acad. Sci. USA* **76**, 939.

Baynes, R., Bezwoda, W., Bothwell, T., Khan, Q. & Mansoor, N. (1986) The non-immune inflammatory response: serial changes in plasma iron, iron-binding capacity, lactoferrin, ferritin and C-reactive protein. *Scand. J. Clin. Lab. Invest.* **46**, 695.

Baysal, E. & Huisman, T.H.J. (1994) Detection of common deletional α-thalassemia-2 determinants by PCR. *Am. J. Hematol.* **46**, 208.

Baysal, E., Indrak, K., Bozkurt, G. *et al.* (1992) The β-thalassaemia mutations in the population of Cyprus. *Br. J. Haematol.* **81**, 607.

Beard, M.J., Necheles, T.F. & Allen, D.M. (1969) Clinical experience with intensive transfusion in Cooley's anemia. *Ann. N. Y. Acad. Sci.* **165**, 415.

Beaudry, M.A., Ferguson, D.J., Pearse, K., Yanofsky, R.A., Rubin, E.M. & Kan, Y.W. (1986) Survival of a hydropic infant with homozygous α-thalassemia-1. *J. Pediatr.* **108**, 713.

Beaven, G.H., Ellis, M.J. & White, J.C. (1960) Studies in human foetal haemoglobin. II. Foetal haemoglobin levels in healthy children and adults and in certain haematological disorders. *Br. J. Haematol.* **6**, 201.

Beaven, G.H., Ellis, M.J. & White, J.C. (1961) Studies in human foetal haemoglobin. III. The hereditary haemoglobinopathies and thalassaemia. *Br. J. Haematol.* **7**, 169.

Beaven, G.H., Stevens, B.L., Dance, N. & White, J.C. (1963) Occurrence of haemoglobin H in leukaemia. *Nature* **199**, 1297.

Beaven, G.H., Gratzer, W.B., Stevens, B.L. *et al.* (1964) An abnormal haemoglobin (Lepore/Cyprus) resembling haemoglobin Lepore and its interaction with thalassaemia. *Br. J. Haematol.* **10**, 159.

Beaven, G.H., Fox, R.H. & Hornabrook, R.W. (1974) The occurrence of haemoglobin-J (Tongariki) and of thalassaemia on Karkar Island and the Papua New Guinea mainland. *Phil. Trans. Roy. Soc. Lond. B*, **268**, 269.

Beaven, G.H., Coleman, P.N. & White, J.C. (1978) Occurrence of haemoglobin H in leukaemia: a further case of erythroleukaemia. *Acta Haematol.* **59**, 37.

Becker, G.A. & Rossi, E.C. (1966) The interaction of hereditary persistence of fetal hemoglobin and beta thalassemia. *Ann. Intern. Med.* **65**, 1071.

Beet, E.A. (1946) Sickle cell disease in the Balovale District of Northern Rhodesia. *E. Afr. Med. J.* **23**, 75.

Beet, E.A. (1949) The genetics of the sickle-cell trait in a Bantu tribe. *Ann. Eugen.* **14**, 279.

Beguin, Y. (1992) The soluble transferrin receptor: biological aspects and clinical usefulness as quantitative measure of erythropoiesis. *Haematologica* **77**, 1.

Behringer, R.R., Hammer, R.E., Brinster, R.L., Palmiter, R.D. & Townes, T.M. (1987) Two 3′ sequences direct adult erythroid-specific expression of human β-globin genes in transgenic mice. *Proc. Natl Acad. Sci. USA* **84**, 7056.

Behringer, R.R., Ryan, T.M., Palmiter, R.D., Brinster, R.L. & Townes, T.M. (1990) Human γ- to β-globin gene switching in transgenic mice. *Genes Dev.* **4**, 376.

Beldjord, C., Lapoumeroulie, C., Pagnier, J. *et al.* (1988) A novel beta thalassemia gene with a single base mutation in the conserved polypyrimidine sequence at the 3′ end of IVS-II. *Nucl. Acids Res.* **16**, 4927.

Belgrader, P., Cheng, J., Zhou, X., Stephenson, L.S. & Maquat, L.E. (1994) Mammalian nonsense codons can be *cis* effectors of nuclear mRNA half-life. *Mol. Cell. Biol.* **14**, 8219.

Belhani, M., Dahmane, M., Richard, F., Trabuchet, G., Colonna, P. & Labie, D. (1977) Aspectes cliniques et biologiques des bêta-thalassémies. A propos de 176 observations. *Sem. Hôp. Paris*, **53**, 891.

Belhani, M., Morle, L., Godet, J. *et al.* (1984) Sickle cell beta-

thalassaemia compared with sickle cell anaemia in Algeria. *Scand. J. Haematol.* **32**, 346.

Bellingham, A.J. & Huehns, E.R. (1968) Compensation in haemolytic anaemias caused by abnormal haemoglobins. *Nature* **218**, 924.

Bellwood, P.S. (1989) The colonisation of the Pacific: some current hypotheses. In: *The Colonisation of the Pacific: A Genetic Trail* (eds A.V.S. Hill & S.W. Searjeantson), p. 1. Clarendon Press, Oxford.

Ben-Bassat, I., Hertz, M., Selzer, G. & Ramot, B. (1977) Extramedullary hematopoiesis with multiple tumor-simulating mediastinal masses in a patient with β-thalassemia intermedia. *Israel J. Med. Sci.* **13**, 1206.

Benesch, R. & Benesch, R.E. (1967) The effect of organic phosphates from the human erythrocyte on the allosteric properties of hemoglobin. *Biochem. Biophys. Res. Comm.* **26**, 162.

Benesch, R. & Benesch, R.E. (1968) Oxygenation and ion transport in red cells. *Science* **160**, 83.

Benesch, R. & Benesch, R.E. (1969) Intracellular organic phosphates as regulators of oxygen release by haemoglobin. *Nature* **221**, 618.

Benesch, R.E., Ranney, H.M., Benesch, R. & Smith, G.M. (1961) The chemistry of the Bohr effect. II. Some properties of hemoglobin H. *J. Biol. Chem.* **236**, 2926.

Benesch, R., Benesch, R.E. & Enoki, Y. (1968a) The interaction of hemoglobin and its subunits with 2,3-diphosphoglycerate. *Proc. Natl Acad. Sci. USA* **61**, 1102.

Benesch, R., Benesch, R.E. & Yu, C.I. (1968b) Reciprocal binding of oxygen and diphosphoglycerate by human hemoglobin. *Proc. Natl Acad. Sci. USA* **59**, 526.

Bennani, C., Bouhass, R., Perrin-Pecontal, P. *et al.* (1994) Anthropological approach to the heterogeneity of β-thalassemia mutations in Northern Africa. *Hum. Biol.* **66**, 369.

Bennett, J.M., Catovsky, D., Daniel, M.T. *et al.* (1982) Proposals for the classification of the myelodysplastic syndromes. *Br. J. Haematol.* **51**, 189.

Benson, P.J., Peterson, L.C., Hasegawa, D.K. & Smith, C.M. (1990) Abnormality of von Willebrand factor in patients with hemoglobin E-β⁰ thalassemia. *Am. J. Clin. Pathol.* **93**, 395.

Bentley, D.L. (1995) Regulation of transcriptional elongation by RNA polymerase II. *Curr. Opin. Genet. Dev.* **5**, 210.

Benz, E.J. & Forget, B.G. (1971) Defect in messenger RNA for human hemoglobin synthesis in beta thalassemia. *J. Clin. Invest.* **50**, 2755.

Benz, E.J., Swerdlow, P.S. & Forget, B.G. (1973) Globin messenger RNA in hemoglobin H disease. *Blood* **42**, 825.

Benz, E.J., Forget, B.G. & Housman, D. (1974) Molecular genetics of the β thalassemia (-thal) syndromes. *Pediatr. Res.* **8**, 387.

Benz, E.J., Swerdlow, P.S. & Forget, B.G. (1975) Absence of functional messenger RNA activity for beta globin chain synthesis in β⁰ thalassemia. *Blood* **45**, 1.

Benz, E.J., Forget, B.G., Hillman, D.G., Cohen-Solal, M., Pritchard, J. & Cavallesco, C. (1978) Variability in the amount of β globin mRNA in β⁰ thalassemia. *Cell* **14**, 299.

Benz, E.J., Berman, B.W., Tonkonow, B.L. *et al.* (1981) Molecular analysis of the β-thalassemia phenotype associated with inheritance of hemoglobin E ($\alpha_2\beta_2^{26\,Glu\rightarrow Lys}$). *J. Clin. Invest.* **68**, 118.

Benzie, R.J. & Pirani, B.B.K. (1977) Fetoscopy and anterior placentas. *N. Eng. J. Med.* **296**, 573.

Berdoukas, V., Bentley, P., Frost, H. & Schneble, H.P. (1993) Toxicity of oral iron chelator L1. *Lancet* **341**, 1088.

Berg, P.E., Williams, D.M., Qian, R.L., Cohen, R.B., Mittelman, M. & Schechter, A.N. (1989) Proteins binding to regulatory elements 5′ to the human beta-globin gene. *Prog. Clin. Biol. Res.* **316A**, 193.

Berg, P., Mittleman, M., Elion, J., Labie, D. & Schechter, A.N. (1991) Increased protein binding to a −530 mutation of the human β-globin gene associated with decreased β-globin synthesis. *Am. J. Hematol.* **36**, 42.

Bergeron, C. & Kovacs, K. (1978) Pituitary siderosis. A histologic, immunocytologic, and ultrastructural study. *Am. J. Pathol.* **93**, 295.

Bergren, W.R. & Sturgeon, P.H. (1960) Hemoglobin H: some additional findings. In: *Proceedings of the 7th International Congress in Hematology*, p. 488. Grune & Stratton, New York.

Beris, R.P., Miescher, P.A., Diaz-Chico, J.C. *et al.* (1988) Inclusion body β-thalassemia trait in a Swiss family is caused by an abnormal hemoglobin (Geneva) with an altered and extended β chain carboxy-terminus due to a modification in codon β114. *Blood* **72**, 801.

Beris, P., Kitundu, M.N., Baysal, E. *et al.* (1992) Black β-thalassemia homozygotes with specific sequence variations in the 5′ hypersensitive site-2 of the locus control region have high levels of fetal hemoglobin. *Am. J. Hematol.* **41**, 97.

Beris, P., Solenthaler, M., Deutsch, S. *et al.* (1999) Severe inclusion body β-thalassaemia with haemolysis in a patient double heterozygous for β⁰-thalassaemia and quadruplicated α-globin gene arrangement of the anti-4.2 type. *Br. J. Haematol.* **105**, 1074.

Berkovitch, M., Collins, A.F., Papadouric, D. *et al.* (1993) Need for early, low-dose chelation therapy in younger children with transfused homozygous β thalassemia. *Blood* **82**, 359a.

Bernards, R. & Flavell, R.A. (1980) Physical mapping of the globin gene deletion in hereditary persistence of foetal haemoglobin. *Nucl. Acids Res.* **8**, 1521.

Bernards, R., Kooter, J.M. & Flavell, R.A. (1979a) Physical mapping of the globin gene deletion in (δβ)⁰ thalassaemia. *Gene* **6**, 265.

Bernards, R., Little, P.F.R., Annison, G., Williamson, R. & Flavell, R.A. (1979b) Structure of the human ᴳγ-ᴬγ-δ-β-globin gene locus. *Proc. Natl Acad. Sci. USA* **76**, 4827.

Bernet, A., Sabatier, S., Picketts, D.J. *et al.* (1994) Targeted inactivation of the major positive regulatory element (HS −40) of the human α-globin gene locus. *Blood* **86**, 1202.

Bernini, L., Colucci, C.F., de Michele, D., Piomelli, S. & Siniscalco, M. (1962) A possible case of alpha-beta thalassaemia. *Acta Genet. (Basel)* **12**, 202.

Berry, C.L. & Marshall, W.C. (1967) Iron distribution in the liver of patients with thalasaemia major. *Lancet* **i**, 1031.

Berry, M., Grosveld, F. & Dillon, N. (1992) A single point mutation is the cause of the Greek form of hereditary persistence of fetal haemoglobin. *Nature* **358**, 499.

Bertles, J.F. & Milner, P.F.A. (1968) Irreversibly sickled erythrocytes: a consequence of the heterogeneous distribution of hemoglobin types in sickle cell anemia. *J. Clin. Invest.* **47**, 1731.

Bertorello, C.F., Pescetto, T. & Bo, G. (1977) Manifestazioni emorragiche secondarie a coagulopatia da consumo, in paziente affetto da morbo di Cooley. *Min. Pediatr.* **29**, 423.

Bessis, M., Alagille, D. & Breton-Gorius, J. (1958) Particularités des erythroblastes et des erythrocytes dans la maladie de Cooley. Étude au microscope électronique. *Rev. Hematol.* **13**, 538.

Bethlenfalvay, N.C., Motulsky, A.G., Ringelhann, B., Lehmann, H., Humbert, J.R. & Konotey-Ahulu, F.I.D. (1975) Hereditary persistence of fetal hemoglobin, beta thalassemia, and the hemoglobin delta beta locus: further family data and genetic interpretations. *Am. J. Hum. Genet.* **27**, 140.

Betke, K. (1960) Fetal hemoglobin in health and disease. In: *VIII International Congress of Hematology*, p. 1033. Pan Pacific Press, Tokyo.

Betke, K., Marti, H.R. & Schlicht, I. (1959) Estimation of small percentages of foetal haemoglobin. *Nature* **184**, 1877.

Beutler, E., Lang, A. & Lehmann, H. (1974) Hemoglobin Duarte ($\alpha_2\beta_2^{62(E6)Ala \to Pro}$): a new unstable hemoglobin with increased oxygen affinity. *Blood* **43**, 527.

Beutler, E., West, C. & Blume, K.G. (1976) The removal of leukocytes and platelets from whole blood. *J. Lab. Clin. Med.* **88**, 328.

Beutler, E., Matsumoto, F., Powars, D. & Warner, J. (1977) Increased glutathione peroxidase activity in α-thalassemia. *Blood* **50**, 647.

Beutler, E., Lichtman, M.A., Coller, B.S. & Kipps, T.J. (1995) *Williams Hematology*, 5th edn. McGraw-Hill, New York.

Beuzard, Y., Varet, B., Lejeune, J.A., Bouguerra, M., Gaillardon, J. & Rosa, J. (1972) Étude d'une hémoglobine Lepore. Hypothèse de régulation de la synthèse, des chaines Lepore et anti-Lepore. *Nouv. Rev. Fr. Hematol.* **12**, 595.

Bhamapravati, N., Na-Nakorn, S., Wasi, P. & Tuchinda, S. (1967) Pathology of abnormal hemoglobin diseases seen in Thailand. I. Pathology of beta-thalassaemia hemoglobin E disease. *Am. J. Clin. Pathol.* **47**, 745.

Bhavnani, M., Brozovic, M., Old, J.M. & Stephens, A.D. (1994) Guidelines for investigation of the α and β thalassaemia traits. *J. Clin. Pathol.* **47**, 289.

Bianchi, D.W., Beyer, E.C., Stark, A.R., Saffan, D., Sachs, B.P. & Wolfe, L. (1986) Normal long-term survival with α-thalassemia. *J. Pediatr.* **108**, 716.

Bianco, I., Montalenti, G., Silvestroni, E. & Siniscalco, M. (1952) Further data on genetics of microcythemia or thalassaemia minor and Cooley's disease or thalassaemia major. *Ann. Eugen.* **16**, 299.

Bianco, I., Graziani, B., Salvini, P., Mastromonaco, I. & Silvestroni, E. (1972) Fréquence et caractères de l'alpha-microcytémie dans les populations de la Sardaigne septentrionale. Premiers résultats. *Nouv. Rev. Fr. Hematol.* **12**, 191.

Bianco, I., Graziani, B., Mastromonaco, I., Salvini, P. & Silvestroni, E. (1973) Double heterozygosity for alpha- and beta-microcythemias. Its phenotype at the clinical, hematological and biochemical levels. *Hum. Hered.* **23**, 454.

Bianco, I., Graziani, B. & Carboni, C. (1977) Genetic patterns in thalassemia intermedia (constitutional microcytic anemia). Familial, hematologic and biosynthetic studies. *Hum. Hered.* **27**, 257.

Bianco, I., Cappabianca, M.P., Foglietta, E. *et al.* (1997a) Silent thalassemias: genotypes and phenotypes. *Haematologica* **82**, 269.

Bianco, I., Cappabianca, M.P., Lerone, M., Morlupi, L. & Rinaldi, S. (1997b) Hb Siirt [β27(B9) Ala→Gly]: a new, electrophoretically silent, hemoglobin variant. *Hemoglobin* **21**, 495.

Bianco, I., Lerone, M., Foglietta, E. *et al.* (1997c) Phenotypes of individuals with a β thal classical allele associated either with a β thal silent allele or with α globin gene triplicate. *Haematologica* **82**, 513.

Bianco, I., Graziani, B., Lerone, M. *et al.* (1985) Prevention of thalassaemia major in Latium (Italy). *Lancet* **ii**, 888.

Bianco Silvestroni, I.B. (1992) *Microcitemie e Anemia Mediterranea.* Cyanamid Italia, SpA, Catania.

Bienzle, U., Kappes, R., Reimer, A., Feldheim, M., Tischendorf, F.W. & Kohne, E. (1983a) Sickle cell β⁺-thalassemia: a haematological and clinical study in Liberia. *Blut* **47**, 279.

Bienzle, U., Komp, H., Feldheim, M., Reimer, A., Steffen, E. & Guggenmoos-Holzmann, I. (1983b) The distribution and interaction of haemoglobin variants and the β thalassaemia gene in Liberia. *Hum. Genet.* **63**, 400.

Bird, G.W.G., Hasan, M.I., Malhotra, O.P. & Lehmann, H. (1964) Interaction of beta-thalassaemia and hereditary persistence of foetal haemoglobin. *J. Med. Genet.* **1**, 24.

Bissé, E. & Wieland, H. (1988) High performance liquid chromatography, separation of human haemoglobins, simultaneous quantitation of fetal and glycated Hb. *J. Chromatogr.* **434**, 95.

Blackburn, E.H. (1992) Telomerases. *Annu. Rev. Biochem.* **61**, 113.

Blackwell, R.Q., Liu, C.-S., Wang, C.-L., Huang, J.T.-H. & Hung, Y.-O.

(1971) Hereditary persistence of foetal haemoglobin in members of two Chinese families in Taiwan. *Trop. Geogr. Med.* **23**, 145.

Blake, D.R., Winyard, P., Lunec, J. *et al.* (1985) Cerebral and ocular toxicity induced by desferrioxamine. *Quart. J. Med.* **56**, 345.

Blatrix, C., Traverse, P.M., de Coquelet, M.L., Israel, J., Pelletier, P. & Ferrara, G. (1970) Double heterozygotism, hemoglobin C disease-thalassemia in the white race. *Presse Med.* **78**, 1791.

Blau, C.A. (1998) Current status of stem cell therapy and prospects for gene therapy for the disorders of globin synthesis. *Clin. Haematol.* **11**, 257.

Blendis, L.M., Modell, C.B., Bowdler, A.J. & Williams, R. (1974) Some effects of splenectomy in thalassaemia major. *Br. J. Haematol.* **28**, 77.

Bodine, D. (2000) Globin gene therapy: one (seemingly) small vector change, one giant leap in optimism. *Mol. Therapy* **2**, 101.

Bodine, D.M. & Ley, T.J. (1987) An enhancer element lies 3' to the human γ gene. *EMBO J.* **6**, 2997.

Bodmer, W.F. & Cavalli-Sforza, L.L. (1976) *Genes, Evolution and Man.* W.H. Freeman and Co., San Francisco.

Bodmer, W. & McKie, R. (1994) *The Book of Man. The Quest to Discover Our Genetic Heritage.* Little, Brown, London.

Boehm, C.D., Antonarakis, S.E., Phillips, J.A. III, Stetten, G. & Kazazian, H.H. Jr (1983) Prenatal diagnosis using DNA polymorphisms. Report on 95 pregnancies at risk for sickle-cell disease or β-thalassaemia. *N. Eng. J. Med.* **308**, 1054.

Boehm, C.D., Dowling, C.E., Waber, P.G., Giardina, P.J.V. & Kazazian, H.H.J. (1986) Use of oligonucleotide hybridization in the characterization of a β0-thalassaemia gene (β37 TGG →TGA) in a Saudi Arabian family. *Blood* **67**, 1185.

Boehme, W.M., Piira, T.A., Kurnick, J.E. & Bethlenfalvay, N.C. (1978) Acquired hemoglobin H in refractory sideroblastic anemia. *Arch. Intern. Med.* **138**, 603.

Boelaert, J.R., Vergauwe, P.L. & Vandepitte, J.M. (1987) Mucormycosis infections in dialysis patients. *Ann. Intern. Med.* **107**, 782.

de Boer, E., Antoniou, M., Mignotte, V., Wall, L. & Grosveld, F. (1988) The human beta-globin promoter; nuclear protein factors and erythroid specific induction of transcription. *EMBO J.* **7**, 4203.

Bohr, C. (1904) Theoretische Behandlung der quantitativen Verhaltuis der Sauerstoffaufnahine des Hamoglobins. *Zbl. Physiol.* **17**, 682.

Bolton, J.M. & Eng, L.-I.L. (1969) Hb E-beta thalassemia in the West Malaysian Oran Asli (aborigines). *Med. J. Malaysia* **24**, 36.

Bonaventura, J. & Riggs, A. (1968) Hemoglobin Kansas, a human hemoglobin with a neutral amino acid substitution and an abnormal oxygen equilibrium. *J. Biol. Chem.* **243**, 980.

Bond, L.R., Hatty, S.R., Horn, M.E., Dick, M., Meire, H.B. & Bellingham, A.J. (1987) Gall stones in sickle cell disease in the United Kingdom. *Br. Med. J.* **295**, 234.

Bookchin, R.M. & Gallop, P.M. (1968) Structure of hemoglobin A1c: Nature of the N-terminal β-chain blocking group. *Biochem. Biophys. Res. Comm.* **32**, 86.

Bookchin, R.M., Ortiz, O.E., Chalev, O. *et al.* (1988) Calcium transport and ultrastructure of red cells in β-thalassemia intermedia. *Blood* **72**, 1602.

Boonpucknavig, S., Chiewsilp, P., Issarangkura, P., O'Charoen, R. & Akkawat, R. (1988) Immunologic reactivity in thalassemia. *Birth Defects* **23**, 565.

Boontrakoonpoontawee, P., Svasti, J., Fucharoen, S. & Winichagoon, P. (1988) Double heterozygosity for hemoglobin E and a Leporetype hemoglobin found in a Thai woman. *Birth Defects* **23**, 269.

Booth, K. (1966) Haemoglobin H in a Papuan family. *Papua New Guinea Med. J.* **9**, 108.

Booth, K. (1981) Cord blood survey for haemoglobin Barts. *Papua New Guinea Med. J.* **24**, 264.

Borenstein-Ben Yashar, V., Barenholtz, Y., Hy-Am. E., Rachmilewitz, E.A. & Eldor, A. (1993) Phosphatidylserine in the outer leaflet of red blood cells from β-thalassemia patients may explain the chronic hypercoagulable state and thrombotic episodes. *Am. J. Hematol.* **44**, 63.

Boreux, G., Farquet, J.J., Pugin, P., Miescher, P.A. & Klein, D. (1978) Haemoglobinosis C/β-thalassemia double heterozygosity in an Algerian patient with total suppression of haemoglobin A synthesis. *J. Genet. Hum.* **26**, 1.

Borgna-Pignatti, C., De Stefano, P., Bongo, I.G., Avato, F. & Cazzola, M. (1984a) Spleen iron content is low in thalassemia. *Am. J. Pediatr. Hematol. Oncol.* **6**, 340.

Borgna-Pignatti, C., De Stefano, P. & Broglia, A.M. (1984b) Visual loss in patient on high-dose subcutaneous desferrioxamine. *Lancet* **i**, 681.

Borgna-Pignatti, C., de Stefano, P., Zonta, L. *et al.* (1985) Growth and sexual maturation in thalassemia major. *J. Pediatr.* **106**, 150.

Borgna-Pignatti, C., Carneli, V., Caruso, V. *et al.* (1998a) Thromboembolic events in beta thalassemia major: an Italian multicenter study. *Acta Haematol.* **99**, 76.

Borgna-Pignatti, C., Rugolotto, S., De Stefano, P. *et al.* (1998b) Survival and disease complications in thalassemia major. *Ann. N. Y. Acad. Sci.* **850**, 227.

Borow, K.M., Propper, R., Bierman, F.Z., Grady, S. & Inati, A. (1982) The left ventricular end-systolic pressure-dimension relation in patients with thalassemia major. A new non-invasive method for assessing contractile state. *Circulation* **66**, 980.

Bouhass, R., Aguercif, M., Trabuchet, G. & Godet, J. (1990) A new mutation at IVSI nt 2(T→A), in a β-thalassemia from Algeria. *Blood* **76**, 1054.

Bouroncle, B.A. & Doan, C.A. (1964) Cooley's anemia: indications for splenectomy. *Ann. N. Y. Acad. Sci.* **119**, 709.

Bousquet, J., Navarro, M., Robert, G., Aye, P. & Michel, F.B. (1983) Rapid desensitization for desferrioxamine anaphylactoid reactions. *Lancet* **ii**, 859.

Bowden, D.K., Hill, A.V.S., Higgs, D.R., Weatherall, D.J. & Clegg, J.B. (1985) The relative roles of genetic factors, dietary deficiency and infection in anaemia in Vanuatu, southwest Pacific. *Lancet* **ii**, 1025.

Bowden, D.K., Hill, A.V.S., Higgs, D.R., Oppenheimer, S.J., Weatherall, D.J. & Clegg, J.B. (1987a) Different hematologic phenotypes are associated with leftward (−α4.2) and rightward (−α3.7) α+-thalassemia deletions. *J. Clin. Invest.* **79**, 39.

Bowden, D.K., Hill, A.V.S., Weatherall, D.J. & Clegg, J.B. (1987b) High frequency of β thalassaemia in a small island population in Melanesia. *J. Med. Genet.* **24**, 357.

Bowden, D.K., Vickers, M.A. & Higgs, D.R. (1992) A PCR-based strategy to detect the common severe determinants of α thalassaemia. *Br. J. Haematol.* **81**, 104.

Bowdler, A.J. & Huehns, E.R. (1963) Thalassaemia major complicated by excessive iron storage. *Br. J. Haematol.* **9**, 13.

Boyer, S.H. & Dover, G.J. (1979) The *in vivo* biology of F cells in Man. In: *Cellular and Molecular Regulation of Hemoglobin Switching* (eds G. Stamatoyannopoulos & A.W. Nienhuis), p. 47. Grune and Stratton, New York.

Boyer, S.H., Fainer, D.C. & Naughton, M.A. (1963a) Myoglobin: inherited structural variants in man. *Science* **140**, 1228.

Boyer, S.H., Rucknagel, D.L., Weatherall, D.J. & Watson-Williams, E.J. (1963b) Further evidence for linkage between β and δ-loci governing human hemoglobin and the population dynamics of linked genes. *Am. J. Hum. Genet.* **15**, 438.

Boyer, S.H., Belding, T.K., Margolet, L. & Noyes, A.N. (1975) Fetal hemoglobin restriction to a few erythrocytes (F cells) in normal human adults. *Science* **188**, 361.

Boyer, S.H., Margolet, L., Boyer, M.L. *et al.* (1977) Inheritance of

F cell frequency in heterocellular hereditary persistence of fetal hemoglobin: an example of allelic exclusion. *Am. J. Hum. Genet.* **29**, 256.

Bozkurt, G., Dikengil, T., Alimoglu, O. *et al.* (1993) Hepatitis C among Turkish Cypriot thalassemic patients. *Fifth International Conference on Thalassemias and Hemoglobinopathies*, p. 176. Thalassaemia Int. Fed., Nicosia, Cyprus.

Bradley, T.B., Brawner, J.N. & Conley, C.L. (1961) Further observations on an inherited anomaly characterized by persistence of fetal hemoglobin. *Bull. Johns Hopkins Hosp.* **108**, 242.

Bradley, T.B., Wohl, R.C. & Smith, G.J. (1975) Elongation of the α-globin chain in a black family: interaction with HbG Philadelphia. *Clin. Res.* **23**, 1314.

Bradley, D., Newbold, C.I. & Warrell, D.A. (1995) Malaria. In: *The Oxford Textbook of Medicine* (eds D. J. Weatherall, J. G. G. Ledingham & D. A. Warrell), p. 835. Oxford University Press, Oxford.

Brambati, B., Terzian, E. & Tognoni, G. (1991) Randomized clinical trial of transabdominal versus transcervical chorionic villus sampling methods. *Prenat. Diag.* **11**, 285.

Brancati, C. (1961) Diffusione e frequencza della microcitemia e della anemie microcitemiche in Calabria. In: *Proc. Conf. Il Problema Sociale della Microcitemia e del morbo di Cooley*, Rome.

Brancati, C. (1965) Primo caso di omozigosi per la varieta di microcitemia con quota normale di Hb A₂ e quota elevata di Hb F. *Prog. Med. Roma* **21**, 388.

Brancati, C. (1973) Le microcitemie in provincia di Cosenza: aspetti diagnostici ed epidemiologici con particulare riguardo alle forme di α-microcitemie. In: *Atti del V Congresso sulle Microcitemia*, p. 334. Cosenza.

Brancati, C. & Baglioni, C. (1966) Homozygous βδ thalassaemia (βδ-microcythaemia). *Nature* **212**, 262.

Brancati, C. & Puccetti, G. (1964) Microcitemie ed emoglobine abnormi in Calabria. *Il Progr. Med.* **20**, 635.

Brancati, C., Tentori, L., Marinucci, M. & Fontanarosa, P.P. (1978) Double heterozygosis for Hb G San Jose (7 Glu→Gly) and β⁰-thalassaemia in an Italian family. *New Istanbul Contrib. Clin. Sci.* **12**, 238.

Bratu, V. & Predescu, C. (1969) Hemoglobin S, thalassemia and thalassemia association with hemoglobin S in a family from Romania. In: *Vth Congress of the Asian and Pacific Society of Hematology*, p. 69. Kagit Basim Isleri, Turkey.

Braunitzer, G. (1958) Vergliechende Untersuchingen zur Primarstruktur der Protein Komponente emiger Hamoglobine. *Z. Physiol. Chemie* **312**, 78.

Braunitzer, G., Hilschmann, N., Rudloff, V., Hilse, K., Liebold, B. & Muller, R. (1961) The haemoglobin particles. Chemical and genetics aspects of their structure. *Nature* **190**, 480.

Braverman, A.S. & Bank, A. (1969) Changing rates of globin chain synthesis during erythroid cell maturation. *J. Mol. Biol.* **42**, 57.

Braverman, A.S., McCurdy, P.R., Manos, P. & Sherman, A. (1973) Homozygous beta thalassemia in American Blacks: the problem of mild thalassemia. *J. Lab. Clin. Med.* **8**, 857.

Braverman, A.S., Schwartzberg, L. & Berkowitz, R. (1982) Soluble and stroma-bound globin chains in mild and severe β-thalassemia. *Hemoglobin* **6**, 347.

Breathnach, R. & Chambon, R. (1981) Organization and expression of eukaryotic split genes coding for proteins. *Annu. Rev. Biochem.* **50**, 349.

Brennan, S.O., Williamson, D., Smith, M.B., Cauchi, M.N., Macphee, A. & Carrell, R. (1984) Hb A₂ Victoria δ24 (B6) Gly→Asp. A new δ chain variant occurring with β-thalassemia. *Hemoglobin* **8**, 163.

Brennan, S.O., Shaw, J., Allen, J. & George, P.M. (1992) β141 Leu is not deleted in the unstable haemoglobin Atlanta-Coventry but is replaced by a novel amino acid of mass 129 daltons. *Br. J. Haematol.* **81**, 99.

Bridges, K.R. & Hoffman, K.E. (1986) The effects of ascorbic acid on the intracellular metabolism of iron and ferritin. *J. Biol. Chem.* **261**, 14273.

Brill, P.W., Winchester, P., Giardina, P.J. & Cunningham-Rundles, S. (1991) Desferrioxamine-induced bone dysplasia in patients with thalassemia major. *Am. J. Roentgenol.* **156**, 561.

Brimhall, B., Hollan, S., Jones, R.T., Koler, R.D., Stocklen, Z. & Szelenyi, J.G. (1970) Multiple α chain loci for human hemoglobin. *Clin. Res.* **18**, 184.

Brittenham, G.M. (1988) Non-invasive methods for the early detection of hereditary hemochromatosis. *Ann. N. Y. Acad. Sci.* **526**, 199.

Brittenham, G.M. (1990) Pyridoxal isonicotinoyl hydrazone: effective iron chelation after oral administration. *Ann. N. Y. Acad. Sci.* **612**, 315.

Brittenham, G.M. (1992) Development of iron-chelating agents for clinical use. *Blood* **80**, 569.

Brittenham, G.M. (1994) Disorders of iron metabolism: deficiency and overload. In: *Hematology: Basic Principles and Practice* (eds R. Hoffman, E.J., Benz, S.J., Shattil, B. Furie, H.J. Cohen & L.E. Silberstein), p. 492. Churchill Livingstone, New York.

Brittenham, G., Lozoff, B., Harris, J.W., Kan, Y.W., Dozy, A.M. & Nayudu, N.V.S. (1980) Alpha globin gene number: population and restriction endonuclease studies. *Blood* **55**, 706.

Brittenham, G.M., Farrell, D.E., Harris, J.W., Feldman, E.S. & Danish, E.H. (1982) Magnetic-susceptibility measurement of human iron stores. *N. Eng. J. Med.* **307**, 1671.

Brittenham, G.M., Griffith, P.M., Nienhuis, A.W. *et al.* (1994) Efficacy of deferoxamine in preventing complications of iron overload in patients with thalassemia major. *N. Eng. J. Med.* **331**, 567.

Brockelman, C.R., Wongsattayanont, B., Tan-ariya, P. & Fucharoen, S. (1987) Thalassemic erythrocytes inhibit *in vitro* growth of *Plasmodium falciparum. J. Clin. Microbiol.* **25**, 56.

Bronspeigel-Weintrob, N., Olivieri, N.F., Tyler, N.F., Andrews, D., Freedman, M.H. & Holland, F.J. (1990) Effect of age at the start of iron chelation therapy on gonadal function in β-thalassemia major. *N. Eng. J. Med.* **323**, 713.

Brook, C.G., Thompson, E.N., Marshall, W.C. & Whitehouse, R.H. (1969) Growth in children with thalassemia major and effect of two different transfusion regimes. *Arch. Dis. Child.* **44**, 612.

Brosious, E.M., Wright, J.M., Baine, R.M. & Schmidt, R.M. (1978) Microchromatographic methods for hemoglobin A₂ quantitation compared. *Clin. Chem.* **24**, 2196.

Brown, P.J. (1981) New considerations on the distribution of malaria, thalassemia, and glucose-6-phosphate dehydrogenase deficiency in Sardinia. *Hum. Biol.* **53**, 367.

Brown, D.E. & Ober, W.B. (1958) Sickle-cell thalassemia (microdrepanocytic disease) in pregnancy. *Am. J. Obstet. Gynecol.* **75**, 773.

Brown, J.M., Thein, S.L., Mar, K.M. & Weatherall, D.J. (1989) The spectrum of beta-thalassemia in Burma. *Hemoglobin Switching*, 161.

Brown, A.K., Sleeper, L.A., Miller, S.T., Pegelow, C.H., Gill, F.M. & Wacliwiw, M.A. (1994) Reference values and hematologic changes from birth to 5 years in patients with sickle cell disease. *Arch. Pediatr. Adolesc. Med.* **148**, 796.

Browne, P.V., Shalev, O., Kuypers, F.A. *et al.* (1997) Removal of erythrocyte membrane iron *in vivo* ameliorates the pathobiology of murine thalassemia. *J. Clin. Invest.* **100**, 1459.

Brownell, A.I., McSwiggan, D.A., Cubitt, W.D. & Anderson, M.J. (1986) Aplastic and hypoplastic episodes in sickle cell disease and thalassaemia. *J. Clin. Pathol.* **39**, 121.

Bruce-Chwatt, L.J. (1965) Paleogenesis and paleo-epidemiology of primate malaria. *Bull. WHO* **32**, 363.

Bruce-Chwatt, L.J. & de Zulueta, J. (1980) *The Rise and Fall of Malaria in Europe. A Historico-Epidemiological Study.* Oxford University Press, Oxford.

Bruzdzinski, C.J., Sisco, K.L., Ferrucci, S.J. & Rucknagel, D.L. (1984) The occurrence of the $\alpha^{\text{G-Philadelphia}}$-globin allele on a double-locus chromosome. *Am. J. Hum. Genet.* **36**, 101.

Bruzzese, L. D'Avino, A., Frazati, B. & Rotoli, B. (1970) Studies of plasma ^{59}Fe disappearance curves in thalassaemia trait: a manifestation of ineffective erythropoiesis. In: *13th Congress of the International Society of Hematology*, Munich.

Bruzzese, L., D'Avino, A., Frazati, B. & Rotoli, B. (1973) L'eritropoiesi inefficace nelle sindromi Talassemiche eterozigotiche: studi di derrocinetica. In: *14th Congress of the Italian Society of Hematology*, Pavia.

Buckle, V.J. & Kearney, L. (1994) New methods in cytogenetics. *Curr. Opin. Genet. Dev.* **4**, 374.

Buckle, V.J., Higgs, D.R., Wilkie, A.O.M., Super, M. & Weatherall, D.J. (1988) Localisation of human α globin to 16p13.3-pter. *J. Med. Genet.* **25**, 847.

Buja, L.M. & Roberts, W.C. (1971) Iron in the heart: etiology and clinical significance. *Am. J. Med.* **51**, 209.

Bulger, M. & Groudine, M. (1999) Looping versus linking: toward a model for long-distance gene activation. *Genes Dev.* **13**, 2465.

Bulger, M., Hikke von Doorninck, J., Saitoh, N. *et al.* (1999) Conservation of sequence and structure flanking the mouse and human β-globin loci: The β-globin genes are embedded within an array of odorant receptor genes. *Proc. Natl Acad. Sci. USA* **96**, 5129.

Bunch, C., Wood, W.G., Weatherall, D.J., Robinson, J.S. & Corp, M.J. (1981) Haemoglobin synthesis of fetal erythroid cells in adult environment. *Br. J. Haematol.* **49**, 325.

Bunn, H.F. (1987) Subunit assembly of hemoglobin: an important determinant of hematologic phenotype. *Blood* **69**, 1.

Bunn, H.F. (1997) Pathogenesis and treatment of sickle cell disease. *N. Eng. J. Med.* **337**, 762.

Bunn, H.F. (1999) Induction of fetal hemoglobin in sickle cell disease. *Blood* **93**, 1787.

Bunn, H.F. & Forget, B.G. (1986) *Hemoglobin: Molecular, Genetic and Clinical Aspects.* W.B. Saunders, Philadelphia.

Bunn, H.F. & McDonald, M.J. (1983) Electrostatic interactions in the assembly of haemoglobin. *Nature* **306**, 498.

Bunn, H.F., Meriwether, W.D., Balcerzak, S.P. & Rucknagel, D.L. (1972) Oxygen equilibrium of hemoglobin E. *J. Clin. Invest.* **51**, 2984.

Bunn, H.F., Wohl, R.C., Bradley, T.P., Cooley, M. & Gibson, Q.H. (1974) Functional properties of hemoglobin Kempsey. *J. Biol. Chem.* **249**, 7402.

Bunn, H.F., Olaney, D.N., Kain, S., Gabbay, K.H. & Gallop, P.M. (1976) Biosynthesis of hemoglobin A_{Ic} slow glycosylation of hemoglobin *in vivo. J. Clin. Invest.* **57**, 1562.

Bunn, H.F., Forget, B.G. & Ranney, H.M. (1977) *Human Hemoglobins.* W.B. Saunders, Philadelphia.

Bunyaratvej, A., Butthep, P., Sae-Ung, N., Fucharoen, S. & Yuthavong, Y. (1992) Reduced deformability of thalassemic erythrocytes and erythrocytes with abnormal hemoglobins and relation with susceptibility to *Plasmodium falciparum* invasion. *Blood* **79**, 2460.

Bunyaratvej, A., Fucharoen, S., Greenbaum, A. & Mohandas, N. (1994) Hydration of red cells in α and β thalassemias differs. *Am. J. Clin. Pathol.* **102**, 217.

Buonanno, G., Valente, A., Gonnella, F., Cantore, F. & de Bellis, G. (1984) Serum ferritin in β-thalassaemia intermedia. *Scand. J. Haematol.* **32**, 83.

Buratowski, S. (1994) The basics of basal transcription by RNA polymerase II. *Cell* **77**, 1.

Bürgi, W., Schlup, P., Deubelbeiss, K.A., Fischer, S. & Killer, D. (1992) Erworbene hämoglobin H-krankheit im frühstadium einer erythroleukämie. *Schweiz. Med. Wschr.* **122**, 348.

Burka, E.R. & Marks, P.A. (1963) Ribosomes active in protein synthesis in human reticulocytes: a defect in thalassaemia major. *Nature* **199**, 706.

Burr, H. & Lingrel, J.B. (1971) Poly A sequences at the 3' termini of rabbit globin mRNAs. *Nature New Biol.* **233**, 41.

Busslinger, M., Moschanas, N. & Flavell, R.A. (1981) β+ Thalassemia: aberrant splicing results from a single point mutation in an intron. *Cell* **27**, 289.

Butthep, P., Bunyaratvej, P., Kitaguchi, H. & Funahara, S. (1992) Interaction between endothelial cells and thalassaemic red cells *in vitro. Southeast Asian J. Trop. Med. Publ. Hlth* **23**, 101.

Cabannes, R., Baba, S. & Schmidt-Beurrier, A. (1967a) Étude des hémoglobinoses dans la région de Niamey. *Nouv. Rev. Fr. Hematol.* **7**, 309.

Cabannes, R., Baba, S.Y. & Schmitt-Beurrier, A. (1967b) Études des hémoglobines en Côte d'Ivoire. *Med. Afr. Noire* **14**, 367.

Cabannes, R., Larrouy, G., Fernet, P. & Sendrail, A. (1969a) Étude hémotypologique des populations sédentaires de la saoura. *Bull. Mem. Soc. Anthropol. Paris* Serie **12 (4)**, 139.

Cabannes, R., Renaud, R., Boury-Heyler, C., Sangaret, A.M., Clerc, M. & Chesnet, Y. (1969b) Les hémoglobines anormales en milieu obstétrical Ivoirien. *Med. Afr. Noire* **16**, 257.

Cabannes, R., Accurso, A., Nicolas, C. & Arne, D. (1974) Répartition des hémoglobines anormales dans les populations Akan de Côte d'Ivoire. *Ann. Fac. Med.* **8**, 158.

Cabeda, J.M., Correia, C., Estevinho, A. *et al.* (1999) Unexpected pattern of β-globin mutations in β-thalassaemia patients from the North of Portugal. *Br. J. Haematol.* **105**, 68.

Cai, S. & Chehab, F.F. (1996) New frameshift mutation, insertion of A, at codon 95 of the β-globin gene causes β-thalassemia in two Vietnamese families. *Hum. Mutat.* **8**, 293.

Cai, S.P., Zeng, J.Z., Doherty, M. & Kan, Y.W. (1989) A new TATA box mutation detected in prenatal diagnosis. *Am. J. Hum. Genet.* **45**, 112.

Cai, S.P., Chui, D.H.K., Ng, J., Poon, A.O., Freedman, M.H. & Olivieri, N.F. (1991) A new frameshift β⁰-thalassemia mutation (codons 27–28 +C) found in a Chinese family. *Am. J. Hematol.* **37**, 6.

Cai, S.-P., Eng, B., Francombe, W.H. *et al.* (1992) Two novel β-thalassemia mutations in the 5' and 3' noncoding regions of the β-globin gene. *Blood* **79**, 1342.

Cai, S.P., Wall, J., Kan, Y.W. & Chehab, F.F. (1994) Reverse dot blot probes for the screening of β-thalassemia mutations in Asians and American blacks. *Hum. Mutat.* **3**, 59.

Callen, D.F., Hyland, V.J., Baker, E.G. *et al.* (1989) Mapping the short arm of human chromosome 16. *Genomics* **4**, 348.

Callender, S.T. & Weatherall, D.J. (1980) Iron chelation with oral desferrioxamine. *Lancet* **2**, 689.

Camaschella, C. & Cappellini, M.D. (1995) Thalassemia intermedia. *Haematologica* **80**, 58.

Camaschella, C., Ciocca-Vasino, M.A., Guerrasio, A. *et al.* (1979) Biosynthetic studies and γ-chain composition in the Greek type of hereditary persistence of fetal hemoglobin and its association with β-thalassemia. *Acta Haematol.* **61**, 272.

Camaschella, C., Bertero, M.T., Serra, A. *et al.* (1987a) A benign form of thalassaemia intermedia may be determined by the interaction of triplicated α locus and heterozygous β thalassaemia. *Br. J. Haematol.* **66**, 103.

Camaschella, C., Serra, A., Saglio, G. *et al.* (1987b) The 3' ends of the deletions of Spanish δβ⁰-thalassemia and Black HPFH 1 and 1 lie within 17 kilobases. *Blood* **70**, 593.

Camaschella, C., Serra, A., Saglio, G. *et al.* (1988) Meiotic recombination in the β globin gene cluster causing an error in prenatal diagnosis of β thalassaemia. *J. Med. Genet.* **25**, 307.

Camaschella, C., Oggiano, L., Sampietro, M. *et al.* (1989a) The homozygous state of G to A −117 $^{A}\gamma$ hereditary persistence of fetal hemoglobin. *Blood* **73**, 1999.

Camaschella, C., Serra, A., Bertero, M.T. *et al.* (1989b) Molecular characterization of Italian chromosomes carrying the Lepore Boston gene. *Acta Haematol.* **81**, 136.

Camaschella, C., Alfarano, A., Gottardi, E., Serra, A., Revello, D. & Saglio, G. (1990a) The homozygous state for the −87 C→G β⁺ thalassaemia. *Br. J. Haematol.* **75**, 132.

Camaschella, C., Alfarano, A., Gottardi, E. *et al.* (1990b) Prenatal diagnosis of fetal hemoglobin Lepore-Boston disease on maternal peripheral blood. *Blood* **75**, 2102.

Camaschella, C., Serra, A., Gottardi, E. *et al.* (1990c) A new hereditary persistence of fetal hemoglobin deletion has the breakpoint within the 3′ β-globin gene enhancer. *Blood* **75**, 1000.

Camaschella, C., Mazza, U., Roetto, A. *et al.* (1995) Genetic interactions in thalassaemia intermedia: analysis of β-mutations, α-genotype, γ promoters, and β-LCR hypersensitive sites 2 and 4 in Italian patients. *Am. J. Hematol.* **48**, 82.

Camaschella, C., Gonella, S., Calabrese, R. *et al.* (1996) Serum erythropoietin and circulating transferrin receptor in thalassemia intermedia patients with heterogeneous genotypes. *Haematologica* **81**, 397.

Caminopetros, J. (1938a) Recherches sur l'anémia érythroblastique des peuples de la Méditerranée orientale. Premier Memoire: étude nosologique. *Ann. Méd.* **43**, 27.

Caminopetros, J. (1938b) Recherches sur l'anémia érythroblastique infantile des peuples de la Mediterranée orientale. Étude anthropologique, étiologique et pathogénique. La transmission héréditaire de la maladia. *Ann. Méd.* **43**, 104.

Cammisa, M. & Sabella, G. (1967) Clinico-radiological considerations on the pathogenesis of bone changes in thalassemia major. *Nunt. Radiol.* **33**, 77.

Canale, V.C., Steinherz, P., New, M. & Erlandson, M. (1974) Endocrine function in thalassemia major. *Ann. N. Y. Acad. Sci.* **232**, 333.

Cancado, R.D., Guerra, L.G.M., Rosenfeld, M.O.J.A. *et al.* (1993) Prevalence of hepatitis C virus antibody in beta thalassemic patients. *Fifth International Conference on Thalassemia and Hemoglobinopathies*, p. 176. Nicosia, Cyprus.

Cantinieaux, B., Hariga, C., Ferster, A., de-Maertelaere, E., Toppet, M. & Fondu, P. (1987) Neutrophil dysfunctions in thalassaemia major: the role of cell iron overload. *Eur. J. Haematol.* **39**, 28.

Cao, A. (1988) Diagnosis of β-thalassemia intermedia at presentation. *Birth Defects* **23**, 219.

Cao, A. (1994) 1993 William Allan Award Address. *Am. J. Hum. Genet.* **54**, 397.

Cao, A. & Rosatelli, M.C. (1993) Screening and prenatal diagnosis of the haemoglobinopathies. *Clin. Haematol.* **6**, 263.

Cao, A., Galanello, R., Furbetta, M. *et al.* (1978) Thalassaemia types and their incidence in Sardinia. *J. Med. Genet.* **15**, 443.

Cao, A., Galanello, R., Melis, M.A. *et al.* (1981) La nostra esperienza sullo screening e la consultazione genetica delle β-talassemie. *Min. Med.* **72**, 623.

Cao, A., Galanello, R. & Furbetta, M. (1982a) Thalassemia types in Southern Sardinia. *Birth Defects* **18**, 157.

Cao, A., Melis, M.A., Galanello, R. *et al.* (1982b) δβ (F)-thalassaemia in Sardinia. *J. Med. Genet.* **19**, 184.

Cao, A., Goossens, M. & Pirastu, M. (1989) β Thalassaemia mutations in Mediterranean populations. *Br. J. Haematol.* **71**, 309.

Cao, A., Gasperini, D., Podda, A. & Galanello, R. (1990) Molecular pathology of thalassemia intermedia. *Eur. J. Int. Med.* **1**, 227.

Cao, A., Rosatelli, C., Pirastu, M. & Galanello, R. (1991) Thalassemias in Sardinia: molecular pathology, phenotype–genotype correlation and prevention. *Am. J. Pediatr. Hematol. Oncol.* **13**, 179.

Cao, A., Galanello R.M., Rosatelli, M.C., Argiolu, F. & De Virgilis, S. (1996) Clinical experience of management of thalassemia: the Sardinian experience. *Sem. Hematol.* **33**, 66.

Caocci, L., Alberti, M., Burrai, P. & Corda, R. (1978) Screening coagulation tests and clotting factors in homozygous β-thalassemia. *Acta Haematol.* **60**, 358.

Capelli, L. (1966) Major Mediterranean or Cooley's anemia. Radiologic study of 23 cases. *Nunt. Radiol.* **32**, 219.

Capp, G.L., Rigas, D.A. & Jones, R.T. (1967) Haemoglobin Portland 1 — a new human hemoglobin unique in structure. *Science* **157**, 65.

Capp, G.L., Rigas, D.A. & Jones, R.T. (1970) Evidence for a new haemoglobin chain (ζ chain). *Nature* **228**, 278.

Cappellini, M.D., Fiorelli, G. & Bernini, L.F. (1981) Interaction between homozygous β⁰ thalassaemia and the Swiss type of hereditary persistence of fetal haemoglobin. *Br. J. Haematol.* **48**, 561.

Cappellini, M.D., Coppola, R., Robbiolo, L. *et al.* (1996) Procoagulant activity of erythrocytes in thalassemia intermedia. *Blood* **88** (Suppl. 1), 38a.

Cappellini, M.D., Tavazzi, D., Duca, L. *et al.* (1999) Metabolic indicators of oxidative stress correlate with haemochrome attachment to membrane, band 3 aggregation and erythrophagocytosis in β-thalassaemia intermedia. *Br. J. Haematol.* **104**, 504.

Capper, A. (1931) The nature of Von Jaksch's anemia and the effect of splenectomy. *Am. J. Med. Sci.* **181**, 620.

Capua, A. (1998) The Montreal Thalassemia Screening Program. *Ann. N. Y. Acad. Sci.* **850**, 401.

Carcassi, V., Cappellini, R. & Siniscalco, M. (1957a) Il tracciato elettroforetico dell'emoglobina per una migliore discriminizione della talassemie. *Haematologica* **42**, 1635.

Carcassi, V., Ceppellini, R. & Pitzus, F. (1957b) Frequenza della talassemia in quattro popolazioni sarde e suoi rapporti con la distribuzione dei gruppi sanguini e della malaria. *Boll. 1st Sieroter. Mil.* **36**, 206.

Carcassi, U.E.F., Pintus, A., Gravely, M.E. & Huisman, T.H.J. (1980) β⁰-Thalassemia in association with Hb Leslie (α₂β₂ 131Gln→O) in a Sardinian family. *Hemoglobin* **4**, 195.

Cardarelli, A. (1880) Rel. IX Congr. Assoc. Med. It. Genova.

Cardarelli, A. (1890) Nosografia della pseudo-leucemia splenica (indettiva) dei bambini; pelsocioord. Rel. R. Acc. Med. Chir. Napoli. Anno **II**, 17.

Cardia, E., Toscano, S., La Rosa, G. & Zaccone, C., d'Avella, D. & Tomasello, F. (1994) Spinal cord compression in homozygous β-thalassemia intermedia. *Pediatr. Neurosurg.* **20**, 186.

Cardoso, C., Timsit, S., Villard, L., Khrestchatisky, M., Fontès, M. & Colleaux, L. (1998) Specific interaction between the *XNP/ATR-X* gene product and the SET domain of the human EZH2 protein. *Hum. Mol. Genet.* **7**, 679.

Carella, M., D'Ambrosio, L., Totaro, A. *et al.* (1997) Mutation analysis of the HLA-H gene in Italian hemochromatosis patients. *Am. J. Hum. Genet.* **60**, 828.

Carlson, M. & Laurent, B.C. (1994) The SNF/SWI family of global transcriptional activators. *Curr. Opin. Cell. Biol.* **6**, 396.

Carlson, J., Nash, G.B., Gabutti, V., Al-Yaman, F. & Wahlgren, M. (1994) Natural protection against severe *Plasmodium falciparum* malaria due to impaired rosette formation. *Blood* **84**, 3909.

Caroline, L., Kozinn, P.F., Feldman, F., Stiefel, F.M. & Lichtman, H. (1969) Infection and iron overload in thalassemia. *Ann. N. Y. Acad. Sci.* **165**, 148.

Carr, S., Rubin, L., Dixon, D., Star, J. & Dailey, J. (1995) Intrauterine therapy for homozygous α-thalassemia. *Obstet. Gynecol.* **85**, 876.

Carrell, R.W. & Lehmann, H. (1969) The unstable haemoglobin haemolytic anaemias. *Sem. Hematol.* **6**, 116.

Carthew, P., Smith, A.G., Hider, R.C., Dorman, B., Edwards, R.E. & Francis, J.E. (1994) Potentiation of iron accumulation in cardiac myocytes during the treatment of iron overload with the hydroxypyridinine iron chelator CP94. *Biometals* **7**, 267.

Cartwright, G.E., Edwards, C.Q., Kravitz, K. *et al.* (1979) Hereditary hemochromatosis: phenotypic expression of the disease. *N. Eng. J. Med.* **301**, 175.

Caruso-Nicoletti, M., Mancuso, M., Spadaro, G., Samperi, P., Consalvi, C. & Schiliro, G. (1992) Growth and development in white patients with sickle cell diseases. *Am. J. Pediatr. Hematol. Oncol.* **14**, 285.

Casado, A., Pellicer, A., Olmeda, F. *et al.* (1978) Double heterozygosis for hemoglobin C-β thalassemia: description of a Spanish family. *Clin. Genet.* **13**, 265.

Casali, P., Borzini, P., Vergani, D., Mieli-Vergani, G., Masera, G. & Zanussi, C. (1978) Occurrence of circulating immune complexes in β-thalassemia major. *Arch. Dis. Child.* **53**, 141.

Casey, R., Kynoch, P.A.M., Lang, A., Lehmann, H., Nozari, G. & Shinton, K. (1978) Double heterozygosity for two unstable haemoglobins: Hb Sydney (β67 (E11) Val→Ala) and Hb Coventry (β141 (H19) Leu deleted). *Br. J. Haematol.* **38**, 195.

Casoni, I., Perrotta, C.M., Conconi, F., del Senno, L. & Alberti, M.R. (1977) Diminuzione dell'emoglobina O$_{Indonesia}$ in soggetti portatori del gene β-talassermico. Studi biosintetici. In: *13° Riunione del Gruppo di Studio sull'Eritrocita*, Torina.

Castaldi, G. & Zavagli, G. (1972) Anaemia in thalassaemia. *Lancet* **ii**, 1254.

Castaldi, G., Zavagli, G., Ambroso, G., Dallapiccolas, B. & Trotta, F. (1974) Anaemia in beta-thalassaemia carriers. *Br. Med. J.* **i**, 518.

Castaldi, G., Trotta, F., Ambroso, G. *et al.* (1975) L'anemia del beta-talassemico eterozigote. *Prog. Med. Roma* **31**, 1.

Castriota Scanderbeg, A., Izzi, G.C., Butturini, A. & Benaglia, G. (1990) Pulmonary syndrome and intravenous high-dose desferrioxamine. *Lancet* **336**, 1511.

Castro, O., Winter, W.P., Bullock, W.H., Killy, P.N., Gvozden, A.B. & Rucknagel, D.L. (1979) Hemoglobin D Ibadan trait in combination with δβ thalassemia. *Hemoglobin* **3**, 77.

Castro, O., Brambilla, D.J., Thorington, B. *et al.* (1994) The acute chest syndrome in sickle cell disease: incidence and risk factors. The Cooperative Study of Sickle Cell Disease. *Blood* **84**, 643.

de Castro, C.M., Devlin, B., Fleenor, D.E., Lee, M.E. & Kaufman, R.E. (1994) A novel β-globin mutation, βDurham-NC[β114 Leu→Pro], produces a dominant thalassemia-like phenotype. *Blood* **83**, 1109.

Cataldo, F., Varrica, D., Didato, M.A. & Albeggiani, A. (1977) Hemoglobin C and beta-thalassemia in a Sicilian–Sardinian family. *Pediatria* **85**, 312.

Catena, D.L. (1975) Oral manifestations of the hemoglobinopathies. *Dent. Clin. North Am.* **19**, 77.

Caterina, J.J., Ryan, T.M., Pawlik, K.M. *et al.* (1991) Human β-globin locus control region: analysis of the 5' DNase I hypersensitive site HS2 in transgenic mice. *Proc. Natl Acad. Sci. USA* **88**, 1626.

Caterina, J.J., Ciavatta, D.J., Donze, D., Behringer, R.R. & Townes, T.M. (1994) Multiple elements in human β-globin locus control region 5' HS2 are involved in enhancer activity and position-independent, transgene expression. *Nucl. Acids Res.* **22**, 1006.

Cauchi, M.N. (1970) The incidence of glucose-6-phosphate dehydrogenase deficiency and thalassaemia in Malta. *Br. J. Haematol.* **18**, 101.

Cauchi, M.N., Clegg, J.B. & Weatherall, D.J. (1969) Haemoglobin F (Malta): a new foetal haemoglobin variant with a high incidence in Maltese infants. *Nature* **223**, 311.

Cavallo, L., Gurrado, R., Gallo, F., Zacchino, C., de Mattia, D. & Tato, L. (1997) Growth deficiency in polytransfused beta-thalassaemia patients is not growth hormone dependent. *Clin. Endocrinol.* **46**, 701.

Çavdar, A.O. & Arcasoy, A. (1971) The incidence of β-thalassaemia and abnormal hemoglobins in Turkey. *Acta Haematol.* **45**, 312.

Çavdar, A.O. & Arcasoy, A. (1976) Haemoglobin Lepore$_{Boston}$ in a Turkish family. *J. Med. Genet.* **13**, 363.

Cavello-Perin, P., Pacini, B., Cerutti, F. *et al.* (1995) Insulin resistance and hyperinsulinemia in homozygous β-thalassemia. *Metabolism* **44**, 281.

Cavill, I., Ricketts, C., Jacobs, A. & Letsky, E. (1978) Erythropoiesis and the effect of transfusion in homozygous beta-thalassaemia. *N. Eng. J. Med.* **298**, 776.

Cazzetta, R.A. (1990) A patient's perspective. *Ann. N. Y. Acad. Sci.* **612**, 473.

Cazzola, M., Alessandrino, P., Barosi, G., Morandi, S. & Stefanelli, M. (1979) Quantitative evaluation of the mechanisms of the anaemia in heterozygous β-thalassaemia. *Scand. J. Haematol.* **23**, 107.

Cazzola, M., De Stefano, P., Ponchio, L. *et al.* (1995) Relationship between transfusion regimen and suppression of erythropoiesis in β-thalassaemia major. *Br. J. Haematol.* **89**, 473.

Cazzola, M., Borgna-Pignatti, C., Locatelli, F., Ponchio, L., Beguin, Y. & De-Stefano, P. (1997) A moderate transfusion regimen may reduce iron loading in β-thalassaemia major without producing excessive expansion of erythropoiesis. *Transfusion* **37**, 135.

Ceppellini, R. (1959a) Discussion. Biochemistry of human genetics. In: *Ciba Foundation Symposium* (eds G.E.W. Wolstenholme & C.M. O'Connor), p. 133. Little Brown, Boston, MA.

Ceppellini, R. (1959b) L'emoglobina normale lenta A$_2$. *Acta Gen. Med.* **8**, 47.

de Ceulaer, K., Higgs, D.R., Weatherall, D.J., Hayes, R.J., Serjeant, B.E. & Serjeant, G.R. (1983) α-Thalassemia reduces the hemolytic rate in homozygous sickle cell disease. *N. Eng. J. Med.* **309**, 189.

Chada, K., Magram, J. & Costantini, F. (1986) An embryonic pattern of expression of a human fetal globin gene in transgenic mice. *Nature* **319**, 685.

Chakravarti, A., Buetow, K.H., Antonarakis, S.E., Waber, P.G., Boehm, C.D. & Kazazian, H.H. (1984) Nonuniform recombination within the human β-globin gene cluster. *Am. J. Hum. Genet.* **36**, 1239.

Chalevelakis, G., Clegg, J.B. & Weatherall, D.J. (1975) Imbalanced globin chain synthesis in heterozygous β-thalassemia bone marrow. *Proc. Natl Acad. Sci. USA* **72**, 3853.

Chalevelakis, G., Clegg, J.B. & Weatherall, D.J. (1976) Globin synthesis in normal human bone marrow. *Br. J. Haematol.* **34**, 535.

Chan, V., Chan, T.K., Liang, S.T., Ghosh, A., Kan, Y.W. & Todd, D. (1985) Hydrops fetalis due to an unusual form of HbH disease. *Blood* **66**, 224.

Chan, V., Chan, T.K., Cheng, M.Y., Kan, Y.W. & Todd, D. (1986a) Organization of the ζ-α genes in Chinese. *Br. J. Haematol.* **64**, 97.

Chan, V., Chan, T.K., Cheng, M.Y., Leung, N.K., Kan, Y.W. & Todd, D. (1986b) Characteristics and distribution of β thalassemia haplotypes in South China. *Hum. Genet.* **73**, 23.

Chan, V., Chan, T.K., Chebab, F.F. & Todd, D. (1987a) Distribution of β-thalassemia mutations in South China and their association with haplotypes. *Am. J. Hum. Genet.* **41**, 678.

Chan, V., Chan, T.K., Tso, S.C. & Todd, D. (1987b) Combination of three α-globin gene loci deletions and hemoglobin New York results in a severe hemoglobin H syndrome. *Am. J. Hematol.* **24**, 301.

Chan, V., Chan, T.K., Kan, Y.W. & Todd, D. (1988) A novel β-thalassemia frameshift mutation (codon 14/15) detectable by direct visualization of abnormal restriction fragment in amplified genomic DNA. *Blood* **72**, 1420.

Chan, V., Chan, T.K. & Todd, D. (1989) A new codon 71 (+T) mutant resulting in β⁰ thalassemia. *Blood* **74**, 2304.

Chan, V., Chan, T.P.T., Lau, K., Todd, D. & Chan, T.K. (1993) False non-paternity in a family for prenatal diagnosis of β-thalassaemia. *Prenat. Diag.* **13**, 977.

Chan, V., Chan, V.W.Y., Tang, M., Lau, K., Todd, D. & Chan, T.K. (1997) Molecular defects in Hb H hydrops fetalis. *Br. J. Haematol.* **96**, 224.

Chanarin, I. (1980) *The Megaloblastic Anaemias*, 2nd edn. Blackwell Scientific Publications, Oxford.

Chanarin, I. (1989) *Laboratory Haematology*. Churchill Livingstone, London.

Chanarin, I., Dacie, J.V. & Mollin, D.L. (1959) Folic-acid deficiency in haemolytic anaemia. *Br. J. Haematol.* **5**, 245.

Chandcharoensin-Wilde, C., Chairoongruang, S., Jitnuson, P., Fucharoen, S. & Vathanopas, V. (1988) Gallstones in thalassaemia. *Birth Defects* **23**, 263.

Chang, J.C. & Kan, Y.W. (1979) β⁰ Thalassemia, a nonsense mutation in man. *Proc. Natl Acad. Sci. USA* **76**, 2886.

Chang, J.C. & Kan, Y.W. (1981) Antenatal diagnosis of sickle cell anaemia by direct analysis of the sickle mutation. *Lancet* **ii**, 1127.

Chang, J.C. & Kan, Y.W. (1982) A sensitive new prenatal test for sickle-cell anemia. *N. Eng. J. Med.* **307**, 30.

Chang, H., Modell, C.B., Alter, B.P. *et al.* (1975) Expression of the β-thalassemia gene in the first trimester fetus. *Proc. Natl Acad. Sci. USA* **72**, 3633.

Chang, J.C., Temple, G.F., Poon, R., Neumann, K.H. & Kan, Y.W. (1977) The nucleotide sequences of the untranslated 5′ region of human α- and β-globin mRNAs. *Proc. Natl Acad. Sci. USA* **74**, 5145.

Chang, J.C., Poon, R., Neumann, K. & Kan, Y.W. (1978) The nucleotide sequence of the 5′ untranslated region of human γ-globin mRNA. *Nucl. Acids Res.* **5**, 3515.

Chang, J.C., Temple, G.F., Trecartin, R.F. & Kan, Y.W. (1979) Suppression of the nonsense mutation in homozygous β⁰ thalassaemia. *Nature* **281**, 602.

Chang, J.C., Alberti, A. & Kan, Y.W. (1983) A β-thalassemia lesion abolishes the same *Mst* II site as the sickle mutation. *Nucl. Acids Res.* **11**, 7789.

Chang, J.G., Lee, L.S., Lin, C.P., Chen, P.H. & Chen, C.P. (1991) Rapid diagnosis of α-thalassaemia-1 of Southeast Asia type and hydrops fetalis by polymerase chain reaction. *Blood* **78**, 853.

Chang, J.G., Lin, C.-P., Liu, T.-C. *et al.* (1994) Molecular basis of β-thalassaemia minor in Taiwan. *Int. J. Hematol.* **59**, 267.

Chang, J.G., Lu, J.M., Huang, J.M., Chen, J.T., Liu, H.J. & Chang, C.P. (1995a) Rapid diagnosis of β-thalassaemia by mutagenically separated polymerase chain reaction (MS-PCR) and its application to prenatal diagnosis. *Br. J. Haematol.* **91**, 602.

Chang, Y.C., Smith, K.D., Moore, R.D., Serjeant, G.R. & Dover, G.J. (1995b) An analysis of fetal hemoglobin variation in sickle cell disease: the relative contributions of the X-linked factor, β-globin haplotypes, α-globin gene number, gender and age. *Blood* **85**, 1111.

Chanutin, A. & Curnish, R.R. (1967) Effect of organic and inorganic phosphates on the oxygen equilibrium of human erythrocytes. *Arch. Biochem. Biophys.* **121**, 96.

Chapman, S.J., Allison, J.V. & Grimes, A.J. (1973) Abnormal cation movements in human hypochromic red cells incubated *in vitro*. *Scand. J. Haematol.* **10**, 225.

Chapman, R.W.G., Hussein, M.A.M., Gorman, A. *et al.* (1982) Effect of ascorbic acid deficiency on serum ferritin concentrations in patients with β-thalassaemia major and iron overload. *J. Clin. Pathol.* **35**, 487.

Chaptal, J., Jean, R. & Pays, A. (1967) Hémachromatose secondaire de la maladie de Cooley, étude clinique, biologique et anatomique. *Pédiatrie* **19**, 677.

Charache, S. & Conley, C.L. (1969) Hereditary persistence of fetal hemoglobin. *Ann. N. Y. Acad. Sci.* **165**, 37.

Charache, S., Weatherall, D.J. & Clegg, J.B. (1966) Polycythemia associated with a hemoglobinopathy. *J. Clin. Invest.* **45**, 813.

Charache, S., Conley, C.L., Doeblin, T.D. & Bartalos, M. (1974) Thalassemia in Black Americans. *Ann. N. Y. Acad. Sci.* **232**, 125.

Charache, S., Clegg, J.B. & Weatherall, D.J. (1976) The Negro variety of hereditary persistence of fetal haemoglobin is a mild form of thalassaemia. *Br. J. Haematol.* **34**, 527.

Charache, S., Achuff, S., Winslow, R. & Kazazian, H. (1979) Oxygen transport in a woman with hemoglobin Hope/β⁺ thalassemia. *J. Lab. Clin. Med.* **93**, 316.

Charache, S., Dover, G., Smith, K., Talbot, C.C.J., Moyer, M. & Boyer, S. (1983) Treatment of sickle cell anemia with 5-azacytidine results in increased fetal hemoglobin production and is associated with non random hypomethylation of DNA around the gamma-delta-beta-globin gene complex. *Proc. Natl Acad. Sci. USA* **80**, 4842.

Charache, S., Terrin, M.L., Moore, R.D. *et al.* (1995) Effect of hydroxyurea on the frequency of painful crises in sickle cell anemia. *N. Eng. J. Med.* **332**, 1317.

Charache, S., Barton, F.B., Moore, R.D. *et al.* (1996) Fetal hemoglobin, hydroxyurea, and sickle cell anemia: clinical utility of a hemoglobin 'switching' agent. *Medicine* **75**, 300.

Charlton, R.W. & Bothwell, T.H. (1976) Iron, ascorbic acid, and thalassemia. In: *Iron Metabolism and Thalassemia. Birth Defects* (eds D. Bergsma, A. Cerami & C.M. Peterson), p. 63. Alan R. Liss, Inc, New York.

Chatterjea, J.B. (1959) Haemoglobinopathy in India. In: *Abnormal Haemoglobins* (eds J.H.P. Jonxis & J.F. Delafresnaye), p. 322. Blackwell Scientific Publications, Oxford.

Chatterjea, J.B. (1966) Haemoglobinopathies, glucose-6-phosphate dehydrogenase deficiency and allied problems in the Indian subcontinent. *Bull. WHO* **35**, 837.

Chatterjee, R. & Katz, M. (2000) Reversible hypogonadotrophic hypogonadism in sexually infantile male thalassaemic patients with transfusional iron overload. *Clin. Endocrinol.* **53**, 33.

Chatterjee, R., Katz, M., Wonke, B., Hoffbrand, A.V. & Politis, D. (1988) Induction of puberty in patients with beta-thalassemia major. *Birth Defects* **23**, 453.

Chatterjee, R., Katz, M., Cox, T. & Bantock, H. (1993a) Evaluation of growth hormone in thalassaemic boys with failed puberty: spontaneous versus proactive test. *Eur. J. Pediatr.* **152**, 721.

Chatterjee, R., Katz, M., Cox, T.F. & Porter, J.B. (1993b) A prospective study of the hypothalamic–pituitary axis in thalassaemic patients who developed secondary amenorrhoea. *Clin. Endocrinol.* **39**, 287.

Chatterjee, R., Katz, M., Oatridge, A., Bydder, G.M. & Porter, J.B. (1998) Selective loss of anterior pituitary volume with severe pituitary-gonadal insufficiency in poorly compliant male thalassemic patients with pubertal arrest. *Ann. N. Y. Acad. Sci.* **850**, 479.

Chebloune, Y., Pagnier, J., Trabuchet, G. *et al.* (1988) Structural analysis of the 5′ flanking region of the β globin gene in African sickle cell anaemia patients: further evidence for three origins of the sickle mutation in Africa. *Proc. Natl Acad. Sci. USA* **85**, 4431.

Chehab, F.F. & Kan, Y.W. (1989) Detection of specific DNA sequence by fluorescence amplification: a colour complementation assay. *Proc. Natl Acad. Sci. USA* **86**, 9178.

Chehab, F.F., Der Kaloustian, V., Khouri, F.P., Deeb, S.S. & Kan, Y.W. (1987) The molecular basis of β-thalassemia in Lebanon: application to prenatal diagnosis. *Blood* **69**, 1141.

Chehab, F.F., Winterhalter, K.H. & Kan, Y.W. (1989) Characterization of a spontaneous mutation in β-thalassemia associated with advanced paternal age. *Blood* **74**, 852.

Cheng, T.-C., Orkin, S.H., Antonarakis, S.E. *et al.* (1984) β-Thalassemia in Chinese. Use of *in vivo* RNA analysis and oligonucleotide hybridization in systematic characterization of molecular defects. *Proc. Natl Acad. Sci. USA* **81**, 2821.

Chernoff, A.I. (1959) The distribution of the thalassemia gene: a historical review. *Blood* **14**, 899.

Chernoff, A.I. & Pettit, N.M. (1964) The amino acid composition of hemoglobin. III. A qualitative method for identifying abnormalities of the polypeptide chains of hemoglobin. *Blood* **24**, 750.

Chernoff, A.I., Minnich, V. & Chongchareonsuk, S. (1954) Hemoglobin E, a hereditary abnormality of human hemoglobin. *Science* **120**, 605.

Chernoff, A.I., Minnich, V., Na-Nakorn, S., Tuchinda, S., Kashamsant, C. & Chernoff, R.R. (1956) Studies on hemoglobin E: I. The clinical, hematologic, and genetic characteristics of the hemoglobin E syndromes. *J. Lab. Clin. Med.* **47**, 455.

Cheung, M.-C., Goldberg, J.D. & Kan, Y.W. (1996) Prenatal diagnosis of sickle cell anemia and thalassemia by analysis of fetal cells in maternal blood. *Nature Genet.* **14**, 264.

Chiarioni, T., Nardi, E., Papa, G., Sasso, G.F. & Tentori, L. (1974) Une nouvelle hémoglobine anormale (Hb Abruzzo, β 143 His→Arg) a haute affinité pour l'oxygène. *Nouv. Rev. Fr. Hematol.* **14**, 67.

Chibani, J., Vidaud, M., Duquesnoy, P. *et al.* (1988) The peculiar spectrum of β-thalassemia genes in Tunisia. *Hum. Genet.* **78**, 190.

Chim, C.S., Chan, V. & Todd, D. (1998) Hemosiderosis with diabetes mellitus in untransfused Hemoglobin H disease. *Am. J. Hematol.* **57**, 160.

Chini, V. & Valeri, C.M. (1949) Mediterranean hemopathic syndromes. *Blood* **4**, 989.

Chinprasertsuk, S., Wanachiwanawin, W. & Piankijagum, A. (1994) Effect of pyrexia in the formation of intraerythrocytic inclusion bodies and vacuoles in haemolytic crisis of haemoglobin H disease. *Eur. J. Haematol.* **52**, 87.

Chitayat, D., Silver, M.M., O'Brien, K. *et al.* (1997) Limb defects in homozygous α-thalassemia: report of three cases. *Am. J. Med. Genet.* **68**, 162.

Chodirker, B.N., Ray, M., McAlpine, P.J. *et al.* (1988) Developmental delay, short stature and minor facial anomalies in a child with ring chromosome 16. *Am. J. Med. Genet.* **31**, 145.

Choi, O.-R.B. & Engel, J.D. (1988) Developmental regulation of β-globin gene switching. *Cell* **55**, 17.

Choremis, C. & Zannos, L. (1957) Microdrepanocytic disease in Greece. *Blood* **12**, 454.

Choudhury, N.V., Dubey, M.L., Jolly, J.G., Kalra, A., Mahajan, R.C. & Gangury, N.K. (1990) Post-transfusion malaria in thalassaemia patients. *Blut* **61**, 314.

Chouhan, D.M., Sharma, R.S. & Parekh, J.G. (1970) Alpha-thalassaemia in India. *J. Indian Med. Assoc.* **54**, 364.

Chouhan, D.M., Sharma, R.S., Vakil, B.J. & Parekh, J.G. (1971) Haemoglobin Lepore in an Indian family. *J. Indian Med. Assoc.* **56**, 287.

Christakis, J., Vavatsi, N., Hassapopoulou, H. *et al.* (1991) A comparison of sickle cell syndromes in northern Greece. *Br. J. Haematol.* **77**, 386.

Chuansumrit, A., Isarangkura, P., Hathirat, P. & Thirawarapan, S. (1986) A syndrome of post-transfusion hypertension, convulsion and cerebral hemorrhage in β-thalassemia Hb E disease: a case report with high plasma renin activity. *J. Med. Assoc. Thailand* **69**, 1.

Chui, D.H.K. & Waye, J.S. (1998) Hydrops fetalis caused by α-thalassemia: an emerging health care problem. *Blood* **91**, 2213.

Chui, D.H.K., Wong, S.C., Chung, S.-W., Patterson, M., Bhargava, S. & Poon, M.-C. (1986) Embryonic ζ-globin chains in adults: a marker for α-thalassemia-1 haplotype due to a >17.5 kb deletion. *N. Eng. J. Med.* **314**, 76.

Chui, D.H.K., Mentzer, W.C., Patterson, M. *et al.* (1989) Human embryonic ζ-globin chains in fetal and newborn blood. *Blood* **74**, 1409.

Chui, D.H.K., Patterson, M., Dowling, C.E., Kazazian, H.H. Jr & Kendall, A.G. (1990) Hemoglobin Bart's disease in an Italian boy. *N. Eng. J. Med.* **323**, 179.

Chung, S.-W., Wong, S.C., Clarke, B.J., Patterson, M., Walker, W.H.C. & Chui, D.H.K. (1984) Human embryonic ζ-globin chains in adult patients with α-thalassemias. *Proc. Natl Acad. Sci. USA* **81**, 6188.

Chung, J.L., Kao, J.H., Kong, M.S., Yang, C.P., Hung, I.J. & Lin, T.Y. (1997) Hepatitis C and G virus infections in polytransfused children. *Eur. J. Pediatr.* **156**, 546.

Ciechanover, A. (1998) The ubiquitin–proteasome pathway: on protein death and cell life. *EMBO J.* **17**, 7151.

Cin, S., Akar, N., Arcasoy, A., Dedeoglu, S. & Çavdar, A.O. (1984) Prevalance of thalassaemia and G6PD deficiency in North Cyprus. *Acta Haematol.* **71**, 69.

CIOMS (1965) *CIOMS Symposium on Abnormal Haemoglobins in Africa* (ed. J.H.P. Jonxis). Blackwell Scientific Publications, Oxford.

de Ciutiis, A.C., Peterson, C.M., Polley, M.J. & Metakis, L.J. (1978) Alternative pathway activation in sickle cell disease and β-thalassemia major. *J. Natl Med. Assoc.* **70**, 503.

Cividalli, G., Locker, H. & Russell, A. (1971) Increased permeability of erythrocyte membrane in thalassemia. *Blood* **37**, 716.

Cividalli, G., Nathan, D.G., Kan, Y.W., Santamarina, B. & Frigoletto, F. (1974a) Relation of beta to gamma synthesis during the first trimester: an approach to prenatal diagnosis of thalassemia. *Pediatr. Res.* **8**, 553.

Cividalli, G., Nathan, D.G. & Lodish, H.F. (1974b) Translational control of hemoglobin synthesis in thalassemia bone marrow. *J. Clin. Invest.* **53**, 955.

Cividalli, G.G., Antebi, S., Klein, R., Kerem, H. & Rachmilewitz, E.A. (1976) Prenatal diagnosis of heterozygous beta-thalassemia. *Israel J. Med. Sci.* **12**, 1313.

Cividalli, G., Kerem, H., Execkiel, E. & Rachmilewitz, E.A. (1978) β⁰-Thalassemia intermedia. *Blood* **52**, 345.

Cividalli, G., Kerem, H. & Rachmilewitz, E.A. (1979) Globin synthesis in bone marrow cells of patients with sickle anemia and β⁰-thalassemia: contamination of the β-chain with non-globin proteins. *Hemoglobin* **3**, 175.

Clarke, C. & Whitfield, A.G.W. (1977) Deaths from rhesus haemolytic disease in England and Wales 1977; accuracy of records and assessment of anti D prophylaxis. *Br. Med. J.* **i**, 1665.

Clegg, J.B. (1970) Horse haemoglobin polymorphism: evidence for two linked non-allelic α-chain genes. *Proc. Roy. Soc. Lond. (Biol.)* **176**, 235.

Clegg, J.B. (1981) Structure of the human ε and ζ chains. *Texas Reports Biol. Med.* **40**, 23.

Clegg, J.B. (1983) Hemoglobin synthesis. In: *The Thalassemias* (ed. D.J. Weatherall), p. 54. Churchill Livingstone, Edinburgh.

Clegg, J.B. (1987) Can the product of the θ gene be a real globin? *Nature* **329**, 465.

Clegg, J.B. & Gagnon, J. (1981) Structure of the ζ-chain of human embryonic hemoglobin. *Proc. Natl Acad. Sci. USA* **78**, 6076.

Clegg, J.B. & Weatherall, D.J. (1967) Haemoglobin synthesis in alpha-thalassaemia (haemoglobin H disease). *Nature* **215**, 1241.

Clegg, J.B. & Weatherall, D.J. (1972) Haemoglobin synthesis during erythroid maturation in β thalassaemia. *Nature* **240**, 190.

Clegg, J.B. & Weatherall, D.J. (1974) Beta thalassaemia—time for a reappraisal? *Lancet* **ii**, 133.

Clegg, J.B., Naughton, M.A. & Weatherall, D.J. (1965) An improved method for the characterization of human haemoglobin mutants: identification of $\alpha_2\beta_2$ 95Glu, haemoglobin N (Baltimore). *Nature* **207**, 945.

Clegg, J.B., Naughton, M.A. & Weatherall, D.J. (1966) Abnormal human haemoglobins. Separation and characterisation of the α- and β-chains by chromatography, and the determination of two new variants, Hb Chesapeake and Hb J (Bangkok). *J. Mol. Biol.* **19**, 91.

Clegg, J.B., Naughton, M.A. & Weatherall, D.J. (1968a) Separation of the alpha and beta chains of human haemoglobin. *Nature* **219**, 69.

Clegg, J.B., Weatherall, D.J., Na-Nakorn, S. & Wasi, P. (1968b) Haemoglobin synthesis in β-thalassaemia. *Nature* **220**, 664.

Clegg, J.B., Weatherall, D.J. & Eunson, C.E. (1971a) The distribution of nascent globin chains on human reticulocyte polysomes. *Biochim. Biophys. Acta* **247**, 109.

Clegg, J.B., Weatherall, D.J. & Milner, P.F. (1971b) Haemoglobin Constant Spring—a chain termination mutant? *Nature* **234**, 337.

Clegg, J.B., Weatherall, D.J., Contopoulos-Griva, I., Caroutsos, K., Poungouras, P. & Tsevrenis, H. (1974) Haemoglobin Icaria, a new chain termination mutant which causes α-thalassaemia. *Nature* **251**, 245.

Clegg, J.B., Metaxatou-Mavromati, A., Kattamis, C., Sofroniadou, K., Wood, W.G. & Weatherall, D.J. (1979) Occurrence of $^G\gamma$ Hb F in Greek HPFH: analysis of heterozygotes and compound heterozygotes with β thalassaemia. *Br. J. Haematol.* **43**, 521.

Clement, D.H. & Taffel, M. (1955) Splenectomy in Mediterranean anemia. *Pediatr.* **16**, 353.

Clemente, M.G., Congia, M., Lai, M.E. *et al.* (1994) Effect of iron overload on the response to recombinant interferon-alfa treatment in transfusion-dependent patients with thalassaemia major and chronic hepatitis C. *J. Pediatr.* **125**, 123.

Clift, R.A. & Johnson, F.L. (1997) Marrow transplants for thalassemia: the USA experience. *Bone Marrow Transplant.* **19** (Suppl. 2), 57.

Cline, M.J., Stang, H., Mercola, K. *et al.* (1980) Gene transfer in intact animals. *Nature* **284**, 422.

Codrington, J.F., Kutlar, F., Harris, H.F., Wilson, J.B., Stoming, T.A. & Huisman, T.H.J. (1989) Hb A_2-Wrens or $\alpha_2\delta_2$98 (FG5) Val→Met, an unstable δ chain variant identified by sequence analysis of amplified DNA. *Biochim. Biophys. Acta* **1009**, 87.

Codrington, J.F., Li, H.-W., Kutlar, F., Gu, L.-H., Ramachandran, M. & Huisman, T.H.J. (1990) Observations on the levels of Hb A_2 in patients with different β thalassaemia mutations and a δ chain variant. *Blood* **76**, 1246.

Cohen, J. (1996) Infection in the compromised host. In: *Oxford Textbook of Medicine* (eds D.J. Weatherall, J.G.G. Ledingham & D.A. Warrell), p. 1027. Oxford University Press, Oxford.

Cohen, F., Zuelzer, W.W., Neel, J.V. & Robinson, A.R. (1959) Multiple inherited erythrocyte abnormalities in an American Negro family: Hereditary spherocytosis, sickling and thalassemia. *Blood* **14**, 816.

Cohen, A., Markenson, A.L. & Schwartz, E. (1980) Transfusion requirements and splenectomy in thalassemia major. *J. Pediatr.* **97**, 100.

Cohen, A., Cohen, I.J. & Schwartz, E. (1981) Scurvy and altered iron stores in thalassemia major. *N. Eng. J. Med.* **304**, 158.

Cohen, A., Martin, M. & Schwartz, E. (1984a) Depletion of excessive liver iron stores with desferrioxamine. *Br. J. Haematol.* **58**, 369.

Cohen, A.R., Schmidt, J.M., Martin, M.B., Barnsley, W. & Schwartz, E. (1984b) Clinical trial of young red cell transfusions. *J. Pediatr.* **104**, 865.

Cohen, A., Gayer, E. & Mizanin, J. (1989a) Long-term effect of splenectomy on transfusion requirements in thalassemia major. *Am. J. Hematol.* **30**, 254.

Cohen, A.R., Mizanin, J. & Schwartz, E. (1989b) Rapid removal of excessive iron with daily, high-dose intravenous chelation therapy. *J. Pediatr.* **115**, 151.

Cohen, A.R., Martin, M.B. & Schwartz, E. (1995) Hydroxyurea therapy in thalassemia intermedia. In: *Sickle Cell Disease and Thalassemia: New Trends in Therapy* (eds Y. Beuzard, B. Lubin & J. Rosa), p. 193. Colloque INSERM, Paris.

Cohen, A., Galanello, R., Piga, A., Vullo, C. & Tricta, F. (1998) A multi-center safety trial of the oral iron chelator deferiprone. In: *Cooley's Anemia Seventh Symposium* (ed. A. R. Cohen), p. 223. The New York Academy of Sciences, New York.

Coleman, M.B., Steinberg, M.H., Harrell, A.H., Plonczynski, M.W., Walker, A.M. & Adams, J.G. III (1992) The −87 (C→A) β⁺-thalassaemia mutation in a Black family. *Hemoglobin* **16**, 399.

Coleman, M.B., Adams, J.G. III., Steinberg, M.H. *et al.* (1993) $^G\gamma^A\gamma$ (β⁺) Hereditary persistence of fetal hemoglobin: the G gamma −158 C→T mutation in cis to the −175 T→C mutation of the $^A\gamma$-globin gene results in increased $^G\gamma$-globin synthesis. *Am. J. Hematol.* **42**, 186.

Coleman, M.B., Lu, Z.-H., Smith, C.M.I. *et al.* (1995) Two missense mutations in the β-globin gene can cause severe β thalassaemia. Hemoglobin Medicine Lake (β 32[B14]leucine→glutamine; 98 [FG5] valine→methionine). *J. Clin. Invest.* **95**, 503.

Collier, S., Tassabehji, M. & Strachan, T. (1993) A de novo pathological point mutation at the 21-hydroxylase locus: implications for gene conversion in the human genome. *Nature Genet.* **3**, 260.

Collins, F.S., Stoeckert, C.J., Serjeant, G.R., Forget, B.G. & Weissman, S.M. (1984) $^G\gamma\beta^+$ Hereditary persistence of fetal hemoglobin: cosmid cloning and identification of a specific mutation 5′ to the $^G\gamma$ gene. *Proc. Natl Acad. Sci. USA* **81**, 4894.

Collins, F.S., Metherall, J.E., Yamakawa, M., Pan, J., Weissman, S.M. & Forget, B.G. (1985) A point mutation in the $^A\gamma$-globin gene promoter in Greek hereditary persistence of fetal hemoglobin. *Nature* **313**, 325.

Collins, F.S., Cole, J.L., Lockwood, W.K. & Iannuzzi, M.C. (1987) The deletion in both common types of hereditary persistence of fetal hemoglobin is approximately 105 kilobases. *Blood* **70**, 1797.

Collins, A.F., Dias, G.C., Haddad, S. *et al.* (1994) Evaluation of a new neocyte transfusion preparation vs. washed cell transfusion in patients with homozygous beta thalassemia. *Transfusion* **34**, 517.

Collins, A.F., Pearson, H.A., Giardina, P., McDonagh, K.T., Brusilow, S.W. & Dover, G.J. (1995) Oral sodium phenylbutyrate therapy in homozygous beta thalassemia. *Blood* **85**, 43.

Collis, P., Antoniou, M. & Grosveld, F. (1990) Definition of the minimal requirements within the human β-globin gene and the dominant control region for high level expression. *EMBO J.* **9**, 233.

Comi, P., Giglioni, B., Barbarano, L. *et al.* (1977) Transcriptional and post-transcriptional defects in β⁰-thalassaemia. *Eur. J. Biochem.* **79**, 617.

Comings, D.E. & Motulsky, A.G. (1966) Absence of *cis* delta chain synthesis in (δβ) thalassaemia (F-thalassaemia). *Blood* **28**, 54.

Conconi, F. & del Senno, L. (1974) The molecular defect of Ferrara β-thalassaemia. *Ann. N. Y. Acad. Sci.* **232**, 54.

Conconi, F., Bargelessi, A., del Senno, L., Menegatti, E., Pontremoli, S. & Russo, G. (1970) Globin chain synthesis in Sicilian thalassemic subjects. *Br. J. Haematol.* **19**, 469.

Conconi, F., Rowley, P.T., del Senno, L., Pontremoli, S. & Volpato, S. (1972) Induction of β-globin synthesis in the β-thalassaemia of Ferrara. *Nature New Biol.* **238**, 83.

Conconi, F., Alberti, R., Mariuzzi, G.M., Gugluelmini, C., Vullo, C. & del Senno, L. (1978) Decrease of alpha-Hasharon globin in beta-thalassaemia. *Br. J. Haematol.* **39**, 529.

Condon, P.I., Serjeant, G.R. & Ikeda, H. (1973) An unusual chorioretinopathy in sickle-cell disease—a sequel to choroidal infarction. *Br. J. Ophthalmol.* **57**, 81.

Condon, P.I., Gray, R. & Serjeant, G.R. (1974) Ocular findings in children with sickle cell haemoglobin C disease in Jamaica. *Br. J. Ophthalmol.* **58**, 644.

Conley, C.L. (1980) Sickle-cell anemia—the first molecular disease. In: *Blood, Pure and Eloquent* (ed. M.M. Wintrobe), p. 319. McGraw-Hill Book Company, New York.

Conley, C.L. & Wintrobe, M.M. (1976) Thalassemia in the 'D' family: Case Presentation: Mr M.D. *Johns Hopkins Med. J.* **139**, 201.

Conley, C.L., Weatherall, D.J., Richardson, S.N., Shepard, M.K. & Charache, S. (1963) Hereditary persistence of fetal hemoglobin: a study of 79 affected persons in 15 Negro families in Baltimore. *Blood* **21**, 261.

Conner, B.J., Reyes, A.A., Morin, C., Itakura, K., Teplitz, R.L. & Wallace, R.B. (1983) Detection of sickle cell β^S-globin allele by hybridisation with synthetic oligonucleotides. *Proc. Natl Acad. Sci. USA* **80**, 278.

Constantoulakis, M., Panagopoulos, G. & Augoustaki, O. (1975) Stature and longitudinal growth in thalassemia major. A study of 229 Greek patients. *Clin. Pediatr.* **14**, 355.

Constantoulakis, M., Trichopoulos, D., Augoustaki, O. & Economidou, J. (1978) Serum immunoglobulin concentrations before and after splenectomy in patients with homozygous β-thalassaemia. *J. Clin. Pathol.* **31**, 546.

Cook, I.A. & Lehmann, H. (1973) Beta-thalassaemia and some rare haemoglobin variants in the Highlands of Scotland. *Scott. Med. J.* **18**, 14.

Cook, T., Gebelein, B., Mesa, K., Mladek, A. & Urrutia, R. (1998) Molecular cloning and characterization of *TIEG2* reveals a new subfamily of transforming growth factor-β-inducible Sp1-like Zinc finger-encoding genes involved in the regulation of cell growth. *J. Biol. Chem.* **273**, 25929.

Cooley, J.R. & Kitay, D.Z. (1984) Heterozygous β-thalassemia in pregnancy. *J. Reprod. Med.* **29**, 141.

Cooley, T.B. & Lee, P. (1925) A series of cases of splenomegaly in children with anemia and peculiar bone changes. *Trans. Am. Pediatr. Soc.* **37**, 29.

Cooley, T.B. & Lee, P. (1932) Erythroblastic anemia; additional comments. *Am. J. Dis. Child.* **43**, 705.

Cooley, T.B., Witwer, E.R. & Lee, P. (1927) Anemia in children with splenomegaly and peculiar changes in bones; report of cases. *Am. J. Dis. Child.* **34**, 347.

Cooper, A.N. & Krawczak, M. (1993) *Human Gene Mutation*. BIOS Scientific Publishers, Oxford.

Cooper, D.M., Mansell, A.L., Weiner, M.A. *et al.* (1980) Low lung capacity and hypoxemia in children with thalassemia. *Am. Rev. Respir. Dis.* **121**, 639.

Coquelet, M.L., de Traverse, P.N., Israel, J., Pelletier, P. & Blatrix, C. (1970) La double hétérozygotie hémoglobinose C-thalassémie chez les Européens. Étude d'une famille Siciliene. *Nouv. Rev. Fr. Hematol.* **10**, 461.

Coquelet, M.-L., Jaeger, G. & Mullender, N. (1978) Anomalies de l'hémoglobine et données médico-biologiques chez 10000 Africains. *Nouv. Rev. Fr. Hematol.* **20**, 465.

Coquelet, M.-L., Jaeger, G. & Brumpt, L.C. (1983) Dépistage des anomalies de l'hémoglobine chez 35000 boursiers de la coopération. *Bull. Soc. Pathol. Exot.* **76**, 183.

Correra, A., Graziano, J.H., Seaman, C. & Piomelli, S. (1984) Inappropriately low red cell 2,3-diphosphoglycerate and p50 in transfused beta-thalassemia. *Blood* **63**, 803.

Cortesi, S., Vettore, L., Carta, S., Sorcini, M. & de Sandre, G. (1966) Associazione di emoglobinosi D$_{Los Angeles}$ αβ-talassemia in una famiglia Veneta. *Acta Med. Patav.* **26**, 262.

Cosset, F.L. & Russell, S.J. (1996) Targeting retrovirus entry. *Gene Ther.* **3**, 946.

Cossu, P., Toccafondi, C., Vardeu, F. *et al.* (1981) Iron overload and desferrioxamine chelation therapy in beta-thalassemia intermedia. *Eur. J. Pediatr.* **137**, 267.

Costa, F.F., Zago, M.A., Cheng, G., Nechtman, J.F., Stoming, T.A. & Huisman, T.H.J. (1990) The Brazilian type of nondeletional ^{A}γ-fetal hemoglobin has a C-G substitution at nucleotide –195 of the ^{A}γ-globin gene. *Blood* **76**, 1896.

Costagliola, D.G., Girot, R., Rebulla, P. & Lefrère, J.-J. (1992) Incidence of AIDS in HIV-1 infected thalassemia patients. *Br. J. Haematol.* **81**, 109.

Costin, G., Kogut, M.D., Hyman, C. & Ortega, J.A. (1977) Carbohydrate metabolism and pancreatic islet-cell function in thalassemia major. *Diabetes* **26**, 230.

Costin, G., Kogut, M.D., Hyman, C.B. & Ortega, J.A. (1979) Endocrine abnormalities in thalassemia major. *Am. J. Dis. Child.* **133**, 497.

Council for International Organizations of Medical Sciences (1991) *Genetics, Ethics and Human Values. Proceedings of the XXIVth CIOMS Conference*, Geneva.

Cournand, A. (1964) Air and blood. In: *Circulation of the Blood, Men and Ideas* (eds A.W. Fishman & D.W. Richards), p. 3. Oxford University Press, Oxford.

Coutinho Gomes, M.P., Gomes da Costa, M.G., Braga, L.B. *et al.* (1988) β-Thalassemia mutations in the Portuguese population. *Hum. Genet.* **78**, 13.

Craddock, C.F. (1994) *Normal and abnormal regulation of human α globin expression*. D. Phil., University of Oxford.

Craddock, C.F., Vyas, P., Sharpe, J.A., Ayyub, H., Wood, W.G. & Higgs, D.R. (1995) Contrasting effects of α and β globin regulatory elements on chromatin structure may be related to their different chromosomal environments. *EMBO J.* **14**, 1718.

Craig, J.E., Kelly, S.H., Barnetson, R. & Thein, S.L. (1992) Molecular characterization of a novel 10.3 kb deletion causing β-thalassaemia with unusually high Hb A$_2$. *Br. J. Haematol.* **82**, 735.

Craig, J.E., Sheerin, S.M., Barnetson, R. & Thein, S.L. (1993) The molecular basis of HPFH in a British family identified by heteroduplex formation. *Br. J. Haematol.* **84**, 106.

Craig, J.E., Barnetson, R.A., Prior, J., Raven, J.L. & Thein, S.L. (1994) Rapid detection of deletions causing δβ thalassemia and hereditary persistence of fetal hemoglobin by enzymatic amplification. *Blood* **83**, 1673.

Craig, J.E., Efremov, G.D., Fisher, C. & Thein, S.L. (1995) Macedonian (δβ)^0 thalassemia has the same molecular basis as Turkish inversion-deletion (δβ)^0 thalassemia. *Blood* **85**, 1146.

Craig, J.E., Rochette, J. Fisher, C.A. *et al.* (1996) Dissecting the loci controlling fetal haemoglobin production on chromosomes 11p and 6q by the regressive approach. *Nature Genet.* **12**, 58.

Craig, J.E., Rochette, J., Sampietro, M. *et al.* (1997) Genetic heterogeneity in heterocellular hereditary persistence of fetal hemoglobin. *Blood* **90**, 428.

Creighton, T.E. (1997) Proteins. In: *Encyclopedia of Human Biology*, p. 189. Academic Press, New York.

Crosby, W.H. & Akeroyd, J.H. (1952) The limit of hemoglobin synthesis in hereditary hemolytic anemia. *Am. J. Med.* **13**, 273.

Crosby, W.H. & Conrad, M.E. (1964) Iron imbalance in thalassemia minor. A preliminary report. *Ann. N.Y. Acad. Sci.* **119**, 616.

Crosby, W.H. & Dameshek, W. (1951) The significance of hemoglobinuria and associated hemosiderinuria, with particular reference to various types of hemolytic anemia. *J. Lab. Clin. Med.* **38**, 829.

Crout, J.E., McKenna, C.H. & Pettit, R.M. (1976) Symptomatic joint effusions in sickle cell-beta-thalassemia disease. Report of a case. *J.A.M.A.* **235**, 1878.

Crowley, J.P., Metzger, J.B., Merrill, E.W. & Valeri, C.R. (1992) Whole blood viscosity in β thalassemia minor. *Ann. Clin. Lab. Sci.* **22**, 229.

Crystal, R.G., Elson, N.A., Nienhuis, A., Thornton, A.G. & Anderson, W.F. (1973) Initiation of globin synthesis in β thalassemia. *N. Eng. J. Med.* **288**, 1091.

Cumano, A., Dieterlen-Lievre, F. & Godin, I. (1996) Lymphoid potential, probed before circulation in mouse, is restricted to caudal intraembryonic splanchnopleura. *Cell* **86**, 907.

Cumming, R.L.C., Millar, J.A., Smith, J.A. & Goldberg, A. (1969) Clinical and laboratory studies on the action of desferrioxamine. *Br. J. Haematol.* **17**, 257.

Cunningham, T.A. & Vella, F. (1967) Combination of spherocytosis and a variant of beta thalassaemia ('isolated raised Hb A₂'). *J. Med. Genet.* **4**, 109.

Curtain, C.C. (1964) A structural study of abnormal haemoglobins occurring in New Guinea. *Aust. J. Exper. Biol. Med. Sci.* **42**, 89.

Curtin, P., Pirastu, M., Kan, Y.W., Gobert-Jones, J.A., Stephens, A.D. & Lehmann, H. (1985) A distant gene deletion affects β-globin gene function in an atypical γδβ-thalassaemia. *J. Clin. Invest.* **76**, 1554.

Curtin, P.T., Liu, D., Liu, W., Chang, J.C. & Kan, Y.W. (1989) Human β-globin gene expression in transgenic mice is enhanced by a distant DNase I hypersensitive site. *Proc. Natl Acad. Sci. USA* **86**, 7082.

Çürük, M.A., Kutlar, A. & Huisman, T.H.J. (1992a) Hb Shelby α₂β₂ (131) (H9) Gln→Lys]-β⁰-thalassemia [codon 15 (TGG→TGA)] identified by DNA sequencing. *Hemoglobin* **16**, 417.

Çürük, M.A., Yüregir, G.T., Asadov, C.D. *et al.* (1992b) Molecular characterization of β-thalassemia in Azerbaijan. *Hum. Genet.* **90**, 417.

Çürük, M.A., Baysal, E., Gupta, R.B. & Huisman, T.H.J. (1993a) An IVS-I-117 (G→A) acceptor splice site mutation in the α1-globin gene is a nondeletional α-thalassaemia-2 determinant in an Indian population. *Br. J. Haematol.* **85**, 148.

Çürük, M.A., Dimovski, A.J. Baysal, E. *et al.* (1993b) Hb Adana or α₂59 (E8) Gly→Aspβ₂, a severely unstable α₁-globin variant, observed in combination with the −(α) 20.5 kb α-thal-1 deletion in two Turkish patients. *Am. J. Hematol.* **44**, 270.

Çürük, M.A., Molchanova, T.P., Postnikov, Y.V. *et al.* (1994) β-thalassaemia alleles and unstable hemoglobin types among Russian pediatric patients. *Am. J. Hematol.* **46**, 329.

Çürük, M.A., Howard, S.C., Kutlar, A. & Huisman, T.H.J. (1995) A newly discovered β⁰-thalassaemia (IVS-II-850, G→A) mutation in a North European family. *Hemoglobin* **19**, 207.

Cutillo, S. & Meloni, T. (1974) Serum concentrations of haptoglobin and hemopexin in favism and thalassemia. *Acta Haematol.* **52**, 65.

Dacie, J.V. & Lewis, S.M. (1975) *Practical Haematology*, 5th edn. Churchill Livingstone, Edinburgh.

Daiber, A., Pinto, R., Con, I. *et al.* (1976) Hemoglobinopatias: frecuencia en 561 sujetos investigados. *Rev. Med. Chile* **104**, 972.

Dallman, P.R. (1977) The red cell. In: *Blood and Blood-forming Tissues* (ed. P.R. Dallman), p. 1109. Appleton-Century-Crofts, New York.

Dallman, P.R. & Siimes, M.A. (1979) Percentile curves for hemoglobin and red cell volume in infancy and childhood. *J. Pediatr.* **94**, 26.

Dameshek, W. (1940) 'Target cell' anemia. An erythroblastic type of Cooley's erythroblastic anemia. *Am. J. Med. Sci.* **200**, 445.

Dameshek, W. (1943) Familial Mediterranean target–oval cell syndromes. *Am. J. Med. Sci.* **205**, 643.

Dance, N., Huehns, E.R. & Beaven, G.H. (1963) The abnormal haemoglobins in haemoglobin-H disease. *Biochem. J.* **86**, 240.

Dandona, P., Hussain, M.A.M., Varghese, Z., Politis, D., Flynn, D.M. & Hoffbrand, A.V. (1983) Insulin resistance and iron overload. *Ann. Clin. Biochem.* **20**, 77.

Dandona, P., Menon, R.K., Houlder, S., Thomas, M., Hoffbrand, A.V. & Flynn, D.M. (1987) Serum 1,25 dihydroxyvitamin D and osteocalcin concentrations in thalassaemia. *Arch. Dis. Child.* **62**, 474.

Daneshmend, T.K. & Peachey, R.D. (1978) Leg ulcers in α thalassaemia (haemoglobin H disease). *Br. J. Dermatol.* **98**, 233.

Daniels, R.J., Peden, J.F., Lloyd, C. *et al.* (2001) Sequence, structure and pathology of the fully anotated terminal 2 Mb of the short arm of chromosome 16. *Hum. Mol. Genet.* **10**, 339.

Darbellay, R., Mach-Pascual, S., Rose, K., Graf, J. & Beris, P.H. (1995) Haemoglobin Tunis-Bizerte: a new α₁ globin 129 Leu→Pro unstable variant with thalassaemic phenotype. *Br. J. Haematol.* **90**, 71.

Das, B.M. & Deka, R. (1975) Predominance of the haemoglobin E gene in a mongoloid population in Assam (India). *Humangenetik* **30**, 187.

Das, S.R., Das, S.K. & Dawn, C.S. (1973) Haemoglobin Barts in Bengali Hindu Castes studied in Calcutta. *Hum. Hered.* **23**, 381.

Das, B.M., Deka, R. & Das, R. (1980) Haemoglobin E in six populations of Assam. *J. Indian Anthrop. Soc.* **15**, 153.

Dash, S. & Dash, R.J. (1980) Idiopathic myelofibrosis without splenomegaly and with an acquired haemoglobin disorder. *Indian J. Cancer* **17**, 193.

David, C.V. & Balusubramaniam, P. (1983) Paraplegia with thalassemia. *Aust. N.Z. J. Med.* **53**, 283.

Davies, S.C., Marcus, R.E., Hungerford, J.L., Miller, M.H., Arden, G.B. & Huehns, E.R. (1983) Ocular toxicity of high dose intravenous desferrioxamine. *Lancet* **ii**, 181.

Davies, S.C., Luce, P.J., Win, A.A., Riordan, J.F. & Brozovic, M. (1984) Acute chest syndrome in sickle-cell disease. *Lancet* **i**, 36.

Davis, B.A. & Porter J.B. (2000) Longterm outcome of continuous 24-hour deferoxmine infusion via indwelling intravenous catheters in high-risk beta thalassemia. *Blood* **95**, 1229.

De, M., Das, S.K., Bhattacharya, D.K. & Talukder, G. (1997) The occurrence of β-thalassemia mutation and its interaction with hemoglobin E in eastern India. *Int. J. Hematol.* **66**, 31.

De Alarcon, P.A., Donovan, M.E., Forbes, G.B., Landau, S.A. & Stockman, J.A. (1979) Iron absorption in the thalassemia syndromes and its inhibition by tea. *N. Eng. J. Med.* **300**, 5.

De Angioletti, M., Lacerra, G., Castaldo, C. *et al.* (1992) αααα^anti-3.7 type II: a new α-globin gene rearrangement suggesting that the α-globin gene duplication could be caused by intrachromosomal recombination. *Hum. Genet.* **89**, 37.

De Angioletti, M., Lacerra, G. & Carestia, C. (1997) 6th International Conference on Thalassaemia and the Haemoglobinopathies, Abstract 148. Malta.

De Costa, J.L., Loh, Y.S. & Hanam, E. (1974) Extramedullary hemopoiesis with multiple tumor-stimulating mediastinal masses in hemoglobin E-thalassemia. *Chest* **65**, 210.

De Marco, E.V., Crescibene, L., Bagala, A., Brancati, C., Wualitieri, A. & Bria, M. (1994) Hb D-Iran [β22 (B4) Glu→Gln] in southern Italy. *Hemoglobin* **18**, 65.

De Martino, M., Quarta, G., Melpignano, A. *et al.* (1985) Antibodies to HTLV III and the lymphadenopathy syndrome in multitransfused beta-thalassemia patients. *Vox Sang.* **41**, 230.

De Pablos, J.M., Almagro, M., Cabrera, A. & Lopez, P. (1987) Homocigosis para Hb C y doble heteropcigosis Hb C/β⁺ talasemia en una familia espanola. *Sangre-Barc.* **32**, 372.

De Sanctis, V., D'Ascola, G. & Wonke, B.(1986) The development of diabetes mellitus and chronic liver disease in long term chelated β-thalassaemic patients. *Postgrad. Med. J.* **62**, 831.

De Sanctis, V., Vullo, C., Katz, M., Wonke, B., Hoffbrand, A.V. & Bagni, B. (1988a) Hypothalamic–pituitary–gonadal axis in thalassemic patients with secondary amenorrhea. *Obstet. Gynecol.* **72**, 643.

De Sanctis, V., Vullo, C., Katz, M., Wonke, B., Tanas, R. & Bagni, B. (1988b) Gonadal function in patients with beta thalassaemia major. *J. Clin. Pathol.* **41**, 133.

De Sanctis, V., Zurlo, M.G., Senesi, E., Boffa, C., Cavallo, L. & Di Gregorio, F. (1988c) Insulin dependent diabetes in thalassaemia. *Arch. Dis. Child.* **63**, 58.

De Sanctis, V., Vullo, C., Katz, M. *et al.* (1989) Endocrine complications in thalassaemia major. *Prog. Clin. Biol. Res.* **309**, 77.

De Sanctis, V., Vullo, C., Bagni, B. & Chiccoli, L. (1992) Hypoparathyroidism in β-thalassemia major. Clinical and laboratory observations in 24 patients. *Acta Haematol.* **88**, 105.

De Sanctis, V., Katz, M., Vullo, C., Bagni, B., Ughi, M. & Wonke, B. (1994) Effect of different treatment regimes on linear growth and final height in β-thalassaemia major. *Clin. Endocrinol.* **40**, 791.

De Sanctis, V., Pinamonti, A., Di Palma, A. *et al.* (1996) Growth and development in thalassaemia major patients with severe bone lesions due to desferrioxamine. *Eur. J. Pediatr.* **155**, 368.

De Sanctis, V., Galimberti, M., Lucarelli, G. *et al.* (1997) Growth and development in ex-thalassemia patients. *Bone Marrow Transplant.* **19** (Suppl. 2), 126.

De Silva, C.C., Jonxis, J.H.P. & Wickramasinghe, M.R.L. (1959) Haemoglobinopathies in Ceylon. In: *Abnormal Haemoglobins* (eds J.H.P. Jonxis & J.F. Delafresnaye), p. 340. Blackwell Scientific Publications, Oxford.

De Silva, H.J., Senaratne, N.L., Goonetilleke, A.K., de Silva, C. & Jayawickrama, U.S. & Amarasekera, L.R. (1988) Sero-negative rheumatoid arthritis in haemoglobin E thalassaemia. *Ceylon Med. J.* **33**, 131.

De Silva, S., Fisher, C.A., Premawardhena, A. *et al.* (2000) Thalassaemia in Sri Lanka: Implications for the future health burden in Asian populations. *Lancet* **355**, 786.

De Simone, J., Biel, S.I. & Heller, P. (1978) Stimulation of fetal hemoglobin synthesis in baboons by hemolysis and hypoxia. *Proc. Natl Acad. Sci. USA* **75**, 2937.

De Simone, J., Heller, P. & Biel, S.I. (1979) Stimulation of fetal hemoglobin synthesis following stress erythropoiesis. In: *Cellular and Molecular Regulation of Hemoglobin Switching* (eds G. Stamatoyannopoulos & A.W. Nienhuis), p. 139. Grune and Stratton, New York.

De Simone, J., Heller, P., Hall, L. & Zwiers, D. (1982) 5-Azacytidine stimulates fetal hemoglobin synthesis in anemic baboons. *Proc. Natl Acad. Sci. USA* **79**, 4428.

De Virgliis, S., Sanna, G., Carnacchia, G. *et al.* (1980) Serum ferritin, liver iron stores and liver histology in children with thalassaemia. *Arch. Dis. Child.* **55**, 43.

De Virgliis, S., Congia, M., Frau, F. *et al.* (1988) Deferoxamine-induced growth retardation in patients with thalassemia major. *J. Pediatr.* **113**, 661.

Deidda, G., Novelletto, A., Hafez, M. *et al.* (1990) A new β-thalassemia mutation produced by a single nucleotide substitution in the conserved dinucleotide sequence of the IVS-I consensus acceptor site (AG→AA). *Hemoglobin* **14**, 431.

Deidda, G., Novelletto, A., Hafez, M., El-Ziny, M., Terrenato, L. & Felicetti, L. (1991) A new β-thalassaemia frameshift mutation detected by PCR after selective hybridization to immbolized oligonucleotides. *Br. J. Haematol.* **79**, 90.

Deisseroth, A., Nienhuis, A., Turner, P. *et al.* (1977) Localization of the human α-globin structural gene to chromosome 16 in somatic cell hybrids by molecular hybridization. *Cell* **12**, 205.

Deisseroth, A., Nienhuis, A., Lawrence, J., Riles, R., Turner, P. & Ruddle, F. (1978) Chromosomal localization of human β globin gene on chromosome 11 in somatic cell hybrids. *Proc. Natl Acad. Sci. USA* **75**, 1456.

Del Principe, D., Menichelli, A., Di Guilio, S., De Matteis, W., Cianciulli, P. & Papa, G. (1993) PADGEM/GMP-140 expressions on platelet membranes from homozygous beta-thalassaemic patients. *Br. J. Haematol.* **84**, 111.

Delfini, C., Saglio, G., Mazza, U., Muretto, P., Filippetti, A. & Lucarelli, G. (1983) Fetal haemoglobin synthesis following fetal liver transplantation in man. *Br. J. Haematol.* **55**, 609.

Delhanty, J.D.A. (1994) Preimplantation diagnosis. *Prenat. Diag.* **14**, 1217.

Derchi, G., Bellone, P., Forni, G.L. *et al.* (1992) Cardiac involvement in thalassaemia major: altered atrial natriuretic peptide levels in asymptomatic patients. *Eur. Heart J.* **13**, 1368.

Derry, S., Wood, W.G., Pippard, M.J. *et al.* (1984) Hematologic and biosynthetic studies in homozygous hemoglobin Constant Spring. *J. Clin. Invest.* **73**, 1673.

Desai, S., Cohal, R., Gupte, S. & Mohanty, D. (1997) Is cellulose acetate electrophoresis a suitable technique for detection of Hb Bart's at birth? *Hum. Hered.* **47**, 181.

Deutsch, S., Samii, K., Darbellay, R., Kovacsovics, T., Offord, R. & Beris, P. (1998) Nonsense mutations in exon III of β-globin are associated with normal β-thal mRNA production while frameshift mutations lead to a severely decreased amount of β-thal mRNA. *Blood* **92** (Suppl. 1), 334a.

Devi, C.S., Rao, A.N., Laxmidevi, S., Ramaiah, T.Y. & Reddy, C.R. (1969) A case of sickle cell thalassemia. *Israel J. Med. Sci.* **23**, 305.

Dewey, K.W., Grossman, H. & Canale, V.C. (1970) Cholelithiasis in thalassemia major. *Radiology* **96**, 385.

Dhar, V., Nandi, A., Schildkraut, C.L. & Skoultchi, A.I. (1990) Erythroid-specific nuclease-hypersensitive sites flanking the human beta-globin domain. *Mol. Cell. Biol.* **10**, 4324.

Dherte, P., Lehmann, H. & Vandepitte, J. (1959) Haemoglobin P in a family in the Belgian Congo. *Nature* **184**, 1133.

Di Bartolomeo, P., Di Girolamo, G., Olioso, P. *et al.* (1997) The Pescara experience of allogenic bone marrow transplantation in thalassemia. *Bone Marrow Transplant.* **19** (Suppl. 2), 48.

Di Marco, V., Lo Iacono, O., Almasio, P. *et al.* (1997) Long-term efficacy of α-interferon in β-thalassemics with chronic hepatitis C. *Blood* **90**, 2207.

Di Marzo, R., Dowling, C.E., Wong, C., Maggio, A. & Kazazian, H.H. Jr (1988) The spectrum of β-thalassaemia mutations in Sicily. *Br. J. Haematol.* **69**, 393.

Di Rienzo, A., Novelletto, A., Aliquo, M.C. *et al.* (1986) Molecular basis for HbH disease in Italy: Geographical distribution of deletional and non-deletional α-thalassemia haplotypes. *Am. J. Hum. Genet.* **39**, 631.

Diamond, M.P., Cotgreve, I. & Parker, A. (1965) Case of intrauterine death due to α-thalassaemia. *Br. Med. J.* **ii**, 278.

Diaz-Chico, J.C., Yang, K.G., Kutlar, A., Reese, A.L., Aksoy, M. & Huisman, T.H.J. (1987) An ~300 bp deletion involving part of the 5′ β-globin gene region is observed in members of a Turkish family with β-thalassemia. *Blood* **70**, 583.

Diaz-Chico, J.C., Huang, J.H., Juncic, D., Efremov, G.D., Wadsworth, L.D. & Huisman, T.H.J. (1988a) Two new large deletions resulting in εγδβ-thalassemia. *Acta Haematol.* **80**, 79.

Diaz-Chico, J.C., Yang, K.G., Stoming, T.A. *et al.* (1988b) Mild and severe β-thalassemia among homozygotes from Turkey: identification of the types by hybridization of amplified DNA with synthetic probes. *Blood* **71**, 248.

Dickerhoff, R. (1987) Acute aphasia and loss of vision with desferrioxamine overdose. *Am. J. Pediatr. Hematol. Oncol.* **9**, 287.

Diggs, L.W. (1976) Dr. George Hoyt Whipple. *Johns Hopkins Med. J.* **139**, 196.

Diggs, L.W., Kraus, A.O., Morrison, D.B. & Rudnicki, R.P.T. (1954) Intra-erythrocyte crystals in a white patient with hemoglobin C in the absence of other types of hemoglobin. *Blood* **9**, 1172.

Dillon, N. & Grosveld, F. (1991) Human γ-globin genes silenced independently of other genes in β-globin locus. *Nature* **350**, 252.

Dillon, N. & Grosveld, F. (1993) Transcriptional regulation of multigene loci: multilevel control. *Trends Genet.* **9**, 134.

Dillon, N., Trimborn, T., Strouboulis, J., Fraser, P. & Grosveld, F. (1997) The effect of distance on long-range chromatin interactions. *Mol. Cell* **1**, 131.

Dimovski, A.J., Efremov, D.G., Jankovic, L., Plaseska, D., Juricic, D. & Efremov, G.D. (1993) A β^0-thalassaemia due to 1605 base pair deletions of the 5' β-globin gene region. *Br. J. Haematol.* **85**, 143.

Dimovski, A.J., Divoky, V., Adekile, A.D. *et al.* (1994) A novel deletion of ~27 kb including the β-globin gene and the locus control region 3'HS-1 regulatory sequence: β^0-thalassaemia or hereditary persistence of fetal hemoglobin? *Blood* **83**, 822.

Dinçol, G., Aksoy, M. & Erdem, S. (1979) β-thalassaemia with increased haemoglobin A_2 in Turkey. A study of 164 thalassaemic heterozygotes. *Hum. Hered.* **29**, 272.

Dinçol, G., Altay, C., Aksoy, M., Gurgey, A., Felice, A.E. & Huisman, T.H.J. (1981) Clinical and hematological evaluation of two δ^0 β^0-thalassemia homozygotes. *Hemoglobin* **5**, 153.

Dintzis, H.M. (1961) Assembly of the peptide chains of hemoglobin. *Proc. Natl Acad. Sci. USA* **47**, 247.

Divlansky, A., Zaizov, R. & Moses, S. (1976) Sickle cell thalassemia in an Israeli family. *Israel J. Med. Sci.* **12**, 543.

Divoky, V., Bisse, E., Wilson, J.B. *et al.* (1992) Heterozygosity for the IVS-I-5 (G→C) mutation with a G→A change at codon 18 (Val→Met; Hb Baden) *in cis* and a T→G mutation at codon 126 (Val→Gly; Hb Dhonburi) *in trans* resulting in a thalassemia intermedia. *Biochim. Biophys. Acta* **1180**, 173.

Divoky, V., Baysal, E., Schiliro, G., Dibenedetto, S.P. & Huisman, T.H.J. (1993a) A mild type of Hb S-β^+-thalassemia [–92 (C→T)] in a Sicilian family. *Am. J. Hematol.* **42**, 225.

Divoky, V., Gu, L.-H., Indrak, K., Mocikova, K., Zarnovicanova, M. & Huisman, T.H.J. (1993b) A new β^0-thalassaemia nonsense mutation (codon 112, T→A) not associated with a dominant type of thalassaemia in the heterozygote. *Br. J. Haematol.* **83**, 523.

Divoky, V., Svobodova, M., Indrak, K., Chrobak, L., Molchanova, T.P. & Huisman, T.H.J. (1993c) Hb Hradec Kralove (Hb HK) or $\alpha_2\beta_2$ 115 (G17) Ala→Asp, a severely unstable hemoglobin variant resulting in a dominant β-thalassemia trait in a Czech family. *Hemoglobin* **17**, 319.

Divoky, V., Baysal, E., Öner, R. *et al.* (1994) The T→C mutation at position +96 of the untranslated region 3' to the terminating codon of the β-globin gene is a rare polymorphism that does not cause a β-thalassaemia as previously ascribed. *Hum. Genet.* **93**, 77.

Divoky, V., Indrak, K., Mrug, M., Brabec, V., Huisman, T.H.J. & Prchal, J.T. (1996) A novel mechanism of β thalassemia: The insertion of L1 retrotransposable element into β globin IVS II. *Blood* **88**, 148a.

Dmochowski, K., Finegood, D.T., Francombe, W.H., Tyler, B. & Zinman, B. (1993) Factors determining glucose tolerance in patients with thalassemia major. *J. Clin. Endocrinol. Metab.* **77**, 478.

Dobkin, C., Pergolizzi, R.G., Bahre, P. & Bank, A. (1983) Abnormal splice in a mutant β-globin gene not at the site of a mutation. *Proc. Natl Acad. Sci. USA* **80**, 1184.

Dodé, C., Berth, A., Rochette, J., Girot, R. & Labie, D. (1988) Analysis of crossover type in the $\alpha^{-3.7}$ haplotype among sickle cell anemia patients from various parts of Africa. *Hum. Genet.* **78**, 193.

Dodé, C., Krishnamoorthy, R., Lamb, J. & Rochette, J. (1993) Rapid analysis of $-\alpha^{3.7}$ thalassaemia and $\alpha\alpha\alpha^{3.7}$ triplication by enzymatic amplification analysis. *Br. J. Haematol.* **83**, 105.

Dolfin, G., Lumare, A., Tinetti, E., Monetti, C., Jacob, R. & Martoglio, G. (1983) Obstetrical and hematological problems in a pregnant woman with intermediate beta-thalassemia. *Min. Ginecol.* **35**, 227.

Dominski, Z. & Kole, R. (1993) Restoration of correct splicing in thalassemic pre-mRNA by antisense oligonucleotides. *Proc. Natl Acad. Sci. USA* **90**, 8673.

Donald, J.A., Lammi, A. & Trent, R.J. (1988) Hemoglobin F production in heterocellular hereditary persistence of fetal hemoglobin and its linkage to the beta globin gene complex. *Hum. Genet.* **80**, 69.

Donnai, D., Clayton-Smith, J., Gibbons, R.J. & Higgs, D.R. (1991) α Thalassaemia/mental retardation syndrome (non-deletion type): report of a family supporting X linked inheritance. *J. Med. Genet.* **28**, 734.

Donze, D., Townes, T.M. & Bieker, J.J. (1995) Role of erythroid Krüppel-like factor in human γ- to β-globin gene switching. *J. Biol. Chem.* **270**, 1955.

Donze, D., Jeancake, P.H. & Townes, T.M. (1996) Activation of delta-globin gene expression by erythroid Krüppel-like factor: a potential approach for gene therapy of sickle cell disease. *Blood* **88**, 4051.

Dore, F., Bonfigli, S., Pardini, S., Pirozzi, F. & Longinotti, M. (1991) Priapism in thalassemia intermedia. *Haematologica* **76**, 523.

Dore, F., Cianciulli, P., Rovasio, S. *et al.* (1992) Incidence and clinical study of ectopic erythropoiesis in adult patients with thalassemia intermedia. *Ann. Ital. Med. Int.* **7**, 137.

Dore, F., Bonfigli, S., Gaviano, E. *et al.* (1993) Serum erythropoietin levels in thalassemia intermedia. *Ann. Hematol.* **67**, 183.

Dore, F., Bonfigli, S., Pardini, S. & Longinotti, M. (1995) Serum interleukin-8 levels in thalassemia intermedia. *Haematologica* **80**, 431.

Dore, F., Bonfigli, S., Gaviano, E., Pardini, S. & Longinotti, M. (1996) Serum transferrin receptor levels in patients with thalassemia intermedia during rHuEPO administration. *Haematologica* **81**, 37.

Dorléac, E., Morlé, L., Gentilhomme, O., Jaccoud, P., Baudonnet, C. & Delaunay, J. (1984) Thalassaemia-like abnormalities of the red cell membrane in hemoglobin E trait and disease. *Am. J. Hematol.* **16**, 207.

Dormandy, K.M., Lock, S.P. & Lehmann, H. (1961) Haemoglobin Q-alpha-thalassaemia. *Br. Med. J.* **i**, 1582.

Dörmer, P. & Betke, K. (1978) Erythroblast kinetics in homozygous and heterozygous beta-thalassaemia. *Br. J. Haematol.* **38**, 5.

Dover, G.J. & Platt, O.S. (1998) Sickle cell disease. In: *Hematology in Infancy and Childhood* (eds D.G. Nathan & S.H. Orkin), p. 762. W.B. Saunders, Philadelphia.

Dover, G.J., Smith, K.D., Chang, Y.C. *et al.* (1992) Fetal hemoglobin levels in sickle cell disease and normal individuals are partially controlled by an X-linked gene located at Xp22.2. *Blood* **80**, 816.

Dover, G.J., Brusilow, S. & Charache, S. (1994) Induction of fetal hemoglobin production in subjects with sickle cell anemia by oral sodium phenylbutyrate. *Blood* **84**, 339.

Dow, L.W., Terada, M., Natta, C. *et al.* (1973) Globin synthesis in intact cells and activity of isolated mRNA in β-thalassaemia. *Nature New Biol.* **243**, 114.

Dozy, A.M., Kabisch, H., Baker, J. *et al.* (1977) The molecular defects of α thalassemia in the Filipino. *Hemoglobin* **1**, 539.

Dozy, A.M., Forman, E.N., Abuelo, D.N. *et al.* (1979a) Prenatal diagnosis of homozygous α-thalassemia. *J. A. M. A.* **24**, 1610.

Dozy, A.M., Kan, Y.W., Embury, S.H. *et al.* (1979b) α-Globin gene organisation in blacks precludes the severe form of α-thalassaemia. *Nature* **280**, 605.

Drakoulakou, O., Papapanagiotou, E., Loutradi-Anagnostou, A. &

Papadakis, M. (1997) δ-thalassemic phenotype due to two 'novel' δ-globin gene mutations: CD11[GTC→GGC (A8)-HbA$_2$-Pylos] and CD85[TTT→T (F1)-Hb A$_2$-Etolia]. *Hum. Mutat.* **9**, 344.

Dreyfus, J.C., Labie, D., Vibert, M. & Conconi, F. (1972) An attempt at demonstrating the existence of a nonsense mutation in β-thalassemia. *Eur. J. Biochem.* **27**, 291.

Driscoll, M.C., Dobkin, C.S. & Alter, B.P. (1989) γδβ-Thalassemia due to a *de novo* mutation deleting the 5′ β-globin gene activation-region hypersensitive sites. *Proc. Natl Acad. Sci. USA* **86**, 7470.

Drummond, M.R. (1980) *Principles of Economic Appraisal in Health Care.* Oxford Medical Publications, Oxford University Press, Oxford.

Drysdale, H.C. & Higgs, D.R. (1988) α Thalassaemia in an Asian Indian. *Br. J. Haematol.* **68**, 264.

Duma, H., Efremov, G., Sadikario, A. *et al.* (1968) Study of nine families with haemoglobin Lepore. *Br. J. Haematol.* **15**, 161.

Dunn, J.M. & Haynes, R.L. (1967) Sickle cell thalassemia in pregnancy. *Am. J. Obstet. Gynecol.* **97**, 574.

Dyer, M.A., Maidoo, R., Hayes, P.J., Larson, C.J., Verdine, G.L. & Baron, M.H. (1996) A DNA-binding protein interacts with an essential upstream regulatory element of the human embryonic β-like globin gene. *Mol. Cell. Biol.* **16**, 829.

Dzierzak, E., Medvinsky, A. & de Bruijn, M. (1998) Qualitative and quantitative aspects of haematopoietic cell development in the mammalian embryo. *Immunol. Today* **19**, 228.

Eaton, W.A. & Hofrichter, J. (1987) Hemoglobin S gelation and sickle cell disease. *Blood* **70**, 1245.

Eaton, W.A. & Hofrichter, J. (1990) Sickle cell hemoglobin polymerization. *Adv. Protein Chem.* **40**, 63.

Eaton, W.A., Hofrichter, J. & Ross, P.D. (1976) Delay time in gelation: a possible determinant of clinical severity in sickle cell disease. *Blood* **47**, 621.

Eckman, J.R. (1996) Leg ulcers in sickle cell disease. *Hematol./Oncol. Clinics N. Am.* **10**, 1333.

Economidou, J., Augustaki, O., Georgiopoulou, V., Vrettou, H., Parcha, S. & Loukopoulos, D. (1980) Assessment of iron stores in subjects heterozygous for β-thalassenmia based on serum ferritin levels. *Acta Haematol.* **64**, 205.

Economou, E.P., Antonarakis, S.E., Dowling, C.C., Ibarra, B., de la Mora, E. & Kazazian, H.H. Jr (1991) Molecular heterogeneity of β-thalassemia in Mestizo Mexicans. *Genomics* **11**, 474.

Economou-Petersen, E., Aessopos, A., Kladi, A. *et al.* (1998) Apolipoprotein E epsilon 4 allele as a genetic risk factor for left ventricular failure in homozygous beta-thalassemia. *Blood* **92**, 3455.

Edelstein, S.J., Telfrod, J.N. & Crepeau, R.H. (1973) Structure of fibers of sickle cell hemoglobin. *Proc. Natl Acad. Sci. USA* **70**, 1104.

Edington, G.M. & Lehmann, H. (1955) Expression of the sickle-cell gene in Africa. *Br. Med. J.* **i**, 1308.

Edsall, J.T. (1972) Blood and hemoglobin: The evolution of knowledge of functional adaptation in a biochemical system. *J. Histol. Biol.* **5**, 205.

Edsall, J.T. (1980) Hemoglobin and the origins of the concept of allosterism. *Fed. Proc.* **39**, 226.

Efremov, G.D. (1977) An evaluation of the methods for quantitation of hemoglobin A$_2$: results from a survey of 10,663 cases. *Hemoglobin* **1**, 845.

Efremov, G.D. (1978) Hemoglobion Lepore and anti-Lepore. *Hemoglobin* **2**, 197.

Efremov, G.D. (1990) Beta-, delta beta-thalassemia and Hb Lepore among Yugoslav, Bulgarian, Turkish and Albanian. *Haematologica* **75**, 31.

Efremov, G.D. (1992) Hemoglobinopathies in Yugoslavia: an update. *Hemoglobin* **16**, 531.

Efremov, G.D. & Huisman, T.H.J. (1983) The occurrence of α- and β-chain abnormal hemoglobins and β-thalassemia in European countries. In: *Distribution and Evolution of Hemoglobin and Globin Loci* (ed. J.E. Bowman), p. 315. Elsevier, Amsterdam.

Efremov, G.D., Sadikario, A., Stojmirovic, E. *et al.* (1974) Chemical heterogeneity of foetal haemoglobin in the Lepore haemoglobinopathy. *Br. J. Haematol.* **27**, 319.

Efremov, G.D., Nikolov, N., Duma, H., Schroeder, W.A., Miller, A. & Huisman, T.H.J. (1975) δβ-Thalassaemia in two Yugoslavian families. *Scand. J. Haematol.* **14**, 226.

Efremov, G.D., Rudivic, R., Niazi, G.A., Hunter, E., Huisman, T.H.J. & Schroeder, W.A. (1976) An individual with Hb-Lepore-Baltimore-δβ thalassaemia in a Yugoslavian family. *Scand. J. Haematol.* **16**, 81.

Efremov, G.D., Sadikario, A., Stojancov, A., Dojcinov, D. & Huisman, T.H.J. (1977) Homozygous hemoglobin O Arab in a gypsy family in Yugoslavia. *Hemoglobin* **1**, 389.

Efremov, G.D., Mladenovsky, B., Petkov, G. *et al.* (1978) Lepore hemoglobinopathy in Yugoslavia. *New Istanbul Contrib. Clin. Sci.* **12**, 211.

Efremov, G.D., Juricic, D. & Stojanovski, N. (1982) Hemoglobinopathies in Yugoslavia. *Hemoglobin* **6**, 643.

Efremov, G.D., Filipce, V., Gjorgovski, I. *et al.* (1986a) ^{G}γ^{A}γ (δβ)^0-Thalassaemia and a new form of γ globin gene triplication identified in the Yugoslavian population. *Br. J. Haematol.* **63**, 17.

Efremov, G.D., Nikolov, N., Bakioglu, I. & Huisman, T.H.J. (1986b) The 18- to 23-kb deletion of the Macedonian δβ-thalassemia includes the entire δ and β globin genes. *Blood* **68**, 971.

Efremov, G.D., Gjorgovski, I., Stojanovski, N. *et al.* (1987) One haplotype is associated with the Swiss type of HPFH in the Yugoslavian population. *Hum. Genet.* **77**, 132.

Efremov, D.G., Efremov, G.D., Zisovski, N. *et al.* (1988) Variation in clinical severity among patients with Hb Lepore-Boston-β-thalassaemia is related to the type of β-thalassaemia. *Br. J. Haematol.* **68**, 351.

Efremov, G.D., Josifovska, O., Nikolov, N. *et al.* (1990) Hb Icaria-Hb H disease: identification of the Hb Icaria mutation through analysis of amplified DNA. *Br. J. Haematol.* **75**, 250.

Efremov, D., Dimovsky, A., Baysal, E. *et al.* (1994a) Possible factors influencing the haemoglobin and fetal haemoglobin levels in patients with β-thalassaemia due to a homozygosity for the IVS-1-6 (T-C) mutation. *Br. J. Haematol.* **86**, 824.

Efremov, D.G., Dimovski, A.J. & Huisman, T.H.J. (1994b) The −158 (C→T) promoter mutation is responsible for the increased transcription of the 3′ gamma gene in the Atlanta type of heteditary persistence of fetal hemoglobin. *Blood* **83**, 3350.

Ehlers, K.H., Levin, A.R., Markenson, A.L. *et al.* (1980) Longitudinal study of cardiac function in thalassemia major. *Ann. N. Y. Acad. Sci.* **344**, 397.

Eigel, A., Schnee, J., Oehme, R. & Horst, J. (1989) Mutation analysis of β-thalassemia genes in a German family reveals a rare transversion in the first intron. *Hum. Genet.* **81**, 371.

Ein, S.H., Shandling, B., Simpson, J.S. *et al.* (1977) The morbidity and mortality of splenectomy in childhood. *Ann. Surg.* **185**, 307.

Einerhand, M.P.W., Antoniou, M., Zolotukhin, S. *et al.* (1995) Regulated high-level human beta-globin gene expression in erythroid cells following recombinant adeno-associated virus-mediated gene transfer. *Gene Ther.* **2**, 336.

Eisman, J.A. (1996) Vitamin D receptor gene variants: implications for therapy. *Curr. Opin. Genet. Dev.* **6**, 361.

Elder, J.T., Forrester, W.C., Thompson, C. *et al.* (1990) Translocation of an erythroid-specific hypersensitive site in deletion-type hereditary persistence of fetal hemoglobin. *Mol. Cell. Biol.* **10**, 1382.

Eldor, A. (1978a) Abnormal platelet functions in β thalassaemia. *Scand. J. Haematol.* **20**, 447.

Eldor, A. (1978b) Hemorrhagic tendency in β-thalassemia major. *Israel J. Med. Sci.* **14**, 1132.

Eldor, A., Krausz, Y., Atlan, H. *et al.* (1989) Platelet survival in patients with β-thalassemia. *Am. J. Hematol.* **32**, 94.

Eldor, A., Lellouche, F., Goldfarb, A., Rachmilewitz, E.A. & Maclouf, J. (1991) *In vivo* platelet activation in β-thalassemia major reflected by increased platelet-thromboxane urinary metabolites. *Blood* **77**, 1749.

Eldor, A., Durst, R., Hy-Am, E. *et al.* (1999) A chronic hypercoagulable state in patients with β-thalassaemia major is already present in childhood. *Br. J. Haematol.* **107**, 739.

El-Hashimite, N., Petrou, M., Khalifa, A.S., Heshmat, N.M., Rady, M.S. & Delhanty, J.D.A. (1997) Identification of novel Asian Indian and Japanese mutation causing β-thalassaemia in the Egyptian population. *Hum. Genet.* **99**, 271.

El-Hazmi, A.L. (1987) Red cell genetic abnormalities and environmental interactions: a study in Tehamat Aseer. *J. Trop. Med. Hyg.* **90**, 61.

El-Hazmi, M.A. & Al-Swailem, A.R. (1987) Sickle cell-β⁰-thalassaemia in Saudi Arabia. *Hum. Hered.* **37**, 211.

El-Hazmi, M.A.F., Jabbar, F.A., Al-Faleh, F.Z., Al-Swailem, A.R. & Warsy, A.S. (1991) Patterns of sickle cell, thalassaemia and glucose-6-phosphate dehydrogenase deficiency genes in northwestern Saudi Arabia. *Hum. Hered.* **41**, 26.

El-Hazmi, M.A., Warsy, A.S. & Al Fawaz, I. (1994) Iron-endocrine pattern in patients with beta-thalassaemia. *J. Trop. Pediatr.* **40**, 219.

Elion, J., Berg, P.E., Lapoumeroulie, C. *et al.* (1992) DNA sequence variation in a negative control region 5′ to the β-globin gene correlates with the phenotypic expression of the βˢ mutation. *Blood* **79**, 787.

El-Kalla, S. & Mathews, A.R. (1993) Molecular characterization of β-thalassaemia in the United Arab Emirates. *Hemoglobin* **17**, 355.

El-Kalla, S. & Mathews, A.R. (1995) A novel frameshift mutation causing β-thalassaemia in a Sikh. *Hemoglobin* **19**, 183.

El-Kalla, S. & Mathews, A.R. (1997) A significant β-thalassaemia heterogeneity in the United Arab Emirates. *Hemoglobin* **21**, 237.

Ellepola, S.B., Beaven, G.H., Gunasekara, L.S. & Arulanandan, P. (1980) Hb E trait and Hb E-thalassaemia in Sri Lanka. *Ceylon Med. J.* **25**, 29.

Ellis, J.T., Schulman, I. & Smith, C.H. (1954) Generalized siderosis with fibrosis of liver and pancreas in Cooley's (Mediterranean) anemia; with observations on the pathogenesis of the siderosis and fibrosis. *Am. J. Pathol.* **30**, 287.

Ellis, J., Tan-Un, K.C., Harper, A. *et al.* (1996) A dominant chromatin-opening activity in 5′ hypersensitive site 3 of the human β-globin locus control region. *EMBO J.* **15**, 562.

Emanuel, B., Zackai, E., Cryer, D. & Rappaport, E. (1982) Deletion mapping of chromosome 16: phenotypic manifestations and molecular studies of the α-globin complex. *Am. J. Hum. Genet.* **34**, A124.

Embury, S.H. (1995) Advances in the prenatal and molecular diagnosis of the hemoglobinopathies and thalassemias. *Hemoglobin* **19**, 237.

Embury, S.H., Lebo, R.V., Dozy, A.M. & Kan, Y.W. (1979) Organization of the α-globin genes in the Chinese α-thalassemia syndromes. *J. Clin. Invest.* **63**, 1307.

Embury, S.H., Miller, J.A., Dozy, A.M., Kan, Y.W., Chan, V. & Todd, D.

(1980) Two different molecular organizations account for the single α-globin gene of the α-thalassemia-2 genotype. *J. Clin. Invest.* **66**, 1319.

Embury, S.H., Dozy, A.M., Miller, J. *et al.* (1982) Concurrent sickle-cell anemia and α-thalassemia. Effect on severity of anemia. *N. Eng. J. Med.* **306**, 270.

Embury, S.H., Clark, M.R., Monroy, G. & Mohandas, N. (1984) Concurrent sickle-cell anemia and α-thalassemia. Effect on pathological properties of sickle erythrocytes. *J. Clin. Invest.* **73**, 116.

Embury, S.H., Backer, K. & Glader, B.E. (1985a) Monovalent cation changes in sickle erythrocytes: a direct reflection of α-globin gene number. *J. Lab. Clin. Med.* **106**, 75.

Embury, S.H., Gholson, M.A., Gillette, P. & Rieder, R.F. & the National Cooperative Study of Sickle Cell Disease (1985b) The leftward deletion α-Thal-2 haplotype in a black subject with haemoglobin SS. *Blood* **65**, 769.

Embury, S.H., Hebbel, R.P., Mohandes, N. & Stainberg, M.H. (1996) *Sickle Cell Disease: Basic Principles and Clinical Practice.* Raven, New York.

Emond, A.M., Collis, R., Dartvill, D., Higgs, D.R., Maude, G.H. & Serjeant, G.R. (1984) Acute splenic sequestration in homozygous sickle cell disease: natural history and management. *J. Pediatr.* **107**, 201.

Eng, B., Chui, D.H.K., Saunderson, H., Olivieri, N.F. & Waye, J.S. (1993) Identification of two novel β⁰-thalassemia mutations in a Filipino family: frameshift codon 67 (-TG) and a β-globin gene deletion. *Hum. Mutat.* **2**, 375.

Engel, J.D. (1993) Developmental regulation of human β-globin gene transcription: a switch of loyalties? *Trends Genet.* **9**, 304.

Engelhard, D., Cividalli, G. & Rachmilewitz, E.A. (1975) Splenectomy in homozygous beta thalassaemia: a retrospective study of 30 patients. *Br. J. Haematol.* **31**, 39.

England, J.M. & Fraser, P.M. (1979) Discrimination between iron-deficiency and heterozygous-thalassaemia syndromes in differential diagnosis of microcytosis. *Lancet* **i**, 145.

Engle, M.A. (1964) Cardiac involvement in Cooley's anemia. *Ann. N. Y. Acad. Sci.* **119**, 694.

Enver, T., Ebens, A.J., Forrester, W.C. & Stamatoyannopoulos, G. (1989) The human β-globin locus activation region alters the developmental fate of a human fetal globin gene in transgenic mice. *Proc. Natl Acad. Sci. USA* **86**, 7033.

Enver, T., Raich, N., Ebens, A.J., Papayannopoulou, T., Costantini, F. & Stamatoyannopoulos, G. (1990) Developmental regulation of human fetal-to-adult globin gene switching in transgenic mice. *Nature* **344**, 309.

Epner, E., Reik, A., Cimbora, D. *et al.* (1998) The β-globin LCR is not necessary for an open chromatin structure or developmentally regulated transcription of the native mouse β-globin locus. *Mol. Cell* **2**, 447.

Eraklis, A.J., Kevy, S.V., Diamond, L.K. & Gross, R.E. (1967) Hazard of overwhelming infection after splenectomy in childhood. *N. Eng. J. Med.* **276**, 1225.

Erikson, W.D., Burgert, E.O. & Lynn, H.B. (1968) The hazard of infection following splenectomy in children. *Am. J. Dis. Child.* **116**, 1.

Erlandson, M.E., Smith, C.H. & Schulman, I. (1956) Thalassemia-hemoglobin C disease in white siblings. *Pediatr.* **17**, 740.

Erlandson, M.E., Schulman, I., Stern, G. & Smith, C.H. (1958) Studies of congenital hemolytic syndromes. I. Rates of destruction and production of erythrocytes in thalassemia. *Pediatr.* **22**, 910.

Erlandson, M.E., Walden, B., Stern, G., Hilgartner, M.W., Wehman, J. & Smith, C.H. (1962) Studies on congenital hemolytic syndromes. IV Gastrointestinal absorption of iron. *Blood* **19**, 359.

Erlandson, M.E., Brilliant, R. & Smith, C.H. (1964a) Comparison of sixty-six patients with thalassemia major and thirteen patients with thalassemia intermedia: including evaluations of growth, development, maturation and prognosis. *Ann. N. Y. Acad. Sci.* **119**, 727.

Erlandson, M.E., Golubow, J., Wehman, J. & Smith, C.H. (1964b) Metabolism of iron, calcium and magnesium in homozygous thalassemia. *Ann. N. Y. Acad. Sci.* **119**, 769.

Erlandson, M.E., Golubow, J. & Smith, C.H. (1965) Bivalent cations in homozygous thalassemia. *J. Pediatr.* **66**, 637.

Escuredo, E., Duley, J.A., Clegg, J.B., Weatherall, D.J. & Rees, D.C. (2000) A new test for β thalassaemia. *Haemat. J.* **1** (Suppl. 1), 36.

Esposito, L., Ferrara, M., Indolfi, P. & di Gennaro, C. (1976) Various aspects of blood coagulation in thalassemia major. *Pediatria* **84**, 432.

Esposito, L., Ferrara, M. & Ponte, G. (1978) Blood transfusion therapy in thalassemia major. Experience of a 5-year period of activity in the Center for Hemoglobinopathies of the Pediatric Clinic of Naples. *Pediatria* **86**, 537.

Etlinger, J.D. & Goldberg, A.L. (1977) A soluble ATP-dependent proteolytic system responsible for the degradation of abnormal proteins in reticulocytes. *Proc. Natl Acad. Sci. USA* **74**, 54.

European Chromosome 16 Tuberous Sclerosis Consortium (1993) Identification and characterization of the tuberous sclerosis gene on chromosome 16. *Cell* **75**, 1305.

European Commission (1991) Working Group on the ethical, social and legal aspects of human genome analysis, Brussels. Cited in *Genetic Screening: ethical issues* (1993) Nuffield Council on Bioethics, London.

European Polycystic Kidney Disease Consortium (1994) The polycystic kidney disease 1 gene encodes a 14 kb transcript and lies within a duplicated region on chromosome 16. *Cell* **77**, 881.

Faa, V., Rosatelli, M.C., Sardu, R., Meloni, A., Toffoli, C. & Cao, A. (1992) A simple electrophoretic procedure for fetal diagnosis of β-thalassaemia due to short deletions. *Prenat. Diag.* **12**, 903.

Fabbri, G., Petraglia, F., Segre, A. *et al.* (1991) Reduced spinal bone density in young women with amenorrhoea. *Eur. J. Obstet. Gynecol. Reprod. Biol.* **41**, 117.

Fabris, G., Bearzi, A., Beltrami, C.A., Primi, D., di Palma, A. & Berra, B. (1978) Gangliosides, sialoglycoproteins and glucocerebrosides in the spleen and bone marrow of patients with β-thalassemia major. *Ric. Clin. Lab.* **8**, 148.

Factor, J.M., Pottipati, S.R., Rappaport, I., Rosner, I.K., Lesser, M.L. & Giardini, P.J. (1994) Pulmonary function abnormalities in thalassemia major and the role of iron overload. *Am. J. Respir. Crit. Care Med.* **149**, 1570.

Fairbanks, V.F., Warson, M.D. & Beutler, E. (1963) Drugs for iron overload. *Br. Med. J.* **i**, 1414.

Fairbanks, V.F., Gilchrist, G.S., Brimhall, B., Jereb, J.A. & Goldston, E.C. (1979) Hemoglobin E trait reexamined: a cause of microcytosis and erythrocytosis. *Blood* **53**, 109.

Fairbanks, V.F., Oliveros, R., Brandabur, J.H., Willis, R.R. & Fiester, R.F. (1980) Homozygous hemoglobin E mimics β-thalassemia minor without anemia or hemolysis: hematologic, functional, and biosynthetic studies of first North American cases. *Am. J. Hematol.* **8**, 109.

Fairbanks, V.F., McCormick, D.J., Kubik, K.S. *et al.* (1997) Hb S/Hb Lepore with mild sickling symptoms: a hemoglobin variant with mostly δ-chain sequences ameliorates sickle-cell disease. *Am. J. Hematol.* **54**, 164.

Fairweather, D.V.I., Modell, B., Berdoukas, V. *et al.* (1978) Antenatal diagnosis of thalassaemia major. *Br. Med. J.* **i**, 350.

Fairweather, R.B., Chaffee, S., McBride, K.L. *et al.* (1999) Hyperunstable Hb Dartmouth [α2–66(E15)Leu→Pro (CTG→CCG)] in association with α-thalassemia-1 (SE Asian) causes transfusion-dependent α thalassemia. *Blood* **94** (Suppl. 1), 24b.

Falezza, G.C., de Matteis, M.C. & Vettore, L. (1977) Membrane permeability to potassium in hypochromic red blood cells. *Haematologica* **62**, 258.

Faller, D.V. & Perrine, S.P. (1995) Butyrate in the treatment of sickle cell disease and β-thalassemia. *Curr. Opin. Hematol.* **2**, 109.

Falusi, A.G., Esan, G.T.F., Ayyub, H. & Higgs, D.R. (1987) α-Thalassaemia in Nigeria: its interaction with sickle cell disease. *Eur. J. Haematol.* **38**, 370.

Fargion, S., Piperno, A., Panaiotopoulos, N., Taddei, M.T. & Fiorelli, G. (1985) Iron overload in subjects with β-thalassaemia trait: role of idiopathic haemochromatosis gene. *Br. J. Haematol.* **61**, 487.

Farrell, P.J., Balkow, K. & Hunt, T. (1977) Phosphorylation of initiation factor E1F-2 and the control of reticulocyte protein synthesis. *Cell* **11**, 187.

Farzana, F., Zuberi, S.J. & Hashmi, J.A. (1975) Prevalence of abnormal hemoglobins and thalassasemia trait in a group of professional blood donors and hospital staff in Karachi. *J. Pakistan Med. Assoc.* **25**, 237.

Fattoum, S., Guemira, F., Öner, C. *et al.* (1991) β-Thalassemia, Hb S-β-thalassemia and sickle cell anemia among Tunisians. *Hemoglobin* **15**, 11.

Fattoum, S., Guemira, F., Abdennebi, M. & Ben Abdeladhim, A. (1993) HbC/β-thalassemia association. Eleven cases observed in Tunisia. *Ann. Pédiatr.* **40**, 45.

Fatunde, O.J. & Scott, R.B. (1986) Pitted red cell counts in sickle cell disease. Relationship to age, hemoglobin genotype and splenic size. *Am. J. Pediatr. Hematol. Oncol.* **8**, 329.

Faustino, P., Isório-Almeida, L., Barbot, J. *et al.* (1992) Novel promoter and splice junction defects add to the genetic, clinical or geographic heterogeneity of β-thalassaemia in the Portuguese population. *Hum. Genet.* **89**, 573.

al-Fawaz, I., al-Rasheed, S., al-Mugeiren, M. *et al.* (1996) Hepatitis E virus infection in patients from Saudi Arabia with sickle cell anaemia and β-thalassemia major: possible transmission by blood transfusion. *J. Virol. Hepat.* **3**, 203.

Fawdry, A.L. (1944) Erythroblastic anaemia of childhood (Cooley's) anaemia in Cyprus. *Lancet* **i**, 171.

Fearon, E.F., Kazazian, H.H., Waber, P.G. *et al.* (1983) The entire β-globin gene cluster is deleted in a form of γδβ-thalassaemia. *Blood* **61**, 1269.

Feder, J.N., Gnirke, A., Thomas, W. *et al.* (1996) A novel MHC class I-like gene is mutated in patients with hereditary haemochromatosis. *Nature Genet.* **13**, 399.

Feder, J.N., Penny, D.M., Irrinki, A. *et al.* (1998) The hemochromatosis gene product complexes with the transferrin receptor and lowers its affinity for ligand binding. *Proc. Natl Acad. Sci. USA* **95**, 1472.

Fei, Y.J., Fujita, S. & Huisman, T.H.J. (1988a) Two different theta (θ)-globin gene deletions observed among black newborn babies. *Br. J. Haematol.* **68**, 249.

Fei, Y.J., Stoming, T.A., Efremov, G.D. *et al.* (1988b) Beta-thalassemia due to a T→A mutation within the ATA box. *Biochem. Biophys. Res. Comm.* **153**, 741.

Fei, Y.J., Kutlar, F., Harris, H.F. *et al.* (1989a) A search for anomalies in the ζ,α,β,and,γ globin gene arrangements in normal Black, Italian, Turkish and Spanish newborns. *Hemoglobin* **13**, 45.

Fei, Y.J., Stoming, T.A., Kutlar, A., Huisman, T.H.J. & Stamatoyannopoulos, G. (1989b) One form of inclusion body β-thalassemia is due to a GAA→TAA mutation at codon 121 of the β chain. *Blood* **73**, 1075.

Fei, Y.J., Liu, J.C., Walker, E.L.D.I. & Huisman, T.H.J. (1992) A new gene deletion involving the α2-, α1-, and θ1-globin genes in a Black family with HbH disease. *Am. J. Hematol.* **39**, 299.

Feingold, E.A. & Forget, B.G. (1989) The breakpoint of a large deletion causing hereditary persistence of fetal hemoglobin occurs within an erythroid DNA domain remote from the β-globin gene cluster. *Blood* **74**, 2178.

Felbar, B.K., Orkin, S.H. & Hamer, D.H. (1982) Abnormal RNA splicing causes one form of α-thalassemia. *Cell* **29**, 895.

Feldman, R. & Rieder, R.F. (1973) The interaction of hemoglobin E with beta thalassemias: a study of hemoglobin synthesis in a family of mixed Burmese and Iranian origin. *Blood* **42**, 783.

Felice, A.E., Cleek, M.P., McKie, K., McKie, V. & Huisman, T.H.J. (1984) The rare α-thalassemia-1 of Blacks is a ζα-thalassemia-1 associated with deletion of all α- and ζ-globin genes. *Blood* **63**, 1253.

Felice, A.E., Cleek, M.P., Marino, E.M. *et al.* (1986) Different ζ-globin gene deletions among black Americans. *Hum. Genet.* **73**, 221.

Felice, A.E., McKie, K.M., Cleek, M.P., Marino, E.M., Kutlar, A. & McKie, V.C. (1987) Effects of α-thalassemia-2 on the developmental changes of hematological values in children with sickle cell disease from Georgia. *Am. J. Hematol.* **25**, 389.

Felicetti, L., Colombo, B. & Baglioni, C. (1966) Assembly of hemoglobin. *Biochim. Biophys. Acta* **129**, 380.

Feng, W.C., Southwood, C.M. & Bieker, J.J. (1994) Analyses of β-thalassemia mutant DNA interactions with erythroid Krüppel-like factor (EKLF), an erythroid cell-specific transcription factor. *J. Biol. Chem.* **269**, 1493.

Feretis, C.B., Legakis, N.C., Aspostolodis, N.S., Katergiannakis, V.A. & Mhilippakis, M.G. (1985) Prophylactic cholecystectomy during splenectomy for beta thalassemia homozygous in Greece. *Surg. Gynecol. Obstet.* **160**, 9.

Fermi, G., Perutz, M.F., Shaanan, B. & Fourme, B. (1984) The crystal structure of human deoxyhemoglobin at 1.7 Å resolution. *J. Mol. Biol.* **175**, 159.

Ferster, A., Vermylen, C., Cornu, G. *et al.* (1996) Hydroxyurea for treatment of severe sickle cell anemia: a pediatric clinical trial. *Blood* **88**, 1960.

Fessas, P. (1959) Thalassaemia and the alterations of the haemoglobin pattern. In: *Abnormal Haemoglobins* (eds J.H.P. Jonxis & J.F. Delafresnaye), p. 134. Blackwell Scientific Publications, Oxford.

Fessas, P. (1960) Observations on a second haemoglobin abnormality in haemoglobin H disease. In: *Proceedings of the 7th Congress of the European Society of Haematology*, p. 1043. Karger, Basel, London.

Fessas, P. (1961) The beta-chain thalassaemias. In: *Haemoglobin Colloquium, Vienna* (eds H. Lehmann & K. Betke), p. 90. Thieme, Stuttgart.

Fessas, P. (1963) Inclusions of hemoglobin in erythroblasts and erythrocytes of thalassemia. *Blood* **21**, 21.

Fessas, P. (1965) Forms of thalassaemia. In: *Abnormal Haemoglobins in Africa* (ed. J.H.P. Jonxis), p. 71. Blackwell Scientific Publications, Ibadan.

Fessas, P. (1968) The heterogeneity of thalassaemia. In: *Proceedings of the 12th Congress of the International Society of Hematology*, p. 52. Grune and Stratton, New York.

Fessas, P. (1992) Paying a debt: the contribution of Greek medicine to the genetics of inherited disorders of the erythrocyte. In: *Genetics of Hematological Disorders* (eds C.S. Bartsocas & D. Loukopoulos), p. 27. Hemisphere Publishing Corporation, New York.

Fessas, P. & Karaklis, A. (1962) Two-dimensional paper-agar electrophoresis of haemoglobin. *Clin. Chim. Acta* **7**, 133.

Fessas, P. & Loukopoulos, D. (1964) Alpha-chain of human hemoglobin: occurrence *in vivo*. *Science* **143**, 590.

Fessas, P. & Loukopoulos, D. (1974) The β thalassaemias. *Clin. Haematol.* **3**, 411.

Fessas, P. & Mastrokalos, N. (1959) Demonstration of small components in red cell haemolysates by starch-gel electrophoresis. *Nature* **183**, 30.

Fessas, P. & Papaspyrou, A. (1957) A new fast hemoglobin associated with thalassemia. *Science* **126**, 1119.

Fessas, P. & Papayannopoulou, T. (1965) Cytochemical observations on beta-thalassaemia. I. The PAS positive substance of erythroblasts. *Acta Haematol.* **34**, 1.

Fessas, P. & Stamatoyannopoulos, G. (1962) Absence of haemoglobin A₂ in an adult. *Nature* **195**, 1215.

Fessas, P. & Stamatoyannopoulos, G. (1964) Hereditary persistence of fetal haemoglobin in Greece. A study and a comparison. *Blood* **24**, 223.

Fessas, P. & Yataganis, X. (1968) Intraerythroblastic instability of hemoglobin β₄ (Hb H). *Blood* **31**, 323.

Fessas, P., Stamatoyannopoulos, G. & Karaklis, A. (1961) Hereditary persistence of foetal haemoglobin and its combination with alpha and beta-thalassaemia. In: *8th Congress of the European Society of Haematology*, p. 302. Karger, Basel, Vienna.

Fessas, P., Stamatoyannopoulos, G. & Karaklis, A. (1962) Hemoglobin 'Pylos': Study of a hemoglobinopathy resembling thalassemia in the heterozygous, homozygous and double heterozygous state. *Blood* **19**, 1.

Fessas, C., Karaklis, A., Loukopoulos, D., Stamatoyannopoulos, G. & Fessas, P. (1965) Hemoglobin Nicosia: an α-chain variant and its combination with thalassaemia. *Br. J. Haematol.* **11**, 323.

Fessas, P., Loukopoulos, D. & Kaltsoya, A. (1966) Peptide analysis of the inclusions of erythroid cells in β-thalassaemia. *Biochim. Biophys. Acta* **124**, 430.

Fessas, P., Koniavitis, A. & Zeis, P.M. (1969) Urinary beta-aminoisobutyric acid excretion in thalassaemia. *J. Clin. Pathol.* **22**, 154.

Fessas, P., Lie-Injo, L.E., Na-Nakorn, S., Todd, D., Clegg, J.B. & Weatherall, D.J. (1972) Identification of slow-moving haemoglobins in haemoglobin H disease from different racial groups. *Lancet* **i**, 1308.

Fessas, P., Loukopoulos, D., Loutradi-Anagnostou, A. & Komis, G. (1981) 'Silent' β-thalassaemia caused by a 'silent' β-chain mutant: the pathogenesis of a syndrome of thalassaemia intermedia. *Br. J. Haematol.* **51**, 577.

Fichera, M., Rappazzo, G., Spalletta, A. *et al.* (1994) Triplicated α-globin gene locus with translocation of the whole telomeric end in association with β-thalassemia trait, results in a severe syndrome. *Blood* **84**, 260a.

Fichera, M., Spalletta, A., Fiorenza, F. *et al.* (1997) Molecular basis of α-thalassemia in Sicily. *Hum. Genet.* **99**, 381.

Fiering, S., Epner, E., Robinson, K. *et al.* (1995) Targeted deletion of 5′HS2 of the murine β-globin LCR reveals that it is not essential for proper regulation of the β-globin locus. *Genes Dev.* **9**, 2203.

Filon, D., Oron, V., Krichevski, S. *et al.* (1994) Diversity of β-globin mutations in Israeli ethnic groups reflects recent historic events. *Am. J. Hum. Genet.* **54**, 836.

Filon, D., Faerman, M., Smith, P. & Oppenheim, A. (1995) Sequence analysis reveals a β-thalassaemia mutation in the DNA of skeletal remains from the archaeological sites of Akhziv, Israel. *Nature Genet.* **9**, 365.

Finch, C.A., Deubelbeiss, K., Cook, J.D. *et al.* (1970) Ferrokinetics in Man. *Medicine (Baltimore)* **49**, 17.

Finch, J.T., Perutz, M.F., Bertles, J.F. & Dobler, J. (1973) Structure of sickled erythrocytes and of sickle-cell hemoglobin fibers. *Proc. Natl Acad. Sci. USA* **70**, 718.

Fink, H.E. (1964) Transfusion hemochromatosis in Cooley's anemia. *Ann. N.Y. Acad. Sci.* **119**, 680.

Fiorelli, G., Sampietro, M., Romano, M., Albano, M. & Cappellini, M.D. (1988) Clinical features of thalassemia intermedia in Italy. *Birth Defects* **23**, 287.

Fiorelli, G., Fargion, S., Piperno, A., Battafarano, N. & Cappellini, M.D. (1990) Iron metabolism in thalassemia intermedia. *Haematologica* **75**, 89.

Fioretti, G., De Angioletti, M., Masciangelo, F. *et al.* (1992) Origin heterogeneity of Hb Lepore-Boston gene in Italy. *Am. J. Hum. Genet.* **50**, 781.

Fiori, J.G.M. & Mach, B. (1982) A new nonsense mutation as the molecular basis for β⁰ thalassemia. *J. Mol. Biol.* **154**, 531.

Firth, H.V., Boyd, P.A., Chamberlain, P.F., MacKenzie, I.Z., Morriss-Kay, G.M. & Huson, S.M. (1994) Analysis of limb reduction defects in babies exposed to chorionic villus sampling. *Lancet* **343**, 1069.

Fischel-Ghodsian, N., Higgs, D.R. & Beyer, E.C. (1987) Function of a new globin gene. *Nature* **329**, 397.

Fischel-Ghodsian, N., Vickers, M.A., Seip, M., Winichagoon, P. & Higgs, D.R. (1988) Characterization of two deletions that remove the entire human ζ–α globin gene complex (--ᵀʰᵃⁱ and --ᶠⁱˡ). *Br. J. Haematol.* **70**, 233.

Fischer, K.-D. & Nowock, J. (1990) The T→C substitution at −198 of the ᴬγ-globin gene associated with the British form of HPFH generates overlapping recognition sites for two DNA-binding proteins. *Nucl. Acids Res.* **18**, 5685.

Fisher, E. & Scambler, P. (1994) Human haploinsufficiency—one for sorrow, two for joy. *Nature Genet.* **7**, 5.

Fisher, C.A., Premawardhena, A., DeSilva, S. *et al.* (1999) Thalassaemia in Sri Lanka: a molecular basis. *Blood* **94**, (suppl. 1), Abs 1881.

Fitchett, D.H., Coltart, D.J., Littler, W.A. *et al.* (1980) Cardiac involvement in secondary haemochromatosis: a catheter biopsy study and analysis of myocardium. *Cardiovas. Res.* **14**, 719.

Flake, A.W. & Zanjani, E.D. (1999) *In utero* hematopoietic stem cell transplantation: ontogenic opportunities and biologic barriers. *Blood* **94**, 2179.

Flatz, S.D. & Flatz, G. (1980) Population screening for β-thalassaemia. *Lancet* **ii**, 495.

Flatz, G., Pik, C. & Sringam, S. (1965a) Haemoglobin E and β-thalassaemia: their distribution in Thailand. *Ann. Hum. Genet. (London)* **29**, 151.

Flatz, G., Pik, C. & Sringam, S. (1965b) Haemoglobinopathies in Thailand. II. Incidence and distribution of elevations of haemoglobin A₂ and haemoglobin F; a survey of 2,790 people. *Br. J. Haematol.* **11**, 227.

Flatz, G., Chakravartti, M.R., Das, B.M. & Delbrück, H. (1972) Genetic survey in the population of Assam. *Hum. Hered.* **22**, 323.

Flavell, R.A., Kooter, J.M., de Boer, E., Little, P.F.R. & Williamson, R. (1978) Analysis of the β-δ-globin gene loci in normal and Hb Lepore DNA: direct determination of gene linkage and intergene distance. *Cell* **15**, 25.

Flavell, R.A., Bernards, R., Kooter, J.H. *et al.* (1979) The structure of the human β-globin gene in β-thalassaemia. *Nucl. Acids Res.* **6**, 2749.

Fleming, A.F. (1973) Maternal anemia and fetal outcome in pregnancies complicated by thalassemia minor and 'stomatocytosis'. *Am. J. Obstet. Gynecol.* **116**, 309.

Flint, J., Hill, A.V.S., Bowden, D.K. *et al.* (1986) High frequencies of α thalassaemia are the result of natural selection by malaria. *Nature* **321**, 744.

Flint, J., Harding, R.M., Boyce, A.J. & Clegg, J.B. (1993a) The population genetics of the haemoglobinopathies. In: *Baillière's Clinical Haematology; 'Haemoglobinopathies'* (eds D.R. Higgs & D.J. Weatherall), Vol 6: 1, p. 215. Baillière Tindall and W.B. Saunders, London.

Flint, J., Harding, R.M., Clegg, J.B. & Boyce, A.J. (1993b) Why are some genetic diseases common? Distinguishing selection from other processes by molecular analysis of globin gene variants. *Hum. Genet.* **91**, 91.

Flint, J., Craddock, C.F., Villegas, A. *et al.* (1994) Healing of broken human chromosomes by the addition of telomeric repeats. *Am. J. Hum. Genet.* **55**, 505.

Flint, J., Wilkie, A.O.M., Buckle, V.J., Winter, R.M., Holland, A.J. & McDermid, H.E. (1995) The detection of subtelomeric chromosomal rearrangements in idiopathic mental retardation. *Nature Genet.* **9**, 132.

Flint, J., Rochette, J., Craddock, C.F. *et al.* (1996) Chromosomal stabilisation by a subtelomeric rearrangement involving two closely related *Alu* elements. *Hum. Mol. Genet.* **5**, 1163.

Flint, J., Thomas, K., Micklem, G. *et al.* (1997) The relationship between chromosome structure and function at a human telomeric region. *Nature Genet.* **15**, 252.

Flint, J., Harding, R.M., Boyce, A.J. & Clegg, J.B. (1998) The population genetics of the haemoglobinopathies. In: *Baillière's Clinical Haematology; Sickle cell disease and thalassaemia* (ed. G.P. Rodgers), Vol 11: 1, p. 1. Baillière Tindall and W. B. Saunders, London.

Flynn, D.M., Fairney, A., Jackson, D. & Clayton, B.E. (1976) Hormonal changes in thalassemia major. *Arch. Dis. Child.* **51**, 828.

Flynn, T.P., Allen, D.W., Johnson, G.J. & White, J.C. (1983) Oxidant damage of the lipids and proteins of the erythrocyte membranes in unstable hemoglobin disease. *J. Clin. Invest.* **71**, 1215.

Fodde, R., Losekoot, M., van den Broeck, M.N. *et al.* (1988) Prevalence and molecular heterogeneity of alfa⁺ thalassaemia in two tribal populations from Andhra Pradesh, India. *Hum. Genet.* **80**, 157.

Fodde, R., Losekoot, M., Casula, L. & Bernini, L.F. (1990) Nucleotide sequence of the Belgian ᴳγ⁺ (ᴬγδβ)⁰-thalassaemia deletion breakpoint suggests a common mechanism for a number of such recombination events. *Genomics* **8**, 732.

Fodde, R., Harteveld, C.L., Losekoot, M. *et al.* (1991) Multiple recombination events are responsible for the heterogeneity of α⁺-thalassaemia haplotypes among the forest tribes of Andhra Pradesh, India. *Ann. Hum. Genet. (London)* **55**, 43.

Fogarty, W.M., Vedvick, T.S. & Itano, H.A. (1974) Absence of haemoglobin A in an individual simultaneously heterozygous in the genes for hereditary persistence of foetal haemoglobin and beta-thalassaemia. *Br. J. Haematol.* **26**, 527.

Folayan Esan, G.J. (1970) The thalassaemia syndromes in Nigeria. *Br. J. Haematol.* **19**, 47.

Forget, B.G. (1977) Nucleotide sequence of human β globin messenger RNA. *Hemoglobin* **1**, 879.

Forget, B.G. & Hillman, D.G. (1977) β-Globin mRNA in Ferrara β-thalassaemia. *Nature* **269**, 355.

Forget, B.G., Baltimore, D., Benz, E.J. *et al.* (1974a) Globin messenger RNA in the thalassemia syndromes. *Ann. N. Y. Acad. Sci.* **232**, 76.

Forget, B.G., Benz, E.J., Skoultchi, A., Baglioni, C. & Housman, D. (1974b) Absence of messenger RNA for beta globin chain in β⁰ thalassemia. *Nature* **247**, 379.

Forget, B.G., Housman, D., Benz, E.J. & McCaffrey, R.P. (1975) Synthesis of DNA complementary to separated human alpha and beta globin messenger RNAs. *Proc. Natl Acad. Sci. USA* **72**, 984.

Forget, B.G., Hillman, D.G., Lazarus, H. *et al.* (1976) Absence of messenger RNA and gene DNA for β-globin chains in hereditary persistence of fetal hemoglobin. *Cell* **7**, 323.

Forget, B.G., Cavallesco, C., Benz, E.J. *et al.* (1978) Studies of globin chain synthesis and globin mRNA content in a patient homozygous for hemoglobin Lepore. *Hemoglobin* **2**, 117.

Forget, B.G., Cavallesco, C., de Riel, J.K. *et al.* (1979) Structure of the human globin genes. In: *Eukaryotic Gene Regulation* (eds T. Maniatis, R. Axel & C.F. Fox), p. 367. ICN/UCLA Symposium. Academic Press, New York.

Forrester, W.C., Takegawa, S., Papayannopoulou, T., Stamatoyannopoulos, G. & Groudine, M. (1987) Evidence for a locus activation region: the formation of developmentally stable hypersensitive sites in globin-expressing hybrids. *Nucl. Acids Res.* **15**, 10159.

Forrester, W.C., Novak, U., Gelinas, R. & Groudine, M. (1989) Molecular analysis of the human β-globin locus activation region. *Proc. Natl Acad. Sci. USA* **86**, 5439.

Forrester, W.C., Epner, E., Driscoll, M.C. *et al.* (1990) A deletion of the human β-globin locus activation region causes a major alteration in chromatin structure and replication across the entire β-globin locus. *Genes Dev.* **4**, 1637.

Fortina, P., Delgrosso, K., Rappaport, E. *et al.* (1988) A large deletion encompassing the entire α-like globin gene cluster in a family of Northern European extraction. *Nucl. Acids Res.* **16**, 11223.

Fortina, P., Delgrosso, K., Werner, E. *et al.* (1991a) A >200 kb deletion removing the entire β-like globin gene cluster in a family of Irish descent. *Hemoglobin* **15**, 23.

Fortina, P., Dianzani, I., Serra, A. *et al.* (1991b) A newly-characterized α-thalassaemia-1 deletion removes the entire α-like globin gene cluster in an Italian family. *Br. J. Haematol.* **78**, 529.

Fortina, P., Parrella T., Sartore M. *et al.* (1994) Interaction of rare illegitimate recombination event and a poly A addition site mutation resulting in a severe form of alpha thalassemia. *Blood* **83**, 3356.

Fosburg, M.T. & Nathan, D.G. (1990) Treatment of Cooley's anemia. *Blood* **76**, 435.

Fougerousse, F., Meloni, R., Roudaut, C. & Beckmann, J.S. (1992) Dinucleotide repeat polymorphism at the human hemoglobin alpha-1 pseudo-gene (HBAP1). *Nucl. Acids Res.* **20**, 1165.

Fouladi, M., Macmillan, M.L., Nisbet-Brown, E. *et al.* (1998) Hemoglobin E/beta thalassemia: the Canadian experience. *Ann. N. Y. Acad. Sci.* **850**, 410.

Fowler, S.J., Gill, P., Werrett, D.J. & Higgs, D.R. (1988) Individual specific DNA fingerprints from a hypervariable region probe: α-globin 3′HVR. *Hum. Genet.* **79**, 142.

Fowler, J.R.J., Koshy, M., Strub, M. & Chinn, S.K. (1991) Priapism associated with the sickle cell hemoglobinopathies: prevalence, natural history and sequelae. *J. Urol.* **145**, 65.

Fox, P.D., Higgs, D.R. & Searjeant, G.R. (1993) Influence of alpha thalassaemia on the retinopathy of homozygous sickle cell disease. *Br. J. Ophthalmol.* **77**, 89.

Francina, A., Dorleac, E., Aubry, M. *et al.* (1985) Hb Lepore–Hb C and Hb Lepore–β⁰-thalassaemia compound heterozygotes in an Algerian family. *Hemoglobin* **9**, 505.

Fraser, G.R., Stamatoyannopoulos, G., Kattamis, C. *et al.* (1964) Thalassemias, abnormal hemoglobins and glucose-6-phosphate dehydrogenase deficiency in the Arta area of Greece: diagnostic and genetic aspects of complete village studies. *Ann. N. Y. Acad. Sci.* **119**, 415.

Fraser, G.R., Grunwald, P. & Stamatoyannopoulos, G. (1966) Glucose-6-phosphate dehydrogenase (G6PD) deficiency, abnormal haemoglobins, and thalassaemia in Yugoslavia. *J. Med. Genet.* **3**, 35.

Fraser, P., Hurst, J., Collis, P. & Grosveld, F. (1990) DNase I hypersensitive sites 1, 2 and 3 of the human β-globin dominant control region direct position-independent expression. *Nucl. Acids Res.* **18**, 3503.

Fraser, P., Pruzina, S., Antoniou, M. & Grosveld, F. (1993) Each hypersensitive site of the human β-globin locus control region confers a different developmental pattern of expression on the globin genes. *Genes Dev.* **7**, 106.

Frazer, I.D. & Raper, A.B. (1961) Solubility of denatured haemoglobin variants in acid buffers. *Nature* **191**, 355.

Freedman, M.H., Bentur, Y. & Koren, G. (1989) Biological and toxic properties of deferoxamine. In: *Advances and controversies in thalassemia therapy* (eds C.D. Buckner, R.P. Gale & G. Lucarelli), p. 115. Alan R. Liss, New York.

Freedman, M.H., Olivieri, N.F., Grisaru, D., McLuskey, I. & Thorner, P. (1990) Pulmonary syndrome in patients receiving intravenous deferoxamine infusions. *Am. J. Dis. Child.* **144**, 565.

Freeman, A.P., Giles, R.W., Berdoukas, V.A., Walsh, W.F., Choy, D. & Murray, P.C. (1983) Early left ventricular dysfunction and chelation therapy in thalassemia major. *Ann. Intern. Med.* **99**, 450.

Friberg, T.R., Young, C.M. & Milner, P.F. (1986) Incidence of ocular abnormalities in patients with sickle hemoglobinopathies. *Ann. Ophthalmol.* **18**, 150.

Frick, P. (1970) Congenital elliptocytosis. Elliptocytosis and thalassemia in the same family. *Schweiz. Med. Wschr.* **100**, 1009.

Friedman, M.J. (1978) Erythrocytic mechanism of sickle cell resistance to malaria. *Proc. Natl Acad. Sci. USA* **75**, 1994.

Friedman, S. & Schwartz, E. (1976) Hereditary persistence of foetal haemoglobin with β-chain synthesis in cis position (ᴳγ-β⁺-HPFH) in a negro family. *Nature* **259**, 138.

Friedman, S., Oski, F.A. & Schwartz, E. (1972) Bone marrow and peripheral blood globin synthesis in an American Black family with beta thalassemia. *Blood* **39**, 785.

Friedman, S., Atwater, J., Gill, F.M. & Schwartz, E. (1974a) Alpha-thalassemia in Negro infants. *Pediatr. Res.* **8**, 955.

Friedman, S., Schwartz, E., Ahern, V. & Ahern, E. (1974b) Globin synthesis in the Jamaican Negro with beta-thalassaemia. *Br. J. Haematol.* **28**, 505.

Friedman, S., Ozsoylu, S., Luddy, R. & Schwartz, E. (1976a) Heterozygous beta thalassaemia of unusual severity. *Br. J. Haematol.* **32**, 65.

Friedman, S., Schwartz, E., Ahern, E. & Ahern, V. (1976b) Variations in globin chain synthesis in hereditary persistence of fetal haemoglobin. *Br. J. Haematol.* **32**, 357.

Friedman, M.J., Roth, E.F., Nagel, R.L. & Trager, W. (1979) *Plasmodium falciparum*: physiological interactions with the human sickle cell. *Exp. Parasitol.* **47**, 73.

Frigerio, R., Mela, Q., Passiu, G. *et al.* (1984) Iron overload and lysosomal stability in β⁰-thalassaemia intermedia and trait: correlation between serum ferritin and serum N-acetyl-beta-D-glucosaminidase levels. *Scand. J. Haematol.* **33**, 252.

Frischer, H. & Bowman, J. (1975) Hemoglobin E, an oxidatively unstable mutation. *J. Lab. Clin. Med.* **85**, 531.

Fritsch, E.F., Lawn, R.M. & Maniatis, T. (1979) Characterisation of deletions which affect the expression of fetal globin genes in man. *Nature* **279**, 598.

Froster-Iskenius, U. & Baird, P. (1989) Limb reduction defects in over 1,000,000 consecutive livebirths. *Teratology* **39**, 127.

Frumin, A.M., Waldman, S. & Morris, P. (1952) Exogenous hemochromatosis in Mediterranean anemia. *Pediatr.* **9**, 290.

Fucharoen, S. & Winichagoon, P. (1987) Hemoglobinopathies in Southeast Asia. *Hemoglobin* **11**, 65.

Fucharoen, S. & Winichagoon, P. (1992) Thalassemia in Southeast Asia: problems and strategy for prevention and control. *Southeast Asian J. Trop. Med. Publ. Hlth* **23**, 647.

Fucharoen, S. & Winichagoon, P. (1997) Hemoglobinopathies in Southeast Asia: molecular biology and clinical medicine. *Hemoglobin* **21**, 299.

Fucharoen, S., Tunthanavatana, C., Sonakul, D. & Wasi, P. (1981a) Intracranial extramedullary hematopoiesis in β-thalassemia/hemoglobin E disease. *Am. J. Hematol.* **10**, 75.

Fucharoen, S., Youngchaiyud, P. & Wasi, P. (1981b) Hypoxaemia and the effect of aspirin in thalassaemia. *Southeast Asian J. Trop. Med. Publ. Hlth* **12**, 90.

Fucharoen, S., Winichagoon, P., Pootrakul, P. & Wasi, P. (1984) Determination for different severity of anemia in thalassemia: concordance and discordance among sib pairs. *Am. J. Med. Genet.* **19**, 39.

Fucharoen, S., Suthipongchai, S., Poungvarin, N., Ladpli, S., Sonakul, D. & Wasi, P. (1985) Intracranial extramedullary hematopoiesis inducing epilepsy in a patient with β-thalassemia/hemoglobin E. *Arch. Intern. Med.* **145**, 739.

Fucharoen, S., Winichagoon, P., Chaicharoen, S. & Wasi, P. (1987) Different molecular defects of $^G\gamma$ ($^A\gamma\delta\beta$) ^{0}-thalassaemia in Thailand. *Eur. J. Haematol.* **39**, 154.

Fucharoen, S., Winichagoon, P., Pootrakul, P., Piankijagum, A. & Wasi, P. (1988a) Differences between two types of HbH disease, α-thalassaemia 1/α-thalassaemia 2 and α-thalassaemia 1/Hb Constant Spring. *Birth Defects* **23**, 309.

Fucharoen, S., Winichagoon, P., Pootrakul, P., Piankijagum, A. & Wasi, P. (1988b) Variable severity of Southeast Asian β⁰-thalassemia/Hb E disease. *Birth Defects* **23**, 241.

Fucharoen, S., Winichagoon, P., Thonglairuam, V. & Wasi, P. (1988c) EF Bart's disease: interaction of the abnormal α- and β-globin genes. *Eur. J. Haematol.* **40**, 75.

Fucharoen, S., Fucharoen, G., Fucharoen, P. & Fukumaki, Y. (1989a) A novel ochre mutation in the β-thalassemia gene of a Thai. *J. Biol. Chem.* **264**, 7780.

Fucharoen, S., Fucharoen, G., Sriroongrueng, W. *et al.* (1989b) Molecular basis of β-thalassemia in Thailand: analysis of β-thalassemia mutations using the polymerase chain reaction. *Hum. Genet.* **84**, 41.

Fucharoen, G., Fucharoen, S., Jetsrisuparb, A. & Fukumaki, Y. (1990a) Molecular basis of HbE-β-thalassemia and the origin of HbE in northeast Thailand: Identification of one novel mutation using amplified DNA from buffy coat specimens. *Biochem. Biophys. Res. Comm.* **170**, 698.

Fucharoen, S., Fucharoen, G., Ata, K. *et al.* (1990b) Molecular characterization and nonradioactive detection of beta-thalassaemia in Malaysia. *Acta Haematol.* **84**, 82.

Fucharoen, S., Fucharoen, G., Fukumaki, Y. *et al.* (1990c) Three-base deletion in exon 3 of the β-globin gene produced a novel variant (βGunma) with a thalassemia-like phenotype. *Blood* **76**, 1894.

Fucharoen, S., Katsube, T., Fucharoen, G. *et al.* (1990d) Molecular heterogeneity of β-thalassemia in the Japanese: identification of two novel mutations. *Br. J. Haematol.* **74**, 101.

Fucharoen, S., Kobayashi, Y., Fucharoen, G. *et al.* (1990e) A single nucleotide deletion in codon 123 of the β-globin gene causes an inclusion body β-thalassaemia trait: a novel elongated globin chain β^{Makabe}. *Br. J. Haematol.* **75**, 393.

Fucharoen, S., Shimizu, K. & Fukumaki, Y. (1990f) A novel C-T transition within the distal CCAAT motif of the $^G\gamma$-globin gene in the Japanese HPFH: implication of factor binding in elevated fetal globin expression. *Nucl. Acids Res.* **18**, 5245.

Fucharoen, G., Fucharoen, S., Jetsrisuparb, A. & Fukumaki, Y. (1991a) Eight-base deletion of the β-globin gene produced a novel variant (β Khon Kaen) with an inclusion body β-thalassemia trait. *Blood* **78**, 537.

Fucharoen, S., Fucharoen, G., Laosombat, V. & Fukumaki, Y. (1991b) Double heterozygosity of the β-Malay and a novel β-thalassemia gene in a Thai patient. *Am. J. Hematol.* **38**, 142.

Fucharoen, S., Siritanaratkul, N., Winichagoon, P. *et al.* (1996)

Hydroxyurea increases hemoglobin F levels and improves the effectiveness of erythropoiesis in β-thalassemia/hemoglobin E disease. *Blood* **87**, 887.

Fujiwara, Y., Browne, C.P., Cunniff, K., Goff, S.C. & Orkin, S.H. (1996) Arrested development of embryonic red cell precursors in mouse embryos lacking transcription factor GATA-1. *Proc. Natl Acad. Sci. USA* **93**, 12355.

Fukumaki, Y., Ghosh, P.K., Benz, E.J. Jr *et al.* (1982) Abnormally spliced messenger RNA in erythroid cells from patients with β⁺ thalassemia and monkey cells expressing a cloned β⁺-thalassemic gene. *Cell* **28**, 585.

Fukumaki, Y., Fucharoen, S., Fucharoen, G. *et al.* (1992) Molecular heterogeneity of β-thalassemia in Thailand. *Southeast Asian J. Trop. Med. Publ. Hlth* **23**, 14.

Fullerton, S.M., Harding, R.M., Boyce, A.J. & Clegg, J.B. (1994) Molecular and population genetic analysis of allelic sequence diversity at the human β globin locus. *Proc. Natl Acad. Sci. USA* **91**, 1805.

Furbetta, M., Angius, A., Ximines, A. *et al.* (1978) Prenatal diagnosis of β-thalassemia. Experience with 24 cases. *Israel J. Med. Sci.* **14**, 1107.

Furbetta, M., Galanello, R., Ximenes, A. *et al.* (1979) Interaction of alpha and beta thalassaemia genes in two Sardinian families. *Br. J. Haematol.* **41**, 203.

Furbetta, M., Tuveri, T., Rosatacelli, C. *et al.* (1983) Molecular mechanism accounting for milder types of thalassemia major. *J. Pediatr.* **103**, 35.

de Furia, F.G., Miller, D.R. & Canale, V.C. (1974) Red blood cell metabolism and function in transfused β-thalassemia. *Ann. N. Y. Acad. Sci.* **232**, 323.

Gabrielle, O. (1971) Hypoparathyroidism associated with thalassemia. *Southern Med. J.* **64**, 115.

Gabutti, V. & Piga, A. (1996) Results of long-term iron-chelating therapy. *Acta Haematol.* **95**, 26.

Gabuzda, T.G. (1966) Hemoglobin H and the red cell. *Blood* **27**, 568.

Gabuzda, T.G., Nathan, D.G. & Gardner, F.H. (1963) The turnover of hemoglobins A, F and A₂ in the peripheral blood of three patients with thalassemia. *J. Clin. Invest.* **42**, 1678.

Gabuzda, T.G., Nathan, D.G. & Gardner, F.H. (1964) Thalassemia trait. Genetic combinations of increased fetal and A_2 hemoglobins. *N. Eng. J. Med.* **270**, 1212.

Gabuzda, T.G., Nathan, D.G. & Gardner, F.H. (1965) The metabolism of the individual C¹⁴-labeled hemoglobins in patients with H-thalassemia with observation on radiochromate binding to the hemoglobins during red cell survival. *J. Clin. Invest.* **44**, 315.

Gabuzda, T.G., Nathan, D.G., Gardner, F.H., Kreimer-Birnbaum, M. & Bannerman, R.M. (1967) Hemoglobin F and beta-thalassemia. *Science* **157**, 1079.

Gacon, G., Wajcman, H. & Labie, D. (1974) Hemoglobin E: its oxygen affinity in relation with the ionic environment. *FEBS Lett.* **41**, 147.

Gaensler, K.M.L., Kitamura, M. & Kan, Y.W. (1993) Germ-line transmission and developmental regulation of a 150 kb yeast artificial chromosome containing the human β-globin locus in transgenic mice. *Proc. Natl Acad. Sci. USA* **90**, 11381.

Galacteros, F., Delanoe-Garin, J., Monplaisir, N. *et al.* (1984) Two new cases of heterozygosity for hemoglobin Knossos α₂β₂ Ala→Ser detected in the French West Indies and Algeria. *Hemoglobin* **8**, 215.

Galanello, R., Melis, M.A., Ruggeri, R. *et al.* (1979) β⁰ Thalassemia trait in Sardinia. *Hemoglobin* **3**, 33.

Galanello, R., Diana, G., Furbetta, M. *et al.* (1980) α-Thalassaemia in Sardinian infants. *J. Med. Genet.* **17**, 357.

Galanello, R., Melis, M.A., Ruggeri, R. & Cao, A. (1981) Prospective study of red blood cell indices, hemoglobin A_2 and hemoglobin F in infants heterozygous for β-thalassemia. *J. Pediatr.* **99**, 105.

Galanello, R., Melis, M.A., Paglietti, E., Cornacchia, G., de Virgiliis, S. & Cao, A. (1983a) Serum ferritin levels in hemoglobin H disease. *Acta Haematol. (Basel)* **69**, 56.

Galanello, R., Pirastu, M., Melis, M.A., Paglietti, E., Moi, P. & Cao, A. (1983b) Phenotype–genotype correlation in haemoglobin H disease in childhood. *J. Med. Genet.* **20**, 425.

Galanello, R., Ruggeri, R., Paglietti, E., Addis, M., Melis, M.A. & Cao, A. (1983c) A family with segregating triplicated alpha globin loci and beta thalassemia. *Blood* **62**, 1035.

Galanello, R., Paglietti, E., Melis, M.A., Giangu, L. & Cao, A. (1984) Hemoglobin inclusions in heterozygous α-thalassemia according to their α-globin genotype. *Acta Haematol. (Basel)* **72**, 34.

Galanello, R., Dessi, E., Melis, M.A. *et al.* (1989) Molecular analysis of $β^0$-thalassemia intermedia in Sardinia. *Blood* **74**, 823.

Galanello, R., Melis, M.A., Podda, A. *et al.* (1990a) Deletion δ-thalassemia: the 7.2 kb deletion of Corfu δβ-thalassemia in a non-β-thalassemia chromosome. *Blood* **75**, 1747.

Galanello, R., Sanna, M.A., Maccioni, L. *et al.* (1990b) Fetal hydrops in Sardinia: implications for genetic counselling. *Clin. Genet.* **38**, 327.

Galanello, R., Turco, M.P., Barella, S. *et al.* (1990c) Iron stores and iron deficiency anemia in children heterozygous for β-thalassemia. *Haematologica* **75**, 319.

Galanello, R., Lilliu, F., Bertolino, F. & Cao, A. (1991) Percentile curves for red cell indices of $β^0$-thalassaemia heterozygotes in infancy and childhood. *J. Pediatr.* **150**, 413.

Galanello, R., Aru, B., Dessì, C. *et al.* (1992) HbH disease in Sardinia: molecular, haematological and clinical aspects. *Acta Haematol. (Basel)* **88**, 1.

Galanello, R., Barella, S., Ideo, A. *et al.* (1994) Genotype of subjects with borderline hemoglobin A_2 levels: Implication for β-thalassemia carrier screening. *Am. J. Hematol.* **46**, 79.

Galanello, R., Barella, S., Gasperini, D. *et al.* (1995) Evaluation of an automatic HPLC analyser for thalassemia and haemoglobin variants screening. *J. Automat. Chem.* **17**, 73.

Galanello, R., Perseu, L., Melis, M.A. *et al.* (1997) Hyperbilirubinaemia in heterozygous β-thalassemia is related to co-inherited Gilbert's syndrome. *Br. J. Haematol.* **99**, 433.

Gale, R.E., Clegg, J.B. & Huehns, E.R. (1979) Human embryonic haemoglobins Gower 1 and Gower 2. *Nature* **280**, 162.

Galimberti, M., Angelucci, M., Baronciani, D. *et al.* (1997) Bone marrow transplantation in thalassemia: the experience of Pesaro. *Bone Marrow Transplant.* **19** (Suppl. 2), 45.

Gallant, T., Freedman, M.H., Vellend, H. & Francombe, W.H. (1986) *Yersinia* sepsis in patients with iron overload treated with deferoxamine [letter]. *N. Eng. J. Med.* **314**, 1643.

Gallerani, M., Cicognani, I., Ballardini, P. *et al.* (1990) Average life expectancy of heterozygous β thalassemia subjects. *Haematologica* **75**, 224.

Gallerani, M., Scapoli, C., Cicognani, I. *et al.* (1991) Thalassaemia trait and myocardial infarction: low infarction incidence in male subjects confirmed. *J. Intern. Med.* **230**, 109.

Gallo, E., Ricco, G., Mazza, U., Papa, G. & Inglott, G. (1970) Studio su un caso di Hb D Punjab ($α_2β_2$ 121-Glu→Gln). *Boll. Soc. Ital. Biol. Speriment.* **46**, 341.

Gallo, E., Pugliatti, L., Ricco, G., Pich, P.G., Pinna, G. & Mazza, U. (1972) A case of haemoglobin J Sardegna–β-thalassaemia double heterozygosis. *Acta Haematol.* **47**, 311.

Gallo, E., Pich, P.G., Ricco, G., Saglio, G., Camaschella, C. & Mazza, U. (1975) The relationship between anemia, fecal stercobilinogen, erythrocyte survival and globin synthesis in heterozygotes for β-thalassemia. *Blood* **46**, 692.

Gallo, E., Massaro, P., Miniero, R., David, D. & Tarella, C. (1979) The

importance of the genetic picture and globin synthesis in determining the clinical and haematological features of thalassaemia intermedia. *Br. J. Haematol.* **41**, 211.

Gambino, R., Kacian, D.L., Ramirez, F. *et al.* (1974) Decreased globin messenger RNA in thalassemia by hybridisation and biologic activity assays. *Ann. N. Y. Acad. Sci.* **232**, 6.

Gammack, D.B., Huehns, E.R., Lehmann, H. & Shooter, E.M. (1961) The abnormal polypeptide chains in a number of haemoglobin variants. *Acta Haematol.* **11**, 1.

Ganczakowski, M., Bowden, D.K., Maitland, K. *et al.* (1995) Thalassaemia in Vanuatu, SW Pacific: frequency and haematological phenotypes of young children. *Br. J. Haematol.* **89**, 485.

Ganesan, J. & Lie-Injo, L.E. (1978) Interaction of Hb A_2 Indonesia trait with β-thalassemia trait and with Hb E trait. *Acta Haematol.* **59**, 341.

Ganesan, J., George, R. & Lie-Injo, L.E. (1976) Abnormal haemoglobins and hereditary ovalocytosis in the Ulu Jempul district of Kuala Pilah, West Malaysia. *Southeast Asian J. Trop. Med. Publ. Hlth* **7**, 430.

Gardikas, C. (1968) Modes of presentation of thalassaemia minor. *Acta Haematol.* **40**, 34.

Garewal, G., Fearon, C.W., Warren, T.C. *et al.* (1994) The molecular basis of β thalassaemia in Punjabi and Maharashtran Indians includes a multilocus aetiology involving triplicated α-globin loci. *Br. J. Haematol.* **86**, 372.

Garner, C., Mitchell, J., Hatzis, T., Reittie, J., Farrall, M. & Thein, S.L. (1998) Haplotype mapping of a major quantitative-trait locus for fetal hemoglobin production, on chromosome 6q23. *Am. J. Hum. Genet.* **62**, 1468.

Garner, C., Tatu, T., Reittie, J.E. *et al.* (2000) Genetic influences on F cells and other hematologic variables: a twin heritability study. *Blood* **95**, 342.

Gasperini, D., Cao, A., Paderi, L. *et al.* (1993) Normal individuals with high Hb A_2 levels. *Br. J. Haematol.* **84**, 166.

Gasperini, D., Perseu, L., Cossu, P., Podda, R., Cao, A. & Galanello, R. (1994) A novel $δ^0$-thalassemia mutation: TGG→TAG (TRP→STOP) at codon 37. *Hum. Mutat.* **3**, 71.

Gasperini, D., Persue, L., Melis, M.A. *et al.* (1998) Heterozygous β-thalassemia with thalassemia intermedia phenotype. *Am. J. Hematol.* **57**, 43.

Gatti, F., Nicolas, J., van Ros, G. & Vandepitte, J. (1967) Trois cas de β-thalassodrépanocytose avec taus très élevés de l'hémoglobine alcaliresistante dans une famille Congolaise. *Ann. Soc. Belg. Med. Trop.* **47**, 313.

Gatto, I. (1942) Ricerche sui familiari di bambini affetti dá malattia di Cooley. *Arch. Ital. Pediatr. Puer.* **9**, 128.

Gaziev, D.G. (1983) Bart's hemoglobin in the Azerbaijan population (USSR). *Gematol. Transfuziol.* **28**, 47.

Gaziev, D., Polchi, P., Galimberti, M. *et al.* (1997a) Graft-versus-host disease following bone marrow transplantation for thalassemia: an analysis of incidence and risk factors. *Transplantation* **63**, 854.

Gaziev, D.J., Lucarelli, G., Galimberti, M. *et al.* (1997b) Malignancies after bone marrow transplantation for thalassemia. *Bone Marrow Transplant.* **19** (Suppl. 2), 142.

Geever, R.F., Wilson, L.B., Nallaseth, F.S., Milner, P.F. & Wilson, J.T. (1981) Direct identification of sickle cell anemia by blot hybridization. *Proc. Natl Acad. Sci. USA* **78**, 5081.

Geiger, H., Sick, S., Bonifer, C. & Muller, A.M. (1998) Globin gene expression is reprogrammed in chimeras generated by injecting adult hematopoietic stem cells into mouse blastocysts. *Cell* **93**, 1055.

Gelinas, R., Endlich, B., Pfeiffer, C., Yagi, M. & Stamatoyannopoulos, G. (1985) G to A substitution in the distal CCAAT box of the $^Aγ$-globin gene in Greek hereditary persistence of fetal haemoglobin. *Nature* **313**, 323.

Gelinas, R., Bender, M., Lotshaw, C., Waber, P., Kazazian, H.H.J. & Stamatoyannopoulos, G. (1986) Chinese $^A\gamma$ hereditary persistence of fetal hemoglobin: C to T substitution at position –196 of the $^A\gamma$ gene promoter. *Blood* **67**, 1777.

Gelinas, R.E., Rixon, M., Magis, W. & Stamatoyannopoulos, G. (1988) γ Gene promoter and enhancer structure in Seattle variant of hereditary persistence of fetal haemoglobin. *Blood* **71**, 1108.

Genova, R., Bertotto, A., Raimondi, A., Colombo, A. & Gasparini, M. (1975) Evaluation of the phagocytic activity of the neutrophil granulocytes (NBT-test) and the blood immunological level in splenectomized subjects with beta-thalassemia. *Pediatria* **83**, 60.

Genovese, M.G., Neretto, G., Poti, A. & Benincasa, A. (1979) A case of mediastinal extramedullary hemopoiesis (MEH) in a patient with intermediate thalassemia. *Min. Med.* **70**, 981.

Gentilini, M., Richard-Lenoble, D., Danis, M., Ducosson, P. & Volkowa, V. (1975) Les hémoglobinopathies chez l'adulte jeune, Antillais, migrant en métropole. *Bull. Soc. Pathol Exot*, **68**, 210.

Georganda, E.T. (1990) The impact of thalassemia on body image, self-image, and self-esteem. *Ann. N. Y. Acad. Sci.* **612**, 466.

George, E. & Wong, H.B. (1993) Hb E β$^+$ thalassaemia in west Malaysia: clinical features in the most common beta-thalassaemia mutation of the Malays [IVS 1-5 (G→C)]. *Singapore Med. J.* **34**, 500.

George, E., Faridah, K., Trent, R.J., Padanilam, B.J., Huang, H.J. & Huisman, T.H.J. (1986) Homozygosity for a new type of $^G\gamma$ ($^A\gamma\delta\beta$)^0-thalassemia in a Malaysian male. *Hemoglobin* **10**, 353.

George, E., Ferguson, V., Yakas, J., Kornenberg, H. & Trent, R.J. (1989) A molecular marker associated with mild hemoglobin H disease. *Pathol.* **21**, 27.

George, E., Li, H.-J., Fei, Y.-J. *et al.* (1992a) Types of thalassaemia among patients attending a large University clinic in Kuala Lumpur, Malaysia. *Hemoglobin* **16**, 51.

George, P.M., Myles, T., Williamson, D., Higuchi, R. & Symmans, W.A. (1992b) A family with haemolytic anaemia and three β-globins: the deletion in haemoglobin Atlanta-Coventry (β75 Leu→Pro, 141 Leu deleted) is not present at the nucleotide level. *Br. J. Haematol.* **81**, 93.

Gerald, P.S. & Diamond, L.K. (1958) The diagnosis of thalassemia trait by starch block electrophoresis of the hemoglobin. *Blood* **13**, 61.

Gerald, P.S., Efron, M.L. & Diamond, L.K. (1961) A human mutation (the Lepore hemoglobinopathy) possibly involving two cistrons. *Am. J. Dis. Child.* **102**, 514.

Gerhard, D.S., Kidd, K.K., Kidd, J.R., Egeland, J.A. & Housman, D.E. (1984) Identification of a recent recombination event within the human β-globin gene cluster. *Proc. Natl Acad. Sci. USA* **81**, 7875.

Gertner, J.M., Broadus, A.E., Anast, C.S., Grey, M., Pearson, H. & Genel, M. (1979) Impaired parathyroid response to induced hypocalcemia in thalassemia major. *J. Pediatr.* **95**, 210.

Ghaffari, G., Lanyon, W.G., Haghshenas, M. & Connor, J.M. (1997) Molecular characterization of eight β-thalassaemia mutations in the south of Iran. Proceedings of 6th International Conference on Thalassaemia and Haemoglobinopathies, Malta, Abstract no. 49. Thalassaemia International Federation, Cyprus.

Ghanei, M., Adibi, P., Movahedi, M. *et al.* (1997) Pre-marriage prevention of thalassaemia: report of a 100,000 case experience in Asfahan. *Publ. Hlth* **111**, 153.

Ghanem, N., Girodon, E., Vidaud, M. *et al.* (1992) A comprehensive scanning method for rapid detection of β-globin gene mutations and polymorphisms. *Hum. Mutat.* **1**, 229.

Ghosh, K., Shaqalaih, A., Salman, A. & Hassanein, A.A. (1993) Haemoglobinopathies in a large hospital in Kuwait. *Haematologia* **25**, 185.

Giambona, A., Lo-Gioco, P., Marino, M. *et al.* (1995) The great heterogeneity of thalassemia molecular defects in Sicily. *Hum. Genet.* **95**, 526.

Giampaolo, A., Mavilio, F., Massa, A. *et al.* (1984a) Molecular heterogeneity of beta thalassemia in the Italian population. *Br. J. Haematol.* **56**, 79.

Giampaolo, A., Mavilio, F., Sposi, N.M. *et al.* (1984b) Heterocellular HPFH: molecular mechanisms of abnormal γ gene expression in association with β thalassemia and linkage relationship with the β globin gene cluster. *Hum. Genet.* **66**, 151.

Gianni, A.M., Bregni, M., Cappellini, M.D. *et al.* (1983) A gene controlling fetal hemoglobin expression in adults is not linked to the non-α globin cluster. *EMBO J.* **2**, 921.

Giardina, P.J., Schneider, R., Lesser, M. *et al.* (1995) Abnormal bone metabolism in thalassemia. In: *Endocrine Disorders in Thalassemia* (eds S. Ando & C. Brancati), p. 38. Springer, Berlin.

Giardini, C. (1995) Ethical issue of bone marrow transplantation for thalassemia [editorial]. *Bone Marrow Transplant.* **15**, 657.

Giardini, C. (1997) Treatment of β-thalassemia. *Curr. Opin. Hematol.* **4**, 79.

Giardini, C., Galimberti, M., Lucarelli, G. *et al.* (1995) Desferrioxamine therapy accelerates clearance of iron deposits after bone marrow transplantation for thalassaemia. *Br. J. Haematol.* **89**, 868.

Gibbons, R.J. & Higgs, D.R. (2001) The alpha thalassemia/mental retardation syndromes. In: *Disorders of Hemoglobin* (eds B.G. Forget, D.R. Higgs, R.L. Nagel & M.H. Steinberg), p. 470. Cambridge University Press, Cambridge, in press.

Gibbons, R.J., Wilkie, A.O.M., Weatherall, D.J. & Higgs, D.R. (1991) A newly defined X linked mental retardation syndrome associated with α thalassaemia. *J. Med. Genet.* **28**, 729.

Gibbons, R.J., Suthers, G.K., Wilkie, A.O.M., Buckle, V.J. & Higgs, D.R. (1992) X-linked α thalassaemia/mental retardation (ATR-X) syndrome: Localisation to Xq12–21.31 by X-inactivation and linkage analysis. *Am. J. Hum. Genet.* **51**, 1136.

Gibbons, R.J., Brueton, L., Buckle, V.J. *et al.* (1995a) The clinical and hematological features of the X-linked α thalassaemia/mental retardation syndrome (ATR-X). *Am. J. Med. Genet.* **55**, 288.

Gibbons, R.J., Picketts, D.J., Villard, L. & Higgs, D.R. (1995b) Mutations in a putative global transcriptional regulator cause X-linked mental retardation with α-thalassaemia (ATR-X syndrome). *Cell* **80**, 837.

Gibbons, R.J., Bachoo, S., Picketts, D.J. *et al.* (1997) Mutations in transcriptional regulator *ATRX* establish the functional significance of a PHD-like domain. *Nature Genet.* **17**, 146.

Giblett, E.R. & Crookston, M.C. (1964) Agglutinability of red cells by anti-i in patients with thalassaemia major and other haematological disorders. *Nature* **201**, 1138.

Giglioni, B., Casini, C., Mantovani, R. *et al.* (1984) A molecular study of a family with Greek hereditary persistence of fetal hemoglobin and β-thalassemia. *EMBO J.* **3**, 2641.

Gilbert, J.M., Thornton, A.G., Nienhuis, A.W. & Anderson, W.F. (1970) Cell free hemoglobin synthesis in beta-thalassemia. *Proc. Natl Acad. Sci. USA* **67**, 1854.

Gilks, C.F. (1995) Human immunodeficiency virus in the developing world. In: *The Oxford Textbook of Medicine* (eds D.J. Weatherall, J.G.G. Ledingham & D.A. Warrell), p. 483. Oxford University Press, Oxford.

Gill, F.M. & Schwartz, E. (1973) Synthesis of globin chains in sickle β-thalassemia. *J. Clin. Invest.* **52**, 709.

Gill, F., Atwater, J. & Schwartz, E. (1972) Hemoglobin Lepore trait: globin synthesis in bone marrow and peripheral blood. *Science* **178**, 623.

Gill, F.M., Sleeper, L.A., Weiner, S.J. *et al.* (1995) Clinical events in the first decade in a cohort of infants with sickle cell disease. *Blood* **86**, 776.

Gillemans, N., Tewari, R., Lindeboom, F. *et al.* (1998) Altered DNA-binding specificity mutants of EKLF and Sp1 show that EKLF is an activator of the β-globin locus control region *in vivo. Genes Dev.* **12**, 2863.

Gilles, H.M., Fletcher, K.A., Hendrickse, R.G., Linder, R., Reddy, S. & Allan, N. (1967) Glucose-6-phosphate dehydrogenase deficiency, sickling and malaria in African children in South Western Nigeria. *Lancet* **i**, 138.

Gilman, J.G. (1987) The 12.6 kilobase DNA deletion in Dutch β[0]-thalassaemia. *Br. J. Haematol.* **67**, 369.

Gilman, J.G. & Huisman, T.H.J. (1984) Two independent genetic factors in the β-globin gene cluster are associated with high [G]γ-levels in the HbF of SS patients. *Blood* **64**, 452.

Gilman, J.G. & Huisman, T.H.J. (1985) DNA sequence variation associated with elevated fetal [G]γ globin production. *Blood* **66**, 783.

Gilman, J.G., Huisman, T.H.J. & Abels, J. (1984) Dutch β[0]-thalassaemia: a 10 kilobase DNA deletion associated with significant γ-chain production. *Br. J. Haematol.* **56**, 339.

Gilman, J.G., Kutlar, F., Johnson, M.E. & Huisman, T.H.J. (1987) A G to A nucleotide substitution 161 base pairs 5′ of the [G]γ globin gene cap site (–161) in a high [G]γ non-anemic person. *Prog. Clin. Biol. Res.* **251**, 383.

Gilman, J.G., Mishima, N., Wen, X.J., Kutlar, F. & Huisman, T.H.J. (1988a) Upstream promoter mutation associated with a modest elevation of fetal hemoglobin expression in human adults. *Blood* **72**, 78.

Gilman, J.G., Mishima, N., Wen, X.J., Stoming, T.A., Lobel, J. & Huisman, T.H.J. (1988b) Distal CCAAT box deletion in the [A]γ globin gene of two black adolescents with elevated fetal [A]γ globin. *Nucl. Acids Res.* **16**, 10635.

Gilman, J.G., Brinson, E.C. & Mishima, N. (1992) The 32.6 kb Indian δβ-thalassaemia deletion ends in a 3.4 kb L1 element downstream of the β-globin gene. *Br. J. Haematol.* **82**, 417.

Gilsanz, F., Vela, J.G. & Nunez, G.M. (1992) Age and sex matched analysis of Hb Lepore trait in a new population in Spain. *Nouv. Rev. Fr. Hematol.* **34**, 163.

Gimferrer, E. & Baiget, M. (1979) Datos hematologicos de 393 casos de talasemia heteroeigota beta y delta-beta en el hospital de la Santa Creu i Sant Pau de Barcelona. *Biol. Clin. Hematol.* **3**, 251.

Gimferrer, E., Baiget, M., Darbre, P.D. & Lehmann, H. (1976) Haemoglobin Lepore Boston in a Spanish family. *Acta Haematol.* **56**, 234.

Gimferrer, E., Baiget, M. & Rutllant, M.I. (1979) Homozygous δβ-thalassaemia in a Spanish woman. *Acta Haematol.* **61**, 226.

Gimmon, Z., Wexler, M.R. & Rachmilewitz, E.A. (1982) Pathogenesis of juvenile leg ulcers in β-thalassaemia major and intermedia. *Plas. Reconstruct. Surg.* **69**, 320.

Giordano, P.C., Harteveld, C.L., Michiels, J.J. *et al.* (1996) Atypical Hb H disease in a Surinam patient resulting from a combination of the SEA[–18.8] and RW[–3.7] deletions with HbC heterozygosity. *Br. J. Haematol.* **96**, 801.

Giordano, P., Galli, M., Del Vecchio, G.C. *et al.* (1998) Lupus anticoagulant, anticardiolipin antibodies and hepatitis C virus infection in thalassaemia. *Br. J. Haematol.* **102**, 903.

Giri, A.K., Datta, S., Gajra, B. *et al.* (1982) Some genetic markers in tribals of Eastern India. *Acta Anthropogenet.* **6**, 99.

Girodon, E., Ghanem, N., Vidaud, M. *et al.* (1992) Rapid molecular characterization of mutations leading to unstable hemoglobin β-chain variants. *Ann. Hematol.* **65**, 188.

Girot, R., Lefrère, J.J., Schettini, F., Kattamis, C. & Ladis, V. (1991) HIV infection and AIDS in thalassemia. In: *Thalassemia, 1990. 5th Annual Meeting of the COOLEYCARE Group*, p. 69. Centro Trasfusionale Ospedale Naggiore Policlinico Dio Milano Editore, Athens.

Giuzio, E., Bria, M., Bisconte, M.G. *et al.* (1991) Osteoporosis in patients affected with thalassemia. Our experience. *Chir. Organi. Mov.* **76**, 369.

Glasgow, B.G., Goodwin, M.J., Jackson, F. *et al.* (1968) The blood groups, serum groups and haemoglobins of the inhabitants of Lunana and Thimbu, Bhutan. *Vox Sang.* **14**, 31.

Glenn, F., Cornell, G.N., Smith, C.H. & Schulman, I. (1954) Splenectomy in children with idiopathic thrombocytopenic purpura, hereditary spherocytosis and Mediterranean anemia. *Surg. Gynecol. Obstet.* **99**, 689.

Gluckman, E., Rocha, V. & Chastang, C. (1999) Cord blood stem cell transplantation. *Clin. Haematol.* **12**, 279.

Godet, J.V, Erdier, G., Nigon, V. *et al.* (1977) β[0]-Thalassemia from Algeria: genetic and molecular characterization. *Blood* **50**, 463.

Gofstein, R. & Gellis, S.S. (1956) Splenectomy in infancy and childhood: the question of overwhelming infection following operation. *Am. J. Dis. Child.* **91**, 566.

Göksel, V. & Tartaroglu, N. (1961) Hamoglobin C-thalassemie bie zwei Geschwistern von Weißer Rasse. In: *Haemoglobin Colloquium, Vienna* (eds H. Lehmann & K. Betke), p. 55. Thieme, Stuttgart.

Goldberg, M.A. & Schwartz, S.O. (1954) Mediterranean anemia in a Negro complicated by pernicious anemia of pregnancy; report of a case. *Blood* **9**, 648.

Goldberg, J.R., MacIver, J.E. & Went, L.N. (1959) The bone changes in sickle cell anaemia and its genetic variants. *J. Bone Joint Surg.* **41**, 711.

Goldberg, M.A., Brugnara, C., Dover, G.J., Schapira, I., Charache, S. & Bunn, H.F. (1990) Treatment of sickle cell anemia with hydroxyurea and erythropoietin. *N. Eng. J. Med.* **323**, 366.

Golden, N.L., Bilenker, R., Johnson, W.E. & Tischfield, J.A. (1981) Abnormality of chromosome 16 and its phenotypic expression. *Clin. Genet.* **19**, 41.

Golden, C., Styles, L. & Vichinsky, E. (1998) Acute chest syndrome in sickle cell disease. *Curr. Opin. Hematol.* **5**, 89.

Goldfarb, A., Grisaru, D., Gimmon, Z., Okon, E., Lebensart, P. & Rachmilewitz, E.A. (1990) High incidence of cholelithiasis in older patients with homozygous β-thalassemia. *Acta Haematol.* **83**, 120.

Goldsmith, M.E., Humphries, R.K., Ley, T., Cline, A., Kantor, J.A. & Nienhuis, A.W. (1983) Silent substitution in β[+]-thalassemia gene activating a cryptic splice site in β-globin RNA coding sequence. *Proc. Natl Acad. Sci. USA* **80**, 2318.

Goldstein, J., Konigsberg, W. & Hill, R.J. (1963) The structure of human hemoglobin: VI. The sequence of amino acids in the tryptic peptides of the β chain. *J. Biol. Chem.* **238**, 2016.

Gomber, S., Madan, J. & Madan, S. (1997) Validity of Nestroft in screening and diagnosis of beta-thalassemia trait. *J. Trop. Pediatr.* **43**, 363.

Gomori, J.M., Horev, G., Tamary, H. *et al.* (1991) Hepatic iron overload: quantative MR imaging. *Radiology* **179**, 367.

Goni, M.H., Markussis, V. & Tolis, G. (1995) Bone mineral content by single and dual-photon absorptiometry in thalassemic patients. In: *Endocrine Disorders in Thalassemia* (eds S. Ando & C. Brancati), p. 47. Springer-Verlag, Berlin.

Gonzalez-Redondo, J.H., Stoming, T.A., Lanclos, K.D. *et al.* (1988a) Clinical and genetic heterogeneity in Black patients with homozygous β-thalassemia from the Southeastern United States. *Blood* **72**, 1007.

Gonzalez-Redondo, J.M., Kutlar, F., Kutlar, A. *et al.* (1988b) Hb S(C)-β[+]-thalassaemia: different mutations are associated with different levels of normal Hb A. *Br. J. Haematol.* **70**, 85.

Gonzalez-Redondo, J.M., Diaz-Chico, J.C., Malcorra-Azpiazu, J.J., Balda-Aguirre, M.I. & Huisman, T.H.J. (1988c) Characterization of a newly discovered α-thalassaemia-1 in two Spanish patients with HbH disease. *Br. J. Haematol.* **70**, 459.

Gonzalez-Redondo, J.H., Stoming, T.A., Kutlar, A. *et al.* (1989a) A C→T substitution at nt −101 in a conserved DNA sequence of the promoter region of the β-globin gene is associated with 'silent' β-thalassaemia. *Blood* **73**, 1705.

Gonzalez-Redondo, J.M., Kattamis, C. & Huisman, T.H.J. (1989b) Characterization of three types of β⁰-thalassaemia resulting from a partial deletion of the β-globin gene. *Hemoglobin* **13**, 377.

Gonzalez-Redondo, J.M., Stoming, T.A., Kutlar, F. *et al.* (1989c) Hb Monroe or $\alpha_2\beta_2$ 30 (B12) Arg→Thr, a variant associated with β-thalassaemia due to a G→C substitution adjacent to the donor splice site of the first intron. *Hemoglobin* **13**, 67.

Gonzalez-Redondo, J.M., Stoming, T.A., Kutlar, F. *et al.* (1989d) Severe Hb S-β⁰-thalassaemia with a T→C substitution in the donor splice site of the first intron of the β-globin gene. *Br. J. Haematol.* **71**, 113.

Gonzalez-Redondo, J.M., Gilsanz, F. & Ricard, P. (1989e) Characterization of a new α-thalassaemia-1 deletion in a Spanish family. *Hemoglobin* **13**, 103.

Gonzalez-Redondo, J.M., Kutlar, A., McKie, V.C., McKie, K.W., Baysal, E. & Huisman, T.H.J. (1991) Molecular characterization of Hb S(C) β-thalassaemia in American blacks. *Am. J. Hematol.* **38**, 9.

Goodbourn, S.E.Y., Higgs, D.R., Clegg, J.B. & Weatherall, D.J. (1983) Molecular basis of length polymorphism in the human ζ-globin gene complex. *Proc. Natl Acad. Sci. USA* **80**, 5022.

Goossens, M., Dozy, A.M., Embury, S.H. *et al.* (1980) Triplicated α-globin loci in humans. *Proc. Natl Acad. Sci. USA* **77**, 518.

Goossens, M., Lee, K.Y., Liebhaber, S.A. & Kan, Y.W. (1982) Globin structural mutant $\alpha^{125\text{Leu-Pro}}$ is a novel cause of α-thalassaemia. *Nature* **296**, 864.

Goossens, M., Dumez, Y., Kaplan, L. *et al.* (1983) Prenatal diagnosis of sickle-cell anemia in the first trimester of pregnancy. *N. Eng. J. Med.* **309**, 831.

Gorakshakar, A.C., Lulla, C.P., Nadkarni, A.H. *et al.* (1997) Prenatal diagnosis of β-thalassaemia among Indians using denaturing gradient gel electrophoresis. *Hemoglobin* **21**, 4231.

Gottfried, E.L. & Robertson, N.A. (1974) Glycerol lysis time as a screening test for erythrocyte disorders. *J. Lab. Clin. Med.* **83**, 323.

Goueffon, S. & du Saussay, C. (1967) Enquête systématique sur l'hémoglobine E et la glucose-6-phosphate déshydrogénase au Cambodge. *Bull. Soc. Pathol. Exot.* **62**, 1118.

Gourdon, G., Sharpe, J.A., Wells, D., Wood, W.G. & Higgs, D.R. (1994) Analysis of a 70 kb segment of DNA containing the human ζ and α globin genes linked to their regulatory element (HS −40) in transgenic mice. *Nucl. Acids Res.* **22**, 4139.

Gourdon, G., Sharpe, J.A., Higgs, D.R. & Wood, W.G. (1995) The mouse α-globin locus regulatory element. *Blood* **86**, 766.

Gouttas, A., Fessas, P., Tsevrenis, H. & Xefteri, E. (1955) Description d'une nouvelle variété d'anémie hémolytique congénitale. (Étude hématologique, électrophorétique et génétique.) *Sang* **26**, 911.

Gouttas, A., Tsevrenis, H., Rombos, C., Papaspyrou, A. & Garidi, M. (1960) L'hémoglobine E en Grèce. *Sang* **31**, 1.

Grady, R.W., Giardina, P.J., Salbe, A.D. & Hilgartner, M.W. (1993) A clinical trial of HBED: an orally effective iron chelator. *Blood* **82**, 359a.

Gratwick, G.M., Bullough, P.G., Bohne, W.H.O., Markenson, A.L. & Peterson, C.M. (1978) Thalassemia osteoarthropathy. *Ann. Intern. Med.* **88**, 494.

Gray, G.R. & Marion, R.B. (1971) Thalassaemia and G-6-P-D deficiency in Chinese Canadians: admission screening of a hospital population. *Can. Med. Assoc. J.* **105**, 283.

Gray, G.R. & Marion, R.B. (1978) Clinical and hematological studies in a family with hemoglobin Vancouver. *Hemoglobin* **2**, 143.

Gray, G.R., Manson, H.E., Gu, L.-H., Leonova, J.Y. & Huisman, T.H.J. (1995) Hb Lulu Island $(\alpha_2\beta_2$ 107[G9]Gly→Asp)-β⁰-thalassemia (codon 15; TGG→TAG), a form of thalassemia intermedia. *Am. J. Hematol.* **50**, 26.

Graziano, J.H. (1976) Potential usefulness of free radical scavengers in iron overload. In: *Birth Defects: Original Article Series* (eds D. Bergsma, A. Cerami, C.M. Peterson & J.H. Graziano), p. 135. Alan R. Liss, Inc., New York.

Graziano, J.H., Piomelli, S., Hilgartner, M. *et al.* (1981) Chelation therapy in beta-thalassemia major. III. The role of splenectomy in achieving iron balance. *J. Pediatr.* **99**, 695.

Green, N.S. (1992) *Yersinia* infections in patients with homozygous beta-thalassemia associated with iron overload and its treatment. *Pediatr. Hematol. Oncol.* **9**, 247.

Green, J. & Statham, H. (1996) Psychosocial aspects of prenatal screening and diagnosis. In: *The Troubled Helix: Social and Psychological Implications of the New Human Genetics* (eds T. Marteau & M. Richards), p. 140. Cambridge University Press, Cambridge.

Greep, N., Anderson, A.L. & Gallagher, J.C. (1992) Thalassemia minor: a risk for osteoporosis? *Bone Miner.* **16**, 63.

Gregory, R.C., Taxman, D.J., Seshasayee, D., Kensinger, M.H., Bieker, J.J. & Wojchowski, D.M. (1996) Functional interaction of GATA1 with erythroid Krüppel-like factor and Sp1 at defined erythroid promoters. *Blood* **87**, 1793.

Greppi, E. (1928) Ittero emolitico familiare con aumento della resistanza dei globuli. *Min. Med.* **8**, 1.

Gribnau, J., de Boer, E., Trimborn, T. *et al.* (1998) Chromatin interaction mechanism of transcriptional control *in vivo*. *EMBO J.* **17**, 6020.

Grifoni, V., Kamuzora, H., Lehmann, H. & Charlesworth, D. (1975) A new Hb variant: Hb F Sardinia γ75(E19) isoleucine→threonine found in a family with Hb G Philadelphia, β chain deficiency and a Lepore-like haemoglobin indistinguishable from Hb A_2. *Acta Haematol.* **53**, 347.

Griggs, R.C. & Harris, J.W. (1956) Biophysics of the variants of sickle-cell disease. *Arch. Intern. Med.* **97**, 315.

Grinberg, L.N. & Rachmilewitz, E.A. (1995) Oxidative stress in β-thalassemic red blood cells and potential use of antioxidants. In: *Sickle Cell Disease and Thalassaemia: New Trends in Therapy* (eds Y. Beuzard, B. Lubin & J. Rosa), p. 519. Colloque INSERN/John Libby Eurotext Ltd., Paris.

Grinberg, L.N., Rachmilewitz, E.A., Kitrossky, N. & Chevion, M. (1995) Hydroxyl radical generation in β-thalassemic red blood cells. *Free Rad. Biol. Med.* **18**, 611.

Gringras, P., Wonke, B., Old, J. *et al.* (1994) Effect of α thalassaemia trait and enhanced γ chain production on disease severity in β thalassaemia major and intermedia. *Arch. Dis. Child.* **70**, 30.

Grinstein, M., Bannerman, R.M., Vavra, J.D. & Moore, C.V. (1960) Hemoglobin metabolism in thalassemia. *Am. J. Med.* **29**, 18.

Grisaru, D., Rachmilewitz, E.A., Mosseri, M. *et al.* (1990) Cardiopulmonary assessment in beta-thalassemia major. *Chest* **98**, 1138.

Grossbard, E., Terada, M., Dow, L.W. & Bank, A. (1973) Decreased globin messenger RNA activity with polysomes in α thalassaemia. *Nature New Biol.* **241**, 209.

Grosveld, F. (1999) Activation by locus control regions! *Curr. Opin. Genet. Dev.* **9**, 152.

Grosveld, F., van Assendelft, G.B., Breaves, D.R. & Kollias, G. (1987) Position-independent, high-level expression of the human γ-globin gene in transgenic mice. *Cell* **51**, 975.

Grozdea, I., Benegmos, J. & Levêque, M. (1966) Hémoglobines

anormales chez des malades Marocains cancéreux. *Acta Haematol.* **35**, 53.

Grundy, R.G., Woods, R.A., Savage, M.O. & Evans, J.P.M. (1994) Relationship of endocrinopathy to iron chelation status in young patients with thalassaemia major. *Arch. Dis. Child.* **71**, 128.

Gu, Y.C., Landman, H. & Huisman, T.H.J. (1987) Two different quadruplicated α-globin gene arrangements. *Br. J. Haematol.* **66**, 245.

Guerin, A, London, G., Marchais, S., Metivier, F. & Pelisse, J.M. (1985) Acute deafness and desferrioxamine. *Lancet* **ii**, 39.

Guerrini, R., Shanahan, J.L., Carrozzo, R., Bonanni, P., Higgs, D.R. & Gibbons, R.J. (2000) A nonsense mutation of the *ATRX* gene causing mild mental retardation and epilepsy. *Ann. Neurol.* **47**, 117.

Guglielmo, P., Cunsolo, F., Lombardo, T. *et al.* (1984) T-subset abnormalities in thalassaemia intermedia: possible evidence for a thymus functional deficiency. *Acta Haematol.* **72**, 361.

Guida, S., Giglioni, B., Comi, P., Ottolenghi, S., Camaschella, C. & Saglio, G. (1984) The β globin gene in Sardinian δβ⁰ thalassaemia carries a C-T nonsense mutation at codon 39. *EMBO J.* **3**, 785.

Guidotti, G. (1962) *Thalassaemia Conference on Hemoglobin.* Arden House, Columbia University, New York.

Gullo, L., Corcioni, E., Brancati, C., Bria, M., Pezzelli, R. & Sprovieri, G. (1993) Morphologic and functional evaluation of the exocrine pancreas in beta-thalassaemia. *Pancreas* **8**, 176.

Gumruk, F., Gurgey, A., Duru, F. & Altay, C. (1992) Re-evaluation of iron absorption and serum ferritin in β-thalassaemia intermedia. *Pediatr. Hematol. Oncol.* **9**, 359.

Gumucio, D.L., Rood, K.L., Gray, T.A., Riordan, M.F., Sartor, C.I. & Collins, F.S. (1988) Nuclear proteins that bind the human γ-globin gene promoter: alterations in binding produced by point mutations associated with hereditary persistence of fetal hemoglobin. *Mol. Cell. Biol.* **8**, 5310.

Gumucio, D.L., Lockwood, W.K., Weber, J.L. *et al.* (1990) The –175 T-C mutation increases promoter strength in erythroid cells: correlation with evolutionary conservation of binding sites for two *trans*-acting factors. *Blood* **75**, 756.

Gumucio, D.L., Rood, K.L., Blanchard-McQuate, K.L., Gray, T.A., Saulino, A. & Collins, F.S. (1991) Interaction of Sp1 with the human γ globin promoter: binding and transactivation of normal and mutant promoters. *Blood* **78**, 1853.

Gunn, R.B., Silvers, N.D. & Rosse, W.F. (1972) Potassium permeability in β-thalassaemia minor red blood cells. *J. Clin. Invest.* **51**, 1043.

Gupta, S.C., Mehrotra, T.N., Sharma, N.P., Agarwal, A.K., Kapoor, K.K. & Mehrotra, H.K. (1977) Abnormal haemoglobins in Nepali Gorkhas. *Indian J. Med. Res.* **66**, 809.

Gupta, S.C., Goorah, Y.K., Mehrotra, T.N. & Bisht, D. (1979) Abnormal hemoglobins in Gurkhas. *Hemoglobin* **3**, 359.

Gupta, R.B., Tiwary, R.S., Pande, P.L. *et al.* (1991) Hemoglobinopathies among the Gond tribal groups of Central India; interaction of α- and β-thalassaemia with β chain variants. *Hemoglobin* **15**, 441.

Gurgey, A., Altay, C., Beksac, M.S., Bhattacharya, R., Kutlar, F. & Huisman, T.H.J. (1989) Hydrops fetalis due to homozygosity for α-thalassemia-1, (α) –20.5 kb: the first observation in a Turkish family. *Acta Haematol. (Scandinavica)* **81**, 169.

Gurgey, A., Sipahioglu, M. & Aksoy, M. (1990) Compound heterozygosity for Hb E-Saskatoon or α₂β₂22(B4) Glu→Lys and β-thalassaemia type IVS-1-6 (T→C). *Hemoglobin* **14**, 449.

Gutteridge, J.M.C. & Halliwell, B. (1989) Iron toxicity and oxygen radicals. *Clin. Haematol.* **2**, 195.

Gutteridge, J.C.M., Rowley, D.A., Griffiths, E. & Halliwell, B. (1985) Low-molecular-weight iron complexes and oxygen radical reactions in idiopathic haemochromatosis. *Clin. Sci.* **68**, 463.

Guy, G., Coady, D.J., Jansen, V., Snyder, J. & Zinberg, S. (1985) α-

Thalassemia hydrops fetalis: clinical and ultrasonographic considerations. *Am. J. Obstet. Gynecol.* **153**, 500.

Habib, Z. & Böök, J.A. (1982) Thalassaemia in the Egyptian population. *Hereditas* **96**, 149.

Hadjiminas, M., Zachariadis, Z. & Stamatoyannopoulos, G. (1979) α-Thalassaemia in Cyprus. *J. Med. Genet.* **16**, 363.

Haghshenass, M., Ismail-Beigi, F., Clegg, J.B. & Weatherall, D.J. (1977) Mild sickle-cell anaemia in Iran associated with high levels of fetal haemoglobin. *J. Med. Genet.* **14**, 168.

Hahnerman, N. & Mohr, J. (1968) Genetic diagnosis in the embryo by means of biopsy from extra-embryonic membrane. *Bull. Eur. Soc. Hum. Genet.* **2**, 23.

Haji, F., Chadli, A., Fattoum, S., Souilem, J. & Hassine, L. (1985) Double heterozygous Hb O Arab/β-thalassaemia in a Tunisian child. *Arch. Inst. Pasteur Tunis* **62**, 341.

Hajjar, F.M. & Pearson, H.A. (1994) Pharmacologic treatment of thalassemia intermedia with hydroxyurea. *J. Pediatr.* **125**, 490.

Halbrech, I. & Ben-Pora, S. (1971) Incidence of hemoglobin Bart's in the cord blood of Jewish and Arab ethnic groups in Israel. *Kupat-Holim Yearbook (Sick Fund of the General Federation of Labour in Israel)* **1**, 90.

Haldane, J.B.S. (1949a) Disease and evolution. *Ric. Sci.* **19**, 2.

Haldane, J.B.S. (1949b) The rate of mutation of human genes. *Proc. VIII Int. Cong. Genet. Hereditas* **35** (Suppl.), 267.

Hall, J.G. (1990) Genomic imprinting: review and relevance to human diseases. *Am. J. Hum. Genet.* **46**, 857.

Hall, G.W. & Thein, S.L. (1994) Nonsense codon mutations in the terminal exon of the β-globin gene are not associated with a reduction in β-mRNA accumulation: a mechanism for the phenotype of dominant β-thalassaemia. *Blood* **83**, 2031.

Hall, G.W., Franklin, I.M., Sura, T. & Thein, S.L. (1991) A novel mutation (nonsense β 127) in exon 3 of the β globin gene produces a variable thalassaemic phenotype. *Br. J. Haematol.* **79**, 342.

Hall, G.W., Barnetson, R.A. & Thein, S.L. (1992) Beta thalassaemia in the indigenous British population. *Br. J. Haematol.* **82**, 584.

Hall, G.W., Sampietro, M., Barnetson, R., Fitzgerald, J., McCann, S. & Thein, S.L. (1993a) Meiotic recombination in an Irish family with beta-thalassaemia. *Hum. Genet.* **92**, 28.

Hall, G.W., Thein, S.L., Newland, A.C. *et al.* (1993b) A base substitution (T→C) in codon 29 of the α2-globin gene causes α thalassaemia. *Br. J. Haematol.* **85**, 546.

Hall, G.W., Higgs, D.R., Murphy, P., Villegas, A. & de Miguel, A. (1994) A mutation in the polyadenylation signal of the α2 globin gene (AATAAA→AATA−) as a cause of α thalassaemia in Asian Indians. *Br. J. Haematol.* **88**, 225.

Hamilton, R.W., Schwartz, E., Atwater, J. & Erslev, A.J. (1971) Acquired hemoglobin H disease. *N. Eng. J. Med.* **285**, 1217.

Hammond, G.D., Ishikawa, A. & Keighley, G. (1962) Relationship between erythropoietin and severity of anemia in hypoplastic and hemolytic states. In: *Erythropoiesis* (eds L.O. Jacobson & M. Doyle), p. 351. Grune and Stratton, New York.

Hanash, S.M. & Rucknagel, D.L. (1978) Proteolytic activity in erythrocyte precursors. *Proc. Natl Acad. Sci. USA* **75**, 3427.

Handyside, A.H. & Delahunty, J.D. (1997) Preimplantation genetic diagnosis: strategies and surprises. *Trends Genet.* **13**, 270.

Hanscombe, O., Whyatt, D., Fraser, P. *et al.* (1991) Importance of globin gene order for correct developmental expression. *Genes Dev.* **5**, 1387.

Hanslip, J.I., Prescott, E., Lalloz, M., Layton, M. & Wonke, B. (1998) The role of the Sp1 polymorphism in the development of osteoporosis in patients with thalassaemia major. *Br. J. Haematol.* **101**, 26.

Harano, T., Reese, A.L., Ryan, R., Abraham, B.L. & Huisman, T.H.J. (1985) Five haplotypes in Black β-thalassaemia heterozygotes:

three are associated with high and two low $^G\gamma$ values fetal haemoglobin. *Br. J. Haematol.* **59**, 333.

Harkness, M., Harkness, D.R., Kutlar, F. *et al.* (1990) Hb Sun Prairie or α2 130(H13)Ala→Pro-β-2: a new unstable variant occurring in low quantities. *Hemoglobin* **14**, 479.

Harmon, J.V., Osathanondh, R. & Holmes, L.B. (1995) Symmetrical terminal transverse limb defects: report of twenty-week fetus. *Teratology* **51**, 237.

Harris, P.C., Barton, N.J., Higgs, D.R. *et al.* (1990) A long range restriction map between the α-globin complex and a marker linked to the polycystic kidney disease I (PKDI) locus. *Genomics* **7**, 195.

Hart, G.D. (1980) Ancient diseases of the blood. In: *Blood, Pure and Eloquent* (ed. M.M. Wintrobe), p. 33. McGraw-Hill, New York.

Harteveld, C.L. (1998) *The molecular genetics of a-thalassaemia: Structure and expression of the α-globin gene cluster*. PhD thesis, University of Leiden, The Netherlands.

Harteveld, C.L., Losekoot, M., Haak, H., Heister, J.G.A.M., Giordano, P.C. & Bernini, L.F. (1994) A novel polyadenylation signal mutation in the α2-globin gene causing α thalassaemia. *Br. J. Haematol.* **87**, 139.

Harteveld, C.L., Giordano, P.C., Losekoot, M. *et al.* (1996a) Hb Utrecht [α₂ 129(H12)Leu→Pro] a new unstable α2-chain variant in *cis* to a ζ-gene triplication and associated with a mild α-thalassemic phenotype. *Br. J. Haematol.* **94**, 483.

Harteveld, C.L., Heister, A.J.G.A.M., Giordano, P.C., Losekoot, M. & Bernini, L.F. (1996b) Rapid detection of point mutations and polymorphisms of the α-globin genes by DGGE and SSCA. *Hum. Mutat.* **7**, 114.

Harteveld, C.L., Heister, J.G.A.M., Giordano, P.C. *et al.* (1996c) An IVS-1-116 (A→G) acceptor splice site mutation in the α₂-globin gene causing α⁺-thalassaemia in two Dutch families. *Br. J. Haematol.* **95**, 461.

Harteveld, C.L., Losekoot, M., Fodde, R., Giordano, P.C. & Bernini, L.F. (1997a) The involvement of Alu repeats in recombination events at the α-globin gene cluster: characterization of two α⁰-thalassaemia deletion breakpoints. *Hum. Genet.* **99**, 528.

Harteveld, K.L., Losekoot, M., Heister, A.J.G.A.M., Wielen, M.V.D., Giordano, P.C. & Bernini, L.F. (1997b) α-Thalassaemia in The Netherlands: a heterogeneous spectrum of both deletions and point mutations. *Hum. Genet.* **100**, 465.

Hartkamp, M.J., Babyn, P.S. & Olivieri, N.F. (1993) Spinal deformities in deferoxamine-treated beta-thalassemia major patients. *Pediatr. Radiol.* **23**, 525.

Harvey, M.P., Motum, P., Lindeman, R. & Trent, R.J. (1992) An $^A\gamma$ globin promoter (four base-pair deletion) mutant shows linked polymorphic changes throughout the $^A\gamma$ gene. *Exp. Hematol.* **20**, 320.

Hasan, M.F., Marsh, F., Posner, G. *et al.* (1996) Chronic hepatitis C in patients with sickle cell disease. *Am. J. Gastroenterol.* **91**, 1204.

Hashmi, J.A. & Farzana, F. (1976) Thalassaemia trait, abnormal haemoglobins, and raised fetal haemoglobin in Karachi. *Lancet* **2**, 206.

Hassall, O.W., Tillyer, M.L. & Old, J.M. (1998) Prevalence and molecular basis of alpha thalassaemia in British South Asians. *J. Med. Screen.* **5**, 31.

Hathirat, P., Israngkura, P., Sasanakul, W. & Bintadish, P. (1978) Splenectomy in childhood thalassemia. *J. Med. Assoc. Thailand* **61**, 55.

Hatori, M., Sparkman, J., Teixeira, C.C. *et al.* (1995) Effects of deferoxamine on chondrocyte alkaline phosphatase activity: prooxidant role of deferoxamine in thalassemia. *California Tissue Int.* **57**, 229.

Hatton, C., Wilkie, A.O.M., Drysdale, H.C. *et al.* (1990) Alpha thalassemia caused by a large (62 kb) deletion upstream of the human α globin gene cluster. *Blood* **76**, 221.

Hattori, Y., Kutlar, F., Mosley, C.J., Mayson, S.M. & Huisman, T.H.J. (1986) Association of the level of $^G\gamma$ chain in the fetal hemoglobin of normal adults with specific haplotypes. *Hemoglobin* **10**, 185.

Hattori, Y., Yamane, A., Yamashiro, Y. *et al.* (1989) Characterisation of β-thalassemia mutations among the Japanese. *Hemoglobin* **13**, 657.

Hattori, Y., Yamashiro, Y., Ohba, Y. *et al.* (1991) A new β-thalassemia mutation (initiation codon $\underline{A}TG→\underline{G}TG$) found in the Japanese population. *Hemoglobin* **15**, 317.

Hattori, Y., Yamamoto, K., Yamashiro, Y. *et al.* (1992) Three β-thalassemia mutations in the Japanese: IVS-II-1 (G→A), IVS-II-848 (C→G) and codon 90 ($\underline{G}AG→\underline{T}AG$). *Hemoglobin* **16**, 93.

Hattori, Y., Okayama, N., Ohba, Y. *et al.* (1998) A new β-thalassemia allele, codon 26 (GAG→GTAG), found in a Japanese. *Hemoglobin* **22**, 79.

Hayes, R.J., Beckford, M., Grandison, Y., Mason, K., Serjeant, B.E. & Serjeant, G.R. (1985) The haematology of steady state homozygous sickle cell disease. I. Frequency distribution, longitudinal observations, effects of age and sex. *Br. J. Haematol.* **59**, 369.

Hazell, J.W. & Modell, C.B. (1976) E.N.T. complications in thalassaemia major. *J. Laryngol. Otol.* **90**, 877.

Headings, V.E., Winter, W., Reindorf, C. & Castro, O. (1983) Sickle Lepore hemoglobin identified in a black American infant. *Am. J. Pediatr. Hematol. Oncol.* **5**, 259.

Hebbel, R.P. (1985) Auto-oxidation and a membrane-associated 'Fenton Reagent': a possible explanation for development of membrane lesions in sickle erythrocytes. *Clin. Haematol.* **14**, 129.

Hebbel, R.P. (1997) Adhesive interactions of sickle erythrocytes with endothelium. *J. Clin. Invest.* **99**, 2561.

Hebbel, R.P. & Vercellotti, G.M. (1997) The endothelial biology of sickle cell disease. *J. Lab. Clin. Med.* **129**, 288.

Hecht, F., Motulsky, A.G., Lemire, R.J. & Shepard, T.E. (1966) Predominance of hemoglobin Gower 1 in early human embryonic development. *Science* **152**, 91.

Hecht, F., Jones, R.T. & Koler, R.D. (1967) Newborn infants with Hb Portland 1: an indicator of α-chain deficiency. *Ann. Hum. Genet. (London)* **31**, 215.

Hegde, U.M., Khunda, S., Marsh, G.W., Hart, G.H. & White, J.M. (1975) Thalassaemia, iron and pregnancy. *Br. Med. J.* **3**, 509.

Heinrich, H.C., Gabbe, E.E., Oppitz, K.H. *et al.* (1973) Absorption of inorganic and food iron in children with heterozygous and homozygous beta-thalassemia. *Z. Kinderheilkd.* **115**, 1.

Helder, J. & Deisseroth, A. (1987) S1 nuclease analysis of α-globin gene expression in preleukemic patients with acquired hemoglobin H disease after transfer to mouse erythroleukemia cells. *Proc. Natl Acad. Sci. USA* **84**, 2387.

Heller, P., Yakulis, V.J., Rosenweig, A.I., Abildgaard, C.F. & Rucknagel, D.L. (1966) Mild homozygous beta-thalassemia. Further evidence for the heterogeneity of beta-thalassemia. *Ann. Intern. Med.* **64**, 52.

Helley, D., Eldor, A., Girot, R., Ducrocq, R., Guillin, M.C. & Beuzard, A. (1996) Comparison of the procoagulant activity of red blood cells from patients with homozygous sickle cell disease and β-thalassemia. *Thromb. Haemost.* **76**, 322.

Henderson, A.B., Potts, E.B., Burgess, D. & White, F. (1962) Sickle cell thalassemia disease and pregnancy; a case study. *Am. J. Med. Sci.* **244**, 605.

Hendrickse, R.G., Boyo, A.E., Fitzgerald, P.A. & Kuti, S.R. (1960) Studies on the haemoglobin of newborn Nigerians. *Br. Med. J.* **1**, 611.

de Hendrickse, J.P.V., Harrison, K.A., Watson-Williams, E.J., Luzzatto, L. & Ajabor, L.N. (1972) Pregnancy in homozygous sickle-cell anaemia. *J. Obstet. Gynaecol. Br. Commonw.* **79**, 396.

Henni, T., Bachir, D., Tabone, P., Jurdic, P., Godet, J. & Colonna, P. (1981) Hemoglobin Bart's in Northern Algeria. *Acta Haematol.* **65**, 240.

Henni, T., Belhani, M., Morle, F. *et al.* (1985) α-Globin gene triplication in severe heterozygous β-thalassemia. *Acta Haematol.* **74**, 236.

Henry, W.L., Nienhuis, A.W., Wiener, M., Miller, D.R., Canale, V.C. & Piomelli, S. (1978) Echocardiographic abnormalities in patients with transfusion-dependent anemia and secondary myocardial iron deposition. *Am. J. Med.* **64**, 547.

Henson, J. & Huisman, T.H.J. (1978) Possible relationship between the level of Hb Bart's (γ_4) and the relative amount of Hb S or Hb C in Black heterozygous newborn. *Hemoglobin* **2**, 393.

Henthorn, P.S., Smithies, O., Nakatsuji, T. *et al.* (1985) ($^A\gamma\delta\beta$)^0-Thalassaemia in Blacks is due to a deletion of 34 kbp of DNA. *Br. J. Haematol.* **59**, 343.

Henthorn, P.S., Mager, D.K., Huisman, T.H.J. & Smithies, O. (1986) A gene deletion ending within a complex array of repeated sequences 3′ to the human beta-globin gene cluster. *Proc. Natl Acad. Sci. USA* **83**, 5194.

Henthorn, P.S., Smithies, O. & Mager, D.L. (1990) Molecular analysis of deletions in the human β-globin gene cluster: deletion junctions and locations of breakpoints. *Genomics* **6**, 226.

Herington, A.C., Werthe, G.A., Matthews, R.N. & Burger, H.G. (1981) Studies on the possible mechanism for deficiency of nonsuppressible insulin-like activity in thalassemia major. *J. Clin. Endocrinol. Metab.* **52**, 393.

Herman, E.C. & Conley, C.L. (1960) Hereditary persistence of fetal hemoglobin. A family study. *Am. J. Med.* **29**, 9.

Herrick, R.T. & Davis, G.L. (1975) Thalassemia major and non-union of pathologic fractures. *J. LA State Med. Sci.* **127**, 341.

Hershko, C. (1989) Mechanisms of iron toxicity and its possible role in red cell membrane damage. *Sem. Hematol.* **26**, 277.

Hershko, C. & Peto, T.E.A. (1987) Annotation: Non-transferrin iron. *Br. J. Haematol.* **66**, 149.

Hershko, C. & Weatherall, D.J. (1988) Iron-chelating therapy. *CRC Clin. Rev. Clin. Lab. Sci.* **26**, 303.

Hershko, C., Graham, G., Bates, C.W. & Rachmilewitz, E.S. (1978) Non-specific serum iron in thalassemia: an abnormal serum iron fraction of potential toxicity. *Br. J. Haematol.* **40**, 255.

Hershko, C., Peto, T.E.A. & Weatherall, D.J. (1988) Iron and infection. *Br. Med. J.* **296**, 660.

Hershko, C., Konijn, A.M. & Link, G. (1998a) Iron chelators for thalassaemia. *Br. J. Haematol.* **101**, 399.

Hershko, C., Link, G. & Cabantchik, I. (1998b) Pathophysiology of iron overload. *Ann. N. Y. Acad. Sci.* **850**, 191.

Hess, J.F., Schmid, C.W. & Shen, C.-K.J. (1984) A gradient of sequence divergence in the human adult α-globin duplication units. *Science* **226**, 67.

Heuterspreute, M., Derclaye, I., Gala, J.-L. *et al.* (1996) Beta-thalassaemia in indigenous Belgian families: identification of a novel mutation. *Hum. Genet.* **98**, 77.

Heywood, J.D., Karon, M. & Weissman, S. (1965) Asymmetrical incorporation of amino acids into the alpha and beta chains of hemoglobin synthesised in thalassemia reticulocytes. *J. Lab. Clin. Med.* **66**, 476.

Hider, R.C., Kontoghiorghes, G.J. & Silver, J. (1982) UK Patent: GB-2118176.

Hiernaux, J. (1976) Blood polymorphism frequencies in the Sara Majingay of Chad. *Ann. Hum. Biol.* **3**, 127.

Higgs, D.R. (1993) α-Thalassaemia. In: *Baillière's Clinical Haematology: The Haemoglobinopathies* (eds D.R. Higgs & D.J. Weatherall), Vol 6: 1, p. 117. Baillière Tindall, London.

Higgs, D.R. & Weatherall, D.J. (eds) (1993) *The Haemoglobinopathies*, Vol 6: 1. Baillière Tindall, London.

Higgs, D.R., Clegg, J.B., Wood, W.G. & Weatherall, D.J. (1979a) $^G\gamma\beta^+$ type of hereditary persistence of fetal haemoglobin in association with Hb C. *J. Med. Genet.* **16**, 288.

Higgs, D.R., Old, J.M., Clegg, J.B. *et al.* (1979b) Negro α-thalassaemia is caused by deletion of a single α-globin gene. *Lancet* **ii**, 272.

Higgs, D.R., Old, J.M., Pressley, L., Clegg, J.B. & Weatherall, D.J. (1980a) A novel α-globin gene arrangement in man. *Nature* **284**, 632.

Higgs, D.R., Pressley, L., Clegg, J.B., Weatherall, D.J., Carey, P. & Serjeant, G.R. (1980b) Detection of α-thalassaemia in negro infants. *Br. J. Haematol.* **46**, 39.

Higgs, D.R., Pressley, L., Aldridge, B. *et al.* (1981) Genetic and molecular diversity in nondeletion HbH disease. *Proc. Natl Acad. Sci. USA* **78**, 5833.

Higgs, D.R., Aldridge, B.E., Lamb, J. *et al.* (1982) The interaction of alpha-thalassaemia and homozygous sickle-cell disease. *N. Eng. J. Med.* **306**, 1441.

Higgs, D.R., Goodbourn, S.E.Y., Lamb, J., Clegg, J.B., Weatherall, D.J. & Proudfoot, N.J. (1983a) α-Thalassaemia caused by a polyadenylation signal mutation. *Nature* **306**, 398.

Higgs, D.R., Wood, W.G., Barton, C. & Weatherall, D.J. (1983b) Clinical features and molecular analysis of acquired HbH disease. *Am. J. Med.* **75**, 181.

Higgs, D.R., Clegg, J.B., Weatherall, D.J., Serjeant, B.E. & Serjeant, G.R. (1984a) Interaction of the αααα-globin gene haplotype and sickle haemoglobin. *Br. J. Haematol.* **58**, 671.

Higgs, D.R., Hill, A.V.S., Bowden, D.K., Weatherall, D.J. & Clegg, J.B. (1984b) Independent recombination events between duplicated human α-globin genes: Implications for their concerted evolution. *Nucl. Acids Res.* **12**, 6965.

Higgs, D.R., Ayyub, H., Clegg, J.B. *et al.* (1985) α-Thalassaemia in British people. *Br. Med. J.* **290**, 1303.

Higgs, D.R., Wainscoat, J.S., Flint, J. *et al.* (1986) Analysis of the human α-globin gene cluster reveals a highly informative genetic locus. *Proc. Natl Acad. Sci. USA* **83**, 5165.

Higgs, D.R., Vickers, M.A., Wilkie, A.O.M., Pretorius, I.-M., Jarman, A.P. & Weatherall, D.J. (1989) A review of the molecular genetics of the human α-globin gene cluster. *Blood* **73**, 1081.

Higgs, D.R., Wood, W.G., Jarman, A.P. *et al.* (1990) A major positive regulatory region located far upstream of the human α-globin gene locus. *Genes Dev.* **4**, 1588.

Higgs, D.R., Wilkie, A.O.M., Vyas, P., Vickers, M.A., Buckle, V.J. & Harris, P.C. (1993) Characterisation of the telomeric region of human chromosome 16p. *Chromosomes Today* **11**, 35.

Higgs, D.R., Sharpe, J.A. & Wood, W.G. (1998) Understanding α globin gene expression: a step towards effective gene therapy. *Sem. Hematol.* **35**, 93.

Higgs, D.R., Ayyub, H. & Chong, S.S. (1999) The $--^{Thai}$ and $--^{Fil}$ determinants of α thalassaemia in Taiwan. *Am. J. Hematol.* **60**, 80.

Hilgartner, M.W. & Smith, C.H. (1964) Coagulation studies as a measure of liver function in Cooley's anemia. *Ann. N. Y. Acad. Sci.* **119**, 573.

Hill, A.V.S., Nicholls, R.D., Thein, S.L. & Higgs, D.R. (1985) Recombination within the human embryonic ζ-globin locus: a common ζ-ζ chromosome produced by gene conversion of the ψζ gene. *Cell* **42**, 809.

Hill, A.V.S., Gentile, B., Bonnardot, J.M., Roux, A.J., Weatherall, D.J. & Clegg, J.B. (1987a) Polynesian origins and affinities: globin gene variants in Eastern Polynesia. *Am. J. Hum. Genet.* **40**, 453.

Hill, A.V.S., Thein, S.L., Mavo, B., Weatherall, D.J. & Clegg, J.B. (1987b) Non-deletion haemoglobin H disease in Papua New Guinea. *J. Med. Genet.* **24**, 767.

Hill, A.V.S., Bowden, D.K., O'Shaughnessy, D.F., Weatherall, D.J. & Clegg, J.B. (1988) β-Thalassemia in Melanesia: association with malaria and characterization of a common variant (IVSI nt 5 G-C). *Blood* **72**, 9.

Hill, A.V.S., O'Shaughnessy, D.F. & Clegg, J.B. (1989) Haemoglobin and globin gene variants in the Pacific. In: *The Peopling of the Pacific: A Genetic Trail* (eds A.V.S. Hill & S.W. Serjeantson), p. 246. Oxford University Press, Oxford.

Hill, A.V.S., Allsop, C.E.M. & Kwiatkowski, D. (1991) Common west African HLA antigens are associated with protection from severe malaria. *Nature* **352**, 595.

Hillcoat, B.L. & Waters, A.H. (1962) The survival of ^{51}Cr labelled autotransfused red cells in a patient with thalassaemia. *Aust. Med. J.* **11**, 55.

Hillman, R.S. & Giblett, E.R. (1965) Red cell membrane alteration associated with marrow stress. *J. Clin. Invest.* **10**, 1730.

Hinchliffe, R.F., Lilleyman, J.S., Steel, G.J. & Bellamy, G.J. (1995) Usefulness of red cell zinc protoporphyrin concentration in the investigation of microcytosis in children. *Pediatr. Hematol. Oncol.* **12**, 455.

Hiraoka, Y., Kishimoto, C., Takada, H. *et al.* (1993) Role of oxygen derived free radicals in the pathogenesis of coxsackievirus B3 myocarditis in mice. *Cardiovas. Res.* **27**, 957.

Hirsch, R.E., Raventos-Suarex, C., Olson, J.A. & Nagel, R.L. (1985) Ligand state of intraerythrocyte circulating Hb C crystals in homozygous CC patient. *Blood* **66**, 775.

Hirschhorn, J.N., Brown, S.A., Clark, C.D. & Winston, F. (1992) Evidence that SNF2/SWI2 and SNF5 activate transcription in yeast by altering chromatin structure. *Genes Dev.* **6**, 2288.

Hirsh, J. & Dacie, J.V. (1966) Persistent post-splenectomy thrombocytosis and thrombo-embolism. A consequence of continuing anaemia. *Br. J. Haematol.* **12**, 44.

Ho, P.J., Hall, G.W., Nest, N.C., Wimperis, J.Z., Wood, W.G. & Thein, S.L. (1996a) Abnormal accumulation of aberrantly spliced mRNA transcript underlying the unusually severe disease in β thalassaemia. *Blood* **88**, 464a.

Ho, P.J., Rochette, J., Rees, D.C. *et al.* (1996b) Hb Sun Prarie: diagnostic pitfalls in thalassemic hemoglobinopathies. *Hemoglobin* **20**, 103.

Ho, P.J., Rochette, J., Fisher, C.A. *et al.* (1996c) Moderate reduction of β-globin gene transcript by a novel mutation in the 5′ untranslated region: a study of its interaction with other genotypes in two families. *Blood* **87**, 1170.

Ho, P.J., Wickramasinghe, S.N., Rees, D.C., Lee, M.J., Eden, A. & Thein, S.L. (1997) Erythroblastic inclusions in dominantly inherited β thalassaemias. *Blood* **89**, 322.

Ho, P.J., Hall, G.W., Luo, L.Y., Weatherall, D.J. & Thein, S.L. (1998a) Beta thalassaemia intermedia: is it possible to predict phenotype from genotype? *Br. J. Haematol.* **100**, 70.

Ho, P.J., Hall, G.W., Watt, S. *et al.* (1998b) Unusually severe heterozygous β-thalassaemia: evidence for an interacting gene affecting globin translation. *Blood* **92**, 3428.

Ho, P.J., Sloane-Stanley, J., Athanassiadou, A., Wood, W.G. & Thein, S.L. (1999) An *in vitro* system for expression analysis of mutations of the β-globin gene: validation and application to two mutations in the 5′ UTR. *Br. J. Haematol.* **106**, 938.

Hobbins, J.C. & Mahoney, M.J. (1975) Fetal blood drawing. *Lancet* **ii**, 107.

Hobbins, J.C., Mahoney, M.J. & Goldstein, L.A. (1974) New method of intrauterine evaluation by the combined use of fetoscopy and ultrasound. *Am. J. Obstet. Gynecol.* **118**, 1969.

Hocking, I.W. & Ibbotson, R.M. (1966) The effect of the beta thalassaemia trait on pregnancy with particular reference to its complications and outcome. *Med. J. Aust.* **2**, 397.

Hoeper, M.M., Niedermeyer, J., Hoffmeyer, F., Flemming, P. & Fabel, H. (1999) Pulmonary hypertension after splenectomy. *Ann. Intern. Med.* **130**, 506.

Hoffbrand, A.V. (1996) Oral iron chelation. *Sem. Hematol.* **33**, 1.

Hoffbrand, A.V., al-Refaie, F., Davis, B. *et al.* (1998) Long-term trial of deferiprone in 51 transfusion-dependent iron overloaded patients. *Blood* **91**, 295.

Hoffman, J.F., Hillier, J., Parpart, A.K. & Wolman, I.J. (1956) Ultrastructure of erythrocyte membranes in thalassemia major and minor. *Blood* **11**, 946.

Hollenberg, M.D., Kaback, M.M. & Kazazian, H.H. (1971) Adult hemoglobin synthesis by reticulocytes from the human fetus at midtrimester. *Science* **174**, 698.

Holmquist, W.R. & Schroeder, W.A. (1966) A new N-terminal blocking group involving a Schiff base in hemoglobin A_{1c}. *Biochemistry* **5**, 2489.

Holzgreve, W., Curry, C.J.R., Golbus, M.S., Callen, P.W., Filly, R.A. & Smith, J.C. (1984) Investigation of nonimmune hydrops fetalis. *Am. J. Obstet. Gynecol.* **150**, 805.

Honetz, N., Moser, K., Neumann, E. & Seipel, H. (1968) Studies on erythrokinetics and erythrocyte metabolism in thalassemia minor. *Acta Haematol.* **39**, 333.

Honig, G.R., Shamsuddin, M., Mason, R.G. & Vida, L.N. (1978) Hemoglobin Lincoln Park: a βδ fusion (anti-Lepore) variant with an amino acid deletion in the δ chain-derived segment. *Proc. Natl Acad. Sci. USA* **75**, 1475.

Honig, G.R., Shamsuddin, M., Zaizov, R., Steinherz, M., Solar, I. & Kirschman, C. (1981) Hemoglobin Peta Tikvah (α110 Ala-Asp): a new unstable variant with α-thalassaemia-like expression. *Blood* **57**, 705.

Honig, G.R., Shamsuddin, M., Vida, L.N. *et al.* (1984) Hemoglobin Evanston (α14 Trp→Arg): an unstable α-chain variant expressed as α-thalassaemia. *J. Clin. Invest.* **73**, 1740.

Hopmeier, P., Krugluger, W., Gu, L.-H., Smetanina, N.S. & Huisman, T.H.J. (1996) A newly discovered frameshift at codons 120–121 (+A) of the β gene is not associated with a dominant form of β-thalassaemia. *Blood* **87**, 5393.

Horsley, S.W., Daniels, R.J., Anguita, E. *et al.* (2001) Monosomy for the most telomeric, gene-rich region of human chromosome 16p causes minimal phenotypic effects. *Eur. J. Hum. Genet.*, in press.

Horton, B.F. & Huisman, T.H.J. (1963) Linkage of the beta-chain and delta-chain structural genes of human hemoglobins. *Am. J. Hum. Genet.* **15**, 394.

Horton, B.F., Payne, R.A., Bridges, M.T. & Huisman, T.J.H. (1961) Studies on an abnormal minor hemoglobin component (Hb-B$_2$). *Clin. Chim. Acta* **6**, 246.

Horton, B.F., Thompson, R.B., Dozy, A.M., Nechtwan, C.M., Nichols, E. & Huisman, T.H.J. (1962) Inhomogeneity of hemoglobin. VI The minor hemoglobin components of cord blood. *Blood* **20**, 302.

Horton, B.F., Hahn, D.A. & Huisman, T.H.J. (1965) Slight increase in fetal hemoglobin in apparently healthy negroes. *Acta Haematol.* **33**, 312.

Houang, M.T.W., Arozena, X., Skalicka, A., Huehns, E.R. & Shaw, D.G. (1979) Correlation between computed tomographic values and liver iron content in thalassaemia major with iron overload. *Lancet* **i**, 1322.

Housman, D., Forget, B.G., Skoultchi, A. & Benz, E.J. (1973) Quantitative deficiency of chain specific messenger ribonucleic acids in the thalassemia syndromes. *Proc. Natl Acad. Sci. USA* **70**, 1809.

Housman, D., Skoultchi, A., Forget, B.G. & Benz, E.J. (1974) Use of globin cDNA as a hybridization probe for globin mRNA. *Ann. N. Y. Acad. Sci.* **241**, 280.

Hovav, T., Goldfarb, A., Artmann, G., Yedgar, S. & Barshtein, G. (1999) Enhanced adherence of β-thalassaemic erythrocytes to endothelial cells. *Br. J. Haematol.* **106**, 178.

Howell, J. & Wyatt, J.P. (1953) Development of pigmentary cirrhosis in Cooley's anaemia. *Arch. Pathol.* **55**, 423.

Hoyt, R.W., Scarpa, N., Wilmott, R.W., Cohen, A. & Schwartz, E. (1986) Pulmonary function abnormalities in homozygous β-thalassemia. *J. Pediatr.* **109**, 452.

Huang, S.-Z., Wong, C., Antonarakis, S.E., Ro-Lein, T., Lo, W.H.Y. & Kazazian, H.H.J. (1986) The same TATA box β-thalassemia mutation in Chinese and U.S. blacks: another example of independent origins of mutation. *Hum. Genet.* **74**, 162.

Huang, H.J., Stoming, T.A., Harris, H.F., Kutlar, F. & Huisman, T.H.J. (1987) The Greek $^A\gamma\beta^+$-HPFH observed in a large black family. *Am. J. Hematol.* **25**, 401.

Huang, S.-Z., Zhou, X.-D., Zhu, H., Ren, Z.-R. & Zeng, Y.-T. (1990) Detection of β-thalassemia mutations in the Chinese using amplified DNA from dried blood specimens. *Hum. Genet.* **84**, 129.

Huang, S.-Z., Xu, Y.-H., Zeng, F.-Y., Wu, D.-F., Ren, Z.-R. & Zeng, Y.-T. (1991) A novel β-thalassaemia mutation: deletion of 4 bp (-AAAC) in the 5′ transcriptional sequence. *Br. J. Haematol.* **78**, 125.

Huang, S.-Z., Ren, Z.-R., Chen, M.-J. *et al.* (1994) Treatment of β-thalassemia with hydroxyurea. Effects of HU on globin gene expression. *Sci. China (Series B)* **37**, 1350.

Huebers, H.A., Beguin, Y., Pootrakul, P., Einsphar, D. & Finch, C.A. (1990) Intact transferrin receptors in human plasma and their relation to erythropoiesis. *Blood* **75**, 102.

Huehns, E.R., Flynn, F.V., Butler, E.A. & Beaven, G.H. (1960) The occurrence of haemoglobin 'Bart's' in conjunction with haemoglobin H. *Br. J. Haematol.* **6**, 388.

Huehns, E.R., Flynn, F.V., Butler, E.A. & Beaven, G.H. (1961) Two new haemoglobin variants in a very young human embryo. *Nature* **189**, 496.

Huehns, E.R., Beaven, G.H. & Stevens, B.L. (1964a) Recombination studies on haemoglobins at neutral pH. *Biochem. J.* **92**, 440.

Huehns, E.R., Dance, N., Beaven, G.H., Hecht, F. & Motulsky, A.G. (1964b) Human embryonic hemoglobins. *Cold Spring Harbor Sympos. Quant. Biol.* **19**, 327.

Hug, B.A., Wesselschmidt, R.L., Fiering, S. *et al.* (1996) Analysis of mice containing a targeted deletion of beta-globin locus control region 5′ hypersensitive site 3. *Mol. Cell. Biol.* **16**, 2906.

Huisman, T.H.J. (1960a) Genetic aspects of two different minor haemoglobin components found in cord blood samples of Negro babies. *Nature* **188**, 589.

Huisman, T.H.J. (1960b) Properties and inheritance of the new, fast hemoglobin type found in umbilical cord blood samples of Negro babies. *Clin. Chim. Acta* **5**, 709.

Huisman, T.H.J. (1963) Normal and abnormal human hemoglobins. *Adv. Clin. Chem.* **6**, 231.

Huisman, T.H.J. (1990) Frequencies of common β-thalassaemia alleles among different populations: variability in clinical severity. *Br. J. Haematol.* **75**, 454.

Huisman, T.H.J. (1993) The β- and δ-thalassemia Repository (7th edn). *Hemoglobin* **17**, 479.

Huisman, T.H.J. (1997) Compound heterozygosity for Hb S and the hybrid Hbs Lepore, P-Nilotic, and Kenya; comparison of hematological and hemoglobin composition data. *Hemoglobin* **21**, 249.

Huisman, T.H.J. & Jonxis, J.H.P. (1977) *The Hemoglobinopathies: Techniques of Identification.* Marcel Dekker Inc, New York.

Huisman, T.H.J., Prins, H.K. & Van der Schaaf, P.C. (1956) Is alkali-resistant haemoglobin in Cooley's anaemia different from foetal haemoglobin? *Experentia* **12**, 107.

Huisman, T.H.J., Punt, K. & Schaad, J.D.G. (1961) Thalassemia minor associated with hemoglobin B_2 heterozygosity. *Blood* **17**, 747.

Huisman, T.H.J., Wilson, J.B. & Adams, H.R. (1967) The heterogeneity of goat haemoglobin: evidence for the existence of two nonallelic and one allelic α-chain structural genes. *Arch. Biochem. Biophys.* **121**, 528.

Huisman, T.H.J., Schroeder, W.A., Dozy, A.M. *et al.* (1969) Evidence for multiple structural genes for the γ-chain of human fetal hemoglobin in hereditary persistence of fetal hemoglobin. *Ann. N. Y. Acad. Sci.* **165**, 320.

Huisman, T.H.J., Schroeder, W.A., Adams, H.R., Shelton, J.R., Shelton, J.B. & Apell, G. (1970a) A possible subclass of the hereditary persistence of fetal hemoglobin. *Blood* **36**, 1.

Huisman, T.H.J., Schroeder, W.A., Stamatoyannopoulos, G. *et al.* (1970b) Nature of fetal hemoglobin in the Greek type of hereditary persistence of fetal hemoglobin with and without concurrent β-thalassemia. *J. Clin. Invest.* **49**, 1035.

Huisman, T.H.J., Schroeder, W.A., Charache, S. *et al.* (1971) Hereditary persistence of fetal hemoglobin. Heterogeneity of fetal hemoglobin in homozygotes and in conjunction with β-thalassemia. *N. Eng. J. Med.* **285**, 711.

Huisman, T.H.J., Wrightstone, R.N., Wilson, J.B., Schroeder, W.A. & Kendall, A.G. (1972) Hemoglobin Kenya, the product of fusion of γ and β polypeptide chains. *Arch. Biochem. Biophys.* **153**, 850.

Huisman, T.H.J., Schroeder, W.A., Efremov, G.D. *et al.* (1974) The present status of the heterogeneity of fetal hemoglobin in β-thalassemia; an attempt to unify some observations in thalassemia and related conditions. *Ann. N. Y. Acad. Sci.* **232**, 107.

Huisman, T.H.J., Miller, A., Cook, L., Gordon, S. & Schroeder, W.A. (1975a) The molecular heterogeneity of some types of hereditary persistence of fetal hemoglobin (HPFH). In: *International Istanbul Symposium on Abnormal Hemoglobins and Thalassemia* (ed. M. Aksoy), p. 95, TBTAK, Ankara.

Huisman, T.H.J., Miller, A. & Schroeder, W.A. (1975b) A $^G\gamma$ type of the hereditary persistence of fetal hemoglobin with beta chain production in cis. *Am. J. Hum. Genet.* **27**, 765.

Huisman, T.H.J., Gravely, M.E. & Sox, R. (1976) A note on the inheritance of the hereditary persistence of fetal haemoglobin and the delta chain variant HbA_2. *J. Med. Genet.* **13**, 62.

Huisman, T.H.J., Harris, H., Gravely, M. *et al.* (1977) The chemical heterogeneity of the fetal hemoglobin in normal newborn infants and in adults. *Mol. Cell. Biochem.* **17**, 45.

Huisman, T.H.J., Gravely, M.E., Henson, J. *et al.* (1978) Variability in the interaction of β-thalassemia with the α-chain variants Hb G Philadelphia and Hb Rampa. *J. Lab. Clin. Med.* **92**, 311.

Huisman, T.H.J., Efremov, G.D., Reese, A.L. *et al.* (1979) The synthesis of fetal hemoglobin types in red blood cells and in BFU-E derived colonies from peripheral blood of patients with sickle cell anemia, β$^+$ and δβ-thalassemia, various forms of hereditary persistence of fetal hemoglobin, normal adults and newborns. *Hemoglobin* **3**, 223.

Huisman, T.H.J., Gravely, M.E., Webber, B., Okonjo, K., Henson, J. & Reese, A.L. (1981) The gamma chain heterogeneity of fetal hemoglobin in Black β thalassemia and HPFH heterozygotes. *Blood* **51**, 62.

Huisman, T.H., Reese, A.L., Gardiner, M.B. *et al.* (1983) The occurrence of different levels of $^G\gamma$ chain and of the $^A\gamma^T$ variant of fetal hemoglobin in newborn babies from several countries. *Am. J. Hematol.* **14**, 133.

Huisman, T.H.J., Kutlar, F., Nakatsuji, T. *et al.* (1985) The frequency of the γ chain variant $^A\gamma^T$ in different populations, and its use in evaluating γ gene expression in association with thalassemia. *Hum. Genet.* **71**, 127.

Huisman, T.H., Kutlar, F. & Gu, L.H. (1991) Gamma chain abnormalities and gamma-globin gene rearrangements in newborn babies of various populations. *Hemoglobin* **15**, 349.

Huisman, T.H.J., Carver, M.F.H. & Efremov, G.D. (1996) *A Syllabus of Human Hemoglobin Variants*. The Sickle Cell Anemia Foundation, Augusta, GA.

Huisman, T.H.J., Carver, M.F.H. & Baysal, E. (1997) *A Syllabus of Thalassemia Mutations*, p. 309. The Sickle Cell Anemia Foundation, Augusta, GA.

Huisman, T.H.J., Carver, M.F.H. & Efremov, G.D. (1998) *A Syllabus of Human Hemoglobin Variants*, 2nd edn. The Sickle Cell Anemia Foundation, Augusta, GA.

Humphries, R.K., Ley, T.J., Anagnou, N.P., Baur, A.W. & Nienhuis, A.W. (1984) β^0-39 Thalassemia gene: a premature termination codon causes β-mRNA deficiency without affecting cytoplasmic β-mRNA stability. *Blood* **64**, 23.

Hundreiser, J., Sanguansermsri, T., Papp, T. & Flatz, G. (1988) Alpha thalassemia in Northern Thailand. *Hum. Hered.* **38**, 211.

Hundreiser, J., Laig, M., Yongvanit, P. *et al.* (1990) Study of alpha-thalassemia in Northeast Thailand at the DNA level. *Hum. Hered.* **40**, 85.

Hunt, J.A. & Lehmann, H. (1959) Abnormal human haemoglobins. Haemoglobin 'Bart's': a foetal haemoglobin without α chains. *Nature* **184**, 872.

Hunt, R.T., Hunter, A.R. & Munro, A.J. (1968) Control of haemoglobin synthesis: a difference in the size of the polysomes making α and β chains. *Nature* **220**, 481.

Hunt, D.M., Higgs, D.R., Old, J.M., Clegg, J.B., Weatherall, D.J. & Marsh, G.W. (1980) Determination of α thalassaemia phenotypes by messenger RNA analysis. *Br. J. Haematol.* **45**, 53.

Hunt, D.M., Higgs, D.R., Winichagoon, P., Clegg, J.B. & Weatherall, D.J. (1982) Haemoglobin Constant Spring has an unstable α chain messenger RNA. *Br. J. Haematol.* **51**, 405.

Hussain, M.A.M., Green, N. Flynn, D.M., Hussein, S. & Hoffbrand, A.V. (1976) Subcutaneous infusion and intramuscular injection of desferrioxamine in patients with transfusional iron overload. *Lancet* **ii**, 1278.

Hussain, M.A.M., Green, N., Flynn, D.M. & Hoffbrand, A.V. (1977) Effect of dose, time and ascorbate in iron excretion after subcutaneous desferrioxamine. *Lancet* **i**, 977.

Hussain, M.A.M., Myers, A., Wagstaff, D., Flynn, D.M. & Hoffbrand, A.V. (1979) Echocardiographic changes in patients with transfusional iron overload. *Clin. Sci.* **57**, 12.

Hussein, S., Hoffbrand, A.V. & Laulicht, M. (1976) Serum ferritin levels in β-thalassaemia trait. *Br. Med. J.* **ii**, 920.

Hussein, I.R., Temtamy, S.A., El-Beshlawy, A. *et al.* (1993) Molecular characterization of β-thalassaemia in Egyptians. *Hum. Mutat.* **2**, 48.

Hyman, C.B., Landing, B., Alfin-Slater, R., Kozak, L., Weitzman, J. & Ortega, J.A. (1974) D1-alpha-tocopherol, iron and lipofuscin in thalassemia. *Ann. N. Y. Acad. Sci.* **232**, 211.

Hyman, C.B., Ortega, J.A., Costin, G. & Takahashi, M. (1980) The clinical significance of magnesium depletion in thalassaemia. *Ann. N. Y. Acad. Sci.* **344**, 436.

Hynes, M. & Lehmann, H. (1956) Haemoglobin D in a Persian girl: presumably the first case of haemoglobin-D thalassaemia. *Br. Med. J.* **ii**, 923.

Iancu, T.C. (1989) Ultrastructural pathology of iron overload. *Clin. Haematol.* **2**, 475.

Iancu, T.C. & Neustein, H.B. (1977) Ferritin in human liver cells of homozygous β-thalassaemia: ultrastructural observations. *Br. J. Haematol.* **37**, 527.

Iancu, T.C., Landing, B.H. & Neustein, H.B. (1977a) Pathogenic mechanisms in hepatic cirrhosis of thalassemia major: light and electron microscopic studies. *Pathol. Annu.* **12**, 171.

Iancu, T.C., Neustein, H.B. & Landing, B.H. (1977b) The liver in thalassaemia major: ultrastructural observations. In: *Iron Metabolism. Ciba Symposium no. 5*, p. 293. Excerpta Medica, Amsterdam.

Ibbotson, R.N. & Crompton, B.A. (1963) The incidence of β-thalassaemia in Greek and Italian immigrants in Australia and its effects in pregnancy. *Br. J. Haematol.* **9**, 523.

Ibrahim, S.A., Dafalla, A.A. & Lauder, J.R. (1970) A search for abnormal haemoglobins and thalassaemia in the Beni Amer tribe. *Sudan Med. J.* **8**, 88.

Ifediba, T.C., Stern, A., Ibrahim, A. & Rieder, R.F. (1985) *Plasmodium falciparum in vitro*: diminished growth in hemoglobin H disease erythrocytes. *Blood* **65**, 452.

Imai, K., Hamilton, H.B., Miyaji, T. & Shibata, S. (1972) Physicochemical studies of the relation between structure and function in hemoglobin Hiroshima (HC3 β Histidine-Aspartate). *Biochemistry* **11**, 114.

Imamura, T., Sugihara, J., Matsuo, T. *et al.* (1980) Frequency and distribution of structural variants of hemoglobin and thalassemic states in Western Japan. *Hemoglobin* **4**, 409.

Indrák, K., Indrakova, J., Kutlar, F. *et al.* (1991) Compound heterozygosity for a β^0-thalassaemia (frameshift codons 38/39; -C) and a nondeletional Swiss type of HPFH (A$-$C at NT $-$110, $^{G}\gamma$) in a Czechoslovakian family. *Am. J. Hematol.* **63**, 111.

Indrák, K., Brabec, V., Indrakova, J. *et al.* (1992) Molecular characterization of β-thalassemia in Czechoslovakia. *Hum. Genet.* **88**, 399.

Indrák, K., Gu, Y.-C., Novotny, J. & Huisman, T.H.J. (1993) A new α-thalassemia-2 deletion resulting in microcytosis and hypochromia and *in vitro* chain imbalance in the heterozygote. *Am. J. Hematol.* **43**, 144.

Ingram, V.M. (1956) Specific chemical difference between the globins of normal human and sickle-cell anaemia haemoglobin. *Nature* **178**, 792.

Ingram, V.M. (1964) A molecular model for thalassemia. *Ann. N. Y. Acad. Sci.* **119**, 485.

Ingram, V.M. (1989) A case of sickle-cell anaemia: a commentary. *Biochim. Biophys. Acta* **1000**, 147.

Ingram, V.M. & Stretton, A.O.W. (1959) Genetic basis of the thalassemia diseases. *Nature* **184**, 1903.

Ingram, V.M. & Stretton, A.O.W. (1961) Human haemoglobin A$_2$: chemistry, genetics and evolution. *Nature* **190**, 1079.

Intragumtornchai, T., Arjhansiri, K., Posayachinda, M. & Kasantikul, V. (1993) Obstructive uropathy due to extramedullary haematopoiesis in β thalassaemia/haemoglobin E. *Postgrad. Med. J.* **69**, 75.

Intragumtornchai, T., Minaphinant, K., Wanichsawat, C. *et al.* (1994) Echocardiographic features in patients with β thalassemia/hemoglobin E: a combining effect of anemia and iron load. *J. Med. Assoc. Thailand* **77**, 57.

Iolascon, A., Nobili, B., Pinto, L. *et al.* (1982) L'Hb Bart's in neonati della Campania. *La Pediatr.* **90**, 339.

Ion, A., Telvi, L., Chaussain, J.L. *et al.* (1996) A novel mutation in the putative DNA Helicase *XH2* is responsible for male-to-female sex reversal associated with an atypical form of the ATR-X syndrome. *Am. J. Hum. Genet.* **58**, 1185.

di Iorio, E.E., Winterhalter, K.H., Wilson, K., Rosenmund, A. & Marti, H.R. (1975) A Swiss family with hemoglobin P Galveston beta 117 His Arg, including two patients with Hb P/beta thalassemia. *Blut* **31**, 61.

Israngkura, P., Hathirat, P., Sanaskul, W. & Vaivanijkul, P. (1978a) The relationship of growth rate and hemoglobin level in thalassemia. *J. Med. Assoc. Thailand* **61**, 51.

Israngkura, P., Khemapiratana, T. & Tuchinda, P. (1978b) Bone age and bone changes in thalassemia. *J. Med. Assoc. Thailand* **61**, 53.

Israngkura, P., Siripoonya, P., Fucharoen, S. & Hathirat, P. (1987) Hemoglobin Bart's disease without hydrops manifestation. *Birth Defects* **23**, 333.

Israngkura, P., Chantarojanasiri, T., Sudhas Na Ayuthya, P. *et al.* (1988) Studies of cardiopulmonary and platelet function in thalassemic children. *Birth Defects* **23**, 385.

Issaragrisil, S., Piankijagum, A. & Wasi, P. (1981) Spinal cord compression in thalassemia. *Arch. Intern. Med.* **141**, 1033.

Issaragrisil, S., Wanachinwanawin, W., Bhuripanyo, K., Benjasuratwong, Y., Piankijagum, A. & Wasi, P. (1988) Infection in thalassemia: a retrospective study of 1,018 patients with β-thalassemia/Hb E disease. *Birth Defects* **23**, 505.

Italian Working Group on Endocrine Complications in Non-endocrine Diseases (1995) Multicentre study on prevalence of endocrine complications in thalassaemia major. *Clin. Endocrinol.* **42**, 581.

Itano, H.A. (1951) A third abnormal hemoglobin associated with hereditary hemolytic anemia. *Proc. Natl Acad. Sci. USA* **37**, 775.

Itano, H.A. (1953) Qualitative and quantitative control of adult hemoglobin. *Am. J. Hum. Genet.* **5**, 34.

Itano, H.A. (1957) The human hemoglobins: their properties and genetic control. *Adv. Protein Chem.* **12**, 216.

Itano, H.A. & Neel, J.V. (1950) A new inherited abnormality of human hemoglobin. *Proc. Natl Acad. Sci. USA* **36**, 613.

Itano, H.A. & Pauling, L. (1961) Thalassaemia and the abnormal haemoglobins. *Nature* **191**, 398.

Itano, H.A. & Robinson, E.A. (1960) Genetic control of the α and β-chains of hemoglobin. *Proc. Natl Acad. Sci. USA* **46**, 1492.

Izzo, P., Pasculli, D., Schonauer, S. *et al.* (1979) L'alfa thalassemia in Puglia. II. Screening neonatale per l'Hb di Bart. *Boll. Soc. Ital. Biol. Speriment.* **55**, 703.

Jackson, L.G., Wapner, R.J. & Barr, M.A. (1986) Safety of chorionic villus biopsy. *Lancet* **i**, 674.

Jackson, D.N., Strauss, A.A., Groncy, P.K., Bianchi, D.W. & Akabutu, J. (1990a) Outcome of neonatal survivors with homozygous α-thalassemia. *Pediatr. Res.* **27**, 266A.

Jackson, L.G., Wapner, R.J., Grebner, E.E., Barr, M.A. & Davis, G.H. (1990b) Fetal genetic diagnosis by chorionic villus sampling. In: *Human Prenatal Diagnosis* (eds K. Filkins & J.E. Russo), p. 37. Marcel Dekker, Inc., New York.

Jackson, L., Wapner, R.J. & Brambati, B. (1991) Limb abnormalities and chorionic villus sampling. *Lancet* **337**, 1422.

Jackson, L.G., Zachary, J.M., Fowler, S.E. *et al.* (1992) A randomized comparison of transcervical and transabdominal chorionic-villus sampling. The U.S. National Institute of Child Health and Human Development Chorionic-Villus Sampling and Amniocentesis Study Group. *N. Eng. J. Med.* **327**, 594.

Jackson, N., Zaki, M., Rahman, A.R., Nazim, M.N. & Osman, S. (1997) Fatal *Campylobacter jejuni* infection in a patient spelectomised for thalassaemia. *J. Clin. Pathol.* **50**, 436.

Jacob, H.S. (1970) Mechanisms of Heinz body formation and attachment to red cell membrane. *Sem. Hematol.* **7**, 341.

Jacob, F. & Monod, J. (1961) Genetic regulatory mechanisms in the synthesis of proteins. *J. Mol. Biol.* **3**, 318.

Jacob, G.F. & Raper, A.B. (1958) Hereditary persistence of foetal haemoglobin production, and its interaction with the sickle-cell trait. *Br. J. Haematol.* **4**, 138.

Jagadeeswaran, P., Tuan, D., Forget, B.G. & Weissman, S.M. (1982) A gene deletion ending at the midpoint of a repetitive DNA sequence in one form of hereditary persistence of fetal haemoglobin. *Nature* **296**, 469.

Jain, R.C. (1985) Sickle cell and thalassaemic genes in Libya. *Trans. Roy. Soc. Trop. Med. Hyg.* **79**, 132.

Jain, R.C., Andleigh, H.S. & Mehta, J.B. (1970) Haemoglobin D-thalassaemia. *Acta Haematol.* **44**, 124.

Jain, R.C., Andrew, A.M.R. & Choubisa, S.L. (1983) Sickle cell and thalassaemic genes in the tribal population of Rajasthan. *Indian J. Med. Res.* **78**, 836.

Jandl, J.H. & Greenberg, M.S. (1959) Bone marrow failure due to relative nutritional deficiency in Cooley's hemolytic anemia. *N. Eng. J. Med.* **266**, 461.

Jane, S.M. & Cunningham, J.M. (1998) Understanding fetal globin gene expression: a step towards effective HbF reactivation in haemoglobinopathies. *Br. J. Haematol.* **102**, 415.

Jane, S.M., Ney, P.A., Vanin, E.F., Gumucio, D.L. & Nienhuis, A.W. (1992) Identification of a stage selector element in the human γ-globin gene promoter that fosters preferential interaction with the 5′ HS2 enhancer when in competition with the β-promoter. *EMBO J.* **11**, 2961.

Jane, S.M., Gumucio, D.L., Ney, P.A., Cunningham, J.M. & Nienhuis, A.W. (1993) Methylation-enhanced binding of Sp1 to the stage selector element of the human γ-globin gene promoter may regulate developmental specificity of expression. *Mol. Cell. Biol.* **13**, 3272.

Jane, S.M., Nienhuis, A.W. & Cunningham, J.M. (1995) Hemoglobin switching in man and chicken is mediated by a heteromeric complex between the ubiquitous transcription factor CP2 and a developmentally specific protein. *EMBO J.* **14**, 97.

Jankovic, L., Efremov, G.D., Josifovska, O. *et al.* (1990a) An initiation codon mutation as a cause of a β⁰-thalassaemia. *Hemoglobin* **14**, 169.

Jankovic, L., Efremov, G.D., Petkov, G. *et al.* (1990b) Two novel polyadenylation mutations leading to β⁺-thalassaemia. *Br. J. Haematol.* **75**, 122.

Jankovic, L., Dimovski, A.J., Kollia, P., Karageorga, M., Loukopoulos, D. & Huisman, T.H.J. (1991) A C-G mutation at nt position 6 3′ to the terminating codon may be the cause of a silent β-thalassaemia. *Int. J. Hematol.* **54**, 289.

Jankovic, L., Dimovski, A.J., Sukarova, E., Juricic, D. & Efremov, G.D. (1992) A new mutation in the β-globin gene (IVS II-850 G→C) found in a Yugoslavian thalassemia heterozygote. *Haematologica* **77**, 119.

Jankowski, J.A.Z. & Polak, J.M. (1996) *Clinical Gene Analysis and Manipulation.* Cambridge University Press, Cambridge.

Jarman, A.P. & Higgs, D.R. (1988) A new hypervariable marker for the human α-globin gene cluster. *Am. J. Hum. Genet.* **42**, 8.

Jarman, A.P., Nicholls, R.D., Weatherall, D.J., Clegg, J.B. & Higgs, D.R. (1986) Molecular characterization of a hypervariable region downstream of the human α-globin gene cluster. *EMBO J.* **5**, 1857.

Jarman, A.P., Wood, W.G., Sharpe, J.A., Gourdon, G., Ayyub, H. & Higgs, D.R. (1991) Characterization of the major regulatory element upstream of the human α-globin gene cluster. *Mol. Cell. Biol.* **11**, 4679.

Jarolim, P., Lahav, M., Liu, S.C. & Palek, J. (1990) Effect of hemoglobin oxidation products on the stability of red cell membrane skeletons and the association of skeletal protein: correlation with a release of hemin. *Blood* **76**, 2125.

Jauniaux, E., Van Maldergem, L., De Munter, C., Moscoso, G. & Gillerot, Y. (1990) Nonimmune hydrops fetalis associated with genetic abnormalities. *Obstet. Gynecol.* **75**, 568.

Jayabose, S., Tugal, O., Sandoval, C. *et al.* (1996) Clinical and hematologic effects of hydroxyurea in children with sickle cell anemia. *J. Pediatr.* **129**, 559.

Jean, G., Terzoli, S., Mauri, R. *et al.* (1984) Cirrhosis associated with multiple transfusions in thalassemia. *Arch. Dis. Child.* **59**, 67.

Jeffreys, A.J. (1979) DNA sequences in the $^{G}\gamma$-, $^{A}\gamma$-, δ- and β-globin genes of man. *Cell* **18**, 1.

Jeffreys, A.J. (1987) Highly variable minisatellites and DNA fingerprints. *Biochem. Soc. Trans.* **15**, 309.

Jenkins, T. & Stevens, K. (1970) Hereditary persistence of foetal haemoglobin in a South African family. *S. A. Med. J.* **44**, 111.

Jennings, M.W., Jones, R.W., Wood, W.G. & Weatherall, D.J. (1985) Analysis of an inversion within the human beta globin gene cluster. *Nucl. Acids Res.* **13**, 2897.

Jensen, M., Wirtz, A., Walther, J.U., Schemken, E.M., Laryea, M.D. & Driesel, A.J. (1984) Hereditary persistence of fetal haemoglobin (HPFH) in conjunction with a chromosomal translocation involving the haemoglobin beta locus. *Br. J. Haematol.* **56**, 87.

Jensen, C.E., Tuck, S.M., Old, J. *et al.* (1997) Incidence of endocrine complications and clinical disease severity related to genotype analysis and iron overload in patients with β-thalassaemia. *Eur. J. Haematol.* **59**, 76.

Jensen, C.E., Tuck, S.M., Agnew, J.E. *et al.* (1998) High prevalence of low bone mass in thalassaemia major. *Br. J. Haematol.* **103**, 911.

Jessup, M. & Manno, C.S. (1998) Diagnosis and management of iron-induced heart disease in Cooley's anemia. *Ann. N. Y. Acad. Sci.* **850**, 242.

Jewett, J.F. (1976) Sickle-cell trait, thalassemia, G-6-PD deficiency and puerperal pulmonary embolism. *N. Eng. J. Med.* **295**, 1076.

Jiang, N.H., Liang, S., Su, C., Nechtman, J.F. & Stoming, T.A. (1993) A novel β-thalassemia mutation [IVS-II-5 (G→C)] in a Chinese family from Guangxi Province, P.R. China. *Hemoglobin* **17**, 563.

Jimenez, G., Griffiths, S.D., Ford, A.M., Greaves, M.F. & Enver, T. (1992) Activation of the beta-globin locus control region precedes commitment to the erythroid lineage. *Proc. Natl Acad. Sci. USA* **89**, 10618.

Jinks-Robertson, S., Michelitch, M. & Ramcharan, S. (1993) Substrate length requirements for efficient mitotic recombination in *Saccharomyces cerevisiae*. *Mol. Cell. Biol.* **13**, 3937.

Johnsen, J.K., Ibbotson, R.N. & Horwood. J.M. (1966) Thalassaemia minor in Australians of North European extraction: a report of five families. *Aust. Med. J.* **15**, 245.

Johnson, K., Stastny, J.F. & Rucknagel, D.L. (1994) Fat embolism syndrome associated with asthma and sickle cell-β$^{(+)}$-thalassaemia. *Am. J. Hematol.* **46**, 354.

Johnston, F.E. & Roseman, J.M. (1967) The effects of more frequent transfusions upon bone loss in thalassemia major. *Pediatr. Res.* **1**, 479.

Joishy, S.K., Griner, P.F. & Rowley, P.T. (1976) Sickle β-thalassemia: Identical twins differing in severity implicate nongenetic factors influencing course. *Am. J. Hematol.* **1**, 23.

Jonas, M.M. (1999) Hepatitis C infection in children. *N. Eng. J. Med.* **341**, 912.

Jones, R.T. (1964) Structural studies on aminoethylated hemoglobins by automatic peptide chromatography. *Cold Spring Harbor Sympos. Quant. Biol.* **29**, 297.

Jones, R.T. & Schroeder, W.A. (1963) Chemical characterization and subunit hybridization of human hemoglobin H and associated compounds. *Biochemistry* **2**, 1357.

Jones, R.T., Schroeder, W.A., Balog, J.E. & Vinograd, J.R. (1959) Gross structure of hemoglobin A. *J. Am. Chem. Soc.* **81**, 3161.

Jones, R.W., Old, J.M., Trent, R.J., Clegg, J.B. & Weatherall, D.J. (1981a) Major rearrangement in the human β-globin gene cluster. *Nature* **291**, 39.

Jones, R.W., Old, J.M., Trent, R.J., Clegg, J.B. & Weatherall, D.J. (1981b) Restriction mapping of a new deletion responsible for $^{G}\gamma$ (δβ)^0 thalassemia. *Nucl. Acids Res.* **9**, 6813.

Jones, R.W., Old, J.M., Wood, W.G., Clegg, J.B. & Weatherall, D.J. (1982) Restriction endonuclease maps of the β-like globin gene cluster in the British and Greek forms of HPFH, and for one example of $^{G}\gamma\beta^+$ HPFH. *Br. J. Haematol.* **50**, 415.

Jones, S. (1993) *The Language of the Genes.* Harper Collins, London.

de Jong, W.W., Khan, P.M. & Bernini, L.F. (1975) Hemoglobin Koya Dora: high frequency of a chain termination mutant. *Am. J. Hum. Genet.* **27**, 81.

Jonxis, J.H.P. (1965) *Abnormal Haemoglobins in Africa*, p. 67. Blackwell Scientific Publications, Oxford.

Jonxis, J.H.P. & Visser, H.K.A. (1956) Determination of low percentages of fetal hemoglobin in blood of normal children. *Am. J. Dis. Child.* **92**, 588.

Jootar, P. & Fucharoen, S. (1990) Cardiac involvement in β-thalassemia/hemoglobin E disease: clinical and hemodynamic findings. *Southeast Asian J. Trop. Med. Publ. Hlth* **21**, 269.

Josephson, A.M., Masri, M.S., Singer, L., Dworkin, D. & Singer, K. (1958) Starch block electrophoretic studies of human hemoglobin solutions. II. Results in cord blood, thalassemia and other hematologic disorders: comparison with Tiselius electrophoresis. *Blood* **13**, 543.

Joshi, S.R., Mehta, M.M., Mehta, D.M., Bapat, J.B., Baxi, A.J. & Bhatia, H.M. (1978) Genetic studies in three tribal groups of Dadra and Nagar Haveli region in Western India. *Indian J. Phys. Anthrop. Hum. Genet.* **4**, 133.

Jouanolle, A.M., Fergelot, P., Gandon, G., Yaouang, J., Le Gall, J.Y. & David, V. (1997) A candidate gene for hemochromatosis: frequency of the C282Y and H63D mutations. *Hum. Genet.* **100**, 544.

Jullien, A.M., Courouce, A.M., Richard, D., Favre, M., Lefrere, J.J. & Habibi, B. (1988) Transmission of HIV blood from seronegative donors. *Lancet* **2**, 1248.

Juncà, J., Vela, D., Orts, M., Riutort, N. & Feliu, E. (1995) Treating the anaemia of pregnancy with heterozygous β thalassaemia with recombinant human erythropoietin (r-HuEPO). *Eur. J. Haematol.* **55**, 277.

Juricic, D., Crepinko, I., Efremov, G.D. *et al.* (1983) Hb A$_2$-Zagreb or α$_2$δ$_2$ (125)(H3)Gln→Glu, a new δ chain variation in association with δβ-thalassemia. *Hemoglobin* **7**, 443.

Jurkiewicz, M.J., Pearson, H.A. & Furlow, L.T. (1969) Reconstruction of the maxilla in thalassemia. *Ann. N. Y. Acad. Sci.* **165**, 437.

Kacian, D.L., Gambino, R., Dow, L.W. *et al.* (1973) Decreased globin messenger RNA in thalassemia detected by molecular hybridization. *Proc. Natl Acad. Sci. USA* **70**, 1886.

Kadonaga, J.T. (1998) Eukaryotic transcription: an interlaced network of transcription factors and chromatin-modifying machines. *Cell* **92**, 307.

Kaeda, J.S., Saary, M.J., Sauders, S.M., Vulliamy, T.J. & Luzzatto, L. (1992) Dominant β thalassaemia trait due to a novel insertion. *Proceedings of the Thalassaemia Meeting.* Nice, France.

Kahane, I., Polliack, A., Rachmilewitz, E.A., Bayer, E.A. & Skutelsky, E. (1978) Distribution of sialic acids on the red blood cell membrane in β thalassaemia. *Nature* **271**, 674.

Kahn, M.J., Scher, C., Rozans, M., Michaels, R.K., Leissinger, C. & Krause, J. (1997) Factor V Leiden is not responsible for stroke in patients with sickling disorders and is uncommon in African Americans with sickle cell disease. *Am. J. Hematol.* **54**, 12.

Kalaydjieva, L., Eigel, A. & Horst, J. (1989) The molecular basis of β thalassaemia in Bulgaria. *J. Med. Genet.* **26**, 614.

Kalef-Exra, J., Challa, A., Chaliasos, N. *et al.* (1995) Bone minerals in beta-thalassemia minor. *Bone* **16**, 651.

Kalmanti, M., Kalmantis, T., Liacopoulou, T., Tsoumakas, K., Ladis, V.

& Kattamis, C. (1991) Serum erythropoietin in regularly transfused thalassemic patients. *Haematologia-Budap.* **24**, 129.

Kalpravidh, R.W., Komolvanich, S., Wilairat, P. & Fucharoen, S. (1995) Globin chain turnover in reticulocytes from patients with β^0-thalassaemia/Hb E disease. *Eur. J. Haematol.* **55**, 322.

Kaltsoya, A., Fessas, P. & Stavropoulos, A. (1966) Hemoglobins in early human development. *Science* **153**, 1417.

Kamuzora, H., Ringelhann, B., Konotey-Ahulu, F.I.D., Lehmann, H. & Lorkin, P.A. (1974) The γ chain in a Ghanaian adult, homozygous for hereditary persistence of fetal haemoglobin. *Acta Haematol.* **51**, 179.

Kamuzora, H., Ringelhann, B., Konotey-Ahulu, F.I.D., Lehmann, H. & Lorkin, P.A. (1975) Further investigation of the γ-chain in a Ghanaian adult, homozygous for hereditary persistence of fetal haemoglobin. Isolation of γCB3 peptides and $^{G}\gamma^{A}\gamma$ ratio determination in human Hb F. *Acta Haematol.* **53**, 315.

Kan, Y.W. & Dozy, A.M. (1978a) Antenatal diagnosis of sickle cell anaemia by DNA analysis of amniotic-fluid cells. *Lancet* **ii**, 910.

Kan, Y.W. & Dozy, A.M. (1978b) Polymorphism of DNA sequence adjacent to human β-globin structural gene: relationship to sickle mutation. *Proc. Natl Acad. Sci. USA* **75**, 5631.

Kan, Y.W. & Nathan, D.G. (1970) Mild thalassemia: the result of interactions of alpha and beta thalassemia genes. *J. Clin. Invest.* **49**, 635.

Kan, Y.W., Schwartz, E. & Nathan, D.G. (1968) Globin chain synthesis in alpha thalassemia syndromes. *J. Clin. Invest.* **47**, 2515.

Kan, Y.W., Dozy, A.M., Alter, B.P., Frigoletto, F.D. & Nathan, D.G. (1972a) Detection of the sickle gene in the human fetus. Potential for intrauterine diagnosis of sickle-cell anemia. *N. Eng. J. Med.* **287**, 1.

Kan, Y.W., Forget, B.G. & Nathan, D.G. (1972b) Gamma-beta thalassemia: a cause of hemolytic disease of the newborn. *N. Eng. J. Med.* **286**, 129.

Kan, Y.W., Nathan, D.G. & Lodish, H.F. (1972c) Equal synthesis of α and β globin chains in erythroid precursors in heterozygous β thalassemia. *J. Clin. Invest.* **51**, 1906.

Kan, Y.W., Dozy, A.M. & Holland, J.P. (1973) Absence of functional β globin mRNA in homozygous β^0-thalassemia. *Blood* **42**, 991.

Kan, Y.W., Calenti, C., Carnazz, V., Guidotti, R. & Rieder, R.F. (1974a) Fetal blood-sampling *in utero. Lancet* **1**, 79.

Kan, Y.W., Nathan, D.G., Cividalli, G. & Crookston, M.C. (1974b) Concentration of fetal red blood cells of hemoglobinopathies. *Blood* **43**, 411.

Kan, Y.W., Todd, D. & Dozy, A.M. (1974c) Haemoglobin Constant Spring synthesis in red cell precursors. *Br. J. Haematol.* **28**, 103.

Kan, Y.W., Todd, D., Holland, J. & Dozy, A. (1974d) Absence of α globin mRNA in homozygous α-thalassemia. *J. Clin. Invest.* **53**, 37a.

Kan, Y.W., Dozy, A.M., Varmus, H.E. *et al.* (1975a) Deletion of α-globin genes in haemoglobin H disease demonstrates multiple α structural loci. *Nature* **255**, 255.

Kan, Y.W., Golbus, M.S., Klein, P. & Dozy, A.M. (1975b) Successful application of prenatal diagnosis in a pregnancy at risk for homozygous beta-thalassemia. *N. Eng. J. Med.* **292**, 1096.

Kan, Y.W., Golbus, M.S. & Trecartin, R. (1975c) Prenatal diagnosis of homozygous β-thalassaemia. *Lancet* **ii**, 790.

Kan, Y.W., Holland, J.P., Dozy, A.M., Charache, S. & Kazazian, H.H. (1975d) Deletion of β-globin structural gene in hereditary persistence of foetal haemoglobin. *Nature* **258**, 162.

Kan, Y.W., Holland, J.P., Dozy, A.M. & Varmus, H.E. (1975e) Demonstration of non-functional β-globin mRNA in homozygous β^0-thalassemia. *Proc. Natl Acad. Sci. USA* **72**, 5140.

Kan, Y.W., Golbus, M.S. & Dozy, A.M. (1976) Prenatal diagnosis of

α-thalassemia: clinical application of molecular hybridization. *N. Eng. J. Med.* **295**, 1165.

Kan, Y.W., Dozy, A.M., Trecartin, R. & Todd, D. (1977a) Identification of a nondeletion defect in α-thalassemia. *N. Eng. J. Med.* **297**, 1081.

Kan, Y.W., Trecartin, R.F., Golbus, M.S. & Filly, R.A. (1977b) Prenatal diagnosis of β-thalassaemia and sickle cell anaemia. *Lancet* **i**, 269.

Kan, Y.W., Lee, K.Y., Furbetta, M., Angius, A. & Cao, A. (1980) Polymorphism of DNA sequences in the β globin gene region. Application to prenatal diagnosis of β^0 thalassemia in Sardinia. *N. Eng. J. Med.* **302**, 185.

Kanavakis, E., Wainscoat, J.S., Wood, W.G. *et al.* (1982) The interaction of α thalassaemia with heterozygous β thalassaemia. *Br. J. Haematol.* **52**, 465.

Kanavakis, E., Metaxatou-Mavromati, A., Kattamis, C., Wainscoat, J.S. & Wood, W.G. (1983) The triplicated α gene locus and β thalassaemia. *Br. J. Haematol.* **54**, 201.

Kanavakis, E., Tzotzos, S., Liapaki, A., Metaxotou-Mavromati, A. & Kattamis, C. (1986) Frequency of α-thalassemia in Greece. *Am. J. Hematol.* **22**, 225.

Kanavakis, E., Tzotzos, S., Kiapaki, K., Metaxotou-Mavromati, A. & Kattamis, C. (1988) Molecular basis and prevalence of α-thalassemia in Greece. *Birth Defects* **23**, 377.

Kanavakis, E., Traeger-Synodinos, J., Papasotiriou, I. *et al.* (1996) The interaction of α^0 thalassaemia with Hb Icaria: three unusual cases of haemoglobinopathy H. *Br. J. Haematol.* **92**, 332.

Kantchev, K.N., Tcholakov, B.N., Casey, R., Lehmann, H. & El Hazmi, M. (1975) Twelve families with Hb O Arab in the Burgas district of Bulgaria. Observations on sixteen examples of Hb O Arab beta^0 thalassaemia. *Humangenetik* **26**, 93.

Kaplan, E. & Zuelzer, W.W. (1950) Erythrocyte survival studies in childhood. II. Studies in Mediterranean anemia. *J. Lab. Clin. Med.* **36**, 517.

Kar, B.C., Satapathy, R.K., Kulozik, A.E. *et al.* (1986) Sickle cell disease in Orissa State, India. *Lancet* **ii**, 1198.

Karahanyan, E., Stoyaniva, A., Moumdzhiev, I. & Ivanov, I. (1994) Secondary diabetes in children with thalassaemia major (homozygous thalassaemia). *Folia Med. Plovdiv.* **35**, 29.

Karlsson, S., Bodine, D.M., Perry, L., Papayannopoulou, T. & Nienhuis, A.W. (1988) Expression of the human β-globin gene following retroviral-mediated transfer into multipotential hematopoietic progenitors of mice. *Proc. Natl Acad. Sci. USA* **85**, 6062.

Karpathios, T., Nicolaidou, P., Korkas, A. & Thomaidis, T. (1977) The hand–foot syndrome in sickle cell β-thalassemia. *J. A. M. A.* **238**, 1540.

Kattamis, C., Touliatis, N., Chaidis, S. & Matsaniotis, N. (1970) Growth of children with thalassemia. *Arch. Dis. Child.* **45**, 502.

Kattamis, C., Lagos, P., Metaxatou-Mavromati, A. & Matsaniotis, N. (1972) Serum iron and unsaturated iron-binding capacity in the β-thalassaemia trait: their relation to the levels of haemoglobins A, A$_2$ and F. *J. Med. Genet.* **9**, 154.

Kattamis, C., Metataxatou-Mavromati, A., Karamboula, K., Nasika, E. & Lehman, H. (1973) The clinical and haematological findings in children inheriting two types of thalassaemia: high A$_2$ type, beta-thalassaemia and high-F type or delta beta-thalassaemia. *Br. J. Haematol.* **25**, 375.

Kattamis, C., Ladis, V. & Metaxatou-Mavromati, A. (1975) Hemoglobins F and A$_2$ in Greek patients with homozygous β and $\beta/\delta\beta$ thalassaemia. In: *Abnormal Haemoglobins and Thalassaemia: Diagnostic Aspects* (ed. R.M. Schmidt), p. 209. Academic Press, New York.

Kattamis, C., Karambula, K., Metaxatou-Mavromati, A., Ladis, V. &

Constantopoulos, A. (1978) Prevalence of β^0 and β^+thalassemia genes in Greek children with homozygous β-thalassemia. *Hemoglobin* **2**, 29.

Kattamis, C., Metaxatou-Mavromati, A., Wood, W.G., Nash, J.R. & Weatherall, D.J. (1979) The heterogeneity of normal Hb A_2-β thalassaemia in Greece. *Br. J. Haematol.* **42**, 109.

Kattamis, C., Metaxotou-Mavromati, A., Tsiarta, E. *et al.* (1980) Haemoglobin Bart's hydrops syndrome in Greece. *Br. Med. J.* **269**, 268.

Kattamis, C., Efremov, G. & Pootrakul, S. (1981a) Effectiveness of one tube osmotic fragility screening in detecting β-thalassaemia trait. *J. Med. Genet.* **18**, 266.

Kattamis, C., Mallias, A., Metaxatou-Mavromati, A. & Matsaniotis, N. (1981b) Screening for beta-thalassaemias. *Lancet* **ii**, 930.

Kattamis, C., Tzotzos, S., Kanavakis, E., Synodinos, J. & Metaxatou-Mavromati, A. (1988) Correlation of clinical phenotype to genotype in haemoglobin H disease. *Lancet* **i**, 442.

Kattamis, C., Óu, H., Cheng, G. *et al.* (1990) Molecular characterization of β-thalassaemia in 174 Greek patients with thalassaemia major. *Br. J. Haematol.* **74**, 342.

Kaur, P. & Kaur, B. (1995) Thalassemia in Penang. In: *First Asian Congress on Thalassemia*, p. 70. Penang, Malaysia.

Kazazian, H.H. (1990) The thalassemia syndromes: molecular basis and prenatal diagnosis in 1990. *Sem. Hematol.* **27**, 209.

Kazazian, H.H. Jr (1998) Mobile elements and disease. *Curr. Opin. Genet. Dev.* **8**, 343.

Kazazian, H.H. & Boehm, C.D. (1988) Molecular basis and prenatal diagnosis of β-thalassemia. *Blood* **72**, 1107.

Kazazian, H.H. & Woodhead, A.P. (1973) Hemoglobin A synthesis in the developing fetus. *N. Eng. J. Med.* **289**, 58.

Kazazian, H.H. & Woodhead, A.P. (1974) Adult hemoglobin synthesis in the human fetus. *Ann. N. Y. Acad. Sci.* **241**, 691.

Kazazian, H.H., Ginder, G.D., Snyder, P.C., van Beneddan, R.J. & Woodhead, A.P. (1975) Further evidence of a quantitative deficiency of chain specific globin mRNA in the thalassemia syndromes. *Proc. Natl Acad. Sci. USA* **72**, 567.

Kazazian, H.H. Jr, Orkin, S.H., Boehm, C.D., Sexton, J.P. & Antonarakis, S.E. (1983) β-Thalassemia due to deletion of the nucleotide which is substituted in sickle cell anemia. *Am. J. Hum. Genet.* **35**, 1028.

Kazazian, H.H. Jr, Orkin, S.H., Antonarakis, S.E. *et al.* (1984) Molecular characterization of seven β-thalassemia mutations in Asian Indians. *EMBO J.* **3**, 593.

Kazazian, H.H., Dowling, C.E., Waber, P.G., Huang, S. & Lo, W.H.Y. (1986a) The spectrum of β thalassaemia genes in China and Southeast Asia. *Blood* **68**, 964.

Kazazian, H.H., Orkin, S.H., Boehm, C.D. *et al.* (1986b) Characterization of a spontaneous mutation to a β-thalassemia allele. *Am. J. Hum. Genet.* **38**, 860.

Kazazian, H.H., Dowling, C.E., Hurwitz, R.L., Coleman, M. & Adams, J.G. (1989) III. Thalassemia mutations in exon 3 of the β-globin gene often cause a dominant form of thalassemia and show no predilection for malarial-endemic regions of the world. *Am. J. Hum. Genet.* **45**, A242.

Kazazian, H.H. Jr, Dowling, C.E., Hurwitz, R.L., Coleman, M., Stopeck, A. & Adams, J.G. (1992) III. Dominant thalassemia-like phenotypes associated with mutations in exon 3 of the β-globin gene. *Blood* **79**, 3014.

Keberle, H. (1964) The biochemistry of desferrioxamine and its relation to iron metabolism. *Ann. N. Y. Acad. Sci.* **119**, 758.

Keens, T.G., O'Neal, M.H., Ortega, J.A., Hyman, C.B. & Platzker, A.C.G. (1980) Pulmonary function abnormalities in thalassemia patients on a hypertransfusion program. *Pediatr.* **65**, 1013.

Kekwick, J.F. & Lehmann, H. (1960) Sedimentation characteristics of the γ-chain haemoglobin (Haemoglobin 'Bart's'). *Nature* **187**, 158.

Kelemen, E., Calvo, W. & Fliedner, T.M. (1981) *Atlas of Human Hemopoietic Development*. Springer-Verlag, Berlin.

Keller, W. (1995) No end yet to messenger RNA 3′ processing! *Cell* **81**, 829.

Keller, G. & Snodgrass, H.R. (1999) Human embryonic stem cells: the future is now. *Nature Med.* **5**, 151.

Kelly, D.A., Price, E., Jani, B., Wright, V., Rossiter, M. & Walker-Smith, J.A. (1987) *Yersinia enterocolitica* in iron overload. *J. Pediatr. Gastroenterol. Nutr.* **6**, 643.

Kendall, A.G., Ojwang, P.J., Schroeder, W.A. & Huisman, T.H.J. (1973) Hemoglobin Kenya, the product of a γ-β fusion gene: studies of the family. *Am. J. Hum. Genet.* **25**, 548.

Kevles, D.J. (1985) *In the Name of Eugenics*. University of California Press, Berkeley.

Kevles, D.J. & Hood, L. (1992) *The Code of Codes*. Harvard University Press, Cambridge, MA.

Kevy, S.V., Jacobson, M.S., Fosburg, M. *et al.* (1988) A new approach to neocyte transfusion: preliminary report. *J. Clin. Apher.* **4**, 194.

Khan, M.A. (1992) Psycho-social aspects of infection and AIDS in multiple transfused thalassemic children. *Indian J. Pediatr.* **59**, 429.

Khan, S.N. & Riazuddin, S. (1998) Molecular characterisation of β-thalassemia in Pakistan. *Hemoglobin* **22**, 333.

Khanh, N.C., Thu, L.T., Truc, D.B., Hoa, D.P., Hoa, T.T. & Ha, T.H. (1990) Beta-thalassemia/haemoglobin E disease in Vietnam. *J. Trop. Pediatr.* **36**, 43.

Khattak, M.F. & Saleem, M. (1992) Prevalence of heterozygous β-thalassemia in Northern areas of Pakistan. *J. Pakistan Med. Assoc.* **42**, 32.

Kheradpir, M.H. & Albouyeh, M. (1985) Partial splenectomy in the treatment of thalassaemia major. *Kinderchirurgie* **40**, 195.

Kilmartin, J.V. & Clegg, J.B. (1967) Amino-acid replacements in horse haemoglobin. *Nature* **213**, 269.

Kilmartin, J.V. & Rossi-Bernardi, L. (1969) Inhibition of CO_2 combination and reduction of the Bohr effect in haemoglobin chemically modified at its α amino groups. *Nature* **222**, 1243.

Kilmartin, J.V. & Rossi-Bernardi, L. (1971) The binding of carbon dioxide by horse haemoglobin. *Biochem. J.* **124**, 31.

Kimberland, M.L., Boehm, C.D. & Kazazian, H.H. Jr (1995) Two novel β-thalassemia alleles: poly A signal (AATAAA→AAAA) and –92 C→T. *Hum. Mutat.* **5**, 275.

Kimura, A., Matsunaga, E., Takihara, Y., Nakamura, T. & Tagaki, Y. (1983) Structural analysis of a β-thalassemia gene found in Taiwan. *J. Biol. Chem.* **258**, 2748.

King, M.A.R., Wiltshire, B.G., Lehmann, H. & Morimoto, H. (1972) An unstable haemoglobin with a reduced oxygen affinity: Haemoglobin Peterborough β111(G13) Valine→Phenylalanine, its interaction with normal haemoglobin and with haemoglobin Lepore. *Br. J. Haematol.* **22**, 125.

Kinney, T.R., Friedman, S.H., Cifuentes, E., Kim, H.C. & Schwartz, E. (1978) Variations in globin synthesis in delta-beta-thalassaemia. *Br. J. Haematol.* **38**, 15.

Kinniburgh, A.J., Maquat, L.E., Schedl, T., Rachmilewitz, E. & Ross, J. (1982) mRNA-deficient β^0-thalassemia resulting from a single nucleotide deletion. *Nucl. Acids Res.* **10**, 5421.

Kitayaporn, D., Nelson, K.E., Charoenlarp, P. & Pholpothi, T. (1992) Haemoglobin-E in the presence of oxidative substances from fava bean may be protective against *Plasmodium falciparum* malaria. *Trans. Roy. Soc. Trop. Med. Hyg.* **86**, 240.

Klee, G.G. (1980) Role of morphology, and erythrocyte indices in screening and diagnosis. A. The automated hematology group (CBC) as a screen for thalassemias and hemoglobinopathies. In:

Hemoglobinopathies and Thalassemias. Laboratory Methods and Clinical Cases (ed. V.F. Fairbanks), p. 38. Decker, New York.

Kleihauer, E., Braun, H. & Betke, K. (1957) Demonstration von fetealem haemoglobin in den Erythrocyten eines Blutaussttriche. *Klin. Wochenschr.* **35**, 635.

Klein, N., Sen, A., Rusby, J., Ratip, S., Modell, B. & Olivieri, N.F. (1998) The psychosocial burden of Cooley's anemia in affected children and their parents. *Ann. N. Y. Acad. Sci.* **850**, 512.

Kletsky, O.A., Costin, G., Marrs, R.P., Bernstein, G., March, C.M. & Mishell, D.R. (1979) Gonadotrophin insufficiency in patients with thalassemia major. *J. Clin. Endocrinol. Metab.* **48**, 901.

Knox-Macaulay, H.H.M. & Weatherall, D.J. (1974) Studies of red-cell membrane function in heterozygous β thalassaemia and other hypochromic anaemias. *Br. J. Haematol.* **28**, 277.

Knox-Macaulay, H.H.M., Weatherall, D.J., Clegg, J.B., Bradley, J. & Brown, M.J. (1972) Clinical and biosynthetic characterization of αβ-thalassaemia. *Br. J. Haematol.* **22**, 497.

Knox-Macaulay, H.H.M., Weatherall, D.J., Clegg, J.B. & Pembrey, M.E. (1973) Thalassaemia in the British. *Br. Med. J.* **iii**, 150.

Ko, T.-M. & Li, S.-F. (1999) Molecular characterization of the $--^{FIL}$ determinant of alpha-thalassaemia. *Am. J. Hematol.* **60**, 173.

Ko, T.-M., Hsu, P.-M., Chen, C.-J., Hsieh, F.-J., Hsieh, C.-Y. & Lee, T.-Y. (1989) Incidence study of heterozygous β-thalassemia in Northern Taiwan. *J. Formosan Med. Assoc.* **88**, 631.

Ko, T.-M., Hsieh, F.-J., Hsu, P.-M. & Lee, T.-Y. (1991) Molecular characterization of severe α-thalassemias causing hydrops fetalis in Taiwan. *Am. J. Med. Genet.* **39**, 317.

Ko, T.-M., Chen, T.-A., Hsieh, M.-I. *et al.* (1993a) Alpha-thalassemia in the four major aboriginal groups in Taiwan. *Hum. Genet.* **92**, 79.

Ko, T.M., Tseng, L.H., Hsieh, F.J. & Lee, T.Y. (1993b) Prenatal diagnosis of HbH disease due to compound heterozygosity for southeast Asian deletion and Hb Constant Spring by polymerase chain reaction. *Prenat. Diag.* **13**, 143.

Ko, T.-M., Tseng, L.-H., Hsu, P.-M. *et al.* (1997a) Molecular characterization of β-thalassemia in Taiwan and the identification of two new mutations. *Hemoglobin* **21**, 131.

Ko, T.M., Tseng, L.H., Hwa, H.L. *et al.* (1997b) Misdiagnosis of homozygous α-thalassemia 1 may occur if polymerase chain reaction alone is used in prenatal diagnosis. *Prenat. Diag.* **17**, 505.

Ko, T.-M., Tseng, L.-H., Kao, C.-H. *et al.* (1998) Molecular characterization and PCR diagnosis of Thailand deletion of α-globin gene cluster. *Am. J. Hematol.* **57**, 124.

Kobayashi, Y., Fukumaki, Y., Komatsu, N., Ohba, Y., Miyaji, T. & Miura, Y. (1987) A novel globin structural mutant, Showa-Yakushiji (β110 Leu-Pro) causing a β-thalassemia phenotype. *Blood* **70**, 1688.

Koch, L.A. & Shapiro, B. (1932) Erythroblastic anemia; review of cases reported showing roentgenographic changes in bones and 5 additional cases. *Am. J. Dis. Child.* **44**, 318.

Koenig, H.M. & Vedvick, T.S. (1975) Alpha thalassemia in American-born Filipino infants. *J. Pediatr.* **87**, 756.

Kolatat, T. (1964) Oxygen affinity of hemoglobin E Siriraj. *Hosp. Gazette* **16**, 205.

Kollia, P., Gonzalez-Redondo, J.M., Stoming, T.A., Loukopoulos, D., Politis, C. & Huisman, T.H.J. (1989) Frameshift codon 5 [FSC-5 (-CT)] thalassemia; a novel mutation detected in a Greek patient. *Hemoglobin* **13**, 597.

Kollia, P., Voskaridou, E., Rombos, J. *et al.* (1990) Prenatal diagnosis of thalassemia intermedia: is it justified? *Ann. N. Y. Acad. Sci.* **612**, 521.

Kollia, P., Karababa, P.H., Sinopoulou, K. *et al.* (1992) β-Thalassaemia mutations and the underlying β gene cluster haplotypes in the Greek population. *Gene Geograph.* **6**, 59.

Kollias, G., Wrighton, N., Hurst, J. & Grosveld, F. (1986) Regulated

expression of human $^{A}\gamma$-, β-, and hybrid γβ-globin genes in transgenic mice: manipulation of the developmental expression patterns. *Cell* **46**, 89.

Kollias, G., Hurst, J., deBoer, E. & Grosveld, F. (1987) The human β-globin gene contains a downstream developmental specific enhancer. *Nucl. Acids Res.* **15**, 5739.

Kolquist, K.A., Vnencak-Jones, C.L., Swift, L., Page, D.L., Johnson, J.E. & Denison, M.R. (1996) Fatal fat embolism syndrome in a child with undiagnosed hemoglobion S/β⁺ thalassemia: a complication of acute parvovirus B19 infection. *Pediatr. Pathol. Lab. Med.* **16**, 71.

Konigsberg, W., Guidotti, G. & Hill, R.J. (1961) The amino acid sequence of the α-chain of human hemoglobin. *J. Biol. Chem.* **236**, 55.

Konotey-Ahulu, F.I.D. (1973) Effect of environment on sickle cell disease in West Africa: epidemiologic and clinical considerations. In: *Sickle Cell Disease* (eds H. Abramson, J. Bertles & D.L. Wethers), p. 20. Mosby, St Louis.

Konotey-Ahulu, F.I.D. & Ringelhann, B. (1969) Sickle cell anaemia, sickle cell thalassaemia, sickle cell haemoglobin C disease, and asymptomatic haemoglobin C thalassaemia in one Ghanaian family. *Br. Med. J.* **i**, 606.

Kontessis, P., Mayopoulou-Symvoulidis, D., Symvoulidis, A. & Kontopoulou-Griva, I. (1992) Renal involvement in sickle cell-β thalassemia. *Nephron* **61**, 10.

Kontoghiorghes, G.J., Bartlett, A.N., Hoffbrand, A.V. *et al.* (1990) Long-term trial with the oral iron chelator 1,2-dimethyl-3-hydroxypyrid-4-one (L1). *Br. J. Haematol.* **76**, 295.

Korber, E. (1886) Inaugural Dissertation: '*Uber Differenzen Blutforbstoffes*', Dorpat. Cited by H. Bischoff (1926) in *Z. Exp. Med.* **48**, 472.

Koren, A., Garty, I., Antonelli, D. & Katzuni, E. (1987) Right ventricular cardiac dysfunction in β-thalassemia major. *Am. J. Dis. Child.* **141**, 93.

Korovessis, P.G., Milis, Z.T., Spastris, P.M., Urania, P. & Spyropoulos, P. (1990) Acetabular protrusion in thalassemia. A report of four cases. *Clin. Orthop.* **254**, 199.

Kosteas, T., Moschonas, N. & Anagnou, N.P. (1996) The molecular basis for the phenotypic differences between δβ-thalassemia and HPFH: the role of the two silencers upstream of the δ-globin gene. *Blood* **88**, 105a.

Kosteas, T., Palena, A. & Anagnou, N.P. (1997) Molecular cloning of the breakpoints of the hereditary persistence of fetal hemoglobin type-6 (HPFH-6) deletion and sequence analysis of the novel juxtaposed region from the 3' end of the β-globin gene cluster. *Hum. Genet.* **100**, 441.

Kotkow, K.J. & Orkin, S.H. (1995) Dependence of globin gene expression in mouse erythroleukaemia cells on the NF-E2 heterodimer. *Mol. Cell. Biol.* **15**, 4640.

Kotkow, K.J. & Orkin, S.H. (1996) Complexity of the erythroid transcription factor NF-E2 as revealed by gene targeting of the mouse p18 NF-E2 locus. *Proc. Natl Acad. Sci. USA* **93**, 3514.

Kouides, P.A., Slapak, C.A., Rossenwasser, L.J. & Miller, K.B. (1988) *Pneumocystis carinii* pneumonia as a complication of desferrioxamine therapy. *Br. J. Haematol.* **70**, 382.

Kraus, A.P., Koch, B. & Burckett, L. (1961) Two families showing interaction of haemoglobin C or thalassaemia with high foetal haemoglobin in adults. *Br. Med. J.* **i**, 1434.

Kreimer-Birnbaum, M., Pinkerton, P.H., Bannerman, R.M. & Hutchison, H.E. (1966) Urinary 'dipyrroles'; their occurrence and significance in thalassemia and other disorders. *Blood* **28**, 993.

Kreimer-Birnbaum, M., Bannerman, R.M. & Pinkerton, P.H. (1969) Recent studies on pyrrole metabolism in thalassemia. *Ann. N. Y. Acad. Sci.* **165**, 185.

Kreimer-Birnbaum, M., Edwards, J.A., Rusnak, P.A. & Bannerman, R.M. (1975) Mild β-thalassemia in Black subjects. *Johns Hopkins Med. J.* **137**, 257.

Kremastinos, D.T., Tiniakos, G., Theodorakis, G.N., Katritsis, D.G. & Toutouzas, P.K. (1996) Myocarditis in beta-thalassemia major. A cause of heart failure. *Circulation* **91**, 66.

Krishnamurti, L., Chui, D.H.K., Dallaire, M., LeRoy, B., Waye, J.S. & Perentesis, J.P. (1998) Coinheritance of α-thalassemia-1 and hemoglobin E/β⁰-thalassemia: practical implications for neonatal screening and genetic counseling. *J. Pediatr.* **132**, 863.

Kruatrachue, M., Bhaibulaya, M., Klongkamnaunkarn, K. & Harinasuta, C. (1969) Haemoglobinopathies and malaria in Thailand. *Bull. WHO* **40**, 459.

Kruatrachue, M., Sriripanich, B. & Sadudee, N. (1970) Haemoglobinopathies and malaria in Thailand: a comparison of morbidity and mortality rates. *Bull. WHO* **43**, 348.

Kueh, Y.K. (1982) Acute lymphoblastic leukemia with brilliant cresyl blue erythrocytic inclusions—acquired hemoglobin H? *N. Eng. J. Med.* **307**, 193.

Kugler, W., Enssle, J., Hentze, M.W. & Kulozik, A.E. (1995) Nuclear degradation of nonsense mutated β-globin mRNA: a post-transcriptional mechanism to protect heterozygotes from severe clinical manifestation of β-thalassemia? *Nucl. Acids Res.* **23**, 413.

Kühn, L.C. (1994) Molecular regulation of iron proteins. *Clin. Haematol.* **7**, 763.

Kulapongs, P., Jatisatien, K., Romsai, U. & Pintanind, D. (1978) Functional integrity of polymorphonuclear leukocytes of beta thalassemia patients. *J. Med. Assoc. Thailand* **61**, 77.

Kuliev, A.M., Rasulov, I.M.R., Dadasheva, T. *et al.* (1994) Thalassaemia in Azerbaijan. *J. Med. Genet.* **31**, 209.

Kuliev, A., Rechitsky, S., Verlinsky, O. *et al.* (1998) Preimplantation diagnosis of thalassemias. *J. Assist. Reprod. Genet.* **15**, 219.

Kuliev, A., Rechitsky, S., Verlinsky, O. *et al.* (1999) Birth of healthy children after preimplantation diagnosis of thalassaemias. *J. Assist. Reprod. Genet.* **16**, 207.

Kulozik, A.E., Wainscoat, J.S., Serjeant, G.R. *et al.* (1986) Geographical survey of βˢ-globin gene haplotypes: evidence for an independent Asian origin of the sickle-cell mutation. *Am. J. Hum. Genet.* **39**, 239.

Kulozik, A.E., Kar, B.C., Satapathy, R.K., Serjeant, B.E., Serjeant, G.R. & Weatherall, D.J. (1987a) Fetal hemoglobin levels and βˢ globin haplotypes in an Indian population with sickle cell disease. *Blood* **69**, 1742.

Kulozik, A.E., Thein, S.L., Wainscoat, J.S. *et al.* (1987b) Thalassaemia intermedia: interaction of the triple α-globin gene arrangement and heterozygous β-thalassaemia. *Br. J. Haematol.* **66**, 109.

Kulozik, A.E., Kar, B.L., Serjeant, B.E., Serjeant, G.R. & Weatherall, D.J. (1988a) The molecular basis of α-thalassaemia in India. Its interaction with the sickle cell gene. *Blood* **71**, 467.

Kulozik, A., Yarwood, N. & Jones, R.W. (1988b) The Corfu δβ⁰ thalassemia: a small deletion acts at a distance to selectively abolish β globin gene expression. *Blood* **71**, 457.

Kulozik, A.E., Bail, S., Kar, B.C., Serjeant, B.E. & Serjeant, G.E. (1991a) Sickle cell-β⁺ thalassaemia in Orissa State, India. *Br. J. Haematol.* **77**, 215.

Kulozik, A.E., Bellan-Koch, A., Bail, S., Kohne, E. & Kleihauer, E. (1991b) Thalassemia intermedia: moderate reduction of β globin gene transcriptional activity by a novel mutation of the proximal CACCC promoter element. *Blood* **77**, 2054.

Kulozik, A.E., Bellan-Koch, A., Kohne, E. & Kleihauer, E. (1992) A deletion/inversion rearrangement of the β-globin gene cluster in a Turkish family with δβ⁰-thalassemia intermedia. *Blood* **79**, 2455.

Kulozik, A.E., Kohne, E. & Kleihauer, E. (1993) Thalassemia inter-

media: compound heterozygous β⁰/β⁺-thalassemia and co-inherited heterozygous α⁺-thalassemia. *Ann. Hematol.* **66**, 51.

Kumar, R.M. & Khuranna, A. (1998) Pregnancy outcome in women with beta-thalassemia major and HIV infection. *Eur. J. Obstet. Gynecol. Reprod. Biol.* **77**, 163.

Kumar, R., Tandon, R. & Badami, K.G. (1989) Coexisting hereditary methaemoglobinaemia and heterozygous β-thalassaemia. *Acta Paediatr. Scand.* **78**, 149.

Kumar, R.M., Uduman, S., Hamo, I.M., Morrison, J. & Khaurana, A.K. (1994) Incidence and clinical manifestations of HIV-1 infection in multitransfused thalassaemia Indian children. *Trop. Geogr. Med.* **46**, 163.

Kunkel, H.G. & Wallenius, G. (1955) New hemoglobin in normal adult blood. *Science* **122**, 288.

Kunkel, H.G., Ceppellini, R., Müller-Eberhard, U. & Wolf, J. (1957) Observations on the minor basic hemoglobin component in blood of normal individuals and patients with thalassemia. *J. Clin. Invest.* **36**, 1615.

Kuo, B., Zaino, E. & Roginsky, M.S. (1968) Endocrine function in thalassemia. *J. Clin. Endocrinol. Metab.* **28**, 805.

Kuptamethi, S., Pravatmuang, P., Fucharoen, S., Ridthimat, W. & Choopanya, K. (1988) Modified technique for detecting red cells containing inclusion bodies in α-thalassemia trait. *Birth Defects* **23**, 213.

Kutlar, A., Gardiner, M.B., Headlee, M.G. *et al.* (1984) Heterogeneity in the molecular basis of three types of hereditary persistence of fetal hemoglobin and the relative synthesis of the ᴳγ and ᴬγ types of γ chain. *Biochem. Genet.* **22**, 21.

Kutlar, A., Kutlar, F., Aksoy, M. *et al.* (1989a) β-Thalassemia intermedia in two Turkish families is caused by the interaction of Hb Knossos [β27(B9)Ala→Ser] and of Hb City of Hope [β69(E13)Gly→Ser] with β⁰-thalassemia. *Hemoglobin* **13**, 7.

Kutlar, F., Gonzalez-Redondo, J.M., Kutlar, A. *et al.* (1989b) The levels of ζ, γ, and δ chains in patients with HbH disease. *Hum. Genet.* **82**, 179.

Kutlar, A., Kutlar, F., Gu, L.-G., Mayson, S.M. & Huisman, T.H. (1990) Fetal hemoglobin in normal adults and β-thalassemia heterozygotes. *Hum. Genet.* **85**, 106.

Kwan, E.Y.W., Lee, A.C.W., Li, A.M.C. *et al.* (1995) A cross-sectional study of growth, puberty and endocrine function in patients with thalassaemia major in Hong Kong. *J. Paed. Child Health* **31**, 83.

Kwok, S., Kellogg, D.E., McKinney, N. *et al.* (1990) Effects of primer–template mismatches on the polymerase chain reaction: human immunodeficiency virus type I model studies. *Nucl. Acids Res.* **18**, 999.

Kyte, J. (1995) *Structure in Protein Chemistry*. Garland, New York.

La Nasa, G., Vacca, A., Pizzati, A. *et al.* (1997) Role of HLA extended haplotypes in unrelated bone marrow transplantation. *Bone Marrow Transplant.* **19** (Suppl. 2), 186.

Labie, D. & Elion, J. (1996) Sequence polymorphisms of potential functional relevance in the β-globin gene locus. *Hemoglobin* **20**, 85.

Labie, D., Schroeder, W.A. & Huisman, T.H.J. (1966) The amino acid sequence of the δ-β chains of haemoglobin Lepore_Augusta-Lepore_Washington. *Biochim. Biophys. Acta* **127**, 428.

Labie, D., Rosa, J., Tanzer, J. *et al.* (1968) Evidence for β₄ and γ₄ hemoglobins associated with an acute myeloblastic leukemia. In: *Proceedings of the XIIth International Congress in Hematology*, p. 3. Grune & Stratton, New York.

Labie, D., Pagnier, J., Mallarme, J. & Boivin, P. (1971) A case of Lepore hemoglobin in a patient of French origin. *Ann. Biol. Clin. (Paris)* **29**, 343.

Labie, D., Amegnizin, K.P.E., Wajcman, H. *et al.* (1978) Hémoglobinopathies chez les travailleurs de l'Afrique de l'ouest en France. *Sem. Hôp. Paris* **54**, 1343.

Labie, D., Dunda-Belkhodja, O., Rouabhi, F., Pagnier, J., Ragusa A. & Nagel, R.L. (1985a) The −158 site 5′ to the $^{G}\gamma$ gene and $^{G}\gamma$ expression. *Blood* **66**, 1463.

Labie, D., Pagnier, J., Lapoumeroulie, C. *et al.* (1985b) Common haplotype dependency of high $^{G}\gamma$-globin gene expression and high Hb F levels in β-thalassemia and sickle cell anemia patients. *Proc. Natl Acad. Sci. USA* **82**, 2111.

Labie, D., Srinivas, R., Dunda, O. *et al.* (1989) Haplotypes of tribal Indians bearing the sickle gene: evidence for the unicentric origin of the β^{S} mutation and the unicentric origin of the tribal populations of India. *Hum. Genet.* **61**, 479.

Labie, D., Bennani, C. & Beldjord, C. (1990) β-Thalassemia in Algeria. *Ann. N. Y. Acad. Sci.* **612**, 43.

Lacerra, G., Fioretti, G., De Angioletti, M. *et al.* (1991) $(\alpha)\alpha^{5.3}$: a novel α^{+}-thalassemia deletion with the breakpoints in the α2-globin gene and in close proximity to an Alu family repeat between the $\psi\alpha2$- and $\psi\alpha1$-globin genes. *Blood* **78**, 2740.

Lacerra, G., De Angioletti, M., Sabato, V., Schettini, F. & Carestia, C. (1997) South-Italy beta⁰-thalassaemia: A novel deletion, with 3′ breakpoint in a hsRTVL-H element, associated with beta⁰-thalassaemia and HPFH. *6th International Conference on Thalassaemia and the Haemoglobinopathies, Malta.* Abstract 152. Thalassaemia International Federation, Cyprus.

Lacey, D.L., Timms, E., Tan, H.-L. *et al.* (1998) Osteoprotegerin ligand is a cytokine that regulates osteoclast differentiation and activation. *Cell* **93**, 165.

Lachant, N.A. & Tanaka, K.R. (1987) Case report: Dapsone-associated Heinz body hemolytic anemia in a Cambodian woman with hemoglobin E trait. *Am. J. Med. Sci.* **294**, 364.

LaFlamme, S., Acuto, S., Markowitz, D., Vick, L., Landschultz, W. & Bank, A. (1987) Expression of chimeric human beta- and delta-globin genes during erythroid differentiation. *J. Biol. Chem.* **262**, 4819.

Lai, E., Belluzzo, N., Muraca, M.F. *et al.* (1995) The prognosis for adults with thalassemia major. *Blood* **86**, 251a.

Laig, M., Sanguansermsri, T., Wiangnon, S., Hundrieser, J., Pape, M. & Flatz, G. (1989) The spectrum of β-thalassemia mutations in northern and northeastern Thailand. *Hum. Genet.* **84**, 47.

Laig, M., Pape, M., Hundreiser, J. *et al.* (1990a) The distribution of the Hb Constant Spring gene in Southeast Asian populations. *Hum. Genet.* **84**, 188.

Laig, M., Pape, M., Hundreiser, J. & Flatz, G. (1990b) Mediterranean types of β-thalassemia in the German population. *Hum. Genet.* **85**, 135.

Lallemant, M., Galacteros, F., Lallemant-Lecoeur, S. *et al.* (1986) Hemoglobin abnormalities. An evaluation on new-born infants and their mothers in a maternity unit close to Brazzaville (PR Congo). *Hum. Genet.* **74**, 54.

Lam, Y.H. & Tang, M.H.Y. (1997) Prenatal diagnosis of haemoglobin Bart's disease by cordocentesis at 12–14 weeks' gestation. *Prenat. Diag.* **17**, 501.

Lam, V.M.S., Xie, S.S., Tam, J.W.O., Woo, Y.K., Gu, Y.L. & Li, A.M.C. (1990) A new single nucleotide change at the initiation codon (ATG→AGG) identified in amplified genomic DNA of a Chinese β-thalassemic patient. *Blood* **75**, 1207.

Lam, T.-K., Chan, V., Fok, T.-F., Li, C.-K. & Feng, C.-S. (1992) Long-term survival of a baby with homozygous alpha-thalassemia-1. *Acta Haematol.* **88**, 198.

Lamb, J. & Clegg, J.B. (1996) Measurement of aberrant recombination between duplicated globin genes in normal human sperm. *Am. J. Hum. Genet.* **59**, A306.

Lamb, J., Wilkie, A.O.M., Harris, P.C. *et al.* (1989) Detection of break-points in submicroscopic chromosomal translocation, illustrating an important mechanism for genetic disease. *Lancet* **ii**, 819.

Lamb, J., Harris, P.C., Wilkie, A.O.M., Wood, W.G., Dauwerse, J.G. & Higgs, D.R. (1993) De novo truncation of chromosome 16p and healing with $(TTAGGG)_n$ in the α-thalassemia/mental retardation syndrome (ATR-16). *Am. J. Hum. Genet.* **52**, 668.

Lambert, S.M. (1949) *Malariology* (ed. S.M. Boyd), p. 820. W.B. Saunders, Philadelphia.

Lambotte-Legrand, J. & Lambotte-Legrand, C. (1951) L'anémie à hématies falciformes chez l'enfant indigène du Bas-Congo. *Am. Soc. Belg. Med. Trop.* **31**, 207.

Lambotte-Legrand, J., Lambotte-Legrand, C., Ager, J.A.M. & Lehmann, H. (1960) Hemoglobinosis P. Apropos a case of association of hemoglobins P and S. *Rev. Hematol.* **15**, 10.

Lan, N., Howrey, R.P., Lee, S.-W., Smith, C.A. & Sullenger, B.A. (1998) Ribozyme-mediated repair of sickle β-globin mRNAs in erythrocyte precursors. *Science* **280**, 1593.

Lanclos, K.D., Patterson, J., Efremov, G.D. *et al.* (1987) Characterization of chromosomes with hybrid genes for Hb Lepore-Washington, Hb Lepore-Baltimore, Hb P-Nilotic, and Hb Kenya. *Hum. Genet.* **77**, 40.

Lanclos, K.D., Michael, S.K., Gu, T.C., Howard, E.F., Stoming, T.A. & Huisman, T.H.J. (1989) Transient chloramphenicol acetyltransferase expression of the $^{G}\gamma$ globin gene 5′-flanking regions containing substitutions of C→T at position −158, G→A at position −161, and T→A at position −175 in K562 cells. *Biochim. Biophys. Acta* **1008**, 109.

Lanclos, K.D., Oner, C., Dimovski, A.J., Gu, Y.-C. & Huisman, T.H.J. (1991) Sequence variations in the 5′ flanking and IVS-II regions of the $^{G}\gamma$- and $^{A}\gamma$-globin genes of β^{S} chromosomes with five different haplotypes. *Blood* **77**, 2488.

Landau, H., Spitz, I.M., Cividalli, C. & Rachmilewitz, E.A. (1978) Gonadotrophin, thyrotrophin and prolactin reserve in β thalassaemia. *Clin. Endocrinol.* **9**, 163.

Landau, H., Matoth, I., Landau-Cordova, Z., Goldfarb, A., Rachmilewitz, E.A. & Glaser, B. (1993) Cross-sectional and longitudinal study of the pituitary–thyroid axis in patients with thalassaemia major. *Clin. Endocrinol.* **38**, 55.

Landin, B. & Berglund, S. (1996) A novel mutation in the β-globin gene causing β-thalassaemia in a Swedish family. *Eur. J. Haematol.* **57**, 182.

Landin, B. & Rudolphi, O. (1996) A novel mutation in exon 3 of the β-globin gene associated with β-thalassaemia. *Br. J. Haematol.* **93**, 24.

Landin, B., Rudolphi, O. & Ek, B. (1995) Initiation codon mutation (ATG→ATA) of the β-globin gene causing β-thalassaemia in a Swedish family. *Am. J. Hematol.* **48**, 158.

Landing, B.H., Nadorra, R., Hyman, C.B. & Ortega, J.A. (1987) Pulmonary lesions of thalassaemia major. *Perspect. Pediatr. Pathol.* **11**, 82.

Landman, H. (1988) *Haemoglobinopathies and Pregnancy*, p. 250. Van Denderen Printing, Groningen.

Laosombat, V., Panich, V., Surapruk, P. & Pornpatkul, M. (1979) *Abstracts of 3rd Asian Congress on Pediatrics.* Bangkok.

Laosombat, V., Wongchanchailert, M., Kenpatik, K. & Wisitipongpon, V. (1992) Spontaneous platelet aggregation in thalassaemic children and adolescents. *Southeast Asian J. Trop. Med. Publ. Hlth* **23**, 42.

Laosombat, V., Pornpatkul, M., Wongchanchailert, M., Worachat, K. & Wiriyasatienku, A. (1997) The prevalence of hepatitis C virus antibodies in thalassemic patients in the south of Thailand. *Southeast Asian J. Trop. Med. Publ. Hlth* **28**, 149.

Lapouméroulie, C., Pagnier, J., Bank, A., Labie, D. & Kirshnamoorthy, R. (1986) β-Thalassemia due to a novel mutation in IVS-1 sequence donor site consensus sequence creating a restriction site. *Biochem. Biophys. Res. Comm.* **139**, 709.

Lapouméroulie, C., Dunda, O., Ducrocq, R. *et al.* (1992) A novel sickle cell mutation of yet another origin in Africa: the Cameroon type. *Hum. Genet.* **89**, 333.

Larizza, P., Ventura, S., Matioli, G., Sulis, E. & Aresu, G. (1958) Contributo alla conoscenza dell'anemia talassemica; richerche condotte con l'ausilio de Fe⁵⁹. *Haematologica* **43**, 517.

Laros, R.K. & Kalstone, C.E. (1971) Sickle cell-beta thalassaemia and pregnancy. *Obstet. Gynecol.* **37**, 67.

Lasne, Y., Francina, A. & Benzerara, O. (1991) Serum ferritin spectrotypes in patients with heterozygous β-thalassaemia. *Clin. Chim. Acta* **197**, 85.

Lassman, M.N., Genel, M., Wise, J.K., Hendler, R. & Felig, P. (1974a) Carbohydrate homeostasis and pancreatic islet cell function in thalassemia. *Blood* **80**, 65.

Lassman, M.N., O'Brien, R.T., Pearson, H.A. *et al.* (1974b) Endocrine evaluation in thalassemia major. *Ann. N. Y. Acad. Sci.* **232**, 226.

Lattanzi, F., Bellotti, P., Picano, E. *et al.* (1993) Quantitative ultrasonic analysis of myocardium in patients with thalassemia major and iron overload. *Circulation* **87**, 748.

Lau, Y.L., Chow, C.B., Lee, A.C. *et al.* (1993) Hepatitis C virus antibody in multiply transfused Chinese with thalassaemia. *Bone Marrow Transplant.* **12**, 26.

Lauer, J., Shen, C.-K.J. & Maniatis, T. (1980) The chromosomal arrangement of human α-like globin genes: sequence homology and α-globin gene deletions. *Cell* **20**, 119.

Lawn, R.M., Fritsch, E.F., Parker, R.C., Blake, G. & Maniatis, T. (1978) The isolation and characterization of linked δ and β-globin genes from a cloned library of human DNA. *Cell* **15**, 1157.

Lawn, R.M., Efstradiadis, A., O'Connell, C. & Maniatis, T. (1980) The nucleotide sequence of the human β-globin gene. *Cell* **21**, 647.

Le Dourain, B., Nielsen, A.L., Garnier, J.-M. *et al.* (1996) A possible involvement of TIF1α and TIF1β in the epigenetic control of transcription by nuclear receptors. *EMBO J.* **15**, 6701.

Leboulch, P., Huang, G.S., Humphries, R.K. *et al.* (1994) Mutagenesis of retroviral vectors transducing β-globin gene and β-globin locus control region derivates results in stable transmission of an active transcriptional structure. *EMBO J.* **13**, 3065.

Leder, A., Kuo, A., Shen, M.M. & Leder, P. (1992) In situ hybridization reveals co-expression of embryonic and adult α globin genes in the earliest murine erythrocyte progenitors. *Development* **116**, 1041.

Lederberg, J. (1999) J. B. S. Haldane (1949) on infectious disease and evolution. *Genetics* **153**, 1.

Lee, R.C. & Huisman, T.H.J. (1965) β Thalassemia-hemoglobin Dα: a family report. *Am. J. Hum. Genet.* **17**, 148.

Lefort, G., Taib, J., Toutain, A. *et al.* (1993) X-linked α-thalassaemia/mental retardation (ATR-X) syndrome. Report of three male patients in a large French family. *Ann. Génét.* **36**, 200.

Lefrère, J.J., Girot, R., Courouce, A.M., Maier-Redelsperger, M. & Cornu, P. (1986) Familial human parvovirus infection associated with heterozygous β-thalassemia. *J. Infect. Dis.* **153**, 977.

Leger, J., Girot, R., Crosnier, H., Postel-Vinay, M.C. & Rappaport, R. (1989) Normal growth hormone (GH) response to GH-releasing hormone in children with thalassemia major before puberty: a possible age-related effect. *J. Clin. Endocrinol. Metab.* **69**, 453.

Lehmann, H. (1970) Different types of alpha thalassaemia and significance of haemoglobin Bart's in neonates. *Lancet* **ii**, 78.

Lehmann, H. & Carrell, R.W. (1968) Differences between α and β chain mutants of human haemoglobin and between α and β thalassaemia. Possible duplication of the α-chain gene. *Br. Med. J.* **iv**, 748.

Lehmann, H. & Carrell, R. (1969) Variations in the structure of human haemoglobin with particular reference to the unstable haemoglobins. *Br. Med. Bull.* **25**, 14.

Lehmann, H. & Charlesworth, D. (1970) Observations on haemoglobin P (Congo type). *Biochem. J.* **119**, 43.

Lehmann, H. & Kynoch, P.A.M. (1976) *Human Haemoglobin Variants and Their Characteristics.* North Holland Publishing Company, Amsterdam.

Lehmann, H. & Lang, A. (1975) Haemoglobin Q and thalassaemia. *J. Clin. Soc. Thailand* **1**, 41.

Lehmann, H. & Singh, R.B. (1956) Haemoglobin E in Malaya. *Nature* **178**, 695.

Lehmann, H., Story, P. & Thein, H. (1956) Hemoglobin E in Burmese. *Br. Med. J.* **i**, 544.

Lemmens-Zygulska, M., Eigel, A., Helbig, B., Sanguansermsri, T., Horst, J. & Flatz, G. (1996) Prevalence of α-thalassemias in northern Thailand. *Hum. Genet.* **98**, 345.

Lemoine, N.R. & Cooper, D.N. (eds) (1996) *Gene Therapy*, p. 343. BIOS Scientific Publishers, Oxford.

Leon, M.B., Borer, J.S., Bacharach, S.L. *et al.* (1979) Detection of early cardiac dysfunction in patients with severe beta-thalassemia and chronic iron overload. *N. Eng. J. Med.* **301**, 1143.

Leonardi, S., Arcidiacono, G., Colianni, R., DiGregorio, L. & Musumeci, S. (1990) Protein C, protein S, and antithrombin III in thrombotic disease: their role in β-thalassemia major. *Ann. N. Y. Acad. Sci.* **612**, 549.

Leone, L., Monteleone, M., Gabutti, V. & Amione, C. (1985) Reversed-phase high-performance liquid chromatography of human haemoglobin chains. *J. Chromatogr.* **321**, 407.

Letsky, E.A. (1976) A controlled trial of long-term chelation therapy in homozygous β-thalassemia. In: *Birth Defects: Original Article Series* (eds D. Bergsma, A. Cerami, C.M. Peterson & J.H. Graziano), p. 31. Liss, New York.

Letsky, E.A., Flynn, D.M. & Barry, M. (1973) The effect of treatment with long-term chelating agents on iron overload in thalassaemia. *Br. J. Haematol.* **25**, 285.

Letsky, E.A., Miller, F., Worwood, M. & Flynn, D.M. (1974) Serum ferritin in children with thalassaemia regularly transfused. *J. Clin. Pathol.* **27**, 652.

Letvin, N.L., Linch, D.C., Beardsley, G.P., McIntyre, K.W. & Nathan, D.G. (1984) Augmentation of fetal hemoglobin production in anemia monkeys by hydroxyurea. *N. Eng. J. Med.* **310**, 869.

Leung, S.-O., Proudfoot, N.J. & Whitelaw, E. (1987) The gene for θ-globin is transcribed in human fetal erythroid tissues. *Nature* **329**, 551.

Leung, H., Gilbert, A.T., Fleming, P.J. *et al.* (1991) Hb A₂-Parkville or δ47(CD6)Asp→Val, a new δ chain variant. *Hemoglobin* **15**, 407.

Lever, A.M.L. & Goodfellow, P. (1995) Gene therapy. *Br. Med. Bull.* **51**, 1.

Lewin, B. (1997) *Genes VI.* Oxford University Press, Oxford.

Ley, T.J., DeSimone, J., Noguchi, C.T. *et al.* (1983) 5-Azacytidine increases α-globin synthesis and reduces the proportion of dense cells in patients with sickle cell anemia. *Blood* **62**, 370.

Ley, T.J., Maloney, K.A., Gordon, J.I. & Schwartz, A.L. (1989) Globin gene expression in erythroid human fetal liver cells. *J. Clin. Invest.* **83**, 1032.

Li, A.M.C., Lee, F.T. & Todd, D. (1982) The screening of Chinese cord blood for haemoglobinopathies. *Hum. Hered.* **32**, 62.

Li, Q., Clegg, C., Peterson, K., Shaw, S., Raich, N. & Stamatoyannopoulos, G. (1997) Binary transgenic mouse model for studying the *trans* control of globin gene switching: evidence that GATA-1 is an *in vivo* repressor of human ε gene expression. *Proc. Natl Acad. Sci. USA* **94**, 2444.

Liang, S.T., Wong, V.C.W., So, W.W.K., Ma, H.K., Chan, V. & Todd, D. (1985) Homozygous α-thalassaemia: clinical presentation, diagnosis and management. A review of 46 cases. *Br. J. Obstet. Gynaecol.* **92**, 680.

Liang, R., Liang, S., Jiang, N.H. *et al.* (1994) α and β thalassaemia among Chinese children in Guangxi Province, P.R. China: molecular and haematological characterization. *Br. J. Haematol.* **86**, 351.

Lichtman, H.C., Watson, R.J., Feldman, F., Ginsberg, V. & Robinson, J. (1953) Studies on thalassemia. I. An extracorpuscular defect in thalassemia major. II. The effects of splenectomy in thalassemia major with an associated acquired hemolytic anemia. *J. Clin. Invest.* **32**, 1229.

Liebhaber, S.A. & Kan, Y.W. (1981) Differentiation of the mRNA transcripts originating from the α1- and α2-globin loci in normals and α-thalassemics. *J. Clin. Invest.* **68**, 439.

Liebhaber, S.A., Goosens, H. & Kan, Y.W. (1980) Cloning and complete nucleotide sequence of human 5′-α-globin gene. *Proc. Natl Acad. Sci. USA* **77**, 7054.

Liebhaber, S.A., Rappaport, E.F., Cash, F.E., Ballas, S.K., Schwartz, E. & Surrey, S. (1984) Hemoglobin I mutation encoded at both α-globin loci on the same chromosome: concerted evolution in the human genome. *Science* **226**, 1449.

Liebhaber, S.A., Cash, F.E. & Main, D.M. (1985) Compensatory increase in α1-globin gene expression in individuals heterozygous for the α-thalassemia-2 deletion. *J. Clin. Invest.* **76**, 1057.

Liebhaber, S.A., Cash, F.E. & Ballas, S.K. (1986) Human α-globin gene expression. The dominant role of the α2-locus in mRNA and protein synthesis. *J. Biol. Chem.* **261**, 15327.

Liebhaber, S.A., Coleman, M.B., Adams, J.G.I., Cash, F.E. & Steinberg, M.H. (1987) Molecular basis for non-deletion α-thalassemia in American blacks α2$^{116GAG \rightarrow UAG}$. *J. Clin. Invest.* **80**, 154.

Liebhaber, S.A., Griese, E.-U., Weiss, I. *et al.* (1990) Inactivation of human α-globin gene expression by a *de novo* deletion located upstream of the α-globin gene cluster. *Proc. Natl Acad. Sci. USA* **81**, 9431.

Liebhaber, S.A., Wang, Z., Cash, F.E., Monks, B. & Russell, J.E. (1996) Developmental silencing of the embryonic ζ-globin gene: concerted action of the promoter and the 3′-flanking region combined with stage-specific silencing by the transcribed segment. *Mol. Cell. Biol.* **16**, 2637.

Lie-Injo, L.E. (1959a) Haemoglobin of newborn infants in Indonesia. *Nature* **183**, 1125.

Lie-Injo, L.E. (1959b) Pathological haemoglobins in Indonesia. In: *Abnormal Haemoglobins* (eds J.H.P. Jonxis & J.F. Delafresnaye), p. 368. Blackwell Scientific Publications, Oxford.

Lie-Injo, L.E. (1970) Hb H in West Malaysia. *Southeast Asian J. Trop. Med. Publ. Hlth* **1**, 58.

Lie-Injo, L.E. (1973) Haemoglobin Bart's and slow-moving haemoglobin X components in newborns. *Acta Haematol.* **49**, 25.

Lie-Injo, L.E. & Chin, J. (1964) Abnormal haemoglobin and glucose-6-phosphate dehydrogenase deficiency in Malayan aborigines. *Nature* **204**, 291.

Lie-Injo, L.E. & Duraisamy, G. (1972) The slow-moving haemoglobin X components in Malaysians. *Hum. Hered.* **22**, 118.

Lie-Injo, L.E. & de V. Hart, P.L. (1963) Splenectomy in two cases of Hb Q-H-disease (Hb Q-α-thalassaemia) *Acta Haematol.* **29**, 358.

Lie-Injo, L.E. & Jo, B.H. (1960a) A fast moving haemoglobin in hydrops foetalis. *Nature* **185**, 698.

Lie-Injo, L.E. & Jo, B.H. (1960b) Hydrops foetalis with a fast-moving haemoglobin. *Br. Med. J.* **ii**, 1649.

Lie-Injo, L.E. & Ti, T.S. (1961) The fast moving haemoglobin component in healthy newborn babies in Malaya. *Med. J. Malaya* **XVI**, 107.

Lie-Injo, L.E., Lie, H.G., Ager, J.A.M. & Lehmann, H. (1962) α-Thalassaemia as a cause of hydrops foetalis. *Br. J. Haematol.* **8**, 1.

Lie-Injo, L.E., Poey-Oey, H.G. & Mossberger, R.J. (1968) Haptoglobins, transferrins, and hemoglobin B₂ in Indonesians. *Am. J. Hum. Genet.* **20**, 470.

Lie-Injo, L.E., Ganesan, J., Clegg, J.B. & Weatherall, D.J. (1974) Homozygous state for Hb Constant Spring (slow moving Hb X components). *Blood* **43**, 251.

Lie-Injo, L.E., Ganesan, J. & Lopez, C.G. (1975) The clinical, haematological and biochemical expression of hemoglobin Constant Spring and its distribution. In: *Abnormal Haemoglobins and Thalassaemia — Diagnostic Aspects* (ed. R.M. Schmidt), p. 275. Academic Press, New York.

Lie-Injo, L.E., Ganesan, J., Ranhawa, Z.I., Peterson, D. & Kane, J.P. (1977) Hb Leiden-β⁰ thalassemia in a Chinese with severe hemolytic anemia. *Am. J. Hematol.* **2**, 335.

Lie-Injo, L.E., Solai, A., Herrera, A.R. *et al.* (1982) Hb Bart's level in cord blood and deletions of α-globin genes. *Blood* **59**, 370.

Lie-Injo, L.E., Cai, S.-P., Wahidijat, I. *et al.* (1989) β-Thalassemia mutations in Indonesia and their linkage to β haplotypes. *Am. J. Hum. Genet.* **45**, 971.

Lim, L. & Canellakis, E.S. (1970) Adenine-rich polymer associated with rabbit reticulocyte messenger RNA. *Nature* **227**, 710.

Lim, S.K. & Maquat, L.E. (1992) Human β-globin mRNAs that harbor a nonsense codon are degraded in murine erythroid tissues to intermediates lacking regions of exon I or exons I and II that have a cap-like structure at the 5′ termini. *EMBO J.* **11**, 3271.

Lim, S.-K., Sigmund, C.D., Gross, K.W. & Maquat, L.E. (1992) Nonsense codons in human β-globin mRNA result in the production of mRNA degradation products. *Mol. Cell. Biol.* **12**, 1149.

Lin, K.-S., Liu, C.-H., Lee, T.-C, Blackwell. R.Q. & Huang, J.T.-H. (1977) Alpha chain thalassemia in Taiwan. *Clin. Pediatr.* **16**, 71.

Lin, C.K., Peng, H.W., Ho, C.H. & Yung, C.H. (1990) Iron overload in untransfused patients with hemoglobin H disease. *Acta Haematologia (Basel)* **83**, 137.

Lin, L.-I., Lin, K.-S., Lin, K.-H. & Chang, H.-C. (1991) The spectrum of β-thalassemia mutations in Taiwan: Identification of a novel frameshift mutation. *Am. J. Hum. Genet.* **48**, 809.

Lin, C.-K., Lin, J.-S. & Jiang, M.-L. (1992a) Iron absorption is increased in Hemoglobin H disease. *Am. J. Hematol.* **40**, 74.

Lin, L.-I., Lin, K.-S., Lin, K.-H. & Cheng, T.-Y. (1992b) A novel −32 (C-A) mutant identified in amplified genomic DNA of a Chinese β-thalassemic patient. *Am. J. Hum. Genet.* **50**, 237.

Lin, S.-F., Liu, T.-C., Chen, T.-P., Chiou, S.-S., Liu, H.-W. & Chang, J.-G. (1994) Diagnosis of thalassaemia by non-isotope detection of α/β and ζ/α mRNA ratios. *Br. J. Haematol.* **87**, 133.

Lindeman, R., Hu, S.P., Volpato, F. & Trent, R.J. (1991) Polymerase chain reaction (PCR) mutagenesis enabling rapid non-radioactive detection of common β-thalassaemia mutations in Mediterraneans. *Br. J. Haematol.* **78**, 100.

Lindsey, R.J., Jackson, J.M. & Raven, J.L. (1978) Acquired haemoglobin H disease, complicating a myeloproliferative syndrome: a case report. *Pathology* **10**, 329.

Link, G. & Pinson, A. (1985) Heart cells in culture: a model of myocardial iron overload and chelation. *J. Lab. Clin. Med.* **106**, 147.

Link, G., Pinson, A. & Hershko, C. (1994) The ability of orally effective iron chelators dimethyl- and diethyl-hydroxypyrid-4-one and of deferoxamine to restore sarcolemmal thiolic enzyme activity in iron-loaded heart cells. *Blood* **83**, 2692.

Link, G., Tirosh, R., Pinson, A. & Hershko, C. (1996) Role of iron in the potentiation of anthracycline toxicity: identification of heart cell mitochondria as the site of iron–anthracycline interaction. *J. Lab. Clin. Med.* **127**, 272.

Lisker, R. (1981) *Estructura genetica de la poblacion mexicana, aspectos medicos y antropologicos*, p. 71. Salvat Mexicana de Ediciones, Mexico City.

Little, P.F.R., Flavell, R.A., Kooter, J.M., Annison, G. & Williamson, R. (1979) Structure of the human fetal globin gene locus. *Nature* **278**, 227.

Little, P.F.R., Annison, G., Darling, S., Williamson, R., Camba, L. & Modell, B. (1980) Model for antenatal diagnosis of β-thalassaemia and other monogenic disorders by molecular analysis of linked DNA polymorphisms. *Nature* **285**, 144.

Liu, D., Chang, J.C., Flavell, R.A., Moi, P., Liu, W., Kan, Y.W. & Curtin, P.T. (1992) Dissection of the enhancer activity of β-globin 5′ DNase I-hypersensitive site 2 in transgenic mice. *Proc. Natl Acad. Sci. USA* **89**, 3899.

Liu, J.Z., Gao, Q.S., Jiang, Z. *et al.* (1989) Studies of β-thalassemia mutations in families living in three provinces in Southern China. *Hemoglobin* **13**, 585.

Liu, J.-Z., Harano, T., Lanclos, K.D. & Huisman, T.H.J. (1987) The β–δ crossover leading to the beta delta hybrid gene of hemoglobin P-Nilotic is located within 54 base-pairs of the 5′ end of exon 2 or between codons 31 and 50. *Biochim. Biophys. Acta* **909**, 208.

Liu, P. & Olivieri, N. (1994) Iron overload cardiomyopathies: new insights into an old disease. *Cardiovasc. Drugs Ther.* **8**, 101.

Liu, P., Henkelman, M., Joshi, J. *et al.* (1996) Quantitation of cardiac and tissue iron by nuclear magnetic resonance in a novel murine thalassemia–cardiac iron overload model. *Can. J. Cardiol.* **12**, 155.

Liu, Q., Bungert, J. & Engel, J.D. (1997) Mutation of gene-proximal regulatory elements disrupts human ε-, γ- and β-globin expression in yeast artificial chromosome transgenic mice. *Proc. Natl Acad. Sci. USA* **94**, 169.

Liu, Q., Tanimoto, K., Bungert, J. & Engel, J.D. (1998) The ᴬγ-globin 3′ element provides no unique function(s) for human β-globin locus gene regulation. *Proc. Natl Acad. Sci. USA* **95**, 9944.

Liu, S.C., Zhai, S., Lawler, J. & Palek, J. (1985) Hemin-mediated dissociation of erythrocyte membrane skeletal proteins. *J. Biol. Chem.* **260**, 12234.

Liu, T.-C., Chiou, S.-S., Lin, S.-F. *et al.* (1994) Molecular basis and hematological characterization of HbH disease in Southeast Asia. *Am. J. Hematol.* **45**, 293.

Liu, V.W.S., Woo, Y.K., Lam, V.M.S. *et al.* (1988) Molecular studies of β-thalassemic DNA of Chinese patients. *Birth Defects* **23**, 87.

Liu, Y.T., Old, J.M., Miles, K., Fisher, C.A., Weatherall, D.J. & Clegg, J.B. (2000) Rapid detection of α-thalassaemia deletions and α-globin gene triplication by multiplex PCRs. *Br. J. Haematol.* **108**, 295.

Livingstone, F.B. (1967) *Abnormal Hemoglobins in Human Populations*. Aldine, Chicago.

Livingstone, F.B. (1971) Malaria and human polymorphisms. *Annu. Rev. Genet.* **5**, 33.

Livingstone, F.B. (1985) *Frequencies of Hemoglobin Variants*. Oxford University Press, New York.

Llewellyn-Jones, D. (1969) *Fundamentals of Obstetrics and Gynaecology*, Vol. 1. Faber and Faber Ltd., London.

Lloyd, J., Krakowski, J., Crable, S. & Lingrel, J. (1992) Human γ- to β-globin gene switching using a mini construct in transgenic mice. *Mol. Cell. Biol.* **12**, 1561.

Lodish, H.F. (1971) Alpha and beta globin messenger ribonucleic acid. Different amounts and rates of initiation of translation. *J. Biol. Chem.* **246**, 7131.

Lodish, H.F. (1974) Model for the regulation of mRNA. Translation applied to haemoglobin synthesis. *Nature* **251**, 385.

Lodish, H.F. (1976) Translational control of protein synthesis. *Annu. Rev. Biochem.* **45**, 39.

Lodish, H.F. & Jacobsen, M. (1972) Regulation of hemoglobin synthesis. Equal rates of translation and termination of α- and β-globin chains. *J. Biol. Chem.* **247**, 3622.

Logothetis, J., Economidou, J., Constantoulakis, M., Augoustaki, O., Loewenson, R.B. & Bilek, M. (1971a) Cephalofacial deformities in thalassemia major (Cooley's anemia). A correlative study among 138 cases. *Am. J. Dis. Child.* **121**, 300.

Logothetis, J., Haritos-Fatouros, M., Constantoulakis, M., Economidou, J., Augoustaki, P. & Loewensen, R.B. (1971b) Intelligence and behavioural patterns in patients with Cooley's anemia (homozygous beta-thalassemia); a study based on 138 consecutive cases. *Pediatr.* **48**, 740.

Logothetis, J., Constantoulakis, M., Economidou, J. *et al.* (1972a) Thalassemia major (homozygous beta-thalassemia): a survey of 138 cases with emphasis on neurological and muscular aspects. *Neurology* **22**, 294.

Logothetis, J., Loewensen, R.B., Augoustaki, O., Economidou, J. & Constantoulakis, M. (1972b) Body growth in Cooley's anemia (homozygous beta-thalassemia) with a correlative study as to other aspects of the illness in 138 cases. *Pediatr.* **50**, 92.

Lombardo, T., Tamburino, C., Bartoloni, G. *et al.* (1995) Cardiac iron overload in thalassemic patients: an endomyocardial biopsy study. *Ann. Hematol.* **71**, 135.

Lombardo, T., Ferro, G., Frontini, V. & Percolla, S. (1996a) High-dose intravenous desferrioxamine (DFO) delivery in four thalassemic patients allergic to subcutaneous DFO administration. *Am. J. Hematol.* **51**, 90.

Lombardo, T., Frontini, V., Ferro, G., Sergi, P., Guidice, A. & Lombardo, G. (1996b) Laboratory evaluation of a new delivery system to improve patient compliance with chelation therapy. *Clin. Lab. Haematol.* **18**, 13.

Long, J.A.J., Doppman, J.L., Nienhuis, A.W. & Mills, S.T. (1980) Computed tomographic analysis of beta-thalassemic syndromes with hemochromatosis: pathological findings with clinical and laboratory correlations. *J. Comput. Assist. Tomogr.* **4**, 159.

Looareesuwan, S., Suntharasamai, P., Webster, H.K. & Ho, M. (1993) Malaria in splenectomized patients: report of four cases and review. *Clin. Infect. Dis.* **16**, 361.

Lopez, C.G. & Lie-Injo, L.E. (1971) Alpha-thalassaemia in newborns in West Malaysia. *Hum. Hered.* **21**, 185.

Loria, A., Konijn, A.M. & Hershko, C. (1978) Serum ferritin in β thalassemia trait. *Israel J. Med. Sci.* **14**, 1127.

Lorkin, P.A., Stephens, A.D., Beard, M.E.J., Wrigley, P.F.M., Adams, L. & Lehmann, H. (1975) Haemoglobin Rahere (β82 Lys→Thr): a new high affinity haemoglobin associated with decreased 2,3-diphosphoglycerate binding and relative polycythaemia. *Br. Med. J.* **4**, 200.

Losekoot, M., Fodde, R., Giordano, P.C. & Bernini, L.F. (1989) A novel δ⁰-thalassemia arising from a frameshift insertion, detected by direct sequencing of enzymatically amplified DNA. *Hum. Genet.* **83**, 75.

Losekoot, M., Fodde, R., Gerritsen, E.J.A. *et al.* (1991a) Interaction of two different disorders in the β-globin gene cluster associated with an increased hemoglobin F production: a novel deletion type of ᴳγ+(ᴬγδβ)⁰-thalassemia and a δ⁰-hereditary persistence of fetal hemoglobin determinant. *Blood* **77**, 861.

Losekoot, M., Fodde, R., Harteveld, C.L., Van Heeren, H., Giordano, P.C. & Bernini, L.F. (1991b) Denaturing gradient gel electrophoresis and direct sequencing of PCR amplified genomic DNA: a rapid and reliable diagnostic approach to beta thalassaemia. *Br. J. Haematol.* **76**, 269.

Loudianos, G., Cao, A., Ristaldi, M.S. *et al.* (1990) Molecular basis of δβ-thalassemia with normal fetal hemoglobin. *Blood* **75**, 526.

Loudianos, G., Cao, A., Pirastu, M., Vassilopoulos, G., Kollia, P. & Loukopoulos, D. (1991a) Molecular basis of the δ thalassemia in *cis* to hemoglobin Knossos variant. *Blood* **77**, 2087.

Loudianos, G., Murru, S., Kanavakis, E. *et al.* (1991b) A new δ chain variant hemoglobin A₂-Corfu or α₂δ₂ 116 Arg-Cys (G18), detected by δ-globin gene analysis in a Greek family. *Hum. Genet.* **87**, 237.

Loudianos, G., Murru, S., Ristaldi, M.S. *et al.* (1992) A novel δ-thalassaemia mutation. A G→C substitution at codon 30 of the δ-globin gene in a person of Southern Italian origin. *Hum. Mutat.* **1**, 169.

Loudianos, G., Porcu, S., Cossu, P. *et al.* (1993) A new δ-chain variant of hemoglobin A₂-Puglia or α₂δ 26 Glu→Asp (B8) detected by DNA analysis in a family of southern Italian origin. *Hum. Mutat.* **2**, 327.

Loukopoulos, D. (1976) Present status of treatment of thalassemia in Greece. In: *Birth Defects: Original Article Series* (eds D. Bergsma, A. Cerami, C.M. Peterson & J.H. Graziani), p. 1. Liss, New York.

Loukopoulos, D. & Fessas, P. (1965) The distribution of hemoglobin types in thalassemic erythrocytes. *J. Clin. Invest.* **44**, 231.

Loukopoulos, D., Loutradi, A. & Fessas, P. (1978) A unique thalassaemia syndrome: homozygous α-thalassaemia + homozygous β-thalassaemia. *Br. J. Haematol.* **39**, 377.

Loukopoulos, D., Hadji, A., Papadakis, M. *et al.* (1990) Prenatal diagnosis of thalassemia and of the sickle cell syndromes in Greece. *Ann. N. Y. Acad. Sci.* **612**, 226.

Loukopoulos, D., Voskaridou, E., Stamoulakatou, A. *et al.* (1995) Clinical trials with hydroxyurea and recombinant human erythropoietin. In: *The Molecular Biology of Hemoglobin Switching* (eds G. Stamatoyannopoulos & A. W. Nienhuis), p. 365. Alan R. Liss, Inc., New York.

Low, L.C. (1997) Growth, puberty and endocrine function in β-thalassaemia major. *J. Pediatr. Endocrinol. Metab.* **10**, 175.

Low, L.C., Kwan, E.Y.W., Lim, Y.J., Lee, A.C.W., Tam, C.F. & Lam, K.S.L. (1995) Growth hormone treatment of short Chinese children with β-thalassaemia major without growth hormone deficiency. *Clin. Endocrinol.* **42**, 359.

Lowrey, C.H., Bodine, D.M. & Nienhuis, A.W. (1992) Mechanism of DNase I hypersensitive site formation within the human globin locus control region. *Proc. Natl Acad. Sci. USA* **89**, 1143.

Luban, N.L. & Miller, D.R. (1978) Serum inhibitors to granulopoiesis in thalassemia major. *Exp Hematol.* **6**, 185.

Lubin, B.H. (1987) Reference values in infancy and childhood. In: *Hematology of Infancy and Childhood* (eds D.G. Nathan & F.A. Oski), p. 1677. W.B. Saunders, Philadelphia.

Lucarelli, G. & Weatherall, D.J. (1991) For debate: Bone marrow transplantation for severe thalassaemia. *Br. J. Haematol.* **78**, 300.

Lucarelli, G., Galimberti, M., Polchi, P. *et al.* (1990) Bone marrow transplantation in patients with thalassemia. *N. Eng. J. Med.* **322**, 417.

Lucarelli, G., Galimberti, M., Polchi, P. *et al.* (1991) Bone marrow transplantation in thalassemia. *Hematol./Oncol. Clin. N. Am.* **5**, 549.

Lucarelli, G., Galimberti, M., Polchi, P. *et al.* (1992) Bone marrow transplantation in adult thalassemia. *Blood* **80**, 1603.

Lucarelli, G., Galimberti, M., Polchi, P. *et al.* (1993) Marrow transplantation in patients with thalassemia responsive to iron chelation therapy. *N. Eng. J. Med.* **329**, 840.

Lucarelli, G., Giardini, C. & Baronciani, D. (1995) Bone marrow transplantation in β-thalassemia. *Sem. Hematol.* **32**, 297.

Lucarelli, G., Clift, R.A., Galimberti, M. *et al.* (1996) Marrow transplantation for patients with thalassemia: results in class 3 patients. *Blood* **87**, 2082.

Luhby, A.L. & Cooperman, J.M. (1961) Folic acid deficiency in thalassaemia major. *Lancet* **ii**, 490.

Luhby, A.L., Cooperman, J.M., Feldman, R., Ceraolo, J., Herrero, J. & Marley, J.F. (1961) Folic acid deficiency as a limiting factor in the anemias of thalassemia major. *Blood* **18**, 786.

Luhby, A.L., Cooperman, J.M., Lopez, R. & Giorgio, A.J. (1969) Vitamin B₁₂ metabolism in thalassemia major. *Ann. N. Y. Acad. Sci.* **165**, 443.

Lui, P., Henkelman, M., Joshi, J. *et al.* (1996) Quantitation of cardiac and tissue iron by nuclear magnetic resonance in a novel murine thalassemia–cardiac iron overload model. *Can. J. Cardiol.* **12**, 155.

Lukens, J.N. & Neuman, L.A. (1971) Excretion and distribution of iron during chronic deferoxamine therapy. *Blood* **38**, 614.

Luppis, B. & Ventruto, V. (1979) Synthesis of alpha, delta-beta and gamma chains by reticulocytes from two brothers homozygous for haemoglobin Lepore. *Acta Haematol.* **61**, 216.

Lutcher, C.L., Wilson, J.B., Gravely, M.E. *et al.* (1976) Hb Leslie, an unstable hemoglobin due to deletion of glutaminyl residue beta 131 (H9) occurring in association with beta⁰-thalassemia, Hb C and Hb S. *Blood* **47**, 99.

Lux, S.E. & Palek, J. (1995) Disorders of red cell membrane. In: *Blood: Principles and Practice of Hematology* (eds R.I. Handin, S.E. Lux & T.P. Stossel), p. 1701. J.B. Lippincott, Philadelphia.

Luzzatto, L., Nwachiku-Jarrett, E.S. & Reddy, S. (1970) Increased sickling of parasitised erythrocytes as mechanism of resistance against malaria in the sickle-cell trait. *Lancet* **i**, 319.

Luzzi, G.A. & Pasvol, G. (1990) Cytoadherence of *Plasmodium falciparum*-infected α-thalassaemic red cells. *Ann. Trop. Med. Parasitol.* **84**, 413.

Luzzi, G.A., Torii, M., Aikawa, M. & Pasvol, G. (1990) Unrestricted growth of *Plasmodium falciparum* in microcytic erythrocytes in iron deficiency and thalassaemia. *Br. J. Haematol.* **74**, 519.

Luzzi, G.A., Merry, A.H., Newbold, C.I., Marsh, K., Pasvol, G. & Weatherall, D.J. (1991) Surface antigen expression on *Plasmodium falciparum*-infected erythrocytes is modified in α- and β-thalassaemia. *J. Exp. Med.* **173**, 785.

Lyberatos, C., Chalevelakis, G., Platis, A., Stathakis, M., Panani, A. & Gardikis, C. (1972) Erythrocyte content of free protoporphyrin in thalassaemic syndromes. *Acta Haematol.* **47**, 164.

Lynch, J.R., Tate, V.E., Weatherall, D.J. *et al.* (1988) Molecular basis of β-thalassemia in Thailand. *Birth Defects* **23**, 71.

Lynch, J.R., Brown, J.M., Best, S., Jennings, M.W. & Weatherall, D.J. (1991) Characterization of the breakpoint of a 3.5 kb deletion of the β-globin gene. *Genomics* **10**, 509.

Ma, S.K., Chan, A.Y.Y., Ha, S.Y., Chang, G.C.F. & Chan, L.C. (1999) Two novel β-thalassemia alleles in the Chinese: IVSII-2 (-T) β-zero mutation and NT+8 (C→T) silent β-plus mutation. *Blood* **94** (Suppl. 1), 34b.

Maberry, M.C., Mason, R.A., Cunningham, F.G. & Pritchard, J.A. (1990) Pregnancy complicated by hemoglobin CC and C-β-thalassemia disease. *Obstet. Gynecol.* **76**, 324.

Macchia, P., Massei, F., Nardi, M., Favre, C., Brunori, E. & Barba, V. (1990) Thalassemia intermedia and recurrent priapism following splenectomy. *Haematologica* **75**, 486.

MacDonald, V.W. & Charache, S. (1983) Differences in the reaction sequences associated with drug-induced oxidation of hemoglobins E, S, A, and F. *J. Lab. Clin. Med.* **102**, 762.

Machin, G.A. (1981) Differential diagnosis of hydrops fetalis. *Am. J. Med. Genet.* **9**, 341.

MacIver, J.E., Went, L.N. & Irvine, R.A. (1961) Hereditary persistence of foetal haemoglobin: a family study suggesting allelism of the F gene to the S and C haemoglobin genes. *Br. J. Haematol.* **7**, 373.

Macotpet, G., Wilairat, P., Fucharoen, S. & Wasi, P. (1988) Differential expression of erythrocyte calpain and calpastatin activities in β^0-thalassaemia/Hb E disease. *Birth Defects* **23**, 257.

Mager, D.L., Henthorn, P.S. & Smithies, O. (1985) A Chinese $^{G}\gamma+$ $(^{A}\gamma\delta\beta)^0$ thalassemia deletion: comparison to other deletions in the human β-globin gene cluster and sequence analysis of the breakpoints. *Nucl. Acids Res.* **13**, 6559.

Maggio, A., Marcno, R., Cambino, R. *et al.* (1982) What's the significance of Bart's Hb in the Sicilian population? *Haematologica* **67**, 789.

Maggio, A., Giambona, A., Cai, S.P., Wall, J., Kan, Y.W. & Chehab, F.F. (1993) Rapid and simultaneous typing of hemoglobin S, hemoglobin C and seven Mediterranean β-thalassaemia mutations by covalent reverse dot-blot analysis: application to prenatal diagnosis in Sicily. *Blood* **81**, 239.

Magnani, M., Stocchi, V., Camestrari, F. *et al.* (1986) Redox and energetic state of red blood cells in G6PD deficiency, heterozygous β-thalassemia and the combination of both. *Acta Haematol.* **75**, 211.

Magram, J., Chada, K. & Costantini, F. (1985) Developmental regulation of a cloned adult β-globin gene in transgenic mice. *Nature* **315**, 338.

Magro, S., Puzzonia, P., Consarino, C. *et al.* (1990) Hypothyroidism in patients with thalassaemia syndromes. *Acta Haematol.* **84**, 72.

Mainzer, R.A. & O'Connor, W.J. (1958) Evaluation of splenectomy in the treatment of Cooley's anemia. *Ann. Surg.* **148**, 44.

Makler, M.T., Berthrong, M., Locke, H.R. & Dawson, D.L. (1974) A new variant of sickle-cell disease with high levels of foetal haemoglobin homogeneously distributed within red cells. *Br. J. Haematol.* **26**, 519.

Malamos, B., Belcher, E.H., Gyftaki, E. & Binopoulos, D. (1961) Simultaneous studies with Fe^{59} and Cr^{51} in congenital haemolytic anaemias. *Nucl. Med. (Stuttgart)* **2**, 1.

Malamos, B., Fessas, P. & Stamatoyannopoulos, G. (1962) Types of thalassaemia-trait carriers as revealed by a study in their incidence in Greece. *Br. J. Haematol.* **8**, 5.

Malamos, B., Belcher, E.H., Gyftaki, W. & Binopoulos, D. (1963) Simultaneous radioactive tracer studies of erythropoiesis and red-cell destruction in sickle-cell disease and sickle-cell haemoglobin/thalassaemia. *Br. J. Haematol.* **9**, 487.

Malasit, P., Mahasorn, W., Mongkolsapaya, J. *et al.* (1997) Presence of immunoglobulin, C3 and cytolytic C5b-9 complement components on the surface of erythrocytes from patients with β-thalassaemia/Hb E disease. *Br. J. Haematol.* **96**, 507.

Malcorra-Azpiazu, J.J., Wilson, J.B., Molchanova, T.P., Pobedimskaya, D.D. & Huisman, T.H.J. (1993) Hb Porto Allegre or $\alpha_2\beta_2 9(A6)$ Ser→Cys in unrelated families of the Canary Islands. *Hemoglobin* **17**, 457.

Manconi, P.E., Dessi, C., Sanna, G. *et al.* (1998) Human immunodeficiency virus infection in multi-transfused patients with thalassaemia major. *Eur. J. Pediatr.* **147**, 304.

Mancuso, L., Iacona, M.A., Marchi, S., Rigano, P. & Geraci, E. (1985) Severe cardiomyopathy in a woman with intermediate beta-thalassemia. Regression of cardiac failure with desferrioxamine. *G. Ital. Cardiol.* **15**, 916.

Mancuso, P., Zingale, A., Basile, L., Chiaramonte, I. & Tropea, R. (1993) Cauda equina compression syndrome in a patient affected by thalassemia intermedia: complete regression with blood transfusion therapy. *Child. Nerv. Sys.* **9**, 440.

Manganelli, G., Dalfino, G. & Tannoia, N. (1962) Su di un caso associazone tra talassemie e 'persistenza ereditaria de emoglobina fetals'. (On a case of association of thalassemia and 'hereditary persistence of fetal hemoglobin'.) *Haematologica* **47**, 353.

Manglani, M., Lokeshwar, M.R., Vani, V.G., Bhatia, N. & Mhaskar, V. (1997) 'NESTROFT'—an effective screening test for beta thalassemia trait. *Indian Pediatr.* **34**, 702.

Maniatis, A., Bousios, T., Nagel, R.L. *et al.* (1979) Hemoglobin Crete (β129 Ala→Pro): a new high affinity variant interacting with β^0 and $\delta\beta^0$-thalassemia. *Blood* **54**, 54.

Maniatis, G.M., Ramirez, F., Cann, A., Marks, P.A. & Bank, A. (1976) Translation and stability of human globin mRNA in *Xenopus* oocytes. *J. Clin. Invest.* **58**, 1419.

Maniatis, T., Fritsch, E.F., Lauer, J. & Lawn, R.M. (1980) The molecular genetics of human hemoglobins. *Annu. Rev. Genet.* **14**, 145.

Maniatis, T., Fritsch, E.F., Lauer, J. *et al.* (1981) The structure and chromosomal arrangement of human globin genes. In: *Organization and Expression of Globin Genes* (eds G. Stamatoyannopoulos & A.W. Nienhuis), p. 15. Alan R. Liss, Inc., New York.

Mann, J.R., MacNeish, A.S., Bannister, D., Clegg, J.B., Wood, W.G. & Weatherall, D.J. (1972) $\delta\beta$-Thalassaemia in a Chinese family. *Br. J. Haematol.* **23**, 393.

Mannu, F., Arese, P., Cappellini, M.D. *et al.* (1995) Role of hemichrome binding to erythrocyte membrane in the generation of band-3 alterations in β-thalassaemia intermedia erythrocytes. *Blood* **86**, 2014.

Manor, D., Fibach, E., Goldfarb, A. & Rachmilewitz, E.A. (1986) Erythropoietin activity in the serum of beta thalassemic patients. *Scand. J. Haematol.* **37**, 221.

Mantovani, R., Malgaretti, N., Nicolis, S., Ronchi, A., Giglioni, B. & Ottolenghi, S. (1988) The effects of HPFH mutations in the human γ-globin promoter on binding of ubiquitous and erythroid specific nuclear factors. *Nucl. Acids Res.* **16**, 7783.

Maquat, L.E. (1995) When cells stop making sense: effects of nonsense codons on RNA metabolism in vertebrate cells. *RNA* **1**, 453.

Maquat, L.E. (1996) Defects in RNA splicing and the consequence of shortened translational reading frames. *Am. J. Hum. Genet.* **59**, 279.

Maragoudaki, E., Vrettou, C., Kanavakis, E., Traeger-Synodinos, J., Metaxatou-Mavromati, A. & Kattamis, C. (1998) Molecular, haematological and clinical studies of a silent β-gene C→G mutation at 6 bp 3′ to the termination codon (+1480 C→G) in twelve Greek families. *Br. J. Haematol.* **103**, 45.

Maragoudaki, E., Kanavakis, E., Traeger-Synodinos, J. *et al.* (1999) Molecular, haematological and clinical studies of the −101 C→T substitution of the β-globin gene promoter in 25 β-thalassaemia intermedia patients and 45 heterozygotes. *Br. J. Haematol.* **107**, 699.

Marbaix, G., Huez, G. & Burny, A. (1975) Absence of polyadenylate segment in globin messenger RNA accelerates its degradation in *Xenopus* oocytes. *Proc. Natl Acad. Sci. USA* **72**, 3065.

Marcus, R.E., Davies, S.C., Bantock, H.M., Underwood, S.R., Walton, S. & Huehns, E.R. (1984) Desferrioxamine to improve cardiac function in iron-overloaded patients with thalassaemia major. *Lancet* **1**, 373.

Marengo-Rowe, A.J. (1965) Rapid electrophoresis and quantitation of haemoglobins on cellulose acetate. *J. Clin. Pathol.* **18**, 790.

Marengo-Rowe, A.J., McCracken, A.W. & Flanagan, P. (1968) Complete suppression of hemoglobin A synthesis in hemoglobin D Los Angeles-beta thalassemia. *J. Clin. Pathol.* **21**, 508.

Marinone, G. & Bernasconi, C. (1957) Studio elecroforetico quantitavo su blocco d'amido dell'emoglobina normale e dei talassemici. *Haematologica* **42**, 1.

Marinone, G., Bernasconi, C., Gautier, A. & Marcovici, I. (1958) Studi di citologia elettronica nella talassemia. *Haematologica* **43**, 1123.

Marinucci, M., Bruni, E., Tentori, L., de Sandre, G. & Vettore, L. (1977) Double heterozygosis for Hb J Paris and β-thalassemia. *Hemoglobin* **1**, 595.

Marinucci, M., Mavilio, F., Tentori, L. & Alberti, R. (1978a) Hb O Indonesia (α_2 116(GH4) Glu→Lys β_2) in association with β thalassemia. *Hemoglobin* **2**, 59.

Marinucci, M., Mavilio, F., Tentori, L. & Mariuzzi, R.A. (1978b) Hemoglobin O Indonesia (α_2 116(GH4) Glu→Lys β_2) associated with beta-thalassemia in a family from Polosine (Italy). *New Istanbul Contrib. Clin. Sci.* **12**, 272.

Marinucci, M., Mavilio, F., Gabbianelli, M. *et al.* (1979a) Synthesis of Hb Lepore Boston in peripheral blood. *Hemoglobin* **3**, 309.

Marinucci, M., Mavilio, F., Massa, A. *et al.* (1979b) Haemoglobin Lepore trait: haematological and structural studies in the Italian population. *Br. J. Haematol.* **42**, 557.

Mariotti, E., Agostini, E., Angelucci, E., Lucarelli, G. & Sgarbi, E. (1997) Reversal of the initial cardiac damage in thalassemic patients treated with bone marrow transplantation and phlebotomy. *Bone Marrow Transplant.* **19** (Suppl. 2), 139.

Marks, P.A. & Bank, A. (1971) Molecular pathway of thalassemia. *Fed. Proc.* **30**, 977.

Marks, P.A. & Burka, E.R. (1964a) Hemoglobin synthesis in human reticulocytes: a defect in globin formation in thalassemia major. *Ann. N.Y. Acad. Sci.* **119**, 513.

Marks, P.A. & Burka, E.R. (1964b) Hemoglobins A and F: formation in thalassemia and other hemolytic anemias. *Science* **144**, 552.

Marks, P.A., Burka, E.R. & Rifkind, R.A. (1964) Control of protein synthesis in reticulocytes and the formation of hemoglobin A and F in thalassemia syndromes and other hemolytic anemias. *Medicine (Baltimore)* **43**, 769.

Marmont, A. & Bianchi, V. (1948) Mediterranean anaemia: clinical and haematological findings, and pathogenic studies in milder forms of disease (with report of cases). *Acta Haematol.* **1**, 4.

Marotta, C.A., Wilson, J.T., Forget, B.G. & Weissman, S.M. (1977) Human beta-chain messenger RNA. II. Nucleotide sequences derived from complementary DNA. *J. Biol. Chem.* **252**, 5040.

Marsh, M.N., Holbrook, I.B., Clark, C. & Shaffer, J.L. (1981) Tinnitus in a patient with beta-thalassaemia intermedia on long term treatment with desferrioxamine. *Postgrad. Med. J.* **57**, 582.

Marsh, W.L., Rogers, Z.R., Nelson, D.P. & Vedvick, T.S. (1983) Hematologic findings in Southeast Asian immigrants with particular reference to hemoglobin E. *Ann. Clin. Lab. Sci.* **13**, 299.

Marti, H.R. (1963) *Normale und Anormale Menschliche Hamoglobine*, p. 81. Springer, Berlin.

Marti, H.R., Fischer, S. & Killer, D. (1975) The identification and frequency of hemoglobin Lepore. In: *Abnormal Haemoglobins and Thalassaemia; Diagnostic Aspects* (ed. R.M. Schmidt), p. 137. Academic Press, New York.

Martin, D.I.K., Tsai, S.-F. & Orkin, S.H. (1989) Increased γ-globin expression in a nondeletion HPFH mediated by an erythroid-specific DNA-binding factor. *Nature* **338**, 435.

Martin, J., Palacio, A., Petit, J. & Martin, C. (1990) Fatty transformation of thoracic extramedullary hematopoiesis following splenectomy: CT features. *J. Comput. Assist. Tomogr.* **14**, 477.

Martin, D.I., Fiering, S. & Groudine, M. (1996) Regulation of β-globin gene expression: straightening out the locus. *Curr. Opin. Genet. Dev.* **6**, 488.

Martinez, G. & Colombo, B. (1973) Lepore Washington (Boston) hemoglobin and its interaction with beta-thalassemia in a Cuban child. *Rev. Invest Clin.* **25**, 359.

Martinez, G. & Colombo, B. (1974) A new type of hereditary persistence of foetal haemoglobin: is a diffusible factor regulating γ-chain synthesis? *Nature* **252**, 735.

Martinez, G. & Colombo, B. (1976) α-Thalassaemia in Cuba. *Acta Haematol.* **55**, 36.

Martinez, G., Novelletto, A., Di Renzo, A., Felicetti, L. & Colombo, B. (1989) A case of hereditary persistence of fetal hemoglobin caused by a gene not linked to the β-globin cluster. *Hum. Genet.* **82**, 335.

Martínez, G., Ferreira, R., Hernandez, A., Di Rienzo, A., Felicetti, L. & Colombo, B. (1990) Frequency of the –$\alpha^{3.7}$ thalassemia deletion in the non-white Cuban population. *Gene Geograph.* **4**, 65.

Martinson, J.J. (1991) *Genetic variation in South Pacific islanders*. D. Phil. thesis, University of Oxford.

Martinson, J.J., Harding, R.M., Boyce, A.J. & Clegg, J.B. (1994) VNTR alleles associated with the α globin locus are haplotype-and population-related. *Am. J. Hum. Genet.* **55**, 513.

Masala, A., Meloni, T., Gallisai, D. *et al.* (1984) Endocrine function in multitransfused prepubertal patients with homozygous beta-thalassemia. *J. Clin. Endocrinol. Metab.* **58**, 667.

Masera, G., Jean, G., Conter, V., Terzoli, S., Mauri, R.A. & Cazzaniga, M. (1980) Sequential study of liver biopsy in thalassaemia. *Arch. Dis. Child.* **55**, 800.

Masera, G., Monguzzi, W. & Tornotti, G. (1990) Pediatric hematologists and adult thalassemics. *Ann. N.Y. Acad. Sci.* **612**, 461.

Mason, K.P., Grandison, Y., Hayes, R.J. *et al.* (1982) Post-natal decline of fetal haemoglobin in homozygous sickle cell disease: relationship to parental Hb F levels. *Br. J. Haematol.* **52**, 455.

Massa, A., Tannoia, N., Cerquozzi, S. *et al.* (1987) Molecular characterization of α-thalassaemia in Puglia. In: *Thalassaemia Today: The Mediterranean Experience* (eds G. Sirchia & A. Zanella), p. 459. Centro Trasfusionale Ospedale Maggiore Policlinico Di Milano Editore, Milan.

Mathew, C.G. (1991) *Protocols in Human Molecular Genetics. Methods in Molecular Biology* (ed. J.M. Walker), Vol. 9. Humana Press, Clifton, New Jersey.

Mathew, C.G.P., Rousseau, J., Rees, J.S. & Harley, E.H. (1983) The molecular basis of α-thalassaemia in a South African population. *Br. J. Haematol.* **55**, 103.

Matioli, G.T. & del Pianco, E. (1961) Su due casi di talassemia minima a monoespressivitia genica. *Haematologica* **46**, 83.

Matson, G.A., Sutton, H.E., Swanson, J. & Robinson, R. (1963) Distribution of haptoglobin, transferrin, and hemoglobin types among Indians of middle America: Southern Mexico, Guatemala, Honduras and Nicaragua. *Hum. Biol.* **35**, 474.

Matsuda, M., Sakamoto, N. & Fukumaki, Y. (1992) δ-Thalassemia caused by disruption of the site for an erythroid-specific transcription factor, GATA-1, in the δ-globin gene promoter. *Blood* **80**, 1347.

Matsunaga, E., Kimura, A., Yamada, H., Fukumaki, Y. & Takagi, Y. (1985) A novel deletion in δβ-thalassemia found in Japan. *Biochem. Biophys. Res. Comm.* **126**, 185.

Matthay, K.K., Mentzer, W.C. Jr, Dozy, A.M., Kan, Y.W. & Bainton, D.F. (1979) Modification of hemoglobin H disease by sickle trait. *J. Clin. Invest.* **64**, 1024.

Matthews, J.H., Rowlands, D., Wood, J.K. & Wood, W.G. (1981) Homozygous $^{G}\gamma\delta\beta$ thalassaemia. *Clin. Lab. Haematol.* **3**, 121.

Matzner, Y., Goldfarb, A., Abrahamov, A., Drexler, R., Friedberg, A. & Rachmilewitz, E.A. (1993) Impaired neutrophil chemotaxis in patients with thalassaemia major. *Br. J. Haematol.* **85**, 153.

Maude, G.H., Higgs, D.R., Beckford, M. *et al.* (1985) Alpha thalassaemia and the haematology of normal Jamaican children. *Clin. Lab. Haematol.* **7**, 289.

Maungsapaya, W., Winichagoon, P., Fucharoen, S., Pootrakul, S.-N. & Wasi, P. (1985) Improved technic for detecting intraerythrocytic inclusion bodies in α thalassemia trait. *J. Med. Assoc. Thailand* **68**, 43.

Maurer, H.S., Lloyd-Still, J.D., Ingrisano, C., Gonzalez-Crussi, F. & Honig, C.R. (1988) A prospective evaluation of iron chelation therapy in children with severe β-thalassemia: a six-year study. *Am. J. Dis. Child.* **142**, 287.

Mavilio, F., Giampaolo, A., Care, A., Sposi, N.M. & Marinucci, M. (1983) The δβ crossover region in Lepore Boston hemoglobinopathy is restricted to a 59 base pair region around the 5′ splice junction of the large globin gene intervening sequence. *Blood* **62**, 230.

Mazza, U., Saglio, G., Cappio, F.C., Camaschella, C., Neretto, G. & Gallo, E. (1976) Clinical and haematological data in 254 cases of beta-thalassaemia trait in Italy. *Br. J. Haematol.* **33**, 91.

de Mazzoleni, G.Sa. D., Gately, J. & Riddell, R.H. (1991) *Yersinia enterocolitica* infection with ileal perforation associated with iron overload and deferoxamine therapy. *Dig. Dis. Sci.* **36**, 1154.

Mazzone, D. & Distefano, G. (1969) Rivieli colecistografici in case di thalassemia majore e di mallattie drepanocitiche. *Riv. Pediatr. Sicil.* **24**, 74.

Mazzone, D., Romeo, M.A., Fichera, A., Pratico, G., Digregorio, F. & Schiliro, G. (1984) Coagulation parameters in beta thalassaemia major. *Riv. Paediatr. Scienze* **2**, 71.

McCormick, W.F. & Humphreys, E.W. (1960) High fetal-hemoglobin C disease: a new syndrome. *Blood* **16**, 1736.

McCurdy, P.R. & Pearson, H.A. (1961) Genetic study of a family possessing hemoglobins S and C, and classical thalassemia. *Am. J. Hum. Genet.* **13**, 390.

McDonald, M.J., Noble, R.W., Sharma, V.S., Ranney, H.M., Crookston, J.H. & Schegartz, J.M. (1975) A comparison of the functional properties of two Lepore hemoglobins with those of hemoglobin A. *J. Mol. Biol.* **94**, 35.

McDowell, T.L., Gibbons, R.J., Sutherland, H. *et al.* (1999) Localization of a putative transcriptional regulator (ATRX) at pericentromeric heterochromatin and the short arms of acrocentric chromosomes. *Proc. Natl Acad. Sci. USA* **96**, 13983.

McFadzean, A.J.S. & Todd, D. (1971) Cooley's anaemia among the Tanka of South China. *Trans. Roy. Soc. Trop. Med. Hyg.* **65**, 59.

McIntosh, N. (1976a) Beneficial effects of transfusing a patient with non-transfusion-dependent thalassaemia major. *Arch. Dis. Child.* **51**, 471.

McIntosh, N. (1976b) Endocrinopathy in thalassaemia major. *Arch. Dis. Child.* **51**, 195.

McNiel, J.R. (1967) Family studies of thalassemia in Arabia. *Am. J. Hum. Genet.* **19**, 100.

McNiel, J.R. (1968) The inheritance of hemoglobin H disease. Abstracts of the Simultaneous Sessions. In: *XII Congress International and National Society of Hematology*, p. 52. Grune & Stratton, New York.

McNiel, J.R. (1971) Family studies of alpha-thalasemia and hemoglobin H disease in eastern Saudi Arabia. *J. Med. Assoc. Thailand* **54**, 153.

McPherson, E., Clemens, M., Gibbons, R.J. & Higgs, D.R. (1995) X-linked alpha thalassemia/mental retardation (ATR-X) syndrome. A new kindred with severe genital anomalies and mild hematologic expression. *Am. J. Med. Genet.* **55**, 302.

Mears, J.G., Ramirez, F., Liebowitz, D., Nakaura, F., Bloom, A., Konotey-Ahulu, F.I.D. & Bank, A. (1978a) Changes in restricted human cellular DNA fragments containing globin gene sequences in thalassemia and related disorders. *Proc. Natl Acad. Sci. USA* **75**, 1222.

Mears, J.G., Ramirez, F., Leibowitz, D. & Bank, A. (1978b) Organization of human δ- and β-globin genes in cellular DNA and the presence of intragenic inserts. *Cell* **15**, 15.

Mears, J.G., Schoenbrun, M., Schaefer, K.E., Bestak, M. & Radel, E. (1982) Frequent association of alpha thalassemia with splenic sequestration crisis and splenomegaly in sickle cell (SS) subjects. *Blood* **60**, 47a.

Mears, J.G., Lachman, H.M., Labie, D. & Nagel, R.L. (1983) Alpha-thalassemia is related to prolonged survival in sickle cell anemia. *Blood* **62**, 286.

Meduri, D., Notario, A., Tropin, L. & Comin, U. (1973) Analisi delle proteine di membrana nell'eritocita normale ed in quello talassemico. In: *Atti del V⁰ Congresso sulle Microcitemie*, Cosenza, p. 487. Arte Della Stampa, Roma.

Medvinsky, A. & Dzierzak, E. (1996) Definitive hematopoiesis is autonomously initiated by the AGM region. *Cell* **86**, 897.

Mehta, B.C., Dave, V.B., Joshi, S.R., Baxi, A.J., Bhatia, H.M. & Patel, J.C. (1972) Study of hematological and genetical characteristics of Cutchhi Bhanushali community. *Indian J. Med. Res.* **60**, 305.

Meital, V., Izak, G. & Rachmilewitz, M. (1961) L'effet de la grossesse sur la thalassémie. *Nouv. Rev. Fr. Hematol.* **1**, 389.

Mela, Q.S., Cacace, E., Ruggerio, V., Frigerio, R., Pitzus, F. & Carcassi, U. (1988) Virus infection in β-thalassemia intermedia. *Birth Defects* **23**, 557.

Melis, M.A., Pirastu, M., Galanello, R., Furbetta, M., Tuveri, T. & Cao, A. (1983) Phenotypic effect of heterozygous α and β⁰-thalassemia interaction. *Blood* **62**, 226.

Melloni, E., Sparatore, B., Salamino, F., Michetti, M. & Pontremoli, S. (1982) Cytosolic calcium-dependent proteinase of human erythrocytes: formation of an enzyme–natural inhibitor complex induced by Ca^{2+} ions. *Biochem. Biophys. Res. Comm.* **106**, 731.

Meloni, T., Gallisai, D., Dore, A., Forteleoni, G. & Mela, G. (1981) Neonatal screening for hemoglobinopathy in North Sardinia. *Eur. J. Pediatr.* **137**, 195.

Meloni, A., Rosatelli, M.C., Faà, V. *et al.* (1992) Promoter mutations producing mild β-thalassaemia in the Italian population. *Br. J. Haematol.* **80**, 222.

Meloni, A., Demurtas, M., Moi, L., Faà, V., Cao, A. & Rosatelli, M.C. (1994) A novel β-thalassemia mutation: frameshift at codon 59 detected in an Italian carrier. *Hum. Mutat.* **3**, 309.

Menke, W.T. (1973) Mediterranean anaemia in antiquity. *Br. Med. J.* **ii**, 489.

Mentzer, W.C. Jr (1973) Differentiation of iron deficiency from thalassaemia trait. *Lancet* **i**, 882.

Merault, G., Keclard, L., Saint-Martin, C. *et al.* (1985) Hemoglobin Roseau-Pointe a Pitre $\alpha_2\beta_2$90(F6) Glu→Gly: a new hemoglobin variant with slight instability and low oxygen affinity. *FEBS Lett.* **184**, 10.

Merault, G., Keclard, L., Garin, J. *et al.* (1986) Hemoglobin La Desirade $\alpha_2^A\beta_2$ 127(H7) Ala→Val: a new unstable hemoglobin. *Hemoglobin* **10**, 593.

Mercola, K.E., Stang, H.D., Brown, J., Salser, W. & Cline, M.J. (1980) Insertion of a new gene of viral origin into bone marrow cells of mice. *Science* **208**, 1033.

Merghoub, T., Perichon, B., Maier-Redesperger, M. *et al.* (1996) Variation of fetal hemoglobin and F-cell number with the LCR-HS2 polymorphism in nonanemic individuals. *Blood* **87**, 2607.

Merkel, P.A., Simonson, D.C., Amiel, S.A. *et al.* (1988) Insulin resistance and hyperinsulinemia in patients with thalassemia major treated by hypertransfusion. *N. Eng. J. Med.* **318**, 809.

Merritt, D., Jones, R.T., Head, C. *et al.* (1997) Hb Seal Rock [(α2)142 Term→Glu, codon 142 TAA→GAA]: an extended α chain variant associated with anemia, microcytosis, and α-thalassemia-2 (−3.7 kb). *Hemoglobin* **21**, 331.

Merryweather-Clarke, A.T., Pointon, J.J., Shearman, J.D. & Robson, K.J.H. (1997) Global prevalence of putative haemochromatosis mutations. *J. Med. Genet.* **34**, 275.

Meryman, H.T. (1989) Transfusion-induced alloimmunization and immunosuppression and the effect of leukocyte depletion. *Transfus. Med. Review* **3**, 180.

Metaxatou-Mavromati, A.D., Antonopoulou, H.K., Laskari, S.S., Tsiarta, H.K., Ladis, V.A. & Kattamis, C.A. (1982) Developmental changes in hemoglobin F levels during the first two years of life in normal and heterozygous β-thalassemia infants. *Pediatr.* **69**, 734.

Metherall, J.E., Collins, F.S., Pan, J., Weissman, S.M. & Forget, B.G. (1986) β⁰-Thalassaemia caused by a base substitution that creates an alternative splice acceptor site in an intron. *EMBO J.* **5**, 2551.

Metherall, J.E., Gillespie, F.P. & Forget, B.G. (1988) Analyses of linked β-globin genes suggest that nondeletion forms of hereditary persistence of fetal hemoglobin are bona fide switching mutants. *Am. J. Hum. Genet.* **42**, 476.

Metzenberg, A.B., Wurzer, G., Huisman, T.H. & Smithies, O. (1991) Homology requirements for unequal crossing over in humans. *Genetics* **128**, 143.

Mezzadra, G., Guarneri, B. & Schiliro, G. (1974) Contributo allo studio dell'ulcera talassemica. *Rif. Med.* **88**, 8.

Michaeli, J., Mittelman, M., Grisaru, D. & Rachmilewitz, E.A. (1992) Thromboembolic complications in beta thalassemia major. *Acta Haematol.* **87**, 71.

Micheli, F., Penati, F. & Momigliano, L.G. (1935) Ulteriori richerche sulla anemia ipocromica splenomegalica con poichilocitosi. *Haematologica* (Suppl.) **16**, 10.

Michelson, J. & Cohen, A. (1988) Incidence and treatment of fractures in thalassemia. *J. Orthop. Trauma* **2**, 29.

Michelson, A.M. & Orkin, S.H. (1980) The 3′ untranslated regions of the duplicated human α globin genes are unexpectedly divergent. *Cell* **22**, 371.

Michelson, A.M. & Orkin, S.H. (1983) Boundaries of gene conversion within the duplicated human α-globin genes. Concerted evolution by segmental recombination. *J. Biol. Chem.* **258**, 15245.

Middlemis, J.H. & Raper, A.B. (1966) Skeletal changes in the haemogobinopathies. *J. Bone Joint Surg.* **48**, 693.

Mihindukulasuriya, J.C., Chanmugam, D., Machado, V. & Samarasinghe, C.A. (1977) A case of paraparesis due to extramedullary haemopoiesis in Hb E thalassaemia. *Postgrad. Med. J.* **53**, 393.

Milland, M., Bergé-Lefrance, J.L., Lena, D. & Cartouzou, G. (1987) Oligonucleotide screening of β thalassemia mutations in the South East of France. *Hemoglobin* **11**, 317.

Millard, D.P., Mason, K., Serjeant, B.E. & Serjeant, G.R. (1977) Comparison of haematological features of the β⁰ and β⁺ thalassaemia traits in Jamaican Negroes. *Br. J. Haematol.* **36**, 161.

Miller, A.D. (1990) Retrovirus packaging cells. *Hum. Gene Ther.* **1**, 5.

Miller, A.D., Bender, M.A., Harris, E.A.S., Kaleko, M. & Gelinas, R.E. (1988a) Design of retrovirus vector for transfer and expression of the human beta-globin gene. *J. Virol.* **62**, 4337.

Miller, B.A., Salameh, M., Ahmed, M. *et al.* (1987) Analysis of hemoglobin F production in Saudi Arabian families with sickle cell anemia. *Blood* **70**, 716.

Miller, D.R., Weed, R.I., Stamatoyannopoulos, G. & Yoshida, A. (1971) Hemoglobin Koln disease occurring as a fresh mutation: erythrocyte metabolism and survival. *Blood* **38**, 715.

Miller, K.B., Rosenwasser, L.J., Bessette, J.A., Beer, D.J. & Rocklin, R.E. (1981) Rapid desensitisation for desferrioxamine anaphylactic reaction. *Lancet* **i**, 1059.

Miller, S.T., Rieder, R.F., Rao, S.P. & Brown, A.K. (1988b) Cerebrovascular accidents in children with sickle-cell disease and alpha-thalassemia. *J. Pediatr.* **113**, 847.

Milner, P.F. & Huisman, T.H.J. (1976) Studies on the proportion and synthesis of haemoglobin G Philadelphia in red cells of heterozygotes, a homozygote, and a heterozygote for both haemoglobin G and α thalassaemia. *Br. J. Haematol.* **34**, 207.

Milner, P.F. & Wrightstone, R.N. (1981) The unstable hemoglobins: a review. In: *The Function of Red Blood Cells: Erythrocyte Pathobiology* (ed. D.F.H. Wallach), p. 197. Alan R Liss, New York.

Milner, P.F., Clegg, J.B. & Weatherall, D.J. (1971) Haemoglobin H disease due to a unique haemoglobin variant with an elongated α-chain. *Lancet* **i**, 729.

Milner, P.F., Corley, C.C., Pomeroy, W.L., Wilson, J.B., Gravely, M. &

Huisman, T.H.J. (1976) Thalassemia intermedia caused by heterozygosity for both β-thalassemia and hemoglobin Saki (β14(all)Leu→Pro). *Am. J. Hematol.* **1**, 283.

Milner, P.F., Kraus, A.P., Sebes, J.I. *et al.* (1991) Sickle cell disease as a cause of osteonecrosis of the femoral head. *N. Eng. J. Med.* **325**, 1476.

Milner, P.F., Kraus, A.P., Sebes, J.I. *et al.* (1993) Osteonecrosis of the humeral head in sickle cell disease. *Clin. Orthop.* **289**, 136.

Milot, E., Strouboulis, J. Trimborn, T. *et al.* (1996) Heterochromatin effects on the frequency and duration of LCR-mediated gene transcription. *Cell* **87**, 105.

Miniero, R., Rocha, V., Saracco, P. *et al.* (1999) Cord blood transplantation in hemoglobinopathies. *Bone Marrow Transplant.* **22**, 578.

Minnich, V., Na-Nakorn, S., Chongchareonsuk, S. & Kochaseni, S. (1954) Mediterranean anemia: a study of 32 cases in Thailand. *Blood* **9**, 1.

Minnich, V., Na-Nakorn, S., Tuchinda, S., Pravit, W. & Moore, C.V. (1958) Inclusion body anemia in Thailand (Hemoglobin H-thalassemia disease). In: *Proceedings of the 6th International Society of Hematology*, p. 743. Grune and Stratton, Boston.

Minnich, V., Cordonnier, J.K., Williams, W.J. & Moore, C.V. (1962) Alpha, beta and gamma hemoglobin polypeptide chains during the neonatal period with description of fetal form of hemoglobin Dα$_{St. Louis}$. *Blood* **19**, 137.

Miotti, M.L. & Caramello, G.M.T. (1968) Drepanocytic anemia. Presentation of a case with grave bone changes. *Min. Pediatr.* **20**, 700.

Mirabile, E., Testa, R., Consalvo, C., Dickerhoff, R. & Schiliro, G. (1995) Association of Hb S/Hb Lepore and δβ-thalassaemia/Hb Lepore in Sicilian patients: review of the presence of Hb Lepore in Sicily. *Eur. J. Haematol.* **55**, 126.

Mirabile, E., Testa, R., Samperi, P., Consalvo, C., Romano, V. & Schiliro, G. (1997) A mild form of Hb S-β-thalassaemia syndrome is assured in Sicilian patients by β⁺ mutant IVS-1 nt 6 (T→C). *Eur. J. Haematol.* **58**, 67.

Miranda, S.R.P., Figueiredo, M.S., Kerbauy, J., Grotto, H.Z.W., Saad, S.T.O. & Costa, F.F. (1994) Hb Lepore$_{Baltimore}$ (δ50Ser β86Ala) identified by DNA analysis in a Brazilian family. *Acta Haematol.* **91**, 7.

Mirchev, R. & Ferrone, F.A. (1997) The structural link between polymerisation and sickle cell disease. *J. Mol. Biol.* **265**, 475.

Mishima, N., Landman, H., Huisman, T.H.J. & Gilman, J.G. (1989) The DNA deletion in an Indian delta beta-thalassaemia begins one kilobase from the A gamma globin gene and ends in an L1 repetitive sequence. *Br. J. Haematol.* **73**, 375.

Misra, R.C., Ram, B., Mohapatra, B.C., Das, S.N. & Misra, S.C. (1991) High prevalence and heterogenicity of thalassaemias in Orissa. *Indian J. Med. Res.* **94**, 391.

Misteli, T. (1999) RNA splicing: what has phosphorylation got to do with it? *Curr. Biol.* **9**, R198.

Mitchell, J.J., Capua, A., Clow, C. & Scriver, C.R. (1996) Twenty-year outcome analysis of genetic screening programs for Tay–Sachs and β-thalassemia disease carriers in high schools. *Am. J. Hum. Genet.* **59**, 793.

Mitchiner, J.W., Thompson, R.B. & Huisman, T.H.J. (1961) Foetal haemoglobin synthesis in some haemoglobinopathies. *Lancet* **i**, 1169.

Mitra, R., Sarkar, S., Ganguli, S. & De, B.K. (1996) Haemochromatosis in a case of thalassaemia haemoglobin E disease. *J. Indian Med. Assoc.* **94**, 29.

Miyoshi, K., Kaneto, Y., Kawai, H. & Huisman, T.H.J. (1988) X-linked dominant control of F-cells in normal adult life. *Blood* **72**, 1854.

Modell, C.B. (1976) Management of thalassaemia major. *Br. Med. Bull.* **32**, 270.

Modell, C.B. (1977) Total management in thalassaemia major. *Arch. Dis. Child.* **52**, 489.

Modell, B. (1979) Advances in the use of iron-chelating agents for the treatment of iron overload. *Prog. Hematol.* **11**, 267.

Modell, C.B. & Beck, J. (1974) Long-term desferrioxamine therapy in thalassemia. *Ann. N. Y. Acad. Sci.* **232**, 201.

Modell, C.B. & Berdoukas, V.A. (1984) *The Clinical Approach to Thalassaemia*. Grune and Stratton, New York.

Modell, B. & Kuliev, A.M. (1989) Impact of public health on human genetics. *Clin. Genet.* **36**, 286.

Modell, B. & Kuliev, A. (1998) The history of community genetics: the contribution of the haemoglobin disorders. *Comm. Genet.* **1**, 3.

Modell, C.B. & Matthews, R. (1976) Thalassemia in Britain and Australia. In: *Birth Defects: Original Article Series* (eds D. Bergsma, A. Cerami, C.H. Peterson & J.H. Graziano), p. 13. Alan R. Liss, New York.

Modell, C.B. & Petrou, M. (1983) The problem of haemoglobinopathies in India. *Indian J. Haematol.* **1**, 5.

Modell, C.B., Latter, A., Steadman, J.H. & Huehns, E.R. (1969) Haemoglobin synthesis in β-thalassaemia. *Br. J. Haematol.* **17**, 485.

Modell, B., Ward, R.H.T. & Fairweather, D.V.I. (1980) Effect of introducing antenatal diagnosis on reproductive behaviour of families at risk for thalassaemia major. *Br. Med. J.* **280**, 1347.

Modell, B., Petrou, M., Ward, R.H.T. *et al.* (1984) Effect of fetal diagnostic testing on birth-rate of thalassaemia major in Britain. *Lancet* **ii**, 1383.

Modell, B., Petrou, M., Layton, M. *et al.* (1997) Audit of prenatal diagnosis for haemoglobin disorders in the United Kingdom: the first 20 years. *Br. Med. J.* **315**, 779.

Modell, B., Harris, R., Lane, B. *et al.* (2000) Informed choice in genetic screening for thalassaemia during pregnancy: audit from a national confidential inquiry. *Br. Med. J.* **320**, 337.

Modiano, G., Morpurgo, G., Terrenato, L. *et al.* (1991) Protection against malaria morbidity: near fixation of the α thalassaemia gene in a Nepalese population. *Am. J. Hum. Genet.* **48**, 390.

Moi, P., Cash, F.E., Liebhaber, S.A., Cao, A. & Pirastu, M. (1987) An initiation codon mutation (AUG→GUG) of the human α1-globin gene: structural characterization and evidence for a mild thalassemia phenotype. *J. Clin. Invest.* **80**, 1416.

Moi, P., Paglietti, E., Sanna, A. *et al.* (1988) Delineation of the molecular basis of δ- and normal Hb A_2 β-thalassaemia. *Blood* **72**, 530.

Moi, P., Loudianis, G., Lavinha, J. *et al.* (1992) δ-Thalassaemia due to a mutation in an erythroid-specific binding protein sequence 3′ to the δ-globin gene. *Blood* **79**, 512.

Molchanova, T.P. & Huisman, T.H.J. (1997) The levels of abnormal hemoglobin in persons with heterozygosities for an α chain variant and for β-thalassemia. *Hemoglobin* **21**, 173.

Molchanova, T.P. & Huisman, T.H.J. (1998) Hemoglobin abnormalities observed in the populations of the Republics of the Former USSR. *Balkan J. Med. Genet*, **1**, 43.

Molchanova, T.P., Pobedimskaya, D.D. & Huisman, T.H.J. (1994a) The differences in quantities of α2- and α1-globin gene variants in heterozygotes. *Br. J. Haematol.* **88**, 300.

Molchanova, T.P., Pobedimskaya, D.D. & Postnikov, Y.V. (1994b) A simplified procedure for sequencing amplified DNA containing the α-2 or α-1 globin gene. *Hemoglobin* **18**, 251.

Molchanova, T.P., Smetanina, N.S. & Huisman, T.H.J. (1995) A second, elongated, α2-globin mRNA is present in reticulocytes from normal persons and subjects with terminating codon or poly A mutations. *Biochem. Biophys. Res. Comm.* **214**, 1184.

Molina, M.A., Romero, M.J., Abril, E. *et al.* (1994) Frequency of the molecular abnormalities of the β-thalassaemia in Southern Spain and their relationship with the hematologic phenotype. *Sangre* **39**, 253.

de Montalembert, M., Gitor, R., Revillon, Y. *et al.* (1990) Partial splenectomy in homozygous β thalassaemia. *Arch. Dis. Child.* **65**, 304.

Monteiro, C., Rueff, J., Falcao, A.B., Portugal, S., Weatherall, D.J. & Kulozik, A.E. (1989) The frequency and origin of the sickle cell mutation in the district of Coruche/Portugal. *Hum. Genet.* **82**, 255.

Monti, A., Feldhake, C. & Schwartz, S.O. (1964) The S-thalassemia syndrome. *Ann. N. Y. Acad. Sci.* **119**, 474.

Montouri, R., Quattrin, S., Mastrobuoni, A. & Quattrin, N. (1975) Results following splenectomy of 76 cases with Cooley's disease and related syndromes. In: *Proceedings of the International Istanbul Symposium on Abnormal Hemoglobins and Thalassemia*, p. 323, TBTAK, Ankura.

Moo-Penn, W.F., Bechtel, K.C. & Therrell, B.L. (1978a) Hemoglobin P Nilotic in a Mexican-American family. *Hemoglobin* **2**, 65.

Moo-Penn, W.F., Jue, D.L. & Baine, R.M. (1978b) Hemoglobin J Rovigo (α53 Ala→Asp) in association with β-thalassemia. *Hemoglobin* **2**, 443.

Morehouse, L.A., Thomas, C.E. & Aust., S.D. (1984) Superoxide generation of NADPH-Cytochrome P-450 reductase: the effect of iron chelation and the role of superoxide in microsomal lipid peroxidation. *Arch. Biochem. Biophys.* **232**, 366.

Morlé, L., Morlé, F., Dorleac, E. *et al.* (1984) The association of hemoglobin Knossos and hemoglobin Lepore in an Algerian patient. *Hemoglobin* **8**, 229.

Morlé, F., Lopez, B., Henni, T. & Godet, J. (1985) α-Thalassaemia associated with the deletion of two nucleotides at position –2 and –3 preceding the AUG codon. *EMBO J.* **4**, 1245.

Morlé, F., Starck, J. & Godet, J. (1986) α-Thalassaemia due to the deletion of nucleotides –2 and –3 preceding the AUG initiation codon affects translation efficiency both *in vitro* and *in vivo*. *Nucl. Acids Res.* **14**, 3279.

Morlé, F., Francina, A., Ducrocq, R. *et al.* (1995) A new α chain variant Hb Sallanches [α2, 104(G11) Cys→Tyr] associated with HbH disease in one homozygous patient. *Br. J. Haematol.* **91**, 608.

Moseley, J.E. (1962) The thalassemias: Variants and Roentgen bone changes. *J. Mount Sinai Hosp.* **29**, 199.

Moseley, J.E. (1974) Skeletal changes in the anemias. *Sem. Roentgenol.* **9**, 169.

Motta, L. & Polosa, P. (1966) Study of hereditary persistence of fetal hemoglobin (P.H.F.Hb) in a Sicilian family tree. *Haematol. Lat.* **9**, 173.

Motta, M.F.S., Souza, C.A. & Costa, F.F. (1983) Alfa-talassemia em uma populaçao de negros brasileiros. In: *XVI Congresso Brasileiro de Hematologica*. São Paulo, Brazil.

Motulsky, A.G. (1960) Genetic information and the control of protein structure and function. In: *Genetics* (ed. H.E. Sutton), p. 159. Josiah Macy Jr Foundation, New York.

Motulsky, A.G. (1962) Controller genes in synthesis of human haemoglobin. *Nature* **194**, 607.

Motulsky, A.G., Stransky, E. & Fraser, G.R. (1964) Glucose-6-phosphate dehydrogenase (G6PD) deficiency, thalassaemia, and abnormal haemoglobins in the Philippines. *J. Med. Genet.* **1**, 102.

Motum, P.I., Lindeman, R., Hamilton, T.J. & Trent, R.J. (1992) Australian β⁰-thalassaemia: a high haemoglobin A_2 β⁰-thalassaemia due to a 12 kb deletion commencing 5′ to the β-globin gene. *Br. J. Haematol.* **82**, 107.

Motum, P.I., Hamilton, T.J., Lindeman, R., Le, H. & Trent, R.J. (1993a) Molecular characterisation of Vietnamese HPFH. *Hum. Mutat.* **2**, 179.

Motum, P.I., Kearney, A., Hamilton, T.J. & Trent, R.J. (1993b) Filipino

β^0 thalassaemia: a high Hb A_2 β^0 thalassaemia resulting from a large deletion of the 5' β globin gene region. *J. Med. Genet.* **30**, 240.

Motum, P.I., Lindeman, R., Harvey, M.P. & Trent, R.J. (1993c) Comparative studies of nondeletional HPFH γ-globin gene promoters. *Exp. Hematol.* **21**, 852.

Motum, P.I., Deng, Z.-M., Huong, L. & Trent, R.J. (1994) The Australian type of nondeletional $^G\gamma$-HPFH has a C→G substitution at nucleotide −114 of the $^G\gamma$ gene. *Br. J. Haematol.* **86**, 219.

Mount, S.M. (1982) A catalogue of splice junction sequences. *Nucl. Acids Res.* **10**, 459.

Mourant, A.E., Kopec, A.C., Ikin, E.W. *et al.* (1974) The blood groups and haemoglobins of the Kunama and Baria of Eritrea, Ethiopia. *Ann. Hum. Biol.* **1**, 383.

Muirhead, H. & Perutz, M.F. (1963) Structure of haemoglobin A. A three dimensional Fourier synthesis of reduced human haemoglobin at 5.5 Å resolution. *Nature* **199**, 633.

Muklwala, E.C., Branda, J., Siziya, S., Atenyi, J., Fleming, A.F. & Higgs, D.R. (1989) Alpha thalassaemia in Zambian newborn. *Clin. Lab. Haematol.* **11**, 1.

Müller, C.J. (1961) *A comparative study of the structure of mammalian and avian haemoglobins.* Doctoral Thesis, Groningen, Holland. Edited by Can Gorcum & Co., Assen, The Netherlands.

Muller-Eberhard, U., Erlandson, M.E., Ginn, N.E. & Smith, C.N. (1963) Effect of trisodium calcium diethyleneaminopentaacetate on bivalent cations in thalassemia major. *Blood* **22**, 209.

Mulligan, R.C. & Berg, P. (1980) Expression of a bacterial gene in mammalian cells. *Science* **209**, 1422.

Murachi, T., Tanaka, K., Hatanaka, M. & Murakami, T. (1981) Intracellular Ca^{2+}-dependent protease (calpain) and its high-molecular-weight endogenous inhibitor (calpastatin). *Adv. Enzyme Regul.* **19**, 407.

Muretto, P., Del Fiasco, S., Angelucci, E. & Lucarelli, G. (1994) Bone marrow transplantation in thalassemia: modifications of hepatic iron overload and associated lesions after long-term engrafting. *Liver* **14**, 14.

Murru, S., Loudianos, G., Deiana, M. *et al.* (1991) Molecular characterization of β-thalassemia intermedia in patients of Italian descent and identification of three novel β-thalassemia mutations. *Blood* **77**, 1342.

Murru, S., Loudianos, G., Porcu, S. *et al.* (1992) A β-thalassaemia phenotype not linked to the β-globin cluster in an Italian family. *Br. J. Haematol.* **81**, 283.

Musaev, S.K., Iakovleva, G.I., Nasonova, V.A., Smirnov, A.V., Abasov, E. & Efendieva, E.G. (1991) Osteoarthropathy in β-thalassemia. *Ter. Arkh.* **63**, 56.

Musumeci, S., Schiliro, G., Pizzarelli, G., Fischer, A. & Russo, G. (1978) Thalassaemia of intermediate severity resulting from the interaction between α- and β-thalassaemia. *J. Med. Genet.* **15**, 448.

Musumeci, A., Schiliro, G., Pizarelli, G., D'Agate, A., Fischer, A. & Russo, G. (1979a) Alpha thalassaemia in Sicily: haematological and biosynthetic studies. *Br. J. Haematol.* **43**, 413.

Musumeci, S., Schiliro, G., Pizzarelli, G. *et al.* (1979b) Hemoglobin G San José [$\beta_2$7(A4) Glu→Gly α_2], β thalassaemia, and α thalassaemia in a Sicilian family. *Hum. Genet.* **52**, 239.

Musumeci, S., Leonardi, S., Di Dio, R., Fischer, A. & Di Costa, G. (1987) Protein C and antithrombin III in polytransfused patients. *Acta Haematol.* **77**, 30.

Myers, R.M., Tilly, K. & Maniatis, T. (1986) Fine structure genetic analysis of a beta-globin promoter. *Science* **232**, 613.

Nagaratnam, N., Siripala, K.A., Attapatu, A.M., Undevia, J.V. & Sukumaran, P.K. (1971) Hereditary elliptocytosis associated with beta-thalassaemia and a variant of Rh (D). A study in a Singhalese family. *Acta Haematol.* **46**, 232.

Nagel, R.L. (1984) The origin of the hemoglobin S gene: Clinical,

genetic and anthropological consequences. *Einstein Quart. J. Biol. Med.* **2**, 53.

Nagel, R.L. & Bookchin, R.M. (1974) Human haemoglobin mutants with abnormal oxygen binding. *Sem. Hematol.* **11**, 385.

Nagel, R.L. & Ranney, H.M. (1990) Genetic epidemiology of structural mutations of the β globin gene. *Sem. Hematol.* **27**, 342.

Nagel, R.L., Raventos-Suarez, C., Fabry, M.E., Tanowitz, H., Sicard, D. & Labie, D. (1981) Impairment of the growth of *Plasmodium falciparum* in HbEE erythrocytes. *J. Clin. Invest.* **68**, 303.

Najean, Y., Deschryver, F., Henni, T. & Girot, R. (1985) Red cell kinetics in thalassaemia intermedia: its use for a prospective prognosis. *Br. J. Haematol.* **59**, 533.

Nakatsuji, T., Matsumoto, N., Miwa, S. *et al.* (1980) Acquired hemoglobin H disease associated with idiopathic myelofibrosis and hereditary adenosine deaminase deficiency. *Acta Haematol. Japonica* **43**, 92.

Nakatsuji, T., Ohba, Y. & Huisman, T.H.J. (1984) HB F-Yamaguchi (γ 75Thr, γ 80Asn, γ 136Ala) is associated with $^G\gamma$-thalassaemia. *Am. J. Hematol.* **16**, 189.

Nakatsuji, T., Landman, H. & Huisman, T.H.J. (1986) An elongated segment of DNA observed between two human α-globin genes. *Hum. Genet.* **74**, 368.

Nakayama, R., Yamada, D., Steinmiller, V., Hsia, E. & Hale, R.W. (1986) Hydrops fetalis secondary to Bart hemoglobinopathy. *Obstet. Gynecol.* **67**, 176.

Na-Nakorn, S. (1959) Haemoglobinopathies in Thailand. In: *Abnormal Haemoglobins* (eds J.H.P. Jonxis & J.F. Delafresnaye), p. 357. Blackwell Scientific Publications, Oxford.

Na-Nakorn, S. & Wasi, P. (1970) Alpha-thalasemia in Northern Thailand. *Am. J. Hum. Genet.* **22**, 645.

Na-Nakorn, S., Wasi, P. & Suingdumrong, A. (1965) Hemoglobin H disease in Thailand: Clinical and hematological studies in 138 cases. *Israel J. Med. Sci.* **1**, 762.

Na-Nakorn, S., Wasi, P., Pornpatkul, M. & Pootrakul, S. (1969) Further evidence for a genetic basis for haemoglobin H disease from newborn offspring of patients. *Nature* **223**, 59.

Nance, W.E. (1963) Genetic control of hemoglobin synthesis. *Science* **141**, 123.

Naqvi, A., Waye, J.S., Morrow, R., Nisbet-Brown, E. & Olivieri, N.F. (1997) Normal development of an infant with homozygous α-thalassemia. *Blood* **90**, 132A.

Naritomi, Y., Nakashima, H., Kagimoto, M., Naito, Y., Yokota, E. & Imamura, T. (1990) A common Chinese β-thalassemia mutation found in a Japanese family. *Hum. Genet.* **84**, 480.

Nasab, A.H. (1979) Clinical and laboratory findings in the initial diagnoses of homozygous beta thalassaemia in Fars Province, Iran. *Br. J. Haematol.* **43**, 57.

Nash, K.B. (1990) A psychosocial perspective: growing up with thalassemia, a chronic disorder. *Ann. N. Y. Acad. Sci.* **612**, 442.

Nathan, D.G. (1995) *Genes, Blood and Courage. A Boy Called Immortal Sword.* Harvard University Press, Cambridge, MA.

Nathan, D.G. & Benz, E.J. (1976) Pathophysiology of the anaemia of thalassemia. In: *Congenital Disorders of Erythropoiesis* (ed. Ciba Foundation), p. 205. North Holland, Amsterdam.

Nathan, D.G. & Gunn, R.B. (1966) Thalassemia: the consequences of unbalanced hemoglobin synthesis. *Am. J. Med.* **41**, 815.

Nathan, D.G. & Oski, F.A. (1987) *Hematology of Infancy and Childhood*, 3rd edn. W.B. Saunders, Philadelphia.

Nathan, D.G., Stossel, T.B., Gunn, R.B., Zarkowsky, H.S. & Laforet, M.T. (1969) Influence of hemoglobin precipitation on erythrocyte metabolism in alpha and beta thalassemia. *J. Clin. Invest.* **48**, 33.

Natta, C., Banks, J., Niazi, G., Marks, P.A. & Bank, A. (1973) Decreased β globin mRNA activity in bone marrow cells and heterozygous β thalassaemia. *Nature New Biol.* **244**, 280.

Natta, C.L., Niazi, G.A., Ford, S. & Bank, A. (1974) Balanced globin chain synthesis in hereditary persistence of fetal hemoglobin. *J. Clin. Invest.* **54**, 433.

Natta, C.L., Ramirez, F., Wolff, J.A. & Bank, A. (1976) Decreased alpha globin mRNA in nucleated red cell precursors in alpha thalassemia. *Blood* **47**, 899.

Nazarenko, S.A., Nazarenko, L.P. & Baranova, V.A. (1987) Distal 15q trisomy caused by familial balanced translocation t(15;16)(q24;p13) and an unusual mosaicism in the proband's mother. *Tsitol. Genet.* **21**, 434.

Necheles, T.F., Allen, D.M. & Finkel, H.E. (1969) *Clinical Disorders of Hemoglobin Structure and Synthesis.* Appleton Century Crofts, New York.

Necheles, T.F., Chung, S., Sabbah, R. & Whitten, D. (1974) Intensive transfusion therapy in thalassemia major: an eight year follow up. *Ann. N. Y. Acad. Sci.* **232**, 179.

Neeb, H., Beiboer, J.L., Jonxis, J.H.P., Sijpesteijn, J.A.K. & Muller, C.J. (1961) Homozygous Lepore haemoglobin disease appearing as thalassaemia major in two Papuan siblings. *Trop. Geogr. Med.* **13**, 207.

Neel, J.V. (1949) Inheritance of sickle-cell anemia. *Science* **110**, 64.

Neel, J.V. (1950) The population genetics of two inherited blood dyscrasias in man. *Cold Spring Harbor Sympos. Quant. Biol.* **15**, 141.

Neel, J.V. (1994) *Physician to the Gene Pool: Genetic Lessons and Other Stories*, p. 457. John Wiley & Sons, New York.

Neel, J.V. & Valentine, W.N. (1947) Further studies on the genetics of thalassaemia. *Genetics* **32**, 38.

Neel, J.A., Robinson, A.R., Zuelzer, W.W., Livingstone, F.B. & Sutton, H.E. (1961) The frequency of elevations in the A, and fetal hemoglobin fractions in the natives of Liberia and adjacent regions, with data on haptoglobin and transferrin types. *Am. J. Hum. Genet.* **13**, 262.

Neidengard, L. & Sparkes, R.S. (1981) Ring chromosome 16. *Hum. Genet.* **59**, 175.

Newman, A. (1998) RNA splicing. *Curr. Biol.* **8**, R903.

Newton, C.R., Graham, A. & Heptinstall, L.E. (1989) Analysis of any point mutation in DNA. The amplification refractory mutation system (ARMS). *Nucl. Acids Res.* **17**, 2503.

Ney, P.A., Sorrentino, B.P., Lowrey, C.H. & Nienhuis, A.W. (1990a) Inducibility of the HSII enhancer depends on binding of an erythroid specific nuclear protein. *Nucl. Acids Res.* **18**, 6011.

Ney, P.A., Sorrentino, B.P., McDonagh, K.T. & Nienhuis, A.W. (1990b) Tandem AP-1-binding sites within the human β-globin dominant control region function as an inducible enhancer in erythroid cells. *Genes Dev.* **4**, 993.

Ney, P.A., Andrews, N.C., Jane, S.M. *et al.* (1993) Purification of the human NF-E2 complex: cDNA cloning of the hematopoietic cell-specific subunit and evidence for an associated partner. *Mol. Cell. Biol.* **13**, 5604.

Nhonoli, A.M., Kujwalile, J.M., Mmari, P.W. & Shemaghoda, Y. (1979) Haemoglobin Barts in newborn Tanzanians. *Acta Haematol.* **61**, 114.

Nicholls, R.D., Higgs, D.R., Clegg, J.B. & Weatherall, D.J. (1985) α^0-Thalassemia due to recombination between the α1-globin gene and an *Alu*I repeat. *Blood* **65**, 1434.

Nicholls, R.D., Fischel-Ghodsian, N. & Higgs, D.R. (1987) Recombination at the human α-globin gene cluster: sequence features and topological constraints. *Cell* **49**, 369.

Nicolaides, K.H., Rodeck, C.H., Lange, I. *et al.* (1985) Fetoscopy in the assessment of unexplained fetal hydrops. *Br. J. Obstet. Gynaecol.* **92**, 671.

Nicolis, S., Ronchi, A., Malgaretti, N., Mantovani, R., Giglioni, B. & Ottolenghi, S. (1989) Increased erythroid-specific expression of a

mutated HPFH γ globin promoter requires the erythroid factor NFE-1. *Nucl. Acids Res.* **17**, 5509.

Nielsen, K.B., Dyggve, H.V.K.H. & Olsen, J. (1983) A chromosomal survey of an institution for the mentally retarded. *Dan. Med. Bull.* **30**, 5.

Nienhuis, A.W. (1981) Vitamin C and iron. *N. Eng. J. Med.* **304**, 170.

Nienhuis, A.W. & Anderson, W.F. (1971) Isolation and translation of hemoglobin messenger RNA from thalassemia, sickle cell anemia, and normal human reticulocytes. *J. Clin. Invest.* **50**, 2458.

Nienhuis, A.W., Laycock, D.G. & Anderson, W.F. (1971) Translation of rabbit haemoglobin messenger RNA by thalassaemia and non-thalassaemic ribosomes. *Nature* **231**, 205.

Nienhuis, A.W., Canfield, P.H. & Anderson, W.F. (1973) Hemoglobin messenger RNA from human bone marrow: isolation and translation in homozygous and heterozygous β-thalassaemia. *J. Clin. Invest.* **52**, 1735.

Nienhuis, A.W., Delea, C., Aamodt, R., Bartler, F. & Anderson, W.F. (1976) Evaluation of desferrioxamine and ascorbic acid for the treatment of chronic iron overload. In: *Birth Defects: Original Articles Series* (eds D. Bergsma, A. Cerami, C. Peterson & J.H. Graziano), p. 177. Alan R. Liss, New York.

de las Nieves, M.A., de Pablos, J.M. & Garrido, F. (1990) Alpha thalassaemia in a Southern Spanish population. *Br. J. Haematol.* **73**, 282.

Nisli, G., Kavakli, K., Aydinok, Y., Oztop, S. & Cetingul, N. (1997) Serum erythropoietin levels in patients with β thalassemia major and intermedia. *Pediatr. Hematol. Oncol.* **14**, 161.

Noël, P., Tefferi, A., Pierre, R.V., Jenkins, R.B. & Dewald, G.W. (1993) Karyotypic analysis in primary myelodysplastic syndromes. *Blood Rev.* **7**, 10.

Noguchi, C.T. & Schechter, A.N. (1981) The intracellular polymerization of sickle hemoglobin and its relevance to sickle cell disease. *Blood* **58**, 1057.

Noguchi, C.T., Schechter, A.N. & Rodgers, G.P. (1993) Sickle cell disease pathophysiology. *Baillière's Clin. Haematol.* **6**, 57.

Notario, A. & Meduri, D. (1965) I lipidi eritrocitari nelle microcitemie e particolarmente nella talassemia maior. *Giornate di Studio sulla Microcitemia*, Ferrara, p. 3. Istituto Italiano Di Medicine Sociale, Roma.

Notario, A., di Marco, N., Doneda, G. & Zanetti, A. (1964a) Il metabolismo eritrocitario del glucosio-U-14C e dell'acetato-l-14C nel morbo di Cooley. *Haematologica* **49**, 523.

Notario, E., Doneda, G., Zanetti, A. & di Marco, N. (1964b) Il metabolismo eritrocitario della glicina-1–14C, della cristina-35 S nel morbo di Cooley. *Haematologica* **49**, 579.

Notario, E., Comin, U., Meduri, D., Ricetti, M., Frigerio, G. & Bernasconi, P. (1974) Alterazioni eritocitarie di superficie in diverse eritopatie primitive e secondarie. *Min. Med.* **65**, 1.

Notario, A., Comin, U., Ricetti, M., Meduri, D. & Cardena, M.A. (1976) Alterazioni eritocitarie delle proteine di membrana in alcune emoglobinopatie. *Min. Med.* **67**, 1.

Novelletto, A., Hafez, M., Di Rienzo, A. *et al.* (1989) Frequency and molecular types of deletional α-thalassemia in Egypt. *Hum. Genet.* **81**, 211.

Novelletto, A., Hafez, M., Deidda, G. *et al.* (1990) Molecular characterization of β-thalassemia mutations in Egypt. *Hum. Genet.* **85**, 272.

Novikova, E.Z. & Abrakhanova, K.N. (1975) Characteristics of the course of long bone fractures in children with major beta-thalassemia. *Vestn Rentgenol. Radiol.* **3**, 44.

Nowicki, L., Behnken, L. & Martin, H. (1975) Über die häufigkeit von Hämoglobinanomalien und Hämoglobinpathien bei moçambiquanischen Völkerschaften. *Blut* **31**, 283.

Nozari, G., Hyman, C., Chapman, C. & Rahbar, S. (1990) β-

Thalassemia alleles found among Iranians living in Southern California. *Blood* **76**, 71a.

Nozari, G., Rahbar, S., Golshaiyzan, A. & Rahmanzadeh, S. (1995) Molecular analyses of β-thalassemia in Iran. *Hemoglobin* **19**, 425.

Nuez, B., Michalovich, D., Bygrave, A., Ploemacher, R. & Grosveld, F. (1995) Defective haematopoiesis in fetal liver resulting from inactivation of the EKLF gene. *Nature* **375**, 316.

Nuffield Council on Bioethics (1993) *Genetic Screening. Ethical Issues*. Nuffield Council on Bioethics, London.

Nute, P.E., Pararyas, H.A. & Stamatoyannopoulos, G. (1973) The $^G\gamma$ and $^A\gamma$ hemoglobin chains during human fetal development. *Am. J. Hum. Genet.* **25**, 271.

Nute, P.E., Wood, W.G., Stamatoyannopoulos, G., Olweny, C. & Fialkow, P.J. (1976) The Kenya form of hereditary persistence of fetal haemoglobin; structural studies and evidence for homogeneous distribution of haemoglobin F using fluorescent anti-haemoglobin F antibodies. *Br. J. Haematol.* **32**, 55.

O'Brien, R.T. (1973) The effect of iron deficiency on the expression of hemoglobin H. *Blood* **41**, 853.

O'Brien, R.T. (1974) Ascorbic acid enhancement of desferrioxamine induced urinary iron excretion in thalassemia major. *Ann. N. Y. Acad. Sci.* **232**, 221.

O'Brien, R.T., Pearson, H.A. & Spencer, R.P. (1972) Transfusion induced decrease in spleen size in thalassemia major: documentation by radioisotope scan. *J. Pediatr.* **81**, 105.

O'Connell, M.J., Ward, R.J., Baum, H. & Oeters, T.J. (1985) The role of iron in ferritin- and haemosiderin-related peroxidation in liposomes. *Biochem. J.* **229**, 135.

O'Driscoll, A., Mackie, I.J., Porter, J.B. & Machin, S.J. (1995) Low plasma heparin cofactor II levels in thalassaemia syndromes are corrected by chronic blood transfusion. *Br. J. Haematol.* **90**, 65.

O'Neill, O. (1991) Introducing ethics: some current positions. *Bull. Med. Ethics* **73**, 18.

O'Shaughnessy, D.F., Hill, A.V.S., Bowden, D.K., Weatherall, D.J. & Clegg, J.B. with collaborators (1990) Globin genes in Micronesia: origins and affinities of Pacific Island peoples. *Am. J. Hum. Genet.* **46**, 144.

Oberklaid, F. & Seshadri, R. (1975) Hypoparathyroidism and other endocrine dysfunction complicating thalassemia major. *Med. J. Aust.* **1**, 304.

Oggiano, L., Pirastu, M., Moi, P., Longinotti, M., Perseu, L. & Cao, A. (1987) Molecular characterization of a normal Hb A_2 β-thalassaemia determinant in a Sardinian family. *Br. J. Haematol.* **67**, 225.

Oggiano, L., Dore, F., Postidda, P. *et al.* (1988) Homozygous β⁰-39 mutation with thalassemia intermedia in northern Sardinia: clinical, hematological and molecular analysis. *Hemoglobin* **12**, 673.

Oggiano, L., Guiso, L., Frogheri, L. *et al.* (1994) A novel Mediterranean 'δβ-thalassaemia' determinant containing the δ^+27 and β⁰ 39 point mutations in *cis*. *Am. J. Hematol.* **45**, 81.

Ohba, Y., Hattori, Y., Harano, T., Harano, K., Fukumaki, Y. & Ideguchi, H. (1997) β-Thalassemia mutations in Japanese and Koreans. *Hemoglobin* **21**, 191.

Ohsawa, K., Imai, Y., Ito, D. & Kohsaka, S. (1996) Molecular cloning and characterization of annexin V-binding proteins with highly hydrophilic peptide structure. *J. Neurochem.* **67**, 89.

Ohta, Y., Yamaoka, K., Sumida, I., Fujita, S., Fujimura, T. & Yanase, T. (1971a) Homozygous delta-thalassemia first discovered in Japanese family with hereditary persistence of fetal hemoglobin. *Blood* **37**, 706.

Ohta, Y., Yamaoka, K., Sumida, I. & Yanase, T. (1971b) Haemoglobin Miyada, a β-δ fusion peptide (anti-Lepore) type discovered in a Japanese family. *Nature New Biol.* **234**, 218.

Ojwang, P.J., Nakatsuji, T., Gardiner, M.B., Reese, A.L., Gilman, J.G. & Huisman, T.H.J. (1983) Gene deletion as the molecular basis for the Kenya-$^G\gamma$-HPFH condition. *Hemoglobin* **7**, 115.

Ojwang, P.J., Ogada, T., Beris, P. *et al.* (1987) Haplotypes and α globin gene analysis in sickle cell cell anaemia patients from Kenya. *Br. J. Haematol.* **65**, 211.

Okano, M., Bell, D.W., Haber, D.A. & Li, E. (1999) DNA methyltransferases Dnmt3a and Dnmt3b are essential for *de novo* methylation and mammalian development. *Cell* **99**, 247.

Okcuoglu, A., Minnich, V. & Arcasoy, A. (1965) A further example of thalassemia-hemoglobin E disease in Turkey. *Acta Haematol.* **34**, 354.

Okon, E., Levij, I.S. & Rachmilewitz, E.A. (1976) Splenectomy, iron overload and liver cirrhosis in beta-thalassemia major. *Acta Haematol.* **56**, 142.

Okpala, I. (1998) The management of crisis in sickle cell disease. *Eur. J. Haematol.* **60**, 1.

Old, J.M. (1996a) Haemoglobinopathies. *Prenat. Diag.* **16**, 1181.

Old, J.M. (1996b) Haemoglobinopathies. Community clues to mutation detection. In: *Methods in Molecular Medicine, Molecular Diagnosis of Genetic Diseases* (ed. R. Elles), p. 169. Humana Press Inc., Totowa, NJ.

Old, J.M., Longley, J., Wood, W.G., Clegg, J.B. & Weatherall, D.J. (1977) The molecular basis for acquired haemoglobin H disease. *Nature* **269**, 524.

Old, J.M., Clegg, J.B., Weatherall, D.J. & Booth, P.B. (1978a) Haemoglobin J Tongariki is associated with α thalassaemia. *Nature* **273**, 319.

Old, J.M., Proudfoot, N.J., Wood, W.G., Longley, J.I., Clegg, J.B. & Weatherall, D.J. (1978b) Characterization of β-globin mRNA in the β⁰ thalassemias. *Cell* **14**, 289.

Old, J.M., Ayyub, H., Wood, W.G., Clegg, J.B. & Weatherall, D.J. (1982a) Linkage analysis of nondeletion hereditary persistence of fetal hemoglobin. *Science* **215**, 981.

Old, J.M., Ward, R.H.T., Petrou, M., Karagozlu, F., Modell, B. & Weatherall, D.J. (1982b) First-trimester fetal diagnosis for haemoglobinopathies: Three cases. *Lancet* **ii**, 1413.

Old, J.M., Petrou, M., Modell, B. & Weatherall, D.J. (1984) Feasibility of antenatal diagnosis of β thalassaemia by DNA polymorphisms in Asian Indian and Cypriot populations. *Br. J. Haematol.* **57**, 255.

Old, J.M., Fitches, A., Heath, C. *et al.* (1986a) First-trimester fetal diagnosis for haemoglobinopathy: report on 200 cases. *Lancet* **ii**, 763.

Old, J.M., Heath, C., Fitches, A. *et al.* (1986b) Meiotic recombination between two polymorphic restriction sites within the β globin gene cluster. *J. Med. Genet.* **23**, 14.

Old, J.M., Thein, S.L., Weatherall, D.J., Cao, A. & Loukopoulos, D.T. (1989) Prenatal diagnosis of the major haemoglobin disorders. *Mol. Biol. Med.* **6**, 55.

Old, J.M., Varawalla, N.Y. & Weatherall, D.J. (1990) Rapid detection and prenatal diagnosis of β-thalassaemia: studies in Indian and Cypriot populations in the UK. *Lancet* **336**, 834.

Oldrini, R., Salmini, G. & Maioio, A.T. (1972) Studio di un case associazione Hb D-β microcitemia. *Haematologica* **58**, 515.

Olds, R.J., Sura, T., Jackson, B., Wonke, B., Hoffbrand, A.V. & Thein, S.L. (1991) A novel δ⁰ mutation in cis with Hb Knossos: a study of different genetic interactions in three Egyptian families. *Br. J. Haematol.* **78**, 430.

Olesen, E.B., Olesen, K., Livingstone, F.B. *et al.* (1959) Thalassaemia in Liberia. *Br. Med. J.* **i**, 1385.

Oliva, J. & Myerson, R.M. (1961) Hereditary persistence of fetal hemoglobin. *Am. J. Med. Sci.* **241**, 215.

Olivieri, N.F. (1996a) Long-term follow-up of body iron in patients with thalassemia major during therapy with the orally active iron chelator deferiprone (L1). *Blood* **88**, 310a.

Olivieri, N.F. (1996b) Reactivation of fetal hemoglobin in patients with β thalassemia. *Sem. Hematol.* **33**, 24.

Olivieri, N.F. & Brittenham, G.M. (1997) Iron-chelating therapy and the treatment of thalassemia. *Blood* **89**, 739.

Olivieri, N.F. & Weatherall, D.J. (1998) The therapeutic reactivation of fetal haemoglobin. *Hum. Mol. Genet.* **7**, 1655.

Olivieri, N.F., Buncic, J.R., Chew, E. *et al.* (1986) Visual and auditory neurotoxicity in patients receiving subcutaneous deferoxamine infusions. *N. Eng. J. Med.* **314**, 869.

Olivieri, N.F., Chang, L.S., Poon, A.O., Michelson, A.M. & Orkin, S.H. (1987) An α-globin gene initiation codon mutation in a Black family with HbH disease. *Blood* **70**, 729.

Olivieri, N.F., Grisaru, D., Daneman, A., Martin, D.J., Rose, V. & Freedman, M.H. (1989) Computed tomography scanning of the liver to determine efficacy of iron chelation therapy in thalassemia major. *J. Pediatr.* **114**, 427.

Olivieri, N.F., Koren, G., Hermann, C. *et al.* (1990a) Comparison of oral iron chelator L1 and desferrioxamine in iron-loaded patients. *Lancet* **336**, 1275.

Olivieri, N.F., Ramachandran, S., Tyler, B. *et al.* (1990b) Diabetes mellitus in older patients with thalassemia major: Relationship to severity of iron overload and presence of microvascular complications. *Blood* **76**, 72a.

Olivieri, N.F., Berriman, A.M., Davis, S.A., Tyler, B.J., Ingram, J. & Francombe, W.H. (1992a) Continuous intravenous administration of deferoxamine in adults with severe iron overload. *Am. J. Hematol.* **41**, 61.

Olivieri, N.F., Freedman, M., Perrine, S. *et al.* (1992b) Trial of recombinant human erythropoietin in thalassemia intermedia. *Blood* **80**, 3258.

Olivieri, N.F., Koren, G., Harris, J. *et al.* (1992c) Growth failure and bony changes induced by deferoxamine. *Am. J. Pediatr. Hematol. Oncol.* **14**, 48.

Olivieri, N.F., Koren, G., Matsui, D. *et al.* (1992d) Reduction of tissue iron stores and normalization of serum ferritin during treatment with the oral iron chelator L1 in thalassemia intermedia. *Blood* **79**, 2741.

Olivieri, N.F., Liu, P.P., Sher, G.D. *et al.* (1994a) Successful combined cardiac and liver transplantation in an adult with homozygous beta-thalassemia. *N. Eng. J. Med.* **330**, 1127.

Olivieri, N.F., Nathan, D.G., MacMillan, J.H. *et al.* (1994b) Survival of medically treated patients with homozygous β thalassemia. *N. Eng. J. Med.* **331**, 574.

Olivieri, N.F., Basran, R.K., Talbot, A.L., Babyn, P. & Bailey, J.D. (1995a) Abnormal growth in thalassemia major associated with deferoxamine-induced destruction of spinal cartilage and compromise of sitting height. *Blood* **86**, 482a.

Olivieri, N.F., Brittenham, G.M., Matsui, D. *et al.* (1995b) Iron-chelation therapy with oral deferiprone in patients with thalassemia major. *N. Eng. J. Med.* **332**, 918.

Olivieri, N.F., Rees, D.C., Ginder, G.D. *et al.* (1997) Treatment of thalassaemia major with phenylbutyrate and hydroxyurea. *Lancet* **350**, 491.

Olivieri, N.F., Brittenham, G.M., McLaren, C.E. *et al.* (1998a) Long-term safety and effectiveness of iron chelation therapy with deferiprone for thalasemia major. *N. Eng. J. Med.* **339**, 417.

Olivieri, N.F., De Silva, S., Fischer, C. *et al.* (1998b) Natural history study of hemoglobin E/β thalassemia. *Blood* **92**, 10 (Suppl. 1(1), 532a).

Olivieri, N.F., Butany, J., Templeton, D.M. & Brittenhem, G.M. (1998c) Cardiac failure and myocardial fibrosis in a patient with

thalassemia major (TM) treated with long-term deferiprone. *Blood* **92**, 532a.

Olivieri, O., Vitoux, D., Galacteros, F. *et al.* (1992e) Hemoglobin variants and activity of the (K⁺Cl⁻) cotransport system in human erythrocytes. *Blood* **79**, 793.

Olynyk, J.K. & Bacon, B.R. (1995) Hepatitis C. Recent advances in understanding and management. *Postgrad. Med. J.* **98**, 79.

Oman, H. & Wiradisuria, S. (1969) Thalassemia and Hb E thalassemia in Bandung. *Paediatr. Indones.* **9**, 269.

Öner, R., Altay, C., Aksoy, M. *et al.* (1990) β-Thalassemia in Turkey. *Hemoglobin* **14**, 1.

Öner, R., Agarwal, S., Dimovski, A.J. *et al.* (1991a) The G→A mutation at position +22 3′ to the Cap site of the β-globin gene as a possible cause for a β-thalassemia. *Hemoglobin* **15**, 67.

Öner, R., Kutlar, F., Gu, L.-H. & Huisman, T.H. J. (1991b) The Georgia type of nondeletional hereditary persistence of fetal hemoglobin has a C-T mutation at nucleotide –114 of the ᴬγ-globin gene. *Blood* **77**, 1124.

Öner, R., Öner, C., Wilson, J.B., Tamagnini, G.P., Ribeiro, L.M.L. & Huisman, T.H.J. (1991c) Dominant β-thalassaemia trait in a Portuguese family is caused by a deletion of (G)TGGCTGGTGT(G) and an insertion of (G)GCAG(G) in codons 134, 135, 136 and 137 of the β-globin gene. *Br. J. Haematol.* **79**, 306.

Öner, C., Dimovski, A.J., Altay, C. *et al.* (1992) Sequence variations in the 5′ hypersensitive site-2 of the locus control region of βˢ chromosomes are associated with different levels of fetal globin in hemoglobin S homozygotes. *Blood* **79**, 813.

Öner, C., Öner, R., Gürgey, A. & Altay, Ç. (1995) A new Turkish type of β-thalassaemia major with homozygosity for two nonconsecutive 7.6 kb deletions of the ψβ and β genes and an intact δ gene. *Br. J. Haematol.* **89**, 306.

Öner, R., Öner, C., Erdem, G. *et al.* (1996) A novel (δβ)⁰-thalassaemia due to an approximately 30-kb deletion observed in a Turkish family. *Acta Haematol.* **96**, 232.

Öner, R., Gurgey, A., Öner, R. *et al.* (1997) The molecular basis of HbH disease in Turkey. *Hemoglobin* **21**, 41.

Ong, H.C., White, J.C. & Sinnathuray, T.A. (1977) Haemoglobin H disease and pregnancy in a Malaysian woman. *Acta Haematol. (Basel)* **58**, 229.

Ongajyooth, L., Siritanaratkul, N., Pootrakul, P. *et al.* (1995) Glomerulonephritis in β-thalassemia Hb E disease: clinical manifestations, histopathologic studies and outcome. *J. Med. Assoc. Thailand* **78**, 119.

Ongsangkoon, T., Vawesorn, O. & Pootrakul, S.-N. (1978) Pathology of hemoglobin Bart's hydrops fetalis. 1. Gross autopsy findings. *J. Med. Assoc. Thailand* **61**, 71.

d'Onofrio, G., Zini, G., Ricerca, B.M., Mancini, S. & Mango, G. (1992) Automated measurement of red blood cell microcytosis and hypochromia in iron deficiency and β-thalassaemia trait. *Arch. Pathol. Lab. Med.* **116**, 84.

Opartkiattikul, N., Funahara, Y., Fucharoen, S. & Talalak, P. (1992a) Increase in spontaneous platelet aggregation in β-thalassemia/haemoglobin E disease: a consequence of splenectomy. *Southeast Asian J. Trop. Med. Publ. Hlth* **23**, 36.

Opartkiattikul, N., Funahara, Y., Hijikata-Okunomiya, A., Yamaguchi, N., Fucharoen, S. & Talalak, P. (1992b) Detection of PF3 availability in whole blood from volunteers and β-thalassemia/Hb E patients: a promising method for prediction of thrombotic tendency. *Southeast Asian J. Trop. Med. Publ. Hlth* **23**, 52.

Oppenheim, A., Yaari, A., Rund, D. *et al.* (1990) Intrinsic potential for high fetal hemoglobin production in a Druz family with β-thalassemia is due to an unlinked genetic determinant. *Hum. Genet.* **86**, 175.

Oppenheimer, S.J., Higgs, D.R., Weatherall, D.J., Barker, J. & Spark, R.A. (1984) α Thalassaemia in Papua New Guinea. *Lancet* **i**, 424.

Oppenheimer, S.J., Hill, A.V., Gibson, F.D., Macfarlane, S.B., Moody, J.B. & Pringle, J. (1987) The interaction of alpha thalassaemia with malaria. *Trans. Roy. Soc. Trop. Med. Hyg.* **81**, 322.

Orkin, S.H. (1996) Development of the hematopoietic system. *Curr. Opin. Genet. Dev.* **6**, 597.

Orkin, S.H. (1998) Embryonic stem cells and transgenic mice in the study of hematopoiesis. *Int. J. Dev. Biol.* **42**, 927.

Orkin, S.H. & Goff, S.C. (1981a) The duplicated human α-globin genes: their relative expression as measured by RNA analysis. *Cell* **24**, 345.

Orkin, S.H. & Goff, S.C. (1981b) Nonsense and frameshift mutations in β-thalassemia detected in cloned β-globin genes. *J. Biol. Chem.* **256**, 9782.

Orkin, S.H. & Michelson, A. (1980) Partial deletion of the globin structural gene in human α thalassaemia. *Nature* **286**, 538.

Orkin, S.H. & Zon, L.I. (1997) Genetics of erythropoiesis: induced mutations in mice and zebrafish. *Annu. Rev. Genet.* **31**, 33.

Orkin, S.H., Alter, B.P., Altay, C. *et al.* (1978) Application of endonuclease mapping to the analysis and prenatal diagnosis of thalassemias caused by globin-gene deletion. *N. Eng. J. Med.* **299**, 166.

Orkin, S.H., Alter, B.P. & Altay, C. (1979a) Deletion of the $^{A}\gamma$ globin gene in $^{G}\gamma$ δβ-thalassemia. *J. Clin. Invest.* **64**, 866.

Orkin, S.H., Old, J., Lazarus, H. *et al.* (1979b) The molecular basis of α-thalassemias: frequent occurrence of dysfunctional α loci among non-Asians with Hb H disease. *Cell* **17**, 33.

Orkin, S.H., Old, J.M., Weatherall, D.J. & Nathan, D.G. (1979c) Partial deletion of β-globin gene DNA in certain patients with β⁰-thalassemia. *Proc. Natl Acad. Sci. USA* **76**, 2400.

Orkin, S.H., Kolodner, R., Michelson, A. & Husson, R. (1980) Cloning and direct examination of a structurally abnormal human β⁰ thalassemia globin gene. *Proc. Natl Acad. Sci. USA* **77**, 3558.

Orkin, S.H., Goff, S.C. & Hechtman, R.L. (1981a) Mutation in an intervening sequence splice junction in man. *Proc. Natl Acad. Sci. USA* **78**, 5041.

Orkin, S.H., Goff, S.C. & Nathan, D.G. (1981b) Heterogeneity of DNA deletion in γδβ-thalassemia. *J. Clin. Invest.* **67**, 878.

Orkin, S.H., Kazazian, H.H. Jr, Antonarakis, S.E. *et al.* (1982a) Linkage of β-thalassaemia mutations and β-globin gene polymorphisms with DNA polymorphisms in human β-globin gene cluster. *Nature* **296**, 627.

Orkin, S.H., Kazazian, H.H., Antonarakis, S.E., Ostrer, H., Goff, S.C. & Sexton, J.P. (1982b) Abnormal RNA processing due to the exon mutation of βᴱ-globin gene. *Nature* **300**, 768.

Orkin, S.H., Little, P.F.R., Kazazian, H.H. Jr & Boehm, C.D. (1982c) Improved detection of the sickle mutation by DNA analysis. *N. Eng. J. Med.* **307**, 32.

Orkin, S.H., Markham, A.F. & Kazazian, H.H. Jr (1983a) Direct detection of the common Mediterranean β-thalassaemia gene with synthetic DNA probes. An alternative approach for prenatal diagnosis. *J. Clin. Invest.* **71**, 775.

Orkin, S.H., Sexton, J.P., Cheng, T.C. *et al.* (1983b) TATA box transcription mutation in β-thalassemia. *Nucl. Acids Res.* **11**, 4727.

Orkin, S.H., Sexton, J.P., Goff, S.C. & Kazazian, H.H.J. (1983c) Inactivation of an acceptor RNA splice site by a short deletion in β-thalassemia. *J. Biol. Chem.* **258**, 7249.

Orkin, S.H., Antonarakis, S.E. & Kazazian, H.H. Jr (1984a) Base substitution at position –88 in a β-thalassemic globin gene. Further evidence for the role of distal promoter element ACACCC. *J. Biol. Chem.* **259**, 8679.

Orkin, S.H., Antonarakis, S.E. & Loukopoulos, D. (1984b) Abnormal processing of β Knossos RNA. *Blood* **64**, 311.

Orkin, S.H., Cheng, T.-C., Antonarakis, S.E. & Kazazian, H.H. (1985)

Thalassaemia due to a mutation in the cleavage-polyadenylation signal of the human β-globin gene. *EMBO J.* **4**, 453.

Oron, V., Filon, D., Oppenheim, A. & Rund, D. (1994) Severe thalassaemia intermedia caused by interaction of homozygosity for α-globin gene triplication with heterozygosity for β⁰ thalassemia. *Br. J. Haematol.* **86**, 377.

Oron-Karni, V., Filon, D., Rund, D. & Oppenheim, A. (1997) A novel mechanism generating short deletion/insertions following slippage is suggested by a mutation in the human α_2-globin gene. *Hum. Mol. Genet.* **6**, 881.

Orsini, A., Louchet, E., Raybaud, C., Brusquet, Y. & Perrimond, H. (1970) Les péricardites de la maladie de Cooley. *Pédiatrie* **15**, 831.

Orsini, A., Vovan, L. & Vilain, M.L. (1974) Dépistage des hémoglobinases dans le sud-est de la France. Résultats d'une enquête effectuée en milieu obstétrical. *Bull. WHO* **51**, 199.

Orzincolo, C., Scutellari, P.N. & Castaldi, G. (1992) Growth plate injury of the long bones in treated β-thalassemia. *Skeletal Radiol.* **21**, 39.

Orzincolo, C., Castaldi, G., Bariani, L. & Scutellari, P.N. (1994) The evolutionary effects of therapy on the skeletal lesions in β-thalassemia. *Radiol. Med. Torino* **87**, 381.

Oshima, K., Harano, T. & Harano, K. (1996) Japanese β⁰-thalassemia: Molecular characterization of a novel insertion causing a stop codon. *Am. J. Hematol.* **52**, 39.

Ostertag, W. & Smith, E.W. (1969) Hemoglobin Lepore Baltimore, a third type of δβ crossover (δ⁵⁰, β⁸⁶). *Eur. J. Biochem.* **10**, 371.

Ottolenghi, S., Lanyon, W.G., Paul, J. *et al.* (1974) The severe form of α thalassaemia is caused by a haemoglobin gene deletion. *Nature* **251**, 389.

Ottolenghi, S., Lanyon, W.G., Williamson, R., Weatherall, D.J., Clegg, J.B. & Pitcher, C.S. (1975) Human globin synthesis for a patient with β⁰/δβ-thalassemia. *Proc. Natl Acad. Sci. USA* **72**, 2294.

Ottolenghi, S., Comi, P., Giglioni, B. *et al.* (1976) δβ Thalassaemia is due to a gene deletion. *Cell* **9**, 71.

Ottolenghi, S., Comi, P., Giglioni, B., Williamson, R., Vullo, G. & Conconi, F. (1977) Direct demonstration of β-globin mRNA in homozygous β⁰-thalassemia. *Nature* **266**, 231.

Ottolenghi, S., Giglioni, B., Comi, P. *et al.* (1979) Globin gene deletion in HPFH, δ⁰β⁰ thalassaemia and Hb Lepore disease. *Nature* **278**, 654.

Ottolenghi, S., Giglioni, B., Taramelli, R. *et al.* (1982a) Molecular comparison of δβ-thalassemia and hereditary persistence of fetal hemoglobin DNAs: evidence of a regulatory area? *Proc. Natl Acad. Sci. USA* **79**, 2347.

Ottolenghi, S., Giglioni, B., Tarmelli, R., Comi, P. & Gianni, A.M. (1982b) δβ-Thalassemia and HPFH. *Birth Defects* **18**, 65.

Ottolenghi, S., Giglioni, B., Pulazzini, A. *et al.* (1987) Sardinian δβ⁰-thalassemia: a further example of a C to T substitution at position –196 of the $^{A}\gamma$ globin gene promoter. *Blood* **69**, 1058.

Ottolenghi, S., Camaschella, C., Comi, P. *et al.* (1988) A frequent $^{A}\gamma$-hereditary persistence of fetal hemoglobin in northern Sardinia: its molecular basis and hematologic phenotype in heterozygotes and compound heterozygotes with β-thalassemia. *Hum. Genet.* **79**, 13.

Ou, C.N. & Rognerud, C.L. (1993) Rapid analysis of hemoglobin variants by cation-exchange HPLC. *Clin. Chem.* **39**, 820.

Overmoyer, B.A., McLaren, C.E. & Brittenham, G.M. (1987) Uniformity of liver density and nonheme (storage) iron distribution. *Arch. Pathol. Lab. Med.* **111**, 549.

Owen, G.M. & Yanochik-Owen, A. (1977) Should there be a different definition of anemia in Black and White children? *Am. J. Pub. Hlth* **67**, 865.

Özçelik, H., Basak, A.N., Tüzmen, S., Kirdar, B. & Akar, N. (1993) A novel deletion in a Turkish β-thalassemia patient detected by

DGGE and direct sequencing: FSC 22–24 (–7 bp). *Hemoglobin* **17**, 387.

Özsoylu, S., Hisconmez, G. & Altay, C. (1973) Hemoglobin H-beta-thalassemia. *Acta Haematol.* **50**, 184.

Ozsoylu, S., Sipahioglu, G. & Altay, F. (1989) Hemoglobin C Beta⁰ thalassemia. *Isr. J. Med. Sci.* **25**, 410.

Pacheco, P., Peres, M.J., Faustino, P. *et al.* (1995) β-Thalassaemia unlinked to the β-globin gene interacts with sickle-cell trait in a Portuguese family. *Br. J. Haematol.* **91**, 85.

Padanilam, B.J. & Huisman, T.H.J. (1986) The β⁰-thalassemia in an American Black family is due to a single nucleotide substitution in the acceptor splice junction of the second intervening sequence. *Am. J. Hematol.* **22**, 259.

Padanilam, B.J., Felice, A.E. & Huisman, T.H.J. (1984) Partial deletion of the 5′ β-globin gene region causes β⁰-thalassemia in members of an American Black family. *Blood* **64**, 941.

Padmos, M.A., Roberts, G.T., Sackey, K. *et al.* (1991) Two different forms of homozygous sickle cell disease occur in Saudi Arabia. *Br. J. Haematol.* **79**, 93.

Paglietti, E., Galanello, R., Moi, P., Pirastu, M. & Cao, A. (1986) Molecular pathology of haemoglobin H disease in Sardinians. *Br. J. Haematol.* **63**, 485.

Pagnier, J., Wajcman, H. & Labie, D. (1974) Defect in hemoglobin synthesis possibly due to a disturbed association. *FEBS Lett.* **45**, 252.

Pagnier, J., Amegnizin, K.P., Labie, D. & Hayat, M. (1979) Hematological and hemoglobin synthesis studies in a family with δβ-thalassemia trait. *Acta Haematol.* **61**, 27.

Pagnier, T., Dunda-Belkodja, O., Zohoun, I. *et al.* (1984) α-Thalassaemia among sickle cell anemia patients in various African populations. *Hum. Genet.* **68**, 318.

Paik, C.H., Alavi, L., Dunea, G. & Weiner, L. (1970) Thalassemia and gouty arthritis. *J. A. M. A.* **213**, 296.

Palena, A., Blau, A., Stamatoyannopoulos, G. & Anagnou, N.P. (1992) Eastern European (δβ)⁰-Thalassemia: molecular characterization of a novel 9.1-kb deletion resulting in high levels of fetal hemoglobin in the adult. *Blood* **79**, 6a.

Pampana, E.J. (1944) *Epidemiologica della Malaria.* Editrice Nazionale, Rome.

Pande, P.L., Prakash, S., Tiwary, R.S., Kazanetz, E.G., Leonova, J.-Y. & Huisman, T.H.J. (1995) β-Thalassemia intermedia in an Indian female with the Hb Hofu [β 126(H4)Val→Glu]-β⁰-thalassemia [codons 8/9 (+G)] combination. *Hemoglobin* **19**, 301.

Panizon, F. & Vullo, C. (1952) Sulla envoluzione della siderosi e fibrosi epatica nella malattia di Cooley. Studio bioptico su 20 casi. *Acta Paediatr. Lat.* **10**, 71.

Pantelakis, S.N. & Doxiadis, S.A. (1967) Serum lipoproteins in schoolboys in relation to glucose-6-phosphate dehydrogenase deficiency and thalassaemia trait. *Arch. Dis. Child.* **42**, 328.

Paolini, E., Monetti, V.C., Gronieri, E. & Boldrini, P. (1983) Acute cerebrovascular insults in homozygous beta-thalassaemia: a case report. *J. Neurol.* **230**, 37.

Papadakis, M., Papapanagiotou, E. & Loutradi-Anagnostou, A. (1997) Scanning method to identify the molecular heterogeneity of δ-globin gene especially in δ-thalassemias: detection of three novel substitutions in the promoter region of the gene. *Hum. Mutat.* **9**, 465.

Papadimas, J., Mandala, E., Pados, G. *et al.* (1996) Pituitary–testicular axis in men with β-thalassaemia major. *Hum. Reprod.* **11**, 1900.

Papavasiliou, C., Gouliamos, A., Vlahos, L., Trakadas, S., Kalovidouris, A. & Pouliades, G. (1990) CT and MRI of symptomatic spinal involvement by extramedullary haemopoiesis. *Clin. Radiol.* **42**, 91.

Papayannopoulou, T., Buckley, J., Nakamoto, B., Kurachi, S., Nute,

P.E. & Stamatoyannopoulos, G. (1979) Hb F production in endogenous colonies of polycythemia vera. *Blood* **53**, 446.

Papayannopoulou, T., Torrealba de-Ron, A., Veith, R.K. & Stamatoyannopoulos, G. (1984) Arabinosylcytosine induces fetal hemoglobin in baboons by perturbing erythroid cell differentiation kinetics. *Science* **224**, 617.

Papayannopoulou, T., Brice, M. & Stamatoyannopoulos, G. (1986) Analysis of human hemoglobin switching in MEL×human fetal erythroid cell hybrids. *Cell* **46**, 469.

Pardoll, D.M., Charache, S., Hjelle, B.L. *et al.* (1982) Homozygous α thalassaemia/Hb G Philadelphia. *Hemoglobin* **6**, 503.

Parfrey, P.S. & Squier, M. (1978) Thalassaemia minor, iron overload and hepatoma. *Br. Med. J.* **i**, 416.

Park, S.S., Barnetson, R., Kim, S.W., Weatherall, D.J. & Thein, S.L. (1991) A spontaneous deletion of β 33/34 Val in exon 2 of the β globin gene (Hb Korea) produces the phenotype of dominant β thalassaemia. *Br. J. Haematol.* **78**, 581.

Parkes, J.G., Hussain, R.A., Olivieri, N.F. & Templeton, D.M. (1993) Effects of iron loading on uptake, speciation, and chelation of iron in cultured myocardial cells. *J. Lab. Clin. Med.* **122**, 36.

Parkes, J.G., Randell, E.W., Olivieri, N.F. & Templeton, D.M. (1995) Modulation by iron loading and chelation of the uptake of non-transferrin-bound iron by human liver cells. *Biochim. Biophys. Acta* **1243**, 373.

Pasvol, G., Weatherall, D.J. & Wilson, R.J. (1977) Effects of foetal haemoglobin on susceptibility of red cells to *Plasmodium falciparum*. *Nature* **270**, 171.

Pasvol, G., Weatherall, D.J. & Wilson, R.J.M. (1978) A mechanism for the protective effect of haemoglobin S against *P. falciparum*. *Nature* **274**, 701.

Pasvol, G., Weatherall, D.J. & Wilson, R.J. (1980) The increased susceptibility of young red cells to invasion by the malarial parasite *Plasmodium falciparum*. *Br. J. Haematol.* **45**, 285.

Pataryas, H.A. & Stamatoyannopoulos, G. (1972) Hemoglobins in human fetuses: evidence for adult hemoglobin production after the 11th gestational week. *Blood* **39**, 688.

Patrinos, G.P., Kollia, P., Loutradi-Anagnostou, A., Loukopoulos, D. & Papadakis, M.N. (1998) The Cretan type of non-deletional hereditary persistence of fetal hemoglobin [Aγ-158C→T] results from two independent gene conversion events. *Hum. Genet.* **102**, 629.

Pauling, L. (1954) Abnormality of hemoglobin molecules in hereditary hemolytic anemias. In: *The Harvey Lectures 1954–55*, p. 216. Academic Press, New York.

Pauling, L., Itano, H.A., Singer, S.J. & Wells, I.G. (1949) Sickle-cell anemia, a molecular disease. *Science* **110**, 543.

Pavri, R.S., Baxi, A.J., Grover, S. & Parande, R.A. (1977) Study of glycolytic intermediates in hereditary elliptocytosis with thalassemia. *J. Postgrad. Med.* **23**, 189.

Pawar, A.R., Colahn, R.B. & Mohanty, D. (1997) A novel β⁺-thalassemia mutation (codon 10 GCC→GCA) and a rare transcriptional mutation (−28A→G) in Indians. *Blood* **89**, 3888.

Pawlack, A.L. & Kozlowska, F. (1970) Swiss type hereditary persistence of foetal haemoglobin in a case of acquired haemolytic anaemia. *Acta Haematol.* **43**, 184.

Pawlowitzki, I.H., Grobe, H. & Holzgreve, W. (1979) Trisomy 20q due to maternal t(16;20) translocation: first case. *Clin. Genet.* **15**, 167.

Pearson, H.A. (1964) Thalassemia intemedia: genetic and biochemical considerations. *Ann. N. Y. Acad. Sci.* **119**, 390.

Pearson, H.A. (1966) Alpha-beta thalassemia disease in a Negro family. *N. Eng. J. Med.* **275**, 176.

Pearson, H.A. (1969) Hemoglobin S-thalassemia syndrome in Negro children. *Ann. N. Y. Acad. Sci.* **165**, 83.

Pearson, H.A. & Al-Rasheid, A.A. (1987) Sickle cell diseases: comparisons between America and Kuwait. *J. Kuwait Med. Assoc.* **21**, 178.

Pearson, H.A. & McFarland, W. (1962) Erythrokinetics in thalassemias. II. Studies in Lepore trait and hemoglobin H disease. *J. Lab. Clin. Med.* **59**, 147.

Pearson, H.A., Gerald, P.S. & Diamond, L.K. (1959) Thalassemia intermedia due to interaction of Lepore trait with thalassemia trait; report of three cases. *Am. J. Dis. Child.* **97**, 464.

Pearson, H.A., McFarland, W. & King, E.R. (1960) Erythrokinetic studies in thalassemia trait. *J. Lab. Clin. Med.* **56**, 866.

Pearson, H.A., O'Brien, R.T. & McIntosh, S. (1973) Screening for thalassemia trait by electronic measurement of mean corpuscular volume. *N. Eng. J. Med.* **288**, 351.

Pearson, H.A., McPhedran, P., O'Brien, R.T., Aspnes, G.T., McIntosh, S. & Guiliotis, D.K. (1974) Comprehensive testing for thalassemia trait. *Ann. N. Y. Acad. Sci.* **232**, 135.

Pearson, H.A., Motoyama, E., Genel, M., Kramer, M. & Zigas, C. (1977) Intraerythrocytic adaptation (2,3 DPG, P50) in thalassemia minor. *Blood* **49**, 463.

Pearson, H.A., Gallagher, D., Chilcote, R. *et al.* (1985) Developmental pattern of splenic dysfunction in sickle cell disorders. *Pediatr.* **76**, 392.

Pellicer, A. (1967) Frequency of thalassemia in a sample of the Spanish population. *Am. J. Hum. Genet.* **19**, 695.

Pellicer, A. & Casado, A. (1970) Frequency of thalassaemia and G6PD deficiency in five provinces of Spain. *Am. J. Hum. Genet.* **22**, 298.

Pembrey, M.E., McWade, P. & Weatherall, D.J. (1972) Reliable routine estimation of small amounts of foetal haemoglobin by alkali denaturation. *J. Clin. Pathol.* **25**, 738.

Pembrey, M.E., Weatherall, D.J. & Clegg, J.B. (1973) Maternal synthesis of haemoglobin F in pregnancy. *Lancet* **i**, 1350.

Pembrey, M.E., Weatherall, D.J., Clegg, J.B., Bunch, C. & Perrine, R.P. (1975) Haemoglobin Bart's in Saudi Arabia. *Br. J. Haematol.* **29**, 221.

Pembrey, M.E., Wood, W.G., Weatherall, D.J. & Perrine, R.P. (1978) Fetal haemoglobin production and the sickle gene in the oases of Eastern Saudi Arabia. *Br. J. Haematol.* **40**, 415.

Pembrey, M.E., Perrine, R.P., Wood, W.G. & Weatherall, D.J. (1980) Sickle cell β⁰ thalassemia in Eastern Saudi Arabia. *Am. J. Hum. Genet.* **32**, 41.

Penberthy, G.C. & Cooley, T.B. (1935) Results of splenectomy in childhood. *Ann. Surg.* **102**, 645.

Pepe, G., Lupi, L., Mastrobuono, A., Carestia, C., Lania, A. & Luzzatto, L. (1982) The pattern of thalassemia in Naples. In: *Thalassemia: Recent Advances in Detection and Treatment. Birth Defects: Original Article Series* (eds A. Cao, U. Carcassi & P.T. Rowley), p. 177. Alan R. Liss, New York.

Pepe, F., Pepe, L., Greco, L., Sprini, R. & Garozzo, G. (1992) Frequenza della beta-talassemia eterozigote in gravide delle Alta Madonie. *Min. Ginecol.* **44**, 271.

Perabo, V.F. (1954) Uber das vorkommen vou Cooley-anämie in Burma. *Helv. Paediatr. Acta* **9**, 339.

Pereira, J.M., Callado, A.N.A., Monteiro, A.L., Bastos, R.M.N.A., Pinto, A.C. & Lirio, A.S. (1973) Investigaçáo em uma família com alfa talassemia. *Rev. Brasil Pesqu. Med. Biol.* **6**, 349.

Peres, M.J., Romão, L., Carreiro, H. *et al.* (1995) Molecular basis of α-thalassaemia in Portugal. *Hemoglobin* **19**, 343.

Pergament, E., Pietra, M.G.C., Kadotani, T., Sato, H. & Berlow, S. (1970) A ring chromosome no. 16 in an infant with primary hypoparathyroidism. *J. Pediatr.* **76**, 745.

Perignon, F., Brauner, R., Souberbielle, J.C., de Montalembert, M. & Girot, R. (1993) Growth and endocrine function in thalassemia major. *Arch. Fr. Pediatr.* **50**, 657.

Perillie, P.E. & Chernoff, A.I. (1965) Heterozygous beta-thalassemia in association with hereditary elliptocytosis. *Blood* **25**, 494.

Perkins, A.C., Sharpe, A.H. & Orkin, S.H. (1995) Lethal β-thalassaemia in mice lacking the erythroid CACCC-transcription factor EKLF. *Nature* **375**, 318.

Perla, D. & Marmorston, J. (1941) *Natural Resistance and Clinical Medicine*, p. 763. Little Brown & Co, Boston, MA.

Perosa, L. (1949) Il metabolismo del Fe e de la dissociazione ipochromia–ipersideremia nelle sindromi emopatiche Mediterranee. Considerazione patogenotiche. *Rif. Med.* **63**, 807.

Perosa, L., Manganelli, G. & Dalfino, G. (1961) Il primo caso di Hb C-thalassemia descritto in Italia-Rivista sintetica sulla emoglobina C. *Haematologica* **46**, 211.

Perrine, R.P., Brown, M.J., Clegg, J.B., Weatherall, D.J. & May, A. (1972) Benign sickle-cell anaemia. *Lancet* **ii**, 1163.

Perrine, R.P., John, P., Pembrey, M. & Perrine, S. (1981) Sickle cell disease in Saudi Arabs in early childhood. *Arch. Dis. Child.* **56**, 187.

Perrine, S.P., Greene, M.F. & Faller, D.V. (1985) Delay in the fetal globin switch in infants of diabetic mothers. *N. Eng. J. Med.* **312**, 334.

Perrine, S.P., Rudolph, A., Faller, D.V. *et al.* (1988) Butyrate infusions in the ovine fetus delay the biologic clock for globin gene switching. *Proc. Natl Acad. Sci. USA* **85**, 8540.

Perrine, S.P., Ginder, G.D., Faller, D.V. *et al.* (1993) A short-term trial of butyrate to stimulate fetal-globin-gene expression in the β-globin disorders. *N. Eng. J. Med.* **328**, 81.

Persons, D.A. & Nienhuis, A.W. (2000) Gene therapy for the hemoglobin disorders: past, present and future. *Proc. Nat. Acad. Sci. USA*, **97**, 5022.

Perutz, M.F. (1963) X-ray analysis of hemoglobin. *Science* **140**, 863.

Perutz, M.F. (1965) Structure and function of haemoglobin. I. A tentative atomic model of horse haemoglobin. *J. Mol. Biol.* **13**, 646.

Perutz, M.F. (1970a) The Bohr effect and combination with organic phosphates. *Nature* **228**, 734.

Perutz, M.F. (1970b) Stereochemistry of cooperative effects in haemoglobin. *Nature* **228**, 726.

Perutz, M.F. (1972) Nature of haem–haem interaction. *Nature New Biol.* **237**, 495.

Perutz, M.F. (1978) Hemoglobin structure and respiratory transport. *Sci. Am.* **239**, 92.

Perutz, M.F. (1980) Sterochemical mechanism of oxygen transport by haemoglobin. *Proc. Roy. Soc. Lond. (Biol.)* **208**, 135.

Perutz, M.F. (1991) *Protein Structure and Function*. Freeman, New York.

Perutz, M.F. (1998) *I Wish I'd Made You Angry Earlier*. Cold Spring Harbor, New York.

Perutz, M.F., Rossman, M.G., Cullis, A.F., Muirhead, H., Will, G. & North, A.C.T. (1960) Structure of haemoglobin. *Nature* **185**, 416.

Perutz, M.F., Kendrew, J.C. & Watson, H.C. (1965) Structure and function of haemoglobin. II. Some relations between polypeptide chain configuration and amino acid sequence. *J. Mol. Biol.* **13**, 669.

Perutz, M.F., Muirhead, H., Cox, J.M. & Goaman, L.C.G. (1968a) Three-dimensional Fourier synthesis of horse deoxyhaemoglobin at 2.8Å resolution. (2) The atomic model. *Nature* **219**, 131.

Perutz, M.F., Muirhead, H., Cox, J.M. *et al.* (1968b) Three dimensional Fourier synthesis of oxyhaemoglobin at 2.8Å resolution. *Nature* **219**, 29.

Perutz, M.F., Shih, D.T. & Williamson, D. (1994) The chloride effect in human haemoglobin. *J. Mol. Biol.* **239**, 555.

Peschle, C., Migliaccio, A.R., Migliaccio, G. *et al.* (1984) The embryonic→fetal Hb switch in humans: Studies on erythroid bursts generated by embryonic progenitors from yolk sac and liver. *Proc. Natl Acad. Sci. USA* **81**, 2416.

Peschle, C., Mavilio, F., Care, A. *et al.* (1985) Haemoglobin switching in human embryos: asynchrony of ζ–α and ε–γ-globin switches in primitive and definite erythropoietic lineage. *Nature* **313**, 235.

Peterson, C.L. & Herskowitz, I. (1992) Characterisation of the yeast *SWI1*, *SWI2* and *SWI3* genes, which encode a global activator of transcription. *Cell* **68**, 573.

Peterson, K.R. & Stamatoyannopoulos, G. (1993) Role of gene order in developmental control of human γ- and β-globin gene expression. *Mol. Cell. Biol.* **13**, 4836.

Peterson, K.R., Clegg, C.H., Huxley, C. *et al.* (1993) Transgenic mice containing a 248-kb yeast artificial chromosome carrying the human β-globin locus display proper developmental control of human globin genes. *Proc. Natl Acad. Sci. USA* **90**, 7593.

Peterson, K.R., Li, Q.L., Clegg, C.H. *et al.* (1995) Use of yeast artificial chromosomes (YACs) in studies of mammalian development: production of β-globin locus YAC mice carrying human globin developmental mutants. *Proc. Natl Acad. Sci. USA* **92**, 5655.

Petkov, G.H., Efremov, G.D., Efremov, D.G. *et al.* (1990) β-Thalassemia in Bulgaria. *Hemoglobin* **14**, 25.

Petmitr, S., Wilairat, P., Kownkon, J., Winichagoon, P. & Fucharoen, S. (1989) Molecular basis of β⁰-thalassemia/Hb E disease in Thailand. *Biochem. Biophys. Res. Comm.* **162**, 846.

Petrou, M. & Modell, B. (1995) Prenatal screening for haemoglobin disorders. *Prenat. Diag.* **15**, 1275.

Petrou, M., Modell, B., Darr, A., Old, J., Kin, E. & Weatherall, D.J. (1990) Antenatal diagnosis: How to deliver a comprehensive service in the United Kingdom. *Ann. N. Y. Acad. Sci.* **612**, 251.

Pevny, L., Simon, M.C., Robertson, E. *et al.* (1991) Erythroid differentiation in chimaeric mice blocked by a targeted mutation in the gene for transcription factor GATA-1. *Nature* **349**, 257.

Philipsen, S., Talbot, D., Fraser, P. & Grosveld, F. (1990) The β-globin dominant control region: hypersensitive site 2. *EMBO J.* **9**, 2159.

Philipsen, S., Pruzina, S. & Grosveld, F. (1993) The minimal requirements for activity in transgenic mice of hypersensitive site 3 of the β globin locus control region. *EMBO J.* **12**, 1077.

Phillips, J.A., Scott, A.F., Smith, K.D. *et al.* (1979) A molecular basis for hemoglobin-H disease in American Blacks. *Blood* **54**, 1439.

Piankijagum, A., Palungwachira, P. & Lohkoomgunpai, A. (1978) Beta thalassemia, hemoglobin E and hemoglobin H disease. Clinical analysis 1964–1966. *J. Med. Assoc. Thailand* **61**, 50.

Pich, P.G., Gallo, E., Mazza, U. & Ricco, G. (1973) Study on a case of double heterozygosis between Hb C and beta-thalassaemia. *Boll. Soc. Ital. Biol. Speriment.* **49**, 507.

Picketts, D.J., Higgs, D.R., Bachoo, S., Blake, D.J., Quarrell, O.W.J. & Gibbons, R.J. (1996) *ATRX* encodes a novel member of the SNF2 family of proteins: mutations point to a common mechanism underlying the ATR-X syndrome. *Hum. Mol. Genet.* **5**, 1899.

Picketts, D.J., Tastan, A.O., Higgs, D.R. & Gibbons, R.J. (1998) Comparison of the human and murine ATRX gene identifies highly conserved, functionally important domains. *Mammalian Genome* **9**, 400.

Pierce, H.I., Kurachi, S., Sofroniadu, K. & Stamatoyannopoulos, G. (1977) Frequencies of thalassaemia in American Blacks. *Blood* **49**, 981.

Piga, A., Magliano, M., Bianco, L., Capalbo, P., Baccaccini, R. & Gabutti, V. (1987) Compliance with chelation therapy in Torino. In: *Thalassaemia Today: Second Mediterranean Meeting on Thalassaemia*, p. 141. Policlinico di Milano, Milan, Italy.

Piga, A., Luzzatto, L., Capalbo, P., Gambotto, S., Tricta, F. & Gabutti, V. (1988) High-dose desferrioxamine as a cause of growth failure in thalassemic patients. *Eur. J. Haematol.* **40**, 380.

Pik, C., Loos, J.A., Jonxis, J.H.P. & Prins, H.K. (1965) Hereditary and acquired blood factors in the negroid population of Surinam. II.

The incidence of haemoglobin anomalies and the deficiency of glucose-6-phosphate dehydrogenase. *Trop. Geogr. Med.* **1**, 61.

Pinkerton, P.H., Wilson, J.B., Lam, H., Williams, D. & Huisman, T.H.J. (1979) Hemoglobin Riyadh – β⁰ thalassemia in an Indian family. *Hemoglobin* **3**, 451.

Pinto, L., Esposito, L., Vitale, R., Cicale, F., Scarano, G. & Nobili, B. (1978) L'alfa-talassemia in Campania: risultati di una indagine condotta su 319 neonati. *La Pediatr.* **86**, 637.

Pintor, C., Cella, S.G., Manso, P. *et al.* (1986) Impaired growth hormone (GH) response to GH-releasing hormone in thalassemia major. *J. Clin. Endocrinol. Metab.* **62**, 263.

Piomelli, S. (1993) Management of Cooley's anaemia. *Clin. Haematol.* **6**, 287.

Piomelli, S. & Siniscalco, M. (1969) The haematological effects of glucose-6-phosphate dehydrogenase deficiency and thalassaemia trait: interaction between the two genes at the phenotype level. *Br. J. Haematol.* **16**, 537.

Piomelli, S., Danoff, S.J., Becker, M.H., Lipera, M.J. & Travis, S.F. (1969) Prevention of bone malformations and cardiomegaly in Cooley's anemia by early hypertransfusion regimen. *Ann. N. Y. Acad. Sci.* **165**, 427.

Piomelli, S., Karpatkin, M.H., Arzanian, M. *et al.* (1974) Hypertransfusion regimen in patients with Cooley's anemia. *Ann. N. Y. Acad. Sci.* **232**, 186.

Piomelli, S., Seaman, C., Reibman, J., Tyrun, A., Graziano, J. & Tabachnik, N. (1978) Separation of younger red cells with improved survival *in vivo*: an approach to chronic transfusion therapy. *Proc. Natl Acad. Sci. USA* **75**, 3474.

Piomelli, S., Hart, D., Graziano, J., Grant, G., Karpatkin, M. & McCarthy, K. (1985) Current strategies in the management of Cooley's anemia. *Ann. N. Y. Acad. Sci.* **445**, 256.

Piomelli, S., Seaman, C., Cirella, B. *et al.* (1986) Does α-thalassemia protect from early stroke in sickle cell anemia? *Pediatr. Res.* **20**, 285A.

Pippard, M.J. & Wainscoat, J.S. (1987) Erythrokinetics and iron status in heterozygous β thalassaemia, and the effect of interaction with α thalassaemia. *Br. J. Haematol.* **66**, 123.

Pippard, M.J. & Weatherall, D.J. (1984) Iron absorption in non-transfused iron loading anaemias: reduction of risk for iron loading, and response to iron chelation treatment, in β thalassaemia and congenital sideroblastic anaemias. *Haematologica* **17**, 17.

Pippard, M.J., Callender, S.T., Letsky, E.A. & Weatherall, D.J. (1978a) Prevention of iron loading in transfusion-dependent thalassaemia. *Lancet* **i**, 1178.

Pippard, M.J., Callender, S.T. & Weatherall, D.J. (1978b) Intensive iron-chelation therapy with desferrioxamine in iron loading patients. *Clin. Sci. Mol. Med.* **54**, 99.

Pippard, M.J., Warner, G.T., Callender, S.T. & Weatherall, D.J. (1979) Iron absorption and loading in β-thalassaemia intermedia. *Lancet* **ii**, 819.

Pippard, M.J., Callender, S.T. & Finch, C.A. (1982a) Ferrioxamine excretion in iron loaded man. *Blood* **60**, 288.

Pippard, M.J., Rajagopalan, B., Callender, S.T. & Weatherall, D.J. (1982b) Iron loading, chronic anaemia, and erythroid hyperplasia as determinants of the clinical features of β-thalassaemia intermedia. In: *Advances in Red Blood Cell Biology* (eds D.J. Weatherall, G. Fiorelli & S. Gorini), p. 103. Raven Press, New York.

Pippard, M.J. & Weatherall, D.J. (2000) Oral iron chelation therapy for thalassemia: an uncertain scene. *Brit. J. Haematol.* **110**, 1.

Pirastu, M., Lee, K.Y., Dozy, A.M. *et al.* (1982) Alpha-thalassaemia in two Mediterranean populations. *Blood* **60**, 509.

Pirastu, M., Kan, Y.W., Cao, A., Conner, B.J., Teplitz, R.L. & Wallace, R.B. (1983a) Prenatal diagnosis of β-thalassemia. Detection of a single nucleotide mutation in DNA. *N. Eng. J. Med.* **309**, 284.

Pirastu, M., Kan, Y.W., Lin, C.C., Baine, R. & Holbrook, C.T. (1983b) Hemolytic disease of the newborn caused by a new deletion of the entire β-globin cluster. *J. Clin. Invest.* **72**, 602.

Pirastu, M., Kan, Y.W., Galanello, R. & Cao, A. (1984a) Multiple mutations produce (δβ⁰) thalassaemia in Sardinia. *Science* **223**, 929.

Pirastu, M., Saglio, G., Chang, J.C., Cao, A. & Kan, Y.W. (1984b) Initiation codon mutation as a cause of α-thalassaemia. *J. Biol. Chem.* **259**, 12315.

Pirastu, M., Ristaldi, M.S., Loudianos, G. *et al.* (1990) Molecular analysis of atypical β-thalassaemia heterozygotes. *Ann. N. Y. Acad. Sci.* **612**, 90.

Pissard, S. & Beuzard, Y. (1994) A potential regulatory region for the expression of fetal hemoglobin in sickle cell disease. *Blood* **84**, 331.

Pissard, S. M'rad, A., Beuzard, Y. & Roméo, P.-H. (1996) A new type of hereditary persistence of fetal haemoglobin (HPFH): HPFH Tunisia β⁺ (+C-200) ᴳγ. *Br. J. Haematol.* **95**, 67.

Pistidda, P., Frogheri, L., Guiso, L. *et al.* (1997) Maximal γ-globin expression in the compound heterozygous state for –175 ᴳγ HPFH and β⁰39 nonsense thalassaemia: a case study. *Eur. J. Haematol.* **58**, 320.

Pittis, M.G., Estevez, M.E., Diez, R.A., de Miani, S.A. & Sen, L. (1994) Decreased phagolysosomal fusion of peripheral blood monocytes from patients with thalassemia major. *Acta Haematol.* **92**, 66.

Plato, C.C., Rucknagel, D.L. & Gershowitz, H. (1964) Studies on the distribution of glucose-6-phosphate dehydrogenase deficiency, thalassaemia, and other genetic traits in the coastal and mountain villages of Cyprus. *Am. J. Hum. Genet.* **16**, 267.

Platt, O.S. (1994) Membrane proteins. In: *Sickle Cell Disease: Basic Principles and Clinical Practice* (eds S.H. Embury, R.P. Hebbel, N. Mohandas & M.H. Steinberg), p. 125. Raven Press Ltd, New York.

Platt, O.S. & Falcone, J.F. (1988) Membrane protein lesions in erythrocytes with Heinz bodies. *J. Clin. Invest.* **82**, 1051.

Platt, O.S., Orkin, S., Dover, G.J., Beardsley, G.P., Miller, B. & Nathan, D.G. (1984) Hydroxyurea enhances fetal hemoglobin production in sickle cell anemia. *J. Clin. Invest.* **74**, 652.

Platt, O.S., Thorington, B., Branbilla, D. *et al.* (1991) Pain in sickle cell disease. *N. Eng. J. Med.* **325**, 11.

Platt, O.S., Brambilla, D.J., Rosse, W.F. *et al.* (1994) Mortality in sickle cell disease. Life expectancy and risk factors for early death. *N. Eng. J. Med.* **330**, 1639.

Plonczynski, M., Figueiredo, M.S. & Steinberg, M.H. (1997) Fetal hemoglobin in sickle cell anemia: examination of phylogenetically conserved sequences within the locus control region but outside the cores of hypersensitive sites 2 and 3. *Blood Cell. Mol. Dis.* **23**, 188.

Pobedimskaya, D.D., Molchanova, T.P., Streichman, S. & Huisman, T.H.J. (1994) Compound heterozygosity for two α-globin gene defects Hb Taybe (α1; 38 or 39 minus Thr) and a poly A mutation (α2; AATAA<u>A</u>→AATAA<u>G</u>), results in a severe hemolytic anemia. *Am. J. Hematol.* **47**, 198.

Podda, A., Galanello, R., Maccioni, L. *et al.* (1991) Hemoglobin Cagliari (β 60 [E4] Val-Glu): a novel unstable thalassemic hemoglobinopathy. *Blood* **77**, 371.

Politis, C. (1989) Complications of blood transfusion in thalassemia. In: *Advances and Controversies in Thalassemia Therapy: Bone Marrow Transplantation and Other Approaches* (eds C.D. Buckner, R.P. Gale & G. Lucarelli), p. 67. Alan R. Liss, New York.

Politis, C., Roumeliotou, A., Germenis, A. & Papaevangelou, G. (1986) Risk of acquired immune deficiency syndrome in multi-transfused patients with thalassemia major. *Plasma Ther. Transfus. Technol.* **7**, 41.

Politis, C., Spigos, D.G., Georgiopoulou, P. *et al.* (1987) Partial splenic

embolisation for hypersplenism of thalassaemia major: five year follow-up. *Br. Med. J.* **294**, 665.

Polliack, A. & Rachmilewitz, E.A. (1973) Ultrastructural studies in β-thalassaemia major. *Br. J. Haematol.* **24**, 319.

Polliack, A., Yataganas, X. & Rachmilewitz, E.A. (1974a) Ultrastructure of the inclusion bodies and nuclear abnormalities in beta-thalassemic erythroblasts. *Ann. N. Y. Acad. Sci.* **232**, 261.

Polliack, A., Yataganas, X., Thorell, B. & Rachmilewitz, E.A. (1974b) An electron microscopic study of the nuclear abnormalities in erythroblasts in beta-thalassaemia major. *Br. J. Haematol.* **26**, 201.

Polosa, P., Motta, L., Calcagno, G. & Linetta, M. (1966) L'Hb C-thalasemia negli individui di razza bianca. *Haematologica* **51**, 771.

Polosa, P., Motta, L. & Calcagno, G. (1970) Clinical considerations on 7 cases of Hb C-thalassemia. *Haematologica* **55**, 333.

Poncz, M., Ballantine, M., Solowiejczyk, D., Barak, I., Schwartz, E. & Surrey, S. (1983) β-Thalassemia in a Kurdish Jew. *J. Biol. Chem.* **257**, 5994.

Pondel, M.D., Sharpe, J.A., Clark, S., Pearson, L., Wood, W.G. & Proudfoot, N.J. (1996) Proximal promoter elements of the human ζ-globin gene confer embryonic-specific expression on a linked reporter gene in transgenic mice. *Nucl. Acids Res.* **24**, 4158.

Pongsamart, S., Pootrakul, S., Wasi, P. & Na-Nakorn, S. (1975) Hemoglobin Constant Spring: hemoglobin synthesis in heterozygous and homozygous states. *Biochem. Biophys. Res. Comm.* **64**, 681.

Pontremoli, S., Bargellesi, A. & Conconi, F. (1969) Globin chain synthesis in the Ferrara thalassemia population. *Ann. N. Y. Acad. Sci.* **165**, 253.

Pootrakul, S., Wasi, P. & Na-Nakorn, S. (1967a) Haemoglobin Bart's hydrops fetalis in Thailand. *Ann. Hum. Genet. (Lond.)* **30**, 283.

Pootrakul, S., Wasi, P. & Na-Nakorn, S. (1967b) Studies on haemoglobin Bart's (Hb-γ₄) in Thailand: the incidence and the mechanism of occurrence in cord blood. *Ann. Hum. Genet. (Lond.)* **31**, 149.

Pootrakul, S., Wasi, P., Pornpatkul, M. & Na-Nakorn, S. (1970) Incidence of alpha thalassemia in Bangkok. *J. Med. Assoc. Thailand* **53**, 250.

Pootrakul, P., Wasi, P. & Na-Nakorn, S. (1973) Haematological data in 312 cases of β thalassaemia trait in Thailand. *Br. J. Haematol.* **24**, 703.

Pootrakul, S., Sapprapa, S., Wasi, P., Na-Nakorn, S. & Suwanik, R. (1975a) Hemoglobin synthesis in 28 obligatory cases for alpha-thalassemia traits. *Humangenetik* **29**, 121.

Pootrakul, S., Wasi, P., Na-Nakorn, S. & Pravatmuang, P. (1975b) Hemoglobin Bart's and hemoglobin Constant Spring in the cord blood. In: *Istanbul Symposium on Abnormal Hemoglobins and Thalassemia*, p. 111. Ataturk Bulvaria 221, Ankara, Istanbul.

Pootrakul, P., Hungsprenges, S., Fucharoen, S. *et al.* (1981a) Relation between erythropoiesis and bone metabolism in thalassemia. *N. Eng. J. Med.* **304**, 1470.

Pootrakul, P., Vougsmasa, V., Laongpanich, P. & Wasi, P. (1981b) Serum ferritin levels in thalassemias and the effect of splenectomy. *Acta Haematol.* **66**, 244.

Pootrakul, P., Winichagoon, P., Fucharoen, S., Pravatmuang, P., Piankijagum, A. & Wasi, P. (1981c) Homozygous haemoglobin Constant Spring: a need for revision of concept. *Hum. Genet.* **59**, 250.

Pootrakul, P., Kitcharoen, K., Yansukon, P. *et al.* (1988) The effect of erythroid hyperplasia on iron balance. *Blood* **71**, 1124.

Poovorawan, Y., Theamboonlers, A., Chongsrisawat, V. & Jantaradsamee, P. (1998) Prevalence of infection with hepatitis G virus among various groups in Thailand. *Ann. Trop. Med. Parasitol.* **92**, 89.

Popat, N., Wood, W.G., Weatherall, D.J. & Turnbull, A.C. (1977) The pattern of maternal F-cell production during pregnancy. *Lancet* ii, 377.

Popovich, B.W., Rosenblatt, D.S., Kendall, A.G. & Nishioka, Y. (1986) Molecular characterization of an atypical β-thalassaemia caused by a large deletion in the 5′ β-globin gene region. *Am. J. Hum. Genet.* **39**, 797.

Pornpatkul, M., Wasi, P. & Na-Nakorn, S. (1969) Hematologic parameters in obligatory alpha-thalassemia. *J. Med. Assoc. Thailand* **52**, 801.

Pornpatkul, M., Pootrakul, S.-N., Muangsrup, W. & Wasi, P. (1978) Intraerythrocytic inclusion bodies in obligatory alpha thalassemia traits. *J. Med. Assoc. Thailand* **61**, 63.

Pornpatkul, M., Bumrungtrakul, P., Surapruk, P. *et al.* (1980) The incidence of thalassemias and hemoglobin E in Vietnamese. *Southeast Asian J. Trop. Med. Publ. Hlth* **11**, 142.

Porter, J.B. (1996) Evaluation of new iron chelators for clinical use. *Acta Haematol.* **95**, 13.

Porter, J.B. & Huehns, E.R. (1989) The toxic effects of desferrioxamine. *Clin. Haematol.* **2**, 459.

Porter, J.B., East, C.A., Jaswon, M.S. & Huehns, E.R. (1988) Audiometric abnormalities in thalassaemia: risk factor associated with the use of desferrioxamine. *Br. J. Haematol.* **69**, 88.

Porter, J.B., Huehns, E.R. & Hider, R.C. (1989a) The development of iron chelating drugs. *Clin. Haematol.* **2**, 257.

Porter, J.B., Jaswon, M.S., Huehns, E.R., East, C.A. & Hazell, J.W.P. (1989b) Desferrioxamine ototoxicity: evaluation of risk factors in thalassaemia patients and guidelines for safe dosage. *Br. J. Haematol.* **73**, 403.

Porter, J.B., Singh, S., Epemolu, R.O., Ackerman, R., Huehns, E.R. & Hider, R.C. (1991) Oral efficacy and metabolism of 1,2-diethyl-3-hydroxypyridin-4-one in thalassemia major. *Blood* **78**, 207a.

Portier, A., de Traverse, P., Duzer, A., Destaing, F. & Porot, J.F. (1960) L'hémoglobinose C-thalassemia (apropos d'une observation familiale caractéristique). *Presse Med.* **68**, 1760.

Potente, G. (1988) Complicanze asrticolari nella drepanocitosi-talassemia dopo l'ete infantile. *Radiol. Med. Torino* **76**, 409.

Poulik, M.D. (1957) Starch gel electrophoresis in a discontinuous system of buffers. *Nature* **180**, 1477.

Pouya, Y. (1959) Thalassaemia in Iran. In: *Abnormal Haemoglobins* (eds J.H.P. Jonxis & J.F. Delafresnaye), p. 263. Blackwell Scientific Publications, Oxford.

Powell, W.N., Rodarte, J.G. & Neel, J.V. (1950) The occurrence in a family of Sicilian ancestry of the traits for both sickling and thalassemia. *Blood* **5**, 887.

Powers, P.A., Altay, C., Huisman, T.H.J. & Smithies, O. (1984) Two novel arrangements of the human fetal globin genes: $^{G}\gamma$-$^{G}\gamma$ and $^{A}\gamma$-$^{A}\gamma$. *Nucl. Acids Res.* **12**, 7023.

Poynton, H.G. & Davey, K.W. (1968) Thalassemia. Changes visible in radiographs used in dentistry. *Oral Surg.* **25**, 564.

Prankerd, T.A.J. (1963) The spleen and anaemia. *Br. Med. J.* ii, 517.

Prasad, A.S., Diwany, M., Gabr, M., Sandstead, H.H., Mokhtar, N. & El Hefny, A. (1965) Biochemical studies in thalassemia. *Ann. Intern. Med.* **62**, 87.

Prati, D., Zanella, A., Bosoni, P. *et al.* (1998) The incidence and natural course of transfusion-associated GB virus C/hepatitis G virus infection in a cohort of thalassemic patients. The Cooleycare Cooperative Group. *Blood* **91**, 774.

Pratico, G., Di Gregorio, F., Caltabiano, L., Palano, G.M. & Caruso-Nicoletti, M. (1998) Calcium phosphate metabolism in thalassemia. *Pediatr. Med. Chir.* **20**, 265.

Prchal, J.T., Adler, B., Wilson, J.B. *et al.* (1995) Hb Bibba or α-2, 136(H19) Leu→Pro-β-2 in a caucasian family from Alabama. *Hemoglobin* **19**, 151.

Predescu, C., Bratu, V. & Teitel, P. (1968) Apreciari asupra raspindirii talasemies in Romania. *Doc. Haematol.* **1**, 69.

Préhu, M.-O., Préhu, C., Goossens, M., Galactéros, E. & Wajcman, H. (1994) A new anti-Lepore hemoglobin, Hb P India (β87-δ105), found in coincidence with a C→G substitution at position 162 of IVS2 in both the δ and δβ genes, questions on the genetic mechanisms leading to Hbs Lepore and anti-Lepore. *Blood* **83**, 261a.

Pressley, L. (1980) *The genetic and molecular basis of α thalassaemia.* D. Phil. thesis, University of Oxford.

Pressley, L., Higgs, D.R., Aldridge, B., Metaxatou-Mavromati, A., Clegg, J.B. & Weatherall, D.J. (1980a) Characterisation of a new thalassaemia 1 defect due to a partial deletion of the α globin gene complex. *Nucl. Acids Res.* **8**, 4889.

Pressley, L., Higgs, D.R., Clegg, J.B., Perrine, R.P., Pembrey, M.E. & Weatherall, D.J. (1980b) A new genetic basis for hemoglobin-H disease. *N. Eng. J. Med.* **303**, 1383.

Pressley, L., Higgs, D.R., Clegg, J.B. & Weatherall, D.J. (1980c) Gene deletions in α thalassemia prove that the 5′ ζ locus is functional. *Proc. Natl Acad. Sci. USA* **77**, 3586.

Preto, R., Trincao, C., Melo, J., Cordiero Ferreria, N. & Cutinho, B. (1961) Consideracoes sobre numa hemoglobinopatia familia associacae talassemia-hemoglobina D numa familia algarvia. *Boll. Clin. Hosp. Civ. Lisboa* **25**, 483.

Prieto, J., Barry, M. & Sherlock, S. (1974) Serum ferritin in patients with iron overload and with acute and chronic liver disease. *Gut* **15**, 343.

Pritchard, J.A. (1962) Hereditary hypochromic microcytic anemia in obstetrics and gynecology. *Am. J. Obstet. Gynecol.* **83**, 1193.

Pritchard, J., Clegg, J.B., Weatherall, D.J. & Longley, J. (1974) The translation of human globin messenger RNA in heterologous assay systems. *Br. J. Haematol.* **28**, 141.

Pritchard, J., Longley, J., Clegg, J.B. & Weatherall, D.J. (1976) Assay of thalassaemic messenger RNA in the wheatgerm system. *Br. J. Haematol.* **32**, 473.

Promboon, A., Wilairat, P., Fucharoen, S. & Wasi, P. (1988) Determination of variable severity of anemia in thalassemia: erythrocyte proteolytic activity. *Birth Defects* **23**, 249.

Propper, R.D., Shurin, S.B. & Nathan, D.G. (1976) Reassessment of the use of desferrioxamine B in iron overload. *N. Eng. J. Med.* **294**, 1421.

Propper, R.D., Cooper, B., Rufo, R.R. *et al.* (1977) Continuous subcutaneous administration of deferoxamine in patients with iron overload. *N. Eng. J. Med.* **297**, 418.

Propper, R.D., Button, L.N. & Nathan, D.G. (1980) New approaches to the transfusion management of thalassemia. *Blood* **55**, 55.

Proudfoot, N.J. (1977) Complete 3′ non coding region sequences of rabbit and human β-globin messenger RNAs. *Cell* **10**, 559.

Proudfoot, N.J. (1986) Transcriptional interference and termination between duplicated α-globin gene constructs suggests a novel mechanism for gene regulation. *Nature* **322**, 562.

Proudfoot, N.J. & Baralle, F.E. (1979) Molecular cloning of the human ε globin gene. *Proc. Natl Acad. Sci. USA* **76**, 5435.

Proudfoot, N.J. & Longley, J.J. (1976) The 3′ terminal sequences of human α and β globin messenger RNAs: comparison with rabbit globin messenger RNA. *Cell* **9**, 733.

Proudfoot, N.J. & Maniatis, T. (1980) The structure of a human α-globin pseudogene and its relationship to α-globin gene duplication. *Cell* **21**, 537.

Proudfoot, N.J., Shander, M.H.M., Lanley, J.L., Gefter, M.L. & Maniatis, T. (1980) Structure and *in vitro* transcription of human globin genes. *Science* **209**, 1329.

Proudfoot, N.J., Gil, A. & Maniatis, T. (1982) The structure of the human ζ-globin gene and a closely linked, nearly identical pseudogene. *Cell* **31**, 553.

Pruzina, S., Hanscombe, O., Whyatt, D., Grosveld, F. & Philipsen, S.

(1991) Hypersensitive site 4 of the human β globin locus control region. *Nucl. Acids Res.* **19**, 1413.

Psichogiou, M., Tzala, E., Boletis, J. *et al.* (1996) Hepatitis E virus infection in individuals at high risk of transmission of non-A, non-B hepatitis and sexually transmitted diseases. *Scand. J. Infect. Dis.* **28**, 443.

Punt, K. & Van Gool, J. (1957) Thalassaemia-haemoglobin E disease in two Indo-European boys. *Acta Haematol.* **17**, 305.

Purucker, M., Bodine, D., Lin, H., McDonagh, K. & Nienhuis, A.W. (1990) Structure and function of the enhancer 3' to the human $^A\gamma$ globin gene. *Nucl. Acids Res.* **18**, 7407.

Putignano, A., Caruso, G. & Tannoia, N. (1973) Cooley in adulta. Studio clinico e anatomopatologico di un case. In: *Atti del V^0 Congresso Microcitemie*, Cosenza, p. 568. Istituto Italiano di Medicina Sociale, Roma.

Quaife, R., Al-Gazali, L., Abbes, S. *et al.* (1994) The spectrum of β thalassaemia mutations in the UAE national population. *J. Med. Genet.* **31**, 59.

Quattrin, N. & Ventruto, V. (1974) Hemoglobin Lepore: its significance for thalassemia and clinical manifestations. *Ann. N. Y. Acad. Sci.* **232**, 65.

Quattrin, N., Bianchi, P., Cimino, P. *et al.* (1966a) Le microcitemie ed altre emoglobinopatie in Campania. Cinque anni di recherche. *Rif. Med.* **80**, 285.

Quattrin, N., Ventruto, V. & Dini, E. (1966b) Prima osservacione Italian di malattia da omozugosi di Hb Lepore. *Haematologica* **51**, 189.

Quattrin, N., Bianchi, P., Cimino, R., de Rosa, L., Dini, E. & Ventruto, V. (1967) Study on nine families with haemoglobin Lepore in Campania. *Acta Haematol.* **37**, 266.

Quattrin, N., Ventruto, V. & De Rosa, L. (1970) Hemoglobinopathies in Campania with particular reference to the rare and new types. *Blut* **20**, 292.

Quattrin, N., Ventruto, V., Brancaccio, V., Mastrobuoni, A., de Rosa, C. & Cimino, R. (1973) Popolazionistica delle microcitemie ed emoglobinopatie genotipiche in Campania: Quattordici anni de richerche (1960–1973). In: *Atti del V^0 Congresso Microcitemie*, Cosenza, p. 281. Istituto Italiano di Medicina Sociale, Roma.

Quattrin, N., Luzzatto, L. & Quattrin, S. (1980) New clinical and biochemical findings from 235 patients with hemoglobin Lepore. *Ann. N. Y. Acad. Sci.* **344**, 364.

Quintana, A., Sordo, M.T., Estevez, C., Ludena, M.C. & San Roman, C. (1983) 16 Ring chromosome. *Clin. Genet.* **23**, 243.

Rachmilewitz, E.A. (1969) Formation of hemichromes from oxidised hemoglobin subunits. *Ann. N. Y. Acad. Sci.* **165**, 171.

Rachmilewitz, E.A. (1974) Denaturation of the normal and abnormal hemoglobin molecule. *Sem. Hematol.* **11**, 441.

Rachmilewitz, E.A. (1976) The role of intracellular hemoglobin precipitation, low MCHC and iron overload on red blood cell membrane peroxidation in thalassemia. In: *Birth Defects: Original Articles Series* (eds D. Bergsma, A. Cerami, C.M. Peterson & J.H. Graziano), p. 123. Alan R. Liss, New York.

Rachmilewitz, E.A. & Harari, E. (1972) Slow rate of haemichrome formation from oxidized haemoglobin Bart's (γ_4): a possible explanation for the unequal quantities of haemoglobins H (β_4) and Bart's in alpha thalassaemia. *Br. J. Haematol.* **22**, 357.

Rachmilewitz, E.A. & Thorell, B. (1972) Hemichromes in single inclusion bodies in red cells of beta thalassemia. *Blood* **39**, 794.

Rachmilewitz, E.A., Peisach, J., Bradley, T.B. & Blumberg, W.E. (1969) Role of haemichromes in the formation of inclusion bodies in haemoglobin H disease. *Nature* **222**, 248.

Rachmilewitz, E.A., Huisman, T.H.J. & Schroeder, W.A. (1973) Heterogeneity of fetal hemoglobin among Israeli families with beta thalassemia. *Israel J. Med. Sci.* **9**, 1464.

Rachmilewitz, E.A., Shifter, A. & Kahane, I. (1979) Vitamin E deficiency in β-thalassemia major: changes in hematological and biochemical parameters after a therapeutic trial with α-tocopherol. *Am. J. Clin. Nutr.* **32**, 1850.

Rachmilewitz, E.A., Shinar, E., Shalev, O., Galili, U. & Schrier, S.L. (1985) Erythrocyte membrane alterations in beta-thalassaemia. *Clin. Haematol.* **14**, 163.

Rachmilewitz, E.A., Goldfarb, A. & Dover, G. (1991) Administration of erythropoietin to patients with β-thalassemia intermedia: a preliminary trial. *Blood* **78**, 1145.

Rachmilewitz, E.A., Aker, M., Perry, D. & Dover, G. (1995) Sustained increase in haemoglobin and RBC following long-term administration of recombinant human erythropoietin to patients with homozygous β-thalassaemia. *Br. J. Haematol.* **90**, 341.

Rack, K.A., Harris, P.C., MacCarthy, A.B. *et al.* (1993) Characterization of three de novo derivative chromosomes 16 by 'reverse chromosome painting' and molecular analysis. *Am. J. Hum. Genet.* **52**, 987.

Raghaven, K., Lokeshwar, M.R., Birewar, N., Nigam, V., Manglani, M.V. & Raju, N.B. (1991) Evaluation of naked eye single tube red cell osmotic fragility test in detecting beta-thalassemia trait. *Indian Pediatr.* **28**, 469.

Ragusa A., Lombardo, M., Sortino, G., Lombardo, T., Nagel, R.L. & Labie, D. (1988) β^S in Sicily is in linkage disequilibrium with the Benin haplotype: implications for gene flow. *Am. J. Hematol.* **27**, 139.

Rahbar, S. & Bunn, H.F. (1987) Association of hemoglobin H disease with Hb J-Iran (β77 His→Asp): impact on subunit assembly. *Blood* **70**, 1790.

Rahbar, S., Golban-Moghadam, N. & Saoodi, H. (1974) Hemoglobin Lepore$_{Boston}$ in two Iranian families. *Blood* **43**, 79.

Rahbar, S., Azizi, M. & Nowzari, G. (1975) A case of homozygous haemoglobin Lepore Boston in Iran. *Acta Haematol.* **53**, 60.

Rahko, P.S., Salerni, R. & Uretsky, B.F. (1986) Successful reversal by chelation therapy of congestive cardiomyopathy due to iron overload. *J. Am. Coll. Cardiol.* **8**, 426.

Raich, N., Enver, T., Nakamoto, B., Josephson, B., Papayannopoulou, T. & Stamatoyannopoulos, G. (1990) Autonomous developmental control of human embryonic globin gene switching in transgenic mice. *Science* **250**, 1147.

Raich, N., Papayannopoulou, T., Stamatoyannopoulos, G. & Enver, T. (1992) Demonstration of a human epsilon-globin gene silencer with studies in transgenic mice. *Blood* **79**, 861.

Raich, N., Clegg, C.H., Grofti, J., Roméo, P.-H. & Stamatoyannopoulos, G. (1995) GATA1 and YY1 are developmental repressors of the human ε-globin gene. *EMBO J.* **14**, 801.

Rajevska, D., Beksedic, M., Kuzmaovic, M. & Lehmann, H. (1978) Le cas du double hétérozygote: L'hémoglobine O Arabia dans la combinaison avec l'hémoglobine Lepore. In: *17th Congress of the International Society of Hematology*, Paris (abstract).

Rakshit, M.M., Chatterjea, J.B. & Mitra, S.S. (1973) Observations on the intraerythrocytic distribution of foetal haemoglobin in Hb E-thalassaemia disease. *Indian J. Pathol. Bact.* **16**, 41.

Ramirez, F., Natta, C., O'Donnell, J.V. *et al.* (1975) Relative numbers of human globin genes assayed with purified α and β complementary human DNA. *Proc. Natl Acad. Sci. USA* **72**, 1550.

Ramirez, F., O'Donnell, J.V., Marks, P.A. *et al.* (1976) Abnormal or absent mRNA in β^0 Ferrara and gene deletion in δβ thalassaemia. *Nature* **263**, 471.

Ramirez, F., Starkman, D., Bank, A., Kerem, H., Cividalli, G. & Rachmilewitz, E.A. (1978) Absence of β mRNA in β^0 thalassemia in Kurdish Jews. *Blood* **52**, 735.

Ramot, B., Sheba, C., Fisher, S., Ager, J.A.M. & Lehmann, H. (1959)

Haemoglobin H disease with persistent 'Bart's' in an oriental Jewess and her daughter. *Br. Med. J.* **ii**, 1228.

Ramot, B., Abrahamov, A., Frayer, Z. & Gafni, D. (1964) The incidence and types of thalassaemia-trait carriers in Israel. *Br. J. Haematol.* **10**, 155.

Ramot, B., Ben-Bassat, I., Garni, D. & Zaanoon, R. (1970) A family with three δβ-thalassemia homozygotes. *Blood* **35**, 158.

Ramot, B., Ben-Bassat, I., Mozel, M. & Shacked, N. (1973) Globin synthesis in alpha- and beta-thalassaemia. *Israel J. Med. Sci.* **9**, 1469.

Ramsay, M. & Jenkins, T. (1987) Globin gene-associated restriction fragment-length polymorphisms in South African peoples. *Am. J. Hum. Genet.* **41**, 1132.

Rand, C., Pearson, T.C. & Heatley, F.W. (1987) Avascular necrosis of the femoral head in sickle cell syndrome: a report of 5 cases. *Acta Haematol.* **78**, 186.

Randell, E.W., Parkes, J.G., Olivieri, N.F. & Templeton, D.M. (1994) Uptake of non-transferrin-bound iron by both reductive and nonreductive processes is modulated by intracellular iron. *J. Biol. Chem.* **269**, 16046.

Randhawa, Z.I., Jones, R.T. & Lie-Injo, L.E. (1984) Human hemoglobin Portland II ($\zeta_2\beta_2$). *J. Biol. Chem.* **259**, 7325.

Ranney, H.M. (1954) Observations on the inheritance of sickle-cell hemoglobin and hemoglobin C. *J. Clin. Invest.* **33**, 1634.

Ranney, H.M. & Jacobs, A.S. (1964) Simultaneous occurrence of haemoglobins C and Lepore in an Afro-American. *Nature* **204**, 163.

Ranney, H.M., Jacobs, A.S., Bradley, T.B.J. & Cordova, F.A. (1963) A 'new' variant of haemoglobin A₂ and its segregation in a family with haemoglobin S. *Nature* **197**, 164.

Ranney, H.M., Jacobs, A.S., Ramot, B. & Bradley, T.B. (1969) Hemoglobin NYU, a δ chain variant, $\alpha_2\delta_2^{12Lys}$. *J. Clin. Invest.* **48**, 2057.

Rao, A.V., Bai, K.I. & Ramanujiah, D. (1972) Hypertriglyceridaemia in thalassaemia major. *J. Indian Med. Assoc.* **59**, 15.

Rao, M., Mukhopadhyay, S. & Bhargava, S. (1989) Unusual manifestation of extramedullary haematopoiesis in thalassaemia major (report of 2 cases). *Australas. Radiol.* **33**, 187.

Rao, V.B., Natrajan, P.G., Lulla, C.P. & Bandodkar, S.B. (1997) Rapid mid-trimester prenatal diagnosis of β-thalassaemia and other haemoglobinopathies using a non-radioactive anion exchange HPLC technique—an Indian experience. *Prenat. Diag.* **17**, 725.

Raper, A.B., Gammack, D.B., Huehns, E.R. & Shooter, E.M. (1960) Four haemoglobins in one individual: a study of the genetic interaction of Hb G and Hb C. *Br. Med. J.* **2**, 1257.

Rappaport, E.F., Schwartz, E., Poncz, M. & Surrey, S. (1984) Frequent occurrence of a ζ-globin region deletion in American Blacks accounts for a previously-described restriction site polymorphism. *Biochem. Biophys. Res. Comm.* **125**, 817.

Rashkov, R. (1978) *Characteristics and distribution of normal and mutant haemoglobins and some haemoglobinopathies in Bulgaria.* Doctoral Dissertation, Sofia.

Raskó, I. & Downes, C.S. (1995) *Genes in Medicine.* Chapman & Hall, London.

Ray, P.F. & Handyside, A.H. (1996) Increasing the denaturation temperature during the first cycles of amplification reduces allele dropout from single cells for preimplantation genetic diagnosis. *Mol. Hum. Reprod.* **2**, 213.

Reddy, P.H., Petrou, M., Reddy, P.A., Tiurory, R.S. & Modell, B. (1995) Hereditary anaemias and iron deficiency in a tribal population (the Baiga) of central India. *Eur. J. Haematol.* **55**, 103.

Reed, R.E., Winter, W.P. & Rucknagel, D.L. (1974) Haemoglobin Inkster ($\alpha_2^{85}Asp{\rightarrow}Val\ \beta_2$) coexisting with beta-thalassaemia in a Caucasian family. *Br. J. Haematol.* **26**, 475.

Reemsta, K. & Elliot, R.H. (1956) Splenectomy in Mediterranean anemia: an evaluation of long-term results. *Ann. Surg.* **144**, 999.

Rees, M.I., Worwood, M., Thompson, P.W., Gilbertson, C. & May, A. (1994) Red cell dimorphism in a young man with a constitutional chromosomal translocation t(11;22) (p15.5;q11.21). *Br. J. Haematol.* **87**, 386.

Rees, D.C., Duley, J., Simmonds, H.A. *et al.* (1996) Interaction of hemoglobin E and pyrimidine 5' nucleotidase deficiency. *Blood* **88**, 2761.

Rees, D.C., Clegg, J.B. & Weatherall, D.J. (1998a) Is hemoglobin instability important in the interaction between hemoglobin E and β thalassaemia? *Blood* **92**, 2141.

Rees, D.C., Porter, J.B., Clegg, J.B. & Weatherall, D.J. (1998b) Insights into causes of increased Hb F production in Hb E/β thalassaemia—the effects of blood transfusion. *Blood* **92**, 10 (Suppl. 1(1), 697a).

Rees, D.C., Styles, J., Vichinsky, E.P., Clegg, J.B. & Weatherall, D.J. (1998c) The hemoglobin E syndromes. *Ann. N. Y. Acad. Sci.* **850**, 334.

Rehman, Z.-U., Saleem, M., Alvi, A.A., Anwar, M., Ahmed, P.A. & Ahmad, M. (1991) α-Thalassaemia: prevalence and pattern in Northern Pakistan. *J. Pakistan Med. Assoc.* **41**, 246.

Reik, A., Telling, A., Zitnik, G., Cimbora, D., Epner, E. & Groudine, M. (1998) The locus control region is necessary for gene expression in the human β-globin locus but not the maintenance of an open chromatin structure in erythroid cells. *Mol. Cell. Biol.* **18**, 5992.

Reismann, K.R., Ruth, W.E. & Nomura, T. (1961) A human hemoglobin with lowered oxygen affinity and impaired heme–heme interactions. *J. Clin. Invest.* **40**, 1826.

Reiss, G., Ranney, H.M. & Shaklai, N. (1982) The association of hemoglobin C with red cell ghosts. *J. Clin. Invest.* **70**, 946.

Renda, M., Maggio, A., Warren, T.C. & Kazazian, H.H. (1992a) Detection of an IVS-1 3' end (G-C) β-thalassaemia mutation in the AG invariant dinucleotide of the acceptor splice site in a Sicilian subject. *Genomics* **13**, 234.

Renda, M., Piazza, T., Ciaccio, C. & Maggio, A. (1992b) δ⁺ 27 Homozygosis in a Sicilian family. *Haematologica* **77**, 82.

Repka, T., Shalev, O., Reddy, R. *et al.* (1993) Nonrandom association of free iron with membranes of sickle and β-thalassemic erythrocytes. *Blood* **82**, 3204.

Resegotti, L., Dalforno, S., Infelise, V. & Rossi, M. (1974) Gaucher-like cells in the spleen of an adult with Cooley's anaemia. *Panmin. Med.* **16**, 261.

Resegotti, L., Dalforno, S., Rossi, M. & Infelise, V. (1975) Gaucher-like cells in the spleen of an adult subject with Cooley's disease. *Min. Med.* **66**, 1156.

Restrepo, A. (1971) Frequency and distribution of abnormal haemoglobins and thalassaemia in Colombia, South America. In: *Genetical, Functional, and Physical Studies of Hemoglobins* (eds T. Arends, G. Bemski & R.L. Nagel), p. 39. Karger, Basel.

Revel, M. & Groner, Y. (1978) Post-transcriptional and translational controls of gene expression in eukaryotes. *Annu. Rev. Biochem.* **47**, 1079.

Revillon, Y. & Girot, R. (1985) Désartérialisation partielle de la rate et splénectomie partielle chez l'enfant. *Presse Med.* **14**, 423.

Reyes, G.R., Pina-Camara, A., Felice, A.E., Gravely, M.E. & Huisman, T.H.J. (1978) δβ Thalassaemia in a Mexican family: clinical differences among homozygotes. *Hemoglobin* **2**, 513.

Rhinesmith, H.S., Schroeder, W.A. & Pauling, L. (1957) A quantitative study of hydrolysis of human dinitrophenyl (DNP) globin: the number and kind of polypeptide chains in normal adult human hemoglobin. *J. Am. Chem. Soc.* **79**, 4682.

Ribeiro, M.L.S., Baysal, E., Kutlar, F. *et al.* (1992) A novel β⁰-thalassaemia mutation (codon 15, TGG→TGA) is prevalent in a population of Central Portugal. *Br. J. Haematol.* **80**, 567.

Ribeiro, M.L., Cunha, E., Goncalves, P. *et al.* (1997) Hb Lepore-

Baltimore (δ^{68Leu}-β^{84Thr}) and Hb Lepore-Washington-Boston (δ^{87Gln}-$\beta^{IVS-II-8}$) in Central Portugal and Spanish Alta Extremadura. *Hum. Genet.* **99**, 669.

Ribio Perez, P., Sanchez Sanchez, L., Aguirre Jaca, M. & Merchante Inglesias, A. (1976) Radiological changes of the skeleton in patients with thalassemia. *Rev. Clin. Esp.* **143**, 235.

Ricci, G., Scutellari, P.N., Franceschini, F. & Gualandi, G. (1982) A new case of hemoglobin Lepore-beta-thalassemia disease. *Min. Med.* **73**, 191.

Rich, A. (1952) Studies on the hemoglobin of Cooley's anemia and Cooley's trait. *Proc. Natl Acad. Sci. USA* **38**, 187.

Rieder, R.F. & Weatherall, D.J. (1965) Studies on hemoglobin biosynthesis: asynchronous synthesis of hemoglobin A and A$_2$ by human erythrocyte precursors. *J. Clin. Invest.* **44**, 42.

Rieder, R.F., Woodbury, D.H. & Rucknagel, D.L. (1976) The interaction of α-thalassaemia and haemoglobin G Philadelphia. *Br. J. Haematol.* **32**, 159.

Rieder, R.F., Ibrahim, A. & Etlinger, J.D. (1988) ATP-dependent proteolysis in red blood cell precursors. *Birth Defects* **23**, 263.

Rietti, F. (1925) Ittero emolitico primitivo. *Atti Acad. Sci. Med. Nar. Ferrara* **2**, 14.

Rifkind, R.A. (1966) Destruction of injured red cells *in vivo*. *Am. J. Med.* **41**, 711.

Rigano, P., Manfré, L., La Galla, R. *et al.* (1997) Clinical and hematologic response to hydroxyurea in a patient with Hb Lepore/β-thalassemia. *Hemoglobin* **21**, 219.

Rigas, D.A. & Koler, R.D. (1961) Decreased erythrocyte survival in hemoglobin H disease as a result of the abnormal properties of hemoglobin H: the benefit of splenectomy. *Blood* **18**, 1.

Rigas, D.A., Kohler, R.D. & Osgood, E.E. (1955) New hemoglobin possessing a higher electrophoretic mobility than normal adult hemoglobin. *Science* **121**, 372.

Ringelhann, B., Dodu, S.R.A., Konotey-Ahulu, F.I.D. & Lehmann, H. (1968) A survey for haemoglobin variants, thalassaemia and glucose-6-phosphate dehydrogenase deficiency in Northern Ghana. *Ghana Med. J.* **7**, 120.

Ringelhann, B., Konotey-Ahulu, F.I.D., Lehmann, H. & Lorkin, P.A. (1970) A Ghanaian adult, homozygous for hereditary persistence of foetal haemoglobin and heterozygous for elliptocytosis. *Acta Haematol.* **43**, 100.

Ringelhann, B., Acquaye, C.T.A., Oldham, J.H. *et al.* (1977) Homozygotes for the hereditary persistence of fetal hemoglobin: the ratio of $^G\gamma$ to $^A\gamma$ chains and biosynthetic studies. *Biochem. Genet.* **15**, 1083.

Ringelhann, B., Efremov, G.D., Csak, E. & Reviczky, A. (1979) Hemoglobin Lepore Washington and hemochromatosis in a Hungarian patient. *Hemoglobin* **3**, 193.

Ringelhann, B., Szelenyi, J.G., Horanyi, M. *et al.* (1993) Molecular characterization of β-thalassaemia in Hungary. *Hum. Genet.* **92**, 385.

Rioja, L., Girot, R., Garabedian, M. & Cournot-Witmer, G. (1990) Bone disease in children with homozygous beta-thalassemia. *Bone Miner.* **8**, 69.

Riou, J., Godart, C., Hurtrel, D. *et al.* (1997) Cation-exchange HPLC evaluated for presumptive identification of hemoglobin variants. *Clin. Chem.* **43**, 34.

Risdon, A.R., Barry, M. & Fynn, D.M. (1975) Transfusional iron overload: the relationship between tissue iron concentration and hepatic fibrosis in man. *J. Pathol.* **116**, 83.

Ristaldi, M.S., Pirastu, M., Rosatelli, C. & Cao, A. (1989) Prenatal diagnosis of β-thalassaemia in Mediterranean populations by dot blot analysis with DNA amplification and allele specific oligonucleotide probes. *Prenat. Diag.* **9**, 629.

Ristaldi, M.S., Murru, S., Loudianos, G. *et al.* (1990a) The C-T substitution in the distal CACCC box of the β-globin gene promoter is a common cause of silent β thalassaemia in the Italian population. *Br. J. Haematol.* **74**, 480.

Ristaldi, M.S., Pirastu, M., Murru, S. *et al.* (1990b) A spontaneous mutation produced a novel elongated β^0 globin chain structural variant (Hb Agnana) with a thalassaemia-like phenotyope. *Blood* **75**, 1378.

Rixon, M.W. & Gelinas, R.E. (1988) A fetal globin gene mutation in $^A\gamma$ nondeletion HPFH increases promoter strength in a non-erythroid cell. *Mol. Cell. Biol.* **8**, 713.

Robert-Guroff, M., Giardina, P.J., Robey, W.G. *et al.* (1987) HTLV III neutralizing antibody development in transfusion-dependent seropositive patients with β-thalassemia. *J. Immunol.* **138**, 3731.

Roberts, I.A.G. (1994) Meeting report: bone marrow transplantation in children: current results and controversies. *Bone Marrow Transplant.* **14**, 197.

Roberts, A.V., Weatherall, D.J. & Clegg, J.B. (1972) The synthesis of human haemoglobin A$_2$ during erythroid maturation. *Biochem. Biophys. Res. Comm.* **47**, 81.

Roberts, A.V., Clegg, J.B. & Weatherall, D.J. (1973) Synthesis *in vitro* of anti-Lepore haemoglobin. *Nature New Biol.* **245**, 23.

Roberts, I.A.G., Darbyshire, P.J. & Will, A.M. (1997a) B.M.T. for children with β-thalassaemia major in the U.K. *Bone Marrow Transplant.* **19** (Suppl. 2), 60.

Roberts, N.A., Sloane-Stanley, J.A., Sharpe, J.A., Stanworth, S.J. & Wood, W.G. (1997b) Globin gene switching in transgenic mice carrying HS2-globin gene constructs. *Blood* **89**, 713.

Roberts-Thomson, J.M., Martinson, J.J., Norwich, J.T., Harding, R.M., Clegg, J.B. & Boettcher, B. (1996) An ancient common origin of aboriginal Australians and New Guinea highlanders is supported by alpha-globin haplotype analysis. *Am. J. Hum. Genet.* **58**, 1017.

Robins-Browne, R.M. & Prpic, J.K. (1985) Effects of iron and desferrioxamine in infections with *Yersinia enterocolitica*. *Infect. Immunol.* **47**, 774.

Robinson, R.F. (1976) Subacute combined system degeneration in Cooley's anemia: excessive vitamin B$_{12}$ utilization producing a relative deficiency combined system degeneration. *J. Indiana State Med. Assoc.* **69**, 735.

Roche, J., Derrien, Y., Diancono, G. & Roques, M. (1953) Sur les hémoglobines humains au cours des thalasssémies mineure, (maladie de Rietti–Greppi–Micheli) et majeure (anémie de Cooley). *C. R. Soc. Biol. Paris* **147**, 771.

Roche, J., Derrien, Y., Diancono, G. *et al.* (1956) Coexistence des tares sicklémique et thalassémique dans une famille Tunisienne; conséquences hématologiques. *Rev. Hematol.* **11**, 26.

Rochette, J., Barnetson, R., Kiger, L. *et al.* (1994) Association of a novel high oxygen affinity haemoglobin variant with δβ thalassaemia. *Br. J. Haematol.* **86**, 118.

Rochette, J., Barnetson, R., Varet, B., Valensi, F. & Thein, S.L. (1995) Hb Questembert is due to a base substitution (T→C) in codon 131 of the α$_2$-globin gene and has an α-thalassemia biosynthetic ratio. *Am. J. Hematol.* **48**, 289.

Rodan, G.A. (1998) Bone homeostasis. *Proc. Natl Acad. Sci. USA* **95**, 13361.

Rodda, C.P., Reid, E.D., Johnson, S., Doery, J., Matthews, R. & Bowden, D.K. (1995) Short stature in homozygous β-thalassaemia is due to disproportionate truncal shortening. *Clin. Endocrinol.* **42**, 587.

Rodeck, C.H. (1980) Fetoscopy guided by real-time ultrasound for pure fetal blood samples, fetal skin samples, and examination of the fetus *in utero*. *Br. J. Obstet. Gynaecol.* **87**, 449.

Rodeck, C.H. & Morsman, J.M. (1983) First-trimester chorion biopsy. *Br. Med. Bull.* **39**, 338.

Rodgers, G.P., Dover, G.J., Uyesaka, N., Noguchi, C.T., Schechter, A.N. & Nienhuis, A.W. (1993) Augmentation by erythropoietin of the fetal-hemoglobin response to hydroxyurea in sickle cell disease. *N. Eng. J. Med.* **328**, 73.

Roeser, H.P., Halliday, J.W. & Sizemore, D.E.A. (1980) Serum ferritin in ascorbic acid deficiency. *Br. J. Haematol.* **45**, 457.

Rohne, R.A., Sharma, C.A. & Ranney, H.M. (1973) Hemoglobin D Iran $\alpha^A\beta^{22\ Glu\to Gln}$ in association with thalassemia. *Blood* **42**, 455.

Romana, M., Keclard, L., Guillemin, G. *et al.* (1996) Molecular characterization of β-thalassemia mutations in Guadeloupe. *Am. J. Hematol.* **53**, 228.

Rombos, J., Voskaridou, E., Vayenas, C., Boussiou, M., Papadakis, M. & Loukopoulos, D. (1989) Hemoglobin H in association with the Greek type of HPFH. In: *International Congress on Thalassemia*, Sardinia, p. 19. Thalassemia International Fed., Cyprus.

Romero, C., Gonzalez, C., Gasalla, R., Martin Villar, J. & Hurtado, T. (1976) A case of double heterozygosity for (beta delta)⁰ thalassaemia and beta thalassaemia. *Sangre* **21**, 847.

Romero, C., Fernandez-Fuertes, I., Hernandez-Jodra, M. & Navarro, J.L. (1983) Association of Hb Lepore Boston and β⁺ thalassemia in a Spanish family. *Sangre* **28**, 348.

Romero, C., Fernandez-Fuertes, I., Quintana, A. *et al.* (1985) Hb G-Szuhu or $\alpha_2\beta_2(80)(EF4)$ Asn→Lys, in combination with β⁰-thalassemia in a Spanish family. *Hemoglobin* **9**, 535.

Rona, R., Rozovski, J. & Stekel, A. (1973) Sickle-thalassemia: study of a Chilean generation. *Rev. Med. Chile* **101**, 237.

Ronchi, A., Nicolis, S., Santoro, C. & Ottolenghi, S. (1989) Increased Sp1 binding mediates erythroid-specific overexpression of a mutated (HPFH) γ-globin promoter. *Nucl. Acids Res.* **17**, 10231.

Ronchi, A., Berry, M., Raguz, S. *et al.* (1996) Role of the duplicated CCAAT box region in γ-globin gene regulation and hereditary persistence of fetal haemoglobin. *EMBO J.* **15**, 143.

Rönich, P. & Kleihauer, E. (1967) Alpha-thalassämie mit HbH und Hb Bart's in einer deutschen Familie. *Klin. Wochenschr.* **45**, S1193.

Ros, G., Seynhaeve, V. & Fiasse, L. (1976) Beta⁺-thalassaemia, haemoglobin A and hereditary elliptocytosis in a Zairian family. Ischaemic costal necroses in a child with sickle-cell beta⁺ thalassaemia. *Acta Haematol.* **56**, 241.

Rosatelli, C., Falchi, A.M., Scalas, M.T., Tuveri, T., Furbetta, M. & Cao, A. (1984) Hematological phenotype of double heterozygous state for alpha and beta thalassaemia. *Hemoglobin* **8**, 25.

Rosatelli, C., Falchi, A.M., Tuveri, T. *et al.* (1985) Prenatal diagnosis of beta-thalassaemia with the synthetic-oligomer technique. *Lancet* **i**, 241.

Rosatelli, C., Oggiano, L., Leoni, G.B. *et al.* (1989) Thalassemia intermedia resulting from a mild beta-thalassemia mutation. *Blood* **73**, 601.

Rosatelli, C., Leoni, G.B., Tuveri, T. *et al.* (1992a) Heterozygous β-thalassemia: relationship between the hematological phenotype and the type of β-thalassemia mutation. *Am. J. Hematol.* **39**, 1.

Rosatelli, M.C., Dozy, A., Faà, V. *et al.* (1992b) Molecular characterization of β-thalassemia in the Sardinian population. *Am. J. Hum. Genet.* **50**, 422.

Rosatelli, M.C., Tuveri, T., Scalas, M.T. *et al.* (1992c) Molecular screening and fetal diagnosis of β-thalassemia in the Italian population. *Hum. Genet.* **89**, 585.

Rosatelli, M.C., Pischedda, A., Meloni, A. *et al.* (1994) Homozygous β-thalassaemia resulting in the β-thalassaemia carrier state phenotype. *Br. J. Haematol.* **88**, 562.

Rosatelli, M.C., Faà, V., Meloni, A. *et al.* (1995) A promoter mutation,

C→T at position –92, leading to silent β-thalassaemia. *Br. J. Haematol.* **90**, 483.

Rosenzweig, A.I., Heywood, J.D., Motulsky, A.G. & Finch, C.A. (1968) Hemoglobin H as an acquired defect of alpha-chain synthesis. *Acta Haematol.* **39**, 91.

Rosmino, G.C., Norelli, M.T. & Ghidella, G. (1968) Blood uric acid levels in childhood. 3. In patients with Cooley's disease. *Min. Pediatr.* **20**, 313.

Ross, J. (1995) mRNA stability in mammalian cells. *Microbiol. Rev.* **59**, 423.

Ross, D.W., Ayscue, L.H., Watson, J. & Bentley, S.A. (1988) Stability of hematologic parameters in healthy subjects. *Am. J. Clin. Pathol.* **90**, 262.

Roth, C., Pekrun, A., Bartz, M. *et al.* (1997) Short stature and failure of pubertal development in thalassaemia major: evidence for hypothalamic neurosecretory dysfunction of growth hormone secretion and defective pituitary gonadotropin secretion. *Eur. J. Pediatr.* **156**, 777.

Rothschild, H., Bickers, J. & Marcus, R. (1976) Regulation of the β- and δ-hemoglobin genes. A family with hereditary persistence of fetal hemoglobin and β-thalassemia. *Acta Haematol.* **56**, 285.

Rotoli, B. (1976) Thalassemia in Italy: Treatment of Cooley's disease and iron kinetics in heterozygotes. In: *Birth Defects: Original Article Series* (eds D. Bergsma, A. Cerami, C.M. Peterson & J.H. Graziano), p. 53. Alan R. Liss, New York.

Rouyer-Fessard, P., Garel, M.-C., Domenget, C. *et al.* (1989) A study of membrane protein defects and α hemoglobin chains of red blood cells in human β thalassemia. *J. Biol. Chem.* **264**, 19092.

Rowley, P.T. & Jacobs, M. (1972) Hypersplenic thrombocytopenia in sickle cell-beta thalassemia. *Am. J. Med. Sci.* **264**, 489.

Rowley, P.T., Barnes, F. & Williams, E. (1969) A Lepore hemoglobin in a Rumanian. *Hum. Hered.* **19**, 48.

Rowley, P.T., Loader, S. & Walden, M.E. (1985) Toward providing parents the option of avoiding the birth of the first child with Cooley's anemia: response to hemoglobinopathy screening and counseling during pregnancy. *Ann. N. Y. Acad. Sci.* **445**, 408.

Rowley, P.T., Loader, S. & Sutera, C.J. (1990) Feasibility of routine prenatal testing for β-thalassemia trait. *Ann. N. Y. Acad. Sci.* **812**, 524.

Roy, R.N., Banerjee, D., Chakraborty, K.N. & Basu, S.P. (1971) Observations on radiological changes of bones in thalassaemia syndrome. *J. Indian Med. Assoc.* **57**, 90.

Rubin, R.B., Barton, A.L., Banner, B.F. & Bonkovsky, H.L. (1995) Iron and chronic viral hepatitis: emerging evidence for an important interaction. *Dig. Dis.* **13**, 223.

Rucknagel, D.L. & Neel, J.V. (1961) The hemoglobinopathies. *Prog. Med. Genet.* **1**, 158.

Rudivic, R., Efremov, G.D., Juricic, D., Rolovic, Z., Ruzdic, I. & Pendic, S. (1975) Hemoglobin Beograd $(\alpha_2\beta_2 121\ Glu\to Val)$ interacting with β-thalassaemia. *Acta Haematol.* **54**, 180.

Ruenwongsa, P. & Yuthavong, Y. (1975) Studies on the subunit dissociation of the abnormal haemoglobins E and New York. *J. Med. Assoc. Thailand* **58**, 253.

Ruf, A., Pick, M., Deutsch, V. *et al.* (1997) *In vivo* platelet activation correlates with red cell anionic phospholipid exposure in patients with β-thalassaemia major. *Br. J. Haematol.* **98**, 51.

Ruiz Reyes, G. (1983) Hemoglobin variants in Mexico. *Hemoglobin* **7**, 603.

Rund, D. & Rachmilewitz, E. (1995) Advances in the pathophysiology and treatment of thalassemia. *Crit. Rev. Oncol./Hematol.* **20**, 237.

Rund, D., Filon, D., Dowling, C., Kazazian, H.H.J., Rachmilewitz, E.A. & Oppenheim, A. (1990) Molecular studies of β-thalassemia in Israel. Mutational analysis and expression studies. *Ann. N. Y. Acad. Sci.* **612**, 98.

Rund, D., Cohen, T., Filon, D. *et al.* (1991) Evolution of a genetic disease in an ethnic isolate: β-thalassemia in the Jews of Kurdistan. *Proc. Natl Acad. Sci. USA* **88**, 310.

Rund, D., Dowling, C., Najjar, K., Rachmilewitz, E.A., Kazazian, H.H. Jr & Oppenheim, A. (1992) Two mutations in the β-globin polyadenylylation signal reveal extended transcripts and new RNA polyadenylylation sites. *Proc. Natl Acad. Sci. USA* **89**, 4324.

Rund, D., Oron-Karni, V., Filon, D., Goldfarb, A., Rachmilewitz, E. & Oppenheim, A. (1997) Genetic analysis of β-thalassemia intermedia in Israel: diversity of mechanisms and unpredictability of phenotype. *Am. J. Hematol.* **54**, 16.

Russell, D.A., Wigley, S.L., Vincin, D.R., Scott, G.C., Booth, P.B. & Simmons, R.T. (1971) Blood groups and salivary ABH secretion of inhabitants of the Karimui plateau and adjoining areas of the New Guinea highlands. *Hum. Biol. Oceania* **1**, 79.

Russell, J.E., Morales, J., Makeyev, A.V. & Liebhaber, S.A. (1998) Sequence divergence in the 3′ untranslated regions of human zeta- and alpha-globin mRNAs mediates a difference in their stabilities and contributes to efficient alpha-to-zeta gene development switching. *Mol. Cell. Biol.* **18**, 2173.

Russo, G., La Grutta, A. & Mollica, F. (1963) Sulla eterogenetica della thalassemia. Contributo casistico ed interpretazione biochemica e genetica. *Riv. Pediatr. Sicil.* **P18**, 239.

Russo, G., Musumeci, S., Schiliro, G., D'Agate, A. & Pizzarelli, G. (1973a) Hemoglobin synthesis in δβ-thalassemia. In: *Atti del V° Congresso sulle Microcitemia*, Cozenza. Arte Della Stampa, Roma.

Russo, G., Schiliro, G., Musumeci, S., D'Agate, A. & Pizzarelli, G. (1973b) Hemoglobin synthesis in α-thalassemia. In: *Atti del V° Congresso sulle Microcitemia*, Cozenza. Arte Della Stampa, Roma.

Rutland, P.C., Pembrey, M.E. & Davies, T. (1983) The estimation of fetal haemoglobin in healthy adults by radioimmunoassay. *Br. J. Haematol.* **53**, 673.

Rutter, M. & Graham, P. (1968) The reliability and validity of psychiatric assessment of the child: Interview with the child. *Br. J. Psych.* **114**, 581.

Ruymann, F.B., Popejoy, L.A. & Brouillard, R.B. (1978) Splenic sequestration and ineffective erythropoiesis in hemoglobin E-β-thalassemia disease. *Pediatr. Res.* **12**, 1020.

Ryan, B.P.K. (1961) Thalassaemia, report of a case in Papua. *Med. J. Aust.* **2**, 753.

Ryan, B.P.K., Campbell, A.L. & Brain, P. (1961) Haemoglobin H disease in a Papuan. *Med. J. Aust.* **2**, 901.

Ryan, T.M., Behringer, R.R., Martin, N.C., Townes, T.M., Palmiter, R.D. & Brinster, R.L. (1989) A single erythroid-specific DNase I super-hypersensitive site activates high levels of human β-globin gene expression in transgenic mice. *Genes Dev.* **3**, 314.

Saarinen, U.M., Chorba, T.L., Tattersall, P. *et al.* (1986) Human parvovirus B19-induced epidemic acute red cell aplasia in patients with hereditary haemolytic anaemia. *Blood* **67**, 1411.

Saba, L., Meloni, A., Sardu, R. *et al.* (1992) A novel β-thalassaemia mutation (G→A) at the initiation codon of the β-globin gene. *Hum. Mutat.* **1**, 420.

Sabath, D.E., Spangler, E.A., Rubin, E.M. & Stamatoyannopoulos, G. (1993) Analysis of the human ζ-globin gene promoter in transgenic mice. *Blood* **82**, 2899.

Sabath, D.E., Detter, J.C. & Tait, J.F. (1994) A novel deletion of the entire α globin locus causing α-thalassaemia-1 in a Northern European family. *Am. J. Clin. Pathol.* **102**, 650.

Sabato, A., De Sanctis, V., Atti, G., Capra, L., Bagni, L. & Vullo, C.

(1983) Primary hypothyroidism and the low T_3 syndrome in thalassemia major. *Arch. Dis. Child.* **58**, 120.

Sachs, A.B. (1993) Messenger RNA degradation in eukaryotes. *Cell* **74**, 413.

Sadelain, M. (1997) Genetic treatment of the haemoglobinopathies: recombinations and new combinations. *Br. J. Haematol.* **98**, 247.

Sadelain, M., Wang, C.-H.J., Antoniou, M., Grosveld, F. & Mulligan, R.C. (1995) Generation of a high-titer retroviral vector capable of expressing high levels of the human beta-globin gene. *Proc. Natl Acad. Sci. USA* **92**, 6728.

Sadikario, A., Duma, H., Efremov, G. *et al.* (1969) Thalassaemias and abnormal haemoglobins in SR Macedonia. *Acta Haematol.* **41**, 162.

Sadiq, M.F.G. & Huisman, T.H.J. (1994) Molecular characterization of β-thalassemia in North Jordan. *Hemoglobin* **18**, 325.

Saenger, P., Schwartz, E., Markenson, A.L. *et al.* (1980) Depressed serum somatomedin activity in beta-thalassemia. *J. Pediatr.* **96**, 214.

Safaya, S. & Rieder, R.F. (1988) Dysfunctional α-globin gene in hemoglobin H disease in blacks. *J. Biol. Chem.* **263**, 4328.

Safaya, S., Rieder, R.F., Dowling, C.E., Kazazian, H.H. Jr & Adams, J.G. (1989) Homozygous β-thalassemia without anemia. *Blood* **73**, 324.

Saglio, G., Camaschella, C., Serra, A. *et al.* (1986) Italian type of deletional hereditary persistence of fetal hemoglobin. *Blood* **68**, 646.

Saha, N. & Banerjee, B. (1973) Haemoglobinopathies in the Indian sub-continent. *Acta Genet. Med. Gemellol. (Roma)* **22**, 117.

Saha, N., Samuel, A.P.W., Omer, A., Ahmed, M.A., Hussein, A.A. & Gaddoura, E.N. (1978) A study of some genetic characteristics of the population of the Sudan. *Ann. Hum. Biol.* **5**, 569.

Saichua, S., Sathiropas, P. & Rompruk, A. (1983) Prevalence of thalassemia in Srinagarind Hospital. *J. Med. Techn. Assoc. Thailand* **11**, 1.

Saiki, R.K., Scharf, S., Faloona, F. *et al.* (1985) Enzymatic amplification of β-globin genomic sequences and restriction site analysis for diagnosis of sickle cell anemia. *Science* **230**, 1350.

Saiki, R.K., Chang, C.A., Levenson, C.H. *et al.* (1988) Diagnosis of sickle cell anemia and beta-thalassaemia with enzymatically amplified DNA and nonradioactive allele specific olignucleotide probes. *N. Eng. J. Med.* **319**, 537.

Saiki, R.K., Walsh, P.S., Levenson, C.H. & Erlich, H.A. (1989) Genetic analysis of amplified DNA with immobilized sequence-specific oligonucleotide probes. *Proc. Natl Acad. Sci. USA* **86**, 6230.

Salihu, H.M. (1997) Genetic counselling among Muslims: questions remain unanswered. *Lancet* **350**, 1035.

Salkie, M.L., Gordon, P.A., Rigal, W.M. *et al.* (1982) Hb A_2-Canada or $\alpha_2\delta_299(G1)$ Asp→Asn, a newly discovered δ chain variant with increased oxygen affinity occurring in *cis* to β-thalassemia. *Hemoglobin* **6**, 223.

Salzano, F.M. & Tondo, C.V. (1982) Hemoglobin types in Brazilian populations. *Hemoglobin* **6**, 85.

Sampietro, M., Cazzola, M., Cappellini, M.D. & Fiorelli, G. (1983) The triplicated alpha-gene locus and heterozygous beta thalassemia: a case of thalassaemia intermedia. *Br. J. Haematol.* **55**, 709.

Sampietro, M., Thein, S.L., Contreras, M. & Pazmany, L. (1992) Variation of Hb F and F-cell number in the $^{G}\gamma$ *Xmn* I polymorphism in normal individuals. *Blood* **79**, 832.

Sampietro, M., Lupica, L., Perrero, L. *et al.* (1997) The expression of uridine diphosphate glucuronosyltransferase gene is a major determinant of bilirubin level in heterozygous β-thalassaemia and in glucose-6-phosphate dehydrogenase deficiency. *Br. J. Haematol.* **99**, 437.

Samuels, M.P., Stebbens, V.A., Davies, S.C., Picton-Jones, E. &

Southall, D.P. (1992) Sleep related upper airway obstruction and hypoxaemia in sickle cell disease. *Arch. Dis. Child.* **67**, 925.

Sancar, G.B., Tatsis, B., Cedeno, M.M. & Rieder, R.F. (1980) Proportion of hemoglobin G Philadelphia ($\alpha_2^{68\text{Asn-Lys}}\beta_2$) in heterozygotes is determined by α-globin gene deletions. *Proc. Natl Acad. Sci. USA* **77**, 6874.

Sandhaus, L.M., Smith, C.M.N. & Peterson, L. (1983) Hb E disorders in a Minnesota Southeast Asian immigrant population: morphology, indices, electrophoretic patterns and clinical manifestations. *Minn. Med.* **66**, 163.

Sanguansermsri, T., Matragoon, S., Changloah, L. & Flatz, G. (1979) Hemoglobin Suan-Dok ($\alpha_2^{109(G16)\,\text{Leu-Arg}}\beta_2$): an unstable variant associated with α-thalassaemia. *Hemoglobin* **3**, 161.

Sanguansermsri, T., Flatz, G. & Flatz, S.D. (1987) Distribution of hemoglobin E and β thalassaemia in Kampuchaea (Cambodia). *Hemoglobin* **11**, 481.

Sanna, G., Frau, F., Melis, M.A., Galanello, R., de Virgiliis, S. & Cao, A. (1980) Interaction between glucose-6-phosphate dehydrogenase deficiency and thalassaemia genes at phenotype level. *Br. J. Haematol.* **44**, 555.

Sansone, G., Russo, C., Zunin, C. & Salomone, P. (1955) Studio clinico ed anatomo-patologico di due banbini con anemia di Cooley deceduti per reazione transfusionale. *Min. Pediatr.* **7**, 1005.

Sansone, G., Vallarino, G. & Centa, A. (1967) Association of a triple genetic erythrocyte defect: thalassemia, sickle cell disease and glucose-6-phosphate dehydrogenase deficiency in a child of Calabro-Sardinian origin. *Haematologica* **52**, 479.

Santamaria, F., Villa, M.P., Werner, B., Cutrera, R., Barreto, M. & Ronchetti, R. (1994) The effect of transfusion on pulmonary function in patients with thalassemia major. *Pediatr. Pulmon.* **18**, 139.

Saraya, A.K., Kumar, R., Kailash, S. & Sehgal, A.K. (1984) Vitamin B_{12} and folic acid deficiency in β-heterozygous thalassaemia. *Indian J. Med. Res.* **79**, 783.

Sassa, S. (1995) The porphyrias. In: *Hematology* (eds E. Beutler, M.A. Lichtman, B.S. Coller & T.J. Kipps), p. 726. McGraw-Hill, New York.

Sasso, C.F., Marinucci, M., Crema, A., Massa, A., Tagliamonte, L. & Nardi, E. (1975) La doppia eterozugozi emoglobinopatia Lepore/β-thalassemia. *Experientia* **31**, 788.

Satta, S., Bernard, O. & Yann, L. (1970) Résultats préliminaires d'une étude des rapports existant entre l'hémoglobine E (Hb E) et le paludisme au Cambodge. *Nouv. Rev. Fr. Hematol.* **10**, 317.

Saudek, C.D., Hemm, R.M. & Peterson, C.M. (1977) Abnormal glucose tolerance in beta-thalassemia major. *Metabolism* **26**, 43.

Savage, D.A., Wood, N.A.P., Bidwell, J.L., Fitches, A., Old, J.M. & Hui, K.M. (1995) Detection of β-thalassaemia mutations using DNA heteroduplex generator molecules. *Br. J. Haematol.* **90**, 564.

Saxena, R., Jain, P.K., Thomas, E. & Verma, I.C. (1998) Prenatal diagnosis of β-thalassaemia: experience in a developing country. *Prenat. Diag.* **18**, 1.

Saxon, B.R., Brittenham, G.M., Nisbet-Brown, E. *et al.* (1997) Liver biopsy is safe and provides quantitative guidelines for initiation of chelating therapy in children with thalassaemia major. *Blood* **90** (Suppl. 1), 130a.

Saxon, B.R., Rees, D. & Olivieri, N.F. (1998) Regression of extramedullary haemopoiesis and augmentation of fetal haemoglobin concentration during hydroxyurea therapy in β thalassaemia. *Br. J. Haematol.* **101**, 416.

Scacchi, M., Damesi, L., De Martin, M. *et al.* (1991) Treatment with biosynthetic growth hormone of short thalassaemic patients with impaired growth hormone secretion. *Clin. Endocrinol.* **35**, 335.

Scerri, C.A., Abela, W., Galdies, R., Pizzuto, M., Grech, J.L. & Felice, A.E. (1993) The β^+ IVS, I-NT no. 6 (T→C) thalassaemia in heterozygotes with an associated Hb Valetta or Hb S heterozygosity in homozygotes from Malta. *Br. J. Haematol.* **83**, 669.

Schanfield, M.S., Scalise, G., Economidou, I., Modell, C.B., Bate, C. & Zuckerman, A.J. (1975) Immunogenetic factors in thalassemia and hepatitis B infection. A multicentre study. *Dev. Biol. Stand.* **30**, 257.

Schellhammer, P.F., Engle, M.A. & Hagstrom, J.W.C. (1967) Histochemical studies of the myocardium and conduction system in acquired iron-storage disease. *Circulation* **35**, 631.

Schettini, F., de Mautone, A. & Lucia, I. (1974) 2,3-Diphosphoglycerate content of erythrocytes in the thalassaemic trait. *Boll. Soc. Ital. Biol. Speriment.* **50**, 215.

Schiliro, G. (1978) Sicily: the world reservoir for thalassaemias and haemoglobinopathies. *Nature* **276**, 761.

Schiliro, G. (1987) Epidemiology of thalassemia and hemoglobinopathies in Sicilia in a historic perspective. In: *Thalassaemia Today*, p. 474. Centro Trasfusionale, Ospedale Maggiore Policlinico di Milano, Milano.

Schiliro, G., Musumeci, S., Pizzarelli, G. *et al.* (1976) A new alkali resistant haemoglobin $\alpha^{\text{J Oxford}}\gamma^{\text{F}}$ in a Sicilian baby girl with homozygous β^0 thalassaemia. *Blood* **48**, 639.

Schiliro, G., Musumeci, S., Pizzarelli, G., Fischer, A., Romero, M.A. & Russo, G. (1980) Haemoglobin Lepore Boston-Washington in Sicily: clinical, haematological and biosynthetic studies. *J. Med. Genet.* **17**, 179.

Schiliro, G., Musumeci, S., Romeo, M.A. *et al.* (1983) Unusual combination of genetic defects in a Sicilian family. *Br. J. Haematol.* **55**, 473.

Schiliro, G., Spena, M., Giambelluca, E. & Maggio, A. (1990) Sickle hemoglobinopathies in Sicily. *Am. J. Hematol.* **33**, 81.

Schiliro, G., Russo-Mancuso, G., Dibenedetto, S.P. *et al.* (1991) Six rare hemoglobin variants found in Sicily. *Hemoglobin* **15**, 431.

Schiliro, G., di-Gregorio, F., Samperi, P. *et al.* (1995) Genetic heterogeneity of β-thalassemia in southeast Sicily. *Am. J. Hematol.* **48**, 5.

Schizas, N., Tegos, K., Ventsadakis, A. *et al.* (1977) The frequency and distribution of β-thalassemia and abnormal hemoglobins in Greece. A study of 15 500 recruits. *Hellenic Armed Forces Med. Rev.* **11** (Suppl.), 197.

Schmaier, A.H., Maurer, H.M., Johnson, C.L. & Scott, R.B. (1973) Alpha thalassemia screening in neonates by mean corpuscular volume and mean corpuscular hemoglobin concentration. *J. Pediatr.* **83**, 794.

Schmidt, R.M. & Brosious, E.M. (1979) Quantitation of hemoglobin A_2. An interlaboratory study. *Am. J. Clin. Pathol.* **71**, 534.

Schmidt, R.M. & Huisman, T.H.J. (1974) *The Detection of Hemoglobinopathies*. CRC Press, Cleveland.

Schmidt, R.M., Rucknagel, D.L. & Necheles, T.F. (1975) Comparison of methodologies for thalassemia screening by Hb A_2 estimation. *J. Lab. Clin. Med.* **86**, 873.

Schnee, J., Griese, E.V., Eigel, A. & Horst, J. (1989) β-Thalassemia gene analysis in a Turkish family reveals a 7 bp deletion in the coding region. *Blood* **73**, 2224.

Schneider, R.G., Levin, W.C. & Everett, C. (1961) A family with S and C hemoglobins and the hereditary persistence of F hemoglobin. *N. Eng. J. Med.* **265**, 1278.

Schneider, R.G., Ueda, S., Alperin, J.B., Levin, W.C., Jones, R.T. & Brimhall, B. (1968) Hemoglobin D Los Angeles in two Caucasian families: hemoglobin SD disease and hemoglobin D thalassemia. *Blood* **32**, 250.

Schneider, A.S., Bischoff, F.Z., McCaskill, C., Coady, M.L., Stopfer, J.E. & Shaffer, L.G. (1996) Comprehensive 4-year follow-up on a case of maternal heterodisomy for chromosome 16. *Am. J. Med. Genet.* **66**, 204.

Schoentag, R., Pedersen, J. & Ballard, H. (1985) Double heterozygosity for hemoglobins C and Lepore in an American black man. *Arch. Pathol Lab. Med.* **109**, 777.

Schokker, R.C., Went, L.N. & Bok, J. (1966) A new genetic variant of beta-thalassaemia. *Nature* **209**, 44.

Schorr, J.B. & Radel, E. (1964) Transfusion therapy and its complications in patients with Cooley's anemia. *Ann. N. Y. Acad. Sci.* **119**, 703.

Schrier, S.L. (1994) Thalassemia: pathophysiology of red cell changes. *Ann. Rev. Med.* **45**, 211.

Schrier, S.L. (1997) Pathobiology of thalassemic erythrocytes. *Curr. Opin. Hematol.* **4**, 75.

Schrier, S.L., Rachmilewitz, E.A. & Mohandas, N. (1989) Cellular and membrane properties of alpha and beta thalassemia erythrocytes are different: implication for differences in clinical manifestations. *Blood* **74**, 2194.

Schrier, S.L., Bunyaratvej, A., Khukapinant, A. *et al.* (1997) The unusual pathobiology of hemoglobin Constant Spring red blood cells. *Blood* **89**, 1762.

Schroeder, W.A. & Huisman, T.H.J. (1970) Nonallelic structural genes and hemoglobin synthesis. In: *XIIth International Congress of Hematology*, Plenary Sessions, p. 26. Lehmanns, Munich.

Schroeder, W.A. & Matsuda, G.J. (1958) N-terminal residues of human fetal hemoglobin. *J. Am. Chem. Soc.* **80**, 1521.

Schroeder, W.A., Cua, J.T., Matsuda, G. & Fenninger, W.D. (1962) Hemoglobin F_1, an acetyl-containing hemoglobin. *Biochim. Biophys. Acta* **63**, 532.

Schroeder, W.A., Shelton, J.R., Shelton, J.B., Cormack, J. & Jones, R.T. (1963) The amino acid sequence of the γ-chain of human fetal hemoglobin. *Biochemistry* **2**, 992.

Schroeder, W.A., Huisman, T.H.J., Shelton, J.R. *et al.* (1968) Evidence for multiple structural genes for the γ-chain of human fetal hemoglobin. *Proc. Natl Acad. Sci. USA* **60**, 537.

Schroeder, W.A., Huisman, T.H.J., Hyman, C., Chelton, J.R. & Apell, G. (1973a) An individual with 'Miyada'-like hemoglobin indistinguishable from hemoglobin A. *Biochem. Genet.* **10**, 135.

Schroeder, W.A., Huisman, T.H.J. & Sukumaran, P.K. (1973b) A second type of hereditary persistence of foetal haemoglobin in India. *Br. J. Haematol.* **25**, 131.

Schroeder, W.A., Huisman, T.H.J., Shelton, J.R. *et al.* (1974) On the structure of the hemoglobins A, A_2 and F in a Negro with homozygous beta-thalassemia. *Biochem. Med.* **10**, 276.

Schuman, J.E., Tanser, C.L., de Peloquin, R. & Leeuw, N.K.M. (1973) The erythropoietic response to pregnancy in β thalassaemia minor. *Br. J. Haematol.* **25**, 249.

Schwartz, E. (1969) The silent carrier of beta thalassaemia. *N. Eng. J. Med.* **281**, 1327.

Schwartz, E. (1970) Heterozygous beta thalassemia: balanced globin synthesis in bone marrow cells. *Science* **167**, 1513.

Schwartz, E. & Atwater, J. (1972) α-Thalassemia in the American Negro. *J. Clin. Invest.* **51**, 412.

Schwartz, E., Kan, Y.W. & Nathan, D.G. (1969) Unbalanced globin chain synthesis in alpha-thalassemia heterozygotes. *Ann. N. Y. Acad. Sci.* **165**, 288.

Schwartz, E., Cohen, A. & Surrey, S. (1988) Overview of the β thalassemias: genetic and clinical aspects. *Hemoglobin* **12**, 551.

Schwartz, E., Goltsov, A.A., Kaboaev, O.K. *et al.* (1989) A novel frameshift mutation causing β-thalassemia in Azerbaijan. *Nucl. Acids Res.* **17**, 3997.

Schwartz, S.O. & Hartz, W.H. (1955) Mediterranean anemia in the Negro. *Blood* **10**, 1256.

Schwartz-Tiene, E., Corda, G. & Careddu, P. (1953) Modificazioni del metabolismo dei lipidi e delle porfirine nell'anemia mediterranea. *Min. Pediatr.* **5**, 829.

Scott, R.B., Ferguson, A.D. & Jenkins, M.E. (1962) Thalassemia major (Mediterranean or Cooley's anemia). *Am. J. Dis. Child.* **104**, 74.

Scott, G.L., Rasbridge, M.R. & Grimes, A.J. (1970) *In vitro* studies of red cell metabolism in haemoglobin H disease. *Br. J. Haematol.* **18**, 13.

Scott, M.D., Rouyer-Fessard, P., Lubin, B. & Beuzard, Y. (1990) Entrapment of purified α-hemoglobin chains in normal erythrocytes. A model for β-thalassemia. *J. Biol. Chem.* **265**, 17953.

Scott, M.D., Rouyer-Fessard, P., Ba, M.S., Lubin, B.H. & Beuzard, Y. (1992) α- and β-haemoglobin chain induced changes in normal erythrocyte deformability: comparison to β thalassaemia intermedia and Hb H disease. *Br. J. Haematol.* **80**, 519.

Scott, M.D., van den Berg, J., Repka, T. *et al.* (1993) Effect of excess α-hemoglobin chains on cellular and membrane oxidation in model β-thalassemic erythrocytes. *J. Clin. Invest.* **91**, 1706.

Scott, J.P., Hillery, C.A., Brown, E.R., Misiewicz, V.M. & Labotka, R.J. (1996) Hydroxyurea therapy in children severely affected with sickle cell disease. *J. Pediatr.* **128**, 820.

Scriver, C.R., Bardanis, M., Cartier, L., Clow, C.L., Lancaster, G.A. & Ostrowsky, J.T. (1984) β-Thalassemia disease prevention: genetic medicine applied. *Am. J. Hum. Genet.* **36**, 1024.

Seltzer, W.K., Abshire, T.C., Lane, P.A., Roloff, J.S. & Githens, J.H. (1992) Molecular genetic studies in black families with sickle cell anemia and unusually high levels of fetal hemoglobin. *Hemoglobin* **16**, 363.

Selwyn, J.G. (1953) Cited by Dacie, J.V. (1960) in *The Haemolytic Anaemias*, 2nd edn, p. 206. Churchill, London.

Selwyn, J.G. & Dacie, J.V. (1954) Autohemolysis and other changes resulting from the incubation *in vitro* of red cells from patients with congenital hemolytic anemia. *Blood* **9**, 414.

Semenza, G.L., Delgrosso, K., Poncz, M., Mallidi, P., Schwartz, E. & Surrey, S. (1984) The silent carrier allele: β thalassemia without a mutation in the β-globin gene or its immediate flanking regions. *Cell* **39**, 123.

Semenza, G.L., Dowling, C.E. & Kazazian, H.H. Jr (1989) Hinf I polymorphisms 3′ to the human β globin gene detected by the polymerase chain reaction (PCR). *Nucl. Acids Res.* **17**, 2376.

Sen, S., Mishra, N.M., Giri, T. *et al.* (1993) Acquired immunodeficiency syndrome (AIDS) in multitransfused children with thalassemia. *Indian Pediatr.* **30**, 455.

del Senno, L., Bernardi, F., Bruno, M.R. *et al.* (1979) Reduced levels of variant α-globins in β-thalassaemia. *Haematologica* **64**, 278.

Senok, A.C., Li, K., Nelson, E.A., Yu, L.M., Tian, L.P. & Oppenheimer, S.J. (1997) Invasion and growth of *Plasmodium falciparum* is inhibited in fractionated thalassaemic erythrocytes. *Trans. Roy. Soc. Trop. Med. Hyg.* **91**, 138.

Sephton-Smith, R. (1962) Iron excretion in thalassaemia major after administration of chelating agents. *Br. Med. J.* **ii**, 1577.

Sephton-Smith, R. (1964) Chelating agents in the diagnosis and treatment of iron overload. *Ann. N. Y. Acad. Sci.* **119**, 776.

Seracchioli, R., Porcu, E., Colombi, C. *et al.* (1994) Transfusion-dependent homozygous β-thalassaemia major: successful twin pregnancy following *in vitro* fertilization and tubal embryo transfer. *Hum. Reprod.* **9**, 1964.

Sergiacomi, G., Palma, E., Cianciulli, P., Forte, L., Papa, G. & Simonetti, G. (1993) Correlazioni clinico-radiologiche nella talassemia intermedia. *Radiol. Med. Torino* **85**, 570.

Serirodom, S., Bhasuwakul, T. & Bovornkitti, S. (1972) Tuberculin sensitivity and resistance to tuberculosis in thalassaemic patients. *Siriraj Hosp. Gaz.* **24**, 1294.

Serjeant, G.R. (1985) *Sickle Cell Disease*. Oxford University Press, Oxford.

Serjeant, G.R. (1992) *Sickle Cell Disease*, 2nd edn. Oxford University Press, New York.

Serjeant, G.R. & Ashcroft, M.T. (1973) Delayed skeletal maturation in sickle cell anaemia in Jamaicans. *Johns Hopkins Med. J.* **132**, 95.

Serjeant, G.R. & Serjeant, B.E. (1972) A comparison of erythrocyte characteristics in sickle cell syndromes in Jamaica. *Br. J. Haematol.* **23**, 205.

Serjeant, G.R. & Serjeant, B.E. (1982) Comparison of sickle cell-β^0 thalassemia and sickle cell-β^+ thalassemia in Black populations. In: *Thalassemia: Recent Advances in Detection and Treatment* (eds A. Cao, U. Carcassi & P.T. Rowley), p. 223. Alan R. Liss, New York.

Serjeant, G.R., Serjeant, B.E. & Condon, P.I. (1972) The conjunctival sign in sickle cell anemia. *J. A. M. A.* **219**, 1428.

Serjeant, G.R., Ashcroft, M.Y., Serjeant, B.E. & Milner, P.F. (1973) The clinical features of sickle-cell β thalassaemia in Jamaica. *Br. J. Haematol.* **24**, 19.

Serjeant, G.R., Serjeant, B.E. & Mason, K. (1977) Heterocellular hereditary persistence of fetal haemoglobin and homozygous sickle-cell disease. *Lancet* **i**, 795.

Serjeant, G.R., Sommereux, A.M., Stevenson, M., Mason, K. & Serjeant, B.E. (1979) Comparison of sickle cell-β^0 thalassaemia with homozygous sickle cell disease. *Br. J. Haematol.* **41**, 83.

Serjeant, G.R., Serjeant, B.E., Forbes, M., Hayes, R.J., Higgs, D.R. & Lehmann, H. (1986) Haemoglobin frequencies in the Jamaican population: a study in 100,000 newborns. *Br. J. Haematol.* **64**, 253.

Serjeant, G., Serjeant, B., Stephens, A. *et al.* (1996) Determinants of haemoglobin level in steady-state homozygous sickle cell disease. *Br. J. Haematol.* **92**, 143.

Seward, D.P., Ware, R.E. & Kinney, T.R. (1993) Hemoglobin Sickle-Lepore: report of two siblings and review of the literature. *Am. J. Hematol.* **44**, 192.

Shaeffer, J.R. (1983) Turnover of excess hemoglobin α-chains in β-thalassaemic cells is ATP-dependent. *J. Biol. Chem.* **258**, 13172.

Shaeffer, J.R. (1988) ATP-dependent proteolysis of hemoglobin alpha chains in beta-thalassemic hemolysates is ubiquitin-dependent. *J. Biol. Chem.* **263**, 13663.

Shaeffer, J.R. & Cohen, R.E. (1997) Ubiquitin aldehyde increases adenosine triphosphate-dependent proteolysis of hemoglobin alpha-subunits in beta-thalassemic hemolysates. *Blood* **90**, 1300.

Shaeffer, J.R. & Moake, J.L. (1975) Sickle-cell beta^0 thalassemia variant with high hemoglobin F and mild clinical course. *Am. J. Med.* **61**, 437.

Shaffer, C.D., Wallrath, L.L. & Elgin, S.C.R. (1993) Regulating genes by packaging domains: bits of heterochromatin in euchromatin? *Trends Genet.* **9**, 35.

Shafritz, D.A., Weinstein, J.A., Sofer, B. *et al.* (1976) Evidence for role of m^7G^5-phosphate group in recognition of eukaryotic mRNA by initiation factor IF-M$_3$. *Nature* **261**, 291.

Shahid, M.J. & Abu Haydar, N. (1967) Absorption of inorganic iron in thalassaemia. *Br. J. Haematol.* **13**, 713.

Shahid, M.J., Khouri, F.P. & Sahli, I.F. (1974) Haemoglobin H disease and beta-thalassaemia. Clinical, haematological and electrophoretic studies in a family from South Lebanon. *J. Med. Genet.* **11**, 275.

Shakin, S.H. & Liebhaber, S.A. (1986) Translational profiles of $\alpha 1$-, $\alpha 2$-, and β-globin messenger ribonucleic acids in human reticulocytes. *J. Clin. Invest.* **78**, 1125.

Shalev, O., Mogilner, S., Shinar, E., Rachmilewitz, E.A. & Schrier, S.L. (1984) Impaired erythrocyte calcium homeostasis in β-thalassemia. *Blood* **64**, 564.

Shalev, O., Repka, T., Goldfarb, A. *et al.* (1995) Deferiprone (L1) chelates pathologic iron deposits from membranes of intact thalassemic and sickle red blood cells both *in vitro* and *in vivo*. *Blood* **86**, 2008.

Shalev, O., Shinar, E. & Lux, S.E. (1996) Isolated beta-globin chains reproduce, in normal red cell membranes, the defective binding of spectrin to alpha-thalassaemic membranes. *Br. J. Haematol.* **94**, 273.

Shalit, M., Tedeschi, A., Miadonna, A. & Levi-Shaffer, A. (1991) Desferal (desferrioxamine). A novel activator of connective tissue-type mast cells. *J. Allergy Clin. Immunol.* **6**, 854.

Shalmon, L., Kirschmann, C. & Zaizov, R. (1994) A new deletional α-thalassemia detected in Yemenites with Hemoglobin H disease. *Am. J. Hematol.* **45**, 201.

Sharma, R.S., Kabir, S.M.S., Baxi, A.J., Shanbaug, S.R. & Bhatia, H.M. (1971) Haematological and genetic studies in the Saraswat and Lohna communities. In: *Proceedings of the Annual Meeting of the Indian Society of Haematology and Blood Transfusion*, p. 27. Bangalore, India.

Sharma, R.S., Williams, L., Wilson, J.B. & Huisman, T.H.J. (1975) Hemoglobin A$_2$-Coburg or $\alpha_2\delta_2 116$ Arg leads to His (G18). *Biochim. Biophys. Acta* **393**, 379.

Sharma, R.S., Yu, V. & Walters, W.A.W. (1979) Haemoglobin Bart's hydrops fetalis syndrome in an infant of Greek origin and prenatal diagnosis of alpha-thalassemia. *Med. J. Aust.* **2**, 404.

Sharpe, J.A., Chan-Thomas, P.S., Lida, J., Ayyub, H., Wood, W.G. & Higgs, D.R. (1992) Analysis of the human α globin upstream regulatory element (HS –40) in transgenic mice. *EMBO J.* **11**, 4565.

Sharpe, J., Wells, D.J., Whitelaw, E., Vyas, P., Higgs, D.R. & Wood, W.G. (1993) Analysis of the human α-globin gene cluster in transgenic mice. *Proc. Natl Acad. Sci. USA* **90**, 11262.

Shatkin, A.J. (1976) Capping of eukaryotic mRNAs. *Cell* **9**, 645.

Shchory, M. & Ramot, B. (1972) Globin chain synthesis in the marrow and reticulocytes of beta thalassemia, hemoglobin H disease and delta beta thalassemia. *Blood* **40**, 105.

Shehadeh, N., Hazani, A., Rudolf, M.C.J., Benderly, A. & Hochberg, Z. (1990) Neurosecretory dysfunction of growth hormone secretion in thalassaemia major. *Acta Paediatr. Scand.* **79**, 790.

Shen, S.H., Slightom, J.L. & Smithies, O. (1981) A history of the human fetal globin gene duplication. *Cell* **26**, 191.

Shepherd, M.K., Weatherall, D.J. & Conley, C.L. (1962) Semi-quantitative estimation of the distribution of fetal hemoglobin in red cell populations. *Bull. Johns Hopkins Hosp.* **110**, 293.

Sher, G.D., Belluzzo, N., Babyn, P., Collins, A.F., Bailey, J.D. & Olivieri, N.F. (1993) Improvement in deferoxamine-induced bony abnormalities in transfusion-dependent patients following withdrawal or reduction of deferoxamine and initiation of the oral chelator. *Blood* **82**, 360a.

Sher, G.D., Ginder, G., Little, J.A., Wang, S.Y., Dover, G. & Olivieri, N.F. (1995) Extended therapy with arginine butyrate in patients with thalassemia and sickle cell disease. *N. Eng. J. Med.* **332**, 106.

Sheridan, B.L., Weatherall, D.J., Clegg, J.B. *et al.* (1976) The patterns of fetal haemoglobin production in leukaemia. *Br. J. Haematol.* **32**, 487.

Sherlock, S., Dick, R. & van-Leeuwen, D.J. (1985) Liver biopsy today. The Royal Free Hospital experience. *J. Hepatol.* **1**, 75.

Shesely, E.G., Kim, H.-S., Shehee, W.R., Papayannopoulou, T., Smithies, O. & Popovich, B.W. (1991) Correction of a human β^S-globin gene by gene targeting. *Proc. Natl Acad. Sci. USA* **88**, 4294.

Shi, Y.-P., Alpers, M.P., Povoa, M.M. & Lai, A.A. (1992) Diversity in the immunodominant determinants of the circumsporozoite protein of *Plasmodium falciparum* parasites from malaria-endemic regions of Papua New Guinea and Brazil. *Am. J. Trop. Med. Hyg.* **47**, 844.

Shih, D.M., Wall, R.J. & Shapiro, S.G. (1993) A 5′ control region of the human ε-globin gene is sufficient for embryonic specificity in transgenic mice. *J. Biol. Chem.* **268**, 3066.

Shinar, E. & Rachmilewitz, E.A. (1990a) Differences in the pathophysiology of hemolysis of α- and β-thalassemic red blood cells. *Ann. N. Y. Acad. Sci.* **612**, 118.

Shinar, E. & Rachmilewitz, E.A. (1990b) Oxidative denaturation of red blood cells in thalassemia. *Sem. Hematol.* **27**, 70.

Shinar, E. & Rachmilewitz, E.A. (1993) Haemoglobinopathies and red cell membrane function. *Clin. Haematol.* **6**, 357.

Shinar, E., Shalev, O., Rachmilewitz, R.A. & Schrier, S.L. (1987) Erythrocyte membrane skeleton abnormalities in severe β-thalassemia. *Blood* **70**, 158.

Shinar, E., Rachmilewitz, E.A. & Lux, S.E. (1989) Different erythrocyte membrane skeletal protein defects in alpha and beta thalassemia. *J. Clin. Invest.* **83**, 1190.

Shiokawa, S., Yamada, H., Takihara, Y. *et al.* (1988) Molecular analysis of Japanese δβ-thalassemia. *Blood* **72**, 1771.

Shirahata, A., Funahara, Y., Opartkiattikul, N., Fucharoen, S., Laosombat, V. & Yamada, K. (1992) Protein C and S deficiency in thalassaemic patients. *Southeast Asian J. Trop. Med. Publ. Hlth* **23**, 65.

Shivdasani, R.A., Rosenblatt, M.F., Zucker-Franklin, D. *et al.* (1995) Transcription factor NF-E2 is required for platelet formation independent of the actions of thrombopoietin/MGDF in megakaryocyte development. *Cell* **81**, 695.

Shooter, E.M., Skinner, E.R., Garlick, J.P. & Barnicot, N.A. (1960) The electrophoretic characterization of haemoglobin G and a new minor haemoglobin, G$_2$. *Br. J. Haematol.* **6**, 140.

Short, E.M., Winkle, R.A. & Billingham, M.E. (1981) Myocardial involvement in idiopathic hemochromatosis. Morphologic and clinical improvement following venisection. *Am. J. Med.* **70**, 1275.

Shulman, H.M. & Hinterberger, W. (1992) Hepatic veno-occlusive disease—liver toxicity syndrome after bone marrow transplantation. *Bone Marrow Transplant.* **10**, 197.

Shyamala, M., Kiefer, C.R., Moscoso, H. & Garver, F.A. (1991) Application of a monoclonal antibody specific for the delta chain of hemoglobin A$_2$ in the diagnosis of beta thalassemia. *Am. J. Hematol.* **38**, 214.

Sicard, D., Lieurzou, Y., Lapoumeroulie, C. & Labie, D. (1979) High genetic polymorphism of hemoglobin disorders in Laos. *Hum. Genet.* **50**, 327.

Sicuranza, B.J., Tisdall, L.H., Sarreck, R. & DeStefano, R. (1978) Thalassemia minor. Cause of complications in pregnant Black and Hispanic women. *N. Y. State J. Med.* **78**, 1691.

Siegel, W., Cox, R., Schroeder, W.A., Huisman, T.H.J., Penner, O. & Rowley, P.T. (1970) An adult homozygous for persistent fetal hemoglobin. *Ann. Intern. Med.* **72**, 533.

Signorelli, S. (1966) Thalassaemia-sickle cell disease (thalasso-drepanocytosis) in Sicily. *Haematol. Lat.* **9**, 151.

Silprasert, A., Laokuldilok, T. & Kulapongs, P. (1998) Zinc deficiency in β-thalassemic children. *Birth Defects* **23**, 473.

Silva, A.E. & Varella-Garcia, M. (1989) Plasma folate and vitamin B$_{12}$ levels in β-thalassemia heterozygotes. *Braz. J. Med. Biol. Res.* **22**, 1225.

Silvestroni, E. (1949) Microcitemia e malattie a substrato microcitemico; falcemia e malattie falcemiche. In: *50° Congresso della Societa di Medicina Internationale*, p. 108. Ed. Pozzi, Roma.

Silvestroni, E. & Bianco, I. (1944) La resistenza osmotica delle emazie nei soggetti normali e prime osservazioni di resistenze globulari aumentate in soggetti sani. *Pont. Acad. Sci. Comm.* **8**, 633.

Silvestroni, E. & Bianco, I. (1944–45) Microdrepanocitoanemia, in un sogetto di razza bianca. *Boll. Atti Acad. Med.* **70**, 347.

Silvestroni, E. & Bianco, I. (1945) Dimostrazione nell'uomo di una particolare anomalia ematologica costituzionale e rapporti fra questa anolalia e l'anemia microcitica costituzionale. *Policlinico* **52**, 1.

Silvestroni, E. & Bianco, I. (1946a) Ricerche sui familiari sani di malati di morbo di Cooley. *Ric. Morfol.* **22**, 217.

Silvestroni, E. & Bianco, I. (1946b) Una nova entita nosologica: La malatia microdrepanocitica. *Haematologica* **29**, 455.

Silvestroni, E. & Bianco, I. (1947) Sulla frequenza dei porta tori di malatia di morbo di Cooley e primi observazioni sulla frequenza dei portatore di microcitemia nel Ferrarese e inakune regioni limitrofe. *Boll. Atti Acad. Med.* **72**, 32.

Silvestroni, E. & Bianco, I. (1948) Ricerche cliniche, genetiche ed ematologiche sui malati di anemia microcitica costituzionale e di morbo di Cooley. *Haematologica* **31**, 1.

Silvestroni, E. & Bianco, I. (1951) L'anemia microcitica costituzionale. *Medicina* **3**, 343.

Silvestroni, E. & Bianco, I. (1952) Genetic aspects of sickle cell anemia and microdrepanocytic disease. *Blood* **7**, 429.

Silvestroni, E. & Bianco, I. (1955a) *La Malattia Microdrepanocitica*. Il Pensiero Scientifico, Rome.

Silvestroni, E. & Bianco, I. (1955b) New data on microdrepanocytic disease. *Blood* **10**, 623.

Silvestroni, E. & Bianco, I. (1959) The distribution of the microcythaemias (or thalassaemias) in Italy. Some aspects of the haematological and haemoglobinic picture in these haemopathies. In: *Abnormal Haemoglobins* (eds J.H.P. Jonxis & J.F. Delafresnaye), p. 242. Blackwell Scientific Publications, Oxford.

Silvestroni, E. & Bianco, I. (1962) Haemoglobin Bart's in Italy. *Nature* **195**, 394.

Silvestroni, E. & Bianco, I. (1963) *Le Emoglobine Umane: Biochimica, genetica, popolazionistica patologia e clinica.* Istituto 'Gregorio Mendel', Roma.

Silvestroni, E. & Bianco, I. (1964) Un caso di malattia microdrepanocitica da Hb E e varieta di microcitemia con quota normale di Hb A$_2$ e quota elevata di Hb F. *Prog. Med. Roma* **20**, 509.

Silvestroni, E. & Bianco, I. (1966) Pluralita delle microcitemia (O thalassemie). *Policlinico* **73**, 41.

Silvestroni, E. & Bianco, I. (1968) La microcitemia: contributi personali in 25 anni di lavoro e di studio. *Policlinico* **75**, 1645.

Silvestroni, E. & Bianco, I. (1969) La malattia microdrepanocitica e sue varianti cliniche e genetiche. *Policlinico* **76**, 1.

Silvestroni, E. & Bianco, I. (1975) Screening for microcytemia in Italy: analysis of data collected in the past 30 years. *Am. J. Hum. Genet.* **27**, 198.

Silvestroni, E., Bianco, I. & Montalenti, G. (1949) On genetics and geographical distribution of a human blood disease. *Proc. VIII Int. Cong. Genet. Hereditas*, **35** (Suppl.), 662.

Silvestroni, E., Bianco, I., Muzzolini, M., Modiano, G. & Vallisneri, E. (1957) Studio biochimico, elettroforetica e spettrofotometrico dell'emoglobina di malati di anemia microcitica costituzionale e di morbo di Cooley. *Experientia* **13**, 705.

Silvestroni, E., Bianco, I., Lucci, R. & Soffriti, E. (1960) Il quadro ematologico nei portatori di Hb L individual nel Ferrarese: associazione e rapporti con la microcitemia. *Experientia* **16**, 553.

Silvestroni, E., Bianco, I. & Brancati, C. (1964) Presenza di microcitemia con quota normale di emoglobina A$_2$ e quota elevata di emoglobina F in una famiglia Calabrese. *Policlinico* **71**, 1543.

Silvestroni, E., Bianco, I. & Baglioni, C. (1965a) Interaction of hemoglobin Lepore with sickle cell trait and microcythemia (thalassemia) in a Southern Italian family. *Blood* **25**, 457.

Silvestroni, E., Bianco, I. & Muratore, F. (1965b) Frequenza dei vari tipi di microcitemia e di emoglobine abnormi nella provincia di Lecce. *Il Progr. Med.* **21**, 211.

Silvestroni, E., Bianco, I. & Graziani, B. (1968a) The haemoglobin picture in Cooley's disease. *Br. J. Haematol.* **14**, 303.

Silvestroni, E., Bianco, I. & Reitano, G. (1968b) Three cases of homozygous δβ-thalassaemia (or microcythemia) with high haemoglobin F in a Sicilian family. *Acta Haematol.* **40**, 220.

Silvestroni, E., Bianco, I., Graziani, B., Carboni, C. & D'Acra, S.U. (1978) First premarital screening of thalassaemia carriers in intermediate schools in Latium. *J. Med. Genet.* **15**, 202.

Silvestroni, E., Bianco, I., Graziani, B., Carboni, C., Valente, M. & Lerone, M. (1981a) La frequenza della microcitemie nel Lazio. Provincia di Roma. *Min. Med.* **72**, 672.

Silvestroni, E., Bianco, I., Graziani, B. *et al.* (1981b) Screening delle microcitemie nella popolazione scolastica del Lazio. *Min. Med.* **72**, 677.

Simon, G. (1972) Hyperosmolar diabetic state with sickle thalassemia. *N. Y. State J. Med.* **72**, 486.

Simon, T.L., Sohmer, P. & Nelson, E.F. (1989) Extended survival of neocytes produced by a new system. *Transfusion* **29**, 221.

Simonet, W.S., Lacey, D.L., Dunstan, C.R. *et al.* (1997) Osteoprotegerin: a novel secreted protein involved in the regulation of bone density. *Cell* **89**, 309.

Simpson, J.L. & Elias, S. (1994) Isolating fetal cells in maternal circulation for prenatal diagnosis. *Prenat. Diag.* **14**, 1229.

Singer, K. & Fisher, B. (1952) Studies on abnormal hemoglobins. V. The distribution of type S (sickle cell) hemoglobin and type F (alkali resistant) hemoglobin within the red cell population in sickle cell anemia. *Blood* **7**, 1216.

Singer, S.T. & Vichinsky, E.P. (1999) Deferoxamine treatment during pregnancy: is it harmful? *Am. J. Hematol.* **60**, 24.

Singer, K., Chernoff, A.I. & Singer, L. (1951) Studies on abnormal hemoglobin. I. Their demonstration in sickle cell anemia and other hematologic disorders by means of alkali denaturation. *Blood* **6**, 413.

Singer, K., Kraus, A.P., Singer, L., Rubinstein, H.M. & Goldberg, S.R. (1954) Studies on abnormal hemoglobins. X. A new syndrome: hemoglobin C-thalassemia disease. *Blood* **9**, 1032.

Singer, K., Singer, L. & Goldberg, S.R. (1955) Studies on abnormal hemoglobins. XI. Sickle cell-thalassemia disease in the Negro. The significance of the S+A+F and S+A patterns obtained in hemoglobin analysis. *Blood* **10**, 405.

Singer, K., Josephson, A.M., Singer, L., Heller, P. & Simmerman, H.J. (1957) Studies on abnormal hemoglobins. XIII. Hemoglobin S-thalassemia disease and hemoglobin C-thalassemia. *Blood* **12**, 593.

Siniscalco, M., Bernini, L., Filippi, G., Latte, B., Khan, M., Piomeli, S. & Rattazi, M. (1966) Population genetics of haemoglobin variants, thalassaemia and glucose-6-phosphate dehydrogenase deficiency, with particular reference to the malaria hypothesis. *Bull. WHO* **34**, 379.

Sinniah, D., Vegnaendra, V. & Kammaruddin, A. (1977) Neurological complications of beta-thalassaemia major. *Arch. Dis. Child.* **52**, 977.

Sippel, A.E., Stavrianopoulos, J.G., Schutz, G. & Feigelson, P. (1974) Translational properties of rabbit globin mRNA after specific removal of poly (A) with ribonuclease H. *Proc. Natl Acad. Sci. USA* **71**, 4635.

Sitarz, A.L., Ultmann, J.E. & Wolff, J.A. (1963) Erythrocyte life-span and sites of destruction in thalassemia major. *Acta Haematol.* **30**, 204.

Skarsgard, E., Doski, J., Jaksic, T. *et al.* (1993) Thrombosis of the portal venous system after splenectomy for pediatric hematologic disease. *J. Pediatr. Surg.* **28**, 1109.

Sklar, C.A., Lew, L.Q., Yoon, D.J. & David, R. (1987) Adrenal function in thalassemia major following long-term treatment with multiple transfusions and chelation therapy. Evidence for dissociation of cortisol and adrenal androgen secretion. *Am. J. Dis. Child.* **141**, 327.

Slater, T.F. (1984) Free radical mechanisms in tissue injury. *Biochem. J.* **222**, 1.

Slater, L.M., Muir, W.A. & Weed, R.I. (1968) Influence of splenectomy on insoluble hemoglobin inclusion bodies in β-thalassemic erythrocytes. *Blood* **31**, 766.

Slightom, J.L., Blechl, A.E. & Smithies, O. (1980) Human $^G\gamma$- and $^A\gamma$-globin genes: complete nucleotide sequences suggest that DNA can be exchanged between these duplicated genes. *Cell* **21**, 627.

Smetanina, N.S., Leonova, J.Y., Levy, N. & Huisman, T.H.J. (1996) The α/β and α2/α1-globin mRNA ratios in different forms of α-thalassaemia. *Biochim. Biophys. Acta* **1315**, 188.

Smidt-Jensen, S., Hahnemann, N., Hariri, J. (1986) Transabdominal chorionic villi sampling for first trimester fetal diagnosis: First 26 pregnancies followed to term. *Prenat. Diag.* **6**, 125.

Smith, C.H. (1948) Detection of mild types of Mediterranean (Cooley's) anemia. *Am. J. Dis. Child.* **75**, 505.

Smith, C.H., Sisson, T.R.C., Floyd, W.H.J. & Siegal, S. (1950) Serum iron and iron binding capacity of the serum in children with severe Mediterranean (Cooley's) anemia. *Pediatr.* **5**, 799.

Smith, C.H., Schulman, I., Ando, R.E. & Stern, G. (1955) Studies in Mediterranean (Cooley's) anemia. I. Clinical and hematologic aspects of splenectomy with special reference to fetal hemoglobin synthesis. *Blood* **10**, 582.

Smith, C.H., Erlandson, M.E., Schulman, I. & Stern, G. (1957) Hazard of severe infections in splenectomized infants and children. *Am. J. Med.* **22**, 390.

Smith, C.H., Erlandson, M.E., Stern, G. & Scholman, I. (1960) The role of splenectomy in the management of thalassemia. *Blood* **15**, 197.

Smith, C.H., Erlandson, M.E., Stern, G. & Hilgartner, M.W. (1962) Postsplenectomy infection in Cooley's anemia. An appraisal of the problem in this and other blood disorders, with consideration of prophylaxis. *N. Eng. J. Med.* **266**, 737.

Smith, C.H., Erlandson, M.E., Stern, G. & Hilgartner, H. (1964) Postsplenectomy infection in Cooley's anemia. *Ann. N. Y. Acad. Sci.* **119**, 748.

Smith, D.H., Clegg, J.B., Weatherall, D.J. & Gilles, H.M. (1973) Hereditary persistence of foetal haemoglobin associated with a γβ fusion variant, Haemoglobin Kenya. *Nature New Biol.* **246**, 184.

Smith, E.W. & Conley, C.L. (1954) Clinical features of the genetic variants of sickle cell disease. *Bull. Johns Hopkins Hosp.* **94**, 289.

Smith, E.W. & Krevans, J.R. (1959) Clinical manifestations of haemoglobin C disorders. *Bull. Johns Hopkins Hosp.* **104**, 17.

Smith, E.W. & Torbert, J.V. (1958) Study of two abnormal hemoglobins with evidence for a new genetic locus for hemoglobin formation. *Bull. Johns Hopkins Hosp.* **102**, 38.

Smith, P.R., Manjoney, D.L., Teitcher, J.B., Choi, K.N. & Braverman, A.S. (1988) Massive hemothorax due to intrathoracic extramedullary hematopoiesis in a patient with thalassemia inter-media. *Chest* **94**, 658.

Smith, R. (1996) Disorders of the skeleton. In: *Oxford Textbook of Medicine* (eds D.J. Weatherall, J.G.G. Ledingham & D.A. Warrell), p. 3055. Oxford University Press, Oxford.

Smith, R.A., Ho, P.J., Clegg, J.B., Kidd, J.R. & Thein, S.L. (1998) Recombination breakpoints in the human β-globin gene cluster. *Blood* **92**, 4415.

Smithies, O. (1959) An improved procedure for starch-gel electrophoresis: further variation in the serum proteins of normal individuals. *Biochem. J.* **71**, 585.

Smithies, O. (1964) Chromosomal rearrangements and protein structure. *Cold Spring Harbor Sympos. Quant. Biol.* **29**, 309.

Smithies, O., Connel, G.E. & Dixon, G.H. (1962) Chromosomal rearrangements and the evolution of haptoglobin genes. *Nature* **196**, 232.

Smithies, O., Blechl, A.E., Denniston-Thompson, K. *et al.* (1978) Cloning human fetal γ globin and mouse α-type globin DNA: characterization and partial sequencing. *Science* **202**, 1284.

Sofro, A.S.M. (1995) Molecular pathology of β-thalassemia in Indonesia. *Southeast Asian J. Trop. Med. Publ. Hlth* **26**, 221.

Sofro, A.S.M., Suhorto, S. & Madiyan, M. (1985) Frekuensi trait thalassemia beta pada beberapa kelompok etnik mahasiwa di Yogyakarta. *Laporan Penelitian Proyek PIT no. 287/PIT/DPPM/335.* University of Gadjah Mada, Yogyakarta.

Sofroniadou, K., Wood, W.G., Nute, P.E. & Stamatoyannopoulos, G. (1975) Globin chain synthesis in Greek type (^{A}γ) of hereditary persistence of fetal haemoglobin. *Br. J. Haematol.* **29**, 137.

Solanki, D.L., Kletter, G.G. & Castro, O. (1986) Acute splenic sequestration crises in adults with sickle cell disease. *Am. J. Med.* **80**, 985.

Soliman, A.T., el-Banna, N., Al Salmi, I. & Asfour, M. (1996) Insulin and glucagon responses to provocation with glucose and arginine in prepubertal children with thalassemia major before and after long-term blood transfusion. *J. Trop. Pediatr.* **42**, 291.

van Solinge, W.W., Lind, B., van Wijk, R. & Kraaijenhagen, R.J. (1996) Clinical expression of a rare β-globin gene mutation co-inherited with haemoglobin E disease. *Eur. J. Clin. Chem. Clin. BioChem.* **34**, 949.

Somma, L. (1884) *Arch. It. Patol. Inf. Napoli* 1.

Sonakul, D. (1989) *Pathology of Thalassaemic Diseases.* Amarin Printing Group, Thailand.

Sonakul, D. & Fucharoen, S. (1992) Brain pathology in 6 fatal cases of post-transfusion hypertension, convulsion and cerebral hemorrhage syndrome. *Southeast Asian J. Trop. Med. Publ. Hlth* **23**, 116.

Sonakul, D., Sook-aneak, M. & Pacharee, P. (1978) Pathology of thalassemic diseases in Thailand. *J. Med. Assoc. Thailand* **61**, 72.

Sonakul, D., Pacharee, P., Laohapand, T., Fucharoen, S. & Wasi, P. (1980) Pulmonary artery obstruction in thalassaemia. *Southeast Asian J. Trop. Med. Publ. Hlth* **11**, 516.

Sonakul, D., Pacharee, P., Wasi, P. & Fucharoen, S. (1984) Cardiac pathology in 47 patients with beta thalassaemia/haemoglobin E. *Southeast Asian J. Trop. Med. Publ. Hlth* **15**, 554.

Sonakul, D., Pacharee, P. & Thakerngpol, K. (1988a) Pathologic findings in 76 autopsy cases of thalassemia. *Birth Defects* **23**, 157.

Sonakul, D., Suwananagool, P., Sirivaidyapong, P. & Fucharoen, S. (1988b) Distribution of pulmonary thromboembolic lesions in thalassemic patients. *Birth Defects* **23**, 375.

Sophocleous, T., Higgs, D.R., Aldridge, B. *et al.* (1981) The molecular basis for the haemoglobin Bart's hydrops fetalis syndrome in Cyprus. *Br. J. Haematol.* **47**, 153.

Southern, E.M. (1975) Detection of specific sequences among DNA fragments separated by gel electrophoresis. *J. Mol. Biol.* **98**, 503.

Spangler, E.A., Andrews, K.A. & Rubin, E.M. (1990) Developmental regulation of the human ζ globin gene in transgenic mice. *Nucl. Acids Res.* **18**, 7093.

Spanos, T., Ladis, V., Palamidou, F. *et al.* (1996) The impact of neocyte transfusion in the management of thalasssaemia. *Vox Sang.* **70**, 217.

Speiser, S. & Etlinger, J.D. (1982) Loss of ATP-dependent proteolysis with maturation of reticulocytes and erythrocytes. *J. Biol. Chem.* **257**, 14122.

Spiegelberg, R., Aulehla-Scholz, C., Erlich, H. & Horst, J. (1989) A β-thalassemia gene caused by a 290-base pair deletion: analysis by direct sequencing of enzymatically amplified DNA. *Blood* **73**, 1695.

Spirito, P., Lupi, G., Melevendi, C. & Vecchio, C. (1990) Restrictive diastolic abnormalities identified by Doppler echocardiography in patients with thalassemia major. *Circulation* **82**, 88.

Spitz, I.M., Hirsch, H.J., Landau, H., Zylber-Haran, E., Gross, V. & Rachmilewitz, E.A. (1984) TSH secretion in thalassemia. *J. Endocrinol. Invest.* **7**, 495.

Spritz, R.A., DeRiel, J.K., Forget, B.G. & Weissman, S.M. (1980) Complete nucleotide sequence of the human δ-globin gene. *Cell* **21**, 639.

Spritz, R.A., Jagadeeswaran, P., Choudary, P.V. *et al.* (1981) Base substitution in an intervening sequence of a β⁺ thalassemic human globin gene. *Proc. Natl Acad. Sci. USA* **78**, 2455.

Sproat, I.A., Dobranowski, J., Chen, V., Ali, M. & Woods, D. (1991) Presacral extramedullary hematopoiesis in thalassemia interme-dia. *Can. Assoc. Radiol. J.* **42**, 278.

Srichaikul, T., Tipayasakda, J., Atichartakarn, V., Jootar, S. & Bovornbinyanun, P. (1984) Ferrokinetic and erythrokinetic studies in alpha and beta thalassemia. *Clin. Lab. Haematol.* **6**, 133.

Stallings, M., Abraham, A. & Abraham, E.C. (1983) α-Thalassemia influences the levels of fetal hemoglobin components in new born infants. *Blood* **62**, 75a.

Stamatoyannopoulos, G. & Fessas, P. (1963) Observations of hemoglobin 'Pylos': the hemoglobin Pylos–hemoglobin S combination. *J. Lab. Clin. Med.* **62**, 193.

Stamatoyannopoulos, G. & Fessas, P. (1964) Thalassaemia, glucose-6-phosphate dehydrogenase deficiency sickling, and malarial endemicity of Greece: a study of five areas. *Br. Med. J.* **i**, 875.

Stamatoyannopoulos, G. & Papayannopoulou, T. (1981) The switching from hemoglobin F to hemoglobin A formation in man: parallels between the observations *in vivo* and the findings in erythroid cultures. *Prog. Clin. Biol. Res.* **55**, 665.

Stamatoyannopoulos, G., Sofroniadou, C. & Akrivakis, A. (1967) Absence of hemoglobin A in a double heterozygote for F-thalassemia and hemoglobin S. *Blood* **30**, 772.

Stamatoyannopoulos, G., Fessas, P. & Papayannopoulou, T. (1969a) F-thalassemia: a study of thirty-one families with simple heterozygotes and combination of F-thalassemia and A₂-thalassemia. *Am. J. Med.* **47**, 194.

Stamatoyannopoulos, G., Papayannopoulou, T., Fessas, P. & Motulsky, A.G. (1969b) The beta-delta thalassemias. *Ann. N. Y. Acad. Sci.* **165**, 25.

Stamatoyannopoulos, G., Schroeder, W.A., Huisman, T.H.J. *et al.* (1971) Nature of foetal haemoglobin F-thalassaemia. *Br. J. Haematol.* **21**, 633.

Stamatoyannopoulos, G., Woodson, R., Papayannopoulou, T., Heywood, D. & Kurachi, M.S. (1974) Inclusion-body β-thalasemia trait. A form of β thalassemia producing clinical manifestations in simple heterozygotes. *N. Eng. J. Med.* **290**, 939.

Stamatoyannopoulos, G., Wood, W.G., Papayannopoulou, T. & Nute, P.E. (1975) A new form of hereditary persistence of fetal hemoglobin in Blacks and its association with sickle cell trait. *Blood* **46**, 683.

Stamatoyannopoulos, G., Weitkamp, L.R., Kotsakis, P. & Akrivakis, A. (1977) The linkage relationships of the β and δ hemoglobin genes. *Hemoglobin* **1**, 561.

Stamatoyannopoulos, G., Veith, R.W., Al-Khatti, A., Fritsch, E.F., Goldwasser, E. & Papayannopoulou, Th. (1987) On the induction of fetal hemoglobin in the adult: stress erythropoiesis, cell cycle-specific drugs, and recombinant erythropoietin. In: *Developmental Control of Globin Gene Expression* (eds G. Stamatoyannopoulos & A.W. Nienhuis), p. 443. A.R. Liss, New York.

Stamatoyannopoulos, G., Marjerus, P.W., Perlmutter, R.M. & Varmus, H. (eds) (2001) *Molecular Basis of Blood Diseases*, 2nd edn. W.B. Saunders Company, Philadelphia.

Stamatoyannopoulos, J.A., Goodwin, A., Joyce, T. & Lowrey, C.H. (1995) NF-E2 and GATA binding motifs are required for the formation of DNase 1 hypersensitive site 4 of the human β-globin locus control region. *EMBO J.* **14**, 106.

Stamatoyannopoulos, J.A., Clegg, C.H. & Li, Q. (1997) Sheltering of γ-globin expression from position effects requires both an upstream locus control region and a regulatory element 3′ to the A γ-globin gene. *Mol. Cell. Biol.* **17**, 240.

Stanworth, S.J., Roberts, N.A., Sharpe, J.A., Sloane-Stanley, J. & Wood, W.G. (1995) Established epigenetic modifications determine the expression of developmentally regulated globin genes in somatic cell hybrids. *Mol. Cell. Biol.* **15**, 3969.

Starck, J., Sarkar, R., Romana, M. *et al.* (1994) Developmental regulation of human γ- and β-globin genes in the absence of the locus control region. *Blood* **84**, 1656.

Stark, D.D., Moseley, M.E., Bacon, B.R. & Moss, A.A. (1985) Magnetic resonance imaging and spectroscopy of hepatic iron overload. *Radiology* **154**, 137.

Stayton, C.L., Dabovic, B., Gulisano, M. *et al.* (1994) Cloning and characterisation of a new human Xq13 gene, encoding a putative helicase. *Hum. Mol. Genet.* **3**, 1957.

Stefanis, L., Kanavakis, E., Traeger-Synodinos, J., Tzetis, M., Metaxotou-Mavromati, A. & Kattamis, C. (1994) I: Hematologic phenotype of the mutations IVS1-n6 (T→C), IVS1-n110 (G→A), and CD39 (C→T) in carriers of beta-thalassemia in Greece. *Pediatr. Hematol. Oncol.* **11**, 509.

Stegagno, G.A. & Pollitzer, C. (1963) Richerche citochimiche sui polisaccaridi e lipidi delle cellule ematoche e midollari di bambini effeti da talassemia major (morbo di Cooley). *Arch. Ital. Pediatr. Pueri.* **16**, 247.

Steinberg, M.H. (1991) The interactions of α-thalassemia with hemoglobinopathies. *Hematol./Oncol. Clinics N. Am.* **5**, 453.

Steinberg, M.H. (1993) Case report: effects of iron deficiency and the −88 C→T mutation on Hb A₂ levels in β-thalassemia. *Am. J. Med. Sci.* **305**, 312.

Steinberg, M.H. (1996) Modulation of the phenotypic diversity of sickle cell anemia. *Hemoglobin* **20**, 1.

Steinberg, M.H. (1998) Pathophysiology of sickle cell disease. *Clin. Haematol.* **11**, 163.

Steinberg, M.H. & Adams, J.G. III. (1991) Hemoglobin A₂: origin, evolution and aftermath. *Blood* **78**, 2165.

Steinberg, M.H. & Dreiling, B.J. (1976) Clinical, hematological and biosynthetic studies in sickle cell-beta⁰-thalassemia: a comparison with sickle cell anemia. *Am. J. Hematol.* **1**, 35.

Steinberg, M.H., Adams, J.G. III. & Dreiling, B.J. (1975) Alpha thalassaemia in adults with sickle-cell trait. *Br. J. Haematol.* **30**, 31.

Steinberg, M.H., Rosenstock, W., Coleman, M.B. *et al.* (1984) Effects of thalassemia and microcytosis on the hematologic and vasoocclusive severity of sickle cell anemia. *Blood* **63**, 1353.

Steinberg, M.H., Coleman, M.B., Adams, J.G. III, Hartmann, R.C.,

Saba, H. & Anagnou, N.P. (1986) A new gene deletion in the alpha-like globin gene cluster as the molecular basis for the rare α-thalassemia-1 (−−/αα) in blacks: HbH disease in sickle cell trait. *Blood* **67**, 469.

Steinberg, M.H., Adams, J.G. III, Morrison, W.T. *et al.* (1987) Hemoglobin Mississippi (β⁴⁴Ser→Cys). Studies of the thalassemia phenotype in a mixed heterozygote with β-thalassemia. *J. Clin. Invest.* **79**, 826.

Steinberg, M.H., Forget, B.G., Higggs, D.R. & Nagel, R.L. (2001) *Disorders of Hemoglobin*. Cambridge University Press, New York.

Stella, M., Pinzello, G. & Maggio, A. (1998) Letter to Editor. *N. Eng. J. Med.* **339**, 1712.

Stevens, M.C., Lehmann, H., Mason, K.P., Serjeant, B.E. & Serjeant, G.R. (1982) Sickle cell-Hb Lepore Boston syndrome. Uncommon differential diagnosis to homozygous sickle cell disease. *Am. J. Dis. Child.* **136**, 19.

Stevens, M.C., Maude, G.H., Beckford, M. *et al.* (1985) Haematological change in sickle cell-haemoglobin C disease and in sickle cell β-thalassaemia: a cohort study from birth. *Br. J. Haematol.* **60**, 279.

Stevens, M.C.G., Maude, G.H., Beckford, M. *et al.* (1986) α Thalassemia and the hematology of homozygous sickle cell disease in childhood. *Blood* **67**, 411.

Stohlman, F.J. (1964) Regulation of erythropoiesis. XIV: A model for abnormal erythropoiesis in thalassemia. *Ann. N. Y. Acad. Sci.* **119**, 578.

Stolle, C.A., Penny, L.A., Ivory, S., Forget, B.G. & Benz, E.J.J. (1990) Sequence analysis of the γ-globin gene locus from a patient with the deletion form of hereditary persistence of fetal hemoglobin. *Blood* **75**, 499.

Stoming, T.A., Stoming, G.S., Lanclos, K.D. *et al.* (1989) An ᴬγ type of nondeletional hereditary persistence of fetal hemoglobin with a T→C mutation at position −175 to the cap site of the ᴬγ globin gene. *Blood* **73**, 329.

Strachan, T. & Read, A.P. (1996) *Human Molecular Genetics*. BIOS Scientific Publishers Ltd, Oxford.

Stransky, J. (1996) The discovery of hepatitis G virus. *Cas. Lek. Cesk.* **135**, 99.

Strauss, M.B., Daland, G.A. & Fox, H.J. (1941) Familial microcytic anemia. *Am. J. Med. Sci.* **201**, 30.

Strouboulis, J., Dillon, N. & Grosveld, F. (1992) Developmental regulation of a complete 70-kb human β-globin locus in transgenic mice. *Genes Dev.* **6**, 1857.

Sturgeon, P. & Finch, C.A. (1957) Erythrokinetics in Cooley's anemia. *Blood* **12**, 64.

Sturgeon, P., Itano, H.A. & Valentine, W.N. (1952) Chronic hemolytic anemia associated with thalassemia and sickling trait. *Blood* **7**, 350.

Sturgeon, P., Itano, H.A. & Bergren, W.R. (1955) Genetic and biochemical studies of 'intermediate' types of Cooley's anaemia. *Br. J. Haematol.* **1**, 264.

Sturgeon, P., Chen, L.P.L. & Bergren, W.R. (1958) Free erythrocyte porphyrins in thalassemia: preliminary observation. In: *6th International Congress of the International Society of Hematology*, p. 730. Grune and Stratton, New York.

Sturgeon, P., Jones, R.T., Bergren, W.R. & Schroeder, W.A. (1961) Observations on 'Bart's' and the 'fast' hemoglobins of thalassemia H disease. In: *Proceedings of the 8th International Congress of Hematology*, p. 1041. Pan Pacific Press, Tokyo.

Sturgeon, P., Schroeder, W.A., Jones, R.T. & Bergren, W.R. (1963) The relation of alkali resistant haemoglobin in thalassemia and abnormal haemoglobin syndromes to foetal haemoglobin. *Br. J. Haematol.* **9**, 438.

Styles, L., Foote, D.H., Kleman, K.M., Klumpp, C.J., Heer, N.B. & Vichinsky, E.P. (1997) Hemoglobin H-Constant Spring Disease:

an under recognized, severe form of α thalassemia. *Int. J. Pediatr. Hematol./Oncol.* **4**, 69.

Su, C.W., Liang, S., Liang, R., Wen, X.J. & Tang, C.N. (1992) HbH disease in association with the silent β chain variant Hb Hamilton or $\alpha_2\beta_2$11 (A8) Val→Ile. *Hemoglobin* **16**, 403.

Sukumaran, P.K. (1975) Abnormal haemoglobins in India. In: *Trends in Haematology* (eds N.N. Sen & A.K. Basu), p. 225. Sree Saraswaty Press Ltd, Calcutta.

Sukumaran, P.K. & Master, H.R. (1974) The distribution of abnormal haemoglobins in the Indian population. In: *Proceedings of the First Conference of the Indian Society for Human Genetics; Human Population Genetics in India*, p. 91.

Sukumaran, P.K., Sanghvi, L.D. & Nazreth, F.A. (1960) Haemoglobin D-thalassaemia. A report of two families. *Acta Haematol.* 23, 309.

Sukumaran, P.K., Randella, H.P., Sanghvi, L.D. & Merechant, S.M. (1961) Thalassaemia syndromes in Bombay. *J. Assoc. Phys. Ind.* **9**, 69.

Sukumaran, P.K., Huisman, T.H.J., Schroeder, W.A. *et al.* (1972) A homozygote for the Hb $^G\gamma$ type of foetal haemoglobin in India: a study of two Indian and four Negro families. *Br. J. Haematol.* **23**, 403.

Sukumaran, P.K., Nakatsuji, T., Gardiner, M.B., Reese, A.L., Gilman, J.G. & Huisman, T.H.J. (1983) Gamma thalassaemia resulting from the deletion of a γ-globin gene. *Nucl. Acids Res.* **11**, 4635.

Sumiyoshi, A., Thakerngpol, K. & Sonakul, D. (1992) Pulmonary microthromboemboli in thalassaemia cases. *Southeast Asian J. Trop. Med. Publ. Hlth* **23**, 29.

Summers, M.R., Jacobs, A., Tudway, D., Perera, P. & Ricketts, C. (1979) Studies in desferrioxamine and ferrioxamine metabolism in normal and iron-loaded subjects. *Br. J. Haematol.* **42**, 547.

Sunshine, H.R., Hofrichter, J. & Eaton, W.A. (1979) Gelation of sickle cell haemoglobin in mixtures with normal adult and foetal haemoglobins. *J. Mol. Biol.* **133**, 435.

Superti-Furga, G., Barberis, A., Schaffner, G. & Busslinger, M. (1988) The −117 mutation in Greek HPFH affects the binding of three nuclear factors to the CCAAT region of the γ-globin gene. *EMBO J.* **7**, 3099.

Surrey, S., Delgrosso, K., Malladi, P. & Schwartz, E. (1988) A single-base change at position −175 in the 5′-flanking region of the $^G\gamma$-globin gene from a black with $^G\gamma$-β+ HPFH. *Blood* **71**, 807.

Sutcharitchan, P., Saiki, R., Fucharoen, S., Winichagoon, P., Erlich, H. & Embury, S.H. (1995) Reverse dot-blot detection of Thai β-thalassaemia mutations. *Br. J. Haematol.* **90**, 809.

Suvatte, V., Tuchinda, M., Pongpitat, D., Assateerawatt, A. & Tuchinda, S. (1978) Host defense in thalassemias and the effect of splenectomy. 3. Humoral and cell-mediated immunities. *J. Med. Assoc. Thailand* **61**, 73.

Suzuki, H., Matsumori, A., Matoba, Y. *et al.* (1993) Enhanced expression of superoxide dismutase messenger RNA in viral myocarditis. An SH-dependent reduction of its expression and myocardial injury. *J. Clin. Invest.* **91**, 2727.

Swank, R.A. & Stamatoyannopoulos, G. (1998) Fetal gene reactivation. *Curr. Opin. Genet. Dev.* **8**, 366.

Swarup, S., Ghosh, S.K. & Chatterjea, J.B. (1960a) Glutathione stability test in haemoglobin E thalassaemia disease. *Nature* **188**, 153.

Swarup, S., Ghosh, S.K. & Chatterjea, J.B. (1960b) Observations on autohaemolysis in thalassaemia syndromes. *Proc. Natl Inst. Sci. India* **26B** (Suppl.), 158.

Swarup, S., Chatterjea, J.B., Ghosh, S.K., Hosain, P. & Hosain, F. (1961) Observations on erythropoiesis in Hb E-thalassaemia disease — a study with Cr^{51} and Fe^{59}. *Indian J. Pathol. Bact.* **4**, 1.

Swarup, S., Ghosh, S.K. & Chatterjea, J.B. (1966a) Stability of erythrocytic reduced glutathione and nicotine adenine dinucleotide phosphate in Hb E-thalasaemia disease. *Separ. Exp.* **22**, 580.

Swarup, S., Ghosh, S.K., Dutta, M.C. & Chatterjea, J.B. (1966b) Erythrocytic adenosine triphosphate (ATP) level and its stability in Hb E-thalassaemia. *Bull. Calcutta Sch. Trop. Med.* 14, 3.

Swarup-Mitra, S. (1988) Immunologic status of Hb E-thalassaemia patients. *Birth Defects* **23**, 571.

Swarup-Mitra, S., Ghosh, S.K. & Chatterjea, J.B. (1969) Haemolytic anaemia due to interaction of genes for spherocytosis and beta-thalassaemia. *Indian J. Med. Res.* 57.

Sykes, K. & Kaufman, R. (1990) A naturally occurring gamma globin gene mutation enhances SP1 binding activity. *Mol. Cell. Biol.* **10**, 95.

Szelényi, J., Horányi, M., Földi, J., Ringelhann, B. & Hollán, S. (1983) Hemoglobinopathies in Hungary. *Hemoglobin* **7**, 297.

Tabone, P., Henni, T., Belhani, M., Colonna, P., Verdier, G. & Godet, J. (1981) Hemoglobin H disease from Algeria: genetic and molecular characterisation. *Acta Haematol. (Basel)* **65**, 26.

Tagiev, A.F., Surin, V.L., Gol'tsov, A.A. *et al.* (1993) The spectrum of β-thalassaemia mutations in Azerbaijan. *Hum. Mutat.* **2**, 152.

Tagiev, A.F., Surin, V.L., Luk'yanenko, A.V. *et al.* (1994) The spectrum of DNA haplotypes and β-thalassaemia mutations in Azerbaijan. *Genetika* **30**, 535.

Tai, D.Y.H., Wang, Y.T., Lou, J., Wang, W.Y., Mak, K.H. & Cheng, H.K. (1996) Lungs in thalassaemia major patients receiving regular transfusion. *Eur. Respir.* **9**, 1389.

Taj-Eldin, S., Al-Rabbi, H., Jawad, J. & Fakhri, O. (1968) Thalassaemia in Iraq. *Ann. Trop. Med. Parasitol.* **62**, 147.

Takabayashi, H., Kuwabara, S., Ukita, T., Ikawa, K., Yamafuji, K. & Igarashi, T. (1995) Development of non-invasive fetal DNA diagnosis from maternal blood. *Prenat. Diag.* **15**, 74.

Takeshita, K., Forget, B.G., Scarpa, A. & Benz, E.J. (1984) Intranuclear defect in β-globin mRNA accumulation due to a premature translation termination codon. *Blood* **64**, 13.

Takihara, Y., Matsunaga, E., Nakamura, T. *et al.* (1984) One base substitution in IVS-2 causes a β+-thalassaemia phenotype in a Chinese patient. *Biochem. Biophys. Res. Comm.* **121**, 324.

Takihara, Y., Nakamura, T., Yamada, H., Takagi, Y. & Fukumaki, Y. (1986) A novel mutation in the TATA box in a Japanese patient with β+-thalassaemia. *Blood* **67**, 547.

Talbot, D. & Grosveld, F. (1991) The 5′HS2 of the globin locus control region enhances transcription through the interaction of a multimeric complex binding at two functionally distinct NF-E2 binding sites. *EMBO J.* **10**, 1391.

Talbot, D., Collis, P., Antoniou, M., Vidal, M., Grosveld, F. & Greaves, D.R. (1989) A dominant control region from the human β-globin locus conferring integration site-independent gene expression. *Nature* **338**, 352.

Talbot, D., Philipsen, S., Fraser, P. & Grosveld, F. (1990) Detailed analysis of the site 3 region of the human β-globin dominant control region. *EMBO J.* **9**, 2169.

Tamagnini, G.P., Lopes, M.C., Castanheira, M.E., Wainscoat, J.S. & Wood, W.G. (1983) β+ Thalassaemia — Portuguese type: clinical, haematological and molecular studies of a newly defined form of β thalassaemia. *Br. J. Haematol.* **54**, 189.

Tamagnini, G.P., Gonçalves, P., Ribeiro, M.L.S. *et al.* (1993) β-Thalassaemia mutations in the Portuguese: high frequencies of two alleles in restricted populations. *Hemoglobin* **17**, 31.

Tamary, H., Klinger, G., Shalmon, L. *et al.* (1997) α-Thalassaemia caused by a 16 nt deletion in the 3′ untranslated region of the α2-globin gene including the first nucleotide of the poly A signal sequence. *Hemoglobin* **21**, 121.

Tampakoudis, P., Tsatalas, C., Mamopoulos, M. *et al.* (1997) Transfusion-dependent homozygous β-thalassaemia major: successful pregnancy in five cases. *Eur. J. Obstet. Gynecol. Reprod. Biol.* **74**, 127.

Tan, T.G., Jim, R.T. & Blackwell. R.Q. (1978) Hemoglobin G Waimanalo β thalassemia. *Hawaii Med. J.* **37**, 235.

Tan, S.L., Tseng, A.M.P. & Thong, P.-W. (1989) Bart's hydrops fetalis — clinical presentation and management — an analysis of 25 cases. *Aust. N. Z. J. Obstet. Gynaecol.* **3**, 233.

Tan, J.A.M.A., Tay, J.S.H., Lin, L.I. *et al.* (1994) The amplification refractory mutation system (ARMS): a rapid and direct prenatal diagnostic techniques for β-thalassaemia in Singapore. *Prenat. Diag.* **14**, 1077.

Tanaka, M., Fujiwara, Y. & Hirota, Y. (1979) Globin chain synthesis in acquired hemoglobin H disease. *Acta Haematol. Japonica* **42**, 9.

Tang, W., Luo, H.-Y., Albitar, M. *et al.* (1992) Human embryonic ζ-globin expression in deletional α-thalassemias. *Blood* **80**, 517.

Tang, D.C., Ebb, D., Hardison, R.C. & Rodgers, G.P.F. (1997) Restoration of the CCAAT box or insertion of the CACCC motif activate δ-globin gene expression. *Blood* **90**, 421.

Tanner, J.M. & Whitehouse, R.H. (1976) Clinical longitudinal standards for height, weight, height velocity, weight velocity, and stages of puberty. *Arch. Dis. Child.* **51**, 170.

Tannoia, N., Ciavarella, N. & Putignano, A. (1968) Presence in a pedigree of Mediterranean anemia and of Pelger–Huet's leukocyte abnormality. *Haematologica* **53**, 394.

Tanphaichitr, P., Mekanandha, V. & Phuwastein, P. (1973) N.B.T. test in thalassaemia. *Asian J. Med.* **9**, 205.

Tanphaichitr, V., Suvatte, V., Mahasandana, C. & Tuchinda, S. (1978) Host defense in thalassemias and the effects of splenectomy. I. Incidence of mild and severe infections. *J. Med. Assoc. Thailand* **61**, 66.

Tanphaichitr, V.S., Pung-amritt, P., Puchaiwatanon, O. *et al.* (1985) Studies on haemoglobin Bart's and deletion of α-globin genes from cord blood in Thailand. *Abstracts of the International Congress on Thalassaemia*, p. 95. Medical Media, Bangkok.

Taramelli, R., Kioussis, D., Vanin, E. *et al.* (1986) γδβ-Thalassaemias 1 and 2 are the result of a 100 kbp deletion in the human β-globin cluster. *Nucl. Acids Res.* **14**, 7017.

Tas, I., Smith, P. & Cohen, T. (1976) Metric and morphologic characteristics of the dentition in beta thalassemia major in man. *Arch. Oral Biol.* **21**, 583.

Tasheva, E.S., Toshkov, S.A. & Dobreva, A.M. (1987) Hemoglobinopathies in Bulgaria. *Hemoglobin* **11**, 523.

Tate, V.E., Wood, W.G. & Weatherall, D.J. (1986) The British form of hereditary persistence of fetal haemoglobin results from a single base mutation adjacent to an S1 hypersensitive site 5′ to the ^Aγ globin gene. *Blood* **68**, 1389.

Tatsis, B. (1978) Hereditary persistence of fetal hemoglobin (HPFH) with β-chain production in *cis*: a new case in interaction with α-thalassemia. *Blood* **52** (Suppl.), 119.

Tatsumi, N., Tsuda, I., Funahara, Y. *et al.* (1992) Size distribution curves of blood cells in thalassemias and hemoglobin H. *Southeast Asian J. Trop. Med. Publ. Hlth* **23**, 79.

Tayebi, B. & Labie, D. (1974) Fréquence et diffusion de l'hémoglobine lepore. Intérêt d'une méthode simple d'analyse structurale. *Nouv. Rev. Fr. Hematol.* **14**, 677.

Tayles, N. (1996) Anemia, genetic diseases, and malaria in prehistoric mainland Southeast Asia. *Am. J. Physiol. Anthrop.* **101**, 11.

Taylor, J.M., Dozy, A., Kan, Y.W. *et al.* (1974) Genetic lesion in homozygous α-thalassemia (hydrops foetalis). *Nature* **251**, 392.

Tegos, C., Voutsadakis, A., Paleologou, N. *et al.* (1987) The incidence and distribution of thalassaemias in Greece (a study on 64,814 recruits). *Hellenic Armed Forces Med. Rev.* **21**, 27.

Telfer, P.T., Garson, J.A., Whitby, K. *et al.* (1997) Combination therapy with interferon alpha and ribavirin for chronic hepatitis C infection in thalassaemic patients. *Br. J. Haematol.* **98**, 850.

Temin, H.M. & Mizutani, S. (1970) RNA-dependent DNA polymerase in virions of Rous sarcoma virus. *Nature* **226**, 1211.

Temple, G.F., Chang, J.C. & Kan, Y.W. (1977) Authentic β-globin mRNA sequences in homozygous β⁰ thalassemia. *Proc. Natl Acad. Sci. USA* **74**, 3047.

Tenenbein, M., Kowalski, S., Sienko, A., Bowden, D.H. & Adamson, I.Y.R. (1992) Pulmonary toxic effects of continuous desferrioxamine administration in acute iron poisoning. *Lancet* **339**, 699.

Tentori, L., Bruni, E. & Marinucci, M. (1975) Three examples of association between beta-thalassemia and rare hemoglobin variants. In: *International Istanbul Symposium on Abnormal Hemoglobins and Thalassemia* (ed. M. Aksoy), p. 53. Ataturk, Ankara.

Terrenato, L., Shrestha, S., Dixit, K.A. *et al.* (1988) Decreased malaria morbidity in the Tharu people compared to sympatric populations in Nepal. *Ann. Trop. Med. Parasitol.* **82**, 1.

Testa, U., Dubart, A., Hinard, N. *et al.* (1980) Beta⁰-thalassaemia/Hb E association. Hemoglobin synthesis in blood reticulocytes and bone marrow cells fractionated by density gradient and in blood erythroid colonies in culture. *Acta Haematol.* **64**, 42.

Tewari, R., Gillemans, N., Wijgerde, M. *et al.* (1998) Erythroid Krüppel-like factor (EKLF) is active in primitive and definitive erythroid cells and is required for the function of 5′HS3 of the β-globin locus control region. *EMBO J.* **17**, 2334.

Thakerngpol, K., Fucharoen, S., Sumiyoshi, A. & Stitnimankarn, T. (1992) Liver tissue injury secondary to iron overload in β-thalassemia/hemoglobin E disease. *Southeast Asian J. Trop. Med. Publ. Hlth* **23**, 110.

Thakerngpol, K., Fucharoen, S., Boonyaphipat, P. *et al.* (1996) Liver injury due to iron overload in thalassemia: histopathologic and ultrastructural studies. *Biometals* **9**, 177.

Thein, S.L. (1993) β-Thalassaemia. In: *Baillière's Clinical Haematology. International Practice and Research: The Haemoglobinopathies* (eds D.R. Higgs & D.J. Weatherall), p. 151. Baillière Tindall, London.

Thein, S.L. (1999) Is it dominantly inherited β thalassaemia or just a β-chain variant that is highly unstable? *Br. J. Haematol.* **107**, 12.

Thein, S.L. & Weatherall, D.J. (1989) A non-deletion hereditary persistence of fetal hemoglobin (HPFH) determinant not linked to the β-globin gene complex. In: *Hemoglobin Switching. Part B: Cellular and Molecular Mechanisms* (series eds G. Stamatoyannopoulos & A.W. Nienhuis), p. 97. Alan R. Liss, New York.

Thein, S.L., Al-Hakim, I. & Hoffbrand, A.V. (1984a) Thalassaemia intermedia: a new molecular basis. *Br. J. Haematol.* **56**, 333.

Thein, S.L., Old, J.M., Wainscoat, J.S., Petrou, M. & Modell, B. (1984b) Population and genetic studies suggest a single origin for the Indian deletion β⁰ thalassaemia. *Br. J. Haematol.* **57**, 271.

Thein, S.L., Wainscoat, J.S., Old, J.M. *et al.* (1985) Feasibility of prenatal diagnosis of β-thalassaemia with synthetic DNA probes in two Mediterranean populations. *Lancet* **ii**, 345.

Thein, S.L., Lynch, J.R., Old, J.M. & Weatherall, D.J. (1987a) Direct detection of haemoglobin E with Mnl I. *J. Med. Genet.* **24**, 110.

Thein, S.L., Sampietro, M., Old, J.M. *et al.* (1987b) Association of thalassaemia intermedia with a beta-globin gene haplotype. *Br. J. Haematol.* **65**, 370.

Thein, S.L., Hesketh, C., Wallace, R.B. & Weatherall, D.J. (1988a) The molecular basis of thalassaemia major and thalassaemia intermedia in Asian Indians: application to prenatal diagnosis. *Br. J. Haematol.* **70**, 225.

Thein, S.L., Wallace, R.B., Pressley, L., Clegg, J.B., Weatherall, D.J. & Higgs, D.R. (1988b) The polyadenylation site mutation in the α-globin gene cluster. *Blood* **71**, 313.

Thein, S.L., Hesketh, C., Brown, J.M., Anstey, A.V. & Weatherall, D.J. (1989) Molecular characterization of a high A₂ β thalassemia by direct sequencing of single strand enriched amplified genomic DNA. *Blood* **73**, 924.

Thein, S.L., Hesketh, C., Taylor, P. *et al.* (1990a) Molecular basis for dominantly inherited inclusion body β thalassemia. *Proc. Natl Acad. Sci. USA* **87**, 3924.

Thein, S.L., Winichagoon, P., Hesketh, C., Fucharoen, S., Wasi, P. & Weatherall, D.J. (1990b) The molecular basis of β-thalassemia in Thailand: application to prenatal diagnosis. *Am. J. Hum. Genet.* **47**, 369.

Thein, S.L., Best, S., Sharpe, J., Paul, B., Clark, D.J. & Brown, M.J. (1991) Hemoglobin Chesterfield (β 28 Leu→Arg) produces the phenotype of inclusion body β thalassemia. *Blood* **77**, 2791.

Thein, S.L., Barnetson, R. & Abdalla, S. (1992) A β-thalassemia variant associated with unusually high Hb A₂ in an Iranian family. *Blood* **79**, 2801.

Thein, S.L., Wood, W.G., Wickramasinghe, S.N. & Galvin, M.C. (1993) β-Thalassemia unlinked to the β-globin gene in an English family. *Blood* **82**, 961.

Thein, S.L., Sampietro, M., Rohde, K., Weatherall, D.J., Lathrop, G.M. & Demenais, F. (1994) Detection of a major gene for heterocellular HPFH after accounting for genetic modifiers. *Am. J. Hum. Genet.* **54**, 214.

Thermann, R., Neu-Yilik, G., Deters, A. *et al.* (1998) Binary specification of nonsense codons by splicing and cytoplasmic translation. *EMBO J.* **17**, 3484.

Thillet, J., Cohen-Solal, M., Seligmann, M. & Rosa, J. (1976) Functional and physiochemical studies of hemoglobin St. Louis β28 (B10) Leu→Gln. A variant with ferric β heme iron. *J. Clin. Invest.* **58**, 1098.

Thirawarapan, S.S., Snongchart, N., Fucharoen, S., Tanphaichitr, V.S. & Dhorranintra, B. (1989) Study of mechanisms of posttransfusion hypertension in thalassaemic patients. *Southeast Asian J. Trop. Med. Publ. Hlth* **20**, 471.

Thomas, E.D., Buckner, C.D., Sanders, J.E. *et al.* (1982) Marrow transplantation for thalassaemia. *Lancet* **ii**, 227.

Thompson, G.R. & Lehmann, H. (1962) Combinations of high levels of haemoglobin F with haemoglobins A, S and C in Ghana. *Br. Med. J.* **i**, 1521.

Thompson, R.B., Mitchner, J.W. & Huisman, T.H.J. (1961) Studies on the fetal hemoglobin in the persistent high Hb-F anomaly. *Blood* **18**, 267.

Thompson, R.B., Warrington, R., Odom, J. & Bell, W.N. (1965) Interaction between genes for delta thalassemia and hereditary persistence of fetal hemoglobin. *Acta Haematol.* **15**, 190.

Thompson, R.B., Odom, J., Ard, E. & Bell, W.N. (1966) Interaction between beta and delta thalassemia and hemoglobin D. *Acta Genet. (Basel)* **16**, 340.

Thompson, C.C., Ali, M.A. & Vacovsky, M. (1989) The interaction of anti 3.7 type quadruplicated α-globin genes and heterozygous β-thalassemia. *Hemoglobin* **13**, 125.

Thonglairuam, V., Winichagoon, P., Fucharoen, S. & Wasi, P. (1989) The molecular basis of AE-Bart's disease. *Hemoglobin* **13**, 117.

Thool, A.A., Walde, M.S., Shrikhande, A.V. & Talib, V.H. (1998) A simple screening test for the detection of heterozygous beta thalassemia. *Indian J. Pathol. Microbiol.* **41**, 423.

Thorpe, S.J., Thein, S.L., Sampietro, M., Craig, J.E., Mahon, B. & Huehns, E.R. (1994) Immunochemical estimation of haemoglobin types in red blood cells by FACS analysis. *Br. J. Haematol.* **87**, 125.

Thumasathit, B., Nondasuta, A., Silpisornkosol, S., Lousuebsakul, B., Unchalipongse, P. & Mangkornkanok, M. (1968) Hydrops fetalis associated with Bart's hemoglobin in northern Thailand. *J. Pediatr.* **73**, 132.

Ting, Y.L., Naccarato, S., Qualtieri, A., Chidichimo, G. & Brancati, C. (1994) *In vivo* metabolic studies of glucose, ATP and 2,3-DPG in β-thalassaemia intermedia, heterozygous β-thalassaemic and normal erythrocytes: ¹³C and ³¹P MRS studies. *Br. J. Haematol.* **88**, 547.

Titus, E.A.B., Hsia, Y.E. & Hunt, J.A. (1988) α-Thalassemia screening reveals quadruple ζ-globin genes in a Laotian family. *Hemoglobin* **12**, 539.

Toccafondi, R., Maioli, M. & Meloni, T. (1970a) The plasma HGH and 11-OHCS response to insulin induced hypoglycaemia in children affected by thalassemia major. *Riv. Clin. Med.* **70**, 102.

Toccafondi, R., Maioli, M. & Meloni, T. (1970b) Plasma insulin response to oral carbohydrate in Cooley's anemia. *Riv. Clin. Med.* **70**, 96.

Todd, D. (1978) Genes, beans and Marco Polo. *University of Hong Kong Gaz.* **XXVI**, 1.

Todd, D., Lai, M.C.S. & Braga, C.A. (1967) Thalassaemia and hydrops foetalis—family studies. *Br. Med. J.* **iii**, 347.

Todd, D., Lai, M.C.S., Braga, C.A. & Soo, H.N. (1969) Alpha-thalassaemia in Chinese: Cord blood studies. *Br. J. Haematol.* **16**, 551.

Todd, D., Lai, M.C.S., Beaven, G.H. & Huehns, E.R. (1970) The abnormal haemoglobins in homozygous α-thalassaemia. *Br. J. Haematol.* **19**, 27.

Tokarev, Y.N. & Spivak, V.A. (1982) Heterogeneity and distribution of hemoglobinopathies in some parts of the USSR. *Hemoglobin* **6**, 653.

Tokuda, K., Kyoshoin, K., Kitajima, K. *et al.* (1984) A case of sideroblastic anemia associated with acquired hemoglobin H. *Acta Haematol. (Japan)* **47**, 1396.

Tolis, G., Politis, C., Kontopoulou, I. *et al.* (1988) Pituitary somatotropic and corticotropic function in patients with β-thalassaemia on iron chelation therapy. *Birth Defects* **23**, 449.

Tolot, F., Bocquet, B. & Baron, M. (1970) Hemochromatosis and pigmentary cirrhosis in minor thalassemia in adults. *J. Med. Lyon* **51**, 655.

Tolstoshev, P., Mitchell, J., Lanyon, G. *et al.* (1976) Presence of gene for β globin in homozygous β⁰ thalassaemia. *Nature* **259**, 95.

Tondury, P., Kontoghiorghes, G.J., Ridolfi-Luthy, A.R. *et al.* (1990) L1 (1,2-dimethyl-3-hydroxypyrid-4-one) for oral iron chelation in patients with beta-thalassaemia major. *Br. J. Haematol.* **76**, 550.

Tondury, P., Zimmermann, A., Nielsen, P. & Hirt, A. (1998) Liver iron and fibrosis during long-term treatment with deferiprone in Swiss thalassaemic patients. *Br. J. Haematol.* **101**, 413.

Toselli, G., Bertoni, G., Alessio, L. & Mannucci, P.M. (1969) High incidence of thalassaemia in patients with intraocular haemorrhages. *Ophthalmologica* **157**, 343.

Tovo, P.A., Miniero, R. & Pontone, A. (1977) NBT test in thalassemia. *J. Pediatr.* **90**, 666.

Townes, T.M. & Behringer, R.R. (1990) Human globin locus activation region (LAR): Role in temporal control. *Trends Genet.* **6**, 219.

Townes, T.M., Lingrel, J.B., Chen, H.Y., Brinster, R.L. & Palmiter, R.D. (1985) Erythroid-specific expression of human β-globin genes in transgenic mice. *EMBO J.* **4**, 1715.

Trabuchet, G., Pagnier, J., Benabadji, M. & Labie, D. (1976–77) Homozygous cases for hemoglobin J Mexico (α⁵⁴(E3) Gln→Glu). Evidence for a duplicated α gene with unequal expression. *Hemoglobin* **1**, 13.

Trabuchet, G., Belhani, M., Richard, F., Hanladji, R., Benebadji, M. & Colonna, P. (1977a) Premières observations d'alpha-thalassémie en Algérie: 12 cas de hémoglobinase H. *Sem. Hôp. Paris* **53**, 885.

Trabuchet, G., Dahmane, M. & Benabadji, M. (1977b) Hemoglobin anormales en Algerie. *Sem. Hôp. Paris* **52**, 879.

Traeger, J., Wood, W.G., Clegg, J.B., Weatherall, D.J. & Wasi, P. (1980) Defective synthesis of Hb E is due to reduced levels of βᴱ mRNA. *Nature* **288**, 497.

Traeger, J., Winichagoon, P. & Wood, W.G. (1982) Instability of β^E-messenger RNA during erythroid cell maturation in hemoglobin E homozygotes. *J. Clin. Invest.* **69**, 1050.

Traeger-Synodinos, J., Tzetis, M., Kanavakis, E., Metaxotou-Mavromati, A. & Kattamis, C. (1991) The Corfu $\delta\beta$ thalassaemia mutation in Greece: haematological phenotype and prevalence. *Br. J. Haematol.* **79**, 302.

Traeger-Synodinos, J., Kanavakis, E., Tzetis, M., Kattamis, A. & Kattamis, C. (1993) Characterization of nondeletion α-thalassemia mutations in the Greek population. *Am. J. Hematol.* **44**, 162.

Traeger-Synodinos, J., Kanavakis, E., Vrettou, C. *et al.* (1996) The triplicated α-globin gene locus in β-thalassaemia heterozygotes: clinical, haematological, biosynthetic and molecular studies. *Br. J. Haematol.* **95**, 467.

Tran, K.C., Webb, D.J. & Pootrakul, P. (1990a) β-Thalassaemia/haemoglobin E tissue ferritins. II: A comparison of heart and pancreas ferritins with those of liver and spleen. *Biol.-Met.* **3**, 227.

Tran, K.C., Webb, J., Macey, D.J., Pootrakul, P. & Yansukon, P. (1990b) β-Thalassaemia/haemoglobin E tissue ferritins. I: Purification and partial characterization of liver and spleen ferritins. *Biol.-Met.* **3**, 222.

de Traverse, P.-M., Chat, L.X. & Coquelet, M.L. (1959) Les hémoglobinopathies au Viet-nam. In: *Proceedings of the Seventh Congress of the European Society of Haematology*, p. 1053. S. Karger, Basel.

Trecartin, R.F., Liebhaber, S.A., Chang, J.C., Lee, Y.W. & Kan, Y.W. (1981) β^0-Thalassaemia in Sardinia is caused by a nonsense mutation. *J. Clin. Invest.* **68**, 1012.

Treisman, R., Proudfoot, N.J., Shander, M. & Maniatis, T. (1982) A single base change at a splice site in a β^0-thalassemic gene causes abnormal RNA splicing. *Cell* **29**, 903.

Treisman, R., Orkin, S.H. & Maniatis, T. (1983) Specific transcription and RNA splicing defects in five cloned β-thalassaemia genes. *Nature* **302**, 591.

Trent, R.J., Higgs, D.R., Clegg, J.B. & Weatherall, D.J. (1981) A new triplicated α-globin gene arrangement in man. *Br. J. Haematol.* **49**, 149.

Trent, R.J., Davis, B., Wilkinson, T. & Kronenberg, H. (1984a) Identification of β variant hemoglobins by DNA restriction endonuclease mapping. *Hemoglobin* **8**, 443.

Trent, R.J., Jones, R.W., Clegg, J.B., Weatherall, D.J., Davidson, R. & Wood, W.G. (1984b) ($^A\gamma\delta\beta$) Thalassaemia: similarity of phenotype in four different molecular defects, including one newly described. *Br. J. Haematol.* **57**, 279.

Trent, R.J., Mickleson, K.N.P., Wilkinson, T. *et al.* (1985) α Globin gene rearrangements in Polynesians are not associated with malaria. *Am. J. Hematol.* **18**, 431.

Trent, R.J., Mickleson, K.N.P., Wilkinson, T. *et al.* (1986a) Globin genes in Polynesians have many rearrangements including a recently described $\gamma\gamma\gamma$/. *Am. J. Hum. Genet.* **39**, 350.

Trent, R.J., Svirklys, L., Harris, M.G., Hocking, D.R. & Kronenberg, H. (1986b) ($\delta\beta$)^0 Thalassaemia of the Southern Italian type. Its geographical origin and interaction with the sickle cell gene. *Pathology* **18**, 117.

Trent, R.J., Wilkinson, T., Yakas, J., Carter, J., Lammi, A. & Kronenberg, H. (1986c) Molecular defects in 2 examples of severe HbH disease. *Scand. J. Haematol.* **36**, 272.

Trent, R.J., Svirklys, L. & Jones, P. (1988) Thai ($\delta\beta$)^0-thalassaemia and its interaction with γ-thalassaemia. *Hemoglobin* **12**, 101.

Trent, R.J., Williams, B.G., Kearney, A., Wilkinson, T. & Harris, P.C. (1990) Molecular and hematologic characterization of Scottish-Irish type ($\epsilon\gamma\delta\beta$)^0 thalassaemia. *Blood* **76**, 2132.

Trepicchio, W.L., Dyer, M.A. & Baron, M.H. (1993) Developmental regulation of the human embryonic β-like globin gene is mediated by synergistic interactions among multiple tissue- and stage-specific elements. *Mol. Cell. Biol.* **13**, 7457.

Trepicchio, W.L., Dyer, M.A. & Baron, M.H. (1994) A novel developmental regulatory motif required for stage-specific activation of the epsilon-globin gene and nuclear factor binding in embryonic erythroid cells. *Mol. Cell. Biol.* **14**, 3763.

Trifillis, P., Ioannou, P., Schwartz, E. & Surrey, S. (1991) Identification of four novel δ-globin gene mutations in Greek Cypriots using polymerase chain reaction and automated fluorescence-based DNA sequence analysis. *Blood* **78**, 3298.

Trifillis, P., Kyrri, A., Kalogirou, E. *et al.* (1993) Analysis of δ-globin gene mutations in Greek Cypriots. *Blood* **82**, 1647.

Trimborn, T., Gribnau, J., Grosveld, F. & Fraser, P. (1999) Mechanisms of developmental control of transcription in the murine α- and β-globin loci. *Genes Dev.* **13**, 112.

Trudel, M. & Costantini, F. (1987) A 3′ enhancer contributes to the stage-specific expression of the human β-globin gene. *Genes Dev.* **1**, 954.

Tsiantis, J. (1990) Family reactions and relationships in thalassemia. *Ann. N. Y. Acad. Sci.* **612**, 451.

Tsistrakis, G.A., Amarantos, S.P. & Konkouris, L.L. (1974) Homozygous $\beta\delta$-thalassaemia. *Acta Haematol.* **51**, 185.

Tsistrakis, G.A., Scampardonis, G.J., Clonizakis, J.P. & Concouris, L.L. (1975) Haemoglobin D and β thalassaemia. A family report comprising 18 members. *Acta Haematol.* **54**, 172.

Tso, S.C., Chan, T.K. & Todd, D. (1982) Venous thrombosis in haemoglobin H disease after splenectomy. *Aust. N. Z. J. Med.* **12**, 635.

Tso, S.C., Loh, T.T. & Todd, D. (1984) Iron overload in patients with haemoglobin H disease. *Scand. J. Haematol.* **32**, 391.

Tsukamoto, H., Horne, W., Kamimura, S. *et al.* (1995) Experimental liver cirrhosis induced by alcohol and iron. *J. Clin. Invest.* **96**, 620.

Tuan, D., Biro, P.A., de Riel, J.K., Lazarus, H. & Forget, B.G. (1979) Restriction endonuclease mapping of the human gamma globin gene loci. *Nucl. Acids Res.* **6**, 2519.

Tuan, D., Murnane, M.J., de Riel, J.K. & Forget, B.G. (1980) Heterogeneity in the molecular basis of hereditary persistence of fetal haemoglobin. *Nature* **285**, 335.

Tuan, D., Feingold, E., Newman, M., Weissman, S.M. & Forget, B.G. (1983) Different 3′ end points of deletions causing $\delta\beta$-thalassemia and hereditary persistence of fetal hemoglobin; implications for the control of γ-globin gene expression in man. *Proc. Natl Acad. Sci. USA* **80**, 6937

Tuan, D.Y.H., Solomon, W.B., Li, Q. & London, I.M. (1985) The 'β-like globin' domain in human erythroid cells. *Proc. Natl Acad. Sci. USA* **82**, 6384.

Tuan, D., Kong, S. & Hu, K. (1992) Transcription of the hypersensitive site HS2 enhancer in erythroid cells. *Proc. Natl Acad. Sci. USA* **89**, 11219.

Tuchinda, S., Vareenil, C., Bhanchit, P. & Minnich, V. (1959) 'Fast' hemoglobin component found in umbilical-cord blood of Thai babies. *Pediatr.* **24**, 43.

Tuchinda, S., Rucknagel, D.L., Minnich, V., Boonyaprakob, U., Balankura, K. & Suvatee, V. (1964) The coexistence of the genes for haemoglobin E and alpha thalassemia in Thais, with resultant suppression of hemoglobin E synthesis. *Am. J. Hum. Genet.* **16**, 311.

Tuchinda, S., Beale, D. & Lehmann, D. (1967) The suppression of haemoglobin E synthesis when haemoglobin H disease and haemoglobin E trait occur together. *Humangenetik* **3**, 312.

Tuchinda, C., Punnakanta, L. & Angsusingha, K. (1978) Endocrine disturbances in thalassemia children. *J. Med. Assoc. Thailand* **61**, 55.

Turrini, F., Arese, P. & Low, P.S. (1991) Clustering of integral membrane proteins of the human erythrocyte membrane stimulates autologous IgS binding, complement deposition and phagocytosis. *J. Biol. Chem.* **266**, 23611.

Turrini, F., Mannu, F., Cappadoro, M., Ulliers, D., Girbaldi, G. & Arese, P. (1994) Binding of natural occurring antibodies to oxidatively and nonoxidatively modified erythrocyte band 3. *Biochim. Biophys. Acta* **1190**, 297.

Tyuma, I. & Shimizu, K. (1969) Different response to organic phosphates of human fetal and adult hemoglobins. *Arch. Biochem. Biophys.* **129**, 404.

Tzetis, M., Traeger-Synodinos, J., Kanavakis, E., Metaxotou-Mavromati, A. & Kattamis, C. (1994) The molecular basis of Hb A$_2$ (type 2) β-thalassemia in Greece. *Hematol. Pathol.* **8**, 25.

Tzotzos, S., Kanavakis, E., Metaxotou-Mavromati, A. & Kattamis, C. (1986) The molecular basis of HbH disease in Greece. *Br. J. Haematol.* **63**, 263.

Udomsangpetch, R., Sueblinvong, T., Pattanapanyasat, K., Dharmkrong-at, A., Kittilayawong, A. & Webster, H.K. (1993) Alteration in cytoadherence and rosetting of *Plasmodium falciparum*-infected thalassemic red blood cells. *Blood* **82**, 3752.

Ulrich, M.J. & Ley, T.J. (1990) Function of normal and mutated γ-globin gene promoters in electroporated K562 erythroleukemia cells. *Blood* **75**, 990.

Ulrich, M.J., Gray, W.J. & Ley, T.J. (1992) An intramolecular DNA triplex is disrupted by point mutations associated with hereditary persistence of fetal hemoglobin. *J. Biol. Chem.* **267**, 18649.

Untario, S. (1988) Trait of thalassaemia and haemoglobin E in Surabaya, Indonesia. *Trop. Geogr. Med.* **40**, 128.

Untario, S., Netty, R.H.T. & Bambang, P. (1986) Trait thalassemia dan hemoglobinopatia pada sekelompok mahasiswa kedokteran dan dokter anak di Surabaya, p. 30. In: *Kongres Nasional V perhimpunan Hematologi dan Transfusi Darah, Indonesia.* Semarang, Indonesia.

Vaeusorn, O., Fucharoen, S., Ruangpiroj, T. *et al.* (1985) Fetal pathology and maternal morbidity in hemoglobin Bart's hydrops fetalis: an analysis of 65 cases. In: *First International Conference on Thalassemia,* Bangkok.

Valassi-Adam, H., Nassika, E., Kattamis, C. & Matsaniotis, N. (1976) Immunoglobulin levels in children with homozygous beta-thalassemia. *Acta Paediatr. Scand.* **65**, 23.

Valenti, C. (1973) Antenatal detection of hemoglobinopathies — a preliminary report. *Am. J. Obstet. Gynecol.* **115**, 851.

Valentine, W.N. & Neel, J.V. (1944) Hematologic and genetic study of transmission of thalassemia (Cooley's anemia: Mediterranean anemia). *Arch. Intern. Med.* **74**, 185.

Valentine, W.N. & Neel, J.V. (1948) A statistical study of the hematologic variables in subjects with thalassemia minor. *Am. J. Med. Sci.* **215**, 456.

Van Baelen, H., Vandepitte, J., Cornu, G. & Eeckels, R. (1969) Routine detection of sickle-cell anaemia and haemoglobin Bart's in Congolese neonates. *Trop. Geogr. Med.* **21**, 412.

Vandenplas, S., Higgs, D.R., Nicholls, R.D., Bester, A.J. & Mathew, C.G.P. (1987) Characterization of a new α^0 thalassaemia defect in the South African population. *Br. J. Haematol.* **66**, 539.

Van der Ploeg, L.H.T., Konings, A., Cort, M., Roos, D., Bernini, L. & Flavell, R.A. (1980) γ-β-Thalassaemia studies showing that deletion of the γ- and δ-genes influences β-globin gene expression in man. *Nature* **283**, 637.

Van der Weyden, M.B., Fong, H., Hallam, L.J. & Harrison, C. (1989) Red cell ferritin and iron overload in heterozygous β-thalassemia. *Am. J. Hematol.* **30**, 201.

Van Slyck, E.J. (1976) Joint effusions in sickle cell-beta-thalassemia disease. *J. A. M. A.* **236**, 2941.

Vanin, E.F., Henthorn, P.S. & Kioussis, D. (1983) Unexpected relationships between four large deletions in the human β-globin gene cluster. *Cell* **35**, 701.

Vannassaeng, S., Ploybutr, S., Visutakul, P., Tandhanand, S., Suwanik, R. & Wasi, P. (1978) Endocrine functions in thalassemia patients. *J. Med. Assoc. Thailand* **61**, 54.

Varawalla, N.Y., Old, J.M., Sarkar, R., Venkatesan, R. & Weatherall, D.J. (1991a) The spectrum of β-thalassaemia mutations on the Indian subcontinent: the basis for prenatal diagnosis. *Br. J. Haematol.* **78**, 242.

Varawalla, N.Y., Old, J.M. & Weatherall, D.J. (1991b) Rare β-thalassaemia mutations in Asian Indians. *Br. J. Haematol.* **79**, 640.

Vassilopoulos, G., Papassotiriou, I., Voskaridou, E. *et al.* (1995) Hb Arta [β45(CD4) Phe→Cys]: a new unstable haemoglobin with reduced oxygen affinity in *trans* with β-thalassaemia. *Br. J. Haematol.* **91**, 595.

Vassilopoulou-Sellin, R., Oyedeji, C.O., Foster, P.L., Thompson, M.M. & Saman, N.A. (1989) Haemoglobin as a direct inhibitor of cartilage growth *in vitro. Horm. Metab. Res.* **21**, 11.

Vatanavicharn, S., Avunatankulchai, M., Na-nakorn, S. & Wasi, P. (1978) Serum and erythrocyte folate levels in thalassemia patients. *J. Med. Assoc. Thailand* **61**, 56.

Vatanavicharn, S., Anuvatanakulchai, M., Na-Nakorn, S. & Wasi, P. (1979) Serum erythrocyte folate levels in thalassaemia patients in Thailand. *Scand. J. Haematol.* **22**, 241.

Vatanavicharn, S., Anuwatanakulchai, M., Tuntawiroon, M., Suwanik, R. & Wasi, P. (1983) Iron absorption in patients with β-thalassemia/haemoglobin E disease and the effect of splenectomy. *Acta Haematol.* **69**, 414.

Vaughan, J. (1936) *The Anaemias,* 2nd edn. Oxford Medical Publications, Oxford University Press, Oxford.

Vaughan, J. (1948) Anaemia associated with trauma and sepsis. *Br. Med. J.* **i**, 35.

Vecchio, F. (1946) Sulla resistenza della emoglobina alla denaturazione alcalina in alcune sindromi emopatiche. *Pediatria* **54**, 545.

Vedovato, M., Salvatorelli, G., Taddei-Masieri, M. & Vullo, C. (1993) Epo serum levels in heterozygous β-thalassemia. *Haematologia-Budap.* **25**, 19.

Veer, A., Kosciolek, B.A., Bauman, A.W. & Rowley, P.T. (1979) Acquired hemoglobin H disease in idiopathic myelofibrosis. *Am. J. Hematol.* **6**, 199.

Velati, C., Sampietro, M., Sciariada, L. *et al.* (1983) Neonatal screening for Hb Bart's in Italian subjects of heterogeneous regional origin born in Lombardy. *Haematologica* **68**, 20.

Velati, C., Sampietro, M., Biassoni, M. *et al.* (1986) Alpha thalassaemia in an Italian population. *Br. J. Haematol.* **63**, 497.

Vella, F. (1958a) Hereditary abnormalities in human haemoglobin synthesis. In: *Proceedings of the Centenary and Bicentenary Congress of Biology,* p. 193. University of Malaya Press, Singapore.

Vella, F. (1958b) The incidence of abnormal haemoglobin variants in Singapore and Malaya. *Indian J. Child Hlth* **7**, 804.

Vella, F. (1959) Haemoglobin A$_2$ estimations by starch block electrophoresis. *Med. J. Malaya* **14**, 31.

Vella, F. (1962a) Abnormal haemoglobins, thalassaemia and erythrocyte glucose-6-phosphate dehydrogenase deficiency in Singapore and Malaya. *Oceania* **32**, 219.

Vella, F. (1962b) The frequency of thalassaemia minor in the Maltese Islands. *Acta Haematol.* **27**, 278.

Vella, F. (1965) The haemoglobinopathies in the Sudan. In: *Abnormal Haemoglobins in Africa* (ed. J.H.P. Jonxis), p. 339. F.A. Davis, Philadelphia.

Vella, F. (1977) Variation in hemoglobin A$_2$. *Hemoglobin* **1**, 619.

Vella, F. & Lehmann, H. (1974) Haemoglobin D Punjab (D Los Angeles). *J. Med. Genet.* **11**, 341.

Vella, F. & Tavaria, D. (1961) Haemoglobin variants in Sarawak and North Borneo. *Nature* **190**, 729.

Vella, F., Wells, R.H.C., Ager, J.A.M. & Lehmann, H. (1958) A haemoglobinopathy involving haemoglobin H and a new (Q) haemoglobin. *Br. Med. J.* **i**, 752.

Vellodi, A., Picton, S., Downie, C.J.C., Eltumi, M., Stevens, R. & Evans, D.I.K. (1994) Bone marrow transplantation for thalassemia: experience of two British centres. *Bone Marrow Transplant.* **13**, 559.

Venkatesan, R., Sarkar, R. & Old, J.M. (1992) β-Thalassaemia mutations and their linkage to β-haplotypes in Tamil Nadu in Southern India. *Clin. Genet.* **42**, 251.

Ventruto, V., Cimino, R., de Rosa, L. & Quatrrin, N. (1967) Disease due to Hb Lepore and δβ-microcythemia. The first observation. *Prog. Med. Roma* **23**, 920.

Ventruto, V., de Rosa, C., Mastrobuoni, A., Cimino, R. & Quattrin, N. (1970) Studio di una famiglia benecetans con emoglobine Lepore e J Oxford. Prima osservaxione di doppia eterozigosi fra Hb Lepore e Hb J Oxford. *Prog. Med. Roma* **26**, 681.

Verma, I.C., Saxena, R., Thomas, E. & Jain, P.K. (1997) Regional distribution of β-thalassemia mutations in India. *Hum. Genet.* **100**, 109.

Vetter, B., Schwarz, C., Kohne, E. & Kulozik, A.E. (1997) Betathalassaemia in the immigrant and non-immigrant German populations. *Br. J. Haematol.* **97**, 266.

Vetter, B., Neu-Yilik, G., Kohne, E. *et al.* (2000) Dominant β-thalassaemia: a highly unstable haemoglobin is caused by a novel 6 bp deletion of the β-globin gene. *Br. J. Haematol.* **108**, 176.

Vettore, L., Falezza, G.C., Cetto, G.L. & de Matteis, M.C. (1974) Cation content and membrane deformability of heterozygous beta-thalassemia red blood cells. *Br. J. Haematol.* **27**, 429.

Vettore, L., Corvi, C. & de Matteis, M.C. (1977a) Rapporti tra permeabilita di membrana al potassio e contenuto in ATP dei globuli rossi ipochrimica. In: *Atti del XXXVI Congresso Nazionale della Societa Italiana di Ematologia*, p. 766.

Vettore, L., de Matteis, M.C. & Antoni, L. (1977b) Permeability of membrane to potassium in hypochromic red cells with different specific density. *Acta Haematol.* **58**, 145.

Vettore, L., de Matteis, M.C. & del Conte, G. (1977c) Effects of dipyridamole on sodium and potassium content of human red blood cells. *Acta Haematol.* **57**, 193.

Vezzoso, B. (1946) Influenza della malaria sulla mortalita infantile per anemia con speciale riguardo al morbo di Cooley. *Riv. Malarial.* **XXV**, 61.

Vichinsky, E.P. (1998) The morbidity of bone disease in thalassemia. *Ann. N. Y. Acad. Sci.* **850**, 344.

Vichinsky, E.P., Haberkern, C.M., Neumayr, L. *et al.* (1995) A comparison of conservative and aggressive transfusion regimens in the perioperative management of sickle cell disease. The Preoperative Transfusion in Sickle Cell Disease Study Group. *N. Eng. J. Med.* **333**, 206.

Vickers, M.A. & Higgs, D.R. (1989) A novel deletion of the entire α-globin gene cluster in a British individual. *Br. J. Haematol.* **72**, 471.

Vidaud, M., Gattoni, R., Stevenin, J. *et al.* (1989) A 5′ splice-region G→C mutation in exon 1 of the human β-globin gene inhibits pre-mRNA splicing: a mechanism for β+-thalassaemia. *Proc. Natl Acad. Sci. USA* **86**, 1041.

Viens, A.M., Sharma, S. & Olivieri, N.F. (1998) Re-assessment of the value of splenectomy in thalassemia major (TM). *Blood* **92**, 533a.

Vigi, V., Volpato, S., Gaburro, D., Conconi, F., Bargellessi, A. & Pontremoli, S. (1969) The correlation between red-cell survival and excess of α-globin synthesis in β-thalassaemia. *Br. J. Haematol.* **16**, 25.

Villard, L., Gecz, J., Mattéi, J.F. *et al.* (1996a) XNP mutation in a large family with Juberg–Marsidi syndrome. *Nature Genet.* **12**, 359.

Villard, L., Lacombe, D. & Fontés, M. (1996b) A point mutation in the XNP gene, associated with an ATR-X phenotype without α-thalassemia. *Eur. J. Hum. Genet.* **4**, 316.

Villard, L., Toutain, A., Lossi, A.-M. *et al.* (1996c) Splicing mutation in the ATR-X gene can lead to a dysmorphic mental retardation phenotype without α-thalassaemia. *Am. J. Hum. Genet.* **58**, 499.

Villari, N., Caramella, D., Lippi, A. & Guazeli, C. (1992) Assessment of liver iron overload in thalassemic patients by MR imaging. *Acta Radiol.* **4**, 347.

Villegas, A., Perez Gutierrez, A., Diaz Mediavilla, J. & Espinos, D. (1979) Observaciones de alfa-talasemia y de hemoglobina H en espanoles. *Sangre* **24**, 1088.

Villegas, A., Calero, F., Vickers, M.A., Ayyub, H. & Higgs, D.R. (1989) α Thalassaemia in two Spanish families. *Eur. J. Haematol.* **44**, 110.

Villegas, A., Sanchez, J. & Sal del Rio, E. (1992) α-Globin genotypes in a Spanish population. *Hemoglobin* **16**, 427.

Villegas, A., Sanchez, J., Ricard, P. *et al.* (1994) Characterization of a new α-thalassemia-1 mutation in a Spanish family. *Hemoglobin* **18**, 29.

Vincent, S.H. (1989) Oxidative effects of heme and porphyrins on proteins and lipids. *Sem. Hematol.* **26**, 105.

Visuphiphan, S., Ketsa-Ard, K., Tumliang, S. & Piankijagum, A. (1994) Significance of blood coagulation and platelet profiles in relation to pulmonary thrombosis in β-thalassemia/Hb E. *Southeast Asian J. Trop. Med. Publ. Hlth* **25**, 449.

Vogel, F. & Motulsky, A.G. (1986) *Human Genetics. Problems and Approaches*, 2nd edn. Springer-Verlag, Berlin.

Vogt, M., Lang, T., Frösner, G. *et al.* (1999) Prevalence and clinical outcome of hepatitis C infection in children who underwent cardiac surgery before the implementation of blood-donor screening. *N. Eng. J. Med.* **341**, 866.

Von Jaksch, R. (1889) Uber Leukaemia und Leukocytose im Kindesalter. *Wein. Klin. Wchnschr.* **2**, 435.

Von Jaksch, R. (1890) Uber Diagnose und Therapie der Erkrankungen des Blutes. *Prog. Med. Wschchr.* **15**, 389.

Voskaridou, E., Kollia, P. & Loukopoulos, D. (1990) Sickle cell thalassemia in Greece: Identification and contribution of the interacting β-thalassemia gene. *Ann. N. Y. Acad. Sci.* **612**, 508.

Voskaridou, E., Konstantopoulos, K., Kollia, P., Papadakis, M. & Loukopoulos, D. (1995) Hb Lepore (Pylos)/Hb S compound heterozygosity in two Greek families. *Am. J. Hematol.* **49**, 131.

Voskaridou, E., Kyrtsonis, M.-C. & Loutradi-Anagnostou, A. (1999) Healing of chronic leg ulcers in the hemoglobinopathies with perilesional injections of granulocyte–macrophage colony-stimulating factor. *Blood* **93**, 3568.

Vullo, C. & Tunioli, A.M. (1958) Survival studies of thalassaemiac erythrocytes transfused into donors, into subjects with thalassaemia minor and into normal and splenectomized subjects. *Blood* **13**, 803.

Vullo, C., De Sanctis, V., Katz, M. *et al.* (1990) Endocrine abnormalities in thalassemia. *Ann. N. Y. Acad. Sci.* **612**, 293.

Vyas, P., Higgs, D.R., Weatherall, D.J., Dunn, D., Serjeant, B.E. & Serjeant, G.R. (1988) The interaction of alpha thalassaemia and sickle cell-beta⁰ thalassaemia. *Br. J. Haematol.* **70**, 449.

Vyas, P., Vickers, M.A., Simmons, D.L., Ayyub, H., Craddock, C.F. & Higgs, D.R. (1992) *Cis*-acting sequences regulating expression of the human α globin cluster lie within constitutively open chromatin. *Cell* **69**, 781.

Vyas, P., Vickers, M.A., Picketts, D.J. & Higgs, D.R. (1995) Conservation of position and sequence of a novel, widely expressed gene containing the major human α-globin regulatory element. *Genomics* **29**, 679.

Waber, P.G., Bender, M.A., Gelinas, R.E. et al. (1986) Concordance of a point mutation 5′ to the $^A\gamma$ globin gene in $^A\gamma\beta^+$ HPFH in Greeks. Blood 67, 551.

Wada, Y., Fujita, T., Kidoguchi, K. & Hayashi, A. (1986) Fetal hemoglobin variants in 80,000 Japanese neonates: high prevalence of Hb F Yamaguchi ($^A\gamma$T 80 Asp-Asn). Hum. Genet. 72, 196.

Wagstaff, M., Peters, S.W., Jones, B.M. & Jacobs, A. (1985) Free iron and iron toxicity in iron overload. Br. J. Haematol. 61, 566.

Wahidijat, I., Markum, A.H. & Adang, Z.K. (1972) Early splenectomy in the management of thalassemic children in Djakarta. Acta Haematol. 48, 28.

Wahidijat, I., Markum, A.H. & Moeslichan, S. (1974) A case of thalassemia-Hb S disease in Jakarta. Paediatr. Indones. 14, 128.

Wahidiyat, I., Modell, B.C., Muslichan, M. & Abdulsalem, M. (1987) Thalassemia and its problems in Indonesia by the year 2000. In: Thalassemia: Pathophysiology and Management, Part B (eds S. Fucharoen, P.T. Rowley & N.W. Paul), p. 349. Alan R Liss, New York.

Wainscoat, J.S., Kanavakis, E., Weatherall, D.J. et al. (1981) Regional localisation of the human α-globin genes. Lancet 2, 301.

Wainscoat, J.S., Kanavakis, E., Wood, W.G. et al. (1983a) Thalassaemia intermedia in Cyprus—the interaction of α- and β-thalassaemia. Br. J. Haematol. 53, 411.

Wainscoat, J.S., Old, J.M., Weatherall, D.J. & Orkin, S.H. (1983b) The molecular basis for the clinical diversity of β thalassaemia in Cypriots. Lancet i, 1235.

Wainscoat, J.S., Bell, J.I., Thein, S.L. et al. (1983c) Multiple origins of the sickle mutation: evidence from beta S globin gene cluster polymorphisms. Mol. Biol. Med. 1, 191.

Wainscoat, J.S., Old, J.M., Thein, S.L. & Weatherall, D.J. (1984a) A new DNA polymorphism for prenatal diagnosis of β-thalassaemia in Mediterranean populations. Lancet 2, 1299.

Wainscoat, J.S., Old, J.M., Wood, W.G., Trent, R.J. & Weatherall, D.J. (1984b) Characterization of an Indian $(\delta\beta)^0$ thalassaemia. Br. J. Haematol. 58, 353.

Wainscoat, J.S., Thein, S.L., Wood, W.G. et al. (1985) A novel deletion in the β globin gene complex. Ann. N. Y. Acad. Sci. 445, 20.

Wainscoat, J.S., Thein, S.L. & Weatherall, D.J. (1987) Thalassaemia intermedia. Blood Rev. 1, 273.

Walker, J. & Turnbull, E.P.N. (1955) Haemoglobin and red cells in the human foetus. III. Foetal and adult haemoglobins. Arch. Dis. Child. 30, 111.

Walker, E.H., Whelton, M.J. & Beaven, G.H. (1969) Successful pregnancy in a patient with thalassaemia major. J. Obstet. Gynaecol. Br. Commonw. 76, 549.

Wall, L., de Boer, E. & Grosveld, F. (1988) The human beta-globin gene 3′ enhancer contains multiple binding sites for an erythroid-specific protein. Genes Dev. 2, 1089.

Wallace, R.B., Schold, M., Johnson, M.J., Dember, P. & Itakura, K. (1981) Oligonucleotide directed mutagenesis of the human β-globin gene: a general method for producing specific point mutations in cloned DNA. Nucl. Acids Res. 9, 3647.

Walters, M.C. & Thomas, E.D. (1994) Bone marrow transplantation for thalassemia: the United States experience. Am. J. Pediatr. Hematol. Oncol. 16, 1.

Walters, J.H. & Young, N.A. (1954) Micro-drepanocytic disease associated with megaloblastic anbaemia of pregnancy. Trans. Roy. Soc. Trop. Med. Hyg. 48, 253.

Walters, M.C., Patience, M., Leisenring, W. et al. (1996) Bone marrow transplantation for sickle cell disease. N. Eng. J. Med. 335, 369.

Wanachiwanawin, W., Phucharoen, J., Pattanapanyasat, K., Fucharoen, S. & Webster, H.K. (1996) Lymphocytes in β-thalassemia/Hb E: subpopulations and mitogen responses. Eur. J. Haematol. 56, 153.

Wang, Z. & Liebhaber, S.A. (1999) A 3′-flanking NF-κB site mediates developmental silencing of the human ζ-globin gene. EMBO J. 18, 2218.

Wang, C., Tso, S.C. & Todd, D. (1989) Hypogonadotropic hypogonadism in severe beta-thalassemia: effect of chelation and pulsatile gonadotrophin-releasing hormone therapy. J. Clin. Endocrinol. Metab. 68, 511.

Wang, X., Seaman, C., Paik, M., Chen, T., Bank, A. & Piomelli, S. (1994) Experience with 500 prenatal diagnoses of sickle cell diseases: the effect of gestational age on affected pregnancy outcome. Prenat. Diag. 14, 851.

Wapnick, A.A., Lynch, S.R., Charlton, R.W., Seftel, H.C. & Bothwell, T.H. (1969) The effect of ascorbic acid deficiency on desferrioxamine-induced iron excretion. Br. J. Haematol. 17, 563.

Ward, R.H., Modell, B., Petrou, M., Karagozlu, F. & Douratsos, E. (1983) A method of chorionic villi sampling in the first trimester of pregnancy under real time ultrasonic guidance. Brit. Med. J. Clin. Res. Ed. 286, 1542.

Wasi, P. (1970) The alpha thalassemia genes. J. Med. Assoc. Thailand 53, 677.

Wasi, P. (1972) Adverse effects of splenectomy. J. Med. Assoc. Thailand 55, 1.

Wasi, P. (1983) Hemoglobinopathies in Southeast Asia. In: Distribution and Evolution of the Hemoglobin and Globin Loci (ed. J.E. Bowman), p. 179. Elsevier, New York.

Wasi, P. & Fucharoen, S. (1995) The ethics of prenatal diagnosis in different religious and cultural contexts. In: Sickle Cell Disease and Thalassaemias: New Trends in Therapy (eds Y. Beyzard, B. Lubin & J. Rosa), p. 387. Colloque INSERM/John Libbey Eurotext Ltd., Paris.

Wasi, P., Na-Nakorn, S. & Suingdumrong, A. (1964) Haemoglobin H disease in Thailand: a genetical study. Nature 204, 907.

Wasi, P., Na-Nakorn, S. & Suingdumrong, A. (1967) Studies of the distribution of haemoglobin E, thalassaemias and glucose-6-phosphate dehydrogenase deficiency in North-eastern Thailand. Nature 214, 501.

Wasi, P., Disthasongchan, P. & Na-Nakorn, S. (1968a) The effect of iron deficiency on the levels of hemoglobins A_2 and E. J. Lab. Clin. Med. 71, 85.

Wasi, P., Pootrakul, S. & Na-Nakorn, S. (1968b) Hereditary persistence of foetal haemoglobin in a Thai family: the first instance in the mongol race and in association with Haemoglobin E. Br. J. Haematol. 14, 501.

Wasi, P., Na-Nakorn, S., Pootrakul, S. et al. (1969) Alpha- and beta-thalassemia in Thailand. Ann. N. Y. Acad. Sci. 165, 60.

Wasi, C., Wasi, P. & Thongcharoen, P. (1971) Serum immunoglobulin levels in thalassaemia and the effects of splenectomy. Lancet ii, 237.

Wasi, P., Na-Nakorn, S. & Pootrakul, S. (1974) The α thalassaemias. Clin. Haematol. 3, 383.

Wasi, P., Na-Nakorn, S., Pootrakul, P., Sonakul, D., Piankijagum, A. & Pacharee, P. (1978) A syndrome of hypertension, convulsions, and cerebral haemorrhage in thalassaemic patients after multiple blood transfusions. Lancet ii, 602.

Wasi, P., Pravatmuang, P. & Winichagoon, P. (1979) Immunologic diagnosis of α-thalassemia traits. Hemoglobin 3, 21.

Wasi, P., Fucharoen, S., Younghchaiyud, P. & Sonakul, D. (1982) Hypoxemia in thalassemia. Birth Defects 18, 213.

Wasi, P., Pootrakul, P., Fucharoen, S., Winichagoon, P., Wilairat, P. & Promboon, A. (1985) Thalassemia in Southeast Asia: determination of different degrees of severity of anemia in thalassemia. Ann. N. Y. Acad. Sci. 445, 119.

Wasi, C., Kuntang, R., Louisirirotchananakul, S. et al. (1988) Viral infections in β-thalassemia/hemoglobin E patients. *Birth Defects* **23**, 547.

Waters, H.M., Howarth, J.E., Hyde, K. *et al.* (1996) *Evaluation of the Bio-Rad Variant Beta Thalassaemia Short Program.* Medical Devices Agency, London.

Watson-Williams, E.J. (1965) Hereditary persistence of foetal haemoglobin and β-thalassaemia in Nigerians. In: *Abnormal Haemoglobins in Africa* (ed. J.H.P. Jonxis), p. 223. Blackwell Scientific Publications, Oxford.

Waugh, S.M., Walder, J.A. & Low, P.S. (1987) Partial characterization of the copolymerization reaction of erythrocyte membrane band 3 with hemichromes. *Biochemistry* **26**, 1777.

Waxman, H.S. & Brown, E.B. (1969) Clinical usefulness of iron chelating agents. *Prog. Hematol.* **6**, 338.

Waye, J.S., Cai, S.P., Eng, B. *et al.* (1991) High hemoglobin A_2 $β^0$-thalassemia due to a 532-basepair deletion of the 5′ β-globin gene region. *Blood* **77**, 1100.

Waye, J.S., Eng, B. & Chui, D.H.K. (1992) Identification of an extensive ζ-α globin gene deletion in a Chinese individual. *Br. J. Haematol.* **80**, 378.

Waye, J.S., Eng, B., Coleman, M.B., Steinberg, M.H. & Alter, B.P. (1994a) δβ-Thalassemia in an African-American: identification of the deletion endpoints and PCR-based diagnosis. *Hemoglobin* **18**, 389.

Waye, J.S., Eng, B., Hunt, J.A. & Chui, D.H.K. (1994b) Filipino β-thalassemia due to a large deletion: identification of the deletion endpoints and polymerase chain reaction (PCR)-based diagnosis. *Hum. Genet.* **94**, 530.

Waye, J.S., Eng, B., Olivieri, N.F. & Chui, D.H.K. (1994c) Identification of a novel $β^0$-thalassaemia mutation in a Greek family and subsequent prenatal diagnosis. *Prenat. Diag.* **14**, 929.

Waye, J.S., Eng, B., Patterson, M. *et al.* (1994d) Hb E/Hb Lepore-Hollandia in a family from Bangladesh. *Am. J. Hematol.* **47**, 262.

Waye, J.S., Eng, B., Patterson, M. & Chui, D.H.K. (1994e) Identification of a novel termination codon mutation (TAA→TAT, Term→Tyr) in the α2 globin gene of a Laotian girl with Hemoglobin H disease. *Blood* **83**, 3418.

Waye, J.S., Eng, B., Francombe, W.H. & Chui, D.H.K. (1995) Novel seventeen basepair deletion in exon 3 of the β-globin gene. *Hum. Mutat.* **6**, 252.

Waye, J.S., Eng, B., Patterson, M., Chui, D.H.K. & Olivieri, N.F. (1996) Novel mutation of the $α_2$-globin gene initiation codon (ATG→A-G) in a Vietnamese girl with HbH disease. *Blood* **88**, 28b.

Waye, J.S., Eng, B., Patterson, M., Barr, R.D. & Chui, D.H. (1997a) *De novo* mutation of the β-globin gene initiation codon (ATG→AAG) in a Northern European boy. *Am. J. Hematol.* **56**, 179.

Waye, J.S., Eng, B., Patterson, M., Fernandes, B.J. & Chui, D.H.K. (1997b) Novel $β^0$-thalassaemia mutation (codons 72/73-AGTGA +T) in a Canadian woman of British ancestry. *Hemoglobin* **21**, 385.

Waye, J.S., Eng, B., Patterson, M., Chui, D.H. & Fernandes, B.J. (1998) Novel beta-thalassemia mutation in patients of Jewish descent: [β 30(B12) Arg→Gly or IVS-I(-2) (A→G)]. *Hemoglobin* **22**, 83.

Weatherall, D.J. (1963) Abnormal haemoglobins in the neonatal period and their relationship to thalassaemia. *Br. J. Haematol.* **9**, 265.

Weatherall, D.J. (1964a) Biochemical phenotypes of thalassemia in the American Negro populations. *Ann. N. Y. Acad. Sci.* **119**, 450.

Weatherall, D.J. (1964b) Relationship of hemoglobin Bart's and H to alpha thalassemia. *Ann. N. Y. Acad. Sci.* **119**, 463.

Weatherall, D.J. (1965) *The Thalassaemia Syndromes.* Blackwell Scientific Publications, Oxford.

Weatherall, D.J. (1976) Fetal haemoglobin synthesis. In: *Congenital Disorders of Erythropoiesis. Ciba Foundation Symposium*, p. 307. North Holland, Amsterdam.

Weatherall, D.J. (1980) Toward an understanding of the molecular biology of some common inherited anemias: the story of thalassemia. In: *Blood, Pure and Eloquent* (ed. M.M. Wintrobe), p. 373. McGraw-Hill, New York.

Weatherall, D.J. (1991) Prenatal diagnosis of haematological disorders. In: *Fetal and Neonatal Haematology* (eds I.M. Hann, B.E.S. Gibson & E.A. Letsky), p. 285. Baillière Tindall, London.

Weatherall, D.J. (1992) Bone marrow transplantation for thalassemia and other inherited disorders of hemoglobin. *Blood* **80**, 1379.

Weatherall, D.J. (1996) Anaemia: Pathophysiology, classification, and clinical features. In: The Oxford Textbook of Medicine (eds D.J. Weatherall, J.G.G. Ledingham & D.A. Warrel), 3rd edn, p. 3457. Oxford University Press, Oxford.

Weatherall, D.J. (1998a) Gene therapy: Repairing hemoglobin disorders with ribozymes. *Curr. Biol.* **8**, R696.

Weatherall, D.J. (1998b) Hemoglobin E β-thalassemia: an increasingly common disease with some diagnostic pitfalls. *J. Pediatr.* **132**, 765.

Weatherall, D.J. & Baglioni, G. (1962) A fetal hemoglobin variant of unusual genetic interest. *Blood* **20**, 675.

Weatherall, D.J. & Boyer, S.H. (1961) The genetic control of the α chains of human hemoglobins. *Trans. Assoc. Am. Phys.* **74**, 89.

Weatherall, D.J. & Boyer, S.H. (1962) Evidence for the genetic identity of alpha chain determinants in hemoglobins A, A_2 and F. *Bull. Johns Hopkins Hosp.* **110**, 8.

Weatherall, D.J. & Clegg, J.B. (1969) Disorders of globin synthesis in thalassemia. *Ann. N. Y. Acad. Sci.* **165**, 242.

Weatherall, D.J. & Clegg, J.B. (1972) *The Thalassaemia Syndromes*, 2nd edn. Blackwell Scientific Publications, Oxford.

Weatherall, D.J. & Clegg, J.B. (1974) In vitro hemoglobin synthesis in the thalassemia syndromes. *Int. Rev. Exp. Path.* **13**, 117.

Weatherall, D.J. & Clegg, J.B. (1975) The α chain termination mutants and their relationship to thalassaemia. *Phil. Trans. Roy. Soc. Lond. B*, **271**, 411.

Weatherall, D.J. & Clegg, J.B. (1981) *The Thalassaemia Syndromes*, 3rd edn. Blackwell Scientific Publications, Oxford.

Weatherall, D.J. & Clegg, J.B. (1996) Thalassaemia—a global public health problem. *Nature Med.* **2**, 847.

Weatherall, D.J. & Clegg, J.B. (1999) Genetic disorders of hemoglobin. *Sem. Hematol.* **36**, 24.

Weatherall, D.J. & McIntyre, P.A. (1967) Developmental and acquired variations in erythrocyte carbonic anhydrase isozymes. *Br. J. Haematol.* **13**, 106.

Weatherall, D.J. & Vella, F. (1960) Thalassaemia in a Gurkha family. *Br. Med. J.* **i**, 1711.

Weatherall, D.J., Sigler, A.T. & Baglioni, C. (1962) Four hemoglobins in each of three brothers: genetic and biochemical significance. *Bull. Johns Hopkins Hosp.* **111**, 143.

Weatherall, D.J., Clegg, J.B. & Naughton, M.A. (1965) Globin synthesis in thalassemia: an *in vitro* study. *Nature* **208**, 1061.

Weatherall, D.J., Clegg, J.B., Blankson, J. & McNeil, J.R. (1969a) A new sickling disorder resulting from interaction of the genes for haemoglobin S and α-thalassaemia. *Br. J. Haematol.* **17**, 517.

Weatherall, D.J., Clegg, J.B., Na-Nakorn, S. & Wasi, P. (1969b) The pattern of disordered haemoglobin synthesis in homozygous and heterozygous β-thalassaemia. *Br. J. Haematol.* **16**, 251.

Weatherall, D.J., Clegg, J.B. & Boon, W.H. (1970) The haemoglobin constitution of infants with the haemoglobin Bart's hydrops foetalis syndrome. *Br. J. Haematol.* **18**, 357.

Weatherall, D.J., Gilles, H.M., Clegg, J.B. *et al.* (1971) Preliminary surveys for the prevalence of the thalassaemia genes in some African populations. *Ann. Trop. Med. Parasitol.* **65**, 253.

Weatherall, D.J., Clegg, J.B., Knox-Macaulay, H.H.M., Bunch, C., Hopkins, C.R. & Temperley, I.J. (1973) A genetically determined disorder with features of both thalassaemia and congenital dyserythropoietic anaemia. *Br. J. Haematol.* **24**, 681.

Weatherall, D.J., Clegg, J.B., Roberts, A.V. & Knox-Macaulay, H.H.M. (1974a) The clinical and chemical heterogeneity of the β-thalassemias. *Ann. N. Y. Acad. Sci.* **232**, 88.

Weatherall, D.J., Pembrey, M.E. & Pritchard, J. (1974b) Fetal haemoglobin. *Clin. Haematol.* **3**, 467.

Weatherall, D.J., Cartner, R., Clegg, J.B., Wood, W.G., Macrae, I.A. & MacKenzie, A. (1975) A form of hereditary persistence of fetal haemoglobin characterised by uneven cellular distribution of haemoglobin F and the production of haemoglobins A and A$_2$ in homozygotes. *Br. J. Haematol.* **29**, 205.

Weatherall, D.J., Clegg, J.B., Milner, P.F., Marsh, G.W., Bolton, F.G. & Serjeant, G.R. (1976) Linkage relationships between β- and δ-structural loci and African forms of thalassaemia. *J. Med. Genet.* **13**, 20.

Weatherall, D.J., Pippard, M.J. & Callender, S.T. (1977) Iron loading and thalassemia — experimental successes and practical realities. *N. Eng. J. Med.* **297**, 445.

Weatherall, D.J., Old, J., Longley, J. *et al.* (1978) Acquired haemoglobin H disease in leukaemia: pathophysiology and molecular basis. *Br. J. Haematol.* **38**, 305.

Weatherall, D.J., Wood, W.G. & Clegg, J.B. (1979) Genetics of fetal hemoglobin production in adult life. In: *Cellular and Molecular Regulation of Hemoglobin Switching* (eds G. Stamatoyannopoulos & S. W. Nienhuis), p. 3. Grune and Stratton, New York.

Weatherall, D.J., Clegg, J.B., Wood, W.G. *et al.* (1980) The clinical and molecular heterogeneity of the thalassaemia syndromes. *Ann. N. Y. Acad. Sci.* **344**, 83.

Weatherall, D.J., Higgs, D.R., Bunch, C. *et al.* (1981a) Hemoglobin H disease and mental retardation. A new syndrome or a remarkable coincidence? *N. Eng. J. Med.* **305**, 607.

Weatherall, D.J., Pressley, L., Wood, W.G., Higgs, D.R. & Clegg, J.B. (1981b) The molecular basis for mild forms of homozygous β thalassaemia. *Lancet* **i**, 527.

Weatherall, D.J., Old, J.M., Thein, S.L., Wainscoat, J.S. & Clegg, J.B. (1985) Prenatal diagnosis of the common haemoglobin disorders. *J. Med. Genet.* **22**, 422.

Weatherall, D.J., Clegg, J.B. & Kwiatkowski, D. (1997) The role of genomics in studying genetic susceptibility to infectious disease. *Genome Res.* **7**, 967.

Weatherall, D.J., Clegg, J.B., Higgs, D.R. & Wood, W.G. (2001) The hemoglobinopathies. In: *The Metabolic and Molecular Bases of Inherited Disease* (eds C.R. Scriver, A.L. Beaudet, W.S. Sly, D. Valle, B. Childs & B. Vogelstein), p. 471. McGraw-Hill, New York, in press.

Weatherall, D.J. & Letsky, E.A. (2000) Genetic haematological disorders. In: *Antenatal and Neonatal Screening* (ed. N. Wald), 2nd edn, p. 243. Oxford University Press, Oxford.

Weiss, L. (1995) Structure of the spleen. In: *Hematology* (eds E. Beutler, M.A. Lichtman, B.S. Coller & T.J. Kipps), p. 38. McGraw-Hill, New York.

Weiss, H. & Katz, S. (1970) Salmonella paravertebral abscess and cervical osteomyelitis in sickle-thalassemia disease. *Southern Med. J.* **63**, 339.

Weiss, I.M. & Liebhaber, S.A. (1994) Erythroid cell-specific determinants of α-globin mRNA stability. *Mol. Cell. Biol.* **14**, 8123.

Weissman, S.M., Jeffries, I. & Karon, M. (1967) The synthesis of alpha, beta, and delta peptide chains by reticulocytes from subjects with thalassemia or hemoglobin Lepore. *J. Lab. Clin. Med.* **69**, 183.

Weissman, L., Treadwell, M., Foote, D., Heer, N. & Vichinsky, E.P. (1998) Approaches to working with adult thalassemia patients in pediatric settings. *Ann. N. Y. Acad. Sci.* **850**, 516.

Wen, X.-J., Liang, S., Jin, Q. & Lin, W.-X. (1992) The nondeletional types of HbH disease in Guangxi. *Hemoglobin* **16**, 45.

Wennberg, E. & Weiss, L. (1968) Splenic-erythroclasia: an electron microscopic study of hemoglobin H disease. *Blood* **31**, 778.

Went, L.N. & MacIver, J.E. (1958a) An unusual type of hemoglobinopathy resembling sickle cell-thalassemia in a Jamaican family. *Blood* **13**, 559.

Went, L.N. & MacIver, J.E. (1958b) Sickle-cell anaemia in adults and its differentiation from sickle-cell thalassaemia. *Lancet* **ii**, 824.

Went, L.N. & MacIver, J.E. (1961) Thalassaemia in the West Indies. *Blood* **17**, 166.

Went, L.N. & Schokker, R.C. (1965) The genetic variability of thalassaemia. In: *Proceedings of the 10th Congress of the European Society of Haematology*, part II, p. 273.

Went, L.N., de Jong, W.W. & Bos, S.E. (1975) Haemoglobin Lepore Boston and elliptocytosis in a family of Indonesian-German ancestry. *J. Med. Genet.* **12**, 83.

Werther, G.A., Matthews, R.N., Burger, H.G. & Herington, A.C. (1981) Lack of response of nonsuppressible insulin-like activity to short term administration of human growth hormone in thalassemia major. *J. Clin. Endocrinol. Metab.* **53**, 806.

Wessels, R.A., Rogers, B.B., Ou, C.N., Alcorn, R. & Buffone, G.J. (1986) Liquid chromatography used in diagnosis of a rare hemoglobin combination: hemoglobin S/Lepore Boston. *Clin. Chem.* **32**, 903.

Westaway, D. & Williamson, R. (1981) An intron nucleotide sequence variant in a cloned β$^+$ thalassaemia globin gene. *Nucl. Acids Res.* **9**, 1777.

Wheeler, J.T. & Krevans, J.R. (1961) The homozygous state of persistent fetal hemoglobin and the interaction of persistent fetal hemoglobin with thalassemia. *Bull. Johns Hopkins Hosp.* **109**, 217.

Whipple, G.H. & Bradford, W.L. (1932) Racial or familial anemia of children. Associated with fundamental disturbances of bone and pigment metabolism (Cooley–Von Jaksch). *Am. J. Dis. Child.* **44**, 336.

Whipple, G.H. & Bradford, W.L. (1936) Mediterranean disease-thalassemia (erythroblastic anemia of Cooley); associated pigment abnormalities simulating hemochromatosis. *J. Pediatr.* **9**, 279.

Whitcher, B.R. (1930) Erythroblastemia of infants. *Am. J. Med. Sci.* **179**, 1.

White, J.C., Ellis, M., Coleman, P.N. *et al.* (1960) An unstable haemoglobin associated with some cases of leukaemia. *Br. J. Haematol.* **6**, 171.

White, J.M. (1976) The unstable haemoglobins. *Br. Med. Bull.* **32**, 219.

White, J.M. & Dacie, J.V. (1971) The unstable hemoglobins, molecular and clinical features. *Prog. Hematol.* **7**, 69.

White, J.M. & Jones, R.W. (1969) Management of pregnancy in a woman with Hb H disease. *Br. Med. J.* **iv**, 473.

White, J.M., Lang, A. & Lehmann, H. (1972a) Compensation of chain synthesis by the single β chain gene in Hb Lepore trait. *Nature New Biol.* **240**, 271.

White, J.M., Lang, A., Lorkin, P.A., Lehmann, H. & Reeve, J. (1972b) Synthesis of haemoglobin Lepore. *Nature* **235**, 208.

White, J.M., Richards, R., Byrne, M., Buchanan, T., White, Y.S. & Jelenski, G. (1985) Thalassaemia trait and pregnancy. *J. Clin. Pathol.* **38**, 810.

White, J.M., Byrne, M., Richards, R., Buchanan, T., Katsoulis, E. & Weerasingh, K. (1986) Red cell genetic abnormalities in Peninsular Arabs: haemoglobin, G6PD deficiency, and α and β thalassaemia. *J. Med. Genet.* **23**, 245.

White, J.M., Christie, B.S., Nain, D., Daar, S. & Higgs, D.R. (1993) Frequency and clinical significance of erythrocyte genetic abnormalities in Omanis. *J. Med. Genet.* **30**, 396.

Whitten, W.J. & Rucknagel, D.L. (1981) The proportion of Hb A$_2$ is higher in sickle cell trait than in normal homozygotes. *Hemoglobin* **5**, 371.

WHO (1983) Community control of hereditary anaemias. Memorandum from a WHO meeting. *Bull. WHO* **61**, 63.

WHO (1985) *Report of the Third and Fourth Annual Meeting of the WHO Working Group for the Community Control of Hereditary Anaemias* (HMG/WG/85.8). World Health Organization, Geneva.

WHO (1987) *Report of the Vth WHO Working Group on the Feasibility Study on Hereditary Disease Community Control Programmes, Heraklion, Crete, 24–25 October 1987* (WHO/HDP/WG/HA/89.2). World Health Organization, Geneva.

WHO (1989a) *Report of the Vth WHO Working Group on the Feasibility Study on Hereditary Disease Community Control Programmes (Hereditary Anaemias), Cagliari, Sardinia* (WHO/HDP/WG/HA/89.2). World Health Organization, Geneva.

WHO (1989b) *Working Group Feasibility Study on Hereditary Disease Community Control Programmes, Cagliari, Sardinia 8–9 April 1989* (WHO/HDP/HA/WG/89.1). World Health Organization, Geneva.

WHO (1990) *The psychosocial aspects of patients and their families with b-thalassaemia and sickle-cell disease. Summary report, 2nd WHO-sponsored Meeting (Division for Maternal and Child Health), Milan, 1989.* World Health Organization, Geneva.

WHO (1994) *Guidelines for the control of haemoglobin disorders. Report of the VIth Annual Meeting of the WHO Working Group on Haemoglobinopathies, Cagliari, Sardinia, 8–9 April, 1989.* World Health Organization, Geneva.

Wickramasinghe, S.N. (1976) The morphology and kinetics of erythropoiesis in homozygous β-thalassaemia. In: *Congenital Disorders of Erythropoiesis,* Ciba Foundation Symposium, p. 221. North Holland, Amsterdam.

Wickramasinghe, S.N. (1990) Ultrastructural abnormalities and arrest of protein biosynthesis in some erythroblasts from homozygotes for haemoglobin C and double heterozygotes for haemoglobin C and β-thalassaemia. *Clin. Lab. Haematol.* **12**, 401.

Wickramasinghe, S.N. & Bush, V. (1975) Observations on the ultrastructure of erythropoietic cells and reticulum cells in the bone marrow of patients with homozygous β-thalassaemia. *Br. J. Haematol.* **30**, 395.

Wickramasinghe, S.N. & Hughes, M. (1978) Some features of bone marrow macrophages in patients with homozygous β-thalassaemia. *Br. J. Haematol.* **38**, 23.

Wickramasinghe, S.N. & Lee, M.J. (1997) Observations on the relationship between γ-globin chain content and globin chain precipitation in thalassaemic erythroblasts and on the composition of erythroblastic inclusions in Hb E/β-thalassaemia. *Eur. J. Haematol.* **59**, 305.

Wickramasinghe, R.L., Ikin, E.W., Mourant, A.E. & Lehmann, H. (1963) The blood groups and haemoglobins of the Veddahs of Ceylon. *J. Roy. Anthropol. Inst. GB Ireland* **93**, 117.

Wickramasinghe, S.N., Letsky, E. & Moffatt, B. (1973) Effect of α-chain precipitates on bone marrow function in homozygous β-thalassaemia. *Br. J. Haematol.* **25**, 123.

Wickramasinghe, S.N., Hughes, M., Hollan, S.R., Horanyi, M. & Szelenyi, J. (1980) Electron microscopic and high resolution autoradiographic studies of the erythroblasts in haemoglobin H disease. *Br. J. Haematol.* **45**, 401.

Wickramasinghe, S.N., Hughes, M., Wasi, P., Fucharoen, S. & Litwinczuk, R.A. (1984) Ultrastructure and cell cycle distribution of erythropoietic cells in heterozygotes and homozygotes for haemoglobin E. *Br. J. Haematol.* **57**, 685.

Wickramasinghe, S.N., Lee, M.J., Furukawa, T., Eguchi, M. & Reid, C.D.L. (1996) Composition of the intra-erythroblastic precipitates in thalassaemia and congenital dyserythropoietic anaemia (CDA): identification of a new type of CDA with intra-erythroblastic precipitates not reacting with monoclonal antibodies to α- and β-globin chains. *Br. J. Haematol.* **93**, 576.

Wielopolski, L. & Zaino, E.C. (1992) Noninvasive *in-vivo* measurement of hepatic and cardiac iron. *J. Nucl Med.* **33**, 1278.

Wijburg, F.A., ven den Berg, W., van Teunenbroek, A. & Weening, R.S. (1988) Thrombo-embolic complications after splenectomy in Hb E-β-thalassaemia. *Eur. J. Pediatr.* **147**, 444.

Wijgerde, M., Grosveld, F. & Fraser, P. (1995) Transcription complex stability and chromatin dynamics. *Nature* **377**, 209.

Wild, B.J. & Stephens, A.D. (1997) The use of automated HPLC to detect and quantitate haemoglobins. *Clin. Lab. Haematol.* **19**, 171.

Wilkie, A.O.M. (1991) *The α thalassaemia/mental retardation syndromes: model systems for studying the genetic contribution to mental handicap.* DM Thesis, University of Oxford.

Wilkie, A.O.M., Buckle, V.J. Harris, P.C. *et al.* (1990a) Clinical features and molecular analysis of the α thalassaemia/mental retardation syndromes. I. Cases due to deletions involving chromosome band 16p13.3. *Am. J. Hum. Genet.* **46**, 1112.

Wilkie, A.O.M., Lamb, J., Harris, P.C., Finney, R.D. & Higgs, D.R. (1990b) A truncated human chromosome 16 associated with α thalassaemia is stabilized by addition of telomeric repeat (TTAGGG)$_n$. *Nature* **346**, 868.

Wilkie, A.O.M., Zeitlin, H.C., Lindenbaum, R.H. *et al.* (1990c) Clinical features and molecular analysis of the α thalassemia/mental retardation syndromes. II. Cases without detectable abnormality of the α globin complex. *Am. J. Hum. Genet.* **46**, 1127.

Wilkie, A.O.M., Higgs, D.R., Rack, K.A. *et al.* (1991a) Stable length polymorphism of up to 260 kb at the tip of the short arm of human chromosome 16. *Cell* **64**, 595.

Wilkie, A.O.M., Pembrey, M.E., Gibbons, R.J. *et al.* (1991b) The non-deletion type of α thalassaemia/mental retardation: a recognisable dysmorphic syndrome with X-linked inheritance. *J. Med. Genet.* **28**, 724.

Wilkie, T. (1993) *Perilous Knowledge.* Faber and Faber, London.

Wilkinson, T., Kronenberg, H., Isaacs, W.A. & Lehmann, H. (1967) Haemoglobin J Baltimore interacting with beta-thalassaemia in an Australian family. *Med. J. Aust.* **i**, 907.

Wilkinson, T., Gough, P., Owen, M.C., Carrell, R.W. & Kronenberg, H. (1975) The isolation and identification of haemoglobin Lepore Boston (Washington) in an Australian family. *Med. J. Aust.* **ii**, 706.

Willcox, M.C. (1975) Thalassaemia in northern Liberia. A survey in the Mount Nimba area. *J. Med. Genet.* **12**, 55.

Willcox, M. (1983) The haemoglobin pattern of sickle cell and haemoglobin C β⁺-thalassaemia in Liberia. *J. Med. Genet.* **20**, 430.

Willcox, M.C., Björkman, A. & Brohult, J. (1983a) Falciparum malaria and β-thalassaemia trait in northern Liberia. *Ann. Trop. Med. Parasitol.* **77**, 335.

Willcox, M.C., Bjorkman, A., Brohult, J., Persson, P.-O., Rombo, L. & Bengtsson, E. (1983b) A case–control study in northern Liberia of *Plasmodium falciparum* malaria in haemoglobin S and β-thalassaemia traits. *Ann. Trop. Med. Parasitol.* **77**, 239.

Williams, C.E. & Siemsen, A.W. (1968) Hemosiderosis in association with thalassemia minor. *Arch. Intern. Med.* **121**, 356.

Williams, T.N., Maitland, K., Bennett, S. *et al.* (1996a) High incidence of malaria in α-thalassaemic children. *Nature* **383**, 522.

Williams, T.N., Maitland, K., Ganczakowski, M. *et al.* (1996b) Red cell phenotypes in the α⁺ thalassaemias from early childhood to maturity. *Br. J. Haematol.* **95**, 266.

Williamson, D., Brown, K.P., Langdown, J.V. & Baglin, T.P. (1997) Mild thalassemia intermedia resulting from a new insertion/frameshift mutation in the β-globin gene. *Hemoglobin* **21**, 485.

Wilson, D.M. (1966) Haemoglobin SD-beta thalassaemia disease. A case presenting with haematuria. *Med. Servs J. Can.* **22**, 724.

Wilson, J.T., de Riel, J.K., Forget, B.G., Marotta, C.A. & Weissman, S.M. (1977) Nucleotide sequence of 3′ untranslated portion of human α globin mRNA. *Nucl. Acids Res.* **4**, 2356.

Wilson, C.J., Chao, D.M., Imbalzano, A.N., Schnitzler, G.R., Kingston, R.E. & Young, R.A. (1996) DNA polymerase II homoenzyme contains SWI/SNF regulators involved in chromatin remodeling. *Cell* **84**, 235.

Winichagoon, P., Adirojnanon, P. & Wasi, P. (1980) Levels of haemoglobin H and proportions of red cells with inclusion bodies in the two types of haemoglobin H disease. *Br. J. Haematol.* **46**, 507.

Winichagoon, P., Fucharoen, S. & Wasi, P. (1981) Increased circulating platelet aggregates in thalassaemia. *Southeast Asian J. Trop. Med. Publ. Hlth* **12**, 556.

Winichagoon, P., Higgs, D.R., Goodbourn, S.E.Y., Lamb, J., Clegg, J.B. & Weatherall, D.J. (1982) Multiple arrangements of the human embryonic ζ-globin genes. *Nucl. Acids Res.* **10**, 5853.

Winichagoon, P., Higgs, D.R., Goodbourn, S.E.Y., Clegg, J.B., Weatherall, D.J. & Wasi, P. (1984) The molecular basis of α-thalassaemia in Thailand. *EMBO J.* **3**, 1813.

Winichagoon, P., Fucharoen, S., Weatherall, D.J. & Wasi, P. (1985) Concomitant inheritance of α-thalassaemia in β⁰-thalassaemia/Hb E. *Am. J. Hematol.* **20**, 217.

Winichagoon, P., Fucharoen, S., Thoinglairoam, V., Tanapotiwirut, V. & Wasi, P. (1990a) β-Thalassemia in Thailand. *Ann. N. Y. Acad. Sci.* **612**, 31.

Winichagoon, S., Fucharoen, S., Thonglairoam, V. & Wasi, P. (1990b) Thai $^{G}γ$ ($^{A}γδβ$)⁰-thalassaemia and its interaction with a single γ-globin gene on a chromosome carrying β⁰-thalassaemia. *Hemoglobin* **14**, 185.

Winichagoon, P., Fucharoen, S. & Wasi, P. (1992a) The molecular basis of α-thalassaemia in Thailand. *Southeast Asian J. Trop. Med. Publ. Hlth* **23**, 7.

Winichagoon, P., Fucharoen, S., Wilairat, P., Chihara, K., Fukumaki, Y. & Wasi, P. (1992b) Identification of five rare mutations including a novel frameshift mutation causing β⁰-thalassaemia in Thai patients with β⁰-thalassaemia/hemoglobin E disease. *Biochim. Biophys. Acta* **1139**, 280.

Winichagoon, P., Thonglairoam, V., Fucharoen, S., Wilairat, P., Fukimaki, Y. & Wasi, P. (1993) Severity differences in β-thalassaemia haemoglobin E syndromes: implication of genetic factors. *Br. J. Haematol.* **83**, 633.

Winichagoon, P., Fucharoen, S., Wilairat, P., Chihara, K. & Fukumaki, Y. (1994) Nondeletional type of hereditary persistence of fetal haemoglobin: molecular characterization of three unrelated Thai HPFH. *Br. J. Haematol.* **87**, 797.

Winichagoon, P., Fucharoen, S., Kanokpongsakdi, S. & Fukumaki, Y. (1995) Detection of α-thalassemia-1 (Southeast Asian type) and its application for prenatal diagnosis. *Clin. Genet.* **47**, 318.

Winslow, R.M. & Ingram, V.W. (1966) Peptide chain synthesis of human hemoglobins. *J. Biol. Chem.* **241**, 1144.

Winterbourn, C.C. (1990) Oxidative denaturation in congenital hemolytic anemias: the unstable hemoglobins. *Sem. Hematol.* **27**, 41.

Winterbourn, C.C. & Carrell, R.W. (1974) Studies of hemoglobin denaturation and Heinz body formation in the unstable hemoglobins. *J. Clin. Invest.* **54**, 678.

Winterhalter, K.H. & Huehns, E.R. (1964) Preparation, properties and specific recombination of αβ-globin subunits. *J. Biol. Chem.* **239**, 3699.

Winterhalter, K.H., Heywood, J.D., Huehns, E.R. & Finch, C.A. (1969) The free globin in human erythrocytes. *Br. J. Haematol.* **16**, 523.

Wintour, E.M., Smith, M.B., Bell, R.J., McDougall, J.G. & Cauchi, M.N. (1985) The role of fetal adrenal hormones in the switch from fetal to adult globin synthesis in the sheep. *J. Endocrinol.* **104**, 165.

Wintrobe, M.M. (1985) *Hematology, the Blossoming of a Science: A Story of Inspiration and Effort*, p. 353. Lea and Febiger, Philadelphia.

Wintrobe, M.M., Mathews, E., Pollack, R. & Dobyns, B.M. (1940) Familial hemopoietic disorder in Italian adolescents and adults resembling Mediterranean disease (thalassemia). *J. A. M. A.* **114**, 1530.

Wishner, B.C., Ward, K.B., Latman, E.E. & Loue, W.E. (1975) Crystal structure of sickle-cell deoxyhemoglobin at 5 Å resolution. *J. Mol. Biol.* **98**, 179.

Witzleben, C.L. & Wyatt, J.P. (1961) The effect of long-survival on the pathology of thalassaemia major. *J. Pathol. Bact.* **82**, 1.

Wolff, J.A. & Ignatov, V.G. (1963) Heterogeneity of thalassemia major. *Am. J. Dis. Child.* **105**, 235.

Wolff, J.A. & Luke, K.H. (1969) Management of thalassemia: a comparative program. *Ann. N. Y. Acad. Sci.* **165**, 423.

Wolff, J.A., Sitarz, A.L. & VonHofe, F.H. (1960) Effect of splenectomy on thalassemia. *Pediatr.* **26**, 674.

Wollstein, M. & Kreidel, K.V. (1930) Familial hemolytic anemia of childhood — von Jaksch. *Am. J. Dis. Child.* **39**, 115.

Wolman, I.J. (1964) Transfusion therapy in Cooley's anemia: growth and health as related to long-range hemoglobin levels, a progress report. *Ann. N. Y. Acad. Sci.* **119**, 736.

Wolman, I.J. & Ortolani, M. (1969) Some clinical features of Cooley's anemia patients as related to transfusion schedules. *Ann. N. Y. Acad. Sci.* **165**, 407.

Wolstenholme, G.E.W. & O'Connor, C.M. (eds) (1959) *The Biochemistry of Human Genetics*. Ciba Foundation Symposium. Little, Brown, Boston.

Wong, H.B. (1965) Hydrops foetalis in Singapore. *Far East Med. J.* **1**, 8.

Wong, H.B. (1966) *Haemoglobinopathies in Singapore. The First Haridas Memorial Lecture.* Stamford College Press, Singapore.

Wong, H.B. (1971) The genetics of alpha-thalassaemia in Singapore. *J. Singapore Paediatr. Soc.* **13**, 58.

Wong, H.B. (1984) Thalassemias in Singapore. *J. Singapore Paediatr. Soc.* **26**, 1.

Wong, S.C. & Ali, M.A.M. (1982) Hemoglobin E diseases: hematological, analytical, and biosynthetic studies in homozygotes and double heterozygotes for α-thalassaemia. *Am. J. Hematol.* **13**, 15.

Wong, C., Dowling, C.E., Saiki, R.K., Higuchi, R.G., Erlich, H.A. & Kazazian, H.H. Jr (1987) Characterization of β-thalassaemia mutations using direct genomic sequencing of amplified single copy DNA. *Nature* **330**, 384.

Wong, C., Antonarakis, S.E., Goff, S.C. *et al.* (1989a) β-Thalassemia due to two novel nucleotide substitutions in consensus acceptor splice sequences of the β-globin gene. *Blood* **73**, 914.

Wong, S.C., Stoning, T.A., Efremov, G.D. & Huisman, T.H.J. (1989b) High frequencies of a rearrangement (+ATA; –T) at –530 to the β-globin gene in different populations indicate the absence of a correlation with a silent β-thalassaemia determinant. *Hemoglobin* **13**, 1.

Wong, A., Alder, V., Robertson, D. *et al.* (1997) Liver iron depletion and toxicity of the iron chelator deferiprone (L1, CP20) in the guinea pig. *Biometals* **10**, 247.

Wonke, B. (1998) Annotation: Bone disease in β-thalassaemia major. *Br. J. Haematol.* **103**, 897.

Wonke, B., Hoffbrand, A.V., Aldouri, M. *et al.* (1989) Reversal of desferrioxamine induced auditory neurotoxicity during treatment with CaDTPA. *Arch. Dis. Child.* **6**, 77.

Wonke, B., Hoffbrand, V.A., Brown, D. & Dusheiko, G. (1990) Antibody to hepatitis C virus in multiply transfused patients with thalassaemia major. *J. Clin. Pathol.* **43**, 638.

Wonke, B., Hoffbrand, A.V., Bouloux, P., Jensen, C. & Telfer, P. (1998a) New approaches to the management of hepatitis and endocrine disorders in Cooley's anemia. *Ann. N. Y. Acad. Sci.* **850**, 232.

Wonke, B., Wright, C. & Hoffbrand, A.V. (1998b) Combined therapy with deferiprone and desferrioxamine. *Br. J. Haematol.* **103**, 361.

Wood, W.G. (1984) The cellular basis of hemoglobin switching. In: *New Trends in Experimental Hematology* (eds C. Peschle & C. Rizzoli), p. 60. Ares Serono Symposia, Rome.

Wood, W.G. (1989) HbF production in adult life. In: *Hemoglobin Switching, Part B: Cellular and Molecular Mechanisms* (eds G. Stamatoyannopoulos & A.W. Nienhuis), p. 251. A.R. Liss, New York.

Wood, W.G. (1993) Increased HbF in adult life. *Clin. Haematol.* **6**, 177.

Wood, W.G. & Stamatoyannopoulos, G. (1976–77) Globin synthesis during erythroid cell maturation in α thalassaemia. *Hemoglobin* **1**, 135.

Wood, W.G. & Weatherall, D.J. (1973) Haemoglobin synthesis during human foetal development. *Nature* **244**, 162.

Wood, W.G., Stamatoyannopoulos, G., Lim, G. & Nute, P.E. (1975) F-cells in the adult: normal values and levels in individuals with hereditary and acquired elevations of Hb F. *Blood* **46**, 671.

Wood, W.G., Pearce, K., Clegg, J.B. *et al.* (1976a) Switch from foetal to adult haemoglobin synthesis in normal and hypophysectomised sheep. *Nature* **264**, 799.

Wood, W.G., Weatherall, D.J. & Clegg, J.B. (1976b) Interaction of heterocellular hereditary persistence of foetal haemoglobin with β thalassaemia and sickle cell anaemia. *Nature* **264**, 247.

Wood, W.G., Clegg, J.B., Weatherall, D.J. *et al.* (1977a) $^Gγδβ$ Thalassaemia and $^Gγ$ HPFH (Hb Kenya type). Comparison of two new cases. *J. Med. Genet.* **14**, 237.

Wood, W.G., Weatherall, D.J., Clegg, J.B., Hamblin, T.J., Edwards, J.H. & Barlow, A.M. (1977b) Heterocellular hereditary persistence of fetal haemoglobin (heterocellular HPFH) and its interaction with β thalassaemia. *Br. J. Haematol.* **36**, 461.

Wood, W.G., Old, J.M., Roberts, A.V.S., Clegg, J.B., Weatherall, D.J. & Quattrin, N. (1978) Human globin gene expression: control of β, δ and δβ chain production. *Cell* **15**, 437.

Wood, W.G., Clegg, J.B. & Weatherall, D.J. (1979) Hereditary persistence of fetal haemoglobin (HPFH) and δβ-thalassaemia. *Br. J. Haematol.* **43**, 509.

Wood, W.G., Pembrey, M.E., Serjeant, G.R., Perrine, R.P. & Weatherall, D.J. (1980) Hb F synthesis in sickle cell anaemia: a comparison of Saudi Arab cases with those of African origin. *Br. J. Haematol.* **45**, 431.

Wood, W.G., Macrae, I.A., Darbre, P.D., Clegg, J.B. & Weatherall, D.J. (1982a) The British type of non-deletion HPFH: characterisation of developmental changes *in vivo* and erythroid growth *in vitro*. *Br. J. Haematol.* **50**, 401.

Wood, W.G., Weatherall, D.J., Hart, G.H., Bennett, M. & Marsh, G.W. (1982b) Hematologic changes and hemoglobin analysis in β thalassemia heterozygotes during the first year of life. *Pediatr. Res.* **16**, 286.

Wood, W.G., Bunch, C., Kelly, S., Gunn, Y. & Breckon, G. (1985) Control of haemoglobin switching by a developmental clock? *Nature* **313**, 320.

Woodrow, J.C., Noble, R.L. & Martindale, J.H. (1964) Haemoglobin H disease in an English family. *Br. Med. J.* **i**, 36.

World Bank (1993) *World Development Report.* Oxford University Press, Oxford.

Worwood, M., Cragg, S.J., McLaren, C., Ricketts, C. & Economidou, J. (1980) Binding of serum ferritin to concanavalia A: patients with homozygous β thalassaemia and transfusional iron overload. *Br. J. Haematol.* **46**, 409.

Wrightstone, R.N. & Huisman, T.H.J. (1974) Hemoglobins F and A_2 in sickle-cell anemia and some related disorders. *Am. J. Clin. Pathol.* **61**, 375.

Xu, X., Liao, C., Liu, Z. *et al.* (1996) Antenatal screening and fetal diagnosis of β-thalassemia in a Chinese population: prevalence of the β-thalassemia trait in the Guangzhou area of China. *Hum. Genet.* **98**, 199.

Yamak, B. & Ozsoylu, S. (1969) Haptoglobin in thalassemia. *Acta Haematol.* **42**, 176.

Yamak, B., Ozsoylu, S., Altay, C. & Hicsonmez, G. (1973) Hereditary persistence of fetal hemoglobin and β-thalassemia in a Turkish child. *Acta Haematol. (Basel)* **50**, 124.

Yamamoto, K., Yamamoto, K., Hattori, Y. *et al.* (1992) Two β-thalassemia mutations in Japan: Codon 121 (G̲AA→T̲AA) and IVS-I-130 (G→C). *Hemoglobin* **16**, 295.

Yanase, T., Hanada, M., Seita, M. *et al.* (1968) Molecular basis or morbidity from a series of studies of haemogobinopathies in Western Japan. *Japan J. Hum. Genet.* **13**, 40.

Yang, T.Y., Yang, X.Y., Ch'en, W.C. *et al.* (1985) Thalassaemia in China. *Ann. N. Y. Acad. Sci.* **445**, 92.

Yang, K.G., Liu, J.Z., Kutlar, F. *et al.* (1986) $β^0$-Thalassaemia in association with a γ-globin gene quadruplication. *Blood* **68**, 1394.

Yang, K.G., Stoming, T.A., Fei, Y.J. *et al.* (1988) Identification of base substitutions in the promoter regions of the $^Aγ$- and $^Gγ$-globin genes in $^Aγ$- (or $^Gγ$)β$^+$-HPFH heterozygotes using the DNA-amplification–synthetic oligonucleotide procedure. *Blood* **71**, 1414.

Yang, K.G., Kutlar, F., George, E. *et al.* (1989) Molecular characterization of β-globin gene mutations in Malay patients with Hb E-β-thalassaemia and thalassaemia major. *Br. J. Haematol.* **72**, 73.

Yasukawa, M., Saito, S., Fujita, S. *et al.* (1980) Five families with homozygous δ-thalassaemia in Japan. *Br. J. Haematol.* **46**, 199.

Yataganas, X. & Fessas, P. (1969) The pattern of hemoglobin precipitation in thalassemia and its significance. *Ann. N. Y. Acad. Sci.* **165**, 270.

Yataganas, X., Fessas, P. & Gahrton, G. (1972) Quantification of α-chain excess in erythrocytes in β-thalassemia by microinterferometry. *Br. J. Haematol.* **2**, 117.

Yataganas, X., Gahrton, G., Fessas, P., Kesse-Elias, M. & Thorell, B. (1973) Proliferative activity and glycogen accumulation of erythroblasts in β-thalassemia. *Br. J. Haematol.* **24**, 651.

Yataganas, X., Gahrton, G. & Thorell, B. (1974) Intranuclear hemoglobin in erythroblasts of β-thalassemia. *Blood* **43**, 243.

Yates, S.N.R. (1995) *Human genetic diversity and selection by malaria.* D. Phil. thesis, University of Oxford.

Yenchitsomanus, P., Summers, K.M., Board, P.G. *et al.* (1986) Alpha-thalassemia in Papua New Guinea. *Hum. Genet.* **74**, 432.

Yipintsoi, T., Haraphongse, M., Wasi, P. & Na-Nakorn, S. (1968) Cardiological examinations in hemoglobin E and thalassemia diseases. *J. Med. Assoc. Thailand* **51**, 131.

Yoo, D., Schechter, G.P., Amigable, A.N. & Nienhuis, A.W. (1980) Myeloproliferative syndrome with sideroblastic anemia and acquired hemoglobin H disease. *Cancer* **45**, 78.

Yoshida, N., Horikoshi, A., Kanemaru, M. *et al.* (1990) An erythremia with acquired HbH disease and chromosomal abnormality. *Rinsho Ketsueki* **31**, 963.

Youngchaiyud, P., Suthamsmai, T., Fucharoen, S., Udompanich, V., Pushpakon, R. & Wasi, P. (1988) Lung function tests in splenectomized β-thalassemia/Hb E patients. In: *Thalassemia: Pathophysiology and Management, Part A* (eds S. Fucharoen, P.T. Rowley & N.W. Paul) *Birth Defects* **23**, 361. Alan R. Liss, New York.

Yu, Y.C., Kao, E.L., Chou, S.H., Lin, T.J. & Chien, C.H. (1991) Intrathoracic extramedullary hematopoiesis simulating posterior mediastinal mass—report of a case in a patient with beta-thalassemia intermedia. *Kao Hsiung I Hsueh Ko Hsueh Tsa Chih* **7**, 43.

Yuan, J., Angelucci, E., Lucarelli, G., Aljurf, H., Ma, L. & Schrier, S.L. (1992a) Abnormal assembly of membrane proteins in erythroid progenitors of patients with beta thalassemia. *Blood* **80**, 18a.

Yuan, J., Kannan, R., Shinar, E., Rachmilewitz, E.A. & Low, P.S. (1992b) Isolation, characterization, and immunoprecipitation studies of immune complexes from membranes of beta-thalassemic erythrocytes. *Blood* **79**, 3007.

Yuan, J., Angelucci, E., Lucarelli, G. *et al.* (1993) Accelerated programmed cell death (apoptosis) in erythroid precursors of patients with severe beta-thalassemia (Cooley's anemia). *Blood* **82**, 374.

Yuan, J., Bunyaratvej, A., Fucharoen, S., Fung, C., Shinar, E. & Schrier, S.L. (1995) The instability of the membrane skeleton in thalassemic red blood cells. *Blood* **86**, 3945.

Yüregir, G.T., Aksoy, K., Çürük, M.A. *et al.* (1992) HbH in a Turkish family resulting from the interaction of a deletional α-thalassaemia-1 and a newly discovered poly A mutation. *Br. J. Haematol.* **80**, 527.

Yuthavong, Y., Ruenwongsa, P., Benyajati, C. & Suttimool, W. (1975) Studies on the structural stability of haemoglobin E. *J. Med. Assoc. Thailand* **58**, 351.

Yuthavong, Y., Butthep, P., Bunyaratvej, A. & Fucharoen, S. (1987) Inhibitory effect of beta zero-thalassaemia/haemoglobin E erythrocytes on *Plasmodium falciparum* growth *in vitro*. *Trans. Roy. Soc. Trop. Med. Hyg.* **81**, 903.

Yuthavong, Y., Butthep, P., Bunyaratvej, A., Fucharoen, S. & Khurmith, S. (1988) Impaired parasite growth and increased susceptibility to phagocytosis of *Plasmodium falciparum* infected alpha-thalassemia and hemoglobin Constant Spring red blood cells. *Am. J. Clin. Pathol.* **89**, 521.

Zachariadis, Z., Nute, P.E. & Stamatoyannopoulos, G. (1975) Haemoglobin Lepore in Cyprus. *J. Med. Genet.* **12**, 275.

Zago, M.A. & Costa, F.F. (1985) Hereditary haemoglobin disorders in Brazil. *Trans. Roy. Soc. Trop. Med. Hyg.* **79**, 385.

Zago, M.A., Wood, W.G., Clegg, J.B., Weatherall, D.J., O'Sullivan, M. & Gunson, H.H. (1979) Genetic control of F-cells in human adults. *Blood* **53**, 977.

Zago, M.A., Costa, F.F., Tone, L.G. & Bottura, C. (1983) Hereditary hemoglobin disorders in a Brazilian population. *Hum. Hered.* **33**, 125.

Zahed, L., Talhouk, R., Saleh, M., Abou-Jaoudeh, R., Fisher, C. & Old, J. (1997) The spectrum of beta-thalassaemia mutations in the Lebanon. *Hum. Hered.* **47**, 241.

Zaidi, Y., Sivakumaran, M., Graham, C. & Hutchinson, R.M. (1996) Fatal bone marrow embolism in a patient with sickle cell β⁺ thalassaemia. *J. Clin. Pathol.* **49**, 774.

Zaizov, R. & Matoth, Y. (1972) α-Thalassaemia in Yemenite and Iraqi Jews. *Israel J. Med. Sci.* **8**, 11.

Zaino, E.C. & Rossi, M.B. (1974) Ultrastructure of the erythrocytes in β-thalassemia. *Ann. N. Y. Acad. Sci.* **232**, 238.

Zaino, E.C. & Yang, T.Y. (1981) Hemoglobinopathy and thalassemia in China. *N. Eng. J. Med.* **305**, 766.

Zaino, E.C., Kuo, B. & Roginsky, M.S. (1969) Growth retardation in thalassemia major. *Ann. N. Y. Acad. Sci.* **165**, 394.

Zaino, E.C., Rossi, M.B., Pham, T.D. & Azar, H.A. (1971) Gaucher's cells in thalassemia. *Blood* **38**, 457.

Zanella, A., Mozzi, F., Ferroni, P. & Sirchia, G. (1986) Anti-HTLV III

screening in multi-transfused thalassaemia patients. *Vox Sang.* **50**, 192.

Zani, B., Di Palma, A. & Vullo, C. (1995) Psychosocial aspects of chronic illness in adolescents with thalassaemia major. *J. Adolescence* **18**, 387.

Zanjani, E.D., McGlave, P.B., Bhakthavathsalan, A. & Stamatoyannopoulos, G. (1979) Sheep fetal haematopoietic cells produce adult haemoglobin when transplanted in the adult animal. *Nature* **280**, 495.

Zanjani, E.D., Lim, G., McGlave, P.B. *et al.* (1982) Adult haematopoietic cells transplanted to sheep fetuses continue to produce adult globins. *Nature* **295**, 244.

Zelkowitz, L., Torres, C., Bhoopalan, N., Yakulis, V.J. & Heller, P. (1972) Double heterozygous βδ-thalassemia in Negroes. *Arch. Intern. Med.* **129**, 975.

Zemel, R., Dickman, R., Tamary, H., Bukh, J., Zaizov, R. & Tur-Kaspa, R. (1998) Viremia, genetic heterogeneity, and immunity to hepatitis G/GB-C virus in multiply transfused patients with thalassemia. *Transfusion* **38**, 301.

Zeng, Y.-T. (1981) Hemoglobinopathies in China mainland. *Hemoglobin* **5**, 517.

Zeng, Y.-T. & Huang, S.-Z. (1982) Hemoglobin New York (α₂β₂ 113(G15) Val→Glu) in China. *Hemoglobin* **6**, 61.

Zeng, Y.-T. & Huang, S.-Z. (1987) Disorders of haemoglobin in China. *J. Med. Genet.* **24**, 578.

Zeng, Y.-T., Huang, S.-Z., Chen, B. *et al.* (1985a) Hereditary persistence of fetal hemoglobin or (δβ)⁰-thalassemia: three types observed in South-Chinese families. *Blood* **66**, 1430.

Zeng, Y.-T., Huang, S.-Z., Nakatsuji, T. & Huisman, T.H.J. (1985b) ᴳγᴬγ-Thalassaemia and ζ-chain variants in Chinese newborn babies. *Am. J. Hematol.* **18**, 235.

Zeng, Y.T., Huang, S.Z., Ren, Z.R. *et al.* (1995) Hydroxyurea therapy in β-thalassaemia intermedia: improvement in haematological parameters due to enhanced β-globin synthesis. *Br. J. Haematol.* **90**, 557.

Zhang, J.-W., Stamatoyannopoulos, G. & Anagnou, N.P. (1988a) Laotian (δβ)⁰-thalassemia: molecular characterization of a novel deletion associated with increased production of fetal hemoglobin. *Blood* **72**, 983.

Zhang, J.-Z., Cai, S.-P., He, X. *et al.* (1988b) Molecular basis of β thalassemia in South China. *Hum. Genet.* **78**, 37.

Zhang, J.-W., Song, W.-F., Zhao, Y.-J. *et al.* (1993) Molecular characterization of a novel form of (ᴬγδβ)⁰ thalassemia deletion in a Chinese family. *Blood* **81**, 1624.

Zhang, J., Sun, X., Qian, Y. & Maquat, L.E. (1998a) Intron function in the nonsense-mediated decay of β-globin mRNA: Indications that pre-mRNA splicing in the nucleus can influence mRNA translation in the cytoplasm. *RNA* **4**, 801.

Zhang, Y., LeRoy, G., Seelig, H.-P., Lane, W.S. & Reinberg, D. (1998b) The dermatomyositis-specific autoantigen Mi2 is a component of a complex containing histone deacetylase and nucleosome remodeling activities. *Cell* **95**, 279.

Zhao, W., Zhang, J., Wang, N.S. & Deng, P. (1988) The relationship between Hb Bart's levels in cord blood and the deletions of α-globin genes. *Hemoglobin* **12**, 519.

Zhao, J.-B., Zhao, L., Fei, Y.-J., Liu, J.-C. & Huisman, T.H.J. (1991) A novel α-thalassemia-2 (–2.7 kb) observed in a Chinese patient with HbH disease. *Am. J. Hematol.* **38**, 248.

Zhao, J.-B., Zhao, L., Gu, Y.-C. & Huisman, T.H.J. (1992) Types of α-globin gene deficiencies in Chinese newborn babies in the Guangxi region, P.R. China. *Hemoglobin* **16**, 325.

Zhou, W., Clouston, D.R., Wang, X., Cerruti, L., Cunningham, J.M. & Jane, S.M. (2000) Induction of human fetal globin gene expression by a novel erythroid factor, NF-E4. *Mol. Cell Biol.* **20**, 7661.

Ziegler, G. & Marti, H.R. (1966) Protoporphyrin and coproporphyrin of erythrocytes in heterozygotic thalassemia. *Schweiz. Med. Wschr.* **96**, 1272.

Zimmer, E.A., Martin, S.L., Beverley, S.M., Kan, Y.W. & Wilson, A.C. (1980) Rapid duplication and loss of genes coding for the α chains of hemoglobin. *Proc. Natl Acad. Sci. USA* **77**, 2158.

Zoratto, E., Norelli, M.T. & Lumare, A. (1969) Hemolytic anemia caused by association of a double anomaly beta-thalassemia and deficiency of G6PD. *Min. Pediatr.* **21**, 605.

Zschocke, J. & Graham, C.A. (1995) A fluorescent multiplex ARMS method for rapid mutation analysis. *Mol. Cell. Probes* **9**, 447.

Zuckerkandl, E. (1964) Controller-gene diseases: the operon model as applied to β-thalassemia, familial fetal hemoglobinemia and the normal switch from the production of fetal hemoglobin to that of adult hemoglobin. *J. Mol. Biol.* **8**, 128.

Zuelzer, W.W. (1956) Thomas B. Cooley (1871–1948). *J. Pediatr.* **49**, 642.

Zuelzer, W.W. & Kaplan, E. (1954) Thalassemia hemoglobin C-disease: a new syndrome presumably due to the combination of the genes for thalassemia and hemoglobin C. *Blood* **9**, 1047.

Zuelzer, W.W., Neel, J.V. & Robinson, A.R. (1956) Abnormal hemoglobins. *Prog. Hematol.* **1**, 91.

Zuelzer, W.W., Robinson, A.R. & Booker, C.R. (1961) Reciprocal relationship of hemoglobins A_2 and F in beta chain thalassemias, a key to the genetic control of hemoglobin F. *Blood* **17**, 393.

Zuppinger, K., Molinari, B., Hirt, A. *et al.* (1979) Increased risk of diabetes mellitus in beta-thalassaemia major. *Hel. Paediatr. Acta* **4**, 197.

Zurlo, M.F., De Stefano, P., Borgna-Pignatti, C. *et al.* (1989) Survival and causes of death in thalassaemia major. *Lancet* **ii**, 27.

Appendix
Addresses of patient support
organizations (WHO, 1994)

INTERNATIONAL

Thalassaemia International
    Federation (TIF),
PO Box 28807
2083 Nicosia, Cyprus
Fax: +357 2 314552
Email: thalassaemia@cytanet.com.cy

NATIONAL

Argentina

Dra Aurora Feliu Torres
Hospital de Pediatria Dr JP
    Garrahan
Haemato-Oncologia
Pichincha 1850
Buenos Aires
Tel: +54 1 941 8532

Australia

Miss Christine Savva
Thalassaemia Society of Victoria
6 Tiernan Street
Footscray 3001, VA
Tel: +61 3 687 4777
Fax: +61 3 687 4295

Ms Patricia Fleming
Australian Thalassaemia Association
Haematology Department
ICPMR, Westmead Hospital
Westmead, NSW 2145
Tel: +61 2 633 7034
Fax: +61 2 891 5376

Miss Jenny Kelly
Thalassaemia Society of New South
    Wales
PO Box 80
Marrickville, NSW 2204
Tel: +61 2 871 1701

Dr Sylvia Barber — President
Australian Thalassaemia
    Association
c/o The Queen Elizabeth Hospital
28 Woodville Road
Woodville South, SA 2204
Tel: +61 8 450 222
Fax: +61 8 243 6806

Miss Irene Triantafillidis
Thalassaemia Society of South
    Australia
288 Franklin Street
Adelaide, SA 5000
Tel: +61 8 231 1132

Azerbaijan

INSAN
Social and Charitable Centre
Azerbaijan Thalassaemia Society
ab/box N70
Baku Centre 370000
Tel: +7 8922 663 048
Fax: + 7 8922 923 297

Bahrain

Mr Abdulla Saif
President
Bahrain National Hereditary
    Anaemia Society
PO Box 11399
Manama
Tel: +9 73 529 500
Fax: +9 73 643 579

Belgium

Mrs Oriella di Stefano
President
Ligue des Jeunes Thalassémiques
88/5 Rue Waleffe
4220 Seraing-Jemeppe
Tel: +32 41 333 977

Brazil

Mrs Neuza C. Cattassini — President
Abrasta Associacao Brasileira dos
    Talassemicos
113 Rua da Quitanda
6 andar, Sala 62
CEP 01012-010
São Paulo SP
Tel: +55 11 366 151
Fax: +55 11 524 902/341 712

Mr Luis Carlos Salvaterra
Associacao de Pais e Amigos dos
    Thalassemicos
R Parana 203
Bairo Sao Benardo
Campinas SP 13030
Tel: +55 192 391 301

Canada

Ms Naushy Mullani
Ontario Thalassaemia Association
3 Massey Square, No. 2901
Toronto, Ontario
Tel: +1 416 694 6796 (home)

Mrs Mary Sammarco
The Vancouver Thalassaemia Society
    of BC
6620 Bouchard Court
Richmond, British Columbia
BC V7C 5H5
Tel: +1 604 274 1052

Mrs A.C. Kritikos
Quebec Society of Thalassaemia
    Inc.
505 Jean Talon East
Montreal, Quebec
H2R 1T6

824   *Appendix*

Cyprus

The Cyprus Thalassaemia Association
1 Philippou Hadjigeorgiou
Flat 5
PO Box 8503
Nicosia
Tel: +357 2 429 141
Fax: +357 2 315 792

Egypt

Dr M. Gadalla
Egyptian Thalassaemic Friends
 Association
c/o Ciba-Geigy Scientific Office
PO Box 1071
Cairo 11511
Tel: +20 2 919 388 / 917 143
Fax: +20 2 919 388

France

Mr Louis Thiemongue
President
France Hémoglobinoses
(Alpes-Maritimes)
Centre de Transfusion Sanguine
Avenue de Docteur Donat
F-06700 Saint Laurent du Var
Tel: +33 932 23750
Fax: +33 932 23783

Mr Elias Benamou
Association France Hémoglobinoses
86 Avenue du Rove, Bât. D
F-13015 Marseille
Tel: +33 91 60 91 00

Greece

Mr Dimitris Paspalis
Association of Parents and Patients of
 Thessaloniki
T. Papageorgiou 2
Thessaloniki 54 631
Tel: +30 31 228 931

Miss Evaenia Georganda
Panhellenic Thalassaemia Patients'
 Association
1 Tzavella Street
GR-106 81 Athens
Tel: +30 1 364 4682
Fax: +30 1 645 0510

Costas Papageorgiou
Panhellenic Association for the
 Protection of Thalassaemia Patients
Akadimias 64
T.T. 106 79 Athens
Tel: +30 1 362 5102 / 325 2547
Fax: +30 1 323 6115

Mr Elias Sofianos
President
Panhellenic Thalassaemia Federation
Tzavella 1
Z.P. 106 81 Athens
Tel: +30 1 364 4682
Fax: +30 1 645 0510

Mr Karnaros
Panellina Kinisi yia ti Mesogiaki
 Anemia
PO Box 70014
16610 Glyfada
Athens
Tel: +30 1 894 7395 / 681 5605

Thalassaemia Parents' Association
Kassavitti 4
KA 38221
Magnisia

Mr Anastasios Eliopoulos
Thalassaemia Parents' Association
Antonopoulos 98
KA 38221
Volos

Miss Georgia Galanopoulou
Sylogos Pashontou apo Mesogiakin
Iera Metropoli Korinthou
Metropoliticos Naos Ayiou Pavlou
PO Box 303
Korinthos 20 100
Tel: +30 741 23324

Hong Kong

Mrs Ngan-Wah Yeung
The Cooley's Anemia Foundation of
 Hong Kong
PO Box 44379
Block A, Flat G, 21st Floor
Shau Ki Won Centre
9 Factory Street
Shau Ki Won

India

Mr Tapas Sengupta
The Thalassaemia Society of India
1/B Grant Street (Nr. Chandni
 Market)
Calcutta 700 013

Mr Varsha Bihani
Bhoruka Research Centre for
 Haematology and Blood
 Transfusion
Futnani Chambers, Gat 4
Corporation Place
Calcutta 87
Tel: +91 33 449 619 / 448 902

Mr Thakorbhai B. Desai
Parents' Association Thalassaemic
 Trust Unit
Kanji Khetshi New Building, 3rd
 Floor
Tatya Gharpure Marg
Bombay 400 004
Tel: +91 22 363 347

Mr M.B. Agarwal
Thalassaemia & Sickle Cell Society of
 Bombay
Vijay Sadan, Flat No 1
168B Dr Ambedkar Road
Dadar TT, Bombay
Tel: +91 22 414 2272 / 4453
Fax: +91 22 414 0058

Mr Chandrakant Koticha
Rajkot Voluntary Blood Bank and
 Research Centre
c/o Jayshree Traders 'Ajay
 Mansion'
PO Box 508
Malaviya Road
Rajkot 360002
Tel: +91 281 82636 / 82176
Fax: +91 281 47015 / 47016

Dr J.S. Arora
National Thalassaemia Welfare
 Society
KG 1/97
Vikas Puri
New Delhi 110018
Tel: +91 11 550 7483

Dr S.M. Merchant
Research Laboratories BJ Wadia
   Hospital for Children
Acharya Donde Marg
Parel
Bombay 400 012
Tel: +91 22 413 7000 / 412 9786

Mr C.L. Juneja
The Thalassaemia Foundation of India
181/B, MIG
DDA Flats
Rajouri Garden Extension
New Delhi 110027
Tel: +91 11 502 367

Mr Guninder Singh Chandok
Thalassaemia and Sickle Cell Society
   of Bangalore
Jai Rattan Nivas
11 A/22, Cunningham Road
Bangalore 560 002
Tel: +91 812 258 661

Mr M.S. Rekhi
Thalassaemia Children Welfare
   Association
3047, Sector 20-D
Chandigarh

Mr Deepak Chopra
Thalassaemics India (Regd)
C-1/59 Safdarjung Development Area
New Delhi 110016

Indonesia

Mr Ruswandi
Yayasan Thalassaemia Indonesia
J1 Melat No. 40
Gilandak Barat
Jakarta Selatan 12430
Tel: +21 750 0788 / 799 5936

Iran

Dr Mina Izadyar
Director
Iranian Thalassaemia Society
Apt. 10, No 113
Ghaem Farahani Avenue
PO Box 15875 6156
Teheran
Tel: +98 21 646 2977
Fax: +98 21 677 094

Israel

Mr Gilad Silberstein
M. Jakobsohn Ltd.
38 Kalisher St.
PO Box 29096
Tel Aviv 61290
Tel: +972 3 510 3131
Fax: +972 3 517 3585

Italy

Mr Silvano Fassio
Lega Italiana per la Lotta Contro
   le Emopatie e Tumori
   dell'Infanzia
Via Giobert 27
I-14100 Asti
Tel/Fax: +39 141 557 034

Ms Silvia Olla
President
Nuiva Associazione Talassemici
   Italiani
Lungotevere Flaminio, 48
I-00 196 Rome
Tel: +39 6 322 4823
Fax: +39 6 482 0974 / 503 7923

Kuwait

Dr Laila Al-Fezae
Pediatric Department
Sabah Hospital
PO Box 25328
13114 Safat
Tel: +965 254 3377 / 531 2400
Fax: +965 531 9533

Lebanon

Mrs Randa Daouk
Chronic Care Center
PO Box 213
Hazmieh
Beirut
Tel: +961 1 868 109
Fax: +961 1 866 301 / 866 302

Mr Samih Shahine
Lebanese Association
Mea Eng Department
Lim, Beirut
Tel: +961 1 316 316 Ext 2854

Malaysia

Malaysian Association of
   Thalassaemia
Jabatan Pediatrik
University Kebangsaan Malaysia
Salam reja Mude
50300 Kuala Lumpur

Ms Khee Swee Hong
President
Pertubuhan Thalassaemia Pulau
   Pinang
56 Jalan Gen Guan He
11400 Penang
Tel: +60 4 686 412

Rep. of Maldives

Dr Naila Firdous
Society for Health Education
M Kothanmaage (South)
Maaveyo Magu
Male 20-03
Tel: +960 327 117
Fax: +960 322 221

Malta

Mrs Simone Buhagiar
President
Thalassaemia Awareness Maltese
   Association
Comprehensive Genetics
   Programme
University of Malta
Tal-Qroqq
Msida
Tel: +356 314 392 /239 807
Fax: +356 310 577

Pakistan

Mr Amin Bandhani
Fatimid Thalassaemia Centre
393 Britto Road, Garden East
PO Box 3412 (New Town)
Karachi
Tel: +92 21 716 733

Lt. Gen. (Rtd) Fahim Ahmad
   Khan
Pakistan Thalassaemia Welfare
   Society (Regd)
22 Ata-ul-Haq Road
Westridge-I
Rawalpindi
Tel: +92 51 862 227 / 862 393
Fax: +92 51 565 206

Romania

Mrs Michaela Dogaru
Asociata Romania Pentrou
   Protectia
Bolnavilor de Thalasemie Majora
50 Vioiceni Street
Bloc A 15 bis, so 1
Ap 18, Sector 2
73418 Bucharest

Russia

Professor Yuri N. Tokarev
Research Institute for Pediatric
   Haematology
Ministry of Health of the Russian
   Federation
113 Leninsky Drive
Moscow 117513
Tel: +7 095 434 8141
Fax: +7 095 434 8678

Saudi Arabia

Professor Mohsen A.F. El-Hazmi
National Working Group
WHO Collaborating Centre
College of Medicine and King Khalid
   University Hospital
PO Box 2925
Riyadh 11461
Tel: +966 1 467 0830
Fax: +966 1 467 2575

Saudi Thalassaemia Friend's
   Society
King Abdulaziz University
King Fahd Medical Research
   Centre
PO Box 9029
Jeddah 21413
Tel: +966 2 688 1821 / 2057

South Africa

Mr D Brijball
President
South African Thalassaemia
   Association
26 Robin Street
Kharwastan, Durban 4092
Tel: +27 31 413 442

Thailand

Prof. Voravarn S. Tanphaichitr
Secretary
Thalassaemia Foundation of Thailand
Department of Pediatrics
Siriraj Hospital
Bangkok 10700
Tel: +66 2 411 3010
Fax: +66 2 412 1371

Tunisia

Professor Slaheddine Fattoum
A.L.P.H.A.T.T.
Hôpital d'Enfants
Bab Saadoun-1007
Tunis
Tel: +1 262 521 / 663 500 / 664 125
Fax: +1 262 521 / 572 572

Turkey

Professor Ayten Arcasoy
Ankara Thalassaemia Society
Kibris Sok 10/5
Guvenevieri
Asagni Ayranci
Ankara
Tel: +9 319 1440

Opr Dr Duru Malyali
TADAD
Thalassemi Dayanisma Dernegi
Posta Kutusu 403
Kadikoy
81310 Istanbul
Tel: +1 358 0071 / 512 6819
Fax: +1 339 9496 / 991 1934

Professor Huseyin Sipohioglu
President
Akdeniz Talasemi Dernegi
Anafartalar 15/8
07050 Antalya
Tel: +31 124 400 / 128 158

United Kingdom

Mr Costa Paul
United Kingdom Thalassaemia
   Society
107 Nightingale Lane
London N8 7QY
Tel: +44 208 348 2553
Fax: +44 208 348 0437

United States of America

Lucille Gash
President, Thalassemia Action
   Group
c/o Daniele
25 Bassett Lane
Palm Coast, 33137-8823
Tel: +1 904 446 3442
Fax: +1 201 935 3366

Mr Robert Ficarra
Cooley's Anemia Foundation,
   Inc.
Suite 911
105 East 22nd Street
New York, NY 10010
Tel: +1 212 598 0911
Fax: +1 212 944 7327

West Indies

Mrs I. Ramapaul
The Society for Inherited and Severe
   Blood Disorders (Trinidad &
   Tobago) Ltd.
Haematology Treatment Centre
General Hospital
PO Box 421
Port of Spain
Trinidad
Tel/Fax: +1 809 625 4765

Mrs L. Bhagwandin
Thalassaemia Association of Trinidad
   & Tobago Ltd.
352 Southern Main Road
Enterprise, Chaguanas
Trinidad

Index

Page numbers in *italic* refer to Figures and those in **bold** refer to Tables

adolescents 662
adrenal insufficiency 302, 306
Africa
  α thalassaemia distribution 271–2
  β thalassaemia distribution 243–4
    molecular variants 247
  HbS distribution 273, 280, *281*
  public health issues 598
  sickle cell disease/malaria frequency
    studies 273
agar gel electrophoresis 694–5
  buffer system 694
  methods 694–5
AIDS
  management 660
  see also human immunodeficiency virus
    (HIV)
Algeria
  α thalassaemia distribution 272
  β thalassaemia distribution 243
allele-specific oligonucleotide hybridization
  (ASO)
  β thalassaemia mutations analysis 710
  haemoglobin variants detection 717, 718
  prenatal diagnosis 619–20, 621, 622, 623
alleles 133
allostery 67, 77, 80
α chain
  α1:α2 production ratio 101–2, 107
  α thalassaemia
    defective synthesis 122
    genetic classification 123–4
    messenger RNA analysis 50
  assembly 46, *47*
  β chain interactions 21, 22, **72**, *72*
    oxygen binding 78
    oxygenation/deoxygenation
     movements 77, 79
  β thalassaemia excess production *see* β
    thalassaemia
  δ chain association 22
  γ chain association (fetal haemoglobin)
    21, 22
  haem interactions 100
  haemoglobin tetrameric associations **72**,
    72
  historical aspects 15, 18
  red-cell inclusions *see* red-cell inclusion
    bodies
  structure
    primary 73, 74
    three dimensional *75*, 75
  synthesis
    mRNA translation 98–9
    thalassaemias 34, 35–6

variants 23, 108
  α thalassaemia co-inheritance 130,
    518, 518–19
  haemoglobin expression levels 130
  heterozygous β thalassaemia co-
    inheritance **447**, 447–8
  homozygous β thalassaemia co-
    inheritance *445*, 445–7
  notation 130
  unstable 149–50, **150**
  see also α-chain genes, mutations
α-chain genes
  α1 gene 82, 84
    gene product 98, 99
  α2 gene 82, 84
    gene product 98, 99
  chromosomal location 23
  chromosomal organization 23
  evolutionary aspects 80
  gene conversions 84
  historical aspects 15
  homologous unequal recombination 135
  HS–40 (major regulatory element) 92–3
  increased number 82–3, 130–1
    β thalassaemia heterozygous states co-
     inheritance 355, 570–2
    dominant β thalassaemia heterozygous
     state co-inheritance 572
    homozygous β thalassaemia
     (thalassaemia intermedia
     phenotype) co-inheritance 571
  inheritance patterns *126*, 126
  mutations 30–1, 108
    chain termination 29–30, 148–9, *149*
    frameshift 148
    non-deletional 144, **146–7**
    nonsense 148
    point 136
    poly(A) addition 145, **146**
    regulatory element deletions 141–4,
     143
    RNA splicing 144–5
    translation initiation 145, **146**, 148
    unstable α globin variants 149–50, **150**
    see also deletions
  number 23, 31
  structure *88*, 88
  switching (developmental change
    regulation) 22, 107
  see also α-globin gene cluster
α-globin gene cluster 81–5
  CpA repeats 83
  deletions 85
  gene conversion 84–5
  globin gene number variation 82–3

haplotypes 83, *84*
insertions 85
normal variation 82, 83–4
polymorphic base substitutions 83–4
structure *81*, 81–2
  Alu repeats 85
  pseudogenes 82
  ζ globin gene 82
  translocations 82
  variable number tandem repeats
    (VNTRs) 83, *84*
α helix 66
  haemoglobin molecule 75
α interferon therapy 659, 666
α thalassaemia 123, 484–525
  acquired form with myelodysplasia *see* α
    thalassaemia/myelodysplasia
    syndrome
  allele interactions **485**
  α-chain termination mutations 29–30,
    148–9, *149*, 515
  see also Hb Constant Spring
  anaemia 231–2
    mechanism 228–9
    milder α thalassaemias 507, 516
  β thalassaemia co-inheritance 235, 560
    pathophysiology 565
    see also thalassaemia intermedia
  classification 31
    genetic (α globin haplotype) 123–4
    molecular 125
  DNA analysis 706–8
  genetic aspects 29–31
  genotype notation 124
  genotype/phenotype relations 233–4
  geographical distribution *238*, 262–73
    global distribution *264*, **265**
    malaria endemicity relationship *277*,
     277–8
    migration/founder effects 278–9
  globin gene deletions *see* deletions
  globin gene mapping 55–7
  globin messenger RNA analysis 50–1
  haemoglobin Bart's *see* haemoglobin
    Bart's
  haemoglobin homotetramers
    formation 122, 224, 226, 484
    properties 226, 228
  haemoglobin patterns *122*, 122
    secondary changes 126, 232–3
  haemoglobin structural variant
    interactions 28–9, 127–30, **518**,
    518–25, **519**
    α chain **518**, 518–19
    β chain *see* β-chain structural variants

α thalassaemia (*cont.*)
  HbH disease *see* haemoglobin H disease
  heterozygous state
    diagnosis 689, 691
    malaria protection 277, 277–8, 278, 282
    neonatal detection 226
  historical background 17–18, 27–31
  inheritance patterns 126, 126
  iron loading 231–2
  management 672–4
  mental retardation association 526
    prenatal diagnosis 624
    see also ATR-16 syndrome; ATR-X
      syndrome
  milder phenotypes 507–18
    clinical heterogeneity 513–15
    diagnostic problems 515–18
    genotypes 507
    globin synthesis 512–13
    haematological findings 508–10
    haemoglobin analysis 510–12
  molecular pathology 136–50
  older notation (1 and 2) 29, 30, 31, 124
  pathophysiology 223–34, 224, **231**
  prenatal counselling 516–17
  prenatal diagnosis 611, 612, 615, 619, 622
    programme strategies 623–4
  red-cell damage 229–31
  red-cell inclusion bodies 228–9
  sickle cell β thalassaemia co-inheritance
    409
  sickle cell disease co-inheritance 128–9
    haemoglobin expression patterns 128,
      129
    inheritance patterns 128–9, *129*
  terminology 31, 124
  unbalanced globin synthesis 121, 224–6
  unstable α globin variants 149–50, **150**
  see also α⁺ thalassaemia; α⁰ thalassaemia
α⁺ thalassaemia 31, 124, 136, 224, 484
  α⁰ thalassaemia interactions 126, 126
  carrier states 126
  deletional forms (-α/αα;-α/-α) 55–6, 124,
    137, 137–9, 138, 224, 484
    adult haemoglobin values 508
    developmental changes 508, 509,
      510–11, 511
    diagnosis 689
    globin mRNA synthesis 512, 513, 513
    haemoglobin analysis 510–11
    pregnancy-associated changes 508,
      509
  deletional/non-deletional compound
    heterozygotes (αᵀα/-α)
    haematological changes 509
    haemoglobin analysis 511–12
  deletions *see* deletions
  globin synthesis, heterozygotes 226
  milder phenotypes 507
  molecular designations 125
  mRNA analysis 50
  non-deletional (αᵀ) types 56, 124, 144,
    146–7, 224, 484
  non-deletional heterozygotes (αᵀα/αα)
    diagnosis 689
    haematological changes 508–9
    haemoglobin analysis 511–12

non-deletional homozygotes (αᵀα/αᵀα)
    509–10
  clinical heterogeneity 513
  PCR analysis 707–8
α⁰ thalassaemia 31, 124, 125, 136, 224, 484
  --MEDs 125, 139, 141, 142, **707**
  --SEAs 125, 139, **707**
  α⁺ thalassaemia interactions 126, 126
  deletions *see* deletions
  gap PCR detection 706–7, **707**
  globin mRNA analysis 50, 51
  heterogeneity 56
  heterozygous state (--/αα)
    adult haemoglobin values 508
    developmental changes 508, 509,
      510–11, 511
    diagnosis 689
    globin synthesis 226, 262–3, 512, 513,
      513
    haemoglobin analysis 510–11
    pregnancy-associated changes 508, 509
  mental retardation association 139, 624
  milder phenotypes 507
  molecular analysis 139–41, 140, 141
  Southern blot analysis 708–9, 709
α thalassaemia/myelodysplasia syndrome
    541, **544–5**
  clinical features 546
  globin synthesis 546, 548
  haematological findings 546, 546
    blood film 546, 547
  haemoglobin analysis 546, 548
  molecular pathology 547–9
Alu repeats 136, 187
  α-globin-gene cluster 85
  α-globin-gene deletions association 141
    HS –40 deletions 143
  β-globin-gene cluster 86
  recombination events 141
amino acids
  classification 66
  codes **66**
  protein primary structure 65–6, 66
amniotic fluid analysis 615
  Hb Bart's hydrops diagnosis 493
amplification refractory mutation system
    (ARMS)
  β-thalassaemia mutations analysis
    710–11, **711, 712**
  method 718–21, 719
  prenatal diagnosis 620–1, 621, 622, 623
amplification-created restriction sites
    (ACRS) 712
anaemia
  α thalassaemia 228–9, 231–2
    milder forms 507, 516
  β thalassaemia 192, 201–2, 231–2, 319,
    686, 687
    compensatory mechanisms 223
    erythropoietin response 207–9
    heterozygotes 334, **335**, 339, 350
    hyperkinetic response 223
  δβ thalassaemia
    (ᴬγδβ)⁰ homozygous state 383, 388
    (δβ)⁰/(ᴬγδβ)⁰ β thalassaemia
      compound heterozygotes 385–6
  (εγδβ)⁰ thalassaemia 390–1

Hb Bart's hydrops fetalis 493
Hb Lepore homozygous state 361, 363
HbE β thalassaemia 422, 435
  aplastic crises 429
  megaloblastic 429
  HbH disease 494, 506
  thalassaemia intermedia 551, 576, 577
  treatment initiation 630–1
  see also haemolytic anaemia; ineffective
    erythropoiesis
anaemia infantum pseudoleucaemica 5
androgen replacement therapy 656
antibiotics, postsplenectomy infections 658
anticoagulaton 672
anti-i reactivity 327
antioxidant systems **212**, 212
antithrombin III 218
aplastic crisis
  HbE β thalassaemia 429
  sickle cell anaemia 113
apolipoprotein E4 300, 301
Arab populations
  α thalassaemia distribution 267
  β thalassaemia distribution 241–2
Artemisia annua 660
artemisin (qinghaosu) 660
ascorbic acid
  β-thalassaemia-associated deficiency 316
  desferrioxamine co-administration 641,
    641
aspirin 431, 672, 674
Atlanta type heterocellular HPFH **476**, 479
ATR-16 syndrome 82, 527–34, **528**, 541
  chromosomal abnormalities 527, 527,
    530, 530–1, 532, 533
    phenotypic associations 531, 533
  clinical features 527, **529**, 531, 534
  inheritance patterns 527, 530, 530
ATR-X syndrome 534–41
  ATR-X mutations 540, **542–3**
  ATR-X protein intracellular distribution
    539–40
  clinical features 534–6, **535**, 535, 536
  haematological findings 536, 537
  molecular analysis 537–9, 538
  phenotype/genotype relationships 540–1
  X-linkage 536–7
Australian ᴳγβ⁺ HPFH -144C→G **468**, 470
autosomes 133
avoidance measures 597–629, 728, 729
5-azacytidine 677

behavioural impact 317–18
Belgian (ᴬγδβ)⁰ thalassaemia 178
Benin 272
β chain
  α chain interactions 21, 22
    oxygen binding 78
    oxygenation/deoxygenation
      movements 77, 79
  assembly 46, 47, 48
  β thalassaemia 25, 121, 122, 192
    messenger RNA analysis 49–50
  fetal synthesis 36–7
  haem interactions 100
  haemoglobin tetrameric associations **72**,
    72

historical aspects 15
homotetramers formation 16, 122, 224
structural variants *see* β-chain structural
    variants
structure
    primary 73, 74
    three dimensional 75, *76*
synthesis
    heterozygotes 36
    mRNA translation 98
    thalassaemia 34, 35–6
β-chain structural variants 108
    α thalassaemia co-inheritance **519**,
        519–25
    α+ homozygotes/heterozygotes 520–1,
        521
    clinical phenotype 520
    HbE 521–3, **522**
    HbH disease 521
    HbS 520, 521, **523**, 523–5
    pathophysiology 519–20
    cis to β-thalassaemia mutation 444–5
    thalassaemia co-inheritance 127–30
β-chain-gene 85
    chromosomal location 23
    chromosomal organization 22
    chromosomal translocation 86
    deletions *see* deletions
    developmental change (switching) 22,
        102, 105
    evolutionary aspects 80
    fusion variants 86–7
    historical aspects 15
    locus-control region *91*, 91–2
    premature termination mutations 117
    promoter 90
    structure *88*, 88
    see also β-globin-gene cluster
β-globin-gene cluster 23, *81*, *85*, 85–7
    chromosomal translocations 86
    gene conversions 87
    haplotypes *87*, 87
    HbF enhanced production determinants
        184–5, 566–7, **567**
    point mutations 184
    rearrangements 184
    RFLPs 185
    thalassaemia intermedia phenotype
        568–9
    heterocellular HPFH **476**, 479–80
    locus-control region (LCR) 85
    mutations 52, 151, *152–3*, **155–60**
    C–T at position -101 154, 165
    chain termination 164–5, *165*
    consensus sequence 161–2
    cryptic splice-site *162*, 162–4
    deletions *see* deletions
    HbF production effects 184–5
    insertions 151
    mRNA processing 161
    mRNA translation 164–5
    point 150, 184
    poly(A) addition site 164
    promoter region 154, *161*
    splice junction 161
    5' UTR 161, 166
    3' UTR 164, 166

number variation 86–7
polymorphic base substitutions 87
RFLPs *87*, 87, 185
    analysis 714–15, **716**
structure 86–7
    Alu repeats 86
    L1 repeats 86
    microsatelite repeats 86
β sheet 66
β strand 66
β thalassaemia 123
    α chain excess 35, 36, 122, 192, 194–6, *196*,
        198–9, *200*, *201*, 331
    proteolytic degradation 194–5, *196*,
        198, 199, 204, 206
    shortened red-cell survival 202, 203,
        204, 206–7
    α thalassaemia co-inheritance 235, 560
        pathophysiology 565
    see also thalassaemia intermedia
    α-globin variant co-inheritance
        numerical variants 131
        structural variants 130
    anaemia 192, 201–2, 231–2
        compensatory mechanisms 223
        erythropoietin response 207–9
    anti-Lepore Hb interaction 375–6
    β+ (HbA-producing) 25, 124, 287
        gene sequencing 57–8
    β++ (high HbA-producing) 25, 124,
        287
    β0 (non-HbA-producing) 25, 124, 287
        β-globin mRNA analysis 49–50
        Ferrara form 48
        HbE/α thalassaemia interactions
            521–3
    β chain deficit 24, 25, 36, 121, 122, 192
    carrier state *see* β thalassaemia
        heterozygous states
    classification 287–8, **288**
        clinical 123
        genetic 124
        molecular 125
    clinical features 287–356
        see also β thalassaemia major;
            thalassaemia intermedia
    δ thalassaemia co-inheritance 378
    diagnosis 686–7
        DNA analysis 709–15, 718–21
        haemoglobin variants co-inheritance
            692, **693**
    differential diagnosis 687
    dominant forms 117, 123, *165*, 167, **168–9**,
        170, 287, 572–4
        blood film *590*, 590
        chain termination mutants *165*, 170,
            572
        clinical features 590, 592
        distribution 170
        genotype/phenotype relationships
            572, *573*
        haemoglobin constitution 588, **589**
        historical background 572
        phenotypic diversity 572, 573–4
        red-cell inclusion bodies 590, *591*
    Dutch form 354, 568, 588
    gene mutations 57–8, 150, **151**

see also β-globin-gene cluster;
    molecular pathology
genetic heterogeneity 24–7
genotype/phenotype relations 287–8
geographical distribution 239–47
    common alleles **263**
    global surveys *238*, 247
    mild β+ alleles 592–3, *593*
    molecular variants 247, **248–61**, *262*,
        262
globin messenger RNA analysis 49–50,
    52
haemoglobin
    constitution *327*, 327–31
    in vitro synthesis 331–3, **332**, *332*
    patterns 121–2, *122*
    haemoglobin variants co-inheritance
        127–30
    abnormal oxygen affinity 444
    α-chain variants *445*, 445–8, *446*, **447**
    β-chain variants in *cis* 444–5
    δ-chain variants 448–9, **449**
    rare variants 440–1, **442–3**
    unstable variants 444
Hb Lepore compound heterozygotes
    369–70
HbA 331
HbA2 24, 26–7, 121, 124, 329–31, **330**
    haemoglobin Knossos 166–7
    high variants 166, 376
    mild β thalassaemia alleles 552
    molecular mechanisms 151
    normal variant type 1 (silent β
        thalassaemia) 27, 124, 166, 552
    normal variant type 2 27, 124, 166
    normal variants 27, 124, 166, 167, 287
HbE 18, *19*
    see also haemoglobin E β thalassaemia
HbF *see* haemoglobin F
    historical backgound 8, 13, 17–18
    HPFH relationship 125
    inheritance patterns 25, 125–6
    milder forms
        alleles **346**, 346, **347**, **552**, 552, 592–3,
            593
    see also β thalassaemia heterozygous
        states; thalassaemia intermedia
molecular pathology 150–70
    mutations unlinked to β-globin-gene
        complex 355–6
    undefined disorders 356
pathophysiology 192–223, *194*, **231**
    modifying factors 235–6, *236*
Portuguese variant 161–2, 558
prenatal diagnosis *see* prenatal diagnosis
red-cell damage 208, **209**
    bone marrow phagocytosis 204, *205*
    haemichrome formation 204, 207
    membrane damage 203, 204, 206–7
    premature destruction 203, 204, 206–7
    red-cell inclusion bodies 39–40, 198–9,
        200, *201*, 320, *322*, 590, *591*
severe form *see* β thalassaemia major
sickle cell thalassaemia *see* sickle cell β
    thalassaemia
silent forms 13, 27, 287, 288
    alleles **552**, 552

β thalassaemia (*cont.*)
    molecular basis 165–6, *166*
    trans-acting genes 165
    unbalanced globin synthesis 35–6, 39–40,
        121–2, 192, 193–8, *195, 196*
        modifying factors 234–5, **235**
    see also δβ thalassaemia
β thalassaemia heterozygous states 287,
    333–56
    additional α-globin genes co-inheritance
        355
        thalassaemia intermedia phenotype
            570–2
    α thalassaemia co-inheritance
        pathophysiology 565
        thalassaemia intermedia phenotype
            560–3, **561**, *561, 562*
    anaemia 334, 339, 350
    biochemical changes 345
    classification **288**, 333
    clinical features 333–4
        unusually severe course 355
        see also β thalassaemia dominant
            forms
    complications 339–41
    δ thalassaemia compound heterozygotes
        352, 352–3
    $(\delta\beta)^0/(^A\gamma\delta\beta)^0$ thalassaemia compound
        heterozygotes 385–7
    diagnosis 688
        differentiation from iron deficiency
            688–9, 691
        problems 341
        screening procedures 691
    folic acid deficiency 340–1
    Gilbert's syndrome co-inheritance 350
    globin synthesis 345
    glucose-6-phosphate dehydrogenase
        (G6PD) deficiency co-inheritance
        350
    haematology **335**
        bone marrow 337
        red-cell indices 334, **335**, 336
        reticulocyte count 336
    haemoglobin constitution 341–5
        developmental changes 348–9, *349*
        HbA_2 16, 17, 24, 166, 287, 333, 341–3, **342**,
            343
            borderline levels 353–4
            deletional forms 347–8, **348**
            δ chain synthesis 342–3
            developmental changes 348–9, *349*
            elevation 341–3, **342**, *342*
            normal variant phenocopies 353
            normal variant type 1 (silent β
                thalassaemia) 351, 352
            normal variant type 2 351, **352**, 352–3
            specific mutations **347**, 347
            unusually high levels 166, 354
    HbF *see* haemoglobin F
    hereditary elliptocytosis co-inheritance
        350–1
    hereditary haemochromatosis co-
        inheritance 338
    hereditary methaemoglobinaemia co-
        inheritance 351
    hereditary spherocytosis co-inheritance
        351
HPFH compound heterozygotes 344, 354
    Black/Sardinian $^G\gamma\beta^+$ HPFH -175T→C
        469
    British $^A\gamma\beta^+$ HPFH ($^A\gamma$ -198T→C) 473
    $(\delta\beta)^0$ *see* $(\delta\beta)^0$ HPFH
    Greek/Sardinian/Black $^A\gamma\beta^+$ HPFH
        ($^A\gamma$-117 G→A) 471–2
infection susceptibility 341
iron metabolism 337–9
    absorption 338
    ferrokinetics/erythrokinetics 339
    iron loading 338
    iron status 337–8
life expectancy 341
molecular forms, phenotype relationships
    345–8, **346, 347**
pathophysiology 350
Pelger–Huet abnormality co-inheritance
    351
pregnancy 334, 339–40, **340**
pyruvate kinase deficiency co-inheritance
    351
red cells
    metabolism 345
    morphology 336–7, *337*
    survival 337
β thalassaemia major 287, 288–333
    age at presentation 288, **289**
    autopsy findings 318–19
        tissue iron concentrations **319**
    behavioural patterns 317–18
    biochemical changes 325–6
    bleeding tendency 217
    blood transfusion *see* blood transfusion
    bone disease 192, 216–17, 306–7
    bone marrow expansion 192, 209
    cardiac disease *214*, 214–15, 291, 295, *296*,
        296–300, **297**, *298*
    clinical features
        impact of iron chelation therapy 291
        inadequately transfused patients *290*,
            290–1, *291*
        well-transfused patients 291
    complications 292
    diagnosis 289–90, 686–7
    endocrine dysfunction 215, 291, 302–6
        adrenal insufficiency 306
        delayed puberty 304–5
        diabetes mellitus 305
        growth retardation 302–4, **303**
        hypoparathyroidism 306
        hypothalamic/pituitary axis
            dysfunction 304–5
        hypothyroidism 306
    exocrine pancreatic damage 315
    gallstones 317
    genotypes 287
    gout 317
    haematology 319–24
        bone marrow 321, *322*, 323
        serological changes 327
        well-transfused patients 320
    haemoglobin constitution *327*, 327–33
    haemoglobin Lepore/β thalassaemia
        compound heterozygotes 369
    hypersplenism/splenomegaly 192,
        209–10, 293–5, *294*
        see also splenectomy
    ineffective erythropoiesis 192, 199, 201,
        325
        mechanisms 202–4
    infection susceptibility 218–20, 307–11
    intelligence 317–18
    iron metabolism 324–6
        absorption 324–5
    iron overload *see* iron overload
    liver disease 311–15
    lung disease 215–16, 300–1
    management *see* Chapter 15
    neuromuscular abnormalities 317
    plasma volume expansion 210, 294, 295
    platelets 320
    pregnancy 318
    presenting symptoms 288–9
    red cells 319–20, *320, 321*
        metabolism 324
        survival 323–4
    thrombotic complications 217–18, 301–2
    vitamin/trace metal deficiencies 316–17
        folate 315
        vitamin B_{12} 315–16
    white cells 320
β thalassaemia minor *see* β thalassaemia
    heterozygous states
β thalassaemia trait *see* β thalassaemia
    heterozygous states
bilirubin metabolism 325
Black $^A\gamma\beta^+$ HPFH ($^A\gamma$ -114 to -102 deletion)
    468, 475
Black $^A\gamma\beta^+$ HPFH ($^A\gamma$ -175 T→C) **468**, 475
Black $^A\gamma\beta^+$ HPFH ($^A\gamma$ -202 C→T) **468**,
    473–4
Black $(^A\gamma\delta\beta)^0$ thalassaemia 178
Black Americans, β thalassaemia frequency
    246
Black $(\delta\beta)^0$ HPFH (HPFH 1) 180, 187, 188,
    189, 452, 453
    HbC compound heterozygotes **459**, 461
    HbF structure 454
    HbS compound heterozygotes **459**, 459
Black $(\delta\beta)^0$ thalassaemia 177
Black $^G\gamma\beta^+$ HPFH -202C→G 467, **468**
Black Sea area 241
Black/Sardinian $^G\gamma\beta^+$ HPFH -175T→C **468**,
    469
    β^0 compound heterozygotes 469
    HbS compound heterozygotes 469
    heterozygous state 469
bleeding tendency
    β thalassaemia 217, 290
    sickle cell β thalassaemia 403
blood filters 633
blood products 633–4
blood transfusion 41–2, 288, 289, 293,
    633–6, 729
    blood products 633–4
    dangers 635–6
    donor screening programmes 636
    Hb Bart's hydrops fetalis
        prenatal/neonatal therapy 673
    HbH disease 673
    historical aspects 41
    information for parents 632

initiation of treatment 631, 633
  haemoglobin levels 633
iron overload *see* iron overload
malaria transmission 311, 636
neocytes 633–4
red-cell life expectancy 633
regimens 634
  infection susceptibility impact 307–8
sickle cell β thalassaemia 676
target haemoglobin levels 634–5, 729
  minimal levels 635
thalassaemia intermedia 669, 671
transfusion haemochromatosis 42
transfusion reactions 635–6
viral blood-borne infection 308, 309, 310,
  311, 635, 636
blood-borne infections 307, 312, 635, 730
  treatment 659–61
Bohr effect 77, 79–80
  high oxygen-affinity haemoglobin
    variants 118
bone density measurement 657
bone disease 730
  β thalassaemia major 192, 216–17, 290,
    293, 306–7
    pathophysiology 216–17
  Hb Lepore homozygous state 361
  HbE β thalassaemia 434
  historical studies 4–5
  management 657, 671–2
  sickle cell β thalassaemia 396, 397, 398,
    399, **400**, *400*
  thalassaemia intermedia 581, *583*, 583,
    671–2
    bone pain 581
bone marrow
  β thalassaemia heterozygous states 337
  fetal erythropoesis 100, 102
  phagocytic activity 321, 323
  sickle cell β thalassaemia 400–1
bone-marrow expansion/erythroid
  hyperplasia 38, 41
  β thalassaemia 192, 209, 321, *323*, 323
    heterozygous states 337
  Hb Bart's hydrops fetalis 488
  HbE β thalassaemia 429, *430*
  HbH disease 499–500
  sickle cell β thalassaemia 405
  thalassaemia intermedia 587
bone-marrow transplantation 663–7, 728,
  730
  busulphan toxicity 666
  ethical aspects 667
  graft-versus-host disease 665–6
  historical background 663
  indications 666–7
  iron loading management following 666
  malignant disease long-term risk 666, 667
  mixed chimerism 666
  peripheral blood stem cells 667
  practical aspects 667
  results 663–5, *664*, *665*
  sickle cell β thalassaemia 676
  unrelated matched donors 666
  viral hepatitis management following
    666
Bosnia Herzegovina 241

brain syndrome
  sickle cell anaemia 113
  sickle cell β thalassaemia 398
Brazil 281
  α thalassaemia distribution 272–3
Brazilian ^Aγβ^+ HPFH (-195 C→G) **468**, 474
British ^Aγβ^+ HPFH (^Aγ-198T→C) **468**,
  472–3, *474*
  β thalassaemia compound heterozygotes
    473
  heterozygous state 472, *473*
  homozygous state 472
Buddhism 601–2
Burma 31
  β thalassaemia distribution 244
busulphan toxicity 666
butyrate compounds 677

CA repetitive sequences 83, 86, 136
calcium supplements 657, 671
Cambodia
  β thalassaemia distribution 244–5
  HbE distribution 245
Caminopetros 11, *12*
Campylobacter jejuni 428
Cantonese (^Aγδβ)^0 thalassaemia 179
CAP structure 69
  globin gene messenger RNA 95, 97
capping
  globin genes RNA processing 95
  point mutation effects 134–5
carbamate ion formation 80
carbon dioxide transport 80
cardiac disease
  β thalassaemia major *214*, 214–15, 295,
    296, 296–300, **297**
    clinical features 299
    detection 299–300
    pathology 297–8, *298*
    pathophysiology 298–9
    risk assessment 300
  desferrioxamine in prevention 637–8,
    638
  HbE β thalassaemia 431, 433
  iron deposition damage *214*, 214–15, 291,
    295, *296*, 296
    chelation therapy protective effect
      297, 300
    mechanisms 296–7
  management 657
  myocarditis 297, 299
  pericarditis 297
  pulmonary hypertension 297
  thalassaemia intermedia 580–1
cardiac failure
  β thalassaemia major 299
  HbE β thalassaemia 431
  thalassaemia intermedia 580, 581
cardiac transplantation 657
Caribbean
  α thalassaemia distribution 272–3
  HbS origins 281
cDNA/DNA hybridization experiments
  51–2, *52*
ceftriaxone 658
cellulose acetate haemoglobin
  electrophoresis 687, 688, 689, 694

buffer systems 694
  method 694
  screening procedures 691, 692
Central Europe 241
Chad 243
chain termination mutations
  α thalassaemia 29–30, 148–9, *149*, 515
    see also Hb Constant Spring
  β thalassaemia 164–5, *165*
    dominantly inherited forms *165*, 170,
      572
chelation therapy 291, 636–51, 729–30
  body iron burden
    assessment **644**, 644–5
    optimal level 640
  cardiac complications protective effect
    297, 300
  deferiprone 649–51
  historical aspects 42–3
  information for parents 632
  liver disease impact 314
  thalassaemia intermedia 671
  see also desferrioxamine
Chile 273
China
  α thalassaemia distribution 269–70
  β thalassaemia distribution 245
  prenatal diagnosis programmes 621
Chinese (^Aγδβ)^0 thalassaemia 178
  clinical features 378
chloride effect 80
chloroquine 660
cholecystectomy 656
chorionic villus sampling 59, *611*, 611,
  616–17, 624
  complications 616
  DNA yield 616, *617*
  Hb Bart's hydrops diagnosis 493
  maternal tissue contamination 622, 626
chromatin 70, 71
  decondensation 93
chromosomal translocations
  α-globin genes 82
  β-globin-gene cluster 86
chromosomes 70, *71*, 133
  normal karyotype *72*
cis position
  β-chain structural variants β thalassaemia
    co-inheritance 444–5
  DNA regulatory elements 71
  haemoglobin switching regulation 103–
    4
  sickle cell β thalassaemia haemoglobin
    expression patterns 127–8, *129*
citrate agar haemoglobin electrophoresis
  687
  screening procedures 692
co-dominance 126, 133
COLIAI polymorphism 307
column chromatography 688
  HbA$_2$ estimation 695–6
Congo 272
consensus sequence mutations 161–2
control at population level 597–629, 728,
  729
  ethical aspects 598–604
Cooley, Thomas B. 5, *6*, 8

Cooley's anaemia 8, 9, 10, 11, 12, 13
   haemoglobin studies 16
   see also β thalassaemia major
copper levels 316, 317
cord-blood stem-cell bone-marrow
     transplantation 667
Corfu δβ thalassaemia 167, 171, 176
   clinical features 377–8
co-trimoxazole 658
counselling 598, 662
   post-screening test 608–9, 610–11
   prenatal 516–17
   see also genetic counselling
coxsackie B virus 428
Cretan type heterocellular HPFH **476**, 479
Crete 240
Croatia 241
Cuba 273
cyanosis, congenital 119
cyclophosphamide 666
cyclosporin 663
Cyprus 33
   α thalassaemia distribution 266
   β thalassaemia distribution 240
   historical aspects 6–7
   prenatal diagnosis programme 614, 618,
     627
   public health issues 597
   screening programme 601, 605, 606
cytoarabinoside 677
cytomegalovirus 635, 663
Czech type heterocellular HPFH **476**, 479
Czechoslovakia 241

Dahomey 243
deferiprone 649–51
   effectiveness 649–50
   pharmacology 649
   toxicity 650–1
delayed development 304–5
   desferrioxamine-treated patients 639
   management 656–7
   pubertal growth delay 302, 303
deletions 135
   α-chain genes 51, *52*, 137
     α⁺ thalassaemias *137*, 137–9, *138*
     α⁰ thalassaemias 139–41, *140*, *141*, *142*
     α globin expression 139
     in-frame 148
     regulatory elements 141–4, *143*
   α-globin-gene cluster 85
     downstream region 144
   α thalassaemia 51–2, *52*, 55–6
   α⁺ thalassaemia *137*, 137–9, *138*
   α⁰ thalassaemia 55, 56, 139–41, *140*, *141*
     designation 125
     extent 139, *141*
     functional consequences 139–41
     HS –40 regulatory element 141–4, *142*
     mental retardation association 139
     recombinational rearrangements 141,
       142
     telomeric repair events 141
   β-globin-gene cluster 52, 53, 150, 151, *154*
     (δβ)⁰ HPFH 452
     enhancer sequences *189*, 189
     (εᴳγᴬγδβ)⁰ thalassaemia 190

mechanisms 186–7
β thalassaemia 57, 150
   β-globin-gene cluster 150, 151, *154*
   LCR 150
breakpoint characterisitics 186–7
δ-chain gene 52, 53
δβ thalassaemia 52–3, 57, 171, *174*, 186
HbH 51, 55, 224, 494
HPFH 52–3, 57, 171–2, **173**, *174*, 179, 180
mapping, prenatal diagnosis 618–19
ζ-chain gene 139–40
δ amino laevulinic acid (ALA) synthase 99
δ chain
   α chain association 22
   in β thalassaemia 35
     heterozygous states 342–3
   haemoglobin tetrameric associations **72**,
     72
   historical aspects 15
   primary structure 73, 74
   synthesis 360, 361
     α thalassaemia 233
   variants 108
     β thalassaemia/δβ thalassaemia co-
       inheritance 448–9
     thalassaemia co-inheritance *129*, 129
δ-chain gene 15, 85
   chromosomal location 23
   chromosomal organization 22
   deletions 52, 53
   evolutionary aspects 80
   mutations 108, 171, **172**
   promoter region 361
   regulation 22
   transcription 360
δ thalassaemia 391–2
   β thalassaemia co-inheritance 378
   β thalassaemia compound heterozygotes
     352, 352–3
   δ⁺ 124, 171
   δ⁰ 124, 171
   (δβ)⁰ HPFH compound heterozygotes
     465
   genetic classification 124
   haematology 392
   haemoglobin analysis 392
   HPFH co-inheritance 391
   molecular pathology 171, **172**
δβ fusion genes
   (δβ)⁺ thalassaemia *173*, 175
   Hb Lepore 22, 26, 357
     inefficient globin synthesis 370
     see also haemoglobin Lepore
       Washington Boston
   Hb Parchman 376
   mechanism *175*, 175
   potential crossover variants **376**, 376–7
(δβ)⁰ HPFH 125, 171, 179–80, 452–65
   β thalassaemia compound heterozygotes
     462–4
   clinical/haematological findings 463
   haemoglobin constitution **459**, 463–4
   haemoglobin synthesis 464
   HbF structure 464
   inheritance *456*, 464
   pathophysiology 464
   Black (HPFH 1) 86, 180, 187, 188, 189,

452, 453, 454, **459**, 459, 461
classification **452**
δ thalassaemia compound heterozygotes
   465
Ghanaian (HPFH 2) 180, 187, 188, 189,
   452, 453, 454, **459**, 459, 460, 461
HbB₂ (HbA₂') compound heterozygotes
   464–5
HbC compound heterozygotes 454, **459**,
   461–2
   clinical/haematological findings 462
   haemoglobin constitution 454, 462
   Hb F structure 462
   inheritance 462
HbE compound heterozygotes 462
HbS compound heterozygotes 458–61,
   459
   clinical features 459
   haematological findings 459
   haemoglobin cellular distribution *460*,
     460, 461
   haemoglobin constitution 454, 460
   haemoglobin synthesis 460–1
   HbF structure 461
   inheritance 461
   pathophysiology compared with sickle
     cell disease 461
heterozygous state 456–8
   haematological findings 456, **457**
   haemoglobin constitution *457*, 457, *458*
   haemoglobin synthesis 457–8
   HbF cellular distribution 457, *458*
   HbF structure 458
homozygous state 453–6
   clinical features 453
   haematological findings **453**, 453–4
   haemoglobin analysis *454*, 454
   haemoglobin synthesis 454–5, *455*
   HbF structure 454
   inheritance *456*, 456
   pathophysiology 455–6
   red-cell properties 455
Indian (HPFH 3) 180, 188, 452, 464
Italian (HPFH 4) 180, 453
relationship to (δβ)⁰ thalassaemia 456,
   482, 482, *483*
Sicilian (HPFH 5) 180, 453
south-east Asian 180, 453
structural haemoglobin variant
   compound heterozygotes 464
δβ thalassaemia 25, 123
   classification **358**, 358
   genetic 124
   clinical features 357–92
   Corfu form (normal HbA₂) 167, 171, 176,
     377–8
   β thalassaemia trait phenocopies 353
   deletions 52–3, 57, 171, *174*, 186
   (δβ)⁺ *see* haemoglobin Lepore
     Washington Boston
   diagnosis 687–8, 691
   haemoglobin variants co-inheritance
     692, **693**
   DNA analysis 715
   gap PCR **707**, 712, *714*
   geographical distribution 240, 389–90
   haemoglobin variants co-inheritance 448

δ-chain variants 449
HbC association 420–1
HbE interactions 439–40
heterogeneity 26
heterozygous states
  diagnosis 688–9, 691
  differentiation from iron deficiency
    688–9
historical background 357
HPFH relationship 125
molecular pathology 171–2
pathophysiology 387–9
prenatal diagnosis 619, 622
Sardinian 176, 377
sickle cell gene interactions 411–15
south-east Asian 176–7
terminology 357
see also (^{A}γδβ)^0 thalassaemia; (δβ)^0
  thalassaemia
(δβ)^0 thalassaemia 124, 171, 357, 358, 378
β thalassaemia compound heterozygotes
    385–7
  clinical features 385–6, 388
  complications 386
  haematology 385–6
  haemoglobin constitution 386
  haemoglobin synthesis 387
  HbF 386–7
deletions 186
diagnosis 687
eastern European 177
geographical distribution 378–9
Hb Lepore compound heterozygotes 370
heterozygous state 380–2
  clinical features 380
  geographical distribution 380
  haematological findings 380, **381**
  haemoglobin analysis 380–1, **381**
  haemoglobin synthesis 382
  HbF 381, *382*
homozygous state 379–80, *380*
  clinical features 379, 387
  haematological findings 379
  haemoglobin analysis 379
  haemoglobin synthesis 380, 380
  HbF 379–80, 387
Indian 177
Japanese 177
Laotian 176–7
molecular pathology 176–8
Sicilian 176
Spanish 177
Turkish-2 178
Turkish/Macedonian 177
(^{A}γδβ)^0 thalassaemia 124, 171, 357, 358, 378,
    382–7
β thalassaemia compound heterozygotes
    385–7
  clinical features 385–6, 388
  complications 386
  haematology 385–6
  haemoglobin constitution 386
  haemoglobin synthesis 387
  HbF 386–7
Belgian 178
Black 178
Chinese 178, 378

deletions 196
diagnosis 687
German 179
heterozygous state **384**, 384–5
homozygous state 383–4
  clinical features 383, 388
  haematological findings 383–4
  haemoglobin analysis/synthesis 384
Italian 178
Malaysian 2 178–9
molecular pathology 178–9
south-east Asian 179
Turkish 179
Yunnanese 178
denaturing gradient gel electrophoresis
    (DGGE) 708, 710
β thalassaemia, unknown mutations
    analysis 712–13
dental deformity 216
  management 661
desferrioxamine 42–3, 44, 729–30
  administration methods 43, 636–7, 641,
      648
    prolonged subcutaneous infusion
      636–7, *637*
    pumps/infusers 637, 641, 648
  ascorbate co-administration *641*, 641
  clinical effectiveness 637–9, *639*
    cardiac complications 300, 637–8, *638*
    diabetes mellitus 639
    endocrine function 639
    liver disease *638*, 638
  initiation of treatment 640–1
  pharmacology 636
  practical aspects of treatment **642–3**
  pregnancy 647–8
  reversal of iron-induced organ damage
    640, 648, 657
  thalassaemia intermedia 671
  toxicity 645–7
    allergic reactions 645
    chronic systemic side-effects 646–7,
      647
    dose relationship 640
    growth retardation 303, 304
    local cutaneous reactions 645
    monitoring **648**
    prevention 649
    treatment monitoring 644–5
  see also chelation therapy
diabetes mellitus
  β thalassaemia major 302, 305
    pancreatic iron deposition 215
  desferrioxamine in prevention 639
  HbE β thalassaemia 434
  thalassaemia intermedia 579, 580
2,3-diphosphoglycerate (2,3-DPG)
  β thalassaemia, increased level 223
  clinical conditions affecting level **79**
  haemoglobin function modification 77,
    79
  HbH oxygen dissociation curve 226, 504
  high oxygen-affinity haemoglobin variant
    binding 118
direct DNA sequencing 708
dissociation constants 67
DNA analysis 706–23

α thalassaemia 706–8, **707**, *709*
β thalassaemia **707**, 709–15
δβ thalassaemia **707**, 712, *714*, 715
haemoglobin variants 715–18
Hb Lepore **707**, 715
HPFH **707**, 712, 715
laboratory methods 718–23
DNA regulatory elements 71
DNA structure 67–8, *68*
DNA transcription 68
DNase 71
dominance 126, 133

eastern Europe 241
eastern European (δβ)^0 thalassaemia 177
echocardiography 299
EF-1 98
EF-2 98
Egypt 272
EKLF 94, 95, 106
  δ-globin-gene binding site 360, 361
  knockout mice 95
  promoter mutation effects 154
eIF-2 98, 99
elongation mutations **120**, 120, 164–5
embryonic haemoglobins 22, **72**, 72–3, 100,
    101
  evolutionary aspects 80
  globin-chain tetrameric associations **72**,
    72
  haematopoietic tissues 100, 102
  Hb Bart's hydrops fetalis 490
  switch to fetal haemoglobin 102
endocrine dysfunction 730
  β thalassaemia major 215, 291, 302–6
  desferrioxamine in prevention 639
  HbE β thalassaemia 433–4
  iron deposition damage 215, 291, 302–6
  thalassaemia intermedia 579–80
endothelial interactions, sickle cell red cells
    110–11
enhancers 71
  globin genes 89, 90
  HbF, deletion-associated increased
    production 188–9, *189*
ε chain
  embryonic haemoglobin tetrameric
    associations **72**, 72–3
  historical aspects 22
  primary structure 73–4
ε-chain gene 85
  chromosomal location 23
  developmental change (switching) 104–5
  evolutionary aspects 80
(εγδβ)^0 thalassaemia 123
  β thalassaemia trait phenocopies 353
  clinical features 390–1
  genetic classification 124
  haematology 391
  haemoglobin analysis 391
  molecular pathology 190–1
  pathophysiology 390
erythroid-specific transcription elements
    93–5, **94**
  β-globin-locus-control region binding
    sites 91
  globin-gene-promoter binding sites 90

stage-specific factors 106
erythron 211
erythropoietin
    β thalassaemia 207–9
    thalassaemia intermedia 587
Escherichia coli 428
ethical issues 598–604
    bone-marrow transplantation 667
    dysgenic effects of interventions 602–3
    eugenic concerns 598–600
    experimental therapies 684–5
    prenatal diagnosis 600, 603–4
    religious beliefs 600–2
    screening 600, 603–4
Ethiopia 243
eugenics issues 598–600
Europe
    α thalassaemia distribution 263–6
    β thalassaemia distribution 239–41
        molecular variants 247
evolution of globin genes 80
exocrine pancreatic damage 215, 315
exons 68, 69
    cryptic splice-site β-globin-gene
        mutations *163*, 163–4
exons (*cont.*)
    globin genes 88
expressivity 127
extramedullary haemopoietic masses
    β thalassaemia major 290
    HbE β thalassaemia 429, *430*
    HbH disease 496
    neurological complications 669–70
    thalassaemia intermedia *584*, 584–5
        management 669–70, *670*

F cells 101, *102*, 220, 221
    fluorescence-activated cell sorting
        (FACS) 703–4
    genetic control 476–7
    HPFH/δβ thalassaemia screening
        procedures 691–2
    immunofluorescence staining 701–2, *702*
    normal adults 476
    sickle cell β thalassaemia 408
F thalassaemia *see* δβ thalassaemia
facial appearance
    β thalassaemia major 216, 290, *291*
    thalassaemia intermedia *582*
fat embolism 400–1
FC locus 476
Ferrara β⁰ thalassaemia 48
ferritin 212
ferritin serum level
    β thalassaemia *295*, 295, 325
        heterozygous states 337–8
    body iron burden assessment 644, 645
    HbH disease 504, *505*
    thalassaemia intermedia *577*, 577, 670
fetal blood sampling, prenatal diagnosis
    612, 613–14, **614**, **615**
fetal DNA analysis 611, 614–17
    allele-specific oligonucleotide
        hybridization (ASO) 619–20, 621,
        622, 623
    amniotic fibroblast DNA 615
    amplification refractory mutation system

    (ARMS) 620–1, *621*, 622, 623
    chorionic villus DNA 616–17
    deletion mapping 618–19
    fetal cells in maternal blood 628
    gap PCR 621–2, 624
    methods **617**
    polymerase chain reaction (PCR)-based
        methods 620, 624, 626
    prenatal diagnosis programme strategies
        622, **623**
    programmes in developing countries **621**
    reliability 624, **625**, 626
    restriction enzyme analysis 619
    restriction fragment length
        polymorphism linkage analysis
        617–18, *618*, *619*
    reverse dot blotting 621, 622, 626
    sources of error 622
    Southern blot analysis 624
fetoscopy 37
FKLF 95
fluorescence-activated cell sorting (FACS)
    703–4
folate deficiency
    β thalassaemia 315
        heterozygous states 340–1
        pregnant heterozygotes **340**, 340
    HbE β thalassaemia 429
    HbH disease 495
    sickle cell β thalassaemia 402
    thalassaemia intermedia 581, 672
folate supplements 658
    HbH disease 673
    sickle cell β thalassaemia 674
    thalassaemia intermedia 672
fractures, pathological
    β thalassaemia 290, *293*, 306
        management 661
    thalassaemia intermedia 581
frameshift mutations 134, *135*, 135
    α-globin-gene 148
France 240
free radical damage
    antioxidant systems **212**, 212
    β thalassaemia red-cell membranes 204,
        206
    iron overload 211–12
        cardiac complications 298
        liver 311
Fuller kindred 14, *15*, 15
fusion genes
    homologous unequal recombination 135
    see also δβ fusion genes

gallstones
    β thalassaemia 317
    HbE β thalassaemia 434
    HbH disease 494, 495
    prophylactic cholecystectomy 656
    sickle cell β thalassaemia 402
    thalassaemia intermedia 581
        management 672
Gambia 272
γ chain
    ᴬγ deletions 53
    α thalassaemia
        homotetramer formation 17, 122, 224

    persistent production 122, 232–3
    β thalassaemia 194, 195, 196, 198, 202
        persistent production 121, 122
        red-cell-precursor selective survival
            221, 222
    δβ thalassaemias
        ᴳγ and ᴬγ 357
        ᴳγ only 357
        terminology 357
    developmental changes 100
    fetal production 37, 100
        ᴳγ:ᴬγ ratio 100
    Hb Bart's hydrops fetalis 490
    haemoglobin tetrameric associations **72**,
        72
    historical aspects 15
    primary structure 73, 74
    reactivation of production 676
    structural variants 22
        ᴬγ chains 23, 73
        ᴳγ chains 22, 73
    γ-chain genes 15, 85
        chromosomal location 22, 23
        developmental change (switching) 102,
            105
        evolutionary aspects 80
        gene conversions 87
        HPFH 181–2, **182**, *182*
            ᴬγ 181
            ᴳγ 181
        mutations 108
            HbF production effects 184–5
        numerical variation 86, 131
    γ thalassaemia 392
        genetic classification 124–5
    γβ fusion gene, haemoglobin Kenya 23
    gap PCR
        β thalassaemia mutations analysis **707**,
            712, *714*
        δβ thalassaemia mutations analysis **707**,
            712, *714*, 715
        HPFH mutations analysis **707**, 712, 715
        method 722–3
        prenatal diagnosis 621–2, 624
        thalassaemia deletion mutations **707**
            α thalassaemias **707**, 707
    GATA-1 90, 94
        β-globin locus-control region binding
            sites 91, 92
        globin gene promoter binding sites 94
        HS −40 binding site 92
        knockout mice 94
    GATA-2 94
    GATA-3 94
    gene conversions
        α-globin-gene cluster 84–5
        β-globin-gene cluster 87
    gene frequency studies 31–2
        α thalassaemia 29
        malaria hypothesis 32–3, 273
        Mediterranean region 19–21, *20*
        south-east Asia 18–19, 21
        see also population genetics
    gene therapy 59, 680–4, 728, 730
        bone marrow target cells 683
        gene transfer *682*, 682–3
        globin-gene constructs 681–2

safety 684
transplantation strategies 683
genes 67
  activation 71
  alleles 133
  regulation 69–72
  structure 67–8, *68*
  transcription/messenger RNA processing
    67, 68–9, 71
  translation 67, 69, *70*
genetic code 68, **70**
genetic counselling
  phenotype prediction 609
  screening programmes 608–9
genetic disorders of haemoglobin 107–20
  classification **107**, *107*
genetic recombination 135
  homologous unequal 135
    α^0 thalassaemias *137*, 137–9, *138*, 141
  non-homologous 135
  repetitive sequences 135–6
  transposable elements 136
gentamycin 658
geographical distribution 31, 237–84
  Afro-Americans 19
  α thalassaemia 262–73, 277–9
    global distribution *264*, **265**
    migration effects 278–9
  β thalassaemia 239–47, *262*, 262
    common alleles **263**
    mild β^+ alleles 592–3, *593*
    molecular variants 247, **248–61**, 262
  $\delta\beta$ thalassaemia 389–90
    $(\delta\beta)^0$ 378–9, 380
  Hb Lepore 371–2
  HbC β thalassaemia 419
  HbE β thalassaemia *275*, 276, 439
  HbH disease 493–4
  HbS *275*, 276
    Africa 273, 280, *281*
    Indian subcontinent 242, 243, 247, 262,
      280–1
    Middle East 241
  historical background 18–21
  malaria *274*
    see also malaria hypothesis
  Mediterranean region 19–21
    Greece 19
    Italy 19, *20*
  population migrations 278–9, 280–1
  sickle cell β thalassaemia 409–10
  south-east Asia 19
  thalassaemia intermedia 592–4, *593*
  world distribution *238*, 238–9
  see also population genetics
Georgia $^A\gamma\beta^+$ HPFH ($^A\gamma$-114 C→T) **468**,
    475
German ($^A\gamma\delta\beta)^0$ thalassaemia 179
Germany 241
Ghana 244
Ghanaian HPFH (HPFH 2) 180, 187, 188,
    189, 452, 453, 454
  HbC compound heterozygotes **459**, 461
  HbS compound heterozygotes **459**, 459,
    460
Gilbert's syndrome, β thalassaemia trait co-
    inheritance 350

globin chains
  haem intractions/haemoglobin assembly
    99–100
  structure 15
globin genes 3–4, 15
  β thalassaemia 24, 25, 52
  chromosomal location 23
  cloning 57–8
  deletions *see* deletions
  developmental regulation (haemoglobin
    switching) 100–7, *101*
  duplication 22–3, 74, 80
  enhancers 89, 90
  evolutionary aspects 74, 80
  gene product association/assembly 21–
    2
  historical background 15, 22–3
  mapping 55–7
  messenger RNAs *97*, 97
    capping 95, 97
    poly(A) tail 95–6, 97
    processing 95–6
    splicing 96
    transport to cytoplasm 96
  molecular analytical techniques 53–5
  mutations 108
    elongated/shortened chains **120**, 120
    highly unstable globins 117, 572
    see also haemoglobin variants
  organization 22–3, 80–7, *81*
    gene clusters 80–1, *81*
  promoters *89*, 89–90, 94
  regulation of function 89–93
  regulatory elements 71–2, 90–3
    HS –40 92–3
    locus-control region 71, *91*, 91–2
  sequencing 57–8
  structure 54–5, **88**, *88*, 88–9
  transcription 93–5
    basal machinery 93
    erythroid-specific transcription
      elements 93–5, **94**
  transgenic mouse studies 104
globin synthesis 97–9, *195*
  α thalassaemia
    messenger RNA analysis 50–1
    milder types *512*, 512–13
  α thalassaemia/myelodysplasia syndrome
    546, *548*
  anti-Lepore haemoglobins 374–5, *375*
  β thalassaemia 35–6, 39–40, 121–2, 192,
    193–8, *195*, *196*, 234–5, **235**
    $(^A\gamma\delta\beta)^0/(\delta\beta)^0$ compound heterozygotes
      386–7
    α thalassaemia co-inheritance 560,
      562–3
    α-chain variants/homozygous β
      thalassaemia interaction *445*, 445,
      446, 446–7
    heterozygous states 345
    in vitro synthesis 331–3, **332**, *332*
    messenger RNA analysis 49–50
    mild alleles 552
    silent alleles 552
  $(\delta\beta)^0$ HPFH
    β thalassaemia compound
      heterozygotes 464

heterozygous state 382, 457–8
homozygous state *380*, 380, 387–8,
  454–5, *455*
$(\delta\beta)^0$ thalassaemia 387
elongation 98
fetal blood 36–7
Hb Bart's hydrops fetalis 490, *492*
Hb Constant Spring homozygous state
  514, *517*
Hb Kenya *466*, 466
Hb Lepore
  β thalassaemia compound
    heterozygotes 370
  heterozygous state 368
  homozygous state 364
HbC β thalassaemia 418–19
HbE β thalassaemia *438*, 438
HbH disease 35, 224–5, *225*, 504–5
initiation 98
measurement methods 193–4, 704–6
polypeptide chain assembly 46–8, *47*
prenatal diagnosis 37, 612–13, *613*
  errors 624
regulation 98–9
sickle cell β thalassaemia 408–9
termination 98
thalassaemia 34–6, *35*
thalassaemia intermedia 588–90
unbalanced 35–6, 39–40, 121–2, 192,
  193–8, *195*, *196*, 234–5, **235**
  additional α genes 83
  clinical manifestations 38, 39–40
  red-cell heterogeneity in
    haemoglobinization 40
  red-cell inclusion bodies 38–9, *39*, 108,
    198–9, *200*, *201*
glucose-6-phosphate dehydrogenase
  (G6PD) deficiency 350
gonadal dysfunction
  iron deposition damage 215
  osteoporosis 216–17
  see also hypogonadism
gonadotropin-releasing hormone (GnRH)
  303
  pulsatile infusion 657
gout 317, 585
graft-versus-host disease 665–6
Greece 33
  α thalassaemia distribution 265–6
  β thalassaemia distribution 240
  prenatal diagnosis programme 614, **615**
  screening programme 605, *606*
Greek/Sardinian/Black $^A\gamma\beta^+$ HPFH ($^A\gamma$-117
  G→A) **468**, 470–2
  β thalassaemia compound heterozygotes
    471–2
  genetics 472
  heterozygous state 470–1
  homozygous state 470
growth hormone deficiency 302, 303
growth retardation
  β thalassaemia major 290, 302–4,
    303
  endocrine dysfunction 215
  iron overload 291
  desferrioxamine-treated patients 639,
    640

growth retardation (*cont.*)
  HbE β thalassaemia 427
  sickle cell β thalassaemia 397
  thalassaemia intermedia 576

haem 75–6, 77
  β thalassaemia red-cell membrane
      damage 206
  globin association
      haemoglobin assembly 99–100
      unstable haemoglobin variants 115
  haem pocket structure *see* haemoglobin
  haem–haem interactions 77, 78
  synthesis 99, 99
haemichrome formation
  Hb Bart's 228
  HbH 228, 502–3
  thalassaemia intermedia red-cell
      destruction 587
haemin 206
haemoglobin 65, 72–120
  adult **72**, 72–3
  allosteric properties 77, 80
  assembly (haem–globin interactions)
      99–100
  carbon dioxide transport 80
  embryonic 22, **72**, 72–3
  historical background 13–17, *14*, 21–3
      genetic heterogeneity 14–15, 16, 17, 18
      genetic loci 15, 16
      thalassaemia 16–17
  inherited disorders 107–20
      classification **107**, 107
  oxygen binding 77
      Bohr effect 79–80
      chloride effect 80
      conformational change 78–9
      2,3-diphosphoglycerate (2,3-DPG)
          modification 77, **79**, 79
      quaternary states 77
      deoxy (tense; T) 77, 78, 79
      high-affinity haemoglobin variants
          117–18
      oxy (relaxed; R) 77, 79
  solutions preparation for electrophoresis
      692
  structure 73–7
      function relationships 77–80
      haem pocket 75–6, 77, 77
      historical aspects 15, 16
      homotetramers 16–17
      oxygenated/deoxygenated forms 77,
          78–9
      primary 73, 73–4
      subunits 67
      tetramers **72**, 72, 75, 100
      three dimensional 74, 74–7, 75, 76
  switching (developmental change) 100,
      101
      α-globin gene cluster 107
      β-gene expression 105
      cis-active sequences 103–4
      ε-gene expression 104–5
      γ-gene expression 105
      gene order 106
      LCR elements 105–6
      molecular basis 103–7

progenitor cells *103*, 103
timing 102–3
trans-acting factors 106
synthesis 34–7
haemoglobin A **72**, 72
  β thalassaemia 331
  fetal/neonatal production 36, 100
  genetic variants 108
  globin chains 15
  historical aspects 14
  quaternary states 77
  sickle cell β thalassaemia 127, 128, 394,
      395, 395
  tetramer structure 77
haemoglobin A$_{1c}$ 72
haemoglobin A$_2$ **72**, 72
  β thalassaemia *see* β thalassaemia; β
      thalassaemia heterozygous states
  β-chain structural variants/α
      thalassaemia co-inheritance 520
  δ chain variant/β thalassaemia
      heterozygotes 129
  δ thalassaemia 124
  (δβ)^0 HPFH heterozygotes *457*, 457
      β thalassaemia compound
          heterozygotes 463–4, 552
  δβ fusion gene products 376–7
  geographical distribution 20, 21
  globin chains 15
  Hb Kenya *465*, 465
  Hb Lepore HbS compound
      heterozygotes 413
  HbH disease 502
  historical aspects 15
  isolated elevation 354–5
  laboratory estimation methods 695–6,
      699
      screening procedures 690, 691
      interpretation 691
      screening programmes 607–8
      reference laboratories 608
  sickle cell anaemia *113*, 113
  sickle cell β thalassaemia 408
haemoglobin A$_2$ Zagreb 449
haemoglobin A$_2$' *see* haemoglobin B$_2$
haemoglobin A$_3$ 72
haemoglobin Agrinio 512
haemoglobin anti-Kenya 86–7, 186
haemoglobin anti-Lepore 87, *175*, 175, 186,
      372–6, **374**
  β thalassaemia interaction 375–6
  formation mechanism 360
  haematological findings 374
  haemoglobin constitution 374
  haemoglobin synthesis 374–5, *375*
  molecular analysis 374
haemoglobin Atlanta 373
haemoglobin Augusta 1 525
haemoglobin B$_2$ 448
  β thalassaemia co-inheritance 448–9, **449**
  (δβ)^0 HPFH compound heterozygotes
      464–5
  δβ thalassaemia co-inheritance 449
haemoglobin Baden 444
haemoglobin Bart's (γ$_4$) 484
  α thalassaemia 122
      HbE interactions 521–2

heterozygotes 126, 510
α-chain-gene deletions 51, *52*, 55
β-chain structural variants/α
      thalassaemia co-inheritance 520
Hb Constant Spring 514, *515*
HbH disease 232, 502
historical aspects 16–17, 27–8
laboratory methods 695, 698
newborn levels 28, 29, 226, 262–3, 517–18
  Black populations 56
  see also geographical distribution,
      α thalassaemia
oxygen-carrying capacity 228, 493
properties 226, 228
haemoglobin Bart's hydrops fetalis
      syndrome 28, 29, 51, *52*, 126, 126,
          139, 224, 231, 484–91
  clinical features 484, 485–6, *486*
      autopsy findings 486–7, *487*
  developmental abnormalities 485–6, 488,
      493, 672, 673
  diagnosis 492–3, 689
  genetic heterogeneity 490
      geographical frequencies 491
  globin synthesis 36, 224
  haematological findings 488, **490**
      blood film *486*, 488
  haemoglobin constitution 488, 490
      at birth 488, 490, *491*
      during development 490
  haemoglobin synthesis 490, *492*
  long-term survival 487–8, **489**, 673
  management 672–3
      prenatal/neonatal blood transfusion
          673
  maternal complications 487, **488**
  pathophysiology 493
  prenatal counselling 516–17
  prenatal diagnosis 493, 612, 672
haemoglobin Beth Israel 119
haemoglobin C 108, *113*, 114, 276
  α thalassaemia co-inheritance 520, 521
  clinical features 114
  (δβ)^0 HPFH compound heterozygotes
      459, 461–2
      clinical/haematological findings 462
      haemoglobin constitution *454*, 462
      HbF structure 462
      inheritance 462
  distribution 114
  DNA analysis 717–18
  Hb Lepore association 419–20
  HbG double heterozygotes 21
  historical aspects 14
  laboratory methods 695, 698, 699
  prenatal diagnosis 613
  screening procedures 691
haemoglobin C thalassaemia 415–21
  Afro-American populations *415*, 415,
      416
  β$^+$ thalassaemia *415*, 415
      mild form *416*, 416
      severe form 417–18
  β^0 thalassaemia **415**, 415, 416–17
      severe form 417–18
  clinical features 415–18
  δβ thalassaemia 420–1

geographical distribution 419
haemoglobin analysis *406*, 418
haemoglobin studies 16
haemoglobin synthesis 418–19
historical background 415
inheritance 419
Mediterranean populations **415**, 415,
    417–18
pathophysiology 419
haemoglobin Chesterfield 574
haemoglobin Constant Spring 23, 29–30,
    30, 83, 120, 513–15
    chain termination mutation 149, 230
    geographical distribution 270, 271, 273
    HbH disease 29, 30, 234, 506, 513
        haemoglobin analysis 512
    heterozygous state
        haematological findings 514
        haemoglobin constitution *514*, 514, *515*
    homozygous state 513
        clinical features 513
        globin synthesis 514, *517*
        haematological findings 513–14
        haemoglobin constitution *514*, 514
    pathophysiology 514–15
    red-cell membrane abnormalities 230–1
    structure 514, *516*
haemoglobin Coventry 373
haemoglobin Cranston 120
haemoglobin Crete 444, 448
haemoglobin D Ibadan 448
haemoglobin D Los Angeles thalassaemia
    440, **441**
haemoglobin D Punjab 440
    DNA analysis 718
    laboratory methods 698
haemoglobin D screening procedures 691
haemoglobin Dhonburi 444
haemoglobin Duarte 444
haemoglobin E 108, 114–15, 163, 421–2
    allele interactions/thalassaemia
        intermedia 557
    α thalassaemia co-inheritance 521–3,
        522
    clinical features 114–15, 422
    $(\delta\beta)^0$ HPFH compound heterozygotes
        462
    DNA analysis 718
    geographical distribution 114, 239, *275*,
        276
        historical studies 18, 19
        Indian subcontinent 242, 243
        south-east Asia 244–5
    Hb Lepore compound heterozygotes
        439–40
    HbH disease
        haemoglobin production 232–3
        Hb Bart's 233
    molecular pathology 422
    oxygen affinity 421
    prenatal diagnosis 613
    screening procedures 691
haemoglobin E β thalassaemia 18, *19*,
    421–40, 728, 729
    age at diagnosis 427
    α thalassaemia interactions 439, 522–3
    aplastic crises 429

β thalassaemia allele interactions 422,
    423
blood film 435–6, *436*
bone disease 434
bone marrow expansion 429, *430*
    tumour masses 429, *430*, 669
cardiopulmonary dysfunction 431, *432*,
    433
cellular pathophysiology 422–34
clinical features 424–7, *425*, *426*
    heterogeneity 424, 426, 439
coagulation abnormalities 433
complications 427–34
δβ thalassaemias 439–40
    $(^{A}\gamma\delta\beta)^0$ 440
    $(\delta\beta)^0$ 440
diagnosis in newborn 439
endocrine dysfunction 433–4
gallstones 434
geographical distribution 439
growth retardation 427
haematological findings 435–6, **436**,
    436
haemoglobin analysis *437*, 437–8
haemoglobin synthesis 36, *438*, 438
HbF persistent production 222
hepatomegaly 429
historical background 421
hypersplenism 428–9
infection susceptibility 427–8
inheritance 438–9
iron loading 429–31, *431*, 577, 579
leg ulceration 434
myelofibrosis 429
post-transfusion hyperpyrexial reaction
    434
prognosis 434–5
public health issues 597
red-cell metabolic abnormalities 436–7
thrombotic complications 217
    pulmonary manifestations 218, *219*
haemoglobin electrophoresis
    haemoglobin solutions preparation 692
    HbA_2 estimation 695
    screening procedures 690, 691
haemoglobin F 72, *72*, 100
    adult production 101, *102*
        genetic control 476–7
    β thalassaemia 16, 24, 40, 41, 121, 196,
        197, 198, 202, 220–3, **222**, 327–9,
        687
        diagnosis 687
        genetic determinants of level 481–2
        $^{G}\gamma/^{A}\gamma$ ratio 328–9
        molecular mechanisms 151
        oxygen dissociation curve **223**, 223
        persistent production 220–2, *221*
        phenotypic severity relationship 220
        production variation 222–3
    β thalassaemia heterozygous states 333,
        343–5, *344*, 350
        deletional forms **348**, 354
        δβ thalassaemia compound
            heterozygotes 386–7
        developmental changes 348–9, *349*
        specific mutations 348
        very high levels 354

β-chain structural variants/α
    thalassaemia co-inheritance 520
β-gene chromosomal translocation 86
δβ thalassaemias 124, 171, 357
    $(^{A}\gamma\delta\beta)^0$ homozygous state 384
    β thalassaemia compound
        heterozygotes 386–7
    $(\delta\beta)^0$ heterozygous state 381, *382*, 388
    $(\delta\beta)^0$ homozygous state 379–80
developmental changes 100–1
F cells *see* F cells
γ-chain-gene deletions 86
$^{G}\gamma;^{A}\gamma$ ratio 124
Hb Lepore 359
    β thalassaemia compound
        heterozygotes 370
    HbS compound heterozygotes 413
    heterozygous state 367, 368, 371
    homozygous state 364–5, *365*, 371
HbE β thalassaemia 437–8
increased production
    β-globin-gene mutations 184–5
    clinical studies 678–9, *679*
    enhancer sequences 188–9, *189*
    loss of regulatory regions 187–8
    molecular mechanisms 187–90
    therapeutic reactivation 676–80, 730–1
laboratory methods 698, 699
    estimating relative amounts 699–701
    immunological detection 701–3, *702*
    screening procedures 690, 691
    intercellular distribution 691–2
    quantification 691
sickle cell β thalassaemia 395, 406
    cellular distribution 408
    high levels 406–7, *407*
sickle cell disease *113*, 113, 566, 567
    genetic determinants 480–1, *481*
    HbS polymerization inhibition 111
switch from embryonic haemoglobin 102
switch to adult haemoglobin 102
thalassaemia intermedia *see* thalassaemia
    intermedia
see also hereditary persistence of fetal
    haemoglobin
haemoglobin F1 (HbF1) 72
haemoglobin G
    α chain association 21, 22
    HbC double heterozygotes 21
    screening procedures 691
    thalassaemia co-inheritance 130, *131*
haemoglobin G Philadelphia 130, 138, 447,
    448
    α thalassaemia co-inheritance 518–19
    α-globin mutations 148
haemoglobin G Waimanalo 447
haemoglobin Geneva 574
haemoglobin GH disease 130
haemoglobin Gower 1 22, **72**, 72, 100
haemoglobin Gower 2 22, **72**, 72, 73, 100
haemoglobin H 484
    α thalassaemia 122
        carriers 510
    β_4 tetramer formation 225, 226, 505
    genetic aspects 29
    globin gene deletions 51, 55, 224, 494
    haemichrome formation 502–3

haemoglobin H (*cont.*)
  Hb Bart's hydrops fetalis 490
  historical aspects 16, 17, 27–8
  instability 502–3, 506
  laboratory methods 695
  oxygen dissociation curve 78, 226, 503–4
  properties 226, 228, 503–4
  red-cell inclusions 39, 226, 227, 228, 229
    laboratory detection 699
  screening procedures 690, 691
haemoglobin H disease 493–507
  α thalassaemia/β-chain structural
    variants co-inheritance 521
    HbE interactions 522
  α thalassaemia/HbQ co-inheritance 28
  α thalassaemia/myelodysplasia syndrome
    541
  α thalassaemia/unstable α-chain-variants
    co-inheritance 519
  α-chain variants 130, 148
  autopsy findings 507
  β thalassaemia co-inheritance
    heterozygous state 561, 562, 562
    homozygous β⁺ or β⁰ 563–5, 564
  blood transfusion 673
  clinical features 494
    complications 495–6
    course 494
    presentation 494
    variability 233–4, 493
  diagnosis 689
  extramedullary haemopoietic masses
    496
  folate deficiency 495
  gallstones 494, 495
  genetic aspects 29, 30, 31
    inheritance patterns 126, 126
  genotypes 494
    phenotype relationships 234, 505–6
  geographical distribution 493–4
    Africa 272
    Europe 263, 265, 266
    Jamaica 273
    Middle East 266, 267
    south-east Asia 269, 270, 271
  globin synthesis 35, 224–5, 225, 225,
    504–5
  haematological findings 496, **497–9**,
    499–500, 500
    blood film 496, 501
    bone marrow 499–501, 502
    deletional/non-deletional forms 506
  haemoglobin constitution 500, 502, 503,
    506
    developmental changes 502
  haemolytic anaemia 231
  Hb Bart's levels 232, 233
  Hb Constant Spring 29, 30, 234, 506, 512,
    513
  HbE carriers 232–3
  hydrops fetalis 491–2
  hypersplenism 495
  infection susceptibility 495
  iron status 232, 495, 504, 505
  leg ulcers 495
  management 673–4
  mental retardation 56–7

  non-deletional forms 126
  oxygen dissociation curve 504
  pathophysiology 506–7
  pregnancy 496
  prognosis 507
  red-cell damage 229
    membrane changes 230
  red-cell inclusion bodies 39, 227, 229,
    500–1, 502
  red-cell metabolism 505
  red-cell survival 228, 504
  sickle cell disease interactions 524–5
  thromboembolic complications 232,
    495–6
haemoglobin H hydrops fetalis 491–2
  molecular pathology 492
haemoglobin Hamilton 521
haemoglobin Hasheron 130, 445, 445, 447
haemoglobin Headington 448
haemoglobin Hiroshima 118
haemoglobin Hope 444
haemoglobin Hopkins 2 14, 15, 15
haemoglobin I 28, 84
  α thalassaemia co-inheritance 519
haemoglobin Icaria 515, 517
haemoglobin Inkster 447
haemoglobin J Iran 521
haemoglobin J Lome 464
haemoglobin J Mexico 23
haemoglobin J Oxford 448
haemoglobin J Paris 447
haemoglobin J Rovigo 447
haemoglobin J Sardegna 447
haemoglobin J Tongariki 23, 130
haemoglobin J Toronto 518
haemoglobin Kansas 118–19
haemoglobin Kempsey 118
haemoglobin Kenya 53, 86, 175, 186, 187,
    188
  γβ-fusion gene 23
  ᴳγ(γβ)⁺ HPFH 181, 452, 465–6
    clinical/haematological findings 465
    haemoglobin constitution 465, 465–6
    haemoglobin synthesis 466, 466
    HbF structure 466
    HbS compound heterozygous state
      465, 466
  molecular properties 181
haemoglobin Knossos 163, 166–7, 352–3,
    378
  allele interactions/thalassaemia
    intermedia 557–8
  β thalassaemia heterozygous states 336
haemoglobin Koya Dora 23, 268
  heterozygous state 515
  homozygous state 515
haemoglobin L Ferrara 445
haemoglobin Leiden 444
haemoglobin Lepore Baltimore 175, 359,
    360
  geographical distribution 371, 372
  heterozygous state 367, 368
haemoglobin Lepore Hollandia 175, 359,
    360
  heterozygous state 368
  homozygous state 361, **363**, 363, 364
haemoglobin Lepore Pylos 359

haemoglobin Lepore The Bronx 175, 359
haemoglobin Lepore Washington Boston
    26, 87, 108, 124, 135, 171, 173, 175,
    187, 188, 240, 357, 358–78
  β thalassaemia compound heterozygotes
    369–70, 371
    clinical features 369
    haematological findings 369
    haemoglobin analysis 370
    haemoglobin synthesis 370
  β thalassaemia phenotype 360, 362
  (δβ)⁰ thalassaemia compound
    heterozygotes 370
  δβ fusion gene 22, 26, 173, 357
    formation mechanism 175, 175, 186,
      360
    inefficient globin synthesis 370
    product synthesis 359–60, 361
  diagnosis 687–8
    DNA analysis 715
    gap PCR **707**, 715
  geographical distribution 371–2
  haemoglobin constitution 359, 362
  haemoglobin variants co-inheritance 448
  HbC association 419–20
  HbE compound heterozygotes 439–40
  HbF 359
    β thalassaemia compound
      heterozygotes 370
    heterozygous state 367, 368, 371
    homozygous state 364–5, 365, 371
    reactivation therapy 678, 679
  heterozygous state 365–8, 371
    clinical features 366
    haematological findings **366**, 366–7
    haemoglobin analysis 367, 367–8
    haemoglobin synthesis 368
  historical background 358–9
  homozygous state 361, 363–5
    clinical features 361, **363**, 363–4
    haematological findings 364
    haemoglobin analysis 364
    haemoglobin synthesis 364
  Lepore haemoglobin forms 175
  molecular pathology 173, 175
  oxygen affinity 359
  pathophysiology 370–1
  phenocopies 176, 377
  prenatal diagnosis 613, 619
    fetal cells in maternal blood 628
  properties 359
  screening procedures 691
  sickle cell compound heterozygotes
    411–14
    clinical features 411, 413–14
    diagnosis 413
    haematological findings **412**, 413
    haemoglobin pattern 413
  structure 359
haemoglobin Lincoln Park 373, 374
haemoglobin Lleida 512
haemoglobin Lulu Island 444
haemoglobin M 119–20
  clinical features 119–20
  pathophysiology 119
haemoglobin M Boston 119
haemoglobin M Hyde Park 119

haemoglobin M Iwate 119
haemoglobin Malay 164
  allele interactions 557
  β thalassaemia heterozygous states 336
haemoglobin Mississippi 444
haemoglobin Miyada 175, 186, 372–3, 374
  synthesis 374–5, *375*
haemoglobin N Baltimore 520
haemoglobin New York 521
haemoglobin O Arab 441, 448
  DNA analysis 718
  prenatal diagnosis 613
  screening procedures 691
haemoglobin O Indonesia *446*, 446, 447
haemoglobin P Congo 373, 374
haemoglobin P India 374
haemoglobin P Nilotic 175, 186, 373, 374
  β⁰ thalassaemia interaction 375–6
haemoglobin Paksé 515
haemoglobin Parchman 376
haemoglobin Peterborough 448
haemoglobin Portland 22, 56, **72**, 72, 100
  Hb Bart's hydrops fetalis 490, 493
haemoglobin Portland II 490
haemoglobin Pylos 372, 411
haemoglobin Q 130
  HbH disease 28
haemoglobin Q India 447
haemoglobin Q Thailand 447
haemoglobin Quong Sze 270, 518
haemoglobin Rampa 23, 447, 448
haemoglobin S 108, 109
  α thalassaemia co-inheritance 520, 521,
    523, 523–5
  Black/Sardinian ᴳγβ⁺ HPFH -175T→C
    compound heterozygotes 469
  (δβ)⁰ HPFH compound heterozygotes
    458–9, **459**
    clinical features 459
    haematological findings 459
    haemoglobin cellular distribution *460*,
      460, 461
    haemoglobin constitution *454*, 460
    haemoglobin synthesis 460–1
    HbF structure 461
    inheritance 461
    pathophysiology compared with sickle
      cell disease 461
  deoxyhaemoglobin polymer formation
    109–10, *110*, 111
  DNA analysis 716–17, **718**
  expression in sickle cell β thalassaemia
    127, 128
  genetic aspects 15
  geographical distribution 109, *275*, 276
    Africa 273, 280, *281*
    Indian subcontinent 242, 243, 247, 262
    Middle East 241
    population migrations 280–1
  Hb Kenya compound heterozygous state
    465, 466
  heterozygote malaria protection 33,
    273–4
    cellular mechanisms 274–5
  historical aspects 14, *15*, 15
  HPFH co-inheritance 450
  laboratory methods 695, 698, 699

prenatal diagnosis 613, 716–17
screening procedures 691
structure 15
see also sickle cell β thalassaemia; sickle
  cell disease
haemoglobin St Louis 574
haemoglobin St Mandé 119
haemoglobin Saki 444
haemoglobin Sallanches 512
haemoglobin Saverne 120
haemoglobin SC disease 114
haemoglobin Seal Rock 515
haemoglobin Shelby 444
haemoglobin structural variants **107**, 107,
    108–20, 121
  α thalassaemia interactions 28–9, 127–30,
    518, 518–25, **519**
  α thalassaemia phenotype 107, 109
  β thalassaemia co-inheritance 127–30,
    393–449
    abnormal oxygen affinity 444
    α-chain variants *445*, 445–8, *446*, **447**
    β-chain variants in *cis* 444–5
    rare variants 440–1, **442–3**
    unstable variants 444
  classification **108**, 108
  δβ thalassaemia co-inheritance 393, 448
  DNA analysis 715–18
  elongated/shortened globin chains **120**,
    120
  high oxygen-affinity 117–18
    clinical features 118
    pathophysiology 117–18
  laboratory estimation methods 695
  low oxygen-affinity 118–19
  nomenclature 108
  prenatal diagnosis strategies 624
  thalassaemia co-inheritance 127–30
    screening procedures 692, **693**
  thalassaemia phenotype production 108,
    131
  unstable 115–17, *116*
    dominant β thalassaemias 572, *573*, 573
  see also haemoglobin E β thalassaemia;
    sickle cell β thalassaemia
haemoglobin Suan Dok 512
haemoglobin Sydney 373, 374
haemoglobin Tak 120
haemoglobin Vicksburg 444
haemoglobin Wayne 120
haemoglobinopathies *see* haemoglobin
    structural variants
haemolysis 37, 38, 41
  sickle cell red-cells 110
haemolytic anaemia
  α thalassaemias 228–9
  haemoglobin variants 108
  HbC disease 114
  HbH disease 228, 231
  sickle cell anaemia 112
  sickle cell β thalassaemia 396, 397, 403
  unstable haemoglobin variants 116, 117
    dominant β thalassaemias 572, 573
Haemophilus influenzae 308, 654
  postsplenectomy risk 218
  vaccination 655, 674
haemorrhagic complications management

661
hand–foot syndrome 112, 396, 398, *399*
Heinz bodies 115, 117, 149, 198
  HbH disease 229, 499
heparin 672
hepatitis B 307, 308, 428, 585, 635, 659
  diagnosis 659
  treatment 659
  vaccination 635, 674
hepatitis C 307, 309, 428, 585, 635, 659
  diagnosis 659
  thrombotic risk with β thalassaemia 302
  treatment 659–60
hepatitis D 309
hepatitis E 309
hepatitis G 309–10
hepatomegaly 315
  Hb Lepore homozygous state 361
  HbE β thalassaemia 429
  postsplenectomy 655
  thalassaemia intermedia 577
hepatosplenomegaly
  β thalassaemia major *290*, 290
  HbH disease 494
hereditary elliptocytosis 350–1
hereditary haemochromatosis 338
  β thalassaemia trait co-inheritance 338
  gene mutations 338
  optimal body iron burden 640
hereditary methaemoglobinaemia, β
    thalassaemia trait co-inheritance
    351
hereditary persistence of fetal haemoglobin
    (HPFH) 23, 45, 106, 107, 123,
    450–80
  classification 125, 451–2, **452**
  deletional forms *see* (δβ)⁰ HPFH;
    haemoglobin Kenya
  diagnosis 687–8, 691
  DNA analysis 715
    gap PCR **707**, 712, 715
  HbF
    cellular distribution 451
    structure 53
  history 25–6, 450–1
  molecular pathology 52–3, 57, 171–2, *173*,
    174, 179, 180, 186, 467, 468
  non-deletional forms 57, 452, 467–75
    ᴬγβ⁺ 451, **452**, 452
      Black (ᴬγ-114 to -102 deletion) **468**,
        475
      Black (ᴬγ-175 T→C) **468**, 475
      Black (ᴬγ-202 C→T) **468**, 473–4
      Brazilian (ᴬγ-195 C→G) **468**, 474
      British (ᴬγ-198 T→C) **468**, 472–3,
        473, *474*
      Georgia (ᴬγ-114 C→T) **468**, 475
      Greek/Sardinian (ᴬγ-117 G→A)
        468, 470–2
      Italian (ᴬγ-196 C→T) **468**, 474
    ᴳγβ⁺ **452**, 452, 467, **468**, 469–70
      Australian (ᴳγ-144C→G) **468**, 470
      Black (ᴳγ-202C→G) 467
      Black/Sardinian (ᴳγ-175T→C) **468**,
        469
      Japanese (ᴳγ-114C→T) **468**, 469

Tunisian ($^G\gamma$-200+C) **468**,469
hereditary persistence of fetal haemoglobin
(HPFH) (*cont.*)
  heterocellular 451,475–82,**476**,566,
    691,692
    Atlanta type **476**,479
    β thalassaemia amelioration 469–
      70
    β-globin disorder interactions 477,
      478
    β-globin-gene cluster determinants
      476,479–80
    Cretan type **476**,479
    Czech type **476**,479
    family studies 478–9
    Hb S interactions 477–8,*478*
    non-β-globin-gene cluster
      determinants 480
    Seattle type **476**,479
    Swiss type 451,475
  relationship to δβ thalassaemias 450,452,
    456,*482*,482,*483*
  sickle cell β thalassaemia inheritance
    407,407
  unbalanced globin synthesis 52
hereditary spherocytosis, β thalassaemia
  trait co-inheritance 351
heterogeneity of thalassaemia 13,131–2,
  234–6
  haemoglobin studies 14–15,16,17,18
heterozygous state 133
high-performance liquid chromatography
  (HPLC) 688
  HbF estimation 700
  method 698–9
Hinduism 602
histones 70,71
historical aspects 3–62,**60–1**
  α thalassaemia 17–18,27–31
  β thalassaemia 17–18
  δβ thalassaemias 357
  early history 4–11
  genetic transmission patterns 11–13,*12*
  geographical distribution 18–21
  haemoglobin studies 13–17,*14*,21–3
  HbE β thalassaemia 421
  HPFH 25–6,450–1
  Mediterranean region 6,7,**8**
    coexistent childhood
      malaria/malnutrition 6
    Cyprus 6–7
    Greece 11
    Italy 6,7–8,**8**,11
  milder thalassaemias 10–11,12
  molecular pathology 3,4,44–55
  pathophysiology 37–41
  phenotypic variability 13,17
  severe thalassaemia 5,7,8,*9*,10
  sickle cell β thalassaemia 393–4
  terminology 9–10,13
  thalassaemia intermedia 11,550,575–6
  treatment methods 41–4
homologous unequal recombination 135
  α globin genes 135
  gene fusion products 135
homozygous state 133
hormone replacement therapy 656,671

Howel–Jolly bodies 403
HS elements, β-globin locus control region
  91
HS-40 92–3
  deletions 137,141–4,*143*
  erythroid-specific transcription elements
    binding sites 94
  function 92–3
  structure 92
HS-40 knockout mice 143
human immunodeficiency virus (HIV) 307,
  310,310–11,635,636,659,730
  AIDS management 660
Hungary 241
hydroxyurea 670,676
  HbF production stimulation 677,678
hypercoagulable state
  β thalassaemia 217–18
  HbE β thalassaemia 433
  thalassaemia intermedia 672
hypersplenism 41
  β thalassaemia 192,209–10,*290*,290,
    293–5
    complications 294–5
    consequences 210
    mechanisms 209–10
    presentation 289
    transfusion requirement relationship
      293,*294*
  δβ thalassaemia
    ($^A\gamma\delta\beta$)^0 homozygous state 383
    (δβ)^0/($^A\gamma\delta\beta$)^0 β thalassaemia
      compound heterozygotes 385–6
  Hb Lepore homozygous state 361,363
  HbE β thalassaemia 424,*425*,426,427,
    428–9
  HbH disease 495,673
  sickle cell β thalassaemia 397,402
  thalassaemia intermedia 551,576,577
    management 668–9
  unstable haemoglobin variants 116
hyperthyroidism 354
hyperuricaemia 585
hypervariable regions (HVRs) *see* variable
  number tandem repeats (VNTRs)
hypogonadism 662
  β thalassaemia major 215,302,303,304
  desferrioxamine-treated patients 639
  management issues 656–7
  ostoeporosis management/prevention
    657
  thalassaemia intermedia 671
hypoparathyroidism 302,306
hypothalamic/pituitary axis dysfunction
  β thalassaemia major 304–5
  iron overload effects 304,*305*
  management issues 657
hypothyroidism 302,306

immune function 219–20
immunofluorescence, F cell staining 701–2,
  702
in utero haematopoietic stem-cell
  transplantation 680,684
Indian (δβ)^0 thalassaemia 177
Indian HPFH (HPFH 3) 180,452
  β thalassaemia compound heterozygotes

    188,464
Indian subcontinent 31,238
  α thalassaemia distribution 267–8
  β thalassaemia distribution 242–3
    molecular variants 247
  HbS distribution 242,243,247,262,280–1
  prenatal diagnosis programme 614
  public health issues 597
Indonesia 597
  α thalassaemia distribution 270–1
  β thalassaemia distribution 245–6
  HbE distribution 245–6
ineffective erythropoiesis 38
  β thalassaemia 192,199,201
    iron metabolism kinetics 325
  HbE β thalassaemia 422
  highly unstable globins 117
    dominant β thalassaemias 572,*573*
  thalassaemia intermedia 587
infection
  β thalassaemia heterozygous states 341
  β thalassaemia major 218–20,290,307–11
    immune function 219–20
    presentation 289
  HbE β thalassaemia 427–8
  HbH disease 495
  impact of transfusion regimen 307–8
  iron overload relationship 219,220,308
  management 658–61,672
  postsplenectomy 218–19,220,653–4
    prophylaxis 655
  sickle cell β thalassaemia 398,674
  thalassaemia intermedia 585,672
inheritance patterns 125–32
  expressivity/penetrance 127
initiation factors 98
initiation mutations, β-globin-gene cluster
  164
insertions
  α-globin-gene cluster 85
  β-globin-gene cluster 151
insulin-like growth factor (IGF-1) 303
intelligence 317–18
introns (intervening sequences; IVS) 68,69
  globin genes 88,89
inversions 135
Iran
  β thalassaemia distribution 242
  screening programme 601,610,628
Iraq 242
iron metabolism 210–11
  β thalassaemia 324–6
    absorption 324–5
    serum ferritin 325
    serum iron 325
  β thalassaemia heterozygous states
    337–9
    absorption 338
  thalassaemia intermedia 586–7
  see also iron overload
iron overload
  α thalassaemia 231–2
  β thalassaemia 192,210–16,295–300
    heterozygous states 338
    well-transfused patient 291
  blood transfusion regimens 211
  body iron burden

assessment 295, 325, **644**, 644–5
  levels associated with complications
    295, *296*, 296
  optimal level 640
bone disease relationship 216, *217*
cardiac complications *214*, 214–15,
    296–300, 433
  chelation therapy protective effect
    297, 300
  pathology 297–8, *298*
  pathophysiology 298–9
  thalassaemia intermedia 580–1
desferrioxamine in complications
  prevention 637–9, *638*
endocrine dysfunction 215, 291, 302–6,
    433–4
exocrine pancreatic damage 315
growth retardation 302–3
HbE β thalassaemia 429–31, *431*, 433–4,
    435
HbH disease 232, 495, 504
hepatitis C severity influence 659
infection susceptibility 219, 220, 308
liver disease 211, *213*, 213, 311–15, *313*
liver iron levels 325–6
  assessment 312
pathogenesis 41
pituitary dysfunction 304, *305*
post-bone-marrow transplantation
  management 666
postsplenectomy 654
pulmonary pathology 215–16, 433
red-cell membrane damage 204, 206
serum ferritin levels *295*, 295
thalassaemia intermedia *577*, 577–9, **578**,
    578, **579**
  cardiac function 580–1
  management 670–1
tissue damage mechanisms 211–12
tissue iron concentrations (autopsy
    findings) 318–19, **319**
iron, serum levels, β thalassaemia 325
  heterozygous states 337–8
iron-deficiency anaemia
  differentiation from β- and δβ-
    thalassaemia traits 688–9, 691
  historical aspects 4, 6
Islam 601, 602
isoelectric focusing 687, 689
  method 698, 698
  screening procedures 692
Israel 241–2
Italian (ᴬγδβ)⁰ thalassaemia 178
Italian HPFH (HPFH 4) 180, 453
Italian/Chinese ᴬγβ⁺ HPFH (-196 C→T)
    468, 474
Italy 601
  α thalassaemia distribution 263
  β thalassaemia distribution 239–40
  malaria hypothesis 32–3
  screening programme 610
Ivory Coast 243, *244*

J-BP 92
Jamaica 273
Japan 270
Japanese (δβ)⁰ thalassaemia 177

Japanese ᴳγβ⁺ HPFH -114C→T **468**, 469
Jewish populations
  α thalassaemia distribution 266–7
  β thalassaemia distribution 241–2
joint disorders/pain
  sickle cell β thalassaemia 396
  thalassaemia intermedia 581
  management 671–2
Jordan 241

karyotype *72*
Kenya 272
Klebsiella pneumoniae 428
Kleihauer technique 691
  method 700–1
*Kpn*I repeats 136
Kuwait 241

L1 repeats 136, 187
  β-globin-gene cluster 86
  insertions 151
laboratory diagnosis 686, 689–92, **690**
  co-inherited thalassaemias with
    haemoglobin variants 692, **693**
  definitive diagnosis 692
  DNA analysis 706–23
    methods 718–23
  electronic cell counting 690
  flow chart *691*
  methods 692–706
  osmotic fragility tests 690
  primary screen 690
  secondary screen 690–2
Laos 269
Laotian (δβ)⁰ thalassaemia 176–7
Lebanon 241
leg ulceration
  (ᴬγδβ)⁰/(δβ)⁰ β thalassaemia compound
    heterozygotes 386
  HbE β thalassaemia 434
  HbH disease 495
  sickle cell β thalassaemia 396, 401, 675
  thalassaemia intermedia *582*, 585
  management 671
leptocytosis/target cell anaemia 13
Liberia 243
LINES (long interspersed elements) 136
lipid peroxidation 212
liver
  fetal erythropoiesis 100, 102
  iron level assessment 312, 325–6
liver biopsy 325, 644–5, 659, 670
liver disease
  β thalassaemia major 211, *213*, 213,
    311–15
    blood-borne viral infections 312
    iron overload 291, 311–12, *313*
  desferrioxamine in prevention 314, *638*,
    638
  HbE β thalassaemia *431*, 431
liver function tests 314–15
liver transplantation 657
locus-control region (LCR) 71, 85, 91–2
  downregulation mutations 150
  erythroid-specific transcription elements
    binding sites 94
  function 92

γ-chain-gene expression 189
globin gene transcription regulation 93
haemoglobin switching (developmental
    change) 105–6
HS elements 91, 93
  structure *91*, 91
lung disease
  β thalassaemia major 300–1
    iron overload 215–16
  HbE β thalassaemia 218, *219*, 431, *432*,
    433
  lung syndrome in sickle cell β thalassaemia
    398
  management 675
  see also sickle cell disease

Macedonia 241
macrophage respiratory burst 212
magnesium levels 316
magnetic resonance imaging (MRI), iron-
    induced cardiomyopathy 300
malaria
  geographical distribution *274*
  heterozygote resistance 108, 236, 273
    associated genetic polymorphisms **236**
    mechanism 282–4
    sickle cell disease 274–5
    see also malaria hypothesis
  historical aspects
    Italian epidemiology 6, *8*
    Mediterranean region 6, *7*
  impact of control on thalassaemia/sickle
    cell disease 602, *603*
  management 660–1
  prophylaxis 661
  thalassaemic children susceptibility 311
  transfusion-borne infection 311, 636, 660
malaria hypothesis 32–3, 237, 273–82
  α thalassaemia, selection versus
    migration in Melanesia *277*,
    277–8, *278*
  β thalassaemia
    analysis of molecular variants 276–7
    epidemiology 275–7
    selection time-scale 279–80
  gene frequency information 273
  population migrations 278–9, *280*–1
Malattia Rietti–Greppi–Micheli 10, 333,
    550, 575
Malay-1 (ᴬγδβ)⁰ thalassaemia 179
Malaysia
  α thalassaemia 270
  β thalassaemia distribution 245
  HbE distribution 245
Malaysian 2 (ᴬγδβ)⁰ thalassaemia 178–9
Mali 243
Malta 21, 33
  β thalassaemia distribution 240
management 630–85, *631*
  α thalassaemia 672–4
  blood transfusion *see* blood transfusion
  bone disease 657, 661
  bone-marrow transplantation *see* bone-
    marrow transplantation
  cardiac disease 657
  chelation therapy *see* chelation therapy;
    desferrioxamine

management (*cont.*)
  continuity of care 632
  definitive treatment 730–1
  delayed development 656–7
  dental deformity 661
  diagnosis 630–1
    haemoglobin levels assessment 631
  endocrine dysfunction 656–7
  experimental therapies 676–85, **677**
    ethical issues 684–5
    risk–benefit analysis 684
  haemorrhagic complications 661
  historical development 41–4
  infection 658–61
  optimal body iron burden 640
  parent suport
    counselling 662
    early interviews 631–2
    genetic explanations 632
    information-giving 630, 631
  pastoral care 662–3
  prophylactic cholecystectomy 656
  psychological aspects 661–3
    cultural differences 663
  sickle cell β thalassaemia 674–6
  skeletal deformity 661
  social worker support 632
  splenectomy 651–6
  splenic embolization 656
  symptomatic treatment 729–30
  thalassaemia intermedia 668–72
  thalassaemia societies 632, 663
  thrombotic complications 661
  treatment initiation 630–1
  vitamin supplements 658
Mauritania 243
Mediterranean region 31, 238
  historical aspects 5, 10
    childhood illness 6
    malaria 6, 7, **8**
  thalassaemias distribution 19–21, *20*
megaloblastic anaemia 354
  HbE β thalassaemia 429
Melanesia 238
  α thalassaemia distribution 271
    malaria endemicity relationship 277,
      277–8, *278*
  β thalassaemia distribution 246
meningitis 308
mental retardation, α thalassaemia
      association 526
  extent of deletions 139
  see also ATR-16 syndrome; ATR-X
      syndrome
messenger RNA 67
  β-globin-gene cluster translation
      mutations 164–5
  globin genes *97*, 97
    nonsense mutations 96
    transport to cytoplasm 96
  processing 68–9
    β-globin-gene cluster mutations 161
    capping 95
    globin genes 88–9, 95–6
    point mutation effects 134, *135*
    poly(A) addition 95–6
    splicing 96

protein synthesis 69, *70*
methaemoglobin formation 115
methaemoglobinaemia
  haemoglobin M 119
  haemoglobin variants 108
Mexico 281
  β thalassaemia distribution 246
microcytaemia 13
Micronesia 271, 278, 279
microsatellite repeats 83, 86, 136
Middle East 31, 238
  α thalassaemia distribution 266–7
  β thalassaemia distribution 241–2
    molecular variants 247
  sickle cell β thalassaemia 241
mis-sense mutations 134
molecular pathology 133–91
  α thalassaemia 136–50
  β thalassaemia 150–70
    malaria hypothesis 276–7
    molecular variants distribution 247,
      248–61, 262
  clinical applications 58–9
  δ thalassaemia 171, **172**
  δβ thalassaemia 171–9
  εγδβ thalassaemia 190–1
  globin genes 53–5
  historical background 44–55
  HPFH 171–2
  notation 125
  population genetics 237
  thalassaemia classification 125
monocyte function 220
Montreal screening programme 605, 610
Morocco 243
Mozambique 243
mutagenetically separated PCR (MS-PCR)
      711
mutations 133–6
  frequency 133
  functional classification **134**
  large rearrangements 135–6
  point 134–5, *135*
  regulatory 136
  see also molecular pathology
myelofibrosis 429
myocarditis 297, 299

Namibia 272
Neisseria meningitidis 308, 654
  immunization 655
  postsplenectomy risk 218
nested polymerase chain reaction 628
NESTROFT screening procedure 690
neuromuscular abnormalities 317
neutral mutations 134
neutrophil function 220
New Guinea 33
NF-E2 90, 94–5
  β-globin locus-control-region binding
      sites 91, 92
  HS –40 binding site 92
  knockout mice 94–5
Niger 243
Nigeria
  α thalassaemia distribution 272
  β thalassaemia distribution 244

non-homologous recombination 135
nonsense mutations 134, *135*, 135
  see also molecular pathology
north Africa 243
nuclear magnetic resonance analysis,
      protein tertiary structure 66
nucleosome 70–1

Oct-1 90
ocular changes *401*, 401
  ophthalmological monitoring 674
oestrogen replacement therapy 656
olfactory receptor genes 85, 86
Oman 241
operon model 45–6
Orthodox Church 601
osmotic fragility test
  geographical distribution studies *20*,
      20–1
  historical aspects 10, 11, 12, 13
  NESTROFT 690
  screening procedures 606, 690
osteomyelitis 308
  sickle cell β thalassaemia 396, 398
osteoporosis 657
  β thalassaemia major 216–17, 307
  thalassaemia intermedia 671, 672
oxygen affinity of haemoglobin 77, *78*
  β thalassaemia **223**, 223
  (δβ)^0 HPFH homozygous state 455
  Hb Bart's 493
  HbE 421
  HbF 223
  HbH 226, 503–4
  Hb Lepore 359

pancreatic iron deposition 215, 315
Pappenheimer bodies 403
Papua New Guinea 271, 282
paracetamol 674
parvovirus infection 400, 585
pathophysiology 108, 192–236, **193**
  α thalassaemia 223-234, *224*, **231**
  β thalassaemia 192–223, *194*, **231**
    heterozygous states 350
  δβ thalassaemia 387–9
  (εγδβ)^0 thalassaemia 390
  Hb Lepore thalassaemias 370–1
  historical aspects 37–41
Pelger–Huet abnormality 351
penetrance 127
penicillin 655, 658, 674
peptide bonds 65, *66*
pericarditis 297, 308
peripheral blood stem-cell bone-marrow
      transplantation 667, 728, 730
peritonitis 308
Philippines
  α thalassaemia distribution 271
  β thalassaemia distribution 246
pigmentation changes 215, 290, 296
piperacillin 658
pituitary dysfunction
  β thalassaemia major 215
  thalassaemia intermedia 579
  see also hypothalamic/pituitary axis
      dysfunction

plasma volume expansion 210, 294, 295
platelet count
    β thalassaemia major 320
    HbE β thalassaemia 435
    see also splenectomy, complications
platelet function abnormalities 431, 433
pneumonia 218, 308
    sickle cell β thalassaemia 396
point mutations 134–5, *135*
    α thalassaemia alleles 144, **146–7**,
        707–8
    β thalassaemias 150
    β-globin-gene cluster 150, 184
    HbF enhanced production 184, 568–9
    thalassaemia intermedia 568–9
polar body analysis 629
poly(A) addition
    α-globin-gene mutations 145, **146**
    β-globin-gene-cluster mutations 164
    globin genes RNA processing 95–6
    point mutation effects 134–5
poly(A) tail 69
    globin gene messenger RNA 95–6, 97
polycythaemia 108, 117, 118
polymerase chain reaction (PCR) 58
    α thalassaemia alleles
        deletion mutations **707**, 707
        point mutations 707–8
    β thalassaemia 710
        allele-specific oligonucleotides 710
        gap PCR 712
        methods for unknown mutations
            712–14
        primer-specific amplification 710–11,
            711, **712**
        restriction enzyme analysis 711–12,
            713
    δβ thalassaemias diagnosis 687
    HbS detection 716–17
    prenatal diagnosis 611, 614, 620, 624,
        716–17
        errors 624, 626
        nested PCR methods 628
Polynesia
    α thalassaemia distribution 271
        migration/founder effects 278–9
polyribosomes 98
population genetics 31–2, 237–84
    global gene frequency data **239**, 239
    malaria hypothesis *see* malaria hypothesis
    molecular variants analysis 276–7
        migration/founder effects 278–9
    see also geographical distribution
population migrations
    α thalassaemia distribution in Polynesia
        278–9
    HbS distribution 280–1
population screening *see* screening
porotic hyperostosis 4–5
Portugal
    α thalassaemia distribution 266
    β thalassaemia distribution 241
post-transfusion hyperpyrexial reaction
    434
postsplenectomy infection 653–4
    prophylaxis 655
    severe infection treatment 658

pregnancy
    β thalassaemia heterozygous states 334,
        339–40, **340**
    β thalassaemia major 318
    desferrioxamine use 647–8
    HbH disease 496
    milder α thalassaemias 508, *509*
    sickle cell β thalassaemia 402–3
    thalassaemia intermedia 585
preimplantation diagnosis 628–9
prenatal counselling 516–17
prenatal diagnosis 37, 55, 59, 598, 611–29,
        728–9
    α globin-gene haplotypes 84
    β thalassaemia 55
    ethical issues 600, 603–4
    fetal blood sampling 612, 613–14, **614**,
        615
    fetal cells in maternal blood 628
    fetal DNA analysis *see* fetal DNA
        analysis
    globin synthesis measurement 612–13,
        613
    guidelines 603–4
    Hb Bart's hydrops fetalis 493, 672
    PCR techniques 716–17
    population results 626–8, *627*
    preimplantation 628–9
    psychological impact 626
    rare thalassaemias 624
    religious beliefs 600–2
    sickle cell disease 55
    social/psychological pressures 628
    strategies 622–4, **623**
        α thalassaemia 612, 623–4
        β thalassaemia mutations 622–3
    structural haemoglobin variants 624
priapism 398
    management 675
promoter mutations 134
    ^Aγ gene 181
    β-globin-gene cluster 154, *161*
        β thalassaemia Dutch form 354, 568
        HPFH 190
        silent β thalassaemia 165
    ^Gγ gene 181
    HbF enhanced production, thalassaemia
        intermedia phenotype 568, 569
promoters 71
    globin genes *89*, 89–90, 94
protein C 218
protein function 67
protein S 218
protein structure 65–7
    primary 65–6, *66*
    protein function 67
    quaternary 67
    secondary 66–7
    tertiary 66–7
protein synthesis 67–72, *70*
Pseudomonas aeruginosa 428
psychosocial aspects 661–3
    adolescents 662
    cultural differences 663
    infancy/early childhood 662
    pastoral care 662–3
    school problems 662

pubertal growth delay 302, 303
public health issues 597–8, 727–8, 729
    future thalassaemia/sickle cell population
        estimates 598, *599*
pulmonary arterial obstruction 431,
    432
pulmonary embolism 217, 301
    see also thromboembolic complications
pulmonary hypertension
    β thalassaemia major 297
    HbE β thalassaemia 431
    thalassaemia intermedia 581
pyruvate kinase deficiency, β thalassaemia
    trait co-inheritance 351

qinghaosu (artemisin) 660
quinine 660

radionuclide studies, iron-induced
    cardiomyopathy 300
recessivity 126, 133
recombinant growth hormone (rGH)
    therapy 657
red-cell inclusion bodies 38–9, *39*, 108
    α thalassaemia 228–9
    β thalassaemia 198–9, *200*, *201*, 320, 321,
        322, *323*
        diagnosis 686–7
        dominant forms 590, *591*
        heterozygous state 337
    HbE β thalassaemia 435, 436
    HbH disease 39, 226, *227*, 228, 229, 500–1,
        502
    laboratory methods 699
    sickle cell β thalassaemia 405
    see also Heinz bodies
red-cell indices screening 606
red-cell membrane damage
    α thalassaemia 229–31
    β thalassaemia 203, 204, 206–7
    Hb Constant Spring 230–1
    HbH disease 230
red-cell metabolism
    β thalassaemia 324
        heterozygous states 345
    HbH disease 505
red-cell morphology
    β thalassaemia heterozygous states
        336–7, *337*
    β thalassaemia major 319–20, *320*,
        321
red-cell pyrimidine 5' nucleotidase
    activity 607
red-cell survival
    β thalassaemia 323–4
        heterozygous states 337
    HbE β thalassaemia 422
    HbH disease 504
    neocyte transfusions 633
    sickle cell β thalassaemia 405
    thalassaemia intermedia 586
refractory anaemia of pregnancy 334
religious beliefs 600–2
renal disorders 402, 675–6
repetitive sequences 83, 86, 136
    genetic recombination 135–6
research priorities 727–8

restriction endonuclease digestion
  β thalassaemia mutations analysis
    711–12, **713**
  haemoglobin variants detection 717, **718**,
    718
    HbS prenatal diagnosis 717
  method 722
  prenatal diagnosis 619
restriction fragment length polymorphisms
    (RFLPs) 55, 611
  α-globin-gene cluster 83–4, *84*
  β-globin-gene cluster 87, 87, 185, 714–15,
    716
  prenatal diagnosis 617–18, *618, 619*
retrovirus vectors *682*, 682
reverse dot blotting
  HbS detection 717
  prenatal diagnosis 621, 622, 623
    errors 626
Rhodes 240
ribavirin 659
ribosomes 98, 99
Rietti, Fernando 10, *11*
RNA polymerase 68, 71
RNA polymerase II 93
RNA structure 69
Roman Catholicism 600, 601
Romania 241

Salmonella osteomyelitis 398
Sardinia
  α thalassaemia distribution 264–5
  β thalassaemia distribution 240
  prenatal diagnosis programme 617, 623,
    627
  screening programme 601, 605, 610
Sardinian δβ thalassaemia 176, 377
Saudi Arabia
  α thalassaemia distribution 267
  β thalassaemia distribution 241
school problems 662
screening 598, 728–9
  cost-benefit issues 610
  dysgenic effects 602–3
  ethical issues 600, 603–4
  guidelines 603–4
  Hb Bart's hydrops fetalis syndrome 672
  methods 606–8
    audit 608
    further investigations 607–8
    initial screen 606–7
  options for couple at risk 610–11, **611**
  post-test counselling 608–9, 610–11
  procedure 690–2
  programme development criteria 604–5
  programme outcome 609–10
  prospective 605
  psychological impact 626
  public education programmes 605–6
  religious beliefs 600–2
  retrospective 605
  strategy development 606
Seattle type heterocellular HPFH **476**, 479
Senegal
  α thalassaemia distribution 272
  β thalassaemia distribution 243
Serbia 241

severe thalassaemia
  historical aspects 5, 7, 8, *9*, 10
  see also β thalassaemia major
sex chromosomes 133
sexual maturation delay *see* delayed
    development
Sicilian (δβ)⁰ thalassaemia 176
Sicilian HPFH (HPFH 5) 180, 453
Sicily
  α thalassaemia distribution 263–4
  β thalassaemia distribution 240
  prenatal diagnosis programmes 621
sickle cell β thalassaemia 393–411
  α thalassaemia co-inheritance 409
  aplastic crisis management 675
  bleeding tendency 403
  blood film 403, *404*
  bone-marrow/fat embolism 400–1
  bone/joint problems 398, *399*, **400**, *400*
  brain syndrome 398
  βˢ mutation *cis* to β-thalassaemia gene
    410
  childhood course 396
  clinical features 395–7, **396, 397**
    presentation 396
    variability 394, 409–10
  complications 397–8
  fertility 402
  folic acid deficiency 402, 674
  gallstones 402
  genetic counselling 410–11
  geographical distribution 241
  haematological findings 403, *404*, *404*,
    405, *405*
  haemoglobin constitution 405–8
    HbA 16, 17, 394, **395**, 395, 405–6, *406*
    HbA₂ 408
    HbF 395, 406–8, *407*
    HbS 16, 17, 405, *406*
  haemoglobin synthesis 36, 127, 408–9
    cis/trans effects 127–8, *129*
  haemolytic anaemia 396, 397, 403
  hepatic sequestration crisis 675
  historical aspects 4, 16, 24, 25, 28–9, 393–4
  HPFH co-inheritance *407*, 407
  hypersplenism 402, 674
  infection 398
    prevention 674
  inheritance patterns 127–8, *128*, 410
  leg ulcers 401, 675
  lung syndrome 398, 675
  management 674–6
    blood transfusion 676
    bone-marrow transplantation 676
    crises 674–5
    hydroxyurea treatment 676
  metabolic changes 401
  molecular pathology 394–5
  neonatal screening 674
  neurological complications 402, 675
  ocular changes *401*, 401
    ophthalmological monitoring 674
  population distribution 409–10
  post-mortem studies 403
  pregnancy 402–3
  priapism 398, 675
  prognosis 403

renal disorders 402, 675–6
sleep-related upper airway obstruction
    402
splenic sequestration crisis 674
stroke 398, 675
vasocclusive crises 398, 674
sickle cell (δβ)⁰ thalassaemia 414, 415
sickle cell disease (sickle cell anaemia) 4,
    109–14
  α thalassaemia co-inheritance 128–9,
    520, 521, **523**, 523–4
    haemoglobin expression patterns 128,
    129
    impact on symptoms 524
    inheritance patterns 128–9, *129*
  aplastic crisis 113
  brain syndrome 113
  clinical features 112
    sickle cell anaemia 112–14
    sickle cell trait 112
  future population estimates 598, *599*
  gene frequency information 273
  haematological findings *113*, 113
  haemolytic anaemia 112
  hand–foot syndrome 112
  Hb Lepore interactions *see* haemoglobin
    Lepore
  HbF *113*, 113, 566, 567
    genetic determinants 480–1, *481*
    HbS polymerization inhibition 111
    production stimulation 677, 678, 679
  HbH disease 233
  heterozygotes
    HbA levels 127
    malaria protection *see* haemoglobin S
  infection susceptibility 112
  long-term complications 113
  lung crises 112–13
  pathophysiology 109–11, *111*
    haemolysis 110
    red-cell sickling *109*, 109, 110, 111
    vascular endothelial interactions
    110–11
  prenatal diagnosis 37, 55, 59, 615, 616,
    617, 619, 620, 626
    fetal cells in maternal blood 628
  prognosis 113–14
  screening programme outcome 609–10
  splenic sequestration syndrome 113
  vaso-occlusive crisis **112**, 112
  see also haemoglobin SC disease
sickle cell (ᴬγδβ)⁰ thalassaemia 414, 415
silencers 71
silent β thalassaemia 123, 124, 287
  allele interactions 552–5
    β 5'-untranslated region (UTR) +10
    (–T) 554
    β CAP +1 A→C 554
    β CAP +33 C→G 554
    β termination codon +6 C→G 555
    β–101 C→T 554
    IVS2-844 C→G 554–5
  alleles **552**, 552
    β–101 C→T 154, 165
    molecular basis 165–6, *166*
    type 1 (normal HbA₂) 351, 352
SINES (short interspersed elements) 136

single-strand conformation analysis (SSCA) 708
skeletal deformities 41
  β thalassaemia 192, 216–17
  management 661
  see also bone disease
skull changes 290, *292*
  'hair on end' appearance 290, *292*
sleep-related upper airway obstruction 402
south America 238
  α thalassaemia distribution 272–3
  β thalassaemia distribution 246–7
  population studies 281–2
south-east Asia 31, 238
  α thalassaemia distribution 19, 268–71
  β thalassaemia distribution *144*, 244–6
    molecular variants 247
  historical studies 18–19, 21
  public health issues 597, 598
south-east Asian ($^A\gamma\delta\beta)^0$ thalassaemia 179
south-east Asian $(\delta\beta)^0$ HPFH 180, 453
south-east Asian δβ thalassaemia (Laotian $(\delta\beta)^0$ thalassaemia) 176–7
Southern blot analysis 53–4, *54*, 263, 611
  δβ thalassaemias diagnosis 687
  HbS 717
  prenatal diagnosis 617, *618*, 619
    errors 624
Soviet union 242
Sp1 90, 94
  β-globin locus-control region binding sites 91, 92
Spain
  α thalassaemia distribution 266
  β thalassaemia distribution 240–1
Spanish $(\delta\beta)^0$ thalassaemia 177
spinal haemopoietic mass 669–70
splenectomy 43–4, 651–6
  β thalassaemia major 293
  clinical assessment 652–3
  complications 653–5
    preventive measures 655–6
  haematological sequelae 655
  HbH disease 673, 674
  infection risk 218–19, 220, 653–4
    HbE β thalassaemia 428
    prophylaxis 43, 308, 655
  iron loading impact 654
  liver enlargement 315, 655
  partial 656
  prophylactic cholecystectomy 656
  results 653
  thalassaemia intermedia 668–9
  thrombotic disease following 654–5
splenic anaemia of infancy 5
splenic embolization 656
splenomegaly *see* hypersplensim
splice junction mutations 161
splice-site cryptic mutations *162*, 162–4
spliceosome 69, 96
splicing
  α thalassaemia mutations 144–5
  globin genes RNA processing 96
  HbE synthesis disorders 422
  point mutation effects 134, *135*
SQUID magnetometry 325
Sri Lanka 601, 602

starch gel electrophoresis 25, 689, 696–8, *697*
  buffer systems 696
  gel slicing/staining 698
  method 696–8
Streptococcus pneumoniae 308, 428, 654
  postsplenectomy infection 218, 658
  vaccination 674
stroke 398, 675
structure/rate hypothesis 17, 18, 44–5
Sudan 33
  β thalassaemia distribution 243

TAFs (TBP-associated factors) 93
Taiwan 270
Tanzania 272
tap hypothesis 17, 45
target cells
  β thalassaemia heterozygous states 336
  HbE β thalassaemia 435
TATA binding protein (TBP) 93
TEF-2 92
telomeric repair events 141
terminology 9–10, 13
  α thalassaemia 31, 124
  δβ thalassaemia 357
  haemoglobin variants 108
TFIIB 93
TFIIE 93
TFIIF 93
TFIIH 93
Thai ($^A\gamma\delta\beta)^0$ thalassaemia 179
Thailand 33, 597, 601
  α thalassaemia distribution 268–9
  β thalassaemia distribution 244–5
  gene frequency studies 18–19
  HbE distribution 244
  prenatal diagnosis programmes 621
thalassaemia 121
  classification **107**, *107*, 122–5
    clinical 123
    genetic **123**, 123–5
    molecular 125
  definition 121
  future population estimates 597–8, *599*
  globin synthesis 34–6, *35*
  haemoglobin variants 131
  history *see* historical aspects
  inheritance 125–32
    haemoglobin variants co-inheritance 28–9, 127–30
  management *see* management
  origins 33–4
  pathophysiology 108, 192–236
  see also under individual varieties
thalassaemia intermedia 123, 550–94
  age at diagnosis 576
  β thalassaemia dominant forms 572–4
    clinical presentation *590*, 590, *591*, 592
    haemoglobin constitution 588, **589**
    molecular pathology 167
  β thalassaemia heterozygotes with increased α-globin gene number 570–2
    ααα/αα 570–1
    ααα/αα with dominant β thalassaemia 572

ααα/ααα 571
ααααα/αα 571
β thalassaemia homozygote with increased α-globin gene number (ααα/αα) 571
β thalassaemia–α thalassaemia interactions 559–65
β thalassaemia compound heterozygotes 562–3
β thalassaemia homozygotes/HbH disease *564*, 564–5
β thalassaemia homozygous state 562–3
β-thalassaemia trait/α thalassaemia 560–3, **561**, *561*, *562*
  haemoglobin constitution 588
  pathophysiology 565
bone/joint disorders 581, *583*, 583, 671–2
cardiac function 580–1
chelation therapy 671
classification and causes 551
clinical features 575–88
  variability 550, 551
complications 577–86
course 576
definition 551
endocrine function 579–80
erythropoietin response 587
extramedullary erythropoiesis *584*, 584–5, 669–70, *670*
facial appearance *582*, 671
folate deficiency 581, 672
gallstones 581, 672
genetic interactions **551**
genotype/phenotype relationships 574–5, *575*, 668
haematological findings 586
haemoglobin synthesis 588–90
haemoglobin values 551
HbF enhanced production 565–70, 588
  β-globin gene point mutations 568–9
  β-globin-gene cluster determinants 566–7, **567**
  β-thalassaemia deletional alleles 568
  heterocellular HPFH/β thalassaemia interactions 569–70
historical background 10–11, 550, 575–6
hypersplenism 576, 577
  splenectomy 668–9
hyperuricaemia/gout 585
infections 585, 672
iron loading *577*, 577–9, **578**, *578*, **579**
  management 670–1
iron metabolism 586–7
leg ulceration *582*, 585, 671
management 668–72
  blood transfusion 669, 671
  early surveillance 668
  initial assessment 668
  treatment initiation 631
mild β-thalassaemia-allele interactions 552, 555–9
  β CD19 (A*A*C→A*G*C;Asn→Ser;Hb Malay) 557
  β CD26 (GAG→AAG; β 26 Glu→Lys; HbE) 557

thalassaemia intermedia (*cont.*)
  β CD27 (GCC→TCC;Ala→Ser; Hb
    Knossos) 557–8
  β IVS1-6 T→C 558–9
  β–29 A→G 556
  β–30 T→A 556
  β–31 A→G 556
  β–87 C→G 555–6
  β–87 C→T 556
  β–88 C→T 555
  haemoglobin constitution 588
  poly(A);AATAAA→AACAAA 559
  poly(A);AATAAA→AATAAG 559
  poly(A);AATAAA→AATGAA 559
  population variation 592–4, *593*
  pregnancy 585
  red-cell destruction mechanism 587–8
  red-cell survival 586
  silent β-thalassaemia-allele interactions
    β 5'-untranslated region (UTR) +10
      (–T) 554
    β CAP +1 A→C 554
    β CAP +33 C→G 554
    β termination codon +6 C→G 555
    β–101 C→T 554
    IVS2-844 C→G 554–5
  thromboembolic disease 585–6, 672
thalassaemia major
  definition 123
  historical aspects 13
thalassaemia minima, definition 333
thalassaemia minor
  definition 123
  historical aspects 13
thalassaemia societies 632, 663
thromboembolic complications
  β thalassaemia 217–18, 301–2
  HbE β thalassaemia 217–19
  HbH disease 232, 495–6
  management 661, 672
  postsplenectomy 654–5
  thalassaemia intermedia 585–6, 672
Togo 243
trace metal deficiencies 316–17
trans-acting regulatory elements 71
transcription 71
  basal apparatus 93
  globin genes 93–5
  point mutation effects 135
transcription factors 69
transfer RNAs 69, *70*
  globin synthesis 98
transferrin 211, 212
  receptor levels 201
transfusion *see* blood transfusion
transfusion haemochromatosis 42
  see also iron overload
transfusion reactions 635–6
transgenic mouse studies
  β-globin gene cluster expression 104,
    105

ε-gene expression 104
γ-gene expression 105
translation 67, 69, *70*
  globin mRNA 97–9
    elongation 98
    initiation 98
    regulation 98–9
    termination 98
  initiation factors 98
translation mutations
  α-globin-genes 145, **146**, 148
  β-globin-gene cluster 164–5
    elongation 164–5
    initiation 164
  point mutations 134–5
transposable elements 136
  β-globin-gene cluster insertions 151
Tunisia 243
Tunisian $^{G}\gamma\beta^{+}$ -200+C **468**, 469
  heterozygous state 469
  homozygous state 469
Turkey
  α thalassaemia distribution 267
  β thalassaemia distribution 241
Turkish $(^{A}\gamma\delta\beta)^{0}$ thalassaemia 179
Turkish/Macedonian $(\delta\beta)^{0}$ thalassaemia
  177
Turkish 2 $(\delta\beta)^{0}$ thalassaemia 178

UK
  β thalassaemia distribution 241
  prenatal diagnosis methods 618, 620–1,
    621
ultrasound, Hb Bart's hydrops prenatal
  diagnosis 493
United Arab Emirates 241
unstable haemoglobin variants 115–17,
  116
  β thalassaemia co-inheritance 444
  clinical features 116–17
  dominant β thalassaemias 572, *573*, 573
  highly unstable globins 117
  pathophysiology 115–16
Upper Volta
  α thalassaemia distribution 272
  β thalassaemia distribution 243
urine pigments 325
USA 246
USF 94
  β-globin locus-control region binding
    sites 91

vancomycin 658
variable number tandem repeats (VNTRs)
  136
  α globin gene cluster 83, *84*
vasoocclusive episodes
  sickle cell anaemia **112**, 112
  sickle cell β thalassaemia 398
venesection 671
Venezuela 273

Vietnam
  α thalassaemia distribution 269
  β thalassaemia distribution 244–5
vitamin B$_{12}$ deficiency
  β thalassaemia 315–16
    pregnant heterozygotes **340**, 340
  HbE β thalassaemia 429
vitamin D supplements 657, 671
vitamin E deficiency 316
vitamin E supplements 658
vitamin supplements 658
von Jaksch's anaemia 5, 8, 10

warfarin 672
west Africa 243–4
west Asia
  α thalassaemia distribution 266–7
  β thalassaemia distribution 241–2
white cell count 320

X-ray crystallography 66
Xmn-I site polymorphism 154, 184, 185,
  381, 479, 480, 555, 557, 559, 592
  HbF enhanced production relationship
    567, 569

Yemen 241
Yersinia infection 308
  desferrioxamine treatment-associated
    susceptibility 219, 220
  thalassaemia intermedia 585
  treatment 658
yolk sac, embryonic haemoglobin
  production 100, 102
Yunnanese $(^{A}\gamma\delta\beta)^{0}$ thalassaemia 178
YY1 90, 94
  β-globin locus-control region binding
    sites 91
  HS –40 binding site 92

Zambia 272
ζ chain
  α thalassaemia carriers 510
  embryonic haemoglobin tetrameric
    associations **72**, 72
  expression with α^{+} thalassaemia 139, 232
  expression with α^{0} thalassaemia 140
  Hb Bart's hydrops fetalis persistent
    synthesis 490, 493
  historical aspects 22
  primary structure 73–4
ζ-chain gene 82
  chromosomal location 23
  deletions 139–40
  evolutionary aspects 80
  number variation 56, 83
  structure 88
  switching (developmental change
    regulation) 107
  variable number tandem repeats
    (VNTRs) 83
zinc levels in β thalassaemia 316–17